Intensive Care Medicine

Exams are an essential component of one's training pathway in the quest to become a Consultant. For trainees undertaking a career in Intensive Care Medicine (ICM), sadly this is no exception, however, herewith is a suitable text to aid you upon that arduous journey towards the completion of your training – hurrah!

Written in an accessible style, chapters follow a consistent layout throughout, including numerous images and tables, key learning points, and further reading. Experts in all of the main specialties provide specific and detailed knowledge of individual subject areas considered to be fundamental to one's ICM knowledge base. The authors cover a broad spectrum of topics including therapeutic interventions and organ support, paediatric care, comfort and recovery, psychiatric disorders, and end of life care.

An essential preparation textbook and revision aid for exam candidates in Intensive Care Medicine, the book is a useful guide for mentors and trainees too.

Ned (Edward) Gilbert-Kawai, The Royal Liverpool University Hospital, Liverpool

Ned Gilbert-Kawai is a Consultant in Intensive Care Medicine and Anaesthesia at The Royal Liverpool University Hospital. When this book was edited, he was working as an SPR at King's College Hospital, London.

Debsashish Dutta (Dev Dutta), Princess Alexandra Hospital NHS Trust, Essex

Dev Dutta is a Consultant in Anaesthesia and Critical Care Medicine at the Princess Alexandra Hospital NHS Trust in Harlow, Essex.

Carl Waldmann, Royal Berkshire Hospital, Reading

Carl Waldmann is a Consultant in Intensive Care Medicine and Anaesthesia at the Royal Berkshire Hospital in Reading.

Intensive Care Medicine

The Essential Guide

Edited By

Ned (Edward) Gilbert-Kawai
Royal Liverpool University Hospital, Liverpool, UK

Debashish (Dev) Dutta
The Princess Alexandra Hospital, Harlow, UK

Carl Waldmann
Royal Berkshire Hospital, Reading, UK

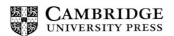

CAMBRIDGE
UNIVERSITY PRESS

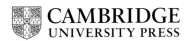

Shaftesbury Road, Cambridge CB2 8EA, United Kingdom

One Liberty Plaza, 20th Floor, New York, NY 10006, USA

477 Williamstown Road, Port Melbourne, VIC 3207, Australia

314–321, 3rd Floor, Plot 3, Splendor Forum, Jasola District Centre, New Delhi – 110025, India

103 Penang Road, #05-06/07, Visioncrest Commercial, Singapore 238467

Cambridge University Press is part of Cambridge University Press & Assessment, a department of the University of Cambridge.

We share the University's mission to contribute to society through the pursuit of education, learning and research at the highest international levels of excellence.

www.cambridge.org
Information on this title: www.cambridge.org/9781108984423
DOI: 10.1017/9781108989060

First published 2023

Printed in Singapore by Markono Print Media Pte Ltd

A catalogue record for this publication is available from the British Library.

Library of Congress Cataloging-in-Publication Data
Names: Gilbert-Kawai, Edward T., editor. | Dutta, Debsashish, editor. | Waldmann, Carl, editor.
Title: Intensive care medicine : the essential guide / edited by Edward Gilbert-Kawai, Debsashish (Dev) Dutta, Carl Waldmann.
Other titles: Intensive care medicine (Gilbert-Kawai)
Description: New York : Cambridge University Press, 2021. | Includes index.
Identifiers: LCCN 2021039837 (print) | LCCN 2021039838 (ebook) | ISBN 9781108984423 (paperback) | ISBN 9781108989060 (ebook)
Subjects: MESH: Critical Care–methods | Emergency Treatment–methods
Classification: LCC RC86.7 (print) | LCC RC86.7 (ebook) | NLM WX 218 | DDC 616.02/8–dc23
LC record available at https://lccn.loc.gov/2021039837
LC ebook record available at https://lccn.loc.gov/2021039838

ISBN 978-1-108-98442-3 Paperback

Dedicated to all our fellow intensive care and hospital staff for their bravery and resilience in the face of this awful pandemic.
Carl, Ned and Dev

To my father Dinesh Chandra Dutta who ignited my passion in life with unrivalled support. Also to my family for the gift of love, patience and support.
Debashish Dutta

To Grace, Arlo and Luxley

They say patience is a virtue, and you have all demonstrated oodles of it.

Thank you, thank you and thank you.
Ned GK

Dedication to Dr Alexander Murray Fletcher

Alex, one of the contributing authors for several of the chapters in this book, brought boundless enthusiasm, laughter and kindness to all those with whom he worked. Greatly valued by his patients, he was able to connect with people from all walks of life with a common-sense approach to medicine.

He was a fantastic clinician, father, husband, brother, son and friend who is missed dearly by his family, friends and colleagues. He touched so many lives, though his was far too brief, and we are so grateful to be able to leave this dedication as a small way of recognising Alex's love for life and his contribution to the world.

Dedication to Dr Kevin Hamilton

This book is also dedicated to Kevin Hamilton, another intensivist whose loss is so keenly felt by the many colleagues and trainees he inspired and encouraged during his too brief life. His great gift was that which is easy to recognise but hard to define, and indeed, this book cannot teach you – 'humanity'. Let this be the chapter he is not here to write. If you cannot understand the lesson, proceed no further with this book – the specialty is not for you.

'Every clinician must be modest enough to question their line of thinking and their decisions made.'
Anonymous

Contents

Contents

Contributors

Authors	Affiliation
Alex Harvey	Senior Lecturer, Department of Clinical Sciences, Brunel University London, London, UK
Alexa Strachan	Consultant Anaesthetist, Royal Free London NHS Foundation Trust, London, UK
Alexander Fletcher	Anaesthetic and Intensive Care Medicine Consultant, Royal Surrey NHS Foundation Trust, Guildford, UK
Alison Pittard	Anaesthetic and Intensive Care Medicine Consultant, Leeds Teaching Hospitals NHS Trust, Leeds, UK
Alistair Connell	Renal Specialist Registrar, University College London Institute for Human Health and Performance, London, UK
Andrew J. Jones	Paediatric Intensive Care Medicine Consultant and Children's Acute Transport Service (CATS) Great Ormond Street Hospital, London, UK
Andy Slack	Nephrology and Intensive Care Medicine Consultant, Guy's and St Thomas' NHS Foundation Trust, London, UK
Andrew Selman	Anaesthetic Specialist Registrar, St George's Hospital, London, UK
Andrew P. Walden	Acute Internal Medicine and Intensive Care Medicine Consultant, Royal Berkshire Hospital, Reading, UK
Anil Dhadwal	Trauma and Orthopaedic Specialist Registrar, Royal Liverpool University Hospital, Liverpool, UK
Anne-Marie Leo	Anaesthetic and Intensive Care Medicine Consultant, Cork University Hospital, Wilton, Cork, Ireland
Anthony O'Dwyer	Anaesthetic Specialist Registrar, London School of Anaesthesia, London, UK
Armine Sefton	Consultant Microbiologist, The Princess Alexandra Hospital NHS Trust/Emerita, Harlow, UK
Arthur W. E. Lieveld	Acute Internal Medicine Consultant, Amsterdam Public Health Research Institute, Amsterdam UMC, Amsterdam, The Netherlands
Arun Krishnamurthy	Anaesthetic and Intensive Care Medicine Consultant, The Princess Alexandra Hospital NHS Trust, Harlow, UK
Audrey Quinn	Consultant Anaesthetist, James Cook University Hospital NHS Trust, Middlesbrough, UK
Behrad Baharlo	Anaesthetic and Intensive Care Medicine Consultant, Queen Elizabeth Hospital, University Hospitals Birmingham, Birmingham, UK
Ben Clevenger	Consultant Anaesthetist, Royal National Orthopaedic Hospital, Stanmore, UK
Benjamin Post	Anaesthetic and Intensive Care Medicine Specialist Registrar, The Royal London Hospital, London, UK
Carl Waldmann	Anaesthetic and Intensive Care Medicine Consultant, Royal Berkshire Hospital, Reading, UK
Caroline Moss	Anaesthetic and Intensive Care Medicine Consultant, Western Sussex Hospitals Foundation Trust, Chichester, UK
Charles M. Oliver	Consultant Anaesthetist, University College London Hospital, London, UK

Charles Rich	Emergency Medicine and Intensive Care Medicine Specialist Registrar, Thames Valley, London, UK
Chris Danbury	Intensive Care Medicine Consultant, Royal Berkshire Hospital and Visiting Fellow in Health Law, University of Reading, Reading, UK
Chris Whitehead	Anaesthetic and Intensive Care Medicine Consultant, The Walton Centre NHS Foundation Trust, Liverpool, UK
Christopher Hellyar	Anaesthetics Core Trainee, The Princess Alexandra Hospital NHS Trust, Harlow, UK
Chun Wah So	Radiology Specialist Registrar, London North West University Healthcare NHS Trust, London, UK
Claire McCann	Anaesthetic Specialist Registrar, Central London School of Anaesthesia, London, UK
Claire Moorthy	Intensive Care Medicine Specialist Registrar, Hospital of St John and St Elizabeth, London, UK
Clare Morkane	Anaesthetic and Intensive Care Medicine Specialist Registrar, Royal Free Hospital NHS Trust, Royal Free Perioperative Research, London, UK
Debashish Dutta	Anaesthetic and Intensive Care Medicine Consultant, The Princess Alexandra Hospital NHS Trust, Harlow, UK
Dominic Moor	Anaesthetic and Intensive Care Medicine Consultant, Basingstoke and North Hampshire Hospital, Basingstoke, UK
Dominik Krzanicki	Consultant Anaesthetist, Royal Free Hospital NHS Trust and Consultant in Pre-hospital Emergency Medicine Barts Health NHS Trust and London's Air Ambulance, London, UK
Dunnya De-Silva	Consultant Haematologist, Maidstone and Tunbridge Wells NHS Trust, Tunbridge Wells, UK
Ed McIlroy	Anaesthetic Specialist Registrar, Royal London Hospital, London, UK
Edward Presswood	Palliative Medicine Consultant, Dorothy House Hospice Care, Bradford-on-Avon, UK
Edward Rintoul	Anaesthetic Specialist Registrar, The Princess Alexandra Hospital NHS Trust, Harlow, UK
Elizabeth Potter	Intensive Care Medicine and Anaesthetic Consultant, Royal Surrey County Hospital, Guildford, UK
Emmar Drasar	Consultant Haematologist, University College London Hospital, London, UK
Eve Corner	Lecturer and Research Physiotherapist, Brunel University London and Imperial College Healthcare NHS Trust, London, UK
Gabor Dudas	Anaesthetic Consultant, Royal Surrey County Hospital NHS Foundation Trust, Guildford, UK
Gary Masterson	Anaesthetic and Intensive Care Medicine Consultant, Royal Liverpool University Hospital, Liverpool, UK
Gursharan Paul Singh Bawa	Anaesthetic and Intensive Care Medicine Consultant, BHR University NHS Trust, Romford, UK
Harish Venkatesh	Anaesthesia and Intensive Care Medicine Specialty Registrar, Royal Berkshire Hospital, Royal Berkshire NHS Foundation Trust, Reading, UK
Harriet Kemp	Anaesthetic and Pain Specialist Registrar, Chelsea and Westminster NHS Foundation Trust, London, UK
Helen Laycock	Anaesthetic and Pain Consultant, Great Ormond Street Hospital, London, UK
Ian Tweedie	Anaesthetic and Intensive Care Medicine Consultant, The Walton Centre NHS Foundation Trust, Liverpool, UK
James McKinlay	Senior Clinical Research Fellow, Royal Surrey NHS Foundation Trust, Guildford, UK
Jeff Phillips	Anaesthetic and Intensive Care Medicine Consultant, The Princess Alexandra Hospital NHS Trust, Harlow, UK

Jenny O'Nions	Consultant Haematologist, University College London Hospital, London, UK
Jeremy Fabes	Anaesthetic Specialist Registrar, Royal Free Hospital NHS Trust, London, UK
Jo Hackney	Anaesthetic Specialist Registrar, The Princess Alexandra Hospital NHS Trust, Harlow, UK
Jo Samanta	Professor of Medical Law, De Montfort University, Leicester, UK
Joel Meyer	Intensive Care Medicine Consultant, Guy's and St Thomas' NHS Foundation Trust, London, UK
John Whittle	Anaesthetic and Intensive Care Medicine Consultant, Duke University Medical School, and Centre for Perioperative Medicine, Durham, NC, USA
Jon Griffiths	Anaesthetic and Intensive Care Medicine Specialty Registrar, Ipswich Hospital, East Suffolk, and North Essex NHS Foundation Trust, Ipswich and Colchester, UK
Jonathan Barnes	Anaesthetic and Intensive Care Medicine Specialist Registrar, Severn Deanery, UK
Jonny Coppel	Anaesthetic Specialist Registrar, University College London, London, UK
Jonny Price	Anaesthetic and Intensive Care Medicine Consultant, Royal United Hospital Bath & Prehospital Care Doctor, Dorset and Somerset Air Ambulance, UK
Julian Howard	Anaesthetic and Intensive Care Medicine Consultant, Royal Free Hospital NHS Trust, London, UK
Julian Millo	Consultant Anaesthetist, Oxford University Hospital, Oxford, UK
Justin Ang	Emergency Medicine Specialist Registrar, Ipswich Hospital, East Suffolk and North Essex NHS Foundation Trust, Ipswich and Colchester, UK
Karim Fouad Alber	Anaesthetic and Intensive Care Medicine Specialist Registrar, Thames Valley, London, UK
Karina Goodwin	Anaesthetic and Intensive Care Medicine Specialist Registrar, Harefield Hospital, Royal Brompton & Harefield NHS Foundation Trust, London, UK
Katarina Lenartova	Anaesthetic and Intensive Care Medicine Consultant, Harefield Hospital, Royal Brompton & Harefield NHS Foundation Trust, London, UK
Kate Tatham	Anaesthetic and Intensive Care Medicine Consultant, Royal Marsden NHS Foundation Trust, London, UK
Katie Samuel	Anaesthetic Consultant, Southmead Hospital, North Bristol NHS Trust, Bristol, UK
Katie Wimble	Anaesthetic Specialist Registrar, Royal Surrey County Hospital, Guildford, UK
Kyron Chambers	Anaesthetic and Intensive Care Medicine Specialist Registrar, Whittington Health NHS Trust, London, UK
Laura Vincent	Intensive Care Medicine Consultant, John Radcliffe Hospital, Oxford, UK
Lee Poole	Anaesthetic and Intensive Care Medicine Consultant, Royal Liverpool University Hospital, Liverpool, UK
Leon Cloherty	Anaesthetic and Intensive Care Medicine Consultant, Whangarei Base Hospital, Northland DHB, Whangarei, New Zealand
Liesl Wandrag	Nutrition & Dietetic Department, Guy's and St Thomas' NHS Foundation Trust, London, UK
Liza Keating	Anaesthetic and Intensive Care Medicine Consultant, Royal Berkshire NHS Foundation Trust, Reading, UK
Lola Loewenthal	Respiratory Specialist Registrar, National Heart and Lung Institute, Imperial College London, London, UK
Louise Swan	Specialist Registrar, Royal Victoria Hospital, Newcastle, UK
Mahmoud Wagih	Anaesthetic and Intensive Care Medicine Consultant, The Princess Alexandra Hospital NHS Trust, Harlow, UK
Mandy Jones	Reader in Physiotherapy, Brunel University, London, UK
Manpreet Bahra	Anaesthetic Specialist Registrar, Royal National Orthopaedic Hospital NHS Trust, London, UK

Marc Wittenberg	Consultant Anaesthetist, Royal Free Hospital NHS Trust and Ex-HEMS Registrar, Essex & Herts Air Ambulance, London, UK
Marc Zentar	Intensive Care Medicine Specialist Registrar, The Royal London Hospital, London, UK
Margaret Presswood	Palliative Medicine Consultant, University Hospital of Wales, Cardiff, UK
Mari Thomas	Consultant Haematologist, University College London Hospital, London, UK
Marlies Ostermann	Nephrology and Intensive Care Medicine Consultant, Guy's and St Thomas' NHS Foundation Trust, London, UK
Matthew Gale	Radiology Specialist Registrar, Nottingham University Hospitals NHS Trust, Nottingham, UK
Megan Fahy	Intensive Care Medicine Specialist Registrar, Queen Elizabeth Hospital Birmingham, University Hospitals Birmingham NHS Foundation Trust, Birmingham, UK
Michael Hoy	Anaesthetic and Intensive Care Medicine Specialist Registrar, Harefield Hospital, Royal Brompton & Harefield NHS Foundation Trust, London, UK
Michael Spiro	Anaesthetic and Intensive Care Medicine Consultant, Royal Free Hospital NHS Trust, London, UK
Mike Peters	Intensive Care Medicine and Renal Specialty Registrar, Thames Valley Deanery, London, UK
Ned Gilbert-Kawai	Consultant in Intensive Care Medicine and Anaesthesia, Royal Liverpool University Hospital, Liverpool, UK
Nick Lees	Anaesthetic and Intensive Care Medicine Consultant, Royal Brompton & Harefield NHS Foundation Trust, London, UK
Nicola Rowe	Respiratory Specialist Registrar, Royal Shrewsbury Hospital, Shrewsbury and Telford Hospital NHS Trust, UK
Niklas Tapper	Anaesthetic and Intensive Care Medicine Consultant, St Vincent's Hospital, Sydney, Australia
Nuttha Lumlertgul	Clinical Research Fellow, Guy's and St Thomas' NHS Foundation Trust and Excellence Center for Critical Care Nephrology and Division of Nephrology, Department of Internal Medicine, King Chulalongkorn Memorial Hospital, Bangkok, Thailand
Oliver Sanders	Otolaryngology Core Surgical Trainee, Southend University Hospital NHS Foundation Trust, Westcliff-on-Sea, UK
Orlanda Allen	Anaesthetic Specialist Registrar, University College London Hospitals, London, UK
Paul Harris	Anaesthetic and Intensive Care Medicine Consultant, Harefield Hospital, Royal Brompton & Harefield NHS Foundation Trust, London, UK
Pete Odor	Consultant Anaesthetist, University College London Hospitals, London, UK
Peter Byrne	Consultant Liaison Psychiatrist, The Royal London Hospital, East London Foundation NHS Trust and Visiting Professor at University of Strathclyde, UK
Peter Remeta	Anaesthetic and Intensive Care Medicine Specialist Registrar, University Hospital of Leicester NHS Trust, Leicester, UK
Raj Saha	Anaesthetic and Intensive Care Medicine Consultant, The Princess Alexandra Hospital NHS Trust, Harlow, UK
Rajamani Sethuraman	Anaesthetic and Intensive Care Medicine Consultant, The Princess Alexandra Hospital, Harlow, UK
Ramprasad Matsa	Intensive Care Medicine Consultant, Royal Stoke University Hospitals, Stoke, UK
Ranil Soysa	Anaesthetic and Intensive Care Medicine Specialist Registrar, Imperial School of Anaesthesia, London, UK
Ravi Bhatia	Consultant Anaesthetist, King's College Hospital NHS Foundation Trust, London, UK

Ravi Kumar	Anaesthetic and Intensive Care Medicine Consultant, Surrey and Sussex NHS Trust, Redhill, UK
Rebecca Brinkler	Anaesthetic Specialist Registrar, London School of Anaesthesia, London, UK
Ruth Taylor	Psychiatry Specialist Registrar, East London Foundation NHS Trust, London, UK
Sachin Mehta	Anaesthetist and Intensive Care Medicine Physician, St Paul's Hospital, Vancouver, Canada, and Honorary Clinical Senior Teaching Fellow, University College London, London, UK
Sam Bampoe	Consultant Anaesthetist, University College London Hospitals, London, UK
Sanjeev Ramachandran	Academic Clinical Fellow in Clinical Radiology, University Hospitals of Leicester NHS Trust, Leicester, UK
Scott Grier	Intensive Care Medicine Consultant, North Bristol NHS Trust and Pre-hospital Care Doctor, Great Western Air Ambulance, Bristol, UK
Selina Ho	Anaesthetic and Intensive Care Medicine Specialist Registrar, Harefield Hospital, Royal Brompton & Harefield NHS Foundation Trust, London, UK
Shankara Nagaraja (Raj Nagaratnam)	Anaesthetic and Intensive Care Medicine Consultant, Liverpool University Hospital NHS Foundation Trust, Liverpool, UK
Shona Johnson	Intensive Care Medicine Specialist Registrar, Milton Keynes University Hospital NHS Foundation Trust, Milton Keynes, UK
Shrijt Nair	Consultant Anaesthetist, St Vincent's University Hospital, Dublin, Republic of Ireland
Simon Mattison	Anaesthetic and Intensive Care Medicine Consultant, Harefield Hospital, Royal Brompton & Harefield NHS Foundation Trust, London, UK
Sridhar Nallapareddy	Anaesthetic and Intensive Care Medicine Consultant, Ipswich Hospital, East Suffolk and North Essex NHS Foundation Trust, Ipswich and Colchester, UK
Stephane Ledot	Intensive Care Medicine Consultant, Royal Brompton & Harefield Foundation Trust, London, UK
Suehana Rahman	Consultant Anaesthetist, Royal Free Hospital, London, UK
Susanna Price	Intensive Care Medicine Consultant, Royal Brompton & Harefield Foundation Trust, London, UK
Tamas Bakonyi	Consultant Anaesthetist, Guy's and St Thomas' NHS Foundation Trust, London, UK
Thomas Brick	Paediatric Intensive Care Medicine Consultant and Children's Acute Transport Service (CATS), Great Ormond Street Hospital, London, UK
Thomas Leith	Anaesthetic and Intensive Care Medicine Specialist Registrar, Royal Marsden Hospital, London, UK
Tim Hartley	Intensive Care Medicine Specialist Registrar, Hospital of St John and St Elizabeth, London, UK
Timothy Snow	Anaesthetic and Intensive Care Medicine Specialist Registrar, The Royal London Hospital, London, UK
Tom Bottomley	Anaesthetic Specialist Registrar, University College London, London, UK
Tom Parker	Anaesthetic and Intensive Care Medicine Specialist Registrar, University College London, London, UK
Valerie Page	Anaesthetic and Intensive Care Medicine Consultant, Watford General Hospital, Watford, UK
Victoria Stables	Consultant Haematologist, Maidstone and Tunbridge Wells NHS Trust, Tunbridge Wells, UK
William Townsend	Consultant Haematologist, University College London Hospital, London, UK
Wilson Fandino	Consultant Anaesthetist, Guy's and St Thomas' NHS Foundation Trust, London, UK

Preface

As practising intensivists involved on both sides of the Intensive Care Medicine examinations 'fence' (the luckier ones of us examined, whilst the unlucky one was being examined!), we fully appreciate the extent of the factual knowledge required of anyone undertaking these examinations. With this in mind, and whilst we recognise that numerous excellent books relating to Critical Care/Intensive Care Medicine already exist, we set ourselves the task of writing a textbook that would have the following unique selling points:

1. It would cover the entire UK FFICM syllabus.

2. It would provide, in a uniform and consistent format, a succinct and digestible summary of each topic (1000–2500 words), rather than an exhaustive, in-depth review.

3. To supplement this approach, Key Learning Points would be listed at the start of every chapter, and it would provide recommendations for further reading should the reader wish to delve deeper into any topic and continue their own self-directed learning.

4. As well as intensivists, the contributing authors would include other affiliated specialists (haematologists, nephrologists, paediatric intensivists, psychiatrists, etc.) who importantly still work on the 'shop floor' on a daily basis, thus ensuring they have up-to-date knowledge and experience of what really is, and is not, important to direct patient care.

To this end, 132 international authors from all fields of medicine were co-opted and the ensuing pages encompass the rich fruits of their labours. Such a multidisciplinary approach will inevitably lead to small overlaps of subject matter, but we have chosen to retain these as an aid to learning and a useful revision tool. Additionally, wishing to avoid the monotony of a uniform textbook, we have also chosen to retain each author's own (and, at times, very different) words and style.

We have undoubtedly learnt a great deal from our colleagues' contributions, and we certainly hope that you too will fill your cup to the brim with the included factual content!

Finally, a word of advice as we leave you to inwardly digest what others far more learned than ourselves have written on the subject of Intensive Care Medicine – remember that when the odd fact or two has slipped your mind, you are never alone because even the best intensivist will also be a 'connexist'. That is to say, someone who is ready to recognise his or her own limitations, and call on the expertise of others when required.

Ned, Dev and Carl
2020

Foreword

Intensive Care Medicine – The Essential Guide lives up to its name. Drs Gilbert-Kawai, Dutta and Waldmann have assembled a sterling cast of 132 intensivists and 'ologists from other specialties to pen 186 chapters covering the breadth of Critical Care. The chapters are brief and to the point, providing a clear overview of each topic, but with further reading suggested for the reader seeking more depth. Importantly, the book mirrors the curriculum for those aiming to become a fellow of the UK Faculty of Intensive Care Medicine. It will also aid those seeking to learn Critical Care or refresh their knowledge, and should appeal to doctors, nurses and other allied healthcare professionals. The varied writing styles have been expressly retained to provide variation and freshness. The editors and authors should be congratulated on delivering such an enjoyable and informative text.

Mervyn Singer
Professor of Intensive Care Medicine
University College London
6 July 2020

Abbreviations

AAD	acute aortic dissection
AAGBI	Association of Anaesthetists of Great Britain and Ireland
AAS	acute aortic syndrome
ABA	American Burn Association
ABG	arterial blood gas
ACC	American College of Cardiology
ACCM	American College of Critical Care Medicine
ACE	angiotensin-converting enzyme
ACE2	angiotensin-converting enzyme 2
ACEI	angiotensin-converting enzyme inhibitor
A4CH	apical four-chamber
ACLF	acute-on-chronic liver failure
ACS	abdominal compartment syndrome; acute coronary syndrome
ACS NSQIP®	American College of Surgeons National Surgical Quality Improvement Program
ACT	activated clotting time
ACTH	adrenocorticotrophic hormone
ADH	anti-diuretic hormone
ADP	adenosine diphosphate
ADRT	advance decision to refuse treatment
AECC	American European Consensus Conference
AECOPD	acute exacerbations of COPD
AED	anti-epileptic drug
AF	atrial fibrillation
AFE	amniotic fluid embolism
AFLP	acute fatty liver of pregnancy
AFM	acute fulminant myocarditis
AHA	American Heart Association
AHT	abusive head trauma
aHUS	atypical haemolytic uraemic syndrome
AHVF	acute hypercapnic ventilatory failure
AI	aortic insufficiency
AIDS	acquired immune deficiency syndrome
AIN	acute interstitial nephritis

AIS	Abbreviated Injury Scale
AKI	acute kidney injury
AKIKI	Artificial Kidney Initiation in Kidney Injury
AKIN	Acute Kidney Injury Network
ALI	acute lung injury
ALL	acute lymphoblastic leukaemia
alloHSCT	allogeneic haematopoietic stem cell transplant
ALP	alkaline phosphatase
ALS	advanced life support
ALT	alanine aminotransferase
AMHP	approved mental health professional
AMI	acute mesenteric ischaemia
AMP	adenosine monophosphate
AmpC	Ambler class C
ANA	anti-nuclear antibody
ANCA	anti-neutrophil cytoplasmic antibody
ANTT	aseptic non-touch technique
AoCKD	acute kidney injury on top of chronic kidney disease
AP	anteroposterior
APACHE	Acute Physiology and Chronic Health Evaluation
aPCC	activated prothrombin complex concentrate
APH	antepartum haemorrhage
APLS	advanced paediatric life support
APRV	airway pressure release ventilation
APTT	activated partial thromboplastin time
AQP	aquaporin
ARAER	ascites-to-rectus abdominis muscle echogenicity ratio
ARB	angiotensin receptor blocker
ARDS	acute respiratory distress syndrome
ARISCAT	Assess Respiratory Risk in Surgical Patients in Catalonia Tool
AS	aortic stenosis
ASA	American Society of Anesthesiologists
ASCI	acute spinal cord injury
ASIA	American Spinal Injury Association
ASO	anti-streptolysin O
ASPEN	American Society for Parenteral and Enteral Nutrition
AST	aspartate aminotransferase
ATC	acute traumatic coagulopathy
ATG	anti-thymocyte globulin
ATLS	advanced trauma life support
ATN	VA/NIH Acute Renal Failure Trial Network

ATP	adenosine triphosphate
ATS	American Thoracic Society
AUC	area under the curve
autoHSCT	autologous haematopoietic stem cell transplant
AV	atrioventricular; arteriovenous
AVNRT	atrioventricular nodal re-entry tachycardia
AVP	arginine vasopressin
AVPR$_2$	vasopressin receptor
AVPU	Alert, responsive to Voice, responsive to Pain, Unresponsive
AVR	aortic valve replacement
AVRT	atrioventricular re-entry tachycardia
AWS	alcohol withdrawal syndrome
AXR	abdominal X-ray
BAL	broncho-alveolar
B-ALL	B cell acute lymphoblastic leukaemia
BAV	balloon aortic valvuloplasty
BBB	bundle branch block
BCNIE	blood culture-negative infective endocarditis
BCPC	bidirectional cavopulmonary connection
BE	base excess
BIA	British Infection Association
BIMDG	British Inherited Metabolic Diseases Group
BiPAP	bi-level positive airway pressure
BIS	bispectral index
BISAP	Bedside Index for Severity in Acute Pancreatitis
BLUE	Bedside Lung Ultrasound in Emergency
BM	bone marrow
BMI	body mass index
BNP	B-type natriuretic peptide
BOS	bronchiolitis obliterans syndrome
bpm	beats per minute
BPS	Behavioral Pain Scale
BRAF	B-rapidly accelerated fibrosarcoma
BSA	body surface area
BSE	British Society of Echocardiography
BSG	British Society of Gastroenterology
BSH	British Society for Haematology
BSPED	British Society for Paediatric Endocrinology and Diabetes
BTS	British Thoracic Society; Blalock–Taussig shunt
BTT	bridge to transplant
BVM	bag–valve–mask

BWPS	Burch–Wartofsky Point Scale
Ca^{2+}	calcium
CABG	coronary artery bypass graft
CABSI	catheter-associated bloodstream infection
CAD	coronary artery disease
CAM-ICU	Confusion Assessment Method for the ICU
CANH	clinically assisted nutrition and hydration
CaO_2	arterial oxygen content
CAP	community-acquired pneumonia
CAR	chimeric antigen receptor
CBF	cerebral blood flow
CBRN	chemical, biological, radiological and nuclear defence
CBT	cognitive behavioural therapy
CCG	Clinical Commissioning Group
CCT	conventional coagulation test; Certificate of Completion of Training
CCU	critical care unit
CDI	cranial diabetes insipidus
CDOP	Child Death Overview Panel
CEI	continuous epidural infusion
$CERO_2$	cerebral oxygen extraction ratio
CF	cystic fibrosis
CFF	citrated functional fibrinogen
CFU	colony-forming units
CHD	congenital heart disease
CICO	Can't Intubate Can't Oxygenate
CIM	critical illness myopathy
CIN	calcineurin inhibitor
CIP	critical illness polyneuropathy
CIPNM	critical illness polyneuromyopathy
CIWA	Clinical Institute Withdrawal Assessment for Alcohol
CJD	Creutzfeldt–Jakob disease
CK	creatine kinase
CKD	chronic kidney disease
Cl^-	chloride
CLF	chronic liver failure
cmH_2O	centimetre of water
CMR	cardiac magnetic resonance
$CMRO_2$	cerebral metabolic rate of oxygen
CMV	cytomegalovirus
CNI	calcineurin inhibitor
CNS	central nervous system

CO	carbon monoxide; cardiac output
CO_2	carbon dioxide
CoBaTrICE	Competency Based Training programme in ICM for Europe and other regions
COHb	carboxyhaemoglobin
COM	cardiac output monitoring
COPD	chronic obstructive pulmonary disease
CoV	coronavirus
COVID	coronavirus disease
COVID-19	coronavirus disease 2019
COX-2	cyclo-oxygenase 2
COX-3	cyclo-oxygenase 3
CPAP	continuous positive airway pressure
CPAx	Chelsea Critical Care Physical Assessment tool
CPB	cardiopulmonary bypass
CPET	cardiopulmonary exercise testing
CPO	cardiogenic pulmonary oedema
CPOT	Critical Care Pain Observation Tool
CPP	cerebral perfusion pressure; child protection plan
CPR	cardiopulmonary resuscitation
CRBSI	catheter-related bloodstream infection
CRCI	critical illness-related corticosteroid insufficiency
CrCl	creatinine clearance
CRE	carbapenem-resistant *Enterobacteriaceae*
CRF	chronic renal failure; corticotrophin-releasing factor
CRP	C-reactive protein
CRRT	continuous renal replacement therapy
CRS	cardio-renal syndrome; cytokine release syndrome
CRT	cardiac resynchronisation therapy; capillary refill time
CRT-D	CRT defibrillator
CRT-P	CRT pacemaker
CS	cardiogenic shock
CSE	convulsive status epilepticus
CSF	cerebrospinal fluid
CSW	cerebral salt wasting
CTG	cardiotocography
CTPA	computed tomography pulmonary angiography
CVA	cerebrovascular accident
CVC	central venous catheter/catheterisation
CVP	central venous pressure
CVR	cerebral vascular resistance
CVS-AKI	cardiac and vascular surgery-associated acute kidney injury

CVVH	continuous veno-venous haemofiltration
CVVHD	continuous veno-venous haemodialysis
CVVHDF	continuous veno-venous haemodiafiltration
CVVHF	continuous veno-venous haemofiltration
CXR	chest X-ray
Da	dalton
DAMP	damage-associated molecular pattern
DAS	Difficult Airway Society
DAT	difficult airway trolley; direct anti-globulin test
DBD	donation after brainstem death
DBP	diastolic blood pressure
DC	direct current
DCD	donation after circulatory death
DCM	dilated cardiomyopathy
DCS	damage control surgery
DDAVP	desmopressin
DE	diaphragmatic excursion
DI	diabetes insipidus
DIC	disseminated intravascular coagulation
DIT	di-iodothyronine
DKA	diabetic ketoacidosis
dl	decilitre
DLCO	diffusion capacity of carbon monoxide
DM	diabetes mellitus
DNA	deoxyribonucleic acid
DNACPR	Do Not Attempt Cardiopulmonary Resuscitation
DOAC	direct oral anticoagulant
DoH	Department of Health
DoLS	Deprivation of Liberty Safeguards
dsDNA	double-stranded deoxyribonucleic acid
DTF	diaphragm thickening fraction
DTs	delirium tremens
DVLA	Driver and Vehicle Licensing Agency
DVT	deep vein thrombosis
EBV	Epstein–Barr virus
ECF	extracellular fluid
Echo	echocardiography
ECLS	extracorporeal life support
ECMO	extracorporeal membrane oxygenation
ECT	electroconvulsive therapy
EDH	extradural haemorrhage

EDTA	ethylene diaminetetraacetic acid
EEG	electroencephalography
eGFR	estimated glomerular filtration rate
EHR	electronic health record
e-ICM	e-learning for intensive care medicine
ELSO	Extracorporeal Life Support Organization
EMB	endomyocardial biopsy
EMC	enhanced maternity care
EMG	electromyography
ENA	extractable nuclear antigen
ENT	ear, nose and throat
ePEEP	extrinsic positive end-expiratory pressure
EPUAP	European Pressure Ulcer Advisory Panel
ERCP	endoscopic retrograde cholangiopancreatography
ERF	Emergency Response Framework
ESA	erythropoietin-stimulating agent
ESBL	extended-spectrum β-lactamase
ESC	European Society of Cardiology
ESICM	European Society of Intensive Care Medicine
ESLD	end-stage liver disease
ESR	erythrocyte sedimentation rate
ESRD	end-stage renal disease
ET	essential thrombocythaemia
ETC	early total care
$ETCO_2$	end-tidal carbon dioxide
ETT	endotracheal tube
EU	European Union
EuroSCORE	European System for Cardiac Operative Risk Evaluation
EVD	external ventricular drain
EWS	Early Warning Score
EXTRIP	EXtracorporeal TReatments In Poisoning
FAST	focussed assessment with sonography in trauma; Face, Arm, Speech, Time
FBC	full blood count
FEAST	Fluid Expansion as Supportive Therapy (trial)
FEEL	focussed echocardiography in emergency life support
FEIBA	factor eight inhibitor bypassing agent
FE_{Na}	fractional excretion of sodium
FEV_1	forced expiratory volume in 1 second
FFP	fresh frozen plasma
FGF	fresh gas flow
FICE	focussed intensive care echocardiography

FICM	Faculty of Intensive Care Medicine
FII	fabricated or induced illness
FiO_2	fraction of inspired oxygen
FOB	fibreoptic bronchoscopy
Fr	French
FRC	functional residual capacity
FSGS	focal segmental glomerulosclerosis
FSS-ICU	Functional Status Scale for ICU
fT3	free T3
fT4	free T4
FVC	forced vital capacity
γGT	gamma-glutamyl transferase
G	gauge
GA	general anaesthetic
GABA	gamma aminobutyric acid
GAS	group A *Streptococcus*
GBM	glomerular basement membrane
GBS	Guillain–Barré syndrome
GCS	Glasgow Coma Score
GDI	gestational diabetes insipidus
GFR	glomerular filtration rate
GHB	gamma hydroxybutyrate
GI	gastrointestinal
GIT	gastrointestinal tract
GMC	General Medical Council
GMP	guanosine monophosphate
GOJ	gastro-oesophageal junction
GOLD	Global Initiative for Chronic Obstructive Lung Disease
GOS	Glasgow Outcome Score
GP	general practitioner
G6PD	glucose-6-phosphate dehydrogenase
GPICS	Guidelines for the Provision of Intensive Care Services
GTN	glyceryl trinitrate
GUCH	grown-up congenital heart disease
GVHD	graft-versus-host disease
GVT	graft-versus-tumour
HAART	highly active anti-retroviral therapy
HAP	hospital-acquired pneumonia
HAPS	Harmless Acute Pancreatitis Score
HAS	human albumin solution
HAT	hepatic artery thrombosis

Hb	haemoglobin
hCG	human chorionic gonadotrophin
HCO$_3$	bicarbonate
Hct	haematocrit
HCV	hepatitis C
HDFN	haemolytic disease of the fetus and newborn
HDU	high dependency unit
HE	hepatic encephalopathy
HELLP	haemolysis, elevated liver enzymes and low platelets
HEMS	helicopter emergency medical services
HF	heart failure
HFNC	high-flow nasal cannulae
HFOV	high-frequency oscillatory ventilation
HFPEF	heart failure with preserved ejection fraction
HFREF	heart failure with reduced ejection fraction
HHS	hyperosmolar hyperglycaemic state
Hib	*Haemophilus influenzae* type b
HIT	heparin-induced thrombocytopenia
HITT	heparin-induced thrombocytopenic thrombosis
HLA	human leucocyte antigen
HLH	haemophagocytic lymphohistiocytosis
HM	haematological malignancy
HME	heat and moisture exchanger
HPA	hypothalamic–pituitary–adrenal
HPS	hepatopulmonary syndrome
hr	hour
H2RB	histamine-2 receptor blocker
HRS	hepatorenal syndrome
hsCRP	high-sensitivity C-reactive protein
HSC	haematopoietic stem cell
HSCT	haematopoietic stem cell transplant
hsTrP	high-sensitivity troponin
HSV	herpes simplex virus
HU	Hounsfield units
HUS	haemolytic uraemic syndrome
Hz	hertz
IA	intrinsic activity
IABP	intra-aortic balloon pump
IAH	intra-abdominal hypertension
IAP	intra-abdominal pressure
IBA	impact brain apnoea

ICANS	immune effector cell-associated neurotoxicity syndrome
ICD	implantable cardioverter–defibrillator; International Statistical Classification of Diseases and Related Health Problems
ICDSC	Intensive Care Delirium Screening Checklist
ICG	International Coordinating Group
ICH	intracerebral haemorrhage
ICM	intensive care medicine
ICNARC	Intensive Care National Audit and Research Centre
ICP	intracranial pressure
ICS	Intensive Care Society; inhaled corticosteroid
ICU-AW	intensive care unit-acquired weakness
ID	infectious disease
IDSA	Infectious Diseases Society of America
IE	infective endocarditis
I:E	inspiratory/expiratory ratio
IEM	inborn errors of metabolism
IgA	immunoglobulin A
IgD	immunoglobulin D
IgE	immunoglobulin E
IGFBP-7	insulin-like growth factor binding protein 7
IgG	immunoglobulin G
IgM	immunoglobulin M
IHD	intermittent haemodialysis; ischaemic heart disease
IIH	idiopathic intracranial hypertension
IJV	internal jugular vein
IL	interleukin
IL-6	interleukin-6
ILD	interstitial lung disease
IM	intramuscular
IMCA	Independent Mental Capacity Advocate
IMER	Ionising Radiation (Medical Exposure) Regulations
IMS	Incident Management System
IMV	invasive mechanical ventilation
INARC	Intensive Care National Audit & Research Centre
INR	international normalised ratio
INTERMACS	Interagency Registry for Mechanically Assisted Circulatory Support
IO	intraosseous
IOCS	intraoperative cell salvage
IPD	intra-pleural distance
IQR	interquartile range
IRIS	immune reconstitution inflammatory syndrome

ISCoS	International Spinal Cord Society
ISS	Injury Severity Score
ISTH	International Society on Thrombosis and Haemostasis
IU	international unit
IV	intravenous
IVC	inferior vena cava
IVDU	intravenous drug user
IVIG	intravenous immunoglobulin
J	joule
JRCALC	Joint Royal Colleges Ambulance Liaison Committee
JVP	jugular venous pressure
K	J(Kell)
K^+	potassium
kcal	kilocalorie
KCl	potassium chloride
KCO	carbon monoxide transfer coefficient
KDIGO	Kidney Disease: Improving Global Outcomes
KIM-1	kidney injury molecule-1
kPa	kilopascal
LA	left atrial/atrium
LABA	long-acting beta-2 agonist
LAD	left axis deviation
LAMA	long-acting muscarinic antagonist
LAP	left atrial pressure
lb	pound
LBBB	left bundle branch block
LBO	large bowel obstruction
LCOS	low cardiac output syndrome
LDH	lactate dehydrogenase
LDL	low-density lipoprotein
L-FAB	liver fatty acid-binding protein
LFT	liver function test
LLN	lower limit of normal
LMWH	low-molecular-weight heparin
LOS	length of stay
LP	lumbar puncture
LPA	lasting power of attorney
LPR	lactate/pyruvate ratio
LRINEC	Laboratory Risk Indicator for Necrotising Fasciitis
LSD	lysergic acid diethylamide
LT	liver transplantation; lung transplant

LTA	light transmission aggregometry
LTi	laryngotracheal injuries
LTOT	long-term oxygen therapy
LV	left ventricular/left ventricle
LVAD	left ventricular assist device
LVEDV	left ventricular end-diastolic volume
LVESD	left ventricular end-systolic diameter
LVESV	left ventricular end-systolic volume
μg	microgram
μmol	micromole
MAHA	microangiopathic haemolytic anaemia
MALDI	matrix-assisted laser desorption/ionisation
MALDI-TOF	matrix-assisted laser desorption/ionisation time-of-flight
MALT	mucosa-associated lymphoid tissue
MAOI	monoamine oxidase inhibitor
MAP	mean arterial pressure
MARS	molecular adsorbent recirculating system
MBC	minimum bactericidal concentration
MBRRACE-UK	Mothers and Babies: Reducing Risk through Audits and Confidential Enquiries across the UK
MCA	Mental Capacity Act
MCS	mechanical circulatory support
MC&S	microscopy, culture and sensitivity
MCV	mean corpuscular volume
MDMA	3,4-methylenedioxymethamphetamine
MDR	multidrug-resistant
MDRD	Modification of Diet in Renal Disease
MDT	multidisciplinary team
MEGX	monoethylglycinexylidide
MELD	Model for End-Stage Liver Disease
MERS	Middle Eastern respiratory syndrome
MERS-CoV	Middle East respiratory syndrome coronavirus
MET	metabolic equivalent
Mg	magnesium
MG	myasthenia gravis
MHA	Mental Health Act
MHC	major histocompatibility complex
MHRA	Medicine and Healthcare products Regulatory Agency
MI	myocardial infarction
MIC	minimum inhibitory concentration
MIP	maximal inspiratory pressure

MIT	mono-iodothyronine
MLSB	macrolides/azalides, lincosamides and the streptogramin B group of antibiotics
M&M	morbidity and mortality
mmHg	millimetres of mercury
mmol	millimole
MODS	Multiple Organ Dysfunction Score; multiple organ dysfunction syndrome
MOF	multiple organ failure
MOH	massive obstetric haemorrhage
mOsm	milliosmole
MOST	multi-organ support therapy
MPC	mutant prevention concentration
MPM	Mortality Prediction Model
MR	mitral regurgitation
MRC	Medical Research Council
MRCP	magnetic resonance cholangiopancreatography
mRNA	messenger ribonucleic acid
MRSA	meticillin-resistant *Staphylococcus aureus*
MS	mitral stenosis
MSCT	multi-slice computed tomography
MSSA	meticillin-sensitive *Staphylococcus aureus*
MSU	midstream urine
MSW	mutant selection window
MTC	major trauma centre
MV	mitral valve
MVF	mean flow velocity
Na$^+$	sodium
NaCl	sodium chloride
NAFLD	non-alcoholic fatty liver disease
NAG	N-acetyl-β-D-glucosaminidase
NAP4	4th National Audit Project
NAPQI	N-acetyl-p-benzoquinone imine
NASH	non-alcoholic steatohepatitis
NCAA	National Cardiac Arrest Audit
NCS	nerve conduction study
NDI	nephrogenic diabetes insipidus
NEWS	National Early Warning Score
NEX	nose, earlobe, xiphisternum
NEXUS	National Emergency X-Radiography Utilisation Study
NF	necrotising fasciitis
NG	nasogastric
NGAL	neutrophil gelatinase-associated lipocalin

NGT	nasogastric tube
NICE	National Institute for Health and Care Excellence
NIHSS	National Institute for Health Stroke Scale
NIV	non-invasive ventilation
NJT	nasojejunal tube
NMBA	neuromuscular-blocking agent
NMDA	N-methyl-D-aspartate
NMES	neuromuscular electrical stimulation
NMS	neuroleptic malignant syndrome
NNBC	National Network for Burn Care
NNT	number needed to treat
NO	nitric oxide
NOAC	novel oral anticoagulant
NOMI	non-occlusive mesenteric ischaemia
NPSA	National Patient Safety Agency
NPUAP	National Pressure Ulcer Advisory Panel
NRLS	National Reporting and Learning System
1/2 NS	0.45% normal saline
NSAID	non-steroidal anti-inflammatory drug
NSTEMI	non-ST-segment elevation myocardial infarction
NT-pro-BNP	N-terminal pro-B-type natriuretic peptide
NTSCI	non-traumatic spinal cord injury
NVE	native valve endocarditis
NYHA	New York Heart Association
OCP	ova, cysts and parasites
OD	overdose
ODS	osmotic demyelination syndrome
OI	oxygenation index
OOHCA	out-of-hospital cardiac arrest
OSI	oxygen saturation index
PA	pulmonary artery; posterior–anterior
P-A	postero-anterior
PABA	para-aminobenzoic acid
PAC	pulmonary artery catheter
$PaCO_2$	partial pressure of carbon dioxide
PACU	post-anaesthesia care unit
PAE	post-antibiotic effect
PAF	platelet-activating factor
PAH	pulmonary arterial hypertension
PAI-1	plasminogen activator inhibitor-1
PALF	paediatric acute liver failure

PAMP	pathogen-associated molecular pattern
PaO_2	partial pressure of oxygen
pARDS	paediatric acute respiratory distress syndrome
PAWP	pulmonary artery wedge pressure
PB	peripheral blood
PBM	patient blood management
PBP	penicillin-binding protein
PBS	protected brush specimen
$PbtO_2$	parenchymal tissue oxygen tension
PCA	patient-controlled analgesia
PCC	prothrombin complex concentrate
PCEA	patient-controlled epidural analgesia
PCI	percutaneous coronary intervention
PCR	polymerase chain reaction
PCT	procalcitonin; Primary Care Trust
PCW	pulmonary capillary wedge
PD	pharmacodynamics
PD-1	programmed death-1
PDOC	prolonged disorders of consciousness
PDPH	post-dural puncture headache
PDT	percutaneous dilatational tracheostomy
PE	pulmonary embolism
PEA	pulseless electrical activity
PEEP	positive end-expiratory pressure
PEF	peak expiratory flow
PEG	percutaneous endoscopic gastrostomy
PEJ	percutaneous endoscopic jejunostomy
PELOD	Pediatric Logistic Organ Dysfunction
$PETCO_2$	partial pressure of end-tidal carbon dioxide
PEX	plasma exchange
PF4	platelet factor 4
PFIT-s	Physical Functional Scale for ICU–score
PGD	primary graft dysfunction
PGE2	prostaglandin E2
PH	portal hypertension; pulmonary hypertension
PICANet	Paediatric Intensive Care Audit Network
PICC	peripherally inserted central catheter
PICS	post-intensive care syndrome
PICS-F	PICS-family
PICU	paediatric intensive care unit
PIM	paediatric index of mortality

PIP	peak inspiratory pressure
PIRRT	prolonged intermittent RRT
PJP	*Pneumocystis jirovecii* pneumonia
PK	pharmacokinetics
PLAPS	posterolateral alveolar and/or pleural syndrome
PLAX	parasternal long axis
PLEX	plasma exchange
pLVAD	percutaneous left ventricular assist device
PMA	paramethoxyamphetamine
PMCS	peri-mortem Caesarean section
PN	parenteral nutrition
PO	orally
PO_4	phosphate
POCT	point-of-care test
PONV	post-operative nausea and vomiting
POPS	Perioperative Care of the Older Person
PPCM	peripartum cardiomyopathy
PPE	personal protective equipment
PPH	post-partum haemorrhage
PPI	proton pump inhibitor
PPM	permanent pacemaker
P-POSSUM	Portsmouth Physiological and Operative Severity Score for the enUmeration of Mortality and morbidity
PRIS	propofol infusion syndrome
PRISM	paediatric risk of mortality
PROPPR	Pragmatic, Randomized, Optimal Platelet and Plasma Ratios (trial)
PRSP	penicillin-resistant *Streptococcus pneumoniae*
PRV	polycythaemic rubra vera
pRVAD	percutaneous right ventricular assist device
PS	performance score
PSAX	parasternal short axis
PSB	protected specimen brush
PSI	Pneumonia Severity Index
PT	prothrombin time
PTH	parathyroid hormone
PT-INR	international normalised ratio
$PtiO_2$	parenchymal tissue oxygen tension
PTP	post-transfusion purpura
PTSD	post-traumatic stress disorder
PTU	propylthiouracil
PVE	prosthetic valve endocarditis

PVR	pulmonary vascular resistance
pVT	pulseless ventricular tachycardia
qSOFA	quick SOFA
RA	right atrium/right atrial
RAAS	renin–angiotensin–aldosterone system
RACHS	Risk Adjustment for Congenital Heart Surgery
RAD	right axis deviation
RAI	renal anginal index
RAP	right atrial pressure
RASS	Richmond Agitation Sedation Scale
RBC	red blood cell
RC	responsible clinician
RCA	regional citrate anticoagulation
RCOG	Royal College of Obstetricians and Gynaecologists
RCP	Royal College of Physicians
RCT	randomised controlled trial
RDT	rapid diagnostic test
REBOA	resuscitative endovascular balloon occlusion of the aorta
RFR	renal functional reserve
Rh	rhesus
RIFLE	Risk, Injury, Failure, Loss, End-stage kidney disease
RIG	radiologically inserted gastrostomy
RMN	registered mental health nurse
ROC	receiver operator characteristic curve
ROSC	return of spontaneous circulation
ROTEM®	rotational thromboelastometry
RRT	renal replacement therapy
rRT-PCR	real-time reverse transcription polymerase chain reaction
RSI	rapid sequence induction
RSV	respiratory syncytial virus
rT3	reverse T3
RTA	road traffic accident
RV	right ventricle; right ventricular; residual volume
RVAD	right ventricular assist device
RVOT	right ventricular outflow tract
RWMA	regional wall motion abnormality
SA	sinoatrial
SAAG	serum–ascites albumin gradient
SA-AKI	sepsis-associated acute kidney injury
SADS	sudden adult death syndrome
SAH	subarachnoid haemorrhage

SALT	speech and language therapy
SAM	systolic anterior motion
SaO_2	arterial oxygen saturation
SAPS	Simplified Acute Physiology Score
SARS	severe acute respiratory syndrome
SARS-CoV	severe acute respiratory syndrome coronavirus
SARS-CoV-1	severe acute respiratory syndrome coronavirus 1
SARS-CoV-2	severe acute respiratory syndrome coronavirus 2
SBO	small bowel obstruction
SBP	systolic blood pressure; spontaneous bacterial peritonitis
SBT	Sengstaken–Blakemore tube
SCAI	Society for Cardiovascular Angiography and Interventions
SCCM	Society of Critical Care Medicine
SCD	sudden cardiac death; sickle cell disease
SCIWORA	spinal cord injury without radiographic abnormality
SCORTEN	SCORe of Toxic Epidermal Necrolysis
SCr	serum creatinine
SCUF	slow continuous ultrafiltration
$ScVO_2$	central venous oxygen saturation
SDD	selective decontamination of the digestive tract
SDH	subdural haemorrhage
SDT	single dilator technique
SGLT-2	sodium–glucose co-transporter 2
SHOT	Serious Hazards of Transfusion
SIADH	syndrome of inappropriate anti-diuretic hormone secretion
S-ICD	subcutaneous implantable cardioverter–defibrillator
SID	strong ion difference
SIDS	sudden infant death syndrome
SIGN	Scottish Intercollegiate Guidelines Network
SIMV	synchronous intermittent mandatory ventilation
SIRS	systemic inflammatory response syndrome
SJS	Stevens–Johnson syndrome
$SjvO_2$	jugular venous oxygen saturation
SLED	slow low-efficiency dialysis
SMR	standardised mortality ratio
SNOD	specialist nurse for organ donation
SNRI	serotonin–noradrenaline reuptake inhibitor
SOAD	second opinion approved doctor
SOD	selective oral decontamination
SOFA	Sequential Organ Failure Assessment
SOP	standard operating procedure

SORT	Surgical Outcome Risk Tool
SpO$_2$	peripheral oxygen saturation
spp.	species
SS	serotonin syndrome
SSI	surgical site infection
SSRI	selective serotonin reuptake inhibitor
ssRNA	single-stranded ribonucleic acid
SSTI	skin and soft tissue infection
ST	surgical tracheostomy
STEC	Shiga-toxin producing *Escherichia coli* infection
STEMI	ST-segment elevation myocardial infarction
SUDEP	sudden unexplained death in epilepsy
SUDI	sudden unexpected death in infancy
SV	stroke volume
SVC	superior vena cava; slow vital capacity
SVCO	superior vena cava obstruction
SvO$_2$	mixed venous oxygen saturation
SVR	systemic vascular resistance
SVV	stroke volume variation
T3	tri-iodothyronine
T4	thyroxine
TACO	transfusion-associated circulatory overload
TAPSE	tricuspid valve annular plane systolic excursion
TAPVD	total anomalous pulmonary venous drainage
TAVI	transcatheter aortic valve implantation
TAVR	transcatheter aortic valve replacement
TB	tuberculosis
TBG	thyroid-binding globulin
TBI	traumatic brain injury
TBSA	total body surface area
TCA	tricyclic antidepressant
TCD	transcranial Doppler ultrasound
TDM	therapeutic drug monitoring
TEG®	thromboelastography
TEN	toxic epidermal necrolysis
TEVAR	thoracic endovascular aortic repair
TF	tissue factor
TGA	transposition of the great arteries
TH	Tandem Heart®
TIC	trauma-induced coagulopathy
TIMP2	tissue inhibitor metalloproteinase

TIPSS	transjugular intrahepatic portosystemic shunt
TLC	total lung capacity
TLCO	transfer factor for carbon monoxide
TLR	Toll-like receptor
TLS	tumour lysis syndrome
TMA	thrombotic microangiopathy
TNF	tumour necrosis factor
TOE	transoesophageal echocardiography
TOF	train-of-four; tetralogy of Fallot
tPA	tissue plasminogen activator
TPN	total parenteral nutrition
TPPPS	Toddler–Preschooler Postoperative Pain Scale
TR	tricuspid regurgitation
TRALI	transfusion-related acute lung injury
TRH	thyrotropin-releasing hormone
TRICC	Transfusion Requirements in Critical Care
TRISS	Trauma Injury Severity Score
TRM	transplant-related mortality
tRNA	transfer ribonucleic acid
TSCI	traumatic spinal cord injury
TSH	thyroid-stimulating hormone
TSS	toxic shock syndrome
TT	thrombin time
TTE	transthoracic echocardiography
TTM	targeted temperature management
TTP	thrombotic thrombocytopenic purpura
TXA	tranexamic acid
U	unit
UA	unstable angina
UAO	upper airway obstruction
U&Es	urea and electrolytes
UF	ultrafiltration
UFH	unfractionated heparin
UGIB	upper gastrointestinal bleeding
UKOSS	UK Obstetric Surveillance System
URL	upper reference limit
USS	ultrasound scanning
VA	alveolar volume; veno-arterial
VAC	vacuum-assisted closure
VAD	ventricular assist device
VA-ECMO	veno-arterial extracorporeal membrane oxygenation

VALI	ventilator-associated lung injury
VAP	ventilator-associated pneumonia
VBG	venous blood gas
VC	vital capacity
V_D	volume of distribution
VET	viscoelastic test
VF	ventricular fibrillation
VHD	valvular heart disease
VILI	ventilator-induced lung injury
VKA	vitamin K antagonist
V/Q	ventilation/perfusion
VRE	vancomycin-resistant *Enterococcus*
Vt	tidal volume
VT	ventricular tachycardia
VTE	venous thromboembolism
VV	veno-venous
VV-ECMO	veno-venous extracorporeal membrane oxygenation
vWF	von Willebrand factor
VZV	varicella-zoster virus
WBC	white blood cell
WCC	white cell count
WHO	World Health Organization
WPW	Wolff–Parkinson–White
WSACS	World Society of the Abdominal Compartment Syndrome

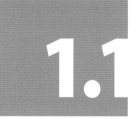

General Introduction to the Recognition, Assessment and Stabilisation of the Acutely Ill Patient with Disordered Physiology

Claire Moorthy

Key Learning Points

1. National Early Warning Scores result in earlier escalation of care and improved outcomes.
2. Approach to assessment, management and stabilisation requires structure and focus.
3. Management of life-threatening conditions is a priority.
4. Initial treatment often precedes diagnosis.
5. Initial assessment, secondary assessment and continued reassessment are required in the critically ill.

Keywords: acutely ill patient, clinical deterioration, assessment, stabilisation, management

Introduction

The initial assessment, stabilisation and management of the acutely unwell patient can be stressful and challenging for both the patient and clinician. Rapid decision-making and actions are required with often limited information and a physiologically unstable patient. The disease process can be unpredictable, and clinical outcome uncertain.

Signs of clinical deterioration are generally similar, regardless of the underlying process, resulting in failure of the respiratory, cardiovascular and central nervous systems. Early recognition and management can potentially prevent the need for ICU admission, cardio-respiratory arrest and ultimately death. Early Warning Score (EWS) systems, and more specifically the National Early Warning Score (NEWS) system (2012), have greatly helped in this regard, resulting in earlier escalation of care and improved outcomes.

Assessment of this group of patients can present a difficult challenge due to physiological instability. A well-structured, iterative approach, much like that used in trauma and cardiopulmonary resuscitation situations, is suggested. Initial assessment, and secondary and continued reassessment, will help to prioritise and simplify the management of life-threatening conditions, abnormal physiology, oxygen delivery and patient safety.

The approach should be:

- Structured
- Systematic
- Focused
- Timely
- Objective

It is important to realise that initial treatment will often precede diagnosis. When the patient has been physiologically stabilised, a more thorough systems-based review can be carried out, and further information gathered. Finally this information, coupled with investigations and imaging, can be used within the clinical context to create a differential diagnosis or a specific diagnosis, which will then permit specific management.

1

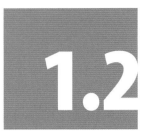

1.2 Management of Cardiopulmonary Resuscitation – Advanced Life Support

Jonny Coppel

Key Learning Points

1. Good leadership during cardiac arrests can significantly impact chances of successful outcomes.
2. Early cardiopulmonary resuscitation (CPR) and defibrillation are the core of good advanced life support (ALS) management.
3. Ventilation should be quickly optimised, with particular emphasis on avoiding overventilating patients.
4. Decisions to end CPR can be difficult but should be based on clinical judgement once reversible causes have been identified.
5. Data from all cardiac arrests are used for a national audit to ensure a widespread provision of a high-quality resus service.

Keywords: cardiac arrest, resuscitation, advanced life support, leadership

Chain of Survival

The Resuscitation Council UK has described a four-step chain of survival to highlight the key elements of a successful resuscitation:

1. Early recognition and call for help
2. Early cardiopulmonary resuscitation (CPR)
3. Early defibrillation
4. Post-resuscitation care

This chapter will not discuss the individual steps of the adult advanced life support (ALS) algorithm (Figure 1.2.1), but instead will discuss some of the leadership and technical principles of effective management of CPR.

Leadership

Good leadership enables safe and efficient management of the cardiac arrest situation which in turn provides the best chances of a successful outcome. The Resuscitation Council UK's set of qualities that ALS providers should have include: situational awareness, task management, decision-making, teamworking and leadership.

Research shows that even in experienced teams, chest compressions are often too slow and too shallow, and the ventilation rate too high. It is therefore important that the leader predicts, recognises and manages these deviations in practice.

Practical Leadership Issues

Ideally, at the beginning of the shift, the resuscitation team should be introduced to each other; a team leader should be appointed, and appropriate responsibilities should be allocated based on skill levels. Leaders should ensure quality CPR is taking place and that CPR providers are not fatiguing and are regularly swapping. 'Time off the chest' should be minimised – especially relevant if following the shockable side of the algorithm. One method to enhance the speed of rhythm checks is to ensure pulse checks only occur if the rhythm is compatible with a pulse. Leaders should monitor the safety of the team, including the need for any personal protective equipment.

Technical

Cardiopulmonary Resuscitation

CPR should have a depth of 5–6 cm and a rate of 100–120 compressions per minute, with rhythm checks occurring after every two-minute cycle. Residual leaning on the chest after each compression by rescuers impairs coronary perfusion pressures. Details of defibrillation and pad positioning are covered in another chapter. Prior to advanced airway management, standard CPR with 30 compressions followed by two breaths should be performed. Pulse checks should

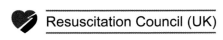 Resuscitation Council (UK) **Adult Advanced Life Support**

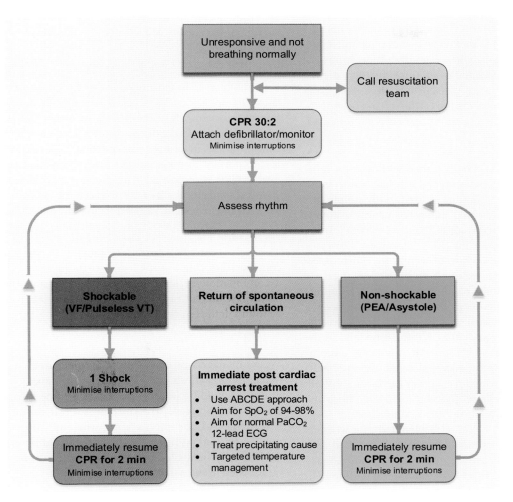

Figure 1.2.1 Adult advanced life support algorithm.
Source: © Resuscitation Council (UK).

be carried out at three different anatomical locations, whilst ensuring both carotids are not checked simultaneously. According to Resuscitation Council UK guidelines, automated mechanical chest compression devices should not be used routinely to replace manual chest compressions. They may, however, enable high-quality compressions when manual compressions are not possible, for example when transporting patients. Precordial thumps are not discussed here, as they carry very low success rates for the cardioversion of shockable rhythms, and their routine use is not recommended.

Ventilation

Airway access should be obtained within a few minutes of starting resuscitation. Initially bag–valve–mask (BVM) ventilation should be used, with simple airway manoeuvres utilised alongside airway adjuncts to maintain patency until a definitive airway can be placed. Endotracheal tube (ETT) placement allows for a definitive airway, suction of secretions, reliable oxygen delivery and protection from inhalation of gastric contents. If possible, avoid stopping chest compressions during laryngoscopy and intubation; however, a brief pause is permissible whilst attempting to pass the ETT between the vocal cords. If intubation fails, or the person is not adequately trained to insert one, a supraglottic airway device (laryngeal mask airway, i-gel®) can be used until a definitive airway can be established. A surgical airway should also be considered if no airway access and ventilation can be established.

Hyperventilation should be avoided as it worsens prognosis. Unnecessarily high tidal volumes and ventilation rates create a mismatch, with poor pulmonary perfusion reduced further by poor cardiac output in CPR. Additionally, excessive BVM ventilation leads to increased intrathoracic pressures, which further decrease venous return and cardiac output.

Tidal volume should be 400–600 ml (approximately one-third of a BVM compression, or sufficient to produce a chest rise over 1 second). Once a definitive airway is *in situ*, chest compressions should continue without a pause for ventilation. Whilst the evidence base for the optimum ventilation rate is poor, a rate of 10 breaths per minute is recommended.

End-Tidal Carbon Dioxide

Measuring end-tidal carbon dioxide plays a key role in cardiac arrests by the following:

1. Indication of correct ETT placement
2. Monitoring ventilation rate during CPR
3. Monitoring the quality of chest compressions
4. Identifying return of spontaneous circulation (ROSC) during CPR
5. Prognostication during CPR (chronically low end-tidal CO_2 is associated with poor outcomes)

Vascular Access

Obtaining access should hinder neither CPR nor defibrillation. If intravenous (IV) access is proving difficult, consider intraosseous (IO) access in the proximal humerus or tibia. IO injection of drugs achieves adequate plasma concentrations in a time comparable with IV injection. It is important to note, however, that circulation time during CPR is prolonged – drugs take approximately 30–60 seconds of quality CPR to reach the central circulation and peripheral vasculature to exert their effects.

The 4 Hs and 4 Ts

The eight reversible causes in Table 1.2.1 must be considered during a cardiac arrest. To do so involves a combination of history and clinical examination, blood gases and ultrasound scanning. More details can be found in the references below.

Special Circumstances

Proper management of a cardiopulmonary arrest must make modifications in special circumstances. One example would be in pregnancy where some form of uterine displacement to reduce aortocaval compression, either of the uterus alone (manual displacement) or by lateral tilt of the pelvis, is recommended. Additionally, defibrillation and drug protocols should be adjusted in cases of hypothermia.

Cessation of CPR

The duration of any resuscitation attempt is a matter of clinical judgement. If appropriately started, it should be continued if the patient remains in identifiable ventricular fibrillation/pulseless ventricular tachycardia, or if there is a potentially reversible cause that can be treated. Asystole for >20 minutes (during ongoing

Table 1.2.1 The 4 Hs and 4 Ts

4 Hs	4 Ts
Hypoxia	Thrombosis
Hypovolaemia	Tension pneumothorax
Hypo-/hyperkalaemia	Tamponade (cardiac)
Hypothermia	Toxins

CPR), in the absence of a reversible cause, provides adequate grounds for stopping further resuscitation attempts. If the decision has been taken to terminate resuscitation, it is essential to allocate time and resources to team debriefing, discussions with the family and ensuring the coroner's obligations are met.

National Audit and Training

The National Cardiac Arrest Audit (NCAA) audits all in-hospital cardiac arrests, allowing national comparisons to be made. This helps monitor adherence to national standards to enable a high-quality resuscitation service. Their core standards can be found in the references below. Any resuscitation-related incidents or equipment problems can be reported to the National Reporting and Learning System (NRLS).

References and Further Reading

Abella BS, Alvarado JP, Myklebust H, *et al.* Quality of cardiopulmonary resuscitation during in-hospital cardiac arrest. *JAMA* 2005;**293**:305–10.

Intensive Care National Audit & Research Centre (INARC) and Resuscitation Council UK. National Cardiac Arrest Audit (NCAA). www.icnarc.org/Our-Audit/ Audits/Ncaa/About

Nolan J, Soar J, Eikeland H. The chain of survival. *Resuscitation* 2006;**71**:270–1.

Resuscitation Council UK. *Advanced Life Support*, 7th edn. London: Resuscitation Council UK; 2016.

Vissers G, Soar J, Monsieurs KG. Ventilation rate in adults with a tracheal tube during cardiopulmonary resuscitation: a systematic review. *Resuscitation* 2017;**119**:5–12.

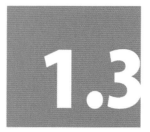

Principles of Management of the Patient Post-resuscitation

Jonny Coppel

Key Learning Points

1. The post-cardiac arrest syndrome is composed of: persistent precipitating pathology, post-cardiac arrest brain injury, post-cardiac arrest myocardial dysfunction and the systemic ischaemic/reperfusion response.
2. Hyperoxia and hypocapnia should be avoided post-return of spontaneous circulation, and oxygen saturations should be titrated to 94–98 per cent.
3. Inotropic support is commonly necessary to support adequate urine output and reducing plasma lactate levels.
4. Targeted temperature management is an important tool in improving outcomes for all cardiac arrest patients who remain unresponsive post-arrest.
5. Post-prognostication is an important opportunity for organ donation evaluation.

Keywords: post-cardiac arrest syndrome, targeted temperature management, prognostication

Introduction

The fourth and final link in the Resuscitation Council UK's chain of survival is post-resuscitation care. After achieving recovery of spontaneous circulation (ROSC), the patient is in a vulnerable state and the subsequent management at this point in part determines the extent of their recovery. Patient management at this stage is best structured in an ABCDE approach in order to appropriately manage post-cardiac arrest syndrome.

Post-cardiac Arrest Syndrome

The hypoxia, ischaemia and reperfusion that occur during and after resuscitation result in damage to multiple organ systems. There are four main components to post-cardiac arrest syndrome:

- Persistent precipitating pathology: the initial cause of the cardiac arrest, unless fully managed, can cause further deterioration of the patient. The most common precipitant is a coronary thrombus, in which case urgent transfer for percutaneous coronary intervention (PCI) must be considered
- Post-cardiac arrest brain injury: reperfusion of the brain after cerebral hypoxia leads to free radical formation and activation of cell death signalling pathways, both of which affect cerebral blood flow autoregulation. This presents itself in a variety of forms, including coma, seizures and other less severe forms of neurological dysfunction. This injury can last for hours to days, and is aggravated by fever, poor glucose control and hypoxia
- Post-cardiac arrest myocardial dysfunction: hypokinesia of cardiac muscles is associated with a reduction in left ventricular ejection fraction. This is most common in the first 24–48 hours after ROSC. It occurs despite adequate coronary blood flow, and manifests itself as tachycardia, hypotension and left ventricular end-diastolic dysfunction
- Systemic ischaemic/reperfusion response: systemic inflammation, endothelial activation and activation of immunologic and coagulation pathways occur. This can present in a similar manner to septic shock, and increases the patient's susceptibility to infection

Airway and Breathing

Normoxia and normocarbia should be aimed for, and hyperventilation must be avoided. Hyperoxia and hypocapnia are independently associated with worse outcomes, and the latter is due to the resulting reduction in cerebral blood flow. In the immediate phase following ROSC, use the highest concentration of oxygen to avoid hypoxia; then once oxygen levels are reliably measured via arterial blood gases, titrate to maintain arterial oxygen saturation (SaO_2) of 94–98 per cent.

After the resuscitation phase, a chest X-ray is warranted to ensure endotracheal tubes are in the correct position, and there are no pneumothoraces secondary to cardiopulmonary resuscitation (CPR). Additionally, check for flail segments and signs of gastric content aspiration. The stomach may need decompressing after bag–mask ventilation.

Circulation

Maintaining perfusion to critical organs is of particular importance post-ROSC. Key parameters to guide treatment are blood pressure, heart rate, urine output, rate of plasma lactate clearance and central venous oxygen saturations. The exact targets for haemodynamic parameters, taking into account co-morbidities, are still undefined. However, a general rule is to target mean arterial blood pressure to achieve a urine output of 1 ml/(kg hr) and normal or reducing plasma lactate values. Inotropic support, commonly using a combination of fluids and noradrenaline (with or without dobutamine), is an effective way of managing post-ROSC hypotension. With regard to the management of acidosis and lactate, bicarbonate should not be given due to its paradoxical effects of increasing intracellular acidosis, unless for certain indications such as hyperkalaemia or tricyclic antidepressant overdoses.

Continuous ECG monitoring is essential, including an early 12-lead ECG and serial cardiac troponins. Direct continuous arterial blood pressure should be used. Echocardiography should be performed at a minimum 24–48 hours post-ROSC to monitor ejection fractions and rule out regional wall motion abnormalities. No routine anti-arrhythmic agent is recommended, but it may be reasonable to continue the infusion of any anti-arrhythmic drug that successfully restored a stable rhythm during resuscitation.

Electrolytes must be monitored. Typically, potassium levels rise post-ROSC, followed by a phase of hypokalaemia secondary to increasing intracellular transport. These both increase the risk of ventricular arrhythmias.

Disability

Seizure Management

Seizures are common post-ROSC. However, routine seizure prophylaxis is not recommended until after the first seizure – assuming precipitating causes have been ruled out. Propofol is often effective to suppress post-anoxic myoclonus.

Targeted Temperature Management

This is recommended for any cardiac arrest patient who remains unresponsive post-arrest. The benefits include:

- A reduction in cerebral metabolic oxygen consumption by 6 per cent for each 1°C reduction in core temperature
- Reducing the cellular effects of reperfusion and decreasing the production of free radicals

It is contraindicated in patients with severe sepsis, coagulopathy and established multi-organ failure.

Core body temperature should be monitored with oesophageal/central venous probes or bladder temperature catheters. A target of 32–36°C should be maintained for 24 hours. Cooling can be achieved by:

- Surface cooling with cooling blankets and ice packs
- Cold infusions
- Evaporative trans-nasal cooling
- Endovascular cooling catheters

Shivering has an adverse effect, and so should need to be controlled with magnesium sulphate and paralytics – which, if used, require neurological monitoring. Patients should be gradually rewarmed at 0.25–0.33°C/hr until normothermic. Rapid rewarming leads to cerebral oedema, seizures and hyperkalaemia. Post-targeted temperature management (TTM) rebound hyperthermia must also be avoided, as it is associated with worse outcomes. One necessary consideration with TTM is that the clearance of sedative drugs and neuromuscular blockers is reduced and thus delays neuro-assessment.

Glycaemic Control

Hyperglycaemia occurs post-ROSC, and also secondary to TTM. It is associated with increased mortality. Glucose levels of 6–10 mmol/l should be targeted.

Exposure

A full detailed history needs to be taken from relatives to determine co-morbidities and the exact circumstances surrounding the cardiac arrest. Furthermore, investigations and more invasive management of the cause of the cardiac arrest should be considered. Appropriate transfer of patients to the most appropriate clinical locations should occur according to

Intensive Care Society UK guidelines. Referral for implantable cardioverter–defibrillator (ICD) assessment should be considered.

Prognostication and Organ Donation

Earliest prognostication in post-ROSC patients is at 72 hours. However, if TTM was used, the earliest time is 72 hours after return to normothermia. After prognostication, organ donation evaluation should be considered.

References and Further Reading

Intensive Care Society. *Guidelines*. www.ics.ac.uk/Society/Guidance/Guidance

Nielsen N, Wetterslev J, Cronberg T, *et al.* Targeted temperature management at 33 degrees C versus 36 degrees C after cardiac arrest. *N Engl J Med* 2013;**369**:2197–206.

Pothiawala FS. Post-resuscitation care. *Singapore Med J* 2017;**58**:404–7.

Resuscitation Council UK. *Advanced Life Support*, 7th edn. London: Resuscitation Council UK; 2016.

Sandroni C, Cariou A, Cavallaro F, *et al.* Prognostication in comatose survivors of cardiac arrest: an advisory statement from the European Resuscitation Council and the European Society of Intensive Care Medicine. *Resuscitation* 2014;**85**:1779–89.

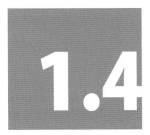# Principles of Triaging and Prioritising Patients Appropriately, Including Timely Admission to ICU

Claire Moorthy

Key Learning Points

1. Prioritise patient admission based on acute clinical needs and potential for deterioration.
2. Ensure daily ICU patient review to allow for appropriate admission and discharge planning.
3. Utilise local hospital policies for admission and discharge planning.
4. There must be a clear plan for escalation of treatment at all levels of care.
5. Patients should not be transferred to another ICU on non-clinical grounds where at all possible.

Keywords: critical care triage, admission criteria, critical care, levels of critical care

Introduction

Triage is a dynamic process of determining the order and priority of patient emergency treatment based on the severity of their condition, and should be undertaken by the senior clinician in charge of the ICU at the time of referral. Decision-making should be explicit and without bias. Ethnic origin, race, sexual orientation and social and financial status should never be considered during the triage process. Definitive treatment is paramount to good outcomes in ICU, and thus delays should be minimised. There should be timely escalation of care with the ideal of consultant-to-consultant referral.

Considerations When Triaging

These include:

- Specific treatment only available in the ICU setting
- Availability of clinical expertise
- Prioritisation based on the patient's clinical condition and potential to deteriorate

- Bed availability
- Potential to benefit from intervention
- Overall prognosis

Age per se is not a barrier for admission to ICU, but because of the potential decline in physiological reserve and decreased ability to recover with increasing age, it is important to consider the following in the very elderly:

- Co-morbidities
- Severity of illness
- Pre-hospital functional status
- Patient preferences

Most hospitals now have local policies in place outlining criteria for patient admission and discharge to ICU. The Department of Health (DoH) developed a classification system focussing on the level of patient dependency, regardless of location within an institution. This classification, although not yet universally employed or nationally validated, is widely used and has formed the basis of *National Guidelines for the Provision of Intensive Care Services* produced by the Faculty of Intensive Care Medicine, which is widely responsible for clinical guidelines nationally in the UK (Table 1.4.1).

Table 1.4.1 Levels of care

Level 0	Patients whose needs can be met through normal ward care in an acute hospital
Level 1	Patients at risk of their condition deteriorating, or those recently relocated from higher levels of care whose needs can be met on an acute ward with additional advice and support from the critical care team
Level 2	Patients requiring more detailed observation or intervention, including support for a single failing organ system or post-operative care, and those 'stepping down' from level 3 care
Level 3	Patients requiring advanced respiratory support alone, or basic respiratory support together with support of at least two organ systems. This level includes all complex patients requiring support for multi-organ failure

Source: The Department of Health (DoH).

9

Admission to ICU Ideals

- There must be clear documentation in patient notes of the time and decision to admit to ICU.
- Unplanned admission must occur within 4 hours of making the decision to admit.
- Patients should not be transferred to another ICU for non-clinical reasons.
- An ICU consultant must be immediately available 24/7, and available to attend within 30 minutes.
- Patients must be seen by an ICU consultant within 12 hours of admission to ICU.
- An ICU consultant-led, multidisciplinary team ward round must occur twice daily.
- A clear and documented treatment plan must be made with the ICU consultant.
- There must be a clear plan for escalation of treatment from level 2 to level 3 for all patients.
- It is acceptable to transfer patients to other specialist facilities, should that specialty be unavailable in the admitting hospital, e.g. neuro- or cardiac ICU.

Discharge Planning

- Should a patient be ready to step down to the high dependency unit (HDU) from ICU, or ward level care from HDU, local policies and procedures should be in place to allow this to be expedited safely.
- Transfer from ICU to the ward must be formalised.
- Handover between medical staff should be standardised with a clear summary of ICU stay, plans for further investigation, management and ongoing treatment.
- Discharge from ICU should occur within 4 hours of making the decision other than in the case of repatriation which will potentially require further planning and organisation.
- Discharge from ICU should ideally occur between 07.00 and 21.59.
- Unplanned readmission to ICU within 48 hours should be investigated.
- A standardised handover procedure must accompany the discharge and is to include:
  - A summary of the critical care stay, including diagnosis, treatment and changes to chronic therapies
  - A monitoring and investigation plan
  - A plan for ongoing treatment
  - Rehabilitation assessment and management incorporating physical, emotional, psychological and communication needs
  - Follow-up arrangements
  - Any treatment limitations
  - Plans for readmission, should it become necessary, including DNACPR (Do Not Attempt Cardiopulmonary Resuscitation)/ treatment escalation plan

Department of Health Guidelines 2000/Updated Review 2011

- Critical care services within NHS trusts should meet the needs of the critically ill or acutely deteriorating patients with the potential to become critically ill. There should be flexibility in the use of available capacity allowing elective and emergency commitments to be fulfilled.
- In order to facilitate this need, all HDU and ICU patients require regular daily review to ascertain continued requirement of this service.
- Should a patient require HDU/ICU facility, every attempt should be made to accommodate that patient within the admitting NHS trust.

References and Further Reading

Department of Health. Comprehensive critical care. London: Department of Health; 2000.

Faculty of Intensive Care Medicine and Intensive Care Society. Section 3.1: Critical care services process – admission, discharge and handover. In: *Guidelines for the provision of intensive care services*, 2nd edn. 2019; pp. 76–9.

General Medical Council. *Good Medical Practice*. London: General Medical Council; 2013.

National Institute for Health and Care Excellence. Acutely ill patients in hospital: Recognition of and response to acute illness in adults in hospital. Clinical guideline [CG50]. London: National Institute for Health and Care Excellence; 2007.

National Institute for Health and Care Excellence. Rehabilitation after critical illness in adults. Clinical guideline [CG83]. London: National Institute for Health and Care Excellence; 2009.

Initial Assessment and Management of the Trauma Patient

1.5

Anil Dhadwal

Key Learning Points

1. Initial assessment and management of a trauma patient require a structured team approach, with good communication and leadership. Often this is best coordinated by someone standing back from the action, and thus able to take account of the whole unfolding scenario.
2. All members should have appropriate personal protection equipment, especially with the recent global coronavirus disease (COVID-19) pandemic.
3. The primary survey using an ABCDE approach is undertaken with the aim to rule out, and treat, any life-threatening injuries.
4. Once the patient has been stabilised with regard to the initial insult, then a full head-to-toe secondary survey examination needs to be performed to identify, treat and document any remaining injuries present.
5. It is important to ask the question: '*Do the patient's treatment needs exceed the capability of this receiving institution?*'. If the answer is yes, then urgent referral should be made to a major trauma centre.

Keywords: ATLS, primary survey, secondary survey, major trauma centre, trauma

Introduction

Managing patients with trauma, especially major trauma, remains a challenge across the world. The recent terrorist attacks in the UK have focussed the service provided by the NHS. Major trauma is traditionally the most common cause of death in men under the age of 40. However, recent literature has indicated that elderly patients with lower-energy injuries are increasing in prevalence and provide their own challenges.

Regardless of the patient demographic, trauma calls and the initial assessment of the patient are paramount to their final recovery. It requires a structured team approach, with good communication and leadership – often best coordinated by someone standing back from the action, and thus able to take account of the whole unfolding scenario.

This chapter provides an introduction to managing trauma patients, their initial assessment and the key parameters specific for intensivists to identify and manage during the initial presentation and beyond.

Pre-arrival Preparation

The whole trauma team (emergency medicine physician, anaesthetist, intensivist, operating department practitioner, general surgeons, trauma surgeons, radiographer and nursing staff, etc.) should be assembled, with their roles identified prior to the arrival of the patient to allow adequate preparation. The trauma team leader should brief the team about the pre-hospital status of the patient, including:

- Demographics (age/sex)
- Special patients (very young/elderly/pregnant)
- Injury (mechanism/severity/how many/timing)
- Injury Severity Score
- Interventions made pre-hospital
- Glasgow Coma Score (GCS)/A-B-C/AMPLE

All members should have appropriate personal protection equipment, especially with the recent global coronavirus disease (COVID-19) pandemic. The anticipated required equipment should be ready, and the roles of who will do what confirmed – with each person ratifying that they have the necessary skills required to manage their role.

The Primary Survey

The patient's immediate status should be confirmed, and a full handover taken from the accompanying medical professionals, which must include any interventions undertaken, medications administered and the patient's current status and observations.

The primary survey is then undertaken, with the aim to rule out and treat any life-threatening injuries. A structured advanced trauma life support (ATLS) ABCDE approach should be undertaken by the team, which, depending on the staff present, may include multiple coordinated assessments at the same time by different team members. Notably, yet still often forgotten, remember that triple immobilisation of the cervical spine is important at all times.

Airway Assessment

- Is the airway patent (verbalising, warmth, noisy breathing, hoarseness, subcutaneous emphysema, increased respiratory effort)?
- Reverse any obstruction (suction ± lateral spinal roll for aspiration; intubation may be necessary or, if intubation unsuccessful, emergency tracheostomy).

Whilst maintenance of cervical spine stability is important and should be ensured at all times, this is not at the expense of a compromised airway. If the patient has reduced or reducing cognitive ability, then it should be presumed their control is compromised and a definitive airway (cuffed and secured) should be inserted.

Breathing and Ventilation

- Inspect, palpate, percuss and auscultate the chest.
- Identify the respiratory rate and oxygen saturations.
- Confirm the position of the endotracheal tube (if inserted).
- Check the position of the trachea.
- Rule out tension pneumothorax/haemothorax/flail chest/open pneumothorax.

If any concern with regard to pneumo- or haemothorax, coordinate needle decompression and/or insertion of a chest drain. Open pneumothorax initially warrants closing the defect with a three-sided sealed sterile dressing.

Circulation with Haemorrhage Control

Haemorrhage is the most common preventable cause of mortality that needs to be managed. Once tension pneumothorax is ruled out as a cause, hypovolaemic shock must be presumed and managed.

- Assess the skin colour (blue, pink, pale or mottled) and temperature.
- Pulse (rate and character), blood pressure and capillary refill time.
- Are there signs of haemorrhage – 'blood on the floor and four more' – chest, abdomen, pelvis and long bones? (Keep the pelvic binder in situ until further imaging. 'First clot is the best clot.')
- Rule out a cardiac tamponade or an abdominal cause (focussed assessment with sonography in trauma (FAST) scan).
- Send bloods and consider full blood count (FBC)/urea and electrolytes (U&Es)/coagulation screen/cross-match. Consider O-negative blood in the immediate setting until type-specific blood available. Other blood products required?
- Prevent, identify and treat coagulopathy (TEG®/ROTEM®/avoid hypothermia –ideally temperature >36°C).
- Consider and give tranexamic acid in severe trauma.
- Take an arterial blood gas (ABG) or venous blood gas (VBG) – what are the pH status, lactic acid and base excess?

Intravenous (IV) access is essential to resuscitate trauma patients. They must have two large-bore (14 or 16 G) cannulae inserted at a minimum, and an early decision has to be made to escalate access measures if peripheral IV access is difficult (e.g. intraosseous (IO) needle/venous cut-down/central line).

If the patient is shocked and bleeding, replace blood with blood and initiate the massive transfusion policy. This varies between establishments, so check local policy, but in essence aims to replace all blood components, not just red cells, thus diminishing the chances of coagulopathy (e.g. a 1:1:1 ratio of red blood cells:platelets:plasma).

Disability

Assess GCS/AVPU, pupils, blood glucose and temperature.

Exposure

Examine the patient fully, ensuring all four limbs are exposed, whilst maintaining modesty and minimising heat loss. Look for any sources of occult blood loss and bony deformity, as well as open injury. A log roll must also always be undertaken, ensuring careful immobilisation of the cervical spine as this occurs.

Imaging

- Chest X-ray (CXR)/pelvic X-ray (traditional)
- Trauma CT (current vogue)

Traditionally, the key imaging obtained in the primary survey was a CXR and pelvic X-ray. In recent times, however, CT scanner availability has improved in most hospitals, especially in major trauma centres, and this is often the first imaging modality used. The decision of whether and when to take the patient for CT should involve all members of the trauma team.

Secondary Survey

Once the patient has been stabilised with regard to the initial insult, then a full head-to-toe examination needs to be performed to identify, treat and document any remaining injuries present. These are commonly musculoskeletal in nature, e.g. distal radius fractures, scaphoid injuries or finger joint dislocations.

Consideration for the Need to Transfer

Having obtained an impression of the patient's injuries, it is important to ask the question: '*Do the patient's treatment needs exceed the capability of this receiving institution?*' If the answer is yes, then urgent referral should be made to a major trauma centre. During this time, it is also essential to work out if the patient is stable enough for transfer (and if so, who will do it), or if not, how you can optimise the patient so that they are safe for transfer. This is often done by anaesthetists or intensivists.

The Multiple Injured Patient – Early Total Care versus Damage Control Surgery

The theory behind early total care (ETC) and damage control surgery (DCS) is to take into consideration, and plan around, the 'second hit' phenomenon. This relates to the patient's physiological response following surgical interventions of their injuries and can directly impact eventual outcome.

ETC proposes all injuries should be surgically managed at one sitting, and then the patient should be subsequently monitored and resuscitated appropriately in the post-operative period. By contrast, in DCS, the patient only undergoes surgical treatment for major life- or limb-threatening injuries (e.g. unstable pelvic fracture) and other injuries are treated conservatively (e.g. splinting closed forearm or long bone fractures).

This allows the patient to be resuscitated in the ICU, recover from the initial stress response of their injury and then receive their definitive surgery when physiologically more stable 2–3 days later.

The decision as to which path a patient follows is usually made intraoperatively among the anaesthetist, the trauma surgeon and the intensivist, and involves prioritisation of injury management: life versus limb versus function.

Parameters for damage control surgery used by the Hanover Group include:

- Injury Severity Score >20 with an associated chest injury
- Polytrauma with abdominal/pelvic trauma and shock (systolic blood pressure <90 mmHg)
- Injury Severity Score >40 with no associated chest injury
- X-ray evidence of bilateral lung contusions
- Mean pulmonary artery pressure >24 mmHg
- Increase of >6 mmHg in pulmonary artery pressure after intramedullary nailing

Clinical parameters associated with poor outcome after multiple injuries include:

- Inadequate initial resuscitation
- Coagulopathy/hypothermia
- Multiple blood transfusions (>25 units)
- Multiple long bone fractures
- Excessive surgical time (>6 hours)
- Metabolic acidosis (pH <7.24)
- Exaggerated inflammatory response measured by interleukin-6 (IL-6) levels (>800 pg/ml)

Conclusion

Managing trauma patients can be a difficult task in a highly stressful environment. It requires a multidisciplinary approach, with clear leadership and repeated assessments for adequacy of resuscitation. The quality of initial assessment and the location of further definitive management are fundamental to the patient's outcome.

References and Further Reading

American College of Surgeons. *Advanced Trauma Life Support*®, 10th edn. Chicago, IL: American College of Surgeons; 2018.

Davenport RA, Brohi K. Cause of trauma-induced coagulopathy. *Curr Opin Anaesthesiol* 2016;**29**:212–19.

Lamb CM, MacGoey P, Navarro AP, Brooks AJ. Damage control surgery in the era of damage control resuscitation. *Br J Anaesth* 2014;**113**:242–9.

1.6 Principles of Assessment and Initial Management of the Patient with Burns

Behrad Baharlo

Key Learning Points

1. Depth and extent of the burn determine management and the need for referral.
2. Lund and Browder charts should be used to estimate the extent of burn (% total body surface area (TBSA)).
3. Increasing age, % TBSA involved and associated inhalation injury correlate with severity.
4. Severe burns require burn shock resuscitation and should be managed in a burns centre.
5. The Parkland formula provides a *guide* to initial resuscitative fluid requirements.

Keywords: burn, Lund–Browder, assessment, Parkland, resuscitation

Assessment

Assessment of burn injuries should establish:
- Type of burn (thermal, chemical, electrical, radiation)
- Depth and extent of burn (% total body surface area (TBSA))
- Associated inhalation injury
- Coexisting conditions
- Possibility of non-accidental injury
- Need for referral

Assessing a burn injury requires an understanding of burn pathophysiology (Table 1.6.1).

Estimating Burn Depth and % TBSA

Estimating burn depth and % TBSA is crucial in the initial management. Resuscitative fluid requirements, severity and the need for referral/transfer to a specialist centre are dependent on this initial assessment.

The preferred method for estimating % TBSA burn is the Lund–Browder chart (applicable in adults and children) (Figure 1.6.1). An alternative (less accurate and unsuitable in children) method is the 'rule of nines' according to the area affected:
- Arm – 9 per cent
- Head – 9 per cent
- Neck – 1 per cent
- Leg – 18 per cent
- Anterior trunk – 18 per cent
- Posterior trunk – 18 per cent

The Mersey Burns app is an electronic alternative that has been evaluated by the National Institute for Health and Care Excellence (NICE).

Table 1.6.1 Burn classification by depth

Degree of burn	Skin depth involved	Involves/affects
First degree	Epidermal	Affects only the epidermis. Red, painful, no blisters
Superficial second degree	Partial thickness (superficial)[a]	Involves the epidermis and part of the papillary dermis. Blistering, swollen and painful. Heals without scarring
Deep second degree	(Deep)[a]	Involves the epidermis and entirety of the dermis. Can be red, white or pink, is less painful and heals with scarring. Would need surgery
Third degree	Full thickness[a]	Destroys the epidermis and dermis and may involve subcutaneous tissue. Appears white and leathery, with no capillary refill. Always needs surgery

[a] Contributes to % TBSA burn.

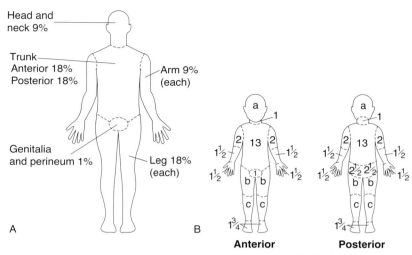

Head and neck 9%

Trunk—
Anterior 18%
Posterior 18%

Arm 9% (each)

Genitalia and perineum 1%

Leg 18% (each)

A

B

Anterior

Posterior

Relative percentage of body surface area (% BSA) affected by growth

Body Part	Age				
	0 yr	1 yr	5 yr	10 yr	15 yr
a = 1/2 of head	9 1/2	8 1/2	6 1/2	5 1/2	4 1/2
b = 1/2 of one thigh	2 3/4	3 1/4	4	4 1/4	4 1/2
c = 1/2 of one lower leg	2 1/2	2 1/2	2 3/4	3	3 1/4

Figure 1.6.1 (a) Rule of nines (for adults) and (b) Lund–Browder chart (for children) for estimating extent of burns
Source: Redrawn from Artz CP, JA Moncrief: *The Treatment of Burns*, ed. 2. Philadelphia, WB Saunders Company, 1969; used with permission.

Regional burn services are organised to care for patients of varying complexity. Criteria exist for referral to specialist burns centres (e.g. guidelines for the admission and transfer of the burn patients in the Midlands).

Severe Burns

A severe burn is defined as one *that requires burn shock resuscitation*. Resuscitation is required if the % TBSA burn exceeds:

- 15 per cent in adults (or 10 per cent if >65 years old)
- 10 per cent in children

Severity correlates with extremes of age, increasing % TBSA burn and associated inhalation injury.

Initial assessment often over- or underestimates % TBSA involved. Therefore, ongoing reassessment is essential as the complete extent (depth and size) may not be clear for 48 hours.

Transfer to a burns centre is necessary for burns requiring resuscitation (severe) where the eventual mean stay is 1 day per % TBSA.

The revised Baux score (age + % TBSA burn + 17 (if inhalation injury present)) is a widely used prognostic score in burns.

Initial Management

This commences in the pre-hospital setting, with fidelity to an ABCDE approach.

Thermal burns should be cooled with water at 12–18°C for 2–3 minutes only (as most temperature reduction occurs within this time). Chemical burns should be irrigated (risk inadvertent hypothermia).

Cling film is applied in layers over the burnt areas to reduce pain and evaporative losses (consider a clear plastic bag for burns to the hand). Administration of analgesia is a priority.

On transfer to hospital, the patient should be managed as per trauma protocols with a methodical primary and secondary survey. Concurrent injuries are frequent and the burn injury has to be prioritised against other injuries elicited on primary and secondary surveys. A full medical history should be taken, including collateral histories from emergency services, as this may be the only opportunity to do so.

The airway should be carefully assessed and burns to the face, neck and mouth or associated inhalation injury should alert the clinician to a potential for airway oedema and compromise. Change in phonation, dyspnoea and stridor may be signs of progressing airway oedema and early intubation may be necessary to obviate a more difficult encounter later. Notably, a third of intubated patients are extubated within 24 hours of admission to a burns centre, suggesting the index intubation was unnecessary. Nevertheless, a cautious approach is advocated.

An uncut endotracheal tube (size ≥8.0 mm) is used in view of potential progressive facial swelling and to service bronchoscopy. Suxamethonium is permissible in the first 24 hours but contraindicated up to 1 year thereafter due to proliferation of extra-junctional acetylcholine receptors and the risk of hyperkalaemia this poses.

Large-bore intravenous (IV) access should be established, though a central venous catheter and an arterial line should be considered early in severe burns. A urinary catheter should also be inserted.

Burns of >15% TBSA require timely resuscitation to maintain perfusion to end-organs and skin (preventing 'burn shock'). Delay in initiating fluid resuscitation of >2 hours has been shown to increase mortality.

Fluid resuscitation should be with crystalloids (lactated Ringers) and utilise the Parkland formula (4 ml/(kg % TBSA)). The Parkland formula is indicated for >15% TBSA burns, or >10 % with concurrent smoke inhalation, and estimates the fluid requirements in the first 24 hours from the time of the burn injury. Half of the total calculated fluid amount should be given in the first 8 hours, and the remainder in the 16 hours thereafter. Fluid already given (e.g. pre-hospital) should be deducted from the calculated requirements. The Parkland formula notoriously overestimates fluid requirements, with the potential for over-resuscitation and poor prognosis associated with excess fluid. Though it remains the most commonly used formula in the UK, such concerns have led to novel concepts of 'permissive hypovolaemia' and the 'half-Parkland' formula (2 ml/(kg % TBSA)) evolving (employed by the military). The Parkland formula is not applicable if the body weight is <30 kg; thus, in children, a modified Parkland of 3 ml/(kg % TBSA) + basal fluid needs is used. In burns of >40% TBSA, the administration of ascorbic acid (vitamin C) at 66 mg/(kg hr) for the first 24 hours may reduce fluid requirements.

An obtunded or agitated patient warrants a CT scan of the brain, measurement of blood glucose and consideration of cyanide or carbon monoxide poisoning. An assessment of the burn should be carefully documented.

Initial investigations include a full blood count, urea, creatinine and electrolytes, creatine kinase

Table 1.6.2 NNBC national burn care referral guidance

All burns >2% TBSA in children or >3% TBSA in adults
All full-thickness burns
All circumferential burns
Inhalational injury
Burns involving the face, hands, feet, genitalia or perineum
Electrical burns, including lightning strike, chemical burns and friction burns
Any cold burns
Any burn not healed within 2 weeks
Burns in patients with a pre-existing medical condition that could complicate management, prolong recovery or affect mortality, e.g. pregnancy, immunosuppression, renal or liver disease
Any burn with associated trauma (or fractures). If the trauma poses the greater initial risk, then the patient should be managed at a trauma centre prior to stabilisation (judgement and communication between the trauma centre and the burns centre are imperative)
Any burn with a predicted or actual need for high dependency unit or intensive care unit
Burn injury in patients assessed to require end-of-life care
Any burn with a suspicion of non-accidental injury in adults or paediatrics (including any burn in a neonate)
Unwell or febrile child with burn

Abbreviations: TBSA = total body surface area.

and an arterial blood gas to include carboxyhaemoglobin (COHb). Further analgesia and a human tetanus immunoglobulin booster should be administered. Referral to regional burns services should be considered.

Criteria for referral to specialist burns services are agreed within regional networks but are generally consistent with those laid down by the National Network for Burn Care (NNBC) (Table 1.6.2).

Acknowledgements

The author would like to thank Dr Tomasz Torlinski, Consultant in Intensive Care Medicine, Queen Elizabeth Hospital, Birmingham for his review of, and suggestions to, this chapter.

References and Further Reading

Guttormsen AB, Berger MM, Sjoberg F, Heisterkamp H. ESICM PACT. Burns injury. 2012. www.yumpu.com/en/document/view/27690157/burns-injury-pact-esicm

Hettiaratchy S, Papini R. ABC of burns. Initial management of a major burn: I–overview. *BMJ* 2004;**328**:1555–7.

Hettiaratchy S, Papini R. ABC of burns. Initial management of a major burn: II–assessment and resuscitation. *BMJ* 2004;**329**:101–3.

National Network for Burn Care. National burn care referral guidance. Version 1. 2012. www.britishburnassociation.org/wp-content/uploads/2018/02/National-Burn-Care-Referral-Guidance-2012.pdf

National Network for Burn Care. National burn care standards. 2013. www.britishburnassociation.org/wp-content/uploads/2017/06/National_Burn_Care_Standards_2013.pdf

1.7 Description and Management of Mass Casualties

Jonny Price and Scott Grier

Key Learning Points

1. Read and understand your organisation's mass casualty plan. Know your role.
2. Plan for a surge in patients, and understand how additional capacity may be created.
3. Anticipate communication difficulties, and introduce redundancies to mitigate this risk.
4. Additional staff will be required for days to weeks afterwards.
5. Care for the physical and psychological health of your staff.

Keywords: mass casualty, medical incidents, command and control, communication

Definitions

A mass casualty incident occurs when the location, number, severity or type of casualties requires extraordinary resources.

Incidents may be classified as:

- Natural (e.g. floods) or man-made (e.g. transport)
- Simple (surrounding infrastructure intact) or compound (damage to infrastructure)
- Compensated (manageable with deployment of additional resources) or decompensated (additional resources are unable to cope)
- Internal (overwhelming organisational pressures requiring alteration of services) or external (incident declared by another organisation)

Globally, the majority of recent incidents are natural, simple and compensated (e.g. earthquakes, hurricanes). In the UK, most incidents in the past decade have been man-made, simple and compensated (e.g. terrorism, rail crashes).

Planning

All healthcare institutions must have a mass casualty plan. In the NHS, this is a statutory requirement.

The plan outlines the roles and actions required of individuals and teams, from senior management to clinical and support staff. All employees must read, understand and be familiar with their organisation's plan in advance.

ICUs should have a dedicated plan describing their role and management within a wider hospital response. Surge capacity is determined by physical space (e.g. beds), resources (e.g. equipment and staff) and disposables.

Many hospitals normally operate at >90 per cent capacity, with ICUs at near maximum capacity on a daily basis. Mass casualty plans must include actions to manage surge capacity under such circumstances. Measures may include expedited discharge of wardable (fit to be discharged to wards) patients from the ICU, cancellation of elective surgery and utilisation of additional facilities (e.g. theatres or recovery rooms) to provide additional critical care capacity.

Hospitals should coordinate within critical care networks to facilitate patient transfers to manage a surge locally. For example, a major trauma centre transferring out existing patients to maintain admission capacity. The logistics of such transfers should be prospectively agreed during planning.

Practice is essential in delivering a successful response. Recent terrorist incidents in Paris, Nice and Manchester demonstrated that increased familiarity improved implementation and practicality of response.

Principles of Treatment in a Mass Casualty Incident

Mass casualty incidents demand a utilitarian approach, aimed at delivering the greatest good for the greatest number. Ultimately, care delivered to an individual patient will be determined by the total number of patients, their arrival rate at the hospital and available resources. Difficult decisions are required to prioritise resources to those most likely to survive.

Declaration of a Mass Casualty Incident

Most incidents are externally declared by emergency medical services. Terminology is important:
- Standby: an incident has occurred, with the potential to escalate
- Declared: an incident has occurred, requiring mass casualty plan activation
- Stand-down: an incident is perceived to be complete

Command and Control

Declaration triggers a multi-faceted response. Three tiers of command are commonly instituted:
- Gold (strategic): usually chaired by the Chief Executive or nominated deputy. Responsible for longer-term consequences of incident (e.g. business continuity) and media liaison
- Silver (tactical): to determine impact of the incident on the organisation. Responsible for making decisions regarding staff deployment and utilisation
- Bronze (operational): departmental level. Responsible for coordinating patient care and flow

Communication is essential. Real and simulated incidents consistently demonstrate saturation and failure of normal communication pathways (e.g. radios or mobile networks). Organisations must expect and plan for such failures, as they can have a significantly deleterious effect on the response delivered. Novel methods such as WhatsApp® messaging have been recently described.

Preparing for Arrival of Casualties

When a mass casualty incident is declared, staff should follow instructions detailed in the organisation's plan. Action cards for individual staff members should be distributed. Declaration of an incident is NOT the time to read the mass casualty plan.

Information gathering and managing resources are the key. The nature of the incident will help predict casualty numbers, type and severity. Incidents involving chemical, biological, radiological or nuclear contamination will require specialist advice, specific treatment priorities (e.g. decontamination) and measures to protect staff.

An initial patient surge will occur in the hours following an incident, and likely require additional staff. Means of staff contact should be described in the mass casualty plan. Ensure that not all staff are utilised immediately, as the next shift and subsequent days to weeks are likely to also require additional resources.

Lessons from Previous Incidents
During the Event
- Record-keeping is difficult. The mass casualty plan will describe a method of patient identification to facilitate laboratory investigations, blood transfusion services, radiology and other treatment. Using a digital voice recorder to keep a contemporaneous record of medical interventions and decisions will help future documentation. Clinicians may be required to describe and justify such decisions many years later in the event of a resulting inquiry or court case.
- Allocating a dedicated scribe to maintain a database of ICU patients admitted, including injuries, outstanding investigations and procedures performed and required, helps organise subsequent care.
- Bottlenecks inevitably occur where resources are limited. The most common are radiology and operating theatres, so it may be necessary for patients to be admitted to the ICU whilst others are being treated elsewhere.

Recovery
- Organisations generally attempt to return to normal too quickly following a mass casualty incident. Increased intensive care workload can last for days to weeks following an incident, with additional theatre visits and radiology transfers. During this phase, it may be necessary to adapt rotas accordingly.
- Debriefing following an incident is essential. This facilitates organisational, team and individual learning from events, outcomes and problems encountered. Most organisations use this opportunity to review their mass casualty plans.

Well-Being
- Do not underestimate the psychological impact of a mass casualty incident on staff. Stress and fatigue are inevitable.
- Many recent events have offered psychology services during and immediately after an incident, in addition to the recovery phase. Encouraging staff to talk, signposting help and normalising attitudes towards well-being all help to minimise longer-term effects.

Long Term

- Months to years following an incident, inquests, criminal or civil trials and public enquiries may occur. It is important that contemporaneous documentation is adequate and thorough. Staff involved in these longer-term events will need appropriate support.

References and Further Reading

Johnson C, Cosgrove JF. Hospital response to a major incident: initial considerations and longer term effects. *BJA Education* 2016;**16**:329–33.

Lowes AJ, Cosgrove JF. Prehospital organisation and management of a mass casualty incident. *BJA Education* 2016;**16**:323–8.

Mahoney EJ, Biffl WL, Cioffi WG. Analytic review: mass-casualty incidents: how does an ICU prepare? *J Intensive Care Med* 2008;**23**:219.

Orban J-C, Quintard H, Ichai C. ICU specialists facing terrorist attack: the Nice experience. *Intensive Care Med* 2017;**43**:683–5.

Shirley P, Mandersloot G. Clinical review: the role of the intensive care physician in mass casualty incidents: planning, organisation and leadership. *Crit Care* 2008;**12**:214.

2.1 Principles of Obtaining a History

Claire Moorthy

Key Learning Points

1. Use a systematic and structured approach to obtain the initial history.
2. Focus on the relevant features of the patient's clinical presentation.
3. Take a more thorough history when the patient is stable.
4. Ensure knowledge of the SBAR approach to communicate among medical professionals.
5. Call for additional help early, especially if there are any life-threatening conditions.

Keywords: clinical history taking, SBAR

Introduction

Obtaining a good initial history is very important and often begins within the referral process. This in itself can present a challenge. The amount of information given may vary and is dependent on the referrer, their experience and the urgency of the situation. Information may be delivered in various formats and can often be unstructured. It is advisable to use a system and structure to prevent missing key information. Writing down details at the time of referral can be very helpful. A structured format can also help to prompt and obtain further appropriate information that you might think important.

The SBAR Tool

The Royal College of Physicians recommends the use of 'SBAR' as a communication tool between healthcare providers when treating patients who are seriously ill or at risk of deterioration (Box 2.1.1). Originally used by the military, aviation industries and eventually, in 2002, rapid response teams in the United States, it has been adopted by many healthcare organisations. The tool allows a simple standardised form of delivery of structured and accurate communication. There is growing evidence that this method of communication is helping to improve outcomes and reduce errors.

Box 2.1.1 SBAR

- **Situation.** Introduce yourself; name the patient and location.
  - Give a concise and brief description of the situation.
  - For example: Mrs A is a 49-year-old woman who was admitted early this morning with shortness of breath. She has a history of asthma and has had nebulisers and steroids, but remains very wheezy and tachycardic, and is now hypotensive.
- **Background.** Briefly state the relevant history relative to the current situation.
  - For example: Mrs A is asthmatic, having had one admission to hospital last year. She has never been in intensive care and is usually managed by her GP. She has no other medical history and no allergies.
- **Assessment.** Summarise the facts. What do you think is going on?
  - For example: we have given the following treatment … Her ABG shows … I have requested an X-ray. I am concerned that she is not responding to the treatment. I think that she may have an infection.
- **Recommendation.** What do you feel needs to happen next? Be specific and give a time frame. This will indicate the urgency of the situation to your colleague. This is your opportunity to give a reason for your referral.
  - For example: please could you come and assess as soon as possible? Is there anything else we can do in the meantime?

Considerations Based on the SBAR

Once adequate information has been obtained and put into context, there are some important questions to be asked:

- Are there any **life-threatening features** within the history and examination?
- Does this patient require **my immediate attendance?** In a busy tertiary referral centre, where there may be three or four referrals at the same time, prioritising and triaging become very important skills.
- Do you need **extra help?** Inform appropriate senior people early (e.g. colleagues, outreach, anaesthetic assistants and senior specialist colleague).
- Is this an **appropriate referral?** If in doubt, go and see for yourself. It is very easy to accept patients, but often more difficult to refuse. Sometimes the referrer may be uncertain of the clinical course and requires a more experienced clinician to assess and give advice on further management.
- In the case of the **dying patient**, often reassurance is needed by the team that this is the case and there is nothing more to be done other than changing the course of the treatment to one of comfort and palliation.

Giving Advice

Following a referral, it may be useful and/or necessary to offer advice to the referring team. In time, this may make your job easier when you eventually review the patient. It may include the following:

- Simple immediate practical advice, e.g. patient positioning, giving oxygen, intravenous (IV) fluid specifics, etc.
- Further tests/management that you think might be required prior to your attendance to save time. There will often be other skilled people who can undertake certain tests, e.g. arterial blood gases, blood cultures, urine dipstick, D-dimer, clotting screen, chest radiograph, 12-lead ECG, etc.
- Always give an expected time of your attendance, and the details of anyone who may attend in your absence on your behalf.
- Give the details of anyone else whom you may have contacted (senior specialist, outreach if you cannot attend).

Further History

On reviewing the patient, a full history should be obtained (Box 2.1.2). Depending on the clinical situation, this may involve conversations with the patient and family, discussions with the medical team and a review of the clinical notes and investigations.

It is important to obtain information that is relevant to the situation. For example, the five previous ophthalmological operations in a patient presenting with acute chest pain will need to be in the written history for completeness eventually, but will be of little relevance in the initial history taking. Of more relevance would be a past medical history of type 2 diabetes mellitus and hypertension.

Box 2.1.2 An Example of an Initial History Template

Date and time of referral
Admitting consultant and specialty
Patient details
Name
DOB
Admission date
Date and time of referral
Original cause for admission It may be different to the current problem
Presenting complaint (PC)/problem list Describe the primary reason for seeking medical attention objectively. Describe the patient's perception of their illness, in their own words if possible. This can also be a problem list if there are multiple problems
History of PC (HPC)/relevant background history Relevant information. Chronological presentation of events leading up to the PC in complicated patients with multiple/previous admissions. Recent illnesses/hospital stays, including ICU admissions
Past medical history (PMH) Initial focused medical/surgical/psychiatric. Assessment of pre-morbid state is important here
Drug and allergy history (DH) Use generic names, doses and timings (saves a great deal of time later). Ascertain the type of allergic reaction
Family history (FH) Relevant information
Social history (SH) Psychosocial dependency, family dynamics
Vital signs or NEWS score Breakdown of the six NEWS parameters

Box 2.1.2 (cont.)

Clinical examination findings Relevant findings. Use an ABCDEFGHI approach or a systems approach. Whichever you use, be systematic to prevent missing important findings

Investigations Relevant previous and recent

Current management and plan

Impression What do you, as the referrer, think?

Anyone else contacted? Other specialties, admitting consultant, family

References and Further Reading

1000 Lives Plus. 2011. Improving clinical communication using SBAR. www.1000livesplus.wales.nhs.uk/ sitesplus/documents/1011/T4I%20%283%29%20 SBAR.pdf

National Institute for Health and Care Excellence. 2007 (updated review 2016). Acutely ill adults in hospital: recognising and responding to deterioration. Clinical guideline [CG50]. www.nice.org.uk/ guidance/cg50

Royal College of Physicians. Acute care toolkit 6. The medical patient at risk: recognition and care of the seriously ill or deteriorating medical patient. London: Royal College of Physicians; 2013.

World Health Organization. Patient safety solutions. Volume 1, solution 3. Geneva: World Health Organization; 2007.

2.2 Principles of Performing an Accurate Clinical Examination

Claire Moorthy

Key Learning Points

1. Use a structured approach to clinical examination.
2. Recognise and immediately treat life-threatening conditions.
3. Complete the initial assessment and reassess regularly.
4. Evaluate the effect of treatment.
5. Recognise the need for additional help early.

Keywords: critical care physiological assessment, life-threatening emergencies, never-miss diagnoses

Introduction

The initial clinical examination should be systematic and structured. There are differing opinions on the best way to carry out a clinical emergency assessment. The traditional systems-based approach is often used in non-emergency and daily review situations.

The focus in this chapter will be on structured physiological assessment. Much like the primary survey in trauma and cardiopulmonary resuscitation, this uses an 'ABCDE' approach, but with a few additional letters/added extras making it the 'ABCDEFGHI' approach (Table 2.2.1).

It is very important to decipher the main clinical features, with the overall aim of treating any life-threatening emergencies (Table 2.2.2) and correcting the acute abnormal physiology. It is also important to try and assess as early as possible the severity of the problem that is presented.

The clinical examination in an acutely unwell or deteriorating patient can be divided into three parts: (1) the initial or primary assessment; (2) the secondary assessment; and (3) continuing assessment.

Initial Primary Assessment
Main Goals

1. Immediate assessment
2. Oxygen delivery to reduce end-organ damage

Table 2.2.1 The 'ABCDEFGHI' approach to performing a structured physiological assessment

Airway and C-spine consideration	Look, listen and feel. Airway patency, positioning, suction, airway manoeuvres/adjuncts needed? Consider early airway protection. Do you need senior/specialist? Call for help early
Breathing	Look, listen and feel. Support breathing. Give oxygen
Circulation	Look, listen and feel. Pulse rate/volume, regularity. Heart sounds/additional sounds. Blood pressure measurement, capillary refill time. Peripheries: warmth, oedema. Obtain IV access. Take bloods, including ABG. Consider fluids – be specific
Disability/drugs	Level of consciousness using AVPU. Moving all four limbs? Facial symmetry, abnormal posturing? Pupillary responses. Do not forget glucose
Exposure/excretion	Expose briefly to check for rashes/covert bleeds. Check catheters and drains
Fluids	Fluid/feed – type, route, volume. Check IV access – patent line?
Gut/general	Examine abdomen – distended/tympanic/rebound or guarding? General – plethoric/pale/jaundiced/temperature
Haematological	Check skin for haematological rashes/bruising/bleeding (check recent bloods, ABG/VBG result)
Infection	Source? Lines/drains – type and location/date of placement. Check wound sites – if possible, take down dressings. Temperature. Review antibiotics early in septic patients/early discussion with microbiologist

Abbreviations: IV = intravenous; ABG = arterial blood gas; VBG = venous blood gas.

Table 2.2.2 Non-exhaustive list of life-threatening emergencies

Respiratory	Respiratory arrest, airway obstruction, hypoxia, hypercarbia
Cardiovascular	Cardiac arrest, acute arrhythmia, acute coronary syndromes, cardiac tamponade. Always consider post-cardiac surgery
Gastrointestinal	Upper/lower gastrointestinal bleed, bowel infarction or ischaemia, acute liver failure, acute severe pancreatitis
Neurological	Refractory seizures, acute bleed/infarct/infections/neurodegenerative conditions
Endocrine/ metabolic	Hypo-/hyperglycaemia, hypertensive crisis – thyroid/phaeochromocytoma, Addisonian crisis
Systemic	Systemic inflammatory response syndrome, sepsis
Immune	Anaphylaxis/anaphylactoid reactions

3. Correct abnormal physiology
4. Reassess regularly
5. Call for early senior help

When entering the domain of a critically ill patient, look for clues and cues around the patient. This may sound old-fashioned, but it is extremely helpful (monitoring, oxygen, nebulisers, patient position). Look, listen and feel at each step of ABC. This assessment should take no longer than 10 minutes to complete, unless there is a complex early intervention needed in the immediate assessment (e.g. relief of an acute airway obstruction other than with simple airway manoeuvres).

It is important during this phase of management to correct problems when found, and to review the responses to your treatment regularly. A 15- to 30-minute review after instigation of initial treatments is useful, and a repeat blood gas to determine patient progress and aid further management/treatment is also often necessary. When the patient has been acutely stabilised, move on to the secondary assessment.

Secondary Assessment
Main Goals

1. Obtain further additional information to explain possible reasons for the abnormal physiology.
2. Re-examine the patient.
3. Use targeted investigations.
4. Formulate a diagnosis or differential diagnosis.
5. Begin definitive treatment.

Methods
History
If not already obtained, take an initial history, focusing on:

1. Acute medical/surgical problem
2. Co-morbidities and pre-morbid state
3. Drugs and allergies
4. Social and collateral history

It is important to know the patient's social situation, specifically psychosocial independence, as this will aid in determining the limitations of treatment. A collateral history may be important and can be obtained via the general practitioner (GP)/family members/carers/recent clinic letters.

Examination
It is important to review and reassess the patient regularly. There may be more time during this phase of assessment to take a systems-based approach and undertake any further examinations more thoroughly. For example:

1. Neurological examination – often initially difficult. Important to look for:
   a. Pupil responses
   b. Localising/lateralising signs
   c. Limb tone
   d. Motor reflexes
   e. Plantars
   f. Full cranial nerves – often not possible in obtunded and critically ill patients, but when resuscitated should be revisited

2. Review of wounds:
   a. Taking down dressings if safe to do so
   b. Surgical review of wounds if recent/complex wounds
   c. Ensuring full examination of the back of the patient – can be easily missed; pressure sores are a potential source of sepsis
   d. Swab wounds – do not forget percutaneous endoscopic gastrostomy (PEG), drain and tracheostomy sites

Investigations
With more information available, it is now time to:
- Chase standard routine tests
- Consider further targeted investigations

25

- Repeat arterial blood gas (ABG)/venous blood gas (VBG) to monitor progress

Procedures

Be meticulous in your planning and undertaking of procedures, ensuring patient safety at all times.
Important considerations include:

1. Further invasive monitoring
    a. Central venous catheter
    b. Arterial catheter
    c. Oesophageal Doppler
    d. Pulmonary artery (PA) catheter
    e. PiCCO/LiDCO
2. X-rays/scans – do not forget contrast-induced nephropathy prevention strategies (refer to local guidance)
3. Therapeutic procedures
    a. Drains
    b. Vascular access for renal replacement therapy
    d. Emergency endoscopy/bronchoscopy

The aims of the secondary assessment are to obtain information, initiate targeted investigations and start forming a diagnosis or a differential diagnosis. The overall goal is to start definitive treatment.

Continuing Assessment
Main Goals

1. To form a treatment plan based on need, the patient and their wishes
2. To review all findings from the secondary assessment
3. To evaluate responses to treatment
4. To aim to form a diagnosis or at least a differential
5. To safely coordinate and support the multidisciplinary team

Iterative Review

- Review all findings from the secondary assessment.

- Obtain further detailed history if not already done.
- Collect and manage laboratory data, linking these to the clinical context.
- Think about other organ involvement. Does this need planning for investigation/further management?
- Plan, monitor and regularly evaluate responses to treatment.

    If poor response, reconsider the diagnosis/evaluate the severity of the disease process.

- If diagnosis remains unclear, formulate a differential diagnosis based on the objective evidence found so far.
- Consider patient location. Do they need to be moved to a safer environment?

Coordinating Teams Involved in Patient Care

- Ensure safety whilst coordinating multidisciplinary teamwork.
- Ensure good communication.
- Be supportive of your team members.
- Obtain information to help formulate a clear treatment plan.
- Ensure adequate and clear documentation.

Treatment Plan

- What are the main problems that need treatment?
- Where is the safest place for treatment?
- Set goals and parameters early.
- Has a diagnosis been made?
- Does everyone know the plan (i.e. patient/family/multidisciplinary team/specialist referrals, etc.)?

References and Further Reading

National Institute for Health and Care Excellence. 2007 (updated review 2016). Acutely ill adults in hospital: recognising and responding to deterioration. Clinical guideline [CG50]. www.nice.org.uk/guidance/cg50

PACT ESICM. Professional development and ethics: clinical examination.

Resuscitation Council UK. The ABCDE approach. www.resus.org.uk.abcde-approach

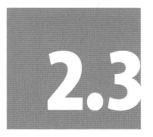

2.3

How to Undertake Timely and Appropriate Investigations

Claire Moorthy

Keywords: critical care, clinical investigation, laboratory monitoring

Introduction

Laboratory tests/investigations must always be carried out within the context of clinical findings. It is rare to establish the presence of disease without doubt. We should aim to use tests with the highest sensitivity and specificity to aid in accurate diagnosis. Predictive values are useful in ascertaining the validity of a test.

Questions to Ask Yourself

1. Are you familiar with the current guidelines for investigation of specific conditions?
2. Have you requested the most appropriate test? If in doubt, check.
3. Is the test requested available in a timely manner?
4. Are there any contraindications to the test (e.g. MRI and metalwork, tests during pregnancy, intravenous (IV) contrast in renal failure, etc.)?

It is important to use investigations to confirm or exclude diagnoses within the clinical context of the patient's presentation. This is especially important in the case of potentially dangerous, rapidly fatal diseases or 'do-not-miss diagnoses'.

Common Immediate Tests

Quick Bedside Tests

Arguably, the single most useful quick bedside test is the arterial blood gas (ABG) or venous blood gas (VBG).

Blood gas analysis aids quicker diagnosis of:

- Hypoxia/hypercarbia
- Acid–base disturbances
- Electrolyte disturbances
- Hyper-/hypoglycaemia
- Anaemia
- Hyperlactataemia

Remember to repeat the ABG/VBG soon after treatment to assess change in condition/adequacy of treatment.

Common Baseline Tests

- Blood tests – ABG/VBG (as above)
- Full blood count (FBC)/C-reactive protein (CRP)/ coagulation screen/liver function tests (LFTs)/urea and electrolytes/magnesium (Mg)/calcium (Ca^{2+})/ phosphate (PO_4)/glucose/group and save*
- Imaging – chest X-ray (CXR)/abdominal X-ray (AXR)/ultrasound scanning (USS)/ echocardiography (Echo)/CT
- 12-Lead ECG
- Urinalysis

* Remember that a full cross-match often takes 45 minutes to perform, and may be longer if there are abnormal antibodies present. If there is an urgent need of blood products, contact your laboratory directly.

Focussed Tests (Examples)

1. Blood tests:
   a. Endocrine: thyroid function tests, adrenal function tests, pancreatic function tests
   b. Cardiac: troponin I, troponin T, high-sensitivity troponin (hsTrP), creatine kinase,

      lipid screens, B-type natriuretic peptide (BNP), N-terminal pro-B-type natriuretic peptide (NT-pro-BNP)

  c. Haematology: thromboelastography (TEG®), activated clotting time (ACT), HbA1c, D-dimer, vasculitic screen, blood film, haptoglobin, Coombs' testing

  d. Biochemistry: drug levels, serum osmolality, procalcitonin, beta d-glucan, beta human chorionic gonadotrophin (hCG)

  e. Immunology: complement, immunoglobulins, autoimmune screen

2. **Microbiology:** microscopy, culture and sensitivity for swabs, blood, sputum, urine, fluid – pleural/peritoneal/drains/joint effusions

3. **Biochemistry:** urine *Legionella* and pneumococcal antigens

4. **Virology:** respiratory viral panel, serology for Epstein–Barr virus (EBV), cytomegalovirus (CMV), varicella-zoster virus (VZV), HIV and herpes simplex virus (HSV), hepatitis screen

5. **Imaging:** CT/CT angiography/MRI/focussed X-rays/angiography

6. **Other:** lumbar puncture (LP) for cerebrospinal fluid (CSF)/bronchoscopy for broncho-alveolar lavage (BAL)

Remember some tests are affected by other disease states; for example, troponin is often raised in renal failure, or thyroid function tests are often deranged in critically ill patients. If in doubt as to which test is best to use to aid/refute a diagnosis (or in complex cases), contact the specific labs or speak to an expert in that field for advice. Use the test that will give you the most timely and accurate result.

A multidisciplinary approach with certain other specialties will often be required, especially in the complex intensive care patient, and lines of communication should be maintained. There will be particular focus on microbiology, pathology and radiology to aid interpretation of results and in order to obtain specialist advice, especially if further time-sensitive investigations may be required and in complicated cases to determine further tests.

Current standards and recommendations include:

1. Clear protocol in place for management of massive haemorrhage

2. Daily input from microbiology senior clinician

3. Antibiotic stewardship with local prescribing guidelines

4. Access to diagnostic radiological services and timely access to a radiologist at all times appropriate to the specialties being cared for

5. Timely imaging investigation reporting followed by a formal written report

6. Clear protocols for access to radiology services that are not available on site (e.g. interventional radiology)

7. Active communication of critical or unexpected microbiology, clinical pathology and radiological investigations to the responsible clinician

8. Urgent clinical chemistry and haematology advice availability within 60 minutes

9. Immediate accessibility to radiologist to support management of critically ill patients

References and Further Reading

Faculty of Intensive Care Medicine and Intensive Care Society. Section 3.5: Interaction with other services: microbiology, pathology, liaison psychiatry and radiology. In: *Guidelines for the Provision of Intensive Care Services*, 2nd edn. 2019; pp. 88–90.

Singer M, Webb AR. Laboratory monitoring. In: M Singer, AR Webb (eds). *Oxford Handbook of Critical Care*, 3rd edn. Oxford: Oxford University Press. 2009; pp. 148–62.

The Association for Clinical Biochemistry & Laboratory Medicine. Lab Tests Online-UK. labtestsonline.org.uk

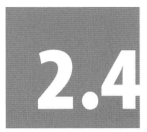

2.4 General Principles of Performing and Interpretation of Electrocardiography Results

Kyron Chambers

Key Learning Points

1. ECGs can be used for monitoring or diagnostic purposes.
2. Classically, in anaesthesia and the intensive care unit, a three-lead configuration is utilised.
3. The cardiac axis describes the summation of myocardial electrical potentials.
4. Classical ECG changes are described for electrolyte abnormalities.
5. The QT interval is dependent on the heart rate, for as the rate increases, the period for diastole decreases.

Keywords: ECG, tachycardias, bradycardia, conduction delays, axis, bundle branch block

ECG Modes and Configurations

ECGs have a standard speed of 25 mm/s, and a calibration of 1 mV/cm. The ECG has two modes:

1. **Monitoring modes.** These have a more limited frequency response, with filters added to reduce environmental artefacts. Filters reduce noise from muscle, and mains current and electromagnetic interference from equipment.
2. **Diagnostic modes.** These have a wider frequency response. Higher frequency limits allow for assessment of ST-segments, QRS morphology and arrhythmias. Low frequency allows for assessment of P waves and ST-segments.

Common Monitoring Configurations
Standard Lead Placement (= Leads I–III)
Classically in anaesthesia and the ICU, a three-lead configuration is utilised. Notably the term 'lead', when applied to an ECG, does not describe the electrical cables connected to the patient, but instead refers to the positioning of the two electrodes being used to detect the electrical activity of the heart. A third electrode acts as a neutral. As only one lead is displayed on the monitor at a time, it is important to choose the lead that yields the most information. Classically, lead II is used as it lies close to the cardiac axis and thus is best for detection of arrhythmias (Figure 2.4.1).

CM5 (Clavicle–Manubrium–V5)
This is best for the detection of ST-segment changes and left ventricular ischaemia.

12-Lead ECG
This is the most accurate method of monitoring the electrical activity of the heart, and a large number of abnormalities can be detected, including arrhythmias, myocardial ischaemia, left ventricular hypertrophy and pericarditis.

Rate

When moving at normal speed, the ECG provides a 10-second snapshot. Heart rate is calculated by multiplying the R–R intervals by 6. Alternatively, divide 300

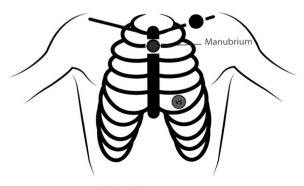

Figure 2.4.1 Standard lead placement.

by the number of 5 mm squares between consecutive QRS complexes. Traditionally, abnormal rates are defined as:

- **Bradycardia:** below 50/min (though cardiac output is compromised below 40/min)
- **Tachycardia:** above 100/min (though symptoms uncommon unless >150/min)

Bradycardias

Myocytes show automaticity, and the rate of their depolarisation is dependent on their location. The heart is controlled by whichever tissue depolarises most frequently:

- **Sinoatrial (SA) node:** depolarises at 70/min
- **Atrioventricular (AV) node:** depolarises at 50/min. If conduction is initiated here, there is loss of the P wave, with a normal QRS complex
- **Ventricles:** depolarise at 30/min. This is a safety mechanism providing a 'ventricular escape'. This results in a broad QRS complex

Tachycardias

These can be further split into:

1. **Supraventricular tachycardias:** initiate above the AV node. These can be further subdivided into:

   a. **Sinus tachycardia:** normal wave morphology

   b. **Atrial fibrillation:** disorganised uncoordinated atrial activity. The P waves are replaced by a wandering baseline, with narrow and irregularly irregular QRS complexes

   c. **Atrial flutter:** re-entry circuit at a rate of 200–400/min. Often associated with an AV block of around 2:1, as the AV node cannot conduct faster than 200/min. Flutter waves are classically described as having a 'sawtooth' appearance

2. **Ventricular tachycardia:** ventricular muscle depolarises with a high frequency, causing rapidly repeating broad QRS complexes

3. **Ventricular fibrillation:** disorganised, independent contraction of the ventricular muscle fibres

4. **Ventricular pre-excitation:** individuals have an abnormal accessory pathway between the atria and ventricles, which allows 1:1 atrial to ventricular conduction. This can be fatal in the presence of supraventricular tachycardias

5. **Atrial tachycardia with aberrant conduction:** the presence of an aberrant conduction through the AV node which is delayed. It is important to differentiate between VT and atrial tachycardia with aberrancy due to bundle branch block (BBB) or Wolff–Parkinson–White (WPW), as the treatment differs. VT may show:

   a. The broader it is, the more likely the complex is to be VT

   b. Likely to be regular

   c. Possible independent dissociated atrial activity

Conduction Delays

Conduction delays can result in ECG abnormalities. These can occur anywhere, including the:

- SA node ≫ AV node ≫ bundle of His ≫ bundle branches

The upper limit for conduction from the SA node to the ventricles is 0.2 seconds (one large square). Any increase is defined as a 'heart block', of which there are three different degrees:

- **First degree:** there is a delay in conduction from the SA node to the ventricles, and this appears as prolongation of the PR interval (i.e. >0.2 seconds)
- **Second degree:** excitations intermittently fail to pass through the AV node or bundle of His. Subtypes include:

  ○ **Mobitz type 1 (Wenckebach's phenomenon):** there is progressive lengthening of the PR interval, followed by failure to conduct atrial beats. This is followed by a conducted beat with a short PR interval, and then the cycle repeats itself

  ○ **Mobitz type 2 (Wenckebach's phenomenon):** excitation fails to pass through the AV node or the bundle of His. Most beats are conducted normally, but occasionally a P wave is seen without a ventricular contraction. Often seen with a 2:1 (alternate conducted and non-conducted beats) or 3:1 (one conducted beat and two non-conducted beats) conduction block

- **Third degree (complete heart block):** there is complete failure of conduction between the atria and ventricles (i.e. no P wave is followed by a normal QRS complex). Ventricular contractions are stimulated by slow escape rhythms

Cardiac Axis

Before understanding the axis, it is important to note that electrical movement towards a lead produces an upward deflection, and that which moves away produces a downward deflection. The axis therefore describes the summation of these electrical potentials. The normal range is −30° and +90°. Each lead views the myocardium at a different angle, and this can be used to calculate the axis as per Figure 2.4.2.

On the ECG, a quick rule of thumb to calculate the cardiac axis may be seen in Table 2.4.1.

Causes of axis deviation include those shown in Table 2.4.2.

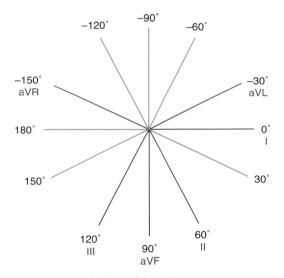

Figure 2.4.2 Calculation of the cardiac axis.

Table 2.4.1 Rule of thumb calculation of the cardiac axis

	Normal axis	Right axis deviation	Left axis deviation
Lead I	Positive	Negative	Positive
Lead II	Positive	Positive or negative	Negative
Lead III	Positive or negative	Positive	Negative

Table 2.4.2 Causes of axis deviation

Left axis deviation (<−30°)	Right axis deviation (>90°)
Normal, e.g. pregnancy	Normal
Left ventricular hypertrophy	Right ventricular hypertrophy
Left bundle branch block	Right bundle branch block
Left anterior hemiblock	Left posterior hemiblock

Bundle Branch Block

If depolarisation reaches the intraventricular septum at a normal rate, the PR interval is subsequently normal. Delays through either bundle branch, however, result in broadening of the QRS (defined as longer than 0.12 seconds).

- **Right BBB:** broad RSR complex in V1, not associated with any change in cardiac axis
- **Left BBB:** in V6, there is a broad, notched complex resembling an 'M'. In V1, the complex resembles a 'W'. Additionally, the left bundle branch has two fascicles:
  - Left anterior hemiblock – results in left axis deviation (LAD)
  - Left posterior hemiblock – results in right axis deviation (RAD)

Blockage to both the right and left bundle branches results in a complete heart block.

QT Interval

This is dependent on the heart rate, for as the rate increases, the period for diastole decreases. It is therefore corrected (QTc) using the formula:

$$QTc = Measured \frac{QT}{\sqrt{(Cycle\ length)}}$$

A prolonged QTc is defined as >440 ms in men, or >460 ms in women. If the QTc is >500 ms, there is an increased risk of torsades de pointe. This is a problem with a number of the drugs encountered in the ICU (e.g. haloperidol, anti-psychotics, quinolones).

Other Abnormalities

- **Capture beats:** atrial contraction causes the QRS complex via the normal route and so the QRS complex has a normal morphology
- **Fusion beats:** ventricles are activated simultaneously by supraventricular and ventricular impulses, with the QRS complex having an intermediate pattern
- **Concordance:** all QRS complexes in the chest leads are predominantly positive or negative.

ST Abnormalities and Ischaemic Changes

- **ST elevation.** This indicates myocardial injury (e.g. infarction or pericarditis). The areas of maximal

Table 2.4.3 ST elevation and area of infarct

Area of infarct	ST elevation
Septal	V1–V2
Anterior	V2–V5
Antero-septal	V1–V4
Anterolateral	I, aVL, V3–V6
Inferior	II, III, aVF
Posterior	ST depression V1–V3 ST elevation V7–V9

elevation classically depict the area of ischaemia (Table 2.4.3).

- **Left bundle branch block.** If new, this indicates pathology – possibly acute infarction. We can use Cabrera's sign or the Sgarbossa criteria to aid diagnosis:
  - ○ **Cabrera's sign:** downward notch of 40 ms in the ascending portion of the S wave in leads V3 and V4. Highly specific, but poorly sensitive to previous myocardial infarction (MI)
  - ○ **Sgarbossa criteria:** a set of ECG findings generally used to identify MI in the presence of a left bundle branch block (Box 2.4.1)
- **Q waves.** They are normal when <3 mm deep and 1 mm across; however, due to lead orientation, they should not occur in leads V1–V3

Electrolyte Abnormalities

ECG changes encountered with electrolyte abnormalities can be seen in Box 2.4.2.

Box 2.4.1 Sgarbossa Criteria

- ST-segment elevation >1 mm and concordant with QRS complex (5 points)
- ST-segment depression >1 mm in leads V1–V3 (3 points)
- ST-segment elevation >5 mm and discordant with QRS complex (2 points)

A score of >3 has a high specificity and low sensitivity for MI.

Box 2.4.2 ECG Electrolyte Abnormalities

Hypokalaemia

- Increase in P wave amplitude
- PR prolongation
- ST depression
- T wave flattening
- U waves (Figure 2.4.3)

Hyperkalaemia

- P wave broadening and reduction in amplitude
- PR elongation
- Broad QRS complex
- Tall, tented T waves (taller than R waves in >1 lead)

Hypocalcaemia

- Long QTc
- T wave inversion
- Heart block

Hypercalcaemia

- Short QT
- Prolonged QRS
- Flat T waves

Inherited Disorders

- **Long QT syndrome.** The QTc is not 100 per cent predictive; therefore, use the Schwartz score to aid diagnosis. Risk of sudden cardiac death (SCD)
- **Brugada syndrome.** Pseudo-right BBB and persistent ST elevation in V1–V3
- **Risk of SCD**
- **WPW.** The presence of an accessory pathway enhancing conduction speed. The PR interval is short (<0.12 seconds), with a delta wave present (Figure 2.4.4)

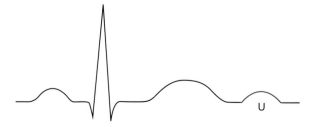

Figure 2.4.3 A 'U' wave.

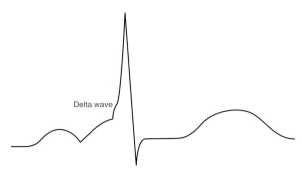

Delta wave

Figure 2.4.4 Delta wave.

References and Further Reading

D'Angelo R, Smiley RM, Riley ET, Segal S. Serious complications related to obstetric anesthesia: the Serious Complication Repository Project of the Society for Obstetric Anesthesia and Perinatology. *Anesthesiol* 2014;**120**:1505–12.

Hampton JR. *The ECG Made Easy*. London: Churchill Livingstone; 2008.

Houghton AR, Gray D. *Making Sense of the ECG: A Hands-On Guide*, 5th edn. Boca Raton, FL: CRC Press; 2020.

Lee J. ECG monitoring in theatre. e-safe-anaesthesia.org/sessions/02_05/pdf/ECG-Monitoring-in-Theatre.pdf

Life in the Fast Lane. lifeinthefastlane.com

Morris F, Edhouse J, Brady WJ, Camm J. *ABC of Clinical Electrocardiography*. London: BMJ Books; 2003.

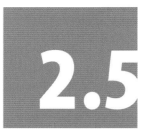

2.5 General Principles of Obtaining Appropriate Microbiological Samples and Interpretation of Results

Tom Bottomley

Key Learning Points

1. Infection is an important cause of morbidity and mortality in the ICU.
2. Invasive devices commonly used in the ICU are a significant cause of nosocomial infections.
3. Replacement of indwelling devices in septic patients is guided by the clinical picture.
4. Surveillance is used to limit spread of these infections.
5. Careful specimen sampling is of utmost importance in achieving clinically relevant microbiological therapy advice.

Keywords: infection, microbiology, interpretation, bacteria, investigation

Introduction

Infection not only can increase ICU length of stay, but it is also an independent predictor for mortality. The incidence of infection in the ICU setting is greatly increased by frequent use of invasive devices such as ventilators, vascular catheters and urinary catheters. These factors are confounded by ICU patients having more acute medical conditions, often with underlying chronic co-morbidities, leading to relative immunosuppression.

The incidence of multidrug-resistant organisms is increasing in the intensive care setting and this comes with a burden of limited treatment options, isolation procedures and increased treatment costs.

This chapter will focus on the types of infection common to ICUs, and on identification and treatment of such infections.

Types of Infection and Related Organisms

Patients in the ICU setting are more susceptible to developing infections, and multidrug-resistant bacteria, such as meticillin-resistant *Staphylococcus aureus* (MRSA), vancomycin-resistant *Enterococcus* (VRE) and carbapenem-resistant *Enterobacteriaceae* (CRE), are increasing in prevalence.

Risk Factors for Colonisation of Multidrug-Resistant Organisms

- Old age
- Co-morbidities: diabetes, cancer, chronic kidney disease, immunosuppressive states
- Length of stay
- Interaction with healthcare professionals caring for large numbers of patients
- Indwelling devices such as central lines, catheters and endotracheal tubes
- Recent surgery
- Multiple interactions with healthcare environments or long stays in medical facilities, e.g. hospitals, nursing homes
- Recent antibiotic therapy prior to ICU

The most common causes of infection are those associated with invasive devices.

- **Ventilator-associated pneumonia (VAP):** lung infection that occurs 48 hours after intubation. It is thought the pathogenesis is due to micro-aspiration of organisms from the oropharynx and gastrointestinal (GI) tract. Treatment is with antibiotics, with coverage for *S. aureus*, *Pseudomonas aeruginosa* and other Gram-negative bacilli. If MRSA is suspected, then vancomycin or linezolid is recommended. If MRSA is not a concern, then piperacillin–tazobactam or meropenem would be appropriate. However, antibiotic choice should be guided by local policy.

- **Catheter-associated urinary tract infection:** most common nosocomial infection. Common causative organisms include *Escherichia coli*, *Enterococcus* species (spp.), *Candida* spp., *P. aeruginosa* and *Klebsiella* spp.

Treatment depends on the clinical picture – antibiotic therapy in asymptomatic patients does not affect outcome. Therapy should be guided by cultures in unwell patients and by local guidelines. As a general rule, in non-severely septic patients, a third-generation cephalosporin would be appropriate (e.g. ceftriaxone). However, if the patient is unwell, more broad-spectrum cover is required, e.g. ciprofloxacin. If on early staining Gram-positive cocci are seen, staphylococci or enterococci could be the causative bacteria, and therefore vancomycin should be started whilst awaiting the final microbiology report.

If the catheter is no longer needed, then it should be removed. When this is not possible, it should be changed at the commencement of antibiotic therapy. It should also be noted that intermittent catheterisation is associated with lower rates of urinary tract infection, and therefore this should be employed if possible.

- **Catheter-related bloodstream infection (CRBSI):** this is becoming increasingly common due to the need for invasive monitoring, increased blood sampling and more intravenous (IV) administration of medications. The sources of infection can be split into:

  1. Skin colonisation
  2. Intraluminal colonisation
  3. Haematogenous seeding (infection originating from another site in the body)
  4. Infusion fluid contamination

Causative bacteria include *S. aureus*, coagulase-negative staphylococci, enterococci, *Candida* spp., *E. coli*, *Klebsiella* spp. and *P. aeruginosa* (especially in burns patients).

- Treatment should again be guided by microbiology results. However, vancomycin is an acceptable agent for empirical therapy, and daptomycin should be used if the unit has high rates of MRSA or if no clinical improvement is seen with vancomycin.

- The catheter should be removed after the diagnosis of a catheter-related infection has been made if there is evidence of severe sepsis or failure of antibiotic therapy after 72 hours. The catheter can, however, be left *in situ* if cultures from the catheter are positive, but peripheral cultures are negative and there is no sign of systemic disease. Additionally, it should be noted that there exists a 'Matching Michigan Bundle' – a group of simple interventions aimed at decreasing central line infections.

Surveillance

Patients admitted to an ICU are screened for multi-drug-resistant organisms: MRSA, VRE and CRE. This serves two purposes – both to indicate which patients need to be isolated and to collect data about the prevalence of these organisms. Along with the screening, there need to be robust reporting systems, so that positive results are flagged up in a timely manner.

Research into active surveillance (mainly focussed around MRSA) suggests that it has limited efficacy in reducing transmission rate – this could be due to the relatively low incidence and because most MRSA-positive patients are colonised prior to admission. One study comparing universal decolonisation for all patients to active surveillance found that MRSA rates were reduced in the decolonisation cohort, when compared to a screening and isolation technique. Emergence of resistance to chlorhexidine and mupirocin, however, is an important consideration which may render universal decolonisation inappropriate.

At present, there is some evidence to suggest that universal contact precautions limit the spread of drug-resistant organisms. With regard to universal precautions for every patient in the ICU, however, this remains controversial, with several large studies reaching different conclusions. Clinicians should therefore be aware that emerging evidence may alter practice in the near future.

General Principles of Sampling

The aim of microbiological sampling is to provide the lab with uncontaminated representative specimens, so that detection of organisms and processing of results are accurate, in order to optimise treatment for the patient. Specimens must be carefully handled in all the steps, from sampling to storage to analysis to disposal.

- **Seek advice from the lab:** site suitability, timings, sample size and to inform the lab of any specific tests
- **Avoid swabs:** tissue and fluid samples provide a much greater yield of organisms and are much less susceptible to contamination
- **Patient consent** (where possible)
- **Aseptic technique:** gloves, gown, mask, visor (where appropriate) and clean field. This reduces the risk of sample contamination from the indigenous flora and of harm to the healthcare professional
- **Safety:** sharps disposal, appropriate packaging, discussion with the lab regarding high-risk samples
- **Timing:** samples should be taken prior to initiation of microbiological therapies
- **Labelling:** demographics, time, date, site, current therapy and whether the sample needs to be divided for pathology. Labelling errors are a common reason for specimen rejection
- **Transfer:** avoid delay in processing. If a delay is unavoidable, then most samples should be refrigerated to preserve the organisms' representative proportions. Exceptions include blood, cerebrospinal fluid (CSF), joint fluid and suspected *Neisseria gonorrhoeae* which should be stored at room temperature

Special Tests – Lumbar Puncture

Lumbar puncture (LP) is used to aid the diagnosis of central nervous system (CNS) infections, subarachnoid haemorrhage and demyelinating diseases. When CNS infection is suspected, an LP is urgent. Interpretation of lab findings has been summarised in Table 2.5.1.

There are contraindications and complications associated with an LP:

- **Contraindications:**
  - Raised intracranial pressure
  - Infection around the proposed puncture site
  - Bleeding diathesis
- **Complications:**
  - Bleeding
  - Infection
  - Failure
  - Nerve damage
  - Back pain
  - Post-dural puncture headache

References and Further Reading

Huang SS, Septimus E, Kleinman K, *et al.* Targeted versus universal decolonization to prevent ICU infection. *N Engl J Med* 2013;**368**:2255–65.

Kalil A, Metersky ML, Klompas M, *et al.* Management of adults with hospital-acquired and ventilator-associated pneumonia: 2016 Clinical Practice Guidelines by the Infectious Diseases Society of America and the American Thoracic Society. *Clin Infect Dis* 2016;**63**:e61–111.

Marchaim D, Kaye K. 2017. Infections and antimicrobial resistance in the intensive care unit: epidemiology and prevention. *UpToDate.* www.uptodate.com/contents/infections-and-antimicrobial-resistance-in-the-intensive-care-unit-epidemiology-and-prevention

O'Grady NP, Alexander M, Burns LA, *et al.* Guidelines for the prevention of intravascular catheter-related infections. *Clin Infect Dis* 2016;**52**:e162–93.

Table 2.5.1 CSF composition in various infectious states

	Pressure (cmH$_2$O)	Leucocytes (/mm³)	Protein (mg/dl)	Glucose (mg/dl)
Normal	6–25	2–4	20–40	40–80
Bacterial meningitis	Increased	100–50,000	100–500	<40
Viral meningitis	Normal or increased	<1000 Mononuclear	20–200	Normal or high
Viral encephalitis	Normal or increased	<1000 Polymorphonuclear initially, then mononuclear	50–200	Normal or high
Tuberculosis meningitis	Increased	10–500 lymphocytes	100–500	Low
Brain abscess	Increased	10–200 lymphocytes	100–500	Normal

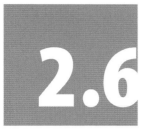

2.6 Obtaining and Interpretation of Results from Blood Gas Samples (Acid–Base Balance and Disorders)

Ed McIlroy

Key Learning Points

1. Whilst the radial artery is a common sample site, 24–27 per cent of patients will have a negative modified Allen's test (no/minimal ulnar supply).
2. Remember to expel air and heparin from the syringe to avoid sample contamination.
3. Errors can be associated with sample collection, machine processing and interpretation.
4. Metabolic acidosis can be high anion gap (MUDPILES) or normal anion gap (PANDA RUSH).
5. Stewart's approach to acid–base disturbance considers the strong ion difference (SID), total weak acid concentration (A_{tot}) and partial pressure of carbon dioxide ($PaCO_2$).

Keywords: ABG, ABG errors, ABG interpretation, Stewart's acid–base approach

Introduction

Arterial blood gas (ABG) sampling is a quick ('snapshot') test used in the assessment of the critically ill or those with chronic lung disease. Therapies and interventions are instituted and titrated according to results. Therefore, correct collection technique, processing and interpretation are paramount. This chapter outlines some of the peri-procedural considerations and some sampling pitfalls, as well a broad overview of ABG interpretation.

Indications for Arterial Blood Gas Samples

- Assessing adequacy of ventilation (spontaneous or ventilated) and response to intervention

- Assessing acid–base disturbances – metabolic, respiratory or mixed
- Assessment of chronic respiratory disease and hypoxia/hypercapnia to consider long-term oxygen therapy (LTOT)
- Carboxyhaemoglobin and methaemoglobinaemia quantification
- Obtaining blood samples in an emergency/difficult access

Contraindications
Absolute

- Local infection/distorted anatomy at the puncture site
- Arteriovenous (AV) fistulae or vessel grafts at the site of sampling
- Known or suspected vascular insufficiency of the limb

Relative

- Severe/acquired (warfarin/heparin/factor X inhibitors) coagulopathy
- Use of thrombolytic agents
- Abnormal Allen test (often cited, but rarely tested or adhered to)

Sampling Sites

1. **Radial** (Figure 2.6.1). This is the most commonly utilised site, as its location and superficial presentation make it easily accessible. Caution in cases of insufficient contralateral (ulnar) arterial supply (24–27 per cent). Consider performing the modified Allen test.
2. **Femoral** (Figure 2.6.2). Midline between the symphysis pubis and the anterior superior iliac crest, 2–4 cm distal to the inguinal ligament. Caution in patients with peripheral arterial disease or bypass grafts. Consider use of ultrasound.

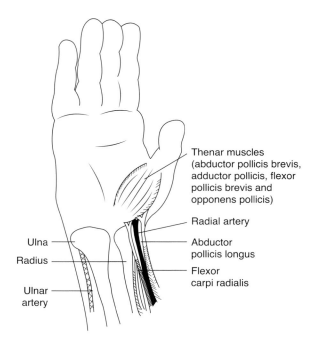

Figure 2.6.1 Location of the radial artery.

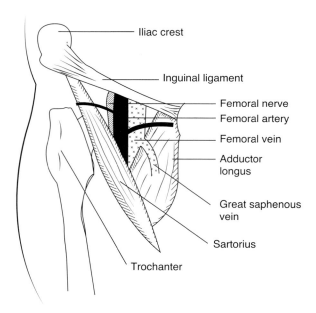

Figure 2.6.2 Location of the femoral artery.

3. **Brachial** (Figure 2.6.3). Commences at the lower
   border of the teres major, and branches into the
   ulnar and radial arteries. Most easily palpated
   between the medial epicondyle of the elbow and
   the tendon of the biceps brachii. There can be

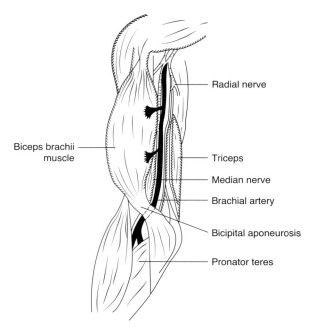

Figure 2.6.3 Location of the brachial artery.

distal implications if a traumatic technique is
employed or if distal pulses are initially difficult to
palpate.

Technique (Follow Local Hospital Procedure)

- Pre-assemble the equipment (syringe, needle,
  gloves, 2% chlorhexidine/skin prep, sterile gauze/
  pack, drape).
- Explain the procedure and obtain consent
  (verbal).
- Position the patient, taking care to optimise
  arterial presentation (i.e. place padding under
  their wrist or elbow to aid palpation of the artery).
- Wear gloves (and consider eye protection).
- Aseptic technique. Apply 2% chlorhexidine skin
  preparation in a circular motion from the centre
  outwards.
- Consider the application of local anaesthetic to the
  needle puncture site (an insulin syringe and needle
  is useful for this).
- Palpate the arterial pulse (using your non-
  dominant index/middle finger) distal to the
  intended puncture site.
- Expel any heparin in the pre-filled heparin
  syringes, and puncture the artery to obtain a
  sample.

- Once obtained, expel all the air/bubbles in the syringe. This avoids dilution of the partial pressure of carbon dioxide ($PaCO_2$) and any increase of partial pressure of oxygen (PaO_2).

Strictly speaking, the sample should be placed on ice (0°C) once taken, as this reduces cellular metabolism – especially important in patients with leucocytosis which consumes oxygen. That said, care should be taken over prolonged chilling, as gases become more soluble in solutions at lower temperatures and thus lower partial pressures will be demonstrated.

Problems

- Uncooperative patient (e.g. cognitive impairment)
- Obesity (excess subcutaneous fat, difficulty with ascertaining anatomy)
- Arteriosclerosis of peripheral arteries, hypovolaemic states, heart failure, multiple previous arterial samplings/lines and vasopressor therapy may make discerning pulses or arterial flow in the syringe difficult to assess

Complications

- Local haematoma
- Artery vasospasm
- Arterial thrombosis/occlusion
- Air/thrombus embolism
- Local anaesthetic anaphylaxis
- Infection at puncture site
- Needlestick injury to health practitioners
- Vessel laceration
- Vasovagal response
- Haemorrhage
- Local pain

Potential Sources of Error

Reasons for errors in ABG sampling and interpretation are plentiful but can be separated into pre-analysis (mostly human error), processing (poor machine calibration) and post-analysis (poor interpretation) errors.

Pre-analytical

- Drawing sample from the wrong patient/ incorrectly labelled sample/results placed in the wrong patient record
- Inadvertently obtaining a non-arterial sample. For example, when arterial and venous pressures may be similar (e.g. in sepsis/heart failure/pulmonary

hypertension), the syringe may be slow to fill. One can compare oxygen saturations between plethysmography and the ABG, and if there is a lack of correlation, venous sampling must be suspected

- Clotting of sample – caution as this will block the blood gas machine
- Haemolysis – e.g. from use of a small needle, prolonged withdrawal of blood sample, prolonged time before analysis
- Incorrect knowledge of the patient's fraction of inspired oxygen (FiO_2) and temperature – can lead to misinterpretation
- Air bubble – alters $PaCO_2$ and PaO_2 (and results are more similar to 'room air' concentrations). The degree of interference depends on the air–blood interface surface area (lots of small bubbles are worse than one big bubble) and the duration of contact (>2 minutes can result in contamination)
- Excessive liquid heparinisation – most syringes use dry heparin, but if liquid heparin is used and not expelled, or a very small blood sample is obtained, this leads to dilution of the sample and:
  - An elevated heparin:blood ratio can decrease haemoglobin (Hb) and haematocrit (Hct) measurements
  - Heparin fully dissociates at physiological pH and is very anionic; thus, even a small amount within the sample may cause metabolic acidosis
  - Dilution with heparin can alter electrolyte concentrations (e.g. increase potassium)
- Delay from collection to analysis – cellular metabolism decreases PaO_2, pH, bicarbonate (HCO_3^-), base excess (BE) and glucose, and $PaCO_2$ and lactate values increase

Processing

- Old or non-calibrated cell electrodes (e.g. the Clark electrode only lasts 3 years)
- Lithium heparin will interfere with sodium (Na^+) measurement
- Chloride (Cl^-) measurement increases in the presence of halogen ions (e.g. during volatile anaesthesia). In salicylate overdose, salicylates can compete for the Cl^- ionophore on the Cl^- electrode
- The ABG machine shreds the erythrocytes (with 30-Hz ultrasound) to release their Hb. It will not therefore notice if there is already free Hb in the

blood sample secondary to haemolysis, and will demonstrate a falsely elevated Hct

- Fetal Hb and carboxyhaemoglobin have similar absorption spectra; therefore, neonatal samples demonstrate a falsely increased carboxyhaemoglobin value. Conversely, in a pregnant woman with carbon monoxide poisoning, fetal–maternal haemorrhage may be masked
- In ethylene glycol poisoning, glycolic acid, a by-product of ethylene glycol metabolism, interferes with the lactate electrode and will give a falsely elevated reading. A laboratory-measured lactate is thus essential in this situation, as it uses a different assay and is correct. Interestingly, a large number of other molecules will interfere with lactate measurement, including ascorbic acid, bilirubin, citrate, ethylene diaminetetraacetic acid (EDTA), ethanol, heparin, glucose, paracetamol, salicylate and urea
- Hyperlipidaemia can interfere with spectrophotometer readings and can cause abnormally high Hb readings (and low carboxyhaemoglobin readings, if present). Equally, a central venous gas taken from a total parenteral nutrition-designated lumen can have the same effect
- Isosulfan/methylene blue can also interfere with spectrometry of Hb

ABG Interpretation

Full interpretation of the ABG requires some knowledge of the patient's history and their FiO_2 and temperature. Most ABG analysers will directly measure: pH, PO_2, pCO_2, Hb, carboxyhaemoglobin, oxygen saturation, Na^+, potassium (K^+), calcium (Ca^{2+}), Cl^-, lactate and glucose. The rest of the acid–base parameters are inferred from the measured variables; for example, the actual HCO_3^- value is derived via the Henderson–Hasselbalch equation (Table 2.6.1).

Table 2.6.1 Normal values of blood gas samples

	Arterial	Venous
pH	7.35–7.45	7.32–7.36
PO_2 (kPa)	10.6–13.3	4.7–5.3
PCO_2 (kPa)	4.6–6.0	5.6–6.1
HCO_3^- (mmol/l)	22–26	24–28
SO_2 (%)	95–100	60–80

Base Excess

The total amount of acid or base (mmols) required to restore 1 litre of blood to a normal pH at PCO_2 of 5.3 kPa at 37°C.

It is a useful indication of the metabolic component of the acid–base disturbance. The ABG machine calculates this value using the Siggaard–Andersen nomogram/Van Slyke equation. A BE more negative than −2 indicates a metabolic acidosis (Table 2.6.2), and a value more than +2 indicates a metabolic alkalosis (Table 2.6.3).

A Quick Approach to Deciphering the ABG

Is There Hypoxia?

Look at the PaO_2. If <8 kPa, this indicates hypoxia and possible imminent respiratory failure. In all cases, the value must be considered in combination with the FiO_2, as the patient may have quite significant hypoxia despite a normal PaO_2.

Look at the pH and PCO_2

Is there acidaemia or alkalaemia? Decide if the PCO_2 is responsible for the pH (e.g. a high PCO_2 and a low pH in respiratory acidosis, or a low PCO_2 and a high pH in respiratory alkalosis). Often more than one acid–base derangement is present.

Strictly speaking, the term acidaemia describes a low arterial pH (pH <7.36 or [H^+] >44 nM), whilst acidosis is used to describe the abnormal processes or condition leading to this state. Conversely, an alkalaemia describes an arterial pH >7.44 ([H^+] <36 nM), and an alkalosis describes the abnormal processes or condition leading to this state.

Table 2.6.2 Causes of high and normal anion gap metabolic acidosis

High anion gap (MUDPILES)	Normal anion gap (PANDA RUSH)
• Methanol/toxic alcohols • Uraemia • Diabetic ketoacidosis • Pyroglutamic acids • Iron overdose • Lactic acidosis • Ethylene glycol • Salicylates	• Pancreatic secretion loss • Acetazolamide • Normal saline intoxication • Diarrhoea • Aldosterone antagonists (spironolactone) • Renal tubular acidosis type 1 • Ureteric diversion • Small bowel fistula • Hyperalimentation (total parenteral nutrition)

Table 2.6.3 Causes of metabolic alkalosis

Metabolic alkalosis
Chloride depletion
• Gastric loss (vomiting/drainage)
• Diuretics: loop/thiazides
• Diarrhoea
• Post-hypercapnic state
• Dietary Cl^- depletion
• Gastrocystoplasty
• Cystic fibrosis (high sweat Cl^- content)
Bicarbonate excess
• Iatrogenic alkalinisation
• Recovery from starvation
• Hypoalbuminaemia
Potassium depletion
• Primary hyperaldosteronism
• Mineralocorticoid over-supplementation
• Liquorice
• Beta-lactam antibiotics
• Liddle syndrome
• Severe hypertension
• Bartter and Gitelman syndromes
• Laxative abuse
• Clay ingestion
Calcium excess
• Hypercalcaemia of malignancy
• Milk-alkali syndrome

Is There Compensation?

- Is there respiratory compensation according to PCO_2?
  - Low pCO_2 compensating for metabolic acidosis
  - High pCO_2 compensating for metabolic alkalosis
- Is there metabolic compensation according to HCO_3^-?

Expect:

- 1 mmol increase with acute respiratory acidosis
- 4 mmol increase with chronic respiratory acidosis
- 2 mmol decrease with acute respiratory alkalosis
- 5 mmol decrease with chronic respiratory alkalosis

Is the Compensation Adequate (i.e. Has the pH Corrected)?

Chronic acid–base disorders may fully compensate for a change in pH. However, acute respiratory and metabolic disorders rarely do so.

Decide on the contribution of extraneous acids/anions to the pH. This can be guided by the **anion gap** (normal value: 8–12 mmol).

$$Anion\ gap = (Na^+ + K^+) - (Cl^- + HCO_3^-)$$

A rise in the anion gap suggests a metabolic acidosis, with HCO_3^- being replaced by unmeasured anions (e.g. lactate, ketones, renal failure, alcohols). When HCO_3^- is lost (e.g. diarrhoea or renal losses), it is lost with Na^+, so there is no change in the anion gap (Table 2.6.2).

Some Caveats

1. **Pregnancy.** ABG changes include: pH increases, $PaCO_2$ decreases, PaO_2 increases and HCO_3^- decreases.
2. **Hypothermia.** Lowering the temperature changes the physicochemical properties of water (H_2O), thus influencing the solubility of gases and auto-ionisation of H_2O to H_3O^+ and OH^-.

For every 1° below 37°C:

- PaO_2 drops by 0.65 kPa
- $PaCO_2$ drops by 0.26 kPa
- pH increases by 0.015

Stewart's Physicochemical Approach to Acid–Base

This more recent approach to acid–base balance applies concepts of physical chemistry to aqueous solutions, and attributes relatively low importance to HCO_3^-. In short, there are independent variables which can be altered from outside the system.

1. **Strong ion difference (SID)**

$$SID = (Na^+ + K^+ + Ca^{2+} + Mg^{2+}) - (Cl^- + other\ strong\ ions\ (e.g.\ SO_4^{2-}, lactate))$$

2. **Total weak acid concentration (A_{tot})**, e.g. albumin
3. **$PaCO_2$** (respiration component)

There are dependent variables (pH and HCO_3^-) that are altered by the above independent variables.

Together, it leads to classifying acid–base disorders as:

- **Respiratory changes:** increased or decreased $PaCO_2$
- **SID changes:** strong ions totally dissociate within water and, in turn, have an impact on ionisation

of other compounds. The SID is usually 40 mEq/l (alkaline), assuming normal protein levels, and if this decreases, there is by definition an acidosis. It may be due to:

- An excess or a deficit of water, causing concentration/dilution change of anions (e.g. dehydration concentrates the alkalinity of the solution)
- An excess or a deficit of strong ions:
  - Decreased Na^+ = decreased SID = acidosis
  - Increased Na^+ = increased SID = alkalosis
  - Increased Cl^- = decreased SID = acidosis
    - Increased inorganic acids (lactate, ketoacids) = decreased SID = acidosis
- **A_{tot} changes:** an excess or a deficit of inorganic phosphate or albumin

References and Further Reading

Baird G. Preanalytical considerations in blood gas analysis. *Biochemia Medica* 2013;**23**:19–27.

Story D. Stewart acid–base: a simple bedside approach. *Anesth Analg* 2016;**123**:511–15.

Yentis S, Hirsch N, Ip J. *Anaesthesia, Intensive Care and Perioperative Medicine A–Z: An Encyclopaedia of Principles and Practice*, 6th edn. Edinburgh: Elsevier; 2018.

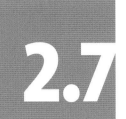

2.7 Principles of Interpreting Imaging Studies (X-ray/CT/MRI)

Chun Wah So and Matthew Gale

Key Learning Points

1. For X-rays, denser tissue (i.e. bone) absorbs more X-rays and therefore is whiter on the final image.
2. In CT imaging, different contrast media are used, depending on the clinical question. Normally oral/nasogastric contrast is given to detect intraluminal bowel pathology, and intravenous contrast is given to delineate the vasculature and lesions.
3. When looking at CT images, the process of windowing is used to optimally display the desired set of tissues. Sequential windows should be reviewed to assess the desired structures.
4. Magnetic resonance imaging works by utilising the magnetic properties of hydrogen ions (protons), which are found in high concentration in water and fat.
5. Different tissues can be characterised by different relaxation times – T1 and T2.

Keywords: radiograph, X-ray, computed tomography, magnetic resonance imaging

Plain Film Radiographs (X-ray)

The principle of plain film radiography is to measure the number of X-rays that pass through a patient to reach the detector. The X-rays will be absorbed to varying degrees by different tissues, depending on their density, which is used to produce an image.

Denser tissue (i.e. bone) = absorbs more X-rays = whiter on the final image

The key radiological densities (from the lowest to the highest densities) are: gas, fat, soft tissue and calcium/bone/metal.

Table 2.7.1 Advantages and disadvantages of radiographs

Advantages	Disadvantages
Relatively low radiation dose compared to CT	Two-dimensional representation of a three-dimensional structure, which can make interpretation challenging
Excellent spatial resolution, best viewed on high-resolution monitors	Poor at assessing soft tissues
Portable chest radiographs	Orthogonal views of bones are mandatory

Advantages and disadvantages of radiographs can be seen in Table 2.7.1.

Computed Tomography

CT uses X-rays to produce a cross-sectional image. An X-ray tube rotates around the patient, with a ring of detectors surrounding the patient measuring the transmitted radiation. The data are processed by a computer to produce the final image in a series of 'slices'. A diagram of a third-generation CT machine can be seen in Figure 2.7.1.

Hounsfield Units and 'Windowing'

The CT image consists of a matrix of pixels, and each pixel is assigned a numerical value relative to the attenuation of water, known as Hounsfield units (HU). On this scale, water is assigned zero; anything less dense will be given a negative value (gas and fat), and anything denser will be given a positive value (soft tissue, blood, contrast, bone).

A CT scan can differentiate among thousands of levels of density, yet the human eye can only distinguish among approximately 20–30 shades of grey. A technique called windowing is therefore used. The selected window will optimally display the desired set of tissues. Therefore, when reviewing a CT scan, the soft tissue, lung and bone windows will be sequentially reviewed to assess the desired structures.

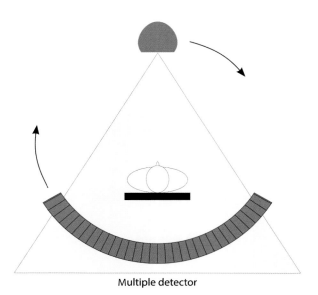

Multiple detector

Figure 2.7.1 Third-generation CT machine.
Source: Image from Abdulla S, Clarke C. *FRCR Physics Notes: Medical imaging physics for the First FRCR examination*. 3rd ed. Nottingham: Radiology Café Publishing, 2020 (ISBN-13: 978–1999988524)

Contrast Medium and Phases

Enhanced CT scans use agents to increase the contrast between two tissues.

Contrast medium is used, depending on the clinical question. Normally, oral/nasogastric (NG) contrast is given to detect intraluminal bowel pathology, and intravenous (IV) contrast is given to delineate the vasculature and lesions.

Following administration of IV contrast, there will be a time interval before starting the scan. This is termed the 'phase' and refers to which area of the body is enhanced when the image is taken. The various phases of scanning include unenhanced (no contrast), arterial, portal venous and delayed (Table 2.7.2). A scan in the 'portal venous phase', for example, refers to when the contrast is in the portal venous system. As different lesions and tissues take up contrast at different times, the radiologist must decide on whether to perform a single or a multi-phase examination, based on the clinical information given and the working diagnosis. It is therefore essential to provide as much information as you can about the suspected pathology or the clinical question when requesting a scan.

Advantages and disadvantages of CT can be seen in Table 2.7.3.

Table 2.7.2 Phases of a CT scan

Phase	Tissues enhanced	Pathology
Unenhanced	None	Intramural haematoma (aorta) Renal/ureteric calculi
Early arterial	Arteries	Pulmonary embolism, dissection, haemorrhage
Late arterial	Arteries, kidneys (outer cortex), pancreas, spleen, bowel	Bowel ischaemia, hypervascular lesions, i.e. hepatocellular carcinoma, haemangiomas
Portal venous	Portal vein, liver parenchyma	Hypovascular lesions (i.e. liver cysts/abscesses/ metastases), collections, abnormal enhancement of abdominopelvic viscera
Delayed	Urinary tract	Renal tract, e.g. ureteric lesions, ileal conduit leak

Table 2.7.3 Advantages and disadvantages of CT

Advantages	Disadvantages
Rapid multi-phase examination technique	High radiation
Good soft tissue contrast and anatomical coverage	Contrast nephropathy, allergy
Three-dimensional volume reconstructions for surgical planning	Not portable
Better for acute intracranial haemorrhage than MRI	Artefact from bone/metal implants

Magnetic Resonance Imaging

MRI works by utilising the magnetic properties of hydrogen ions (protons), which are found in high concentration in water and fat. A powerful magnetic field aligns the hydrogen nuclei and then a radiofrequency pulse displaces the nuclei. The nuclei will then re-align to their lowest energy state. Each tissue type will re-align at different rates, allowing a clever algorithm to create an image of the different tissues.

Tissues can be characterised by different relaxation times – T1 and T2. In T1-weighted sequences, fat, subacute haemorrhage, exudate and gadolinium will appear bright (Figure 2.7.2). On T2-weighted sequences, acute haemorrhage, water, cerebrospinal fluid (CSF) and inflammation will appear bright (Figure 2.7.3).

Advantages and disadvantages of MRI can be seen in Table 2.7.4.

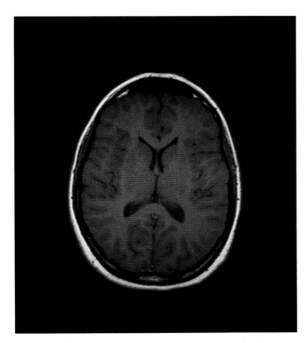

Figure 2.7.2 MRI with T1-weighted sequences. Fat is bright on T1-weighted sequences, and water (CSF) is dark.

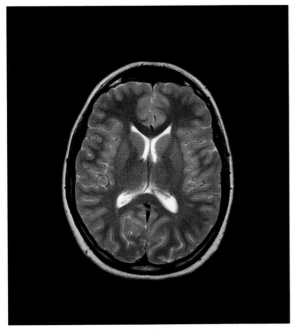

Figure 2.7.3 MRI with T2-weighted sequences. Fluid and fat are bright on T2-weighted sequences. Note the grey matter and white matter have different signal characteristics, compared with the T1-weighted sequence.

Table 2.7.4 Advantages and disadvantages of MRI

Advantages	Disadvantages
No radiation	Claustrophobic and noisy
Excellent soft tissue contrast	Slow (>30 minutes)
Multi-phase	Limited resource, expensive
Arterial type imaging possible without contrast medium administration	Prone to metal and motion artefacts
Main imaging modality for the spine	Contraindicated with some medical devices
	Specific sequences and imaging planes need to be specified in advance, depending on the clinical question
	Unknown impact on the fetus

Radiation

Plain film radiography, fluoroscopy and CT use ionising radiation. The Ionising Radiation (Medical Exposure) Regulations (IRMER) 2000 was created to minimise the potential hazards associated with exposure to ionising radiation. The benefit of performing the examination must outweigh the risks.

Table 2.7.5 shows the average dose per examination, and for reference, the average annual UK

Table 2.7.5 Levels of radiation dose for different imaging modalities

Dose level	Imaging	Radiation dose (mSv)	Equivalent background radiation
High (>2 mSv)	CT abdomen/pelvis	10	4.5 years
	CT chest	8	3.6 years
	CT head	2	1 year
Medium (0.02–2 mSv)	Barium swallow	1.5	8 months
	Lumbar spine	1.3	7 months
	Pelvis anteroposterior (AP)	0.7	4 months
	Abdomen	0.7	4 months
Low (<0.02 mSv)	Chest posteroanterior (PA)	0.015	3 days
	Limbs	<0.01	<1.5 days

Source: Adapted from Public Health England, *Patient dose information: guidance.*

background radiation dose is 2.7 mSv. A single CT chest has over 500 times more radiation than a chest radiograph.

References and Further Reading

Allisy-Roberts P, Williams J. *Farr's Physics for Medical Imaging*, 2nd edn. Edinburgh: Elsevier; 2008.

Darby MJ, Barron D, Hyland RE. *Oxford Handbook for Medical Imaging*. Oxford: Oxford University Press; 2011.

Public Health England. 2008. Patient dose information: guidance. www.gov.uk/government/publications/medical-radiation-patient-doses/patient-dose-information-guidance

Raby N, Berman L, de Lacey G. *Accident & Emergency Radiology: A Survival Guide*, 2nd edn. Edinburgh: Elsevier; 2005.

Radiology Masterclass. 2008. Basics of X-ray physics. www.radiologymasterclass.co.uk/tutorials/physics/x-ray_physics_introduction

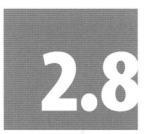

Imaging of the Chest

Chun Wah So and Matthew Gale

Keywords: chest X-ray, endotracheal tube, nasogastric tube, central venous catheter, consolidation

Introduction

The inability of ICU patients to cooperate, combined with the technical limitations of portable radiography, makes it vital for the ICU doctor to be able to accurately interpret a chest X-ray (CXR). A normal CXR can be seen in Figure 2.8.1.

Challenges of Portable Chest Radiography in ICU

- Anteroposterior (AP) films magnify the heart and mediastinum, obscuring the left lower zone.
- Patients are less able to cooperate, with poor inspiration producing a suboptimal image. Patient rotation or beam angulation can simulate mass/consolidation.
- Not all opacities arise from the lungs. Patient clothing, skinfolds, ECG stickers and external tubing/wires can all produce artefacts.

Systematic Assessment of ICU CXRs

There are many different systems for how to interpret a CXR. Many are complex and have multiple steps. However, as the films in the ICU are almost always of poorer quality than those of a healthy outpatient, it may not be feasible to check everything the literature tells you to. The system below is by no means the definitive one, but it may help for developing your own method of interpretation.

The 'LLL' Approach

1. Lines, tubes and drains
2. Lungs and mediastinum
3. Last CXR

Lines, Tubes and Drains

It is important that all lines, tubes and drains are correctly placed, as iatrogenic injury can occur as a result of misplacement.

Central Venous Catheters

For use in ICU, the tip should lie in the superior vena cava (SVC) (Figure 2.8.2). The SVC is not visible on the CXR, so as a rule of thumb, the carina can be used as a landmark, i.e. the tip should lie at the level of the carina to the right of the mediastinum.

If the tip is in the right atrium or ventricle, it may cause an arrhythmia. If the tip is too proximal, it may lead to thrombosis or infection. If the line is malpositioned, there may be a vascular injury that can lead to pneumothorax or infusion of fluid into the pleural space or mediastinum. A misplaced central venous catheter can be seen in Figure 2.8.3.

(a)　　　　　　　　　　　　　　　　(b)

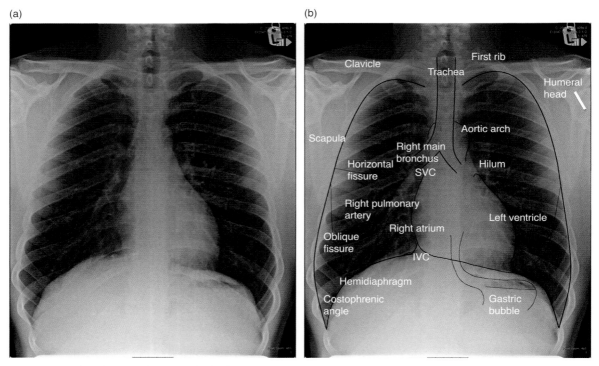

Figure 2.8.1 Normal CXR – without (a) and with labels (b).

(a)　　　　　　　　　　　　　　　　(b)

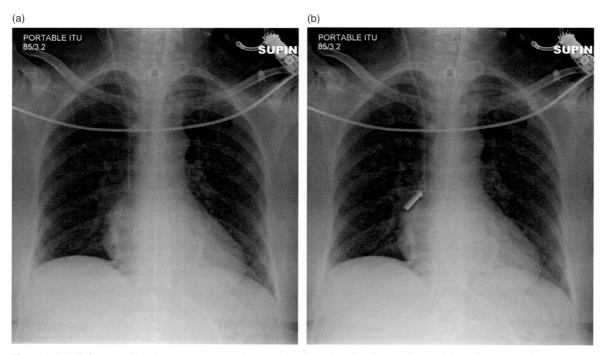

Figure 2.8.2 Right internal jugular central venous catheter – unlabelled (a) and labelled (b). The tip is labelled lying in the SVC.

(a) (b)

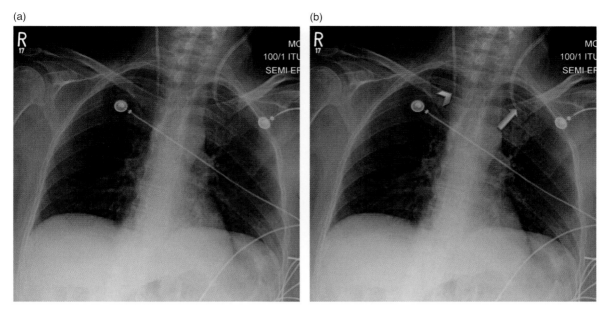

Figure 2.8.3 Misplaced central venous catheter. The left internal jugular central venous catheter (CVC) tip curls left into the left subclavian vein (arrow). The right internal jugular CVC tip is high and probably within the right brachiocephalic vein (arrowhead).

Nasogastric Tube

CXRs are often used when aspiration of a nasogastric (NG) tube is unsuccessful.

In order to be in a satisfactory position, the NG tube must:

- Descend in the midline (on a well-centred CXR) (Figure 2.8.4)
- Bisect the carina/main bronchi (i.e. not follow the course of the main bronchi at the carina)
- Have the tip below the diaphragm, ideally 10 cm distal to the oesophago-gastric junction (some tubes have distal side holes)

Various examples of misplaced NG tubes can be seen in Figure 2.8.5.

Endotracheal Tube

Remember that neck position will affect the location of the endotracheal tube (ETT) tip. Flexion will move it downwards, and extension will move it upwards.

The tip should lie 5–7 cm above the carina. If the carina is not visible, then a good rule of thumb to use is that the carina lies between the 5th and 7th thoracic vertebrae.

If the ETT cannulates a main bronchus, this will lead to collapse of the contralateral lung (Figure 2.8.6). If the tube is in the oesophagus, it can be seen lateral to the tracheal shadow on the CXR, with distension of the stomach evident.

Tracheostomy

The walls of the tracheostomy tube must lie parallel to the tracheal outer margins. The tip is normally positioned halfway between the upper end of the tracheostomy and the carina. Positioning of the tracheostomy can be seen in Figure 2.8.7.

Oesophageal Doppler Probe

Oesophageal Doppler probes are sometimes used to measure cardiac output. The probe should be placed in the mid oesophagus (Figure 2.8.8). Although CXR is not normally used to confirm its placement, you should be familiar with its appearance.

Lungs and Mediastinum

- **Trachea:** central or slightly deviated to the right
  - Tension pneumothorax and effusions will PUSH the trachea
  - Collapse will PULL the trachea

(a)

(b)

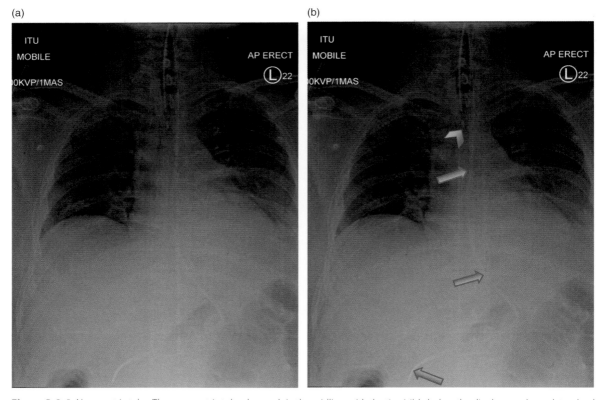

Figure 2.8.4 Nasogastric tube. The nasogastric tube descends in the midline, with the tip visible below the diaphragm. An endotracheal tube can also be seen.

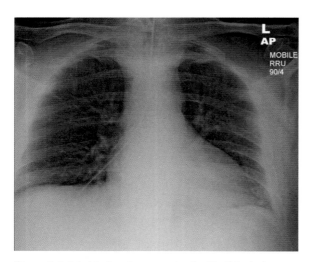

Figure 2.8.5.1 Misplaced nasogastric tube. The NG tube has cannulated the airway and follows the right main bronchus to sit within the lung. The NG tube position at the carina will help determine whether it resides within the airway or the oesophagus. Part of the lower lobes continues posteriorly below the diaphragm, which is difficult to appreciate on a frontal chest radiograph.

- **Hilum:** the left hilum should NEVER be lower than the right. If it is, you must suspect volume loss in the right upper lobe or left lower lobe
- **Lungs:**
  - Divide the lungs into three zones: upper, middle and lower thirds. Compare each side, and check for symmetry
  - Infiltrates (alveolar versus interstitial), masses (Figure 2.8.9)
  - Collapse/atelectasis may cause volume loss (Figure 2.8.10)
  - Pleural effusions are commonly seen in ICU patients due to fluid shifts

(a)　　　　　　　　　　　　　　　　(b)

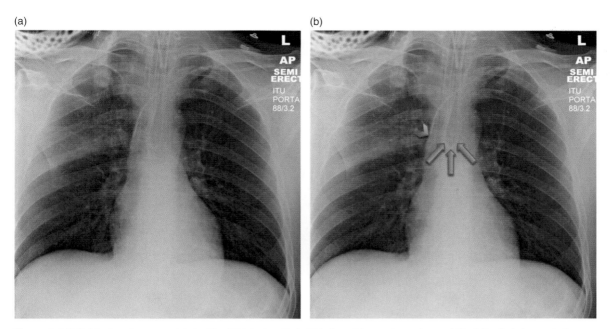

Figure 2.8.5.2 Misplaced nasogastric tube. The NG tube is coiled within the mid oesophagus (arrows). The left subclavian central venous catheter tip is within the SVC.

(a)　　　　　　　　　　　　　　　　(b)

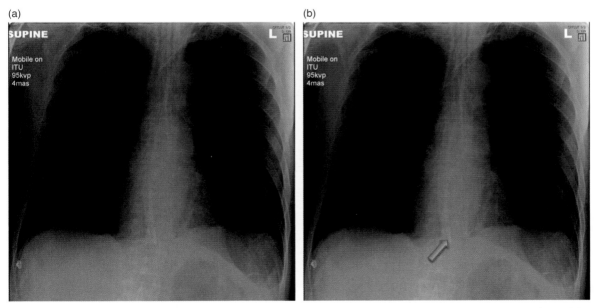

Figure 2.8.5.3 Misplaced nasogastric tube. The NG tube tip is within the distal oesophagus. The tip should ideally be 10 cm beyond the gastro-oesophageal junction.

(a) (b)

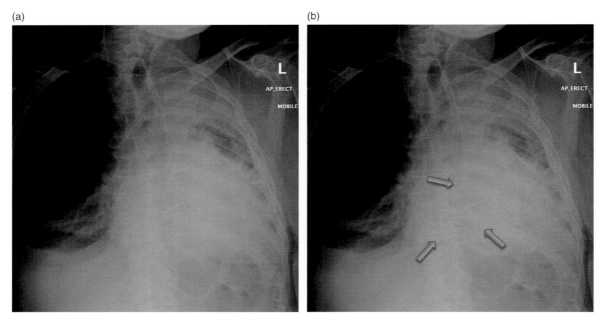

Figure 2.8.5.4 Misplaced nasogastric tube. At first glance, this NG tube appears to be in the left lung. However, this patient has a large diaphragmatic hernia, with the stomach and colon in the thoracic cavity. The NG tube tip is likely to be within the intrathoracic stomach.

(a) (b)

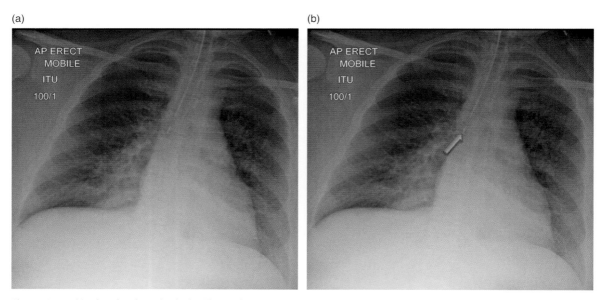

Figure 2.8.6 Misplaced endotracheal tube. The ETT has cannulated the right main bronchus, and the left lung will eventually collapse if nothing is done.

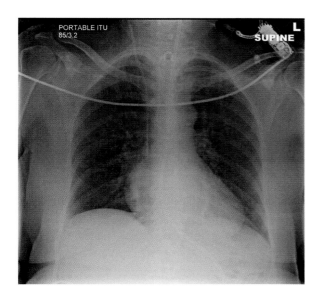

Figure 2.8.7 Tracheostomy. The tracheostomy is positioned in the midline at the trachea in a suitable position. Other lines also are present.

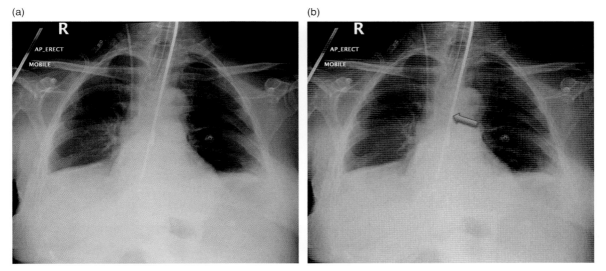

(a) (b)

Figure 2.8.8 Oesophageal Doppler. Oesophageal Doppler probe (arrow), in addition to other lines.

Box 2.8.1 Consolidation

Consolidation refers to small airways and alveoli that have filled with material – pus, fluid, blood or cells. Consolidation is not synonymous with infection as some may think!

Alveolar versus Interstitial Infiltrates – Which Is It?

The pattern of shadowing can often give clues to the underlying pathology. Alveolar shadowing is due to the alveolar air sacs filling with material. Interstitial disease affects the scaffolding of the lungs. Interstitial thickening can be caused by a long list of entities, including fibrosis, inflammation and oedema. CXR properties of alveolar and interstitial infiltrates can be seen in Table 2.8.1.

- **Mediastinum:**
  - The heart will almost always be enlarged on an AP view taken in the ICU
  - Cardiac border definition – may be lost in lesions/consolidation (Boxes 2.8.1 and 2.8.2)

Table 2.8.1 Chest X-ray properties of alveolar and interstitial infiltrates

Alveolar	Interstitial
'Fluffy' or 'blobby'	Small nodules
Ill-defined margins	Linear
Merging	Reticular or 'mesh-like'
Segmental/lobar	Reticulonodular (lines/dots)

(a) (b)

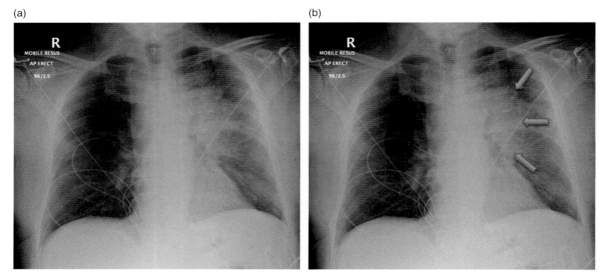

Figure 2.8.9.1 Consolidation. Dense left upper and mid-zone consolidation centred at the left hilum. See subsequent CT scan of the same patient (Figure 2.8.9.2).

(a) (b)

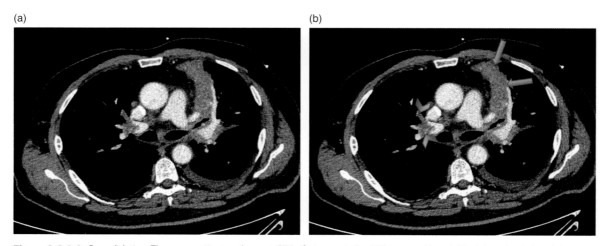

Figure 2.8.9.2 Consolidation. The same patient underwent CT (soft tissue window). The normal lung is black (gas density) and the consolidated lung is grey (soft tissue density). The differential diagnosis would include infection and malignancy. There are also pulmonary emboli within the pulmonary arteries (arrowheads).

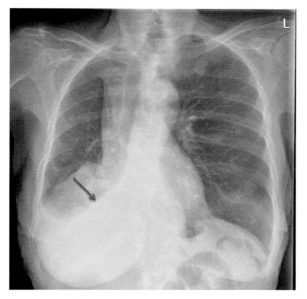

Figure 2.8.10 Right lower zone collapse. The triangular density within the right lower zone represents a right lower lobe collapse. The contour of the right hemidiaphragm is lost.

Box 2.8.2 The Silhouette Sign

The silhouette sign allows subtle pathology to be identified and located (Figure 2.8.11). The term is actually a misnomer and refers to loss of the normal silhouette. Structures such as the heart borders are normally visible because the heart lies adjacent to the aerated lung (with different densities). When there is an abnormal density within the lung, this crisp border is lost and will appear blurred. This helps to localise the lesion.

Table 2.8.2 The silhouette sign – relationship between the border obliterated and the location of the lesion

Border obliterated	Location of lesion
Right heart border/atrium	Middle lobe
Right hemidiaphragm	Right lower lobe
Aortic arch	Left upper lobe
Left ventricle	Lingula
Left hemidiaphragm	Left lower lobe

Source: Adapted from de Lacey G, Morley S, Berman L. *The Chest X-Ray: A Survival Guide*. Elsevier publishing; 2008.

(a)   (b)

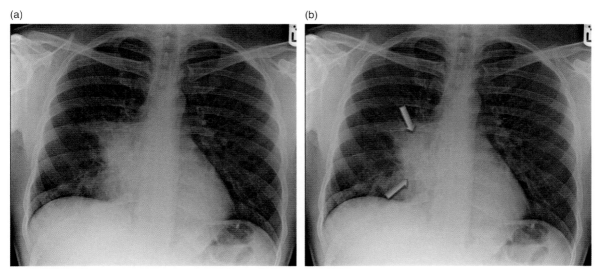

Figure 2.8.11 The silhouette sign. The right heart border is missing, in keeping with middle lobe consolidation. The normally aerated middle lobe is filled with material (e.g. pus/tumour), so the interface between the aerated lung and the heart is lost. In comparison, the left heart border is crisp.

Last Chest X-ray

Detailed systematic assessment of the CXR can be seen in Box 2.8.3. Remember to ALWAYS compare with previous imaging.

Pneumonia versus Pulmonary Oedema versus ARDS – Which Is It?

It can be difficult to differentiate between shadowing caused by pneumonia, pulmonary oedema (Figures 2.8.12.1 and 2.8.12.2) or acute respiratory distress syndrome (ARDS) (Figure 2.8.13). Indeed, they often

coexist in ICU patients. However, there are features that can help you discern between them (Table 2.8.3).

Table 2.8.3 Differentiating between cardiogenic pulmonary oedema and acute respiratory distress syndrome

Cardiogenic pulmonary oedema	Acute respiratory distress syndrome
Perihilar alveolar opacification	Diffuse, uniform alveolar opacification
CXR changes occur with symptoms	CXR changes can occur 12 hours or more post-onset of symptoms
CXR changes clear rapidly in response to treatment	CXR changes can persist despite treatment
Pleural effusions are common	Pleural effusions are rare

Source: Adapted from de Lacey G, Morley S, Berman L. *The Chest X-Ray: A Survival Guide.* Elsevier publishing; 2008.

Complications of Ventilation

Barotrauma is a well-recognised complication of mechanical ventilation, leading to rupture of alveoli, with leakage of air into the pleural space (pneumothorax) (Figures 2.8.14.1, 2.8.14.2 and 2.8.14.3) and/or the mediastinum (pneumomediastinum) (Figure 2.8.15).

Pneumothorax

This is diagnosed upon identifying a pleural edge with absent lung markings peripherally. It is radiolucent, due to less lung tissue absorbing the X-rays, and is easier to see when it is large. Subcutaneous emphysema (gas locules in the soft tissues), should alert you to carefully inspect for a pneumothorax and rib fractures.

On a supine CXR, you will not see the classic pleural edge, because the pleural gas will float up towards the anterior chest wall and therefore cover the entire lung. It may, however, cause one lung to appear more radiolucent (darker) than the other. Other important clues include the 'deep sulcus sign' – where the costophrenic angle is unusually deep due to gas tracking downwards, the hemidiaphragm may appear flattened on the affected side, and the heart, mediastinal and hemidiaphragm borders can appear too sharp/crisp due to gas sitting between these structures and the normal lung.

An important mimic of pneumothorax is bullous disease – critical to be aware of, as insertion of a chest drain into a bulla may have disastrous consequences. The shape of the air cavity, along with detection on previous imaging, may help differentiate between the two. However, CT is sometimes needed for confirmation.

Box 2.8.3 Detailed Systematic Assessment of CXR: ABCDE and Review

This is a more detailed version of the assessment above.

A: Airways
- Trachea and hilar position
- Lungs

B: Bones/Soft Tissues
- Ribs/scapula/humerus for fracture or bone lesions
- Soft tissues – surgical emphysema (Figure 2.8.16), pleural masses

C: Circulation (and Mediastinum)
- Heart size and borders, mediastinal shift
- Aortic size and course

D: Diaphragm
- Right hemidiaphragm higher than the left due to the liver
- Loss of costophrenic angles seen in pleural effusion
- Deep sulcus sign (see later section)
- Flattened in hyperinflation (chronic obstructive pulmonary disease) or tension pneumothorax
- Check for free subdiaphragmatic gas in perforation

Extras
- Lines, tubes, wires and other foreign bodies

Review Areas
- Apices – pneumothorax and tumour (Pancoast)
- Hilum – tumours, lymphadenopathy
- Heart – behind the heart for consolidation; the normal density should be identical on both sides
- Diaphragm – below the diaphragm for mass/free gas
- Bones – bone lesions and fractures

(a)

(b)

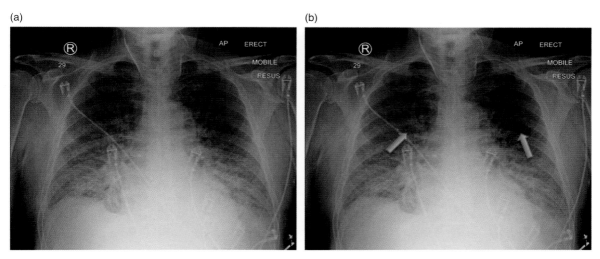

Figure 2.8.12.1 Pulmonary oedema. Perihilar opacification and bronchial wall thickening (arrows) occur due to build-up of interstitial fluid.

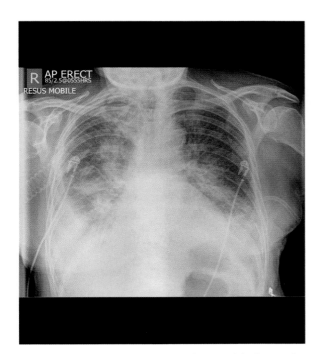

Figure 2.8.12.2 Pulmonary oedema. Classic perihilar (batwing) oedema and pleural effusions.

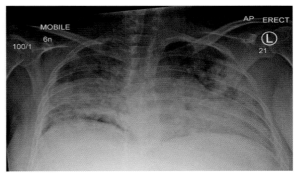

Figure 2.8.13 Acute respiratory distress syndrome. Diffuse and alveolar opacification is consistent with ARDS.

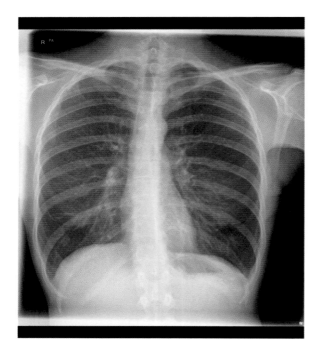

Figure 2.8.14.1 Pneumothorax. A small pneumothorax can be difficult to detect, as shown here in the left upper zone. The pleural edge parallels the chest wall, with absence of lung markings peripherally.

(a)   (b)

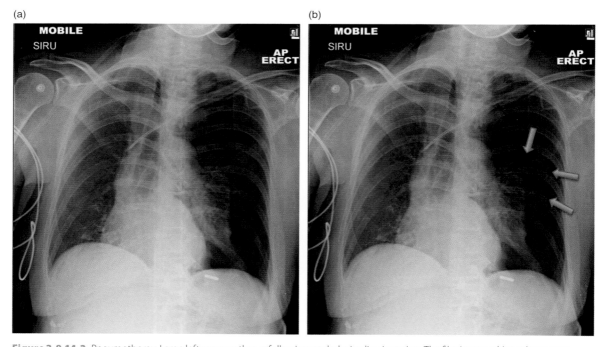

Figure 2.8.14.2 Pneumothorax. Large left pneumothorax following a subclavian line insertion. The film is rotated (vertebrae not in between the medial clavicles), but there is probably some mediastinal shift and flattening of the left hemidiaphragm which are concerning for tension.

(a)

(b)

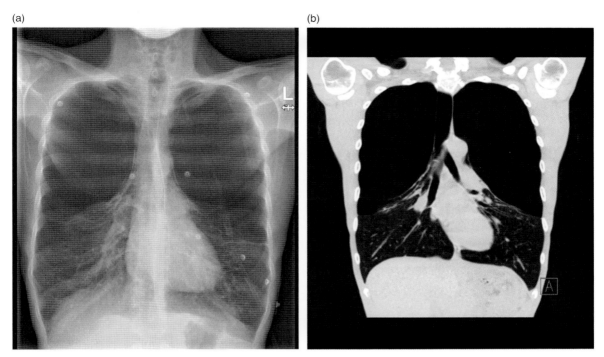

Figure 2.8.14.3 Pneumothorax? There was some diagnostic uncertainty about whether the chest radiograph showed bilateral pneumothoraces or bullae (a). A CT scan was performed, confirming the presence of large bilateral bullae (b). A review of previous chest radiographs is required to confirm the chronicity of bullous disease.

(a)

(b)

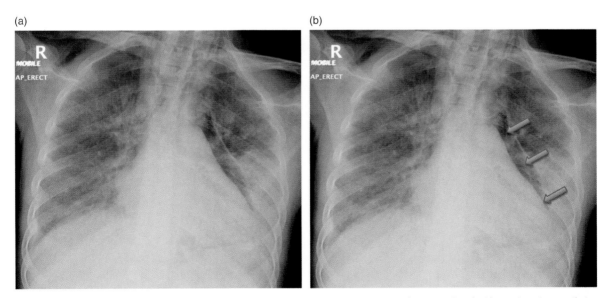

Figure 2.8.15 Pneumomediastinum. This patient has severe pneumocystis pneumonia and was ventilated with non-invasive ventilation, causing extra-luminal mediastinal gas (arrow).

(a) (b)

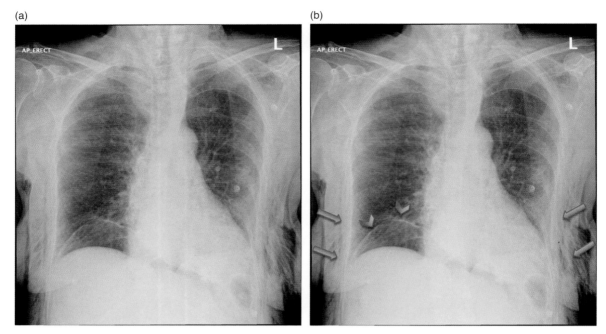

Figure 2.8.16 Surgical emphysema. Recent laparoscopic hysterectomy with expected pneumoperitoneum (arrowheads). The patient also has surgical emphysema over the thorax (arrows) due to apparent aggressive ventilation.

References and Further Reading

de Lacey G, Morley S, Berman L. *The Chest X-Ray: A Survival Guide*. Edinburgh: Elsevier; 2008.

Godoy M, Leitman B, de Groot P, Vlahos I, Naidich D. Chest radiography in the ICU: Part I, evaluation of airway, enteric and pleural tubes. *AJR Am J Roentgenol* 2012;**198**:563–71.

Goodman L. *Felson's Principles of Chest Roentgenology: A Programmed Text*, 3rd edn. Philadelphia, PA: Elsevier; 2007.

Life in the Fast Lane. DRSABCDE of CXR interpretation. litfl.com/drsabcde-of-cxr-interpretation/

Radiology Masterclass. 2019. Chest X-ray – tubes. www.radiologymasterclass.co.uk/tutorials/chest/chest_tubes/chest_xray_tubes_start

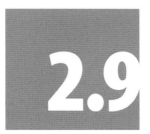

Imaging of the Head

Chun Wah So and Matthew Gale

Key Learning Points

1. Delineation of the lobes on CT is more difficult than on MRI, and instead they are often referred to as 'regions' on CT.
2. Appreciation of the cerebrospinal fluid (CSF) spaces is useful to assess brain volume, mass effect, hydrocephalus and haemorrhage.
3. Subarachnoid haemorrhage (SAH) is commonly seen as abnormal high attenuation within the cerebral sulci, ventricles and/or the basal cisterns.
4. Subdural haematomas (SDH) appear on CT as a concave extra-axial collection (outside the brain parenchyma).
5. Extradural haematomas (EDH) appear as a convex/lens shape and usually underlie a fracture. If the haematoma extends past a suture, it is not extradural.

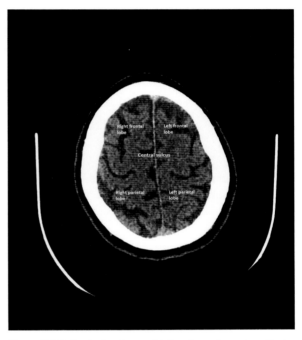

Figure 2.9.1 Cerebral regions - axial slice of superior region of brain.

Keywords: subarachnoid haemorrhage, subdural haematoma, extradural haematoma, ischaemic stroke

Introduction

As is the case with abdominal CT, you are not expected to report CT heads. However, this chapter aims to provide you with a quick checklist of areas to review in order to aid in the recognition of gross pathology.

CT Head Anatomy

Lobes

Delineation of the lobes on CT is more difficult than on MRI, and instead they are often referred to as 'regions' on CT (Figures 2.9.1, 2.9.2 and 2.9.3).

White and grey matter can be differentiated on CT because of the difference in myelin content. White matter contains more myelin (fatty), and grey matter has a higher number of cell bodies. White matter is therefore of a lower density than grey matter and appears darker.

Meninges

The meninges are the dura, arachnoid and pia mater (Figure 2.9.4). The meninges have folds separating the cerebral hemispheres (falx cerebri), and the cerebrum/cerebellum (tentorium cerebelli). Elsewhere they are not visible, but knowledge of their anatomy is crucial to understanding the appearances of intracranial haemorrhages.

Cerebrospinal Fluid Spaces

The cerebrospinal fluid (CSF) surrounds the brain and can be found in the ventricles and basal cisterns. It appears dark/low density on CT due to its water content. Appreciation of the CSF spaces is useful to assess brain volume, mass effect, hydrocephalus and haemorrhage.

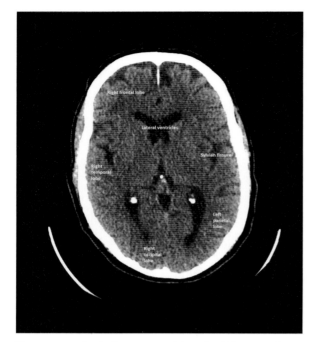

Figure 2.9.2 Cerebral regions - axial slice of middle region of brain.

Figure 2.9.3 Cerebral regions - axial slice of inferior region of brain.

Figures 2.9.1 – 2.9.3 Three axial CT slices starting at the superior, middle and inferior regions of the brain. The central sulcus separates the frontal and parietal lobes (Figure 2.9.1). The ventricles, basal cisterns and sulci are dark due to the water density of the CSF. Grey–white matter differentiation is best appreciated on Figure 2.9.2. Using a stroke window helps accentuate grey–white matter differentiation and identify infarction.

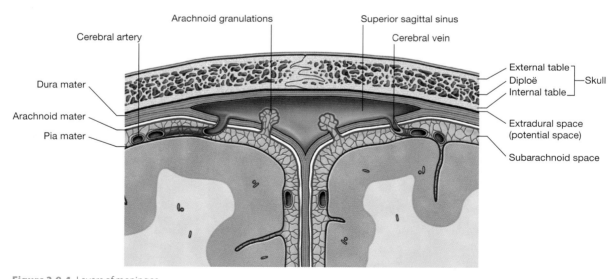

Figure 2.9.4 Layers of meninges.
Source: *Neuroanatomy: An Illustrated Colour Text*, 5e, by AR Crossman and D Neary. © Elsevier.

CT Checklist: 'AB BCS'

1. Asymmetry
2. Blood
3. Brain
4. CSF space
5. Skull/scalp

Asymmetry

Scroll through the slices, checking for asymmetry.

Blood

Acute haemorrhage will usually be denser than the surrounding brain.

- Subarachnoid haemorrhage (SAH) is commonly caused by trauma or a ruptured aneurysm. On CT, there will be abnormal high attenuation within the cerebral sulci, ventricles and/or the basal cisterns (Figure 2.9.5).
- Subdural haematoma (SDH) often occurs due to tearing of the bridging cortical veins, classically in the elderly or anticoagulated patient (Figure 2.9.6). It appears on CT as a concave extra-

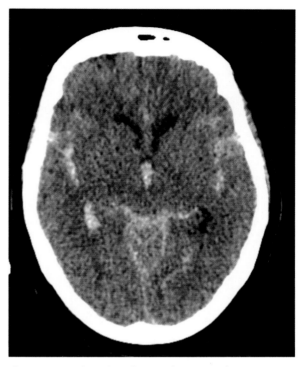

Figure 2.9.5 Subarachnoid haemorrhage. Hyperdense haemorrhage within the ventricles, cisterns and fissures.

(a) (b)

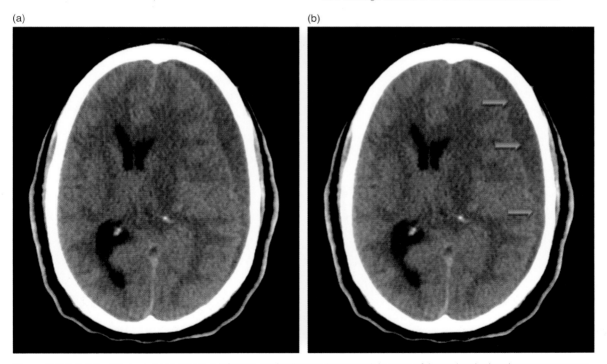

Figure 2.9.6 Subdural haemorrhage. Concave left extra-axial collection (arrow) with layering of dependent higher density suggests an acute-on-chronic process. The haematoma is causing a mass effect, resulting in a shift of midline structures to the right and effacement of the ventricles.

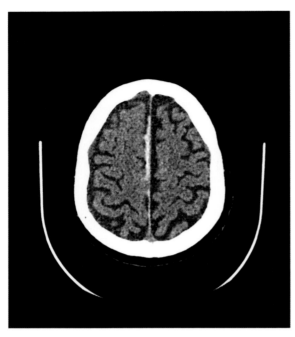

axial collection (outside the brain parenchyma). Acute haematomas are usually of high density and change to lower density, reaching a similar density to that of the CSF, as they mature. SDH can overlie the falx or tentorium, making it challenging to identify (Figure 2.9.7).

- Extradural haematoma (EDH) is a collection of blood between the skull vault and the dura mater. An EDH is caused by arterial haemorrhage (typically the middle meningeal artery) following trauma, and it is this high-pressure bleeding which allows the dura to be peeled away from the skull. It appears as a convex/lens shape and usually underlies a fracture (Figure 2.9.8). If the haematoma extends past a suture, it is not extradural.

Brain
Abnormal Density
- Hyperdense lesions include acute haemorrhage, thrombus and contrast-enhancing lesions.

Figure 2.9.7 Subdural haemorrhage. Parafalcine subdural haemorrhage along the right falx cerebri.

(a) (b)

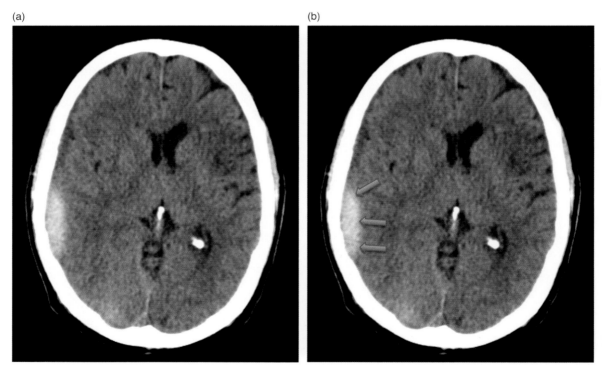

Figure 2.9.8 Extradural haemorrhage. Convex right extra-axial collection in keeping with an EDH. Mass effect is present, with loss of the normal cerebral sulci and a subtle shift of midline structures.

- Hypodense lesions include infarction, oedema, cysts, mature haemorrhage and gas.
- The appearance of a tumour is variable; some require post-contrast imaging to enhance areas of oedema.

Mass Effect

- Causes include, but are not limited to, haemorrhage, tumours, abscesses and cysts.
- Look for a shift of midline structures and a decrease in size (effacement) of the ventricles/basal cisterns and cerebral sulci (Figure 2.9.9).
- Severe mass effect can cause uncal or tonsillar herniation – the latter will cause respiratory depression and death if untreated.

Grey–White Matter Differentiation

- Ischaemia can lead to loss of grey–white matter differentiation (Figures 2.9.10, 2.9.11 and 2.9.12).

CSF Spaces

- Assess the size of the ventricles and cerebral sulci relative to the brain volume. The brain volume can reduce in older age, with secondary enlargement of the ventricles and sulci. However, if the ventricles are enlarged without commensurate loss of brain volume, there may be hydrocephalus (Figure 2.9.13). In this instance, previous imaging is often invaluable.

Skull/Scalp

- Scalp haematomas in the trauma setting are helpful to detect subtle fractures. Knowing the site of impact allows the detection of contrecoup injuries; the brain can hit the skull, causing a contusion injury, most commonly in the inferior frontal and temporal lobes.
- Fluid within the paranasal sinuses and mastoid air cells can represent haemorrhage and should alert you to look for fractures. Sometimes locules of gas

(a)   (b)

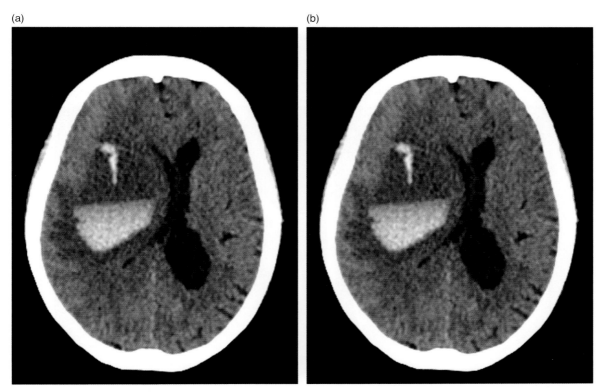

Figure 2.9.9 Mass effect. Large right intra-parenchymal and subarachnoid haemorrhage (high density), with surrounding oedema (low density), causing mass effect. The right cerebral sulci are lost and midline structures have been shifted to the left, with effacement of the lateral ventricles (affecting the right more than the left side).

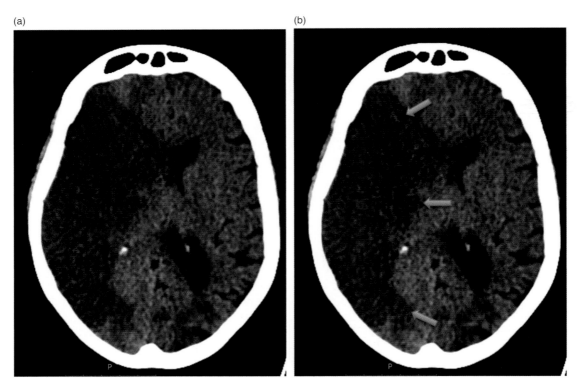

Figure 2.9.10 Ischaemic stroke. Right cerebral low attenuation within the right middle cerebral artery (MCA) territory represents an acute infarct. There is extensive right cerebral oedema, with complete loss of grey–white matter differentiation and mass effect (loss of sulci, left midline shift and ventricular effacement). A search should be made for proximal MCA thrombus leading to a malignant MCA infarct (may require surgery).

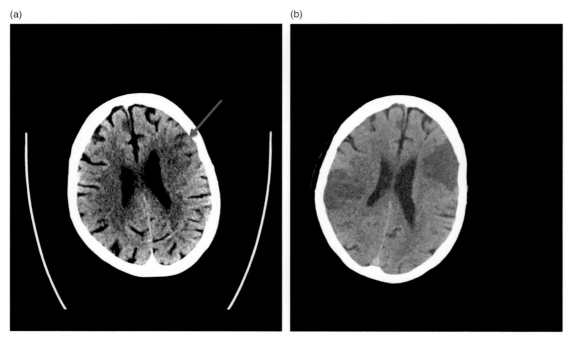

Figure 2.9.11 Ischaemic stroke. Initial CT scan (a) shows subtle loss of grey–white matter differentiation and sulcal effacement within the left frontal lobe (stroke window). The patient was re-imaged within a few hours due to deterioration (b), which shows the left frontal infarct more clearly and the presence of a right middle cerebral artery territory infarct. If scanned early (<6 hours), sometimes no CT changes are present. The main role of CT is to assess for haemorrhage before thrombolysis.

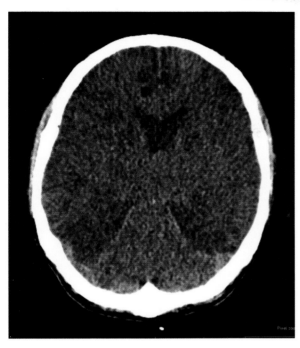

Figure 2.9.12 Hypoxic brain injury. There is generalised loss of grey–white matter differentiation and oedema causing loss of sulci, indicating global ischaemia.

may escape from these sinuses/air cells, resulting in pneumocephalus

- Foreign bodies, such as fragments of glass, can hide under scalp lacerations and can be difficult to detect clinically.

References and Further Reading

Holmes E, Forrest-Hay A, Misra R. *Interpretation of Emergency Head CT: A Practical Handbook*. New York, NY: Cambridge University Press; 2008.

Lewis G, Patel H, Modi S, Hussain S. *On Call Radiology*. Boca Raton, FL: CRC Press; 2016.

Radiology Masterclass. 2008. Acute CT brain. www.radiologymasterclass.co.uk/tutorials/ct/ct_acute_brain/ct_brain_start

(a)   (b)

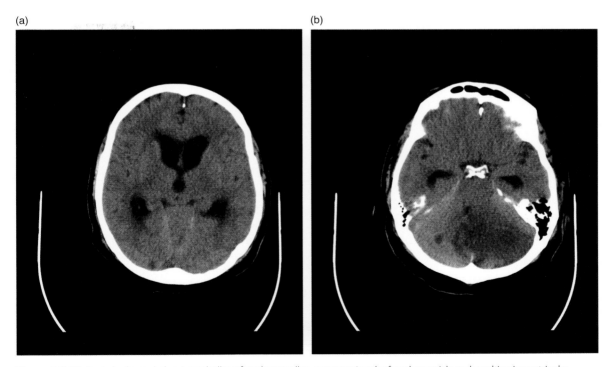

Figure 2.9.13 Acute hydrocephalus. A cerebellar infarct has swollen, compressing the fourth ventricle and resulting in ventricular obstruction. The upstream lateral and third ventricles have become enlarged. The temporal horns of the lateral ventricles are usually the first to enlarge.

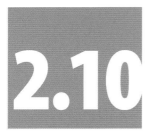

Imaging of the Abdomen

Chun Wah So and Matthew Gale

Key Learning Points

1. On an abdominal X-ray, the bowel is only visible when there is intraluminal gas or an air–fluid level, as the different densities are required to create contrast resolution so they can be perceived on a radiograph.
2. The 3/6/9 rule refers to the maximum size of specific sections of the bowel.
3. On an abdominal X-ray, the small bowel is normally central and valvulae conniventes can be seen. The colon, by contrast, is normally peripheral and has haustral folds which do not completely traverse the lumen.
4. In the early stages of pancreatitis, no abnormalities may be seen on CT imaging.
5. In cholecystitis, ultrasound is more sensitive than CT; however, CT is better at depicting complications such as perforation.

Keywords: abdominal X-ray, CT, obstruction, volvulus

Introduction

Plain abdominal films have limited use due to the advent of CT. Indications include suspected obstruction and foreign bodies. An erect chest radiograph is used for suspected perforation. A normal abdominal X-ray can be seen in Figure 2.10.1.

Systematic Assessment of the Abdominal X-ray: BBC

B: Bowel

- Bowel is only visible when there is intraluminal gas or an air–fluid level, as the different densities are required to create contrast resolution so they can be perceived on a radiograph.

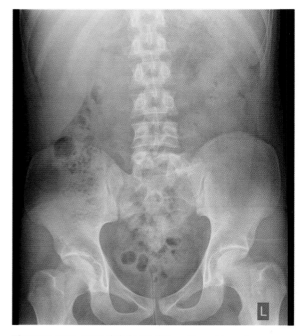

Figure 2.10.1 Normal abdominal X-ray. Normal bowel gas pattern. In addition to reviewing the gas pattern on an abdominal radiograph, it is important to also review the visible lung bases and bones.

- The small and large bowel can be differentiated by:
  - Small bowel: normally central, valvulae conniventes (mucosal folds) that cross the circumference of the bowel
  - Colon: peripheral, except for the transverse colon. The haustral folds do not completely traverse the lumen and may contain faeces that look bubbly due to small locules of gas. Notably, two haustrae can oppose each other, mimicking a small bowel appearance.

The '3/6/9 Rule'

The 3/6/9 rule refers to the maximum size of specific sections of the bowel. The small bowel should be no larger than 3 cm in diameter, the colon no larger than 6 cm and the caecum no larger than 9 cm.

Small Bowel Obstruction

- Causes include: adhesions, herniae and compression from external structures.
- Can be identified on the abdominal X-ray if the small bowel diameter is >3 cm and contains gas (Figure 2.10.2). Fluid-filled bowel will be invisible.
- The 'string of beads' sign is pathognomonic of mechanical small bowel obstruction. Seen on an erect film, it depicts when gas bubbles are trapped between valvulae conniventes in a fluid-filled bowel.
- Most of these patients go on to have a CT scan to locate the transition point, and to check for a closed-loop obstruction which requires surgical management.

Large Bowel Obstruction

- Causes include: colon carcinoma, diverticular disease and volvulus.
- Seen on the abdominal X-ray when colonic diameter >6 cm and contains gas.

- A volvulus is when a loop of bowel twists upon itself and its supporting mesentery, occurring in either the sigmoid colon or the caecum.
  - A sigmoid volvulus often forms an upside-down 'U' shape pointing to the right upper quadrant – likened to a 'coffee bean' (Figure 2.10.3).
  - A caecal volvulus is less common, as the caecum is normally fixed in position. In some patients, however, there is failure of peritoneal fixation, leading to an abnormally mobile caecum. It appears on the abdominal X-ray classically as a distended, gas-filled loop of the colon arising from the right lower quadrant and extending to the epigastrium/left upper quadrant, with a 'kidney bean' appearance (Figure 2.10.4).

Pneumoperitoneum

Normally, only one side of the bowel wall should be visible due to intraluminal gas. In a pneumoperitoneum,

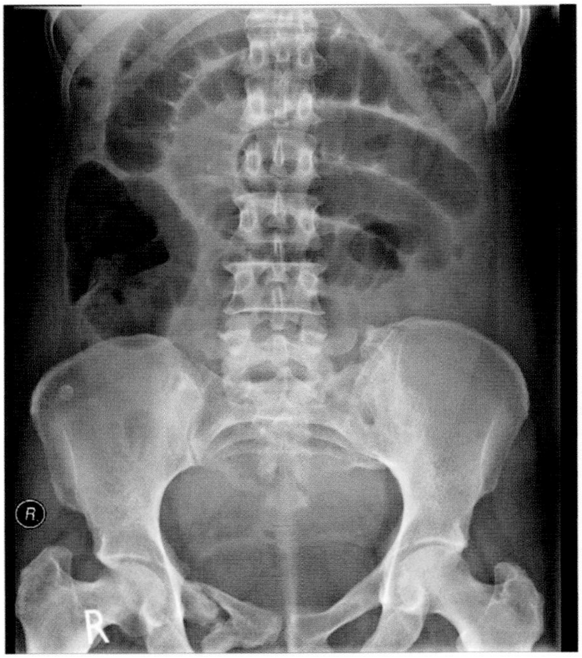

Figure 2.10.2 Small bowel obstruction. Gaseous distension of small bowel loops in keeping with small bowel obstruction, later shown to be adhesional in nature.

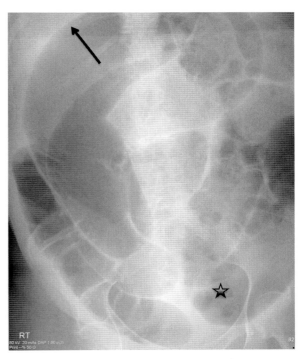

Figure 2.10.3 Sigmoid volvulus. Upside-down 'U' shape pointing towards the diaphragm (arrow) because the twist is located within the left iliac fossa (*).

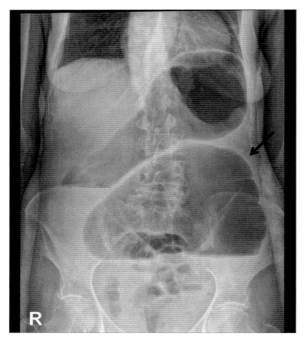

Figure 2.10.4 Caecal volvulus. The U shape points towards the left upper quadrant. Sometimes it is difficult to differentiate between caecal and sigmoid volvulus on radiographs, prompting further imaging with CT. The stomach shows some gaseous distension.

gas will be present on both sides of the bowel wall, so both sides of the wall will be visible. This is known as Rigler's sign or the 'double wall sign' (Figure 2.10.5).

B: Bones/Soft Tissue

- Bones can often yield unexpected pathology. The lumbar spine, lower ribs, pelvis and proximal femurs are normally included.
- Other soft tissues can also be visualised:
  ○ Liver – right upper quadrant
  ○ Spleen – left upper quadrant
  ○ Kidneys – normally at T12–L3
  ○ Lung bases – check for consolidation

C: Calcifications/Artefacts

Various calcifications and artefacts can be seen. These include:

- Renal/ureteric calculi
- Gallstone calculi
- Pancreatic calcification – indicative of chronic pancreatitis (Figure 2.10.6)
- Vascular calcification – check for a calcified abdominal aortic aneurysm
- Surgical clips
- Prior contrast

Abdominal Pathology on CT

Although you are not expected to report abdominal CT scans, this section provides examples of easily interpreted features of common intra-abdominal pathology (Figures 2.10.7 to 2.10.15).

(a)

(b)

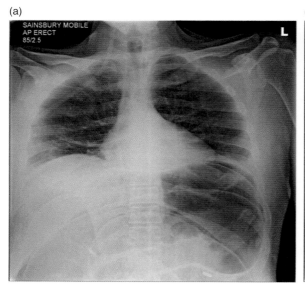
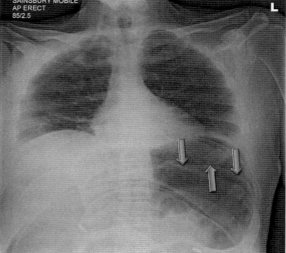

Figure 2.10.5 Pneumoperitoneum – Rigler's sign. Both sides of the bowel wall are visible due to free gas. Normally, only the inner wall should be visible.

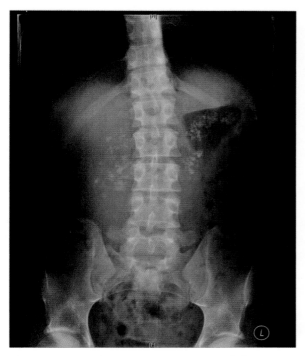

Figure 2.10.6 Calcifications on X-ray. Pancreatic calcification secondary to chronic pancreatitis.

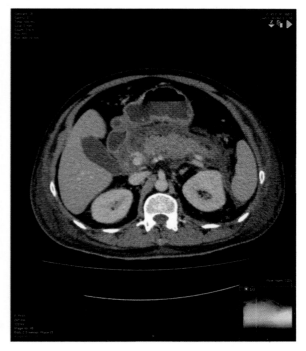

Figure 2.10.7 Pancreatitis. Extensive peri-pancreatic fluid and inflammation. If pancreatitis is scanned very early, no findings may be present.

Figure 2.10.8 Necrotic pancreatitis. There is a focal area of low density within the pancreatic body due to lack of contrast enhancement, indicating necrosis of pancreatic tissue.

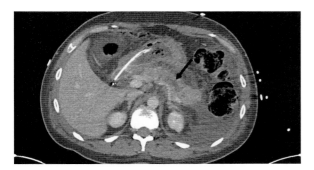

(a)   (b)

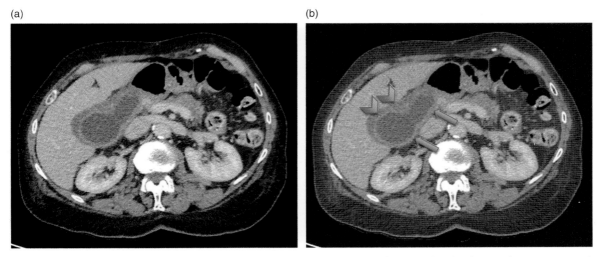

Figure 2.10.9 Cholecystitis. Thickened gall bladder wall (arrows) with peri-cholecystic fluid (arrowheads). Ultrasound is more sensitive than CT; however, CT is better at depicting complications such as perforation.

(a) (b)

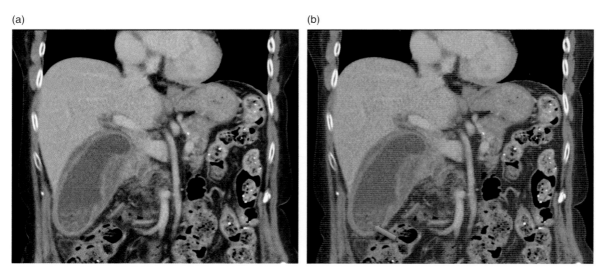

Figure 2.10.10 Cholecystitis. The gall bladder contains multiple stones, with wall thickening and peri-cholecystic fluid. Non-calcified stones may be invisible on CT, which should prompt further assessment with ultrasound.

(a) (b)

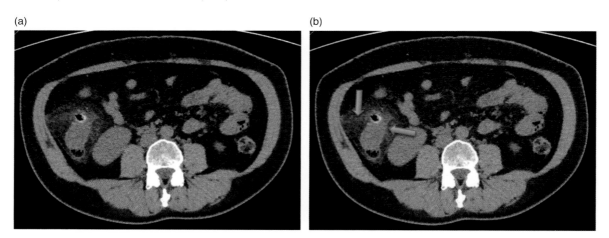

Figure 2.10.11 Diverticulitis. On the right side of the abdomen, there is fat stranding adjacent to a colonic diverticulum, indicating inflammation/infection. Normal fat should appear uniformly dark on soft tissue windows, as shown on the left side of the abdomen.

(a) (b)

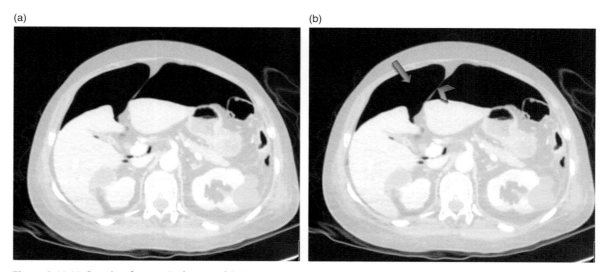

Figure 2.10.12 Bowel perforation. Perforation of the bowel. On lung windowing, there is a large volume of free intra-peritoneal gas (arrow) outside the bowel lumen. The falciform ligament is clearly outlined (arrowhead).

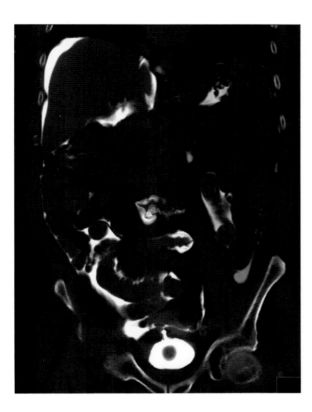

Figure 2.10.13 Bladder perforation. Perforation of the urinary bladder. Contrast medium has been instilled via the urinary catheter. Due to a urinary bladder wall defect, the contrast medium has leaked out and outlines the liver and the bowel.

(a) (b)

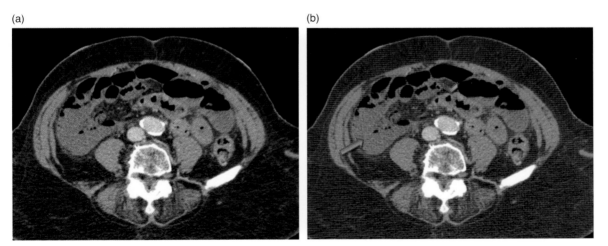

Figure 2.10.14 Bowel ischaemia. Despite intravenous contrast medium, the bowel loops on the right side of the abdomen do not enhance (arrow). Normal bowel wall enhancement is shown in the midline (arrowhead).

(a)

(b)

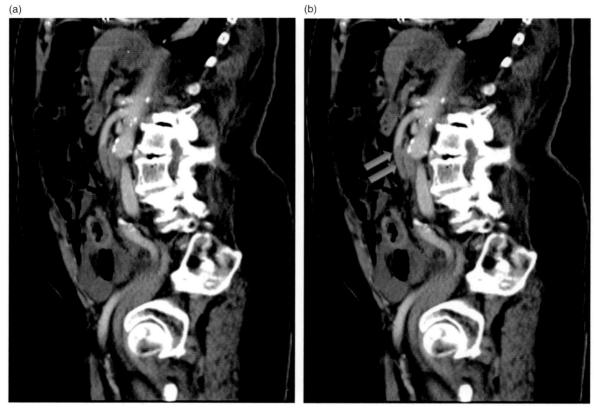

Figure 2.10.15 Bowel ischaemia. A filling defect within the superior mesenteric artery shows an arterial thrombus (arrows).

References and Further Reading

Harvey CJ, Allen S, O'Regan D. Interpretation of the abdominal radiograph: 1. *Br J Hosp Med (Lond)* 2005;**66**:88–90.

Raby N, Berman L, de Lacey G. *Accident and Emergency Radiology: A Survival Guide*, 2nd edn. Edinburgh: Elsevier; 2005.

Radiology Masterclass. 2019. Abdominal X-ray – system and anatomy. www.radiologymasterclass .co.uk/tutorials/abdo/abdomen_x-ray/anatomy_ introduction

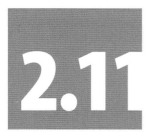

Importance of Monitoring and Responding to Trends in Physiological Variables

2.11

Claire Moorthy

Key Learning Points

1. The aims are to detect clinical deterioration early in all hospitalised patients.
2. Most NHS hospitals use some form of Early Warning Score (EWS).
3. The Royal College of Physicians (RCP) supports the use of a nationally standardised track and trigger system – the National Early Warning Score (NEWS) 2.
4. The NEWS systems aim to support consistent clinical decision-making.
5. A graded clinical response is triggered, dependent on the score, based on simple physiological parameters and their degree of deviation from the normal values.

Keywords: early warning systems, NEWS 2, track and trigger

Introduction

Critical care and acute medical care teams have long realised that patients often deteriorate over a period of time. Previously adopted clinical observation charts would reveal obvious downward trends in clinical parameters, without the necessary guidance to trigger any actions.

Areas such as trauma and cardiopulmonary resuscitation have long established algorithms to aid in diagnosis and management, with a great deal of success. There are currently no standardised protocols or guidelines for the management of the acutely ill or deteriorating patient, largely due to the changing nature and complexity of critical illness over time. A great deal of encouraging work using Early Warning Score (EWS) systems, however, resulted in the Royal College of Physicians (RCP) forming a medical taskforce, which,

in 2012, designed a single standardised National Early Warning Score (NEWS). This was further updated to the NEWS 2 scoring system in 2017 (Figure 2.11.1). This is now commonly used in many NHS hospitals, with recent studies showing a 55.5 per cent uptake in its use and most of the remaining 44.5 per cent using a similar scoring system within their institution. The standardised approach to monitoring and tracking simple vital signs in all patients within the hospital setting allows earlier identification of the sickest patients and triggering of a graded clinical response dependent upon the score (Figure 2.11.2).

Features of NEWS Scoring Systems

- NEWS scoring systems are standardised nationally.
- Uses a track and trigger system – tracks patient observations from time of hospital admission to time of discharge, triggers a graded clinical response dependent upon score.
- Simple scoring system for six clinical observation parameters (Box 2.11.1).
- An uplift of the score by two points for anyone on oxygen.
- Scoring depends upon the magnitude of disturbance from the normal values of each parameter – a highest score of 3 indicates the most extreme variation from the normal.
- Aggregated score used by the observer to trigger a timely response.
- Score range determines the action required (graded clinical response), ensuring change to frequency of monitoring and type of clinical response.
- Higher scores require more urgent escalation response.
- Outline the clinical competencies of the clinical team needed to review the patient.

Figure 2.11.1 National Early Warning Score (NEWS) 2.

Source: Reproduced from: Royal College of Physicians. *National Early Warning Score (NEWS) 2: Standardising the assessment of acute-illness severity in the NHS.* Updated report of a working party. London: RCP, 2017.

NEW score	Frequency of monitoring	Clinical response
0	Minimum 12 hourly	• Continue routine NEWS monitoring
Total 1–4	Minimum 4–6 hourly	• Inform registered nurse, who must assess the patient • Registered nurse decides whether increased frequency of monitoring and/or escalation of care is required
3 in single parameter	Minimum 1 hourly	• Registered nurse to inform medical team caring for the patient, who will review and decide whether escalation of care is necessary
Total 5 or more Urgent response threshold	Minimum 1 hourly	• Registered nurse to immediately inform the medical team caring for the patient • Registered nurse to request urgent assessment by a clinician or team with care competencies in the care of acutely ill patients • Provide clinical care in an environment with monitoring facilities
Total 7 or more Emergency response threshold	Continuous monitoring of vital signs	• Registered nurse to immediately inform the medical team caring for the patient – this should be at least at specialist registrar level • Emergency assessment by a team with critical care competecies, including practitioner(s) with advanced airway management skills • Consider transfer of care to a level 2 or 3 clinical care facility, ie higher-dependency unit of ICU • Clinical care in an environment with monitoring facilities

Figure 2.11.2 Clinical responses to the NEWS trigger threshold (NEWS 2).
Source: Reproduced from: Royal College of Physicians, 2018.

Box 2.11.1 Six Clinical Observation Parameters

- Heart rate
- Respiratory rate
- Oxygen saturation
- Temperature
- Blood pressure
- Level of consciousness or new confusion

Updated NEWS 2 Scoring System

Additional features to the original NEWS chart:

1. Newer format uses the Resuscitation Council UK's ABCDE approach of moving through each parameter systematically.
2. The ranges for the boundaries of each parameter are shown clearly.

3. Recording of the rate of oxygen flow (in litres per minute) and method/device can be documented more clearly.

4. Additional oxygen saturation scale specifically for patients with known hypercapnic respiratory failure (most often due to chronic obstructive pulmonary disease) who have a clinically acceptable oxygen saturation of 88–92 per cent.

5. Recognition of the importance of new-onset confusion, delirium or disorientation as a sign of potential serious clinical deterioration on the new ACVPU scoring scale.

6. Highlighting of a NEWS score of 5 or more as a key threshold for urgent clinical alert, response and review.

7. New colour scheme to avoid any problems for staff with red–green colour blindness.

Advantages

- Aims to reduce variation in care, and improve safety and communication within hospital and pre-hospital care settings
- Tracks the patient from time of admission to hospital until time of discharge from hospital
- Can be used as a surveillance tool for all patients entering hospital
- Aims to detect clinical deterioration early
- Supports consistent clinical decision-making

Disadvantages

- Only suitable for adults aged over 16
- Not suitable for pregnant women over 20 weeks' gestation
- Not suitable for palliative care patients
- Requires users to undergo training

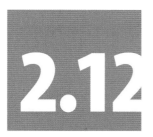

2.12

How to Integrate Clinical Findings with Laboratory Investigations to Form a Differential Diagnosis

Claire Moorthy

Key Learning Points

1. Clinical reasoning is used to interpret and integrate our knowledge into a complete decision-making process.
2. Identify relevant key information from clinical history, examination and investigations using a standardised approach.
3. Describe the problem using this key information to help formulate a diagnosis or clinical syndrome (keeping it relevant and in clinical context).
4. Remember, a clinical syndrome is not the diagnosis. Look for the cause.
5. Structure the problem by applying the key information to a structured framework to create a diagnosis/clinical syndrome/differential.

Keywords: differential diagnosis, clinical reasoning, clinical syndromes, working diagnosis

Introduction

Making a diagnosis is essential to further focussed patient management. In the acutely unwell patient, initial treatment will often precede the diagnosis. A standardised approach should be used to generate a differential diagnosis or ideally a working diagnosis, and to help rule out life-threatening and time-critical conditions. In order to do this, it is important to try to frame key features, eliminating extraneous information and creating a stage for the clinical reasoning that will follow. Ideally this will culminate in a working diagnosis or be aided by the use of clinical syndromes, with the knowledge that some patients will fall out of this structure.

We should aim to understand the type of framework to which key features of a presentation should be applied and know the categories of diagnoses that should be included in a differential. Clinical progress and data should be reviewed, revisiting the clinical context until a diagnosis is reached. If treatment is failing, one must reconsider the diagnosis and re-evaluate the disease severity.

Clinical Reasoning and Critical Thinking

Good clinical reasoning has been shown to impact positively on patient outcomes.

Critical thinking and clinical reasoning are often used interchangeably but are subtly different.

Critical thinking involves key skills of analysis, interpretation, inference and explanation, often in order to aid problem-solving. It involves developing a questioning attitude to formulate a conclusion that is as objective as possible. It is based on evidence and science, and is a cognitive process. It is a fundamentally important concept in medicine.

Clinical reasoning as a concept is as important. It similarly involves the processes of evaluating, integrating and synthesising data from a patient, and utilising factual knowledge relevant to the clinical presentation in that patient. This leads us to interpret the findings and concludes in a decision-making process that hopefully helps to form a diagnosis or differential diagnosis. It is very much dependent on our subjective interpretation of the objective data obtained.

This interpretation can be influenced by many factors, including our individual preconceived ideas, philosophical perspectives and personal attitudes – all of which can to lead to bias and potentially incorrect diagnosis, and hence management. Assumptions and prejudices should be reflected upon by the individual, as they can adversely affect clinical outcomes.

79

Table 2.12.1 Examples of cognitive biases

ANCHORING BIAS	**GIVING EXCESS WEIGHT TO INITIAL INFORMATION TAKEN EARLY IN CONSULTATION**
CONFIRMATION BIAS	Ignoring contradictory evidence whilst focusing only on supporting evidence for a particular diagnosis
AVAILABILITY BIAS	Giving too much weight to a particular diagnosis that has been recently seen or heard about

Cognitive biases to be aware of include those seen in Table 2.12.1.

Critical thinking applied to a clinical situation results in clinical reasoning and here lies the difference.

The Clinical Reasoning Process

This requires:

- Data/information collection, processing and evaluation
- Subjective interpretation of data/information collected
- Determination of relevance of scientific literature specific to a clinical situation and application of biostatistics where appropriate (scoring systems to stratify risk/predict prognosis, e.g. MELD score in end-stage liver disease)
- Use of arguments to accept or refute potential diagnoses
- Knowledge integration, including clinical skills and experience, to help make an informed and complete decision-making process
- That goals are established and acted upon
- Evaluation of outcomes
- That learning is completed by reflection and review of clinical outcomes

Important Steps to Making a Differential Diagnosis

Collect Information/Data

Sources include:

- Full patient history, including detailed drug history
- Findings of clinical examination
- Review of observation charts
- Review of investigations
- Primary and secondary care information/old and new clinic letters/previous relevant investigations

- Collateral history from family/next of kin/friends/carers (with consent of the patient where possible)

Interpret the Data

- Look at the patterns of information found. Do they have a correlation with a known disease or disease process?
- Inferences can be made based on clinical experience and medical knowledge.
- Fact finding with use of reference material – medical textbooks, literature search, studies, Internet and biostatistics.

Identify the Key Information

These are the pieces of data that will help differentiate one diagnosis from another.

This requires:

1. Analysis and processing of the collected data
2. Distinguishing findings that are relevant from those that are irrelevant
3. Determining inconsistencies within the data. It is important to evaluate whether further information is needed. Do you need to go back and ask more questions or to consider a further investigation to accept or refute a potential diagnosis? Always ask: 'Do I have enough basic information about this patient?'
4. Positive and negative findings – both important, and argument for and against a hypothesis will arise, depending on the collected information
5. Avoidance of bias. It is important to keep an open mind and not to give too much weight to any one piece of information too early on in the process (anchoring bias), but to still maintain focus on what is relevant to the patient presentation and clinical situation

Use of good-quality 'qualifiers' helps to turn raw data into medically meaningful information in presenting the key features, e.g. 'I have been vomiting for the past four days. I haven't wanted to eat or drink anything. Vomit looked dark but looks like blood today.' This will be interpreted or qualified by a medical professional as persistent emesis, with recent haematemesis and anorexia.

Organise the Key Information

Create a brief summary statement of the problem using key information. The structure may vary, depending upon your personal presenting style. The aim here is to frame the key important information that is highly relevant to the presenting complaint or primary symptom, eliminate unnecessary information and set the stage for clinical reasoning to hopefully aid diagnosis. An example of key important summarised findings can be seen in Box 2.12.1.

If a diagnosis is not obvious, then synthesise the findings into a clinical syndrome. A single clinical syndrome is a set of clinical signs and symptoms that correlate with each other. It requires inference and deductions using the data, with pattern recognition and matching of the current situation to previous situations and clinical experience.

Remember not to mistake the clinical syndrome for the clinical diagnosis; for example, liver failure, renal failure and cardiac failure are all syndromes. What is the actual cause? If this is known and proven, then this will be the diagnosis.

Create a Structured Framework for Your Information

For any patient, there may be many potential diagnoses. A systematic, structured approach will reduce the risk of missing potential diagnoses.

Frameworks are usually based on a known source of reference. They may be:

- Anatomical (organ-based)
  - For example, chest pain may be due to causes within the heart, lung, abdomen, bone, musculoskeletal system, etc. Each can be

subdivided or split to further hone into a diagnosis
- Physiological (systems-based)
- Pathophysiological (VINDICATE is an example of a useful mnemonic … there are many more!):
  - V – vascular
  - I – infectious
  - N – neoplastic
  - D – drugs/degenerative
  - I – idiopathic
  - C – congenital
  - A – autoimmune
  - T – trauma
  - E – endocrine
- Other classification systems usually adapted from a known source of reference, e.g. liver failure – hyper-acute/acute/subacute; renal failure – pre-renal/renal/post-renal; anaemia – microcytic, macrocytic, normocytic

Apply Key Information to the Structured Framework

This requires further evaluation of the information in order to ascertain relevant information. It is used in reference to the patient presentation. Each piece of key information should be analysed and accepted or refuted. Objective knowledge of the literature and biostatistics appropriate to the potential conditions in the differential and clinical experience are key in this step. The structure is not patient-specific. This will help to form the working or differential diagnosis.

Take a 'Diagnostic Time Out'

Think about the following:
- How did I arrive at this diagnosis?
- Did I accept another clinician's diagnosis without question?
- Did I consider the alternatives?
- Does this diagnosis still fit the clinical situation that presents in front of me?

Remember, time spent looking at how you arrived at your diagnosis or differential is always time well spent.

Important Pointers

- Aim to focus on identifying the key information.
- Include investigations where a likely diagnosis is high.

Box 2.12.1 An Example of Key Important Summarised Findings Focussing on Salient Features of History, Examination and Investigations

- Age
- Gender
- Highly relevant background history
- Presenting complaint with relevant description
- Highly relevant diagnostic data, including pending investigations
- Working diagnosis if obvious/differential diagnosis or clinical syndrome

Summary: Mr X is a 50-year-old man with a history of hypertension and hypercholesterolaemia, presenting with a 20-minute history of central crushing chest pain radiating to his jaw, with associated nausea. He has inferolateral ST depression on the ECG. Blood tests, including troponin, and chest X-ray are pending. The working diagnosis is acute coronary syndrome.

- Include investigations where a diagnosis is dangerous or rapidly fatal ('don't-miss diagnoses').
- Initial list of possible diagnoses explaining the patient's presentation may be broad (this doesn't mean long!).
- Differentials included should only be those relevant to the patient.
- Prioritise your differentials, with the most likely at the top.
- Avoid long lists of differentials – stay focused on the situation.
- Formulate a provisional working diagnosis if possible.
- Remember that atypical presentations of common diseases are more likely than typical presentations of rare conditions.
- Once a treatment plan has been made, act, evaluate and reflect.
- Evaluate and re-evaluate – if a patient is not responding to initial treatment, reconsider your diagnosis or look at the severity of the disease process again.

- Do not be scared to re-formulate the differential diagnosis if necessary.
- Always consider – do I have sufficient understanding of the clinical presentation to offer an opinion? Do I need further specific expert help?

Acknowledgements

I would like to thank Dr Eric Strong for his great teaching videos which have inspired this chapter and my own teaching journey. Although his work is aimed at medical students, it really is suited to all of us at all levels. The basics are always worth revisiting, however senior you may be.

References and Further Reading

Strong E. 2013. How to create a differential diagnosis. Part 1. www.youtube.com/watch?v=qKrLPY_8Cyk

Strong E. 2013. How to create a differential diagnosis. Part 2. www.youtube.com/watch?v=iEbonwYPNVk

Strong E. 2013. How to create a differential diagnosis. Part 3. www.youtube.com/watch?v=n48zY7GLqc0

Victor-Chmil J. Critical thinking vs clinical reasoning vs clinical judgement. *Nurse Educ* 2013;**38**:34–6.

Disease Management: Recognition, Causes and Management

Acute Coronary Syndromes

3.1.1

Michael Hoy

Key Learning Points

1. Acute coronary syndrome (ACS) presentation may be asymptomatic in up to a third of patients and clinical suspicion must be high.
2. Timely intervention has a dramatic change in outcome – percutaneous coronary intervention (PCI) is superior to thrombolysis.
3. Multiple ongoing clinical trials into current intensive care treatment strategies may well change practice.
4. Elevated troponin in the intensive care unit can have multiple non-ischaemic causes.
5. ACS presenting with shock and hypoperfusion carries a mortality of 40 per cent.

Keywords: acute coronary syndrome, cardiogenic shock, complications of ACS, atypical ACS

Introduction

Cardiac ischaemia develops as a consequence of an imbalance between oxygen delivery and myocardial oxygen demand. Ischaemic heart disease conventionally describes a progressive obstructive pathological change within the coronary vessels, increasing the likelihood of symptomatic exercise-induced ischaemia (when demand rises above available supply, as seen in classical angina) potentially developing to the point where resting demand exceeds supply (unstable angina (UA)), with the possibility of sudden complete or critical obstruction precipitating either full-thickness or subendocardial myocardial infarction, leading to ST-segment elevation (STEMI) or non-ST-segment elevation myocardial infarction (NSTEMI).

The acute coronary syndromes (ACS) encompass UA, NSTEMI and STEMI (Table 3.1.1.1). In addition to typical causes of ACS (Table 3.1.1.2), alternative precipitants include coronary artery dissection (spontaneous or iatrogenic), coronary vasospasm/vasculitis and coronary artery embolism – all of which can lead to ACS without a history of ischaemic heart disease. Some major clinical trials are referenced in square brackets.

Table 3.1.1.1 Acute coronary syndrome definitions

ACS definitions	Pathology	Explanation
Unstable angina	Myocardial ischaemia at rest	Development of coronary artery obstruction such that resting myocardial oxygen demand exceeds delivery, with normal ECG and cardiac biomarkers
MI	Acute myocardial injury in the setting of evidence of acute myocardial ischaemia	ECG changes and acute rise in biochemical markers (troponin >99th percentile of upper reference limit). Subendocardial MI manifests as NSTEMI, whereas full-thickness MI causes STEMI or new LBBB
Type 1 MI	Atherosclerotic plaque rupture causing MI	ECG changes, elevation of troponin ± imaging demonstrating RWMA or coronary obstruction at angiography
Type 2 MI	MI unrelated to acute coronary athero-thrombosis (e.g. dissection, embolism, spasm)	ECG changes, elevation of troponin ± imaging demonstrating RWMA
Type 3 MI	Death presumed due to MI, but prior to biochemical confirmation	Cardiac-type chest pain, ischaemic ECG changes or VF, with death prior to confirmation of diagnosis by troponin levels
Type 4 MI	MI associated with percutaneous coronary intervention	Related to acute (e.g. dissection), subacute (in-stent thrombosis) or chronic complication (in-stent restenosis)

Table 3.1.1.1 (cont.)

ACS definitions	Pathology	Explanation
Type 5 MI	CABG-related MI <48 hours after index procedure	Loss of viability either of the new graft or a native vessel following CABG

Abbreviations: ACS = acute coronary syndrome; MI = myocardial infarction; NSTEMI = non-ST-segment elevation myocardial infarction; STEMI = ST-segment elevation myocardial infarction; LBBB = left bundle branch block; RWMA = regional wall motion abnormality; VF = ventricular fibrillation; CABG = coronary artery bypass graft.

Pathophysiology of Atherosclerosis

Transient coronary artery inflammation (present from at least 1 year of age) allows low-density lipoproteins (LDLs) to penetrate the sub-endothelial space of coronary arteries. Vascular smooth muscle cells attract macrophages from the circulation, which then consume LDLs and trigger further local inflammation. Macrophages become 'foam cells' and collectively form a lipid-rich core covered by an endothelial fibrous shell. The effect of this inflammation stimulates thickening of the arterial endothelium and muscle layers – reducing the autoregulatory ability of coronary blood vessels and contributing to mechanical coronary arterial occlusion. If the shell ruptures, it exposes the circulation to the underlying thrombogenic material to which platelets bind, causing either worsening of, or complete, coronary occlusion.

Anticipation of an impending plaque rupture constitutes one of the principal areas of research in cardiovascular medicine, with many implicated biochemical markers – none of which have, as yet, proven to be able to be used as a warning of a forthcoming ACS. As such, management currently involves control of risk factors to reduce atherosclerotic burden (Table 3.1.1.2), pharmacological limitation of oxygen demand, optimisation of coronary artery relaxation and subsequent reactionary treatment of ACS.

Clinical Features

Myocardial ischaemia may cause retrosternal chest pain/tightness, which is classically described as central and heavy, with radiation to the jaw or left arm, although up to a third of patients may be completely asymptomatic. Chest pain can be associated with constitutional symptoms, including nausea and

Table 3.1.1.2 Risk factors for acute coronary syndrome

Conventional cardiac risk factors	Additional risk factors
Male or post-menopausal female	Psychiatric disease
BMI >30	Cocaine usage
Age >50	End-stage renal disease
Hypertension	Ethnicity
Diabetes	Hyperhomocysteinaemia
Hypercholesterolaemia	Lipid-modifying drugs/ diseases – corticosteroids, immunosuppressants, HIV, autoimmune disease
Family history (MI in first-degree relative aged <55)	Pre-eclampsia
Smoking	

Abbreviations: BMI = body mass index; MI = myocardial infarction.

diaphoresis, and demonstrates exertional exacerbation, although in the case of ACS, it will also be present at rest. Other manifestations of myocardial ischaemia relate to cardiogenic shock and include breathlessness with pulmonary oedema, arrhythmias and hypotension.

Investigations

ACS diagnosis originates from the clinical history and is then dependent on ECG changes and biomarkers of cardiomyocyte damage (Figure 3.1.1.1).

A 12-lead ECG should be interpreted with knowledge of coronary artery territories (but notably can be discordant in the setting of long-standing coronary artery disease with retrograde filling via collaterals). Regional ST-segment elevation, new left bundle branch block and cardiogenic shock are indications for emergency revascularisation. Evolution of the ECG occurs over time, as demonstrated in Figure 3.1.1.2.

The subendocardial layer of the myocardium is the most prone to ischaemia or infarction, due to its distance from the coronary arteries, and is typically the area affected during NSTEMI. Troponin, a complex found on the actin filament within skeletal and cardiac muscle, should be measured, though other pathologies can cause a raised value (Table 3.1.1.3). MI diagnosis is based on troponin elevation to >99 times the upper reference limit (URL).

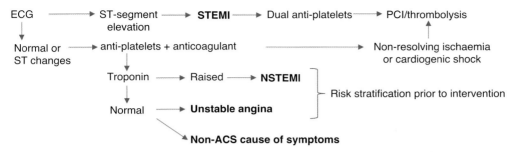

Figure 3.1.1.1 Acute coronary syndrome diagnostic pathway in the setting of clinical suspicion. ACS = acute coronary syndrome; PCI = percutaneous coronary intervention; NSTEMI = non-ST-segment elevation myocardial infarction; STEMI = ST-segment elevation myocardial infarction.
Source: Author's own.

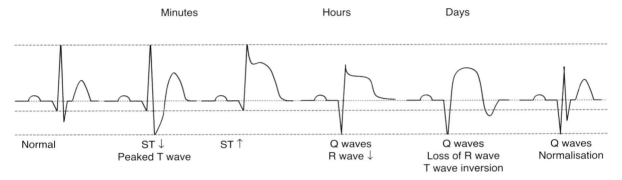

Figure 3.1.1.2 ECG evolution.
Source: Author's own.

Table 3.1.1.3 Non-acute coronary syndrome causes of raised troponin

Non-ACS causes of raised troponin
Acute/chronic heart failure ± arrhythmia
Pulmonary embolism
Myocarditis
Renal failure
Cardiac trauma/surgery
Post-ablation/cardioversion
Post-cardiac transplant
Cardiac transplant graft rejection
Cardiotoxic chemotherapy
Extreme exercise

Management of ACS

ACS management involves diagnosis and risk stratification (Figure 3.1.1.1), revascularisation (Table 3.1.1.4), identification and treatment of complications (Table 3.1.1.5) and longer-term secondary prevention

(Table 3.1.1.6). ICU-specific management is discussed in more detail below.

Table 3.1.1.4 Management of acute coronary syndrome

Pharmacological	
Symptom control	Analgesia Oxygen Nitrates
Anti-platelets	COX inhibition – reduces platelet formation of thromboxane A2 (aspirin) $P2Y_{12}$ ADP (clopidogrel/prasugrel/ticagrelor) Glycoprotein IIb/IIIa (tirofiban)
Anticoagulants	Bivalirudin – a direct thrombin inhibitor Fondaparinux (in normal renal function) is preferred due to better safety profile Low-molecular-weight heparin (particularly enoxaparin) used when fondaparinux contraindicated Unfractionated heparin – used in significant renal impairment
Thrombolysis	Recombinant tissue plasminogen activator (alteplase)

Table 3.1.1.4 (cont.)

Interventional	
Angioplasty	Superior and safer than thrombolysis when delivered in under 90 minutes from symptom onset. UK guidelines support angioplasty over thrombolysis if it can be delivered within 120 minutes of symptom onset. In the event of failed thrombolysis, rescue PCI should be considered

Surgical	
CABG	Surgical revascularisation is indicated in the appropriate patient with three-vessel disease (particularly left main stem) or in those where angiography has failed or would be technically impossible

NB: With the wide variety of medications available, most PCI centres employ their own variations on the above therapies, with no combination proven to have any sustained superiority.
Abbreviations: COX = cyclo-oxygenase; ADP = adenosine diphosphate; PCI = percutaneous coronary intervention.

Table 3.1.1.5 Complications of acute coronary syndrome

Timing	Complications of ACS	Management
Instant	Cardiac arrest	ALS + feperfusion ± ECLS [CHEER trial]
Instant to minutes	Arrhythmias	Cardioversion/pacing ± long-term device
Instant to hours	Cardiogenic shock	Inotropes ± IABP ± ECLS (see main text)
Hours to days	Papillary muscle rupture	Echo to assess severity ± MVR/MitraClip™
Hours to days	Ventricular septal defect	Echo + surgical repair (mortality >50 per cent)
Days to weeks	In-stent thrombosis	Re-angiography/ plasty
Weeks	Pericarditis	NSAIDs, colchicine + investigate for effusion
Weeks to months	LV aneurysm ± thrombus	Echo + anticoagulation ± excision

Abbreviations: ACS = acute coronary syndrome; ALS = advanced life support; IABP = intra-aortic balloon pump; ECLS = extracorporeal life support; MVR = mitral valve repair; NSAID = non-steroidal anti-inflammatory drug; LV = left ventricular.

Table 3.1.1.6 Summary of European Society of Cardiology recommendations for longer-term pharmacotherapy following ACS[a]

Drug	Recommendations
Beta-blocker therapy	Improves intermediate- and long-term survival in the absence of acute heart failure [CAPRICORN]
Lipid-lowering therapy	Improves medium- to long-term survival, regardless of initial cholesterol levels [PROVE IT-TIMI 22, IDEAL]
Nitrates	No evidence for longer-term survival benefit, but useful for angina symptoms
CCBs	Rate-controlling CCBs have shown lowered cardiovascular risk only in those unable to take beta-blockers [DAVIT-II]
ACE-Is/ARBs	Mortality benefit seen within 1 week and recommended to start in all STEMI patients or those with LVEF <40 per cent if no contraindication. ACE-Is have more evidence than ARBs [ISIS-4, CONSENSUS-II, VALIANT]
MRAs	Mortality benefit in patients with LVEF <40 per cent who are already receiving ACE-I and beta-blocker, provided there is no contraindication [EPHESUS, REMINDER, ALBATROSS trials]

[a] Evidence relates to atherosclerotic ischaemic heart disease, rather than to atypical variants.

Abbreviations: CCB = calcium channel blocker; ACE-I = angiotensin-converting enzyme inhibitor; ARB = angiotensin receptor II blocker; STEMI = ST-segment elevation myocardial infarction; LVEF = left ventricular ejection fraction; MRA = mineralocorticoid receptor antagonist.

Acute Coronary Syndromes in Intensive Care

The full role of the ICU in the management of ACS is probably too varied to put into discrete categories, but the simpler presentations are likely to take one of the following forms.

Emergency Admission of Type 1 MI

Approximately 5 per cent of patients presenting with ACS who proceed to PCI will require ventilation, either as a result of low Glasgow Coma Score (GCS) following cardiac arrest or due to cardiogenic shock. In a collapsed patient requiring advanced life support (ALS), early revascularisation should be considered as a part of resuscitation if ACS is considered as a precipitant. Angioplasty can be achieved with minimal delay despite ongoing resuscitation and, where not possible, thrombolysis should be considered.

Cardiogenic shock should be diagnosed and managed (see specific section) with multidisciplinary support, and external referral for mechanical support considered if needed.

The post-out-of-hospital cardiac arrest (OOHCA) patient should be managed in accordance with Resuscitation Council UK guidelines. Specifically, if the clinical presentation is suspicious for ACS (e.g. vascular territory ST-segment elevation), emergent angiography should be considered and neurological status should not be used as grounds to delay intervention. Evidence supports immediate transfer to a primary PCI centre over thrombolysis if initial presentation is to a non-cardiac centre. This evidence holds less true for equivocal clinical histories with mild ECG abnormalities [COACT trial].

Hyperglycaemia should be treated to <11 mmol/l [DAGAMI trial, National Institute for Health and Care Excellence (NICE) guidelines]. Targeted temperature management trials have originated around cardiac causes of cardiac arrest, although they are increasingly broad in their inclusion criteria – local protocols will direct how, and to what degree, hypothermia should be achieved [TTM, HACA, HYPERION].

Type 2 MI

The non-specific presentation of a patient with a markedly raised troponin in the setting of multi-organ failure, or its development during an intensive care admission, can cause significant frustration to managing teams. By definition, a significantly raised (>99 times URL) troponin denotes myocardial damage. Combined with either ECG changes or regional wall motion abnormalities (RWMAs), this can be diagnostic of an MI. Type 2 MI is not uncommon in the ICU, with significant myocardial oxygen demand to compensate for critical illness. In such circumstances, if regional oxygen delivery is insufficient due to, ordinarily, non-critically obstructive lesions, type 2 MI may occur. At angiography, lesions would not usually be considered indicative for PCI and medical management is often employed by cardiologists, pending risk stratification following resolution of the critical illness state. The non-interventionalist approach does not correlate with a lower risk of mortality by comparison with type 1 MI, but is appropriate for the difference in aetiology. Important diagnoses that may present in such a way but might still require intervention are the acute atypical causes of ACS, particularly dissection, embolism and vasospasm.

Acute STEMI in an Otherwise Stable ICU Patient

In a sedated patient, the most common presentations of ACS are haemodynamic deterioration with or without arrhythmia and cardiac arrest. Once a diagnosis is established, the limitation to treatment is often the ability to transfer for PCI versus appropriateness of thrombolytic therapy if transfer is deemed inappropriate. This should be multidisciplinary, involving intensivists, cardiologists and other interested teams. Medical management without any immediate reperfusion therapy is sometimes the consequence.

Prognosis

Uncomplicated ACS presentations carry a good prognosis and patients increasingly are discharged within days. Initial mortality of an uncomplicated NSTEMI is lower than that of a STEMI but mortality is equivalent by 6 months. A recent large analysis summarises the risk of ACS in the deteriorating patient on a clinical stratification. The groups are still being refined, but shocked patients requiring vasoactive drugs to support blood pressure correlates with an approximately 30 per cent intensive care mortality and 40 per cent in-hospital mortality despite full revascularisation and mechanical support.

References and Further Reading

Ibanez B, James S, Agewall S, et al.; ESC Scientific Document Group. 2017 ESC Guidelines for the management of acute myocardial infarction in patients presenting with ST-segment elevation: The Task Force for the management of acute myocardial infarction in patients presenting with ST-segment elevation of the European Society of Cardiology (ESC). *Eur Heart J* 2018;**39**:119–77.

Roffi M, Patrono C, Collet J-P, et al.; ESC Scientific Document Group. 2015 ESC Guidelines for the management of acute coronary syndromes in patients presenting without persistent ST-segment elevation: Task Force for the management of acute coronary syndromes in patients presenting without persistent ST-segment elevation of the European Society of Cardiology (ESC). *Eur Heart J* 2016;**37**:267–315.

Thygesen K, Alpert JS, Jaffe AS, et al.; ESC Scientific Document Group. Fourth universal definition of myocardial infarction (2018). *Eur Heart J* 2019;40: 237–69.

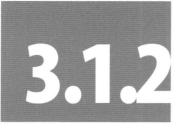

3.1.2 Cardiac Pacing, Implantable Cardioverter–Defibrillators and Cardiac Resynchronisation Therapy

Paul Harris

Key Learning Points

1. Knowledge of both permanent and temporary pacing systems is necessary, as both are encountered in the intensive care environment.
2. A chest X-ray will provide all the information required to identify the type of permanent device *in situ*.
3. All implantable cardioverter–defibrillators (ICDs) have full pacemaker capabilities.
4. Magnets will turn off all anti-tachycardia therapies from an ICD, but not anti-bradycardia therapies.
5. External defibrillator pads must be applied if ICD therapies are turned off.

Keywords: pacemaker, temporary pacing, implantable cardioverter–defibrillators

Introduction

Devices that may be encountered in the intensive care environment can be summarised below.

Temporary

- **Transvenous.** Right ventricular (RV). Inserted for acute symptomatic heart blocks (particularly third-degree) for rapid restoration of the heart rate, as the idioventricular escape rate is normally very slow. Transcutaneous external pacing may be required as an emergency bridging technique. It is also used post-transcatheter aortic valve implantation (TAVI) where oedema around the aortic valve may affect atrioventricular (AV) nodal function.
- **Epicardial.** Right atrial (RA) or RV, or both. Pacing wires are secured, under direct vision, to the heart muscle during cardiac surgery, and then removed 4–5 days post-operatively. Atrial wires provide superior pacing, as late diastolic atrial systole is preserved; however, the risk of cardiac tamponade on removal from the thin-walled chamber is higher than with ventricular wires. They are of no use in atrial fibrillation where the intrinsic atrial rate is over 300/min, as it is impossible to overpace. Atrial pacing alone will fail if heart blocks exist post-surgery. RV wires are easier to insert and safer to remove. Alone, they serve only as emergency treatment for bradycardia; however, in combination with RA pacing, both atrial and ventricular contractility can be maintained. Typical modes are AAI, VVI and DDD (Table 3.1.2.1).

Permanent Transvenous

- **Permanent pacemakers (PPMs).** RA or RV, or both. PPMs are used predominantly for heart blocks and sick sinus syndrome. Whilst sick sinus syndrome can be treated by an atrial lead only, the condition can degenerate to AV node disease, and thus RA and RV leads are often used. As with temporary systems, permanent atrial fibrillation (AF) is a contraindication to atrial pacing wires. Importantly, long-term RV pacing adversely affects systolic function. The number of permanent systems inserted increases yearly, with over 900 per million population inserted in England and Wales alike for 2015–2016.
- **Implantable cardioverter–defibrillator (ICD).** RV lead. ICDs treat life-threatening ventricular arrhythmias. They use complex algorithms to determine malignant rhythms, and treat primarily with anti-tachycardia (overdrive) pacing, cardioversion or defibrillation. Overdrive pacing is often successful, requiring less battery usage, and is better tolerated by patients.

- **Cardiac resynchronisation therapy (CRT).** Biventricular pacing ± RA pacing. CRT is used for patients with impaired left ventricular (LV) systolic function, typically ejection fraction of <35 per cent with left bundle branch block. The left ventricle (LV) is paced via a lead in the coronary sinus via the RA. CRT defibrillator (CRT-D) has ICD capabilities, whilst CRT pacemaker (CRT-P) has pacing modes only. CRT-P is used in New York Heart Association (NYHA) IV patients whose risk of multiple shocks is high and quality of life often poor. The full list of indications for ICDs and CRT can be found in NICE guidelines from 2014.

Miscellaneous

- **Subcutaneous ICD (S-ICD).** This device is used for patients at risk of ventricular arrhythmias, but with contraindications to the transvenous approach, e.g. difficult anatomy. The shock coil is placed subcutaneously along the sternal edge, and the box normally left sub-axillary. It can defibrillate at heart rates of over 170/min, but is limited by no overdrive pacing and no anti-bradycardia pacing (except transient post-shock pacing, which can be very uncomfortable).
- **Leadless pacemaker.** RV wall. This is used for patients with anatomically unsuitable central veins.
- **Implantable loop recorders.** Placed subcutaneously, sensing only; for diagnosis of syncope or palpitations long term.

Every one of the above devices can be confidently identified on a posterior–anterior (PA) chest X-ray, taking into account the number and position of leads and the presence of shock coils of an ICD.

Pacemaker Nomenclature

Table 3.1.2.1 is important in understanding both temporary and permanent pacing systems.

Positions I and II are relatively self-explanatory, remembering that there cannot be dual-chamber pacing or sensing modes if only one lead is present. Position III, 'Inhibited', refers to suppression of pacing by the underlying patient rhythm. Triggering is best demonstrated by A-sense V-pace, whereby if the patient has normal sinus activity, but a degree of heart block, RV pacing is triggered by the patient's own sinus beat. Position IV is adaptive to the patient's physiological need and uses a variety of triggers (e.g. respiratory rate). Position V refers predominantly to CRT, as no bi-atrial systems exist commercially.

Management of Permanent Systems in the ICU

The most important consideration is whether the patient admission to the ICU is related to the device *in situ* or simply to a coincidence that they have a device. The former is more likely in CRT and ICD patients, as the cardiovascular risks will, by definition, already be higher. Advice from the physiology department is essential in interrogating the device function, and the most recent device check should be sought, which may be a challenge if done in another institution. There are only five manufacturers, and the make should be communicated to them as each company has a different portable programmer. Pacing reports will provide the pacing dependence, underlying pathology and implantation date, estimated battery life, mode programmed and sensing and capturing thresholds. ICD reports will also include therapies activated. ICDs are occasionally disabled, particularly in the perioperative period or during resuscitation. It is vital that external defibrillator pads are placed at that time, to avoid delays in defibrillation if an arrhythmia occurs. Care must also be taken with central venous access, which may be challenging, but also because guidewires may produce enough artefact to trigger the device.

Table 3.1.2.1 Pacemaker nomenclature

Position	I	II	III	IV	V
Category	Chamber(s) paced	Chamber(s) sensed	Response to sensing	Rate modulation	Multi-site pacing
	0 = none	0 = none	0 = none	0 = none	0 = none
	A = atrium	A = atrium	T = triggered	R = rate modulation	A = atrium
	V = ventricle	V = ventricle	I = inhibited		V = ventricle
	D = dual (A + V)	D = dual (A + V)	D = dual (A + V)		D = dual (A + V)

Source: 2002 NASPE Position Statement: The Revised NASPE/BPEG Generic Code for Antibradycardia, Adaptive-Rate, and Multisite Pacing.

There is much confusion regarding response to magnets. Magnets will inhibit anti-tachycardia therapies of an ICD and are thus a useful tool when shock functions need disabling (e.g. central venous catheterisation). There is no effect on anti-bradycardia therapies. External pads must be used instead, as, by definition, the patient is already at risk of ventricular arrhythmias. On removal of the magnet, the device must be checked by a physiologist as anti-tachycardia therapies may not be reactivated. Placement of a magnet on a PPM is not a benign event. With all five manufacturers, the magnet will switch the device to an asynchronous mode, e.g. VOO/DOO (depending on the device), at around 100 bpm. If the patient has intrinsic atrial activity, then this may be lost. If there is intrinsic ventricular activity, then this runs the risk of R-on-T as there will be no sensing. It may be a useful mode if the patient has no underlying electrical activity and the device is inhibited by over-sensing.

Management of Temporary Systems in the ICU

It is important to correlate the wires placed with the mode selected. DDD is erroneous if only one wire is placed. Atrial pacing will be ineffective if AF exists. It is preferable to interrogate devices with patients in bed, in case of loss of capture and the need for head-down positioning. It is not advisable to check underlying activity by pausing pacing, although this function does exist on temporary pacing boxes, because of the risk of loss of capture when the pause button is released. A safe approach is as follows:

1. Examine the ECG trace for the presence of atrial and/or ventricular pacing spikes, followed by P waves and wide QRS, respectively. Pacing spikes out of synchronisation suggest sensing or capture problems, or both.

2. Reduce the heart rate to see if the underlying rhythm returns, but not so slow that the underlying rate compromises effective cardiac output. Rhythm and ST changes can then be assessed, and a 12-lead ECG done.

3. Check ventricular lead sensing. Over-sensing (<0.5 mV) will result in under-pacing, as the device will assume all noise is intrinsic activity. This is dangerous if there is insufficient underlying activity. Under-sensing (>3 mV) will result in over-pacing, which is also dangerous, and the device may pace over intrinsic activity, e.g. R-on-T. Optimal sensing is around 1 mV.

4. Check ventricular lead capture. Each pacing spike should produce a wide-paced QRS. If the voltage is too low, it will fail to capture and the spike will have no succeeding QRS. The voltage can be adjusted to find when loss of capture occurs (pacing threshold). It is then programmed at 1.5–2 times this as a safety margin.

5. Repeat for atrial leads, appreciating that atrial sensing may be less than 1 mV. A common phenomenon is a programmed rate of, for example, 80/min, but the device is pacing the ventricle appropriately at a higher rate. Scrutiny of the device may find a faster sinus rate that is triggering the ventricular-paced beat. This may be due to AV nodal block, but it can also be the A–V delay set too low by the pacemaker, e.g. <150 ms. Normal sinus rhythm may be returned by increasing the delay to 200 ms, for example.

References and Further Reading

Holzmeister J, Leclercq C. Implantable cardioverter defibrillators and cardiac resynchronisation therapy. *Lancet* 2011;**378**:722–30.

Jacob S, Panaich SS, Maheshwari P, Haddad JW, Padanilam BJ, John SK. Clinical applications of magnets on cardiac rhythm management devices. *Europace* 2011;**13**:1222–30.

Leyva F. Pacing supplement: cardiac resynchronisation therapy – developments in heart failure management. *Br J Cardiol* 2018;**25**(Suppl 3):S12–19.

National Institute for Health and Care Excellence. 2014. Implantable cardioverter defibrillators and cardiac resynchronisation therapy for arrhythmias and heart failure. www.nice.org.uk/guidance/ta314

3.1.3

Acute Heart Failure

Paul Harris

Key Learning Points

1. Left ventricular failure leads to pulmonary oedema and can occur with preserved contractility.
2. Right ventricular failure increases systemic venous pressures, causing hepatic and renal congestion.
3. Acute coronary syndrome warrants immediate percutaneous coronary intervention.
4. Supportive therapies are primarily oxygen and diuretics, with nitrates and inotropes reserved for decompensated patients.
5. Several mechanical support options exist, requiring referral to specialist cardiac centres.

Keywords: heart failure, PCI, mechanical support

Introduction

Heart failure is the leading cause of admission to hospital in those aged >65, and is responsible for 67,000 hospital admissions per year in England and Wales. It results from any condition that impairs the heart's ability to fill or eject blood. Poor filling of the left ventricle (LV) causes pulmonary oedema, and that of the right ventricle (RV) systemic venous and hepatic congestion. Poor ejection reduces cardiac output, causing inadequate oxygen uptake in the lungs (RV) and inadequate oxygen delivery to the body (LV). ICU management addresses acutely decompensated heart failure, but long-term management of chronic heart failure, as well as preventative management, is equally important.

Causes

Heart failure with reduced ejection fraction (HFREF) is associated with coronary, hypertensive and valvular heart disease, and the underlying cause is important in guiding therapy. Cardiomyopathies (particularly dilated) and cardiotoxic drugs account for a smaller number of presentations.

Heart failure with preserved ejection fraction (HFPEF) is associated with left ventricular (LV) outflow obstruction (e.g. aortic stenosis, hypertrophic obstructive cardiomyopathy) and poor LV compliance (diastolic dysfunction). Contractility is preserved, but high ventricular filling pressures and reduced preload lead to pulmonary oedema.

Right ventricular (RV) systolic dysfunction may occur from the same processes above, but also consider pulmonary hypertension (cor pulmonale, thromboembolic disease), intra-cardiac shunts (left to right) and secondary to LV failure.

Precipitants of Acute Heart Failure

These include acute coronary syndromes, myocarditis, acute valvular degeneration (e.g. endocarditis, ruptured chordae), tachy-arrhythmias (e.g. atrial fibrillation), hypertensive crises, pulmonary embolism and increased oxygen demand from systemic disease (e.g. sepsis, trauma, shock). Acute heart failure can occur post-cardiac surgery, with stunning of ventricular muscle. The underlying cause and precipitants are vital in goal-directed therapy.

Pathophysiology

Cardiac dysfunction reduces oxygen delivery, which activates a range of neurohumoral pathways (i.e sympathetic nervous system, renin–angiotensin–aldosterone system and arginine–vasopressin system), all of which reduce urine output and cause fluid and sodium accumulation. Tissue oedema and venous congestion reduce organ oxygen delivery still further, and the normal renal hydrostatic and oncotic pressure gradient is reduced.

Decompensated Presentation

Poor LV filling increases left atrial (LA) pressure from reduced LV compliance. This causes dyspnoea, orthopnoea and paroxysmal nocturnal dyspnoea. Orthopnoea is caused from an increase in venous return from the extremities and splanchnic bed to the lungs during decumbency. Rales, crackles and wheeze can be auscultated. The patient is tachypnoeic and hypoxic. Chest X-ray shows interstitial and alveolar oedema with pleural effusions.

Poor RV filling increases right atrial (RA) pressure from primary RV failure or secondary to LV failure. Venous congestion distends the jugular veins and raises central venous pressure (CVP). Hepatic congestion causes painful hepatomegaly, with raised liver function tests (LFTs), icterus and cholecystitis. Renal congestion reduces perfusion gradient, causing raised creatinine and reduced urine output. Gut distension causes abdominal pain, nausea and vomiting and malnutrition.

Poor contractility reduces cardiac output, with signs of end-organ hypoperfusion. Dyspnoea and malaise predominate, with hypoxia, raised lactate, acidaemia and reduced venous oxygen saturations (arterial and venous blood gas analysis). ECG changes include myocardial ischaemia or infarction, tachy-arrhythmias or conduction delays and P-mitrale/P-pulmonale. Transthoracic echocardiography (TTE) is the most important test – it is able to quantify RV and LV systolic function (global or regional wall motion abnormalities), LV compliance (diastolic), chamber dilations, valvular integrities, LV outflow obstruction and pulmonary artery (PA) pressure estimation, as well as external pressure (pericardial effusion, cardiac tamponade). Importantly, RV systolic function may be well tolerated as long as pulmonary pressures remain low. PA systolic pressure can be estimated on echocardiography using tricuspid regurgitation velocity with Doppler and the simplified Bernoulli equation (Box 3.1.3.1).

A useful tool is the categorising of patients by congestion ('wet' or 'dry') or hypoperfusion ('warm' or 'cold'). Dry–warm is compensated; wet–warm is congested, but perfused (most common); dry–cold is not perfused, but not congested (rare), with the worst being wet–cold (decompensated).

Box 3.1.3.1 **The Simplified Bernoulli Equation**

$$\text{Pressure} = 4 \times \text{velocity}^2 + \text{CVP}$$

Management

General Measures

The two most important management strategies are immediate support of haemodynamic instability and exclusion of an acute coronary syndrome that requires urgent percutaneous coronary intervention (PCI). Cardiac troponin may be elevated in acute heart failure without ischaemia or infarction. In addition to the tests listed above, with bedside TTE being the most important, other helpful investigations include plasma B-type natriuretic peptide (BNP <100 ng/l or N-terminal pro-BNP <300 mg/l excludes acute decompensated heart failure), cardiac output monitoring (e.g. pulse contour analysis), extravascular lung water (PiCCO$_2$, Volume View/EV 1000) and PA catheterisation. The latter is a more technical intervention but can provide vital information on pulmonary pressures, including pulmonary capillary wedge pressure (may approximate to LA pressure), haemodynamic variables (cardiac output, vascular resistances) and oxygenation parameters (consumption and extraction).

General treatment consists of oxygen and diuretics (e.g. loop). Serial weight and urine output measures are mandatory. Latest National Institute for Health and Care Excellence (NICE) guidelines do not recommend routine use of opiates, nitrates or inotropes unless decompensation has occurred. Treatment should be directed to the underlying cause; thus, antibiotics, anticoagulation and cardiothoracic surgical referral may be warranted. Revascularisation either by PCI or by surgery is the primary consideration in ischaemia. Continuous positive airway pressure (CPAP) is a supportive measure that reduces pulmonary venous return, and may recruit alveoli to reduce atelectasis and improve work of breathing. Again, it should not be used in non-decompensated heart failure. If the above measures fail, sedation, intubation and positive pressure ventilation may be needed. Ultrafiltration is reserved for patients with diuretic resistance or toxicity from levels above daily recommended amounts (as many patients will already be on diuretics pre-admission). Inotrope use should be guided by expert help, and sympathomimetics (e.g. adrenaline, dobutamine) are commonly used. Vasoconstrictors (e.g. noradrenaline, vasopressin) are rarely indicated. Specialist drugs include phosphodiesterase inhibitors (e.g. milrinone) and the calcium-sensitising agent levosimendan, although the value of both is uncertain.

Mechanical Support

Where conservative measures fail, several mechanical therapies exist – although all are invasive and require considerable expertise, in both insertion and subsequent intensive care management.

- **Intra-aortic balloon pump (IABP) counterpulsation.** By inflating during diastole in the descending aorta, this device reduces myocardial oxygen demand (reduces afterload) and increases myocardial oxygen delivery (increases ventricular diastolic perfusion). It serves as a bridging manoeuvre to further definitive therapy or recovery, but its value remains uncertain. It is absolutely contraindicated if aortic regurgitation is present, as it relies on a competent valve to function, and in peripheral vascular disease or descending aortic pathology.

- **Ventricular assist device (VAD).** NICE guidelines 2017 support short-term (30-day) use of the CentriMag external blood pump in both adult and paediatric acute unresponsive heart failure as a bridge to recovery and heart transplantation or to suitable long-term alternatives. The device can support the LV or RV, or both. Inserted surgically, the configuration is normally LA or LV to the ascending aorta (left ventricular assist device (LVAD)) or RA to PA (right ventricular assist device (RVAD)), using cannulae, an external pump and a control console. The motor magnetically levitates the impeller (rotor) and operates without mechanical bearings or seals. The devices still rely on the patient's own lungs to oxygenate the blood sufficiently.

- **Extracorporeal membrane oxygenation (ECMO).** The advantage of ECMO over VADs is the ability to oxygenate blood and the potential avoidance of centrally placed cannulae (by using femoral and jugular vessels). It is important to know that ECMO exists in two configurations, namely veno-venous (VV) for purely intractable respiratory failure, and veno-arterial (VA) for pump failure with hypoxia. Only the latter is useful here.

- **Impella®.** An evolving technology, the Impella® is a short-term VAD, inserted percutaneously (usually femorally), which crosses the aortic valve. It pulls blood from the LV, through a catheter, and delivers it into the ascending aorta, thus increasing cardiac output and relieving LV distension in the failing heart.

- **Cardiac resynchronisation therapy (CRT).** This is not an acute therapy, but worth considering after recovery from the initial decompensation. CRT is a form of cardiac pacing whereby the LV is paced, as well as the RV, to synchronise contractions. This is achieved in the catheter lab by inserting a thin pacing wire into the coronary sinus via the RA. It is considered in patients with low ejection fraction (<35 per cent) and left bundle branch block.

Long-Term Therapies

Goal-directed pharmacological therapy typically includes beta-blockade, angiotensin reduction (angiotensin-converting enzyme inhibition, angiotensin II receptor antagonists), mineralocorticoid receptor antagonists, loop diuretics and statins. Focused therapies include aspirin, anticoagulation and anti-arrhythmic agents.

References and Further Reading

Arrigo M, Parissis J, Akiyama E, Mebazaa A. Understanding acute heart failure: pathophysiology and diagnosis. *Eur Heart J* 2016;**18**(Suppl G):G11–18.

National Institute for Health and Care Excellence. 2014. Acute heart failure: diagnosis and management. www.nice.org.uk/guidance/cg187

National Institute for Health and Care Excellence. 2014. Extracorporeal membrane oxygenation (ECMO) for acute heart failure in adults. www.nice.org.uk/guidance/ipg482

National Institute for Health and Care Excellence. 2017. CentriMag for heart failure. www.nice.org.uk/advice/mib92

Yancy C, Jessup M, Bozkurt B, *et al.* 2013 ACCF/AHA guideline for the management of heart failure. A report of the American College of Cardiology/American Heart Association Task Force on Practice Guidelines. *Circulation* 2013;**128**:e240–327.

Valvular Heart Disease

Katarina Lenartova

Keywords: aortic stenosis, regurgitation, mitral stenosis, diagnosis, treatment

Introduction

Patients with valvular heart disease (VHD) encountered in critical care units typically fall into one of two categories: those who are critically ill because of valvular dysfunction, and those in whom valvular disease represents an important co-morbid condition.

Clinical examination and diagnosis of the patient with VHD are challenging in the settings of critical care, not least due to co-morbidities, stress and infection leading to tachycardia and shorter intervals for evaluation of heart sounds. A delay in recognising the presence of significant valve dysfunction therefore frequently occurs.

Aortic Stenosis

Aetiology and Pathophysiology

Aortic stenosis (AS) is the most prevalent form of cardiovascular disease in the Western world, after hypertension and coronary artery disease. It is usually caused by either degenerative calcification of a tri-leaflet valve or progressive stenosis of a congenital bicuspid valve. Calcific aortic stenosis affects approximately 10 per cent of those older than 75 years. Rheumatic heart disease, the most common aetiology worldwide, is less common in the Western world.

Normal aortic valve area ranges from 3 to 4 cm^2. Significant resistance to outflow does not occur until the valve orifice is reduced by >50 per cent. In practice, as the resistance to outflow rises, the left ventricle (LV) is subject to pressure overload, resulting in compensatory hypertrophy. With progressive hypertrophy, diastolic pressures may rise as LV compliance decreases, resulting in increased LV filling pressures. In addition, the myocardial supply–demand relationship is deleteriously affected by hypertrophy in this setting. With increased wall stress and increased wall mass, myocardial oxygen demand is increased; at the same time, coronary flow reserve is decreased in AS, and in later stages of the disease, diastolic perfusion pressure is lowered.

Physical Examination

In general, in patients with severe AS, the arterial pulse is slow to increase and has a reduced peak (*pulsus parvus et tardus*), which is best appreciated by palpating the carotid pulse. This may not be present in elderly patients because of the rigidity of the vasculature. The characteristic murmur of AS is a crescendo–decrescendo systolic murmur along the left sternal border that radiates to the upper right sternal border and into the carotid arteries. However, it may also radiate to the LV apex (the Gallavardin phenomenon) and may be mistaken for a murmur of mitral regurgitation (MR). Unfortunately, none of these findings has sufficiently high sensitivity or specificity for AS or for differentiating moderate from severe disease.

Diagnostic Testing

Chest Radiography

Cardiac size is often normal in patients with AS, with rounding of the LV border and apex due to LV hypertrophy. Cardiomegaly is a late feature in patients with AS. In patients with heart failure, the heart is enlarged, with congestion of the pulmonary vasculature. In cases of advanced heart failure, the right atrium and right ventricle may also be enlarged.

Echocardiography

Two-dimensional echocardiography demonstrates the morphology of the aortic valve and can often delineate if it is tri-leaflet or bicuspid. The spectrum of calcific aortic valve disease ranges from aortic sclerosis without obstruction to ventricular outflow, to severe AS. The characteristic echocardiographic features of AS are decreased valve leaflet mobility, calcification in all, except congenital AS in adolescents and young adults, and an augmented Doppler velocity that generally allows accurate estimation of the gradient. Doppler signal velocity with peak and mean pressure gradient and valve area by continuity equation provides an accurate overall assessment (Table 3.1.4.1).

The gradient, however, is highly dependent on flow across the valve, and in low-output states, the gradient may result in underestimation of the severity of disease. Conversely, in high-output states, such as in patients with augmented cardiac output caused by inotropic stimulation, endogenous high catecholamine

Table 3.1.4.1 Aortic stenosis severity classification based on American College of Cardiology/American Heart Association and European Society of Cardiology

	Aortic sclerosis	Mild	Moderate	Severe
Aortic jet velocity (m/s)	≤2.5 m/s	2.6–2.9	3.0–4.0	>4.0
Mean gradient (mmHg)	–	<20 (<30[a])	20–40[b] (30–50[a])	>40[b] (>50[a])
Aortic valve area (cm²)	–	>1.5	1.0–1.5	<1
Indexed aortic valve area (cm²/m²)	–	>0.85	0.60–0.85	<0.6
Velocity ratio	–	>0.50	0.25–0.50	<0.25

[a] ESC guideline cut-offs.
[b] ACC/AHA guideline cut-offs.

states and sepsis, the gradient may be disproportionately higher than the severity of stenosis would suggest. Assessing the severity of AS using Doppler criteria is dependent not only on the severity of AS, but also on the aortic flow. In patients with low cardiac output, such as those with LV dysfunction, the calculated gradients and aortic valve area may not be representative of the true severity of stenosis. In such cases of 'low-output, low-gradient' AS, administration of low-dose dobutamine may be needed to truly assess the severity of AS and to differentiate patients with anatomically severe AS from those with 'pseudo' AS.

In AS, the LV cavity is usually of normal size or small. LV hypertrophy is often present, as is left atrial enlargement. LV systolic function is usually normal in early disease. However, if heart failure has developed, the LV may be enlarged and systolic function depressed. The ascending aorta should also be evaluated and measured to detect associated aortic aneurysms, which are more common in patients with bicuspid valves.

Other Imaging Modalities

CT has an established role in evaluating the presence and severity of aortic root and ascending aortic dilation in patients with associated aortic aneurysms. Cardiac magnetic resonance (CMR) is useful for detecting and reliably measuring the anatomic valve area.

Cardiac Catheterisation

Because of the accuracy of echocardiographic assessment of the severity of AS, cardiac catheterisation is currently most often used to identify the presence of associated coronary artery disease (CAD), rather than to define haemodynamic abnormalities. Invasive haemodynamic measurements are, however, helpful in patients in whom non-invasive tests are inconclusive or provide discrepant results regarding the severity of AS.

Treatment

Medical Management

This is predominantly aimed at patient stabilisation because pharmacologic intervention has never been shown to prolong life and can achieve modest haemodynamic improvement at best. In the critical care setting, the approach to the patient with AS normally parallels treatment of corresponding degrees of heart failure, albeit with caution, because the normal therapeutic approach to heart failure can be deleterious or fatal in the setting of severe AS. Traditional heart failure therapies, in particular diuretics and vasodilators, need to be used with care because reduction in preload can cause hypotension, decreased cardiac output and a downward spiral into refractory shock. In patients with small-volume hypertrophic LV, cardiac output is particularly preload-dependent. Atrial arrhythmias, in particular atrial fibrillation (AF), can lead to abrupt and severe decompensation because of loss of the atrial contraction component of LV filling. Vasodilator therapy, as described earlier, results in peripheral vasodilation; however, because of the fixed obstruction to outflow, it may not provide sufficient increase in stroke volume and cardiac output to maintain systemic blood pressure. Inotropic agents are frequently required, and patients with inadequate contractile reserve may show limited improvement. Lipid-lowering therapy and angiotensin-converting enzyme (ACE) inhibitors have been the subject of substantial investigation.

Percutaneous Interventions

1. **Balloon aortic valvuloplasty (BAV).** BAV is a temporising measure for patients who are haemodynamically unstable and are at high risk of aortic valve replacement (AVR).

2. **Transcatheter aortic valve replacement (TAVR).** Tissue valves are sewn to either balloon-expandable or self-expanding stents, which are then crimped onto a catheter and deployed across the stenotic native valve. Whilst data regarding TAVR outcomes appear to be extremely positive, it is also noteworthy that the residual mortality rate in the inoperable TAVR patients remains very high, thus reflecting the severe co-morbid conditions in patients.

3. **AVR.** AVR remains the treatment of choice for severe AS in patients who are considered to have reasonable operable risk. Class I indications include severe AS (valve area <1 cm^2) with symptoms, or symptomless patients who have severe AS and are undergoing coronary artery bypass, surgery to the aorta or other heart valves or who have LV dysfunction. Survival after AVR is excellent if LV function is preserved, with the operative mortality rate in ideal candidates as low as 1 per cent.

Aortic Insufficiency/Regurgitation

Aetiology and Pathophysiology

Aortic insufficiency (AI) results from abnormalities of the aortic leaflets or their supporting structures in the aortic root and annulus, or both. In general, causes of AI have been divided into those that affect the leaflets primarily and those that affect the root and annulus. The former includes bicuspid and other aortic valve abnormalities, endocarditis, rheumatic aortic valve disease, the atherosclerotic process, connective tissue disorders, anti-phospholipid syndrome (Libman–Sacks endocarditis) and toxicity from anorectic drugs. The aortic root and annulus are affected by a variety of co-morbid conditions that dilate the aortic root: Marfan and Ehlers–Danlos syndromes, osteogenesis imperfecta, chronic aortic dissection, syphilitic aortitis, connective tissue disorders and, along with the valve leaflets, ankylosing spondylitis.

In isolated acute AI, sudden onset of regurgitation imposes a large-volume load on the LV in diastole prior to an adaptive process being in place. The abrupt rise in pressure is reflected by parallel development of left atrial and pulmonary vascular hypertension, frequently resulting in pulmonary oedema. In early, compensated severe AR, the LV adapts to the volume overload by development of eccentric hypertrophy. This process is initially reversible, and LV systolic function can improve after restoration of normal loading conditions by AVR. With time, however, myocardial contractile dysfunction may develop, at which point there is a risk of irreversible LV dysfunction. The effective forward stroke volume is therefore low, compensated to some degree by tachycardia, but frequently insufficient to maintain normal cardiac output. Acute severe AI results in approximation of aortic and LV pressures at the end of diastole, with consequent reduction of coronary perfusion of the subendocardium. In contrast, chronic AI features a host of adaptive processes by the LV, including progressive dilation, increased compliance and hypertrophy. In chronic AR, a combined preload and afterload excess is imposed on the LV. The excess preload reflects the volume overload that is directly related to the severity of AR. In addition, the increased stroke volume that is ejected into the high-impedance aorta often creates systolic hypertension, which, in turn, further increases LV afterload. The combination of preload and afterload excess with severe AR ultimately leads to progressive LV dilation, with resultant systolic dysfunction. LV dysfunction may be associated with symptoms of heart failure such as dyspnoea on exertion, orthopnoea and paroxysmal nocturnal dyspnoea.

Physical Examination

Acute AI typically presents with low-cardiac output state, tachycardia, dyspnoea and peripheral vasoconstriction. Typical findings are characteristic for chronic AI, whereby a wide pulse pressure results primarily because of the increased stroke volume augmenting systolic pressure and a low aortic diastolic pressure occurring secondary to volume loss into the LV. Other associated physical findings are bounding carotid and peripheral pulses (Corrigan's, or water hammer, pulse) and Hill's sign (higher systolic blood pressure in the legs than in the arms). The classic murmur of AR is a high-frequency, blowing and decrescendo diastolic murmur, usually heard in the aortic area, but also audible in the left third and fourth intercostal spaces along the sternal border. The Austin–Flint murmur, a mid- to late-diastolic rumble heard best at the apex, is similar to the murmur heard in mitral stenosis (MS) but occurs in patients with no mitral valve (MV) abnormalities.

Diagnostic Testing
Chest Radiography

In patients with acute AR, chest radiography reveals minimal cardiac enlargement. The aortic root and arch are normal. Pulmonary vascular congestion is noted. In patients with chronic AR, chest radiography demonstrates an enlarged cardiac silhouette with LV dilation. The ascending aorta may also be enlarged when an aortic aneurysm or aortic dissection is present. Pulmonary congestion is noted when heart failure has developed.

Echocardiography

Echocardiography is the most widely used diagnostic tool to assess LV dimensions, volumes and ejection fraction. It also allows morphological assessment of the aortic valve, annulus and root, thereby helping to determine the aetiology of AR. Transoesophageal echocardiography (TOE) has superior diagnostic sensitivity to transthoracic echocardiography (TTE) for certain parameters, especially in detecting valvular vegetations. Severity of AI is based on a range of parameters measured, including the width of colour Doppler jet,

Table 3.1.4.2 Aortic regurgitation severity classification based on American College of Cardiology/American Heart Association

Aortic regurgitation	Mild	Moderate	Severe
Qualitative			
Angiographic grade	1+	2+	3–4+
Colour Doppler jet width	Central jet, width <25% of LVOT	Greater than mild, but no signs of severe AR	Central jet, width >65% of LVOT
Doppler vena contracta width (cm)	<0.3	0.3–0.6	>0.6
Quantitative (catheterisation or echocardiography)			
Regurgitant volume (ml/beat)	<30	30–59	>60
Regurgitant fraction (%)	<30	30–49	>50
Regurgitant orifice area (cm^2)	<0.1	0.1–0.29	>0.30
Additional essential criteria			
Left ventricular size	Increased		

Abbreviations: LVOT = left ventricular outflow tract; AR = aortic regurgitation.

compared with the width of the LV outflow tract, width of the vena contracta, regurgitant volume, regurgitant fraction and regurgitant orifice area (Table 3.1.4.2). Additional findings also include the rate of jet velocity deceleration and diastolic flow reversal in the aorta.

The size and function of the LV have been used as thresholds for AVR consideration. The American College of Cardiology (ACC)/American Heart Association (AHA) and the European Society of Cardiology (ESC) guidelines have established slightly different sets of values for class I and II recommendations.

Cardiac Magnetic Resonance Imaging

CMR imaging provides highly accurate assessment of LV volumes and mass and ejection fraction. It can also provide excellent visualisation of the aortic root and ascending aorta.

Cardiac Catheterisation

Cardiac catheterisation is primarily used to assess coronary anatomy before surgery in patients with the appropriate age and risk factor profile.

Treatment

Medical Management

In acute AI, medical management is based on stabilisation pending AVR. Vasodilator therapy and manoeuvres to increase the heart rate are beneficial, as tachycardia decreases the diastolic filling period and therefore reduces regurgitation across the aortic valve. In chronic

AI, the evidence base is incomplete; ACE inhibitors, angiotensin receptor blockers (ARBs) and beta-blockers are useful. In patients with Marfan syndrome, beta-blockers and/or losartan may slow aortic root dilation and reduce the risk of aortic complications, and should be considered before and after surgery.

Aortic Valve Replacement

There are three AHA/ACC class I indications for surgery for patients with severe AI:

1. Patients with symptoms, regardless of LV function
2. Patients with LV ejection fraction of <50 per cent
3. Patients undergoing coronary bypass surgery or any other valve surgery or surgery on the aorta

The ESC describes a fourth class I indication – heart team discussion is recommended in selected patients in whom aortic valve repair may be a feasible alternative to AVR. Surgery results in superior long-term survival over medical treatment alone for symptomatic patients.

Mitral Regurgitation

The mitral valve is the most complex valve of all the heart valves. It consists of the annulus, an anterior and a posterior leaflet, chordae and papillary muscles. MR can be attributed to dysfunction of one or more structures, and geometry of the LV plays a role too. Carpentier classified MR based on leaflet motion (Table 3.1.4.3).

Table 3.1.4.3 Carpentier classification of mitral regurgitation

Mitral regurgitation	Leaflet motion and annulus findings	Lesion	Aetiology
Type I	Normal Dilated annulus	Leaflet perforation Annular dilation	Endocarditis Ischaemic MR ± significant LV dysfunction
Type II	Excessive (prolapse) Normal annulus	Chordae elongation or rupture (flail leaflets) Papillary muscle elongation or rupture	Myxomatous/degenerative disease Endocarditis Trauma Ischaemic cardiomyopathy
Type IIIa	Restricted (diastole and systole) Normal annulus	Leaflet thickening/retraction Leaflet calcification Chordal thickening/retraction/fusion Commissural fusion	Rheumatic heart disease Inflammatory Carcinoid heart disease
Type IIIb	Tethered/restricted (systole) Dilated annulus	LV dilation Papillary muscle displacement Chordae tethering	Dilated ischaemic cardiomyopathy

Abbreviations: MR = mitral regurgitation; LV = left ventricular.

Aetiology and Pathophysiology

MR results in volume overload of the LV. Adaptive changes of the ventricle to volume overload include LV dilation and eccentric hypertrophy. The left atrium also enlarges, thus allowing accommodation of the regurgitant volume at a lower pressure. Unlike AI, the afterload is not increased and overall LV ejection is enhanced. Although patients with compensated chronic MR may remain asymptomatic for many years, decompensation may eventually develop if the regurgitation is sufficiently severe. The LV ejection fraction in chronic MR may be greater than normal because of the increase in preload, and the afterload-reducing effect of ejection into the low-impedance left atrium. The LV ejection fraction can therefore be misleading as a measure of contractile function in this disorder, and advanced myocardial dysfunction may occur whilst LV ejection fraction is still well within the normal range. Consequently, outcome after MV surgery is poorer in patients with a preoperative ejection fraction of <60 per cent.

Physical Examination

In acute MR, sudden left atrial hypertension results in pulmonary oedema, with accompanying clinical findings, and an increase in the pulmonic second sound and paradoxical splitting of the second heart sound. In chronic MR, there are characteristic volume overload features and a prominent precordial pulsation, S3 gallop. The systolic murmur of MR varies according to the aetiology of the regurgitation. The murmur is usually heard best at the apex in the left lateral decubitus position. With severe degenerative MR, the murmur is holosystolic, radiating into the axilla. Early systolic murmurs are typical of acute MR. Late systolic murmurs are typical of MV prolapse or papillary muscle dysfunction.

Diagnostic Testing

Chest Radiography

Cardiomegaly due to LV and left atrial enlargement is common in patients with chronic MR. In patients with pulmonary hypertension, right-sided chamber enlargement is also a common finding. Kerley B lines and interstitial oedema can be seen in patients with acute MR or progressive LV failure.

Echocardiography

This provides information about the mechanism and severity of MR, the size and function of the LV and right ventricle, the size of the left atrium, the degree of pulmonary hypertension and the presence of other associated valve lesions. Doppler evaluation provides quantitative measures of the severity of MR that have been shown to be important predictors of outcome (Table 3.1.4.4).

Table 3.1.4.4 Mitral regurgitation severity classification based on American College of Cardiology/American Heart Association

Mitral regurgitation	Mild	Moderate	Severe
Qualitative			
Angiographic grade	1+	2+	3–4+
Colour Doppler jet area	Small central jet (<4 cm² or 20% of left atrial area)	Signs of MR greater than mild present, but no criteria for severe MR	Vena contracta width >0.7 cm, with large central MR jet (area >40% of left atrial area) or with a wall-impinging jet of any size, swirling in left atrium
Doppler vena contracta width (cm)	<0.3	0.3–0.69	≥0.7
Quantitative (cath or echo)			
Regurgitant volume (ml/beat)	<30	30–59	≥60
Regurgitant fraction (%)	<30	30–59	≥50
Regurgitant orifice area (cm²)	<0.2	0.2–0.39	≥0.4
Additional essential criteria			
Left atrial size	Enlarged		
Left ventricular size	Enlarged		

Abbreviations: MR = mitral regurgitation.

Treatment
Medical Management
For acute severe, symptomatic MR, primary medical therapy consists of aggressive vasodilation to improve aortic flow and decrease left-sided filling pressure. In the setting of MR and shock, a combination of vaso-dilation and intra-aortic balloon pump (IABP) or ino-trope is highly effective.

Mitral Valve Surgery
Urgent surgery is indicated in patients with acute severe MR. In the case of papillary muscle rupture as the underlying disease, valve replacement is, in general, required. Surgery is obviously indicated in sympto-matic patients with severe primary MR. An LV ejection fraction of ≤60 per cent (or LV end-systolic diameter (LVESD) ≥45 mm), AF and/or a systolic pulmonary pressure of ≥50 mmHg predict a worse post-operative outcome, independent of the symptomatic status, and have therefore become triggers for surgery in asympto-matic patients. Transcatheter MV interventions have been developed to correct primary MR, through either a trans-septal or a transapical approach. Amongst the transcatheter procedures, currently only edge-to-edge mitral repair is widely adopted. Despite the absence of a randomised comparison between the results of valve replacement and repair, it is widely accepted that, when feasible, valve repair is the preferred treatment. In sec-ondary MR, the valve leaflets and chordae are structur-ally normal and MR results from an imbalance between closing and tethering forces on the valve secondary to alterations in LV geometry. Surgery is indicated in patients with severe secondary MR undergoing coro-nary artery bypass graft (CABG) and LV ejection frac-tion of >30 per cent.

Mitral Stenosis
Aetiology and Pathophysiology
The most common cause of MS worldwide is rheu-matic fever, and isolated MS is twice as common in women as in men. Other causes of MS are very rare and include congenital anomalies, prior exposure to chest radiation, mucopolysaccharidosis, severe mitral annular calcification and left atrial myxoma. MS is primarily caused by rheumatic deformity scarring the valve leaflets and subvalve region, fusion of the com-missures and annular calcification – all of which cre-ate an obstruction between the left atrium and the LV, resulting in rising left atrial and pulmonary pressures.

A normal MV area is 4.0–5.0 cm², and symptoms usually develop when the valve area decreases below 1.5–2.5 cm². Because antegrade flow occurs entirely during diastole, and the diastolic filling period shortens or lengthens with an increase or decrease in heart rate, respectively, the gradient is highly flow-dependent, and thus maintenance of sinus rhythm is essential to maintain cardiac output. The first symptoms of MS are usually exertional dyspnoea and fatigue. However, patients may also present with pulmonary oedema, AF or an embolic event.

Physical Examination
Classic physical examination findings in patients with MS include a normal apical LV impulse, an accentu-ated S1 and an opening snap, followed by a diastolic rumble with pre-systolic accentuation heard best at the apex in the left lateral decubitus position. These findings, however, may not be present in patients with severe pulmonary hypertension, low cardiac output or a heavily calcified and immobile valve.

Diagnostic Testing
Chest Radiography
The most common chest radiographic finding in patients with severe MS is left atrial enlargement. Enlargement of the right atrium, right ventricle and pulmonary artery also occurs in patients with advanced MS with pulmonary hypertension.

Echocardiography
Echocardiography is the primary imaging tool used to assess patients with MS. The anterior leaflet gener-ally shows a 'hockey stick' deformity because restricted motion of the valve most commonly involves the leaflet tips. The posterior leaflet is often restricted in both systole and diastole. Echocardiography also pro-vides information regarding the size of the left atrium, and the size and function of the LV and right-sided chambers. Doppler examination provides informa-tion about the severity of MS, the presence of other associated valve lesions and the degree of pulmonary hypertension. The MV area can be determined from the diastolic jet velocity across the MV (Table 3.1.4.5).

Cardiac Catheterisation
Routine diagnostic cardiac catheterisation is no longer performed in patients. Diagnostic cardiac catheteri-sation is only necessary when echocardiography is non-conclusive or results are discordant with clinical findings.

Table 3.1.4.5 Mitral stenosis severity classification based on the European Association of Echocardiography (EAE) and the American Society of Echocardiography (ASE)

	Mild	Moderate	Severe
Specific findings			
Valve area (cm²)	>1.5	1.0–1.5	<1.0
Supportive findings			
Mean gradient (mmHg)[a]	<5	5–10	>10
Pulmonary artery pressure (mmHg)	<30	30–50	>50

[a] At heart rates between 60 and 80 bpm and in sinus rhythm.

Treatment

Medical Management

The aim is to maintain a slow sinus rhythm and anticoagulation. Beta-blockade is the preferred option for this. However, if contraindicated, diltiazem and verapamil are sometimes used. AF develops in 30 per cent of patients with MS, and the risk of embolic events is substantially higher than in AF patients without MS.

Mitral Valve Surgery and Percutaneous Intervention

Outcomes for percutaneous balloon mitral valvuloplasty are equivalent, or superior, to surgery in patients with favourable valve anatomy. Symptomatic patients with favourable anatomy, or those with pulmonary hypertension (>50 mmHg at rest), should be considered for percutaneous balloon valvotomy. Surgery should be reserved for patients with unfavourable anatomy, severely thickened or highly calcified MV leaflets and/or subvalvular apparatus, more than mild MR, or persistent thrombus in the left atrium.

Tricuspid Valve Disease and Pulmonary Valve Disease

The tricuspid valve, often regarded as the 'forgotten valve', is the largest and most apically positioned of the four cardiac valves. Tricuspid regurgitation (TR) is more common than tricuspid stenosis, and is usually coincidentally detected during the workup for complaints due to coexisting left-sided heart disease. The aetiology of TR is classified according to the presence of primary tricuspid valve pathology (primary TR), the presence of associated left-sided heart disease (secondary TR) or the presence of AF without any associated left-sided heart disease (isolated TR). Possible causes of primary TR are infective endocarditis (especially in

intravenous drug addicts), rheumatic heart disease, carcinoid syndrome, myxomatous disease, endomyocardial fibrosis, Ebstein's anomaly and congenitally dysplastic valves, drug-induced valve diseases, thoracic trauma and iatrogenic valve damage (transvenous pacing or defibrillator leads, endomyocardial biopsy). In secondary TR, the underlying mechanism is characterised by right ventricular dilation and dysfunction, leading to leaflet tethering, tricuspid annulus dilation and leaflet malcoaptation. Tricuspid stenosis is often combined with TR, most frequently of rheumatic origin. It is therefore almost always associated with left-sided valve lesions, particularly MS, that usually dominate the clinical presentation. Diagnosis is made based on understanding of the tricuspid valve morphology and two-dimensional TTE. Surgery should be carried out sufficiently early to avoid irreversible right ventricular dysfunction. In secondary TR, adding a tricuspid repair, if indicated, during left-sided surgery does not increase the operative risk and has been demonstrated to provide reverse remodelling of the right ventricle.

Pulmonary valve disease is most commonly the result of congenital heart disease. Less common causes are infective endocarditis, carcinoid syndrome and rheumatic heart disease. Treatment options include balloon valvuloplasty – repair or replacement of the valve.

Right Ventricular Function

Assessment of right ventricular function is difficult in VHD because of its complex geometry. Several invasive and non-invasive techniques have been used for estimating right ventricular function. An increase in pulmonary wedge pressure as a result of mitral or aortic valve disease is associated with a rise in mean pulmonary artery pressure. Thus, right ventricular afterload increases as dilation of the right ventricle develops, with a resultant drop in right ventricular ejection fraction. As a consequence, the tricuspid valve annulus dilates and may induce TR, with secondary right ventricular volume overload. Right ventricular ejection fraction was found to be dependent on the pulmonary circulation, with alterations in right ventricular loading conditions, right ventricular geometry and motion of the interventricular septum (ventricular interaction), as well as myocardial structure. Pulmonary artery pressure is usually increased in patients with MV disease, but only slightly altered in patients with aortic valve disease. Irreversible damage to the right ventricle has been described in patients with advanced MV disease, but the point where no normalisation after correction of the valve lesion occurs is difficult to determine.

References and Further Reading

Baumgartner H, Falk V, Bax JJ, *et al.* 2017 ESC/EACTS guidelines for the management of valvular heart disease. *Eur Heart J* 2017;**38**:2739–91.

Bonow RO, Carabello BA, Chatterjee K, *et al.* ACC/AHA 2006 guidelines for the management of patients with valvular heart disease: a report of the American College of Cardiology/American Heart Association Task Force on Practice Guidelines (writing committee to revise the 1998 guidelines for the management of patients with valvular heart disease) developed in collaboration with the Society of Cardiovascular Anesthesiologists and endorsed by the Society for Cardiovascular Angiography and Interventions and the Society of Thoracic Surgeons. *J Am Coll Cardiol* 2006;**48**:e1–148.

Maganti K, Rigolin VH, Sarano ME, Bonow RO. Valvular heart disease: diagnosis and management. *Mayo Clin Proc* 2010;**85**:483–500.

Parrillo JE, Dellinger RP. Valvular heart disease in critical care. In: JE Parrillo, RP Dellinger (eds). *Critical Care Medicine: Principles of Diagnosis and Management in the Adult*, 4th edn. Philadelphia, PA: Elsevier; 2014. pp. 548–75.

Vahanian A, Baumgartner H, Bax J, *et al.*; Task Force on the Management of Valvular Heart Disease of the European Society of Cardiology and ESC Committee for Practice Guidelines. Guidelines on the management of valvular heart disease: The Task Force on the Management of Valvular Heart Disease of the European Society of Cardiology. *Eur Heart J* 2007;**28**:230–68.

3.1.5

Congenital Heart Disease

Anne-Marie Leo

Key Learning Points

1. There are more adults than children with congenital heart disease (CHD).
2. Despite improvements in patient survival, adults with CHD remain at a higher risk of morbidity and death, when compared to the general population.
3. When a patient with CHD presents to the intensive care unit, determine the patient's underlying cardiac condition and any previous intervention, as these will affect the patient's physiology.
4. Patients with CHD may be more sensitive to the effects of critical illness. Consider the interactions between the patient's underlying physiology and their critical care condition.
5. Consider early communication with the patient's cardiac centre to obtain additional patient information and advice regarding management, and to discuss whether the patient requires transfer to a specialist centre.

Keywords: adult congenital heart disease, grown-up congenital heart disease, shunt lesions, tetralogy of Fallot, transposition of the great arteries

Introduction

Due to medical and surgical advancements, there are more adults with congenital heart disease (CHD) than there are children with CHD. It is important for the critical care physician to be aware of this patient group, particularly as these patients can have markedly complex physiologies and early referral to a congenital cardiac centre may be warranted. This chapter describes in brief the types of congenital heart defects that may be present, reviews the most common reasons for these patients to present and provides a template for managing these patients in the ICU. In-depth ICU management of the patient with CHD is beyond the scope of this chapter. If you are in any doubt about how to manage your patient, contact your nearest congenital cardiac centre for advice.

Common Cardiac Conditions Which May Present

It is estimated that 20–25 per cent of grown-up congenital heart disease (GUCH) patients have rare, complex conditions requiring life-long specialist care. A further 35–40 per cent of GUCH patients usually require minimal input from their specialist care team. Therefore, when a GUCH patient presents to the ICU, it is important to ascertain what cardiac condition the patient has, what ongoing specialist input they have (if any) and whether immediate input from a specialist GUCH centre is required. Despite adults with CHD having higher rates of healthcare resource utilisation, when compared to the general population, and 10 per cent of CHD being diagnosed in adulthood, there is surprisingly little information in the literature regarding the distribution of CHD in adults and the reasons why they present to hospital. Table 3.1.5.1 provides data from the Dutch CONCOR registry regarding the prevalence of GUCH.

Table 3.1.5.1 Prevalence of different types of grown-up congenital heart disease

Type of grown-up congenital heart disease	Prevalence (%)
Atrial septal defect	17
Ventricular septal defect	14
Tetralogy of Fallot	11
Aortic coarctation	10
Aortic stenosis	10
Pulmonary stenosis	7
Transposition of the great arteries	5

Table 3.1.5.1 (cont.)

Type of grown-up congenital heart disease	Prevalence (%)
Marfan syndrome	5
Bicuspid aortic valve	4
Pulmonary atresia	2
Ebstein's anomaly	2
Atrioventricular septal defect	2
Congenitally corrected transposition of the great arteries	1
Patent ductus arteriosus	1
Other congenital heart defects	9

Why May a GUCH Patient Present to Hospital and What Causes Their Increased Mortality Rate?

Regarding the reasons why a GUCH patient may present to hospital, the Dutch CONCOR registry found that 61 per cent of GUCH hospital admissions were cardiovascular in nature, one-third of which were due to arrhythmias. Half of all interventions performed were cardiovascular, and half of these interventions were cardioversions. Patients with single ventricles and tricuspid atresia presented the most frequently and had the longest duration of admission. Most non-cardiovascular hospital admissions were obstetric patients. Data from the registry showed that 77 per cent of deaths were cardiovascular in origin, 45 per cent were due to heart failure and 19 per cent were sudden death. Twenty-three per cent of deaths were non-cardiovascular, with 9 per cent due to malignancy and 4 per cent due to pneumonia. Eight per cent of patients died in the peri-surgical period. Conditions associated with the highest mortality were single ventricles, tricuspid atresia and double-outlet right ventricle. Endocarditis, supraventricular arrhythmia, ventricular arrhythmia, conduction disturbances, myocardial infarction and pulmonary hypertension were all associated with an increased risk of all-cause mortality. Nine per cent of adults with CHD also had a moderately to severely impaired glomerular filtration rate (GFR), which is associated with a threefold increase in risk of mortality. Specific cardiac conditions have anticipated sequelae. These are outlined in brief in Table 3.1.5.2.

Table 3.1.5.2 Specific congenital heart disease conditions

Unrepaired ASD	• Left-to-right shunting may result in RV overload • Unrepaired, a large enough ASD will result in exercise intolerance/dyspnoea • Atrial dysrhythmias may develop • Severe PAH develops in approximately 10% of cases • Avoid air emboli as these can pass across the ASD to the left side of the circulation, with neurological sequelae
Repaired ASD	• May be closed surgically or percutaneously (device closure) • Outcomes depend on the patient's age and the presence of pulmonary hypertension at the time of surgery. Patients who are repaired in childhood have similar outcomes to the general population
Unrepaired VSD	• An unrepaired VSD may result in LV volume overload, dilation and failure, excessive left-to-right shunt which can result in pulmonary hypertension and ultimately Eisenmenger syndrome • There is also an association between VSD and aortic regurgitation • Hyperventilation and hyperoxygenation may result in excessive pulmonary blood flow (by encouraging left-to-right shunt through the VSD). This may result in reduced systemic perfusion
Repaired VSD	• Patients with good LV function and functional status pre-operatively and without pulmonary hypertension have relatively normal life expectancies after VSD closure
Unrepaired PDA in an adult	• The PDA connects the left pulmonary artery to the descending aorta, distal to the left subclavian artery • An unrepaired PDA may result in too much pulmonary blood flow, leading to pulmonary vascular damage and pulmonary hypertension • Differential cyanosis may be present (SpO_2 recorded in the feet may be lower than those recorded in the hands) • The PDA wall may be calcified, making ligation difficult. Resection of the adjacent descending aorta using grafting may be required
Repaired coarctation of the aorta	• Coarctation of the aorta describes a narrowing of the aorta • Repaired coarctation of the aorta can result in hypertension, aortic valve dysfunction and premature coronary artery disease

Unrepaired AVSD in an adult	• May have reduced exercise tolerance, elevated pulmonary vascular resistance, atrial dysrhythmias and complete heart block
Adult with previously repaired AVSD	• May have residual septal defects, atrial/ventricular dysrhythmias, valvular regurgitation/stenosis and right heart failure
Adult with previously repaired truncus arteriosus	• Truncus arteriosus describes a single vessel leaving the ventricles, instead of having the aorta from the left ventricle and the pulmonary artery from the right ventricle. A VSD is always present • Ventricular arrhythmias, branch pulmonary stenosis, pulmonary hypertension, insufficiency of the RV–PA conduit, truncal valve insufficiency (may have a valve replacement), RV dysfunction
Adult with previously repaired TOF	• TOF consists of pulmonary stenosis, RV hypertrophy, VSD and an overriding aorta • Patients post-TOF repair have 20-year survival rates exceeding 90 per cent • Pulmonary valve insufficiency, chronic RV volume overload, dilation and failure, tricuspid regurgitation, elevated central venous pressures resulting in hepatomegaly, peripheral oedema and exercise intolerance, atrial/ventricular dysrhythmias
Adult with repaired transposition of the great arteries	• Atrial switch operation (Mustard and Senning procedures). The morphological right ventricle which is supporting the systemic circulation will eventually fail, resulting in CHF and dysrhythmia • Arterial switch operation. The newer version of the above operation; however, the long-term effects are not fully understood. There seems to be an increased incidence of post-operative supravalvular and branch pulmonary arterial stenosis. The neo-aorta may also dilate, resulting in coronary artery distortion and myocardial ischaemia, and there is an increased risk of sudden cardiac death in these patients
Ebstein's anomaly	• In Ebstein's anomaly, the septal and posterior leaflets of the tricuspid valve are displaced towards the apex of the right ventricle, causing downward displacement of the annulus and atrialisation of the right ventricle • These patients are at an increased risk of RV failure and arrhythmias
Fontan circulation	• A Fontan procedure is a palliative surgical procedure that results in redirection of systemic venous blood, so that it flows directly into the pulmonary arteries, rather than returning to the heart. It is often performed after the Glenn operation which connects the SVC to the right pulmonary artery. The Fontan procedure connects the IVC to the pulmonary arteries. This means that blood flow to the lungs depends on passive blood flow. The Fontan procedure is often considered in patients with complex congenital heart disease where a biventricular repair is not possible • Symptoms of heart failure may be present (generalised oedema, ascites, hepatic dysfunction), increased risk of arrhythmias which are poorly tolerated, increased risk of thrombosis and stroke, progressive cyanosis and protein-losing enteropathy • Limited ability to increase stroke volume with exercise due to impaired ventricular function and difficulty with increasing preload • Elevated airway pressures may result in reduced pulmonary blood flow and subsequently reduced venous return to the heart and a reduction in cardiac output • Death occurs most often from heart failure and atrial arrhythmias

Abbreviations: ASD = atrial septal defect; RV = right ventricular; PAH = pulmonary arterial hypertension; VSD = ventricular septal defect; LV = left ventricular; PDA = patent ductus arteriosus; AVSD = atrioventricular septal defect; PA = pulmonary artery; TOF = tetralogy of Fallot; CHF = congestive heart failure; SVC = superior vena cava; IVC = inferior vena cava.

ICU Care

Regarding the need for ICU admission, a study from Quebec reported that 16 per cent of GUCH patients required intensive care, and those with severe CHD had a significantly longer length of ICU stay. Boston Children's Hospital reported that their adult admissions went from 3.6 per cent of total cardiac ICU admissions in 1995 to 9.1 per cent in 2009, demonstrating increasing demands on ICU resources. The Boston data also highlight the ongoing debate between paediatric and adult CHD centres about who is best positioned to care for adults with CHD. Data in 2008 from the United States report that the estimated mortality rate for GUCH patients operated on by paediatric

heart surgeons was significantly lower than that for GUCH patients operated on by non-paediatric heart surgeons. Having a specialised multidisciplinary team for these patients has also been shown to reduce mortality. These debates between CHD centres should serve as a warning to non-CHD centres that early referral of GUCH patients to a CHD centre is important to facilitate management and organise appropriate-level care. This appears to be particularly relevant to medical admissions by GUCH patients to the ICU. Research from The Brompton (UK) has demonstrated that mortality associated with medical admissions for GUCH patients was far higher than for admissions for routine cardiac surgery, highlighting the need for non-CHD

107

centres to refer early, even if congenital surgical intervention is not required. Whilst it is beyond the scope of this chapter to describe the in-depth critical care management of an adult with CHD, a suggested approach is provided in Tables 3.1.5.3 and 3.1.5.4.

History and Clinical Examination

For every GUCH patient presenting to hospital, a thorough and focussed history is required. The patient may have a medical passport or a letter outlining their past medical history, but specific points to consider include the following:

1. What is their exercise tolerance/New York Heart Association (NYHA) class?
   a. How much exertion can the patient tolerate?
   b. Have there been any recent changes in exercise tolerance?
2. Do they have a history of pulmonary hypertension?
   a. Is the patient on home oxygen?
   b. Is the patient on pulmonary vasodilator therapy (calcium channel blockers, endothelin receptor antagonists, phosphodiesterase type 5 inhibitors, prostanoids)?
   c. Is there limited exercise capacity, cyanosis, signs of right ventricular failure or haemoptysis?
3. Do they have a pacemaker/implantable cardioverter–defibrillator?
   a. Is the pacemaker functioning?
   b. When was the last device interrogation?
4. Ask about medications, in particular:
   a. Anticoagulants (a history of venous thrombi may indicate difficult venous access)
   b. Anti-platelets
   c. Pulmonary vasodilators
   d. Oxygen
   e. Anti-arrhythmics
   f. Anti-hypertensives
   g. Infusions (milrinone, prostanoids)

Additionally, on examination, assess for:
- Perfusion:
  ○ Does the patient feel warm or cool peripherally?
  ○ Can you feel peripheral pulses? May require four-limb blood pressure
  ○ What is the rhythm?
  ○ What is the patient's lactate, base excess ± central or mixed venous saturation?
- Left heart failure:
  ○ Pulmonary congestion on chest X-ray
  ○ Pulmonary oedema
  ○ Pleural effusions
  ○ Peripheral hypoperfusion
  ○ Gallop rhythm
- Right heart failure:
  ○ Elevated jugular venous pressure (JVP)/central venous pressure (CVP)
  ○ Hepatomegaly
  ○ Deranged liver function
  ○ Ascites
  ○ Peripheral oedema

Investigations

Table 3.1.5.3 Suggested investigations

Full blood count	• Polycythaemia may indicate the presence of a cyanotic heart defect • Thrombocytopenia may be present in cyanosis
Electrolytes and liver function tests	• Abnormal electrolytes may predispose the patient to arrhythmias • Elevated creatinine/reduced GFR may be long-standing or may indicate systemic hypoperfusion • Elevated liver function tests may indicate right heart failure • Abnormal pre-operative bilirubin, creatinine or thyroid hormone levels have been shown to be highly predictive of mortality
Coagulation	• The patient may be on anticoagulant or anti-platelet therapy (input from haematology may be required if surgery/continued therapy/interruption to usual therapy is expected) • Altered hepatic function and coagulation may indicate right heart failure
ABG and VBG	• Mixed venous or central venous saturations, lactate and base excess can all provide information regarding adequacy of perfusion • Check PaO_2 • $PaCO_2$ may be important in relation to management of pulmonary hypertension
Septic screen	• Consider whether a septic screen needs to be sent • Some patients are at a higher risk of developing infective endocarditis • Many GUCH patients will be less able to tolerate a septic episode

Chest X-ray	• Check for situs inversus • Cardiomegaly • Pulmonary congestion • Pleural or pericardial effusions • Pacemaker/ICD
ECG	• Arrhythmias are often poorly tolerated and require early identification • Is the patient pacemaker-dependent?
Echo	• LV and RV function • Evaluate the connections of the atria and ventricles • Measure pulmonary pressure • Look at heart valve morphology and function • Examine for intra-cardiac shunts and for the presence of thrombi
Cardiac MRI and cardiac catheterisation	• May require GUCH specialists to interpret adequately

Abbreviations: GFR = glomerular filtration rate; ABG = arterial blood gas; VBG = venous blood gas; GUCH = grown-up congenital heart disease; ICD = implantable cardioverter–defibrillator; Echo = echocardiography; LV = left ventricular; RV = right ventricular.

Management

Patients with complex histories may have a medical passport or a letter from their cardiologist/general practitioner outlining the details of their condition. Consider contacting the patient's cardiac centre for information on their clinical condition and for advice regarding management and possible transfer. Many, however, are lost to follow-up or fail to disclose their underlying condition.

Consider the interactions of the ICU condition and the patient's cardiac condition. General points of consideration are shown in Table 3.1.5.4.

Summary

Advances in interventions and perioperative management have led to the majority of children with CHD surviving into adulthood. Adults with CHD have higher rates of healthcare resource utilisation, when compared

Table 3.1.5.4 General points of consideration for congenital heart disease patients

Intubation	• If the patient requires induction, a cautious approach is recommended • Benzodiazepines and propofol may have catastrophic effects on a failing heart
IV access	• Central venous access may be difficult due to multiple prior interventions, surgeries and ICU admissions (re-sternotomy, if required, may also be highly problematic) • Be vigilant to avoid air emboli. The presence of shunts may result in stroke
Arrhythmias	• Some patients are at higher risk of developing an arrhythmia (e.g. patients post-tetralogy of Fallot repair are at an increased risk of ventricular arrhythmia, and 50% of patients with Ebstein's anomaly have Wolff–Parkinson–White syndrome) • Some patients may be very dependent on their atrial kick to maintain adequate cardiac output (e.g. single ventricle patients) • Be cautious if the patient requires cardioversion for an arrhythmia • Unless in an emergent situation, rule out the presence of an intra-cardiac thrombus and obtain advice from the patient's primary team • Management may require transoesophageal echocardiography and input from cardiologists and electrophysiologists specialising in GUCH patients; ultimately, the patient may even require ablation or surgical intervention • Consider early device interrogation, if present
Regional anaesthesia/ CSF sampling	• Be careful with regional techniques (e.g. obtaining CSF samples or providing epidural analgesia for fractured ribs) – the patient may be fully anticoagulated
Infective endocarditis	• Patients with congenital heart disease may be at an increased risk of developing IE • IE may be difficult to identify in patients with complex anatomy • If IE is identified, contact the patient's primary team early to discuss management
Ventilation	• Chronically elevated left atrial pressure (due to ventricular dysfunction), parenchymal lung disease, smoking and chest wall abnormalities from multiple sternotomies may result in the requirement for higher levels of mean airway pressure and PEEP. These may have serious adverse effects when required in the setting of RV failure or in single ventricle physiology • In ARDS, high airway pressures may raise Fontan or right-sided pressures, resulting in reduced venous return to the heart, with resultant reductions in cardiac output • Positive pressure ventilation may, however, be beneficial in a patient with left heart failure
Coagulation	• Some GUCH patients are at high risk of thrombosis (e.g. those with mechanical heart valves or Fontan circulation). It is important to encourage early mobilisation and to liaise with haematology specialists regarding appropriate thromboembolism cover whilst in the ICU. This must also be balanced with increased bleeding risk often seen in these patients (e.g. polycythaemic patients can have reduced platelet function, and right heart failure can result in liver failure and reduced production of clotting factors, etc.)

Table 3.1.5.4 (cont.)

Systemic vascular resistance	• Reduced systemic vascular resistance (e.g. sepsis or anaesthesia) may result in reversal of flow through a shunt (e.g. through an ASD or VSD, etc.), resulting in 'right-to-left' shunt and worsening hypoxia. Increasing systemic vascular resistance may help to return shunt flow to 'left-to-right' and to improve oxygen saturations • Caution is required when increasing vascular resistance in the context of a failing systemic ventricle
Renal	• Patients with cyanotic CHD or Eisenmenger syndrome are more likely to have moderately to severely impaired renal function • Patients with elevated venous pressures (tetralogy of Fallot, Ebstein's anomaly, Fontan circulation) are at risk of renal hypoperfusion when arterial pressure is reduced, e.g. in septic shock • Elevated intra-abdominal pressure (e.g. with severe ascites in a failing Fontan or with RV failure) may also result in renal injury
Liver	• Generalised systemic hypoperfusion may result in acute-on-chronic hepatic failure • Liver congestion can occur in right heart failure • Patients with a Fontan are particularly at risk of developing cirrhosis, portal hypertension and varices
LV failure	• Support cardiac output with adrenaline (± milrinone); support blood pressure with noradrenaline, and ensure adequate oxygen delivery by optimising haematocrit, FiO_2 and volume • Positive pressure ventilation may also be advantageous by reducing work of breathing and LV transmural pressure • Consider emergency control of arrhythmia if thought to be contributing to cardiac failure • Further reducing afterload may be helpful (i.e. with furosemide, opioids and/or nitrates), but this can also result in profound hypotension
RV failure	• Consider oxygen, inhaled nitric oxide and/or milrinone (being aware that milrinone can drop systemic vascular resistance, so additional systemic vascular resistance support may be required) • Heart failure may be best managed in a centre with ECMO, ventricular assist backup and transplant services

Abbreviations: IV = intravenous; GUCH = grown-up congenital heart disease; CSF = cerebrospinal fluid; IE = infective endocarditis; PEEP = positive end-expiratory pressure; RV = right ventricular; ARDS = acute respiratory distress syndrome; ASD = atrial septal defect; VSD = ventricular septal defect; CHD = congenital heart disease; LV = left ventricular; ECMO = extracorporeal membrane oxygenation.

to the general population. The often complex physiology seen with GUCH means that this growing specialty cannot be provided for by every healthcare centre. Experience at non-cardiac and general cardiac centres at times may be limited. It is important that the general critical care physician is aware of issues relevant to the GUCH patient, whether they are presenting with morbidity directly relating to their cardiac condition or due to the usual critical care conditions that affect the general population. If in doubt about how to manage the patient, contact the nearest specialist centre for immediate advice.

References and Further Reading

Allan CK. Intensive care of the adult patient with congenital heart disease. *Progr Cardiovasc Dis* 2011;**53**:274–80.

Andropoulos DB, Stayer SA, Russell IA. *Anesthesia for Congenital Heart Disease*. Hoboken, NJ: Wiley-Blackwell; 2010.

Fraser CD, Kane LC. Congenital heart disease. In: C Townsend, RD Beauchamp, BM Evers, K Mattox (eds). *Sabiston Textbook of Surgery*, 20th edn. Philadelphia, PA: WB Saunders; 2016. pp. 1619–57.

Kelleher A. Adult congenital heart disease (grown-up congenital heart disease). *Contin Educ Anaesth Crit Care Pain* 2012;**12**:28–32.

Webb GD, Smallhorn JF, Therrien J, Redington AN. Congenital heart disease. In: D Mann, D Zipes, P Libby, R Bonow, E Braunwald (eds). *Brawnwald's Heart Disease. A Textbook of Cardiovascular Medicine*, 10th edn. Philadelphia, PA: Elsevier; 2015. pp. 1391–445.

3.1.6

Endocarditis

Selina Ho and Michael Hoy

Key Learning Points

1. Infective endocarditis (IE) is an infection of the endocardial surface of the heart, often affecting the valves of the heart.
2. Its management should involve a collaborative, multidisciplinary 'Endocarditis Team'.
3. For invasive procedures, prophylactic antibiotics are not required for patients deemed at intermediate or low risk.
4. Echocardiography (transthoracic and transoesophageal), positive blood cultures and clinical features remain the cornerstone of IE diagnosis.
5. The Duke criteria are useful but should not replace the clinical judgement of the Endocarditis Team.

Keywords: infective endocarditis, Endocarditis Team, echocardiography, Duke criteria

Introduction

Infective endocarditis (IE) is an infection of the endocardial surface of the heart, often affecting the valves of the heart. It continues to be a serious and deadly disease despite advances in its management. The new European and American guidelines emphasise a collaborative, multidisciplinary 'Endocarditis Team', composed of primary care physicians, cardiologists, cardiac surgeons, microbiologists and infectious disease (ID) specialists.

Prevention

Previous recommendations on antibiotic prophylaxis for IE for invasive procedures was altered for a more restrictive approach in 2002, and in 2008, the National Institute for Health and Care Excellence (NICE) guidelines advised against any antibiotic prophylaxis. However, antibiotic prophylaxis is limited to those patients with the highest risk of IE, as IE in such patients has a worse prognosis and is often associated with devastating outcomes. Prophylactic antibiotics are not required for patients deemed at intermediate or low risk. High-risk patients are those listed in Box 3.1.6.1.

> **Box 3.1.6.1 High-Risk Patients**
>
> - Patients with cardiac prosthetic materials (e.g. prosthetic valves, homografts)
> - Previous endocarditis
> - Untreated cyanotic congenital heart disease
> - Congenital heart disease patients with post-operative palliative shunts/conduits/prostheses

Controversy remains over whether antibiotic prophylaxis is required in cardiac transplant patients, and current European guidelines do not recommend prophylaxis.

The 'Endocarditis Team'

IE is a multi-system disease, with a wide variety of presentations, depending on the organ affected, whether the patient has any underlying cardiac diseases, the microorganism and the presence of complications. IE is therefore best managed with an Endocarditis Team involving practitioners from several specialties with a high level of expertise. Adoption of the Endocarditis Team approach has been shown to significantly reduce 1-year mortality from 18 to 8 per cent.

Diagnosis

Clinical Features

IE remains a diagnostic challenge and should be considered in a wide range of clinical situations. IE can present acutely with rapid progression, subacutely or chronically with a low-grade fever and non-specific symptoms. Table 3.1.6.1 outlines the common clinical presentations of IE.

Twenty-five per cent of patients have embolic complications at the time of diagnosis, which may be the first presenting feature of IE. Emboli are most often seen to the brain, lung or spleen. Hence, IE should be considered as a differential diagnosis in patients presenting with fever and embolic phenomena. Have a low threshold for investigations to rule out IE in high-risk groups and in elderly or immunocompromised patients who may present with atypical features.

Diagnostic Criteria

Echocardiography (transthoracic and transoesophageal), positive blood cultures and clinical features remain the cornerstone of IE diagnosis. Diagnostic classification using the modified Duke criteria is based on clinical, echocardiographic, biological findings and the results of blood cultures and serologies (Tables 3.1.6.2 and 3.1.6.3).

This classification has a sensitivity of approximately 80 per cent.

The modified Duke criteria classify patients into three categories, based on the number of major and minor criteria (Table 3.1.6.4).

The modified Duke criteria have a lower diagnostic accuracy for early diagnosis, particularly in patients with prosthetic valve endocarditis (PVE) and pacemaker lead IE, as echocardiography is inconclusive.

Duke criteria are useful, but they do not replace the clinical judgement of the Endocarditis Team. The additional imaging techniques discussed in this chapter have improved the diagnosis of IE, particularly in difficult cases. Identification of paravalvular lesions on cardiac CT is a major criterion. Recent silent embolic events or mycotic aneurysms on imaging only are only a minor criterion.

Table 3.1.6.1 Clinical presentation of infective endocarditis

	Clinical presentation
CVS	New murmurs in 85% of patients
	Worsening pre-existing murmur
	Coronary embolism
	Heart failure
Respiratory	Pulmonary embolism
	Glomerulonephritis
GI	Splenomegaly
	Hepatic embolism
Immunological	Splinter haemorrhages
	Janeway lesions
	Osler's nodes
	Roth spots
CNS	Neurological symptoms related to cerebral embolism, intracranial haemorrhage or cerebral abscess
Renal	Haematuria
Other	Fever – most common finding
	Anorexia
	Malaise
	Weight loss
	Protracted 'flu-like' course

Abbreviations: CVS = cardiovascular system; GI = gastrointestinal; CNS = central nervous system.

Table 3.1.6.2 Duke major criteria

Positive blood cultures	Typical microorganisms for infective endocarditis from at least two cultures: *Viridans* streptococci, *Streptococcus gallolyticus, Staphylococcus aureus,* HACEK group[a]
	Blood cultures must be consistently positive (>2 positive blood cultures drawn 12 hours apart)
	Single positive blood culture for *Coxiella burnetii*
Positive imaging	Echocardiogram demonstrating vegetation, abscess, pseudoaneurysm, intra-cardiac fistula, valvular perforation, aneurysm, new partial dehiscence of prosthetic valve
	Definite paravalvular lesions by cardiac CT

[a] The acronym HACEK refers to a group of fastidious Gram-negative coccobacillary organisms. HACEK stands for *Haemophilus* species, *Aggregatibacter* species, *Cardiobacterium hominis, Eikenella corrodens* and *Kingella* species.

Table 3.1.6.3 Duke minor criteria

Fever	Temperature >38°C
Predisposition	Predisposing heart condition, intravenous drug use
Vascular phenomena	May include incidental findings on imaging. Major arterial emboli, septic pulmonary infarcts, mycotic aneurysm, intracranial haemorrhage, conjunctival haemorrhages and Janeway lesions
Immunological phenomena	Glomerulonephritis, Osler's nodes, Roth spots and rheumatoid factor
Microbiological evidence	Positive blood culture but does not meet major criterion

Table 3.1.6.4 Modified Duke criteria

Category	Pathological criteria	Clinical criteria
Definite IE	Microorganisms by blood culture Histological examination of vegetation, embolised vegetation or intra-cardiac abscess specimen Active endocarditis on histology	Two major criteria One major and three minor criteria Five minor criteria
Possible IE	Nil	One major and one minor criterion Three minor criteria
Reject IE	No pathological evidence at surgery/autopsy	Firm alternative diagnosis Resolution of symptoms with <4 days of antibiotics Does not meet criteria for possible endocarditis

Abbreviations: IE = infective endocarditis.

Laboratory Investigations

Biomarkers have poor predictive value for IE and are only used for risk stratification – Sequential Organ Failure Assessment (SOFA) score and creatinine clearance (European System for Cardiac Operative Risk Evaluation (EuroSCORE) II).

Imaging Techniques

Diagnosis and management of IE are highly dependent on imaging, particularly echocardiography. Prognostication and follow-up also rely heavily on echocardiography. Using information gathered from imaging allows risk assessments of embolic phenomena. Echocardiography is essential in the diagnosis and management of IE. Other diagnostics that may be helpful include MRI, multi-slice computed tomography (MSCT) and nuclear imaging. These modalities are also helpful in the follow-up and decision-making process. About 50 per cent of IE cases undergo surgery during their hospital stay. Early communication with the cardiac surgical team is essential, particularly in cases of complicated IE.

Echocardiography

Transthoracic (TTE) or transoesophageal echocardiography (TOE) is the imaging modality of choice for the diagnosis of IE. It is also mandatory for follow-up and monitoring of response to treatment. Patients with *Staphylococcus aureus* bacteraemia should have TTE to rule out IE, as the organism causes terrible complications once IE is established.

Echocardiographic diagnostic criteria are vegetation, abscess or pseudoaneurysm, and new dehiscence of a prosthetic valve. Specificity is 90 per cent for both TTE and TOE, and sensitivity for diagnosis is 70 per cent for TTE and 96 per cent for TOE.

Patients with intra-cardiac devices are a challenge to diagnose with echocardiography (TTE or TOE), and other imaging modalities should be considered if IE is still suspected. Small abscesses are difficult to identify, especially in early stages of formation. Repeat TTE/TOE within 5–7 days, in conjunction with other imaging modalities, after a negative echocardiography if suspicion of IE remains high, or in cases of *S. aureus* bacteraemia.

Multi-Slice Computed Tomography

Whilst coronary angiography is often required prior to cardiac surgery, vegetations can embolise during angiography, causing haemodynamic instability. MSCT coronary angiography thus provides a useful non-invasive alternative for such patients. Detecting abscesses and pseudoaneurysms using MSCT is comparable to using TOE, with the added benefit of also providing information regarding the size, extent and anatomy of the lesions, and may reveal concomitant pulmonary disease. MRI is a superior imaging modality for detection of cerebral consequences. However, CT is a more practical alternative for the critically ill patient.

Magnetic Resonance Imaging

Up to 80 per cent of cerebral lesions are ischaemic in nature, regardless of neurological presentations. Frequent small ischaemic lesions are more common than larger infarcts. Only 10 per cent are parenchymal or subarachnoid haemorrhages, abscesses or mycotic aneurysms. Ischaemic lesions are found in half of all IE patients without neurological complaints; thus, systematic cerebral MRI can impact the diagnosis of IE by one minor Duke score in patients without neurological symptoms, and can influence medical and surgical planning in patients with positive neurological signs.

Nuclear Imaging

For patients who fall under the modified Duke category of 'possible IE', nuclear imaging reduces the rate of misdiagnosed IE and improves the detection of embolic and metastatic events.

Microbiological Diagnosis

Healthcare-Associated Infective Endocarditis

Approximately 30 per cent of all IE cases are healthcare-related. It is associated with severe prognosis. Epidemiological studies show an increase in *Staphylococcus* and healthcare-associated IE, and thus infection control measures are of upmost importance.

Blood Culture-Positive Infective Endocarditis

The vast majority of IE cases are due to staphylococci or streptococci. Identifying the causative microorganism is the cornerstone of diagnosis. Three sets of blood cultures, taken at 30-minute intervals, for both sensitivity and culture should be sampled from a peripheral vein to avoid contamination and misinterpretation from a central venous catheter. It is important to obtain cultures before administration of antibiotics. Bacteraemia is constant in IE; therefore, there is no rationale for delaying blood sampling with peaks of pyrexia and, importantly, virtually all blood cultures should test positive. (A single positive result should therefore be interpreted with caution.) Following 48–72 hours of antibiotic treatment, blood cultures should be repeated.

Blood Culture-Negative Infective Endocarditis

Blood culture-negative IE (BCNIE) refers to IE in which no causative microorganism can be identified with conventional blood culture investigations. Up to a third of all IE cases are BCNIE and pose considerable diagnostic and management dilemmas. Mortality is very high (50 per cent), and input from ID specialists and surgical options are recommended. If BCNIE is thought to be a result of previous antibiotic administration, antibiotics may need to be withheld and blood cultures repeated. Other causes are fungi (most frequently observed in PVE, or IE in intravenous drug users (IVDUs) and immunocompromised patients) and fastidious bacteria such as intracellular bacteria. More rare causes of BCNIE include antiphospholipid syndrome and allergic response to porcine bioprosthesis.

Histological Diagnosis

The gold standard diagnostic test for IE is pathological examination of resected valvular tissue or embolic fragments. The specimens should be tested for identification of culprit microorganisms.

Prognostic Assessment

Prognostic assessment should be made at admission and used to aid decision for best clinical management. In-hospital mortality is between 15 and 30 per cent; thus, rapid identification is critical for prognosis. Prognosis is influenced by patient characteristics, the presence or absence of cardiac and non-cardiac complications, the microorganism and echocardiographic findings. Those at highest risk of death are patients with heart failure and periannular complications and *S. aureus* infections, and should be considered for urgent or emergent surgery. Patients with *S. aureus* IE complicated by heart failure and periannular lesions have mortality of up to 80 per cent, highlighting the importance of early diagnosis and management by the Endocarditis Team.

Predictors of poor in-hospital outcome include diabetes, septic shock, ischaemic stroke, brain haemorrhage and the need for renal replacement therapy. Lack of infection control (demonstrated by positive blood cultures 48–72 hours after antibiotic treatment) is an independent risk factor for in-hospital mortality. Approximately half of all IE cases undergo cardiac surgery during their hospital stay. Those who have prohibitive surgical risk have the worst outcome.

Complications of Infective Endocarditis

Indications for Surgery

There are three main indications for early surgery: heart failure, uncontrolled infection and prevention of embolic events. The active phase of IE treatment refers to the duration of antibiotic therapy, and the reason to consider cardiac surgery during this period is to avoid progressive heart failure and irreversible myocardial damage or systemic complications of IE.

Surgery during the active phase of IE is not without significant risk and should be carefully considered, particularly in those with high-risk features. Given the complex decision process, early consultation with a cardiac surgeon is best practice.

Heart Failure

Heart failure is the most common and severe complication of IE and is the most common indication for early surgery. Up to 60 per cent of patients with native valve endocarditis (NVE) develop heart failure, and it is most prevalent with aortic valve IE. Heart failure is a result of worsening severe aortic and mitral regurgitation. However, fistulae and valve obstruction may also occur.

Uncontrolled Infection

Uncontrolled infection is the deadliest complication of IE, and early surgery is required when there is persisting infection with signs of local uncontrolled infection. It is due to resistant or very virulent organisms and/or related perivalvular extension.

Systemic Embolism

Up to half of all IE cases are complicated by embolic phenomena, and this is often the presenting complaint. Once antibiotic therapy is initiated, the incidence of emboli falls dramatically. The risks of embolism are highest during the first 2 weeks of anti-microbial therapy, and the obvious risk factors relate to the size and mobility of the vegetation. In addition to these factors, previous embolism, the type of microorganism and the duration of medical treatment are carefully considered on a bespoke basis before deciding on early cardiac surgery.

Neurological Complications

Symptomatic neurological events develop in up to one-third of all patients with IE, but silent events are also frequently encountered and often go undetected until incidental scanning. Both ischaemic and haemorrhagic strokes are associated with high mortality. Prevention of the first or subsequent neurological complications is achieved by rapid diagnosis and initiation of anti-microbial treatment.

Infectious Aneurysms

Mycotic aneurysms are most commonly located intracranially and have a high tendency to rupture and haemorrhage. Early detection and treatment are therefore pivotal to reducing the high morbidity and mortality associated with rupture. Both CT and MRI accurately detect infectious aneurysms. However, angiography is still the gold standard. Ruptured aneurysms should be managed emergently, and unruptured mycotic aneurysms should be treated with antibiotics and watched carefully with repeated imaging. Consider endovascular interventions prior to cardiac surgery.

Splenic Complications

Consider splenic abscess or rupture in patients with persistent or recurrent fever, abdominal pain and bacteraemia. Splenic infarcts are often asymptomatic and very common.

Myocarditis and Pericarditis

Myocarditis is often associated with abscess formation, immune reactions and cardiac failure. If ventricular arrhythmias are experienced, this is an indicator of poor prognosis and one must urgently reassess for myocardial involvement with echocardiography or cardiac MRI.

Heart Rhythm and Conduction Disturbances

Conduction disturbances are infrequent, but their presence is associated with a worse prognosis and higher mortality. Rhythm disorders occur as a result of spreading infection from the valves to the conduction pathways, so investigate for perivalvular complications.

Musculoskeletal Manifestations

IE can result in complications involving the musculoskeletal system. The more severe complications include vertebral and pyogenic osteomyelitis.

Acute Renal Failure

Acute renal injury is an all too common complication of IE (30 per cent). Its presence worsens the prognosis and is independently associated with an increased risk of in-hospital mortality and perioperative events. The pathophysiology is multifactorial, including:

- Septic emboli resulting in renal infarction
- Immune complex and vasculitic glomerulonephritis
- Malperfusion as a result of heart failure or sepsis
- Nephrotoxics.

Renal replacement therapy may be necessary for management of advanced acute renal injury but carries with it associated mortality.

Infective Endocarditis in the Intensive Care Unit

Patients with IE often require admission to the ICU, especially along the perioperative pathway following cardiac surgery. Indications for admission to the ICU may include haemodynamic instability due to severe sepsis or valvular pathology, overt heart failure and organ failures. Even with recent advances in diagnosis and management of IE, mortality remains especially high in the critically ill patient (80 per cent). Those admitted to the ICU will require a combination of mechanical ventilation (73 per cent), haemodynamic support (40 per cent) and renal replacement therapy.

Right-Sided Infective Endocarditis

Right-sided IE (10 per cent of IE cases) usually affects the tricuspid valve and is mostly seen in IVDUs, particularly if diagnosed with HIV. It is also becoming increasingly encountered in patients with pacemakers, implantable cardioverter–defibrillators (ICDs), central venous catheters and congenital heart defects. *S. aureus* is the causative microbe, accounting for 90 per cent of right-sided IE, and worryingly, methicillin-resistant strains are being detected with ever increasing frequency. In-hospital mortality is approximately 7 per cent. However, surgery is generally avoided in IVDUs due to the high recurrence rate, unless there are intractable symptoms.

Anti-thrombotic Therapy in Infective Endocarditis

Current evidence does not support routine anti-platelet or anticoagulation therapy for IE to prevent embolic phenomena. However, the usual indications for such therapy still apply but must be discussed with the Endocarditis Team on an individual basis.

References and Further Reading

Habib G, Lancellotti P, Atunes MJ, *et al.* 2015 ESC Guidelines for the management of infective endocarditis: The Task Force for the Management of Infective Endocarditis of the European Society of Cardiology (ESC). Endorsed by: European Association for Cardio-Thoracic Surgery (EACTS), the European Association of Nuclear Medicine (EANM). *Eur Heart J* 2015;**36**:3075–128.

Kang D-H, Kim Y-J, Kim S-H, *et al.* Early surgery versus conventional treatment for infective endocarditis. *N Engl J Med* 2012;**366**:2466–73.

National Institute for Health and Care Excellence. 2008. Antimicrobial prophylaxis against infective endocarditis in adults and children undergoing interventional procedures. Clinical guideline [CG64]. www.nice.org.uk/guidance/cg64

Prendergast BD, Tornos P. Surgery for infective endocarditis: who and when? *Circulation* 2010;**121**:1141–52.

Sharma V, Candililo L, Hausenloy DJ. Infective endocarditis: an intensive care perspective. *Trends Anaes Crit Care* 2010;**2**:36–41.

Sonneville R, Mourvillier B, Bouadma L, Wolff M. Management of neurological complications of infective endocarditis in ICU patients. *Ann Intensive Care* 2011;**1**:10.

Thury F, Grisoli D, Collart F, Habib G, Raoult D. Management of infective endocarditis: challenges and perspectives. *Lancet* 2012;**379**:965–75.

Management of Hypertensive Crises

Katarina Lenartova and Anne-Marie Leo

Key Learning Points

1. These patients can present with vague symptoms or no symptoms at all.
2. It is important to establish if there is end-organ damage at an earlier stage in the course of treatment.
3. Distinguishing a hypertensive emergency from hypertensive urgencies helps in guiding acute treatment.
4. Aim to reduce the systolic blood pressure within the first hour according to the appropriate recommended level for the condition involved.
5. The choice of pharmacological agent and target blood pressure should be determined by the underlying pathology.

Keywords: hypertensive emergencies, hypertensive urgencies, end-organ damage, medications

Definitions

Hypertensive crises are defined as elevations in blood pressure >180/120 mmHg and are classified into:

- **Hypertensive emergencies** (in which hypertension is associated with progressive or impending end-organ injury)
- **Hypertensive urgencies** (in which symptoms may be present, but end-organ injury has not yet occurred)

It is important to note that blood pressures lower than this can still result in accelerated end-organ injury. This is particularly important in pregnancy and in children, due to lower blood pressure norms.

Epidemiology

Worldwide, hypertension occurs in approximately 1 billion people and may be responsible for up to 7.5 million deaths annually. Approximately 5 per cent of patients with a history of hypertension will have at least one hypertensive urgency, and 1 per cent will have at least one hypertensive emergency. Hypertension affects men at a slightly higher rate than women, and hypertension and hypertensive emergencies occur more frequently in the black population, when compared to Caucasian or Asian populations.

Presentation of Hypertensive Crises

Patients with hypertensive urgency may be asymptomatic or complain of vague symptoms. Patients with hypertensive emergency (whatever the cause) (Table 3.1.7.1) present with symptoms of end-organ damage, including chest pain, dyspnoea, anxiety, epistaxis, headache, focal neurological deficit, encephalopathy, visual disturbance, altered mental status, nausea, fatigue or dizziness. A large Italian multi-centre study examining emergency department presentations reported that 23 per cent of hypertensive crises occurred in patients with undiagnosed hypertension, and hypertensive emergencies occurred in 25.3 per cent of these crisis episodes. Of these hypertensive emergencies, 55.6 per cent of patients reported non-specific symptoms, and 30.9 per cent had acute pulmonary oedema, 22 per cent stroke, 17.9 per cent myocardial infarction, 7.9 per cent aortic dissection, 5.9 per cent acute renal failure and 4.9 per cent hypertensive encephalopathy. Adverse effects of hypertensive crises can be seen in Table 3.1.7.2.

Table 3.1.7.1 Causes of hypertensive crises

Uncontrolled essential hypertension
Endocrine: • Primary hyperaldosteronism • Phaeochromocytoma • Cushing's syndrome • Renin-secreting adenoma • Hyperparathyroidism or thyroid disease
Sympathomimetic ingestion: • Cocaine • Methamphetamine • Phencyclidine ingestion • Tyramine or sympathomimetic ingestion whilst on monoamine oxidase inhibitors

Table 3.1.7.1 (cont.)

Severe pre-eclampsia (systolic blood pressure >140 mmHg or diastolic blood pressure <90 mmHg) with proteinuria (>300 mg/24 hours) after 20 weeks of gestation

Renal parenchymal disease:
- Glomerulonephritis
- Vasculitis
- Thrombotic thrombocytopenic purpura
- Haemolytic uraemic syndrome

Renovascular disease:
- Renal artery stenosis (seen in 4% of black and 32% of white populations presenting with severe hypertension)

Secondary to end-organ injury:
- Dissecting aortic aneurysm
- Stroke
- Subarachnoid haemorrhage
- Intracranial tumour
- Autonomic hyper-reflexia after spinal cord injury
- Sleep apnoea

Drug-induced (e.g. oral contraceptives, steroids, non-steroidal anti-inflammatory drugs)

Rebound hypertension following discontinuation of medications (clonidine, minoxidil, beta-blockers)

Abrupt withdrawal of alcohol

Perioperative hypertension:
- Adrenergic stimulation from surgical event
- Post-operative pain/anxiety

Coarctation of the aorta

Table 3.1.7.2 Adverse effects of hypertensive crises

Cardiovascular emergencies	Neurological emergencies
Acute coronary syndrome (myocardial infarction, unstable angina)	Cerebral infarction
Aortic dissection	Hypertensive encephalopathy
Acute heart failure	Subarachnoid haemorrhage
Pulmonary oedema	Intracerebral haemorrhage
Hypertensive retinopathy (papilloedema, haemorrhage, retinal oedema)	Eclampsia
Hypertensive nephropathy	

Table 3.1.7.3 Suggested workup for a patient with uncontrolled hypertension

Targeted history and clinical examination	To assess for causes and end-organ injury
Serum creatinine/ glomerular filtration rate	Assessment of renal function
Haemoglobin/Hct	Elevated Hct may indicate sleep apnoea
Electrolytes	Results may indicate glucocorticoid or mineralocorticoid excess Hypokalaemia (suggests Cushing's syndrome or primary aldosteronism) Hyperkalaemia (with normal function and low bicarbonate may suggest Gordon syndrome) Hypernatraemia (suggests primary aldosteronism) Serum bicarbonate (high bicarbonate suggests aldosterone excess) Hypercalcaemia (suggests hyperparathyroidism)
Urinalysis	Proteinuria and haematuria may identify a secondary cause or identify end-organ injury
ECG	May demonstrate LVH and old MI
Serum lipids	To assess for co-risk factors
Glucose	To assess for co-risk factors
Renal duplex ultrasound	Consider for assessment of renal artery stenosis
Fundoscopy	Flame haemorrhages, cotton-wool spots, papilloedema, visual acuity changes
CT brain/CT angiography/ echocardiography	As indicated from clinical examination (stroke, coarctation, aortic dissection, etc.)

Abbreviations: Hct = haematocrit; LVH = left ventricular hypertrophy; MI = myocardial infarction.

Management

Table 3.1.7.3 shows suggested workup for a patient with uncontrolled hypertension. Management of hypertensive crises often requires immediate control of dangerously elevated blood pressure, followed by disease-specific interventions. The 2017 American College of Cardiology (ACC)/American Heart Association (AHA) 'Guideline for the prevention, detection, evaluation, and management for high blood pressure in adults' recommends that patients with hypertensive emergency should be admitted to the ICU. They stratify patients into two groups: (1) those with aortic dissection, severe pre-eclampsia or eclampsia or phaeochromocytoma crisis; and (2) those without. Those with the above pathologies (group 1) are recommended to have their blood pressure lowered to <140 mmHg during the first hour (<120 mmHg in aortic dissection). Those in group 2 (without pathologies) are recommended to have their blood pressure reduced by a maximum of 25 per cent over the first hour, to 160/110 mmHg over the next 2–6 hours and then to normal levels over the next 24–48 hours.

Disease-Specific Management
Neurological Emergencies

- **Hypertensive encephalopathy:** in hypertensive encephalopathy, treatment guidelines state to reduce the mean arterial pressure (MAP) by 25 per cent over an 8-hour period. Labetalol, nicardipine and esmolol are the preferred medications.
- **Acute ischaemic stroke:** withhold anti-hypertensive medications unless the systolic blood pressure (SBP) is above 220 mmHg or the diastolic blood pressure (DBP) is above 120 mmHg, unless the patient is eligible for intravenous tissue plasminogen activator (tPA). If eligible, then aim for a gradual reduction of blood pressure, with an SBP goal of <185 mmHg and a DBP goal of <110 mmHg before initiating thrombolytic therapy. Preferred medications are labetalol and nicardipine.
- **Acute intracerebral haemorrhage:** treatment is based on clinical/radiographic evidence of increased intracranial pressure (ICP). If there are signs of increased ICP, maintain the MAP just below 130 mmHg (or SBP <180 mmHg) for the first 24 hours after onset. In patients without increased ICP, maintain the MAP below 110 mmHg (or SBP <160 mmHg) for the first 24 hours after symptom onset.
- **Subarachnoid haemorrhage:** maintain the SBP below 160 mmHg until the aneurysm is treated or cerebral vasospasm occurs. Although oral nimodipine is used to prevent delayed ischaemic neurological deficits, it is not indicated for treating acute hypertension.

Cardiovascular Emergencies

- **Aortic dissection:** beta-blockers are recommended anti-hypertensive agents in patients with hypertension and thoracic aortic disease. However, avoid beta-blockers if there is aortic valvular regurgitation or suspected cardiac tamponade. For adults with aortic dissection, rapidly lower the SBP to below 120 mmHg.

The preferred agents are esmolol and labetalol. Maintain the SBP below 110 mmHg, unless signs of end-organ hypoperfusion are present. Preferred treatment includes a combination of narcotic analgesics (morphine), beta-blockers (labetalol, esmolol) and vasodilators (nicardipine, nitroprusside).

- **Acute coronary syndrome:** in adults with hypertension at an increased risk of heart failure, the optimal blood pressure should be below 130/80 mmHg. In acute heart failure, the preferred medications are intravenous or sublingual nitroglycerin. Treat with vasodilators (in addition to diuretics), aiming for an SBP of 140 mmHg.
- **Phaeochromocytoma/cocaine toxicity:** phaeochromocytoma treatment guidelines are similar to those of cocaine toxicity. The ACC/AHA recommend lowering the SBP to below 140 mmHg during the first hour with 5 mg boluses of intravenous phentolamine. Additional bolus doses may be given every 10 minutes to achieve target blood pressure. Only after alpha-blockade can beta-blockers to be added for blood pressure control.
- **Pre-eclampsia/eclampsia:** the preferred medications are hydralazine, labetalol and nicardipine. If the platelet count is <100,000 cells/mm³, blood pressure should be maintained below 150/100 mmHg. Patients with eclampsia or pre-eclampsia should also be treated with intravenous magnesium to avoid seizures.

Summary

Hypertensive crises are classified into hypertensive emergencies and hypertensive urgencies. Patients with hypertensive urgency may be asymptomatic or they may complain of vague symptoms. Patients presenting with hypertensive emergency may present with symptoms of end-organ damage. The primary goal is to determine which patients with acute hypertension are at risk of, or have evolving, end-organ damage and, in turn, institute acute therapy promptly. The choice of pharmacological agent and target blood pressure should be determined by the underlying pathology. Parenteral drugs for treatment of hypertensive emergencies are shown in Table 3.1.7.4.

Table 3.1.7.4 Parenteral drugs for treatment of hypertensive emergencies

Drug	Dose	Onset of action	Duration of action	Adverse effects	Special indications
Vasodilators					
Sodium nitroprusside	0.25–10 µg/kg/min as IV infusion (maximal dose for 10 minutes only)	Immediate	1–2 minutes	Nausea, vomiting, muscle twitching, sweating, thiocyanate and cyanide intoxication	Most hypertensive emergencies, caution in patients with high intracranial pressure or azotaemia
Nicardipine hydrochloride	5–15 mg/hr IV	5–10 minutes	1–4 hours	Tachycardia, headache, flushing, local phlebitis	Most hypertensive emergencies, except acute heart failure, caution in patients with coronary ischaemia
Fenoldopam mesylate	0.1–0.3 µg/kg/min as IV infusion	<5 minutes	30 minutes	Tachycardia, headache, nausea, flushing	Most hypertensive emergencies, caution in patients with glaucoma
Nitroglycerin	5–100 µg/min as IV infusion	2–5 minutes	3–5 minutes	Headache, vomiting methaemoglobinaemia, tolerance with prolonged use	Coronary ischaemia
Enalaprilat	1.25–5 mg every 6 hours IV	15–30 minutes	6 hours	Precipitous fall in pressure in high renin states, response variable	Acute left ventricular failure, avoid in patients with acute myocardial infarction
Hydralazine hydrochloride	5–20 mg IV 10–50 mg IM	10–20 minutes 20–30 minutes	3–8 hours	Tachycardia, flushing, headache, vomiting, aggravation of angina	Eclampsia
Diazoxide	50–100 mg as IV bolus, repeated or as 15–30 mg/min infusion	2–4 minutes	6–12 hours	Nausea, flushing, tachycardia, chest pain	Now obsolete, used when intensive monitoring not available
Adrenergic inhibitors					
Labetalol hydrochloride	20–80 mg as IV bolus every 10 minutes or as 0.5–2.0 mg/min IV infusion	5–10 minutes	3–6 hours	Vomiting, scalp tingling, burning in throat, dizziness, nausea, heart block, orthostatic hypotension	Most hypertensive emergencies, except acute heart failure
Esmolol hydrochloride	250–500 µg/kg/min for 1 minute, then 50–100 µg/kg/min for 4 minutes, may repeat sequence	1–2 minutes	10–20 minutes	Hypotension, nausea	Aortic dissection, perioperative
Phentolamine	5–15 mg IV	1–2 minutes	3–10 minutes	Tachycardia, flushing, headache	Catecholamine excess

Abbreviations: IV = intravenous; IM = intramuscular.

References and Further Reading

Babar TB, Basman CL. Hypertension. In: FF Ferri (ed). *Ferri's Clinical Advisor 2017. E-Book*. Philadelphia, PA: Elsevier; 2017. pp. 639–643.e4.

Pinna G, Pascale C, Fornengo P, *et al.* Hospital admissions for hypertensive crisis in emergency departments: a large multicenter Italian study. *PLoS One* 2014;**9**:393542.

Shayne P, Lynch CA. Hypertensive crisis. In: JG Adams, ED Barton, JL Collings, PMC DeBlieux, MA Gisondi, ES Nadel (eds). *Emergency Medicine E-Book Clinical Essentials*, 2nd edn. Philadelphia, PA: Saunders; 2013. pp. 592–601.e1.

Suneja M, Sanders L. Hypertensive emergency. *Med Clin North Am* 2017;**101**:465–78.

Whelton PK, Carey RM, Aornow WS, *et al.* 2017 ACC/AHA/AAPA/ABC/ACPM/AGS/APhA/ASPC/NMA/PCNA guideline for the prevention, detection, evaluation, and management of high blood pressure in adults: a report of the American College of Cardiology/American Heart Association Task Force on Clinical Practice Guidelines. *Hypertension* 2018;**71**:e13–115.

3.1.8 Atrial Fibrillation in the Intensive Care Unit

Paul Harris

Key Learning Points

1. Atrial fibrillation is common in the intensive care unit and may occur in the structurally normal heart.
2. Treatment goals consist of rhythm control, rate control and anticoagulation, as well as addressing the underlying cause.
3. Transoesophageal echocardiography is needed to exclude left atrial clot before electrical or chemical cardioversion if atrial fibrillation is for >48 hours or other risk factors for stroke prevail.
4. Electrical cardioversion is the safest approach where pre-excitation from an accessory pathway occurs.
5. Ventricular arrhythmias are most likely associated with structural heart disease and may be immediately life-threatening.

Keywords: atrial fibrillation, cardioversion, stroke

Introduction

Atrial fibrillation (AF) is characterised by chaotic, varying-amplitude depolarisations of atrial muscle, with irregularly irregular propagation to the ventricles. The rate is 350–600 bpm, which is too fast to be over-drive-paced by intervention. The loss of coordinated atrial systole reduces preload by as much as 30 per cent and, as such, cardiac output. It normally originates from the left atrium (LA), particularly from the origin of the pulmonary veins. Atrial flutter is a re-entry tachycardia normally originating in the right atrium (RA). The principles of management in the ICU are the same. Both arrhythmias, as well as unifocal and multifocal atrial tachycardias, are known as atrioventricular (AV) node-independent.

Causes

AF is the most common arrhythmia, and NHS data suggest at least 1 million people in the UK are affected. It is also very common in critically ill patients (15 per cent). Whilst structural heart disease is an important pre-determinant, acidosis and hypoxia of critical illness produce a less negative cardiomyocyte resting membrane potential. This causes abnormal automaticity and the risk of arrhythmias in an otherwise normal heart. AF adversely affects morbidity and mortality in a number of studies, although this may just be a marker of disease severity.

Important Considerations

- Fluid overload, either from cardiac failure or iatrogenic, causes atrial stretch and increases the risk of AF.
- Impaired homeostatic mechanisms reduce the arrhythmia threshold and, without correction, will limit successful AF management, e.g. acidosis, hypoxia, anaemia, acid–base abnormalities, electrolyte imbalance.
- Structural heart disease is an important cause and may warrant treatment of the underlying cause, e.g. ischaemia, mitral valve disease, hypertension.
- ICU diagnosis is important, e.g. shock, sepsis, thoracic trauma, myocardial infarction.
- ICU therapies may increase the risk of AF, e.g. inotropic support, vasopressors, fluid resuscitation, electrolyte management.

Classification

The longer the length of episodes of AF pre-illness, the more likely it is to occur in the ICU and the greater the challenge in reversing it. In addition, with increasing permanency of AF, the greater likelihood that it has contributed to critical illness onset (Table 3.1.8.1).

Table 3.1.8.1 Classification of atrial fibrillation

Classification	Description
Lone AF	Single episode, often encountered in ICU, eminently treatable
Paroxysmal AF	Non-sustained episodes lasting <7 days, terminating either spontaneously or by intervention, also treatable
Persistent AF	Sustained AF lasting longer than 7 days. In ICU, it may occur in a known AF patient or develop in a long-stay patient. Can be resistant to first-line treatments and up to 18% of ICU-discharged patients will still be in AF
Long-term persistent AF	AF lasting longer than 1 year
Permanent AF	Follows a cardiological decision that rhythm control is likely impossible, so focus dedicated on anticoagulation and rate control

Investigations

Electrocardiography will confirm arrhythmia and rate, demonstrate ischaemia and also rule out pre-excitation, which will influence treatment options. Blood tests are essential, particularly haemoglobin count, inflammatory markers, potassium and magnesium and thyroid function tests. Echocardiography should be undertaken. The transthoracic echocardiography (TTE) approach provides valuable information regarding biventricular and valve function. Stroke risk from an LA appendage clot must be assessed by transoesophageal echocardiography (TOE), as the views are inaccessible by the TTE approach. TOE is not risk-free, as it requires sedation or a ventilated patient and can damage the oesophagus, but it is vital before attempting cardioversion which could dislodge the appendage clot and cause a stroke. Note that removal of a TOE probe will invariably pull out an *in situ* nasogastric tube; thus, this may require re-siting and position check.

Treatment Goals

Treatment goals in the ICU do not differ, in principle, from those for the stable patient, aside from the urgency of restoring haemodynamic instability. Success rate, however, will depend on the management of the underlying cause:

1. Anticoagulation and stroke risk reduction
2. Rate control
3. Rhythm control (cardioversion)
4. Treatment of underlying cause

Anticoagulation

AF risks an embolic stroke, predominantly due to blood stasis in the LA, particularly the appendage. This is irrespective of whether AF is paroxysmal, persistent or permanent. Cardioversion may also cause a stroke by mobilisation of preformed clot. All stable patients should be orally anticoagulated with either warfarin, a novel oral anticoagulant (NOAC) or heparin parenterally. Therapeutic anticoagulation needs to be evidenced for 3 weeks (e.g. international normalised ratio (INR) >2 or no missed NOAC doses) before cardioversion is attempted. If AF is new onset (<48 hours), such as in the ICU, cardioversion can be performed before anticoagulation, but the subsequent risk of a thrombotic event is high. Stroke risk is best assessed using the CHA_2DS_2-VASc score (Table 3.1.8.2) where only a score of zero warrants a decision not to anticoagulate. This should be balanced against the bleeding risk, e.g. HASBLED score (Table 3.1.8.3).

In the ICU, the safest anticoagulation approach is intravenous infusion of unfractionated heparin, due to its relatively short half-life and reversibility with protamine.

Table 3.1.8.2 CHA_2DS_2-VASc score

Risk factor	Points
Congestive heart failure or LV ejection fraction <40%	1
Hypertension	1
Age ≥75	2
Diabetes	1
Stroke/TIA/thromboembolism	2
Vascular disease	1
Age 65–74	1
Sex: female	1

NB: There is a link to a free online calculator (www.mdcalc.com/cha2ds2-vasc-score-atrial-fibrillation-stroke-risk#evidence).

Abbreviations: LV = left ventricular; TIA = transient ischaemic attack.

The adjusted stroke risk (per cent/year) ranges from 1.3 (1 point) to 15.2 (9 points).

Table 3.1.8.3 HASBLED score

Risk factor	Points
Hypertension (uncontrolled)	1
Abnormal renal/liver function	1 or 2
Stroke	1
Bleeding tendency/predisposition	1
Labile INR	1
Elderly (age >65)	1
Drugs, e.g. aspirin, NSAIDs	1

Abbreviations: INR = international normalised ratio; NSAID = non-steroidal anti-inflammatory drug.
Source: www.mdcalc.com/has-bled-score-major-bleeding-risk

The risk of major bleeding (cranial or gastrointestinal) ranges from 1.02–2.8 per cent (1 point) to 7.4–12.5 per cent (5 points), with very few, if any, patients in studies with scores of >5.

Rhythm Control

In terms of all-cause mortality, cardiovascular death, embolism and major bleeding, there may be no advantage of rhythm over rate control. Rhythm control, however, is preferable in younger patients (<65) with heart failure but fewer co-morbidities. Cardioversion may be electrical or chemical. Electrical cardioversion is often performed in the ICU, as this offers rapid return of haemodynamic stability, but does require sedation or anaesthesia to achieve. Defibrillation pads are best applied in the anterior–posterior position and a synchronised high-energy shock (e.g. 150 J) is given, which can be repeated. Success will depend on the underlying cause. Higher energies of up to 360 J and downward pressure on the anterior pad improve success of extra shocks. Atrial flutter typically requires lower energy (e.g. 50 J). Intravenous drugs may be required to prevent regression to AF.

For chemical cardioversion in the ICU setting, the safest intravenous agent is amiodarone, appreciating that the time to work may be as long as 72 hours. It is best given as a loading dose of 300 mg, followed by 24-hour infusions of 900 mg/600 mg/300 mg. It is safe in structural heart disease and is less negatively inotropic than other drugs. The side effect profile from the above regime is favourable, but the decision to continue the drug longer by the enteral route should not be made lightly, as respiratory pathology, thyroid pathology and/or photosensitivity may be irreversible. Other intravenous agents exist, e.g. flecainide, propafenone,

procainamide, but they have risks in structural heart disease and limited availability in the UK and require expert help.

Rate Control

Correction of electrolyte abnormalities should be ensured, and magnesium sulphate has a proven role in both rhythm and rate control, as does prevention of hypokalaemia. They may also improve the success of other treatment modalities.

Ventricular rate control improves cardiovascular haemodynamics, and intravenous titrated beta-blockers (e.g. esmolol, metoprolol) are the primary agents used – unless the patient is in acute heart failure or hypotensive. Non-dihydropyridine calcium channel blockers (e.g. diltiazem, verapamil) are alternatives. If heart failure presides, digoxin is recommended. Amiodarone is also successful, although it must be given centrally.

In Wolff–Parkinson–White (WPW) syndrome, an accessory pathway connects the atria to the ventricles, and AV conduction can bypass the AV node. This is demonstrated by pre-excitation delta waves on the ECG, as dual depolarisations arrive in the ventricles at different rates. AV nodal blockers, e.g. amiodarone, calcium channel blockers, digoxin, adenosine, may be harmful and the American Heart Association (AHA)/American College of Cardiology (ACC) guidelines recommend the use of ibutilide or procainamide. Accessory pathways lack the rate limitation served by the AV node; hence, AV nodal inhibition risks unrestricted accessory conduction and causes ventricular fibrillation. The safest approach is direct current (DC) cardioversion at 100–200 J.

Additional Arrhythmias
Supraventricular Tachycardia (Atrioventricular Node-Dependent Tachycardias)

AV nodal re-entry tachycardia (AVNRT) is a re-entry circuit confined to the AV node, with retrograde conduction via a fast pathway. The heart is structurally normal and presentation in the ICU rare. Acute therapy is by vagal manoeuvres and adenosine. Beta-blockers are useful for rate control.

AV re-entry tachycardia (AVRT) has an accessory pathway that bypasses the AV node. This may produce a delta wave, but in 25 per cent of cases, the accessory pathway has retrograde conduction only. Thus, the pre-excitation is hidden in the QRS. Treatment is as for AVNRT.

The re-entry loop may be orthodromic, in which case QRS will be narrow and the accessory flow retrograde, or instead antidromic, with forward conduction via the accessory pathway and subsequent wide QRS. AV nodal blocking drugs are safe when the action potential origin is not from a distant site, e.g. AF.

Ventricular Tachycardia

Ventricular tachycardia (VT) is a life-threatening condition as it is compromises cardiac output and may degenerate into ventricular fibrillation. The most important risk factor for monomorphic VT (single focus) is structural heart disease. Thus, it will often be a threat in the intensive care setting. In the absence of structural heart disease, a number of channelopathies may present as VT in otherwise fit individuals, e.g. long QT syndromes and Brugada syndrome. VT may be polymorphic (torsades de pointes). Differential diagnosis includes aberrancy (bundle branch block) or antegrade tachycardia via an accessory pathway. Early cardiology advice is essential, as these can be difficult to distinguish. Untreated, sustained VT risks degeneration to VF. On the ECG, VT is favoured by the following:

1. Positive or negative concordance in chest leads, i.e. QRS all positive or all negative
2. Very broad complexes (>160 ms)
3. Positive R wave in aVR (as conduction heading away from ventricles)
4. Absence of an RS wave in all of leads V1–V6
5. Capture beats – occasional normal sinus beat transmitted to ventricle
6. Fusion beats – hybrid complexes from collision of normal sinus beat with VT

TTE is the investigation of choice, providing information on biventricular systolic function, valve integrities and congenital abnormalities, e.g. shunts.

In terms of management, the Resuscitation Council UK algorithm for tachycardia recommends expert help if the arrhythmia is irregular. Haemodynamic instability necessitates immediate synchronised DC cardioversion under sedation – 120–150 J biphasic shock, followed by amiodarone 300 mg IV over 15–20 minutes, and 900 mg over 24 hours. Repeat shocks may be necessary. Pharmacological therapy includes potassium and magnesium replacement and primarily amiodarone as above. Beta-blockers are the first-line therapy in cardiac ischaemia, and only contraindicated in cardiogenic shock and Brugada syndrome. Adenosine can be used with caution to aid diagnosis but may risk VF if the cause is a supraventricular accessory pathway.

Secondary management may involve consideration for an implantable cardioverter–defibrillator (ICD) if the National Institute for Health and Care Excellence (NICE) criteria are fulfilled.

References and Further Reading

Bersten A, Soni N (eds). *Oh's Intensive Care Manual*, 6th edn. Edinburgh: Butterworth Heinemann; 2009.

Caldeira D, David C, Sampaio C. Rate versus rhythm control in atrial fibrillation and clinical outcomes: updated systematic review and meta-analysis of randomized controlled trials. *Arch Cardiovasc Dis* 2012;**105**:226–38.

January CT, Wann LS, Alpert JS, *et al.* 2014 AHA/ACC/HRS guideline for the management of patients with atrial fibrillation: executive summary: a report of the American College of Cardiology/American Heart Association Task Force on practice guidelines and the Heart Rhythm Society. *Circulation* 2014;**130**:2071–104. Erratum in: *Circulation* 2014;**130**:e270–1.

National Institute for Health and Care Excellence. 2014. Implantable cardioverter defibrillators and cardiac resynchronisation therapy for arrhythmias and heart failure. www.nice.org.uk/guidance/ta314/chapter/1-Guidance

Sibley S, Muscedere J. New-onset atrial fibrillation in critically ill patients. *Can Respir J* 2015;**22**:179–82.

3.1.9

Myocarditis

Niklas Tapper

Key Learning Points

1. A high degree of clinical suspicion is required to effectively diagnose and treat myocarditis.
2. Endomyocardial biopsy (EMB) is required to attain a certain diagnosis and direct effective management.
3. Supportive care is the mainstay of medical management if the diagnosis is unclear, and may necessitate the use of inotropic drugs and mechanical assist devices.
4. Complex diagnostic and management issues require a multidisciplinary approach – intensivist, cardiologist, pathologist (trained in myocardial pathology), clinical immunologist and infectious disease specialist.
5. Suspect myocarditis in young patients (<35 years old) with unexplained heart failure or arrhythmia.

Keywords: myocarditis, endomyocardial biopsy, multidisciplinary, heart failure

Definition

Myocarditis has been defined as 'an inflammatory disease of the myocardium diagnosed by established histological, immunological and immunohistochemical criteria'. When myocarditis is associated with systolic and/or diastolic cardiac dysfunction, it is termed 'inflammatory cardiomyopathy'.

Causes

The aetiology of myocarditis is often undetermined. However, there are numerous known causes, which are classified into three main groups.

Infectious

- Viral (parvovirus B19, human herpesvirus 6, enteroviruses and Epstein–Barr virus are the four main types, sometimes found in combination)
- Bacterial, spirochaetal, fungal, protozoal, parasitic, rickettsial

Immune-Mediated

- Allergens (tetanus toxoid, vaccines, serum sickness, drugs)
- Alloantigens (heart transplant rejection)
- Autoantigens (infection-negative lymphocytic, infection-negative giant cell – associated with numerous autoimmune/immune disorders, including sarcoidosis and systemic lupus erythematosus)

Toxic

- Drugs (cocaine, catecholamine, penicillin and numerous others)
- Heavy metals (copper, iron, lead)
- Miscellaneous (insect bites, inhalants)
- Physical agents (radiation, electric shock)

Diagnosis

There is no typical presentation, with symptoms ranging from mild chest pain to cardiogenic shock and ventricular arrhythmias. As such, diagnosis requires a high level of clinical suspicion. Presentations suggestive of myocarditis include acute chest pain, new-onset dyspnoea, fatigue, palpitations, unexplained arrhythmia, syncope and unexplained cardiogenic shock.

First-line tests include electrocardiography (numerous abnormalities are possible) and serum biomarkers (troponin, erythrocyte sedimentation rate (ESR), C-reactive protein (CRP)). Transthoracic echocardiography (TTE) may show new left ventricular (LV) and/or right ventricular (RV) structure and function abnormalities and/or global or regional wall motion abnormalities, with or without ventricular dilation/increased wall thickness/pericardial effusion/endocavity thrombi.

Cardiac magnetic resonance (CMR) in clinically stable presentations may be appropriate and more sensitive than EMB with a pseudoinfarct presentation. Oedema on CMR is possible without inflammatory infiltrate and is not, in itself, diagnostic.

All cases with clinically suspected myocarditis should be considered for coronary angiography and EMB.

EMB is safe, simple, effective and the gold standard for the diagnosis of myocarditis on the basis of histological Dallas criteria and other immunohistochemical criteria. If positive, it will provide the aetiology of the myocarditis, which, in turn, determines treatment. Knowledge of the aetiology is critical, as the specific treatments of infectious and non-infectious myocarditis are diametrically opposed.

Myopericarditis is a term given to predominant pericarditis with myocardial involvement. If there are no symptoms of heart failure and LV function is less than moderately impaired, then the benign prognosis of this disease does not require EMB.

Treatment

- Treat the infectious cause or rule out an infectious cause via EMB.
- Antiviral therapy may be beneficial under guidance of an infectious disease specialist.
- Avoidance of exercise, and conventional medical management for haemodynamic instability and/or arrhythmias.
- Immunosuppression with azathioprine, ciclosporin A, mycophenolate mofetil, alone or in combination with corticosteroids. May need treatment for years, with follow-up serial echocardiography, ECG and occasionally troponins.

- Immunomodulatory therapy, including high-dose intravenous immunoglobulin and immunoadsorption, are promising future therapies, with larger clinical trials still ongoing.

Supportive Management, Veno-arterial Extracorporeal Membrane Oxygenation and Axial Flow Pumps

'Acute fulminant myocarditis (AFM)' describes a rapid-onset, severe haemodynamic compromise with cardiac inflammation. It presents with severe impairment of LV function and is frequently fatal. In addition to specific treatment, aggressive haemodynamic support through use of inotropic agents and mechanical devices is warranted, as survivors of the acute phase have an excellent long-term prognosis. A multi-centre retrospective study of patients with AFM treated with veno-arterial extracorporeal membrane oxygenation (VA-ECMO) between 2008 and 2013 showed a survival rate of 80 per cent in non-arrested patients, and this is consistent with the findings of earlier published studies (survival rate of 60–100 per cent). Four out of 12 patients with AFM in whom VA-ECMO was instituted after cardiac arrest survived. Complication rates related to the institution of VA-ECMO remain high, however, with up to 70 per cent of patients suffering major complications. Axial flow pumps, such as the Impella® systems, used in isolation or in combination with VA-ECMO, have shown promise in case reports as a 'bridge to recovery'. They have the ability to decrease elevated ventricular afterload associated with VA-ECMO, with the potential of reducing inflammation in the hope of avoiding maladaptive cardiac remodelling.

References and Further Reading

Caforio AL, Pankuweit S, Arbustini E, *et al.* Current state of knowledge on aetiology, diagnosis, management, and therapy of myocarditis: a position statement of the European Society of Cardiology Working Group on Myocardial and Pericardial Diseases. *Eur Heart J* 2013;**34**:2636–48, 264848a–d.

3.1.10

Pericardial Disease

Niklas Tapper

Key Learning Points

1. Pericardial effusions may cause haemodynamic compromise if large or rapidly developing.
2. Echocardiography is the most important clinical tool for assessing cardiac tamponade.
3. Typical clinical signs of cardiac tamponade may be absent in post-cardiac surgery patients.
4. Transoesophageal echocardiography is more sensitive than transthoracic echocardiography in post-cardiac surgical patients in the diagnosis of cardiac tamponade.
5. Extreme caution should be taken prior to intubating or initiating positive pressure ventilation in patients with cardiac tamponade.

Keywords: pericardial effusions, pericarditis, cardiac tamponade, TOE, TTE

Pericardial Syndromes

Pericardial disease is commonly divided into four classical pericardial syndromes:

- Pericarditis
- Constrictive pericarditis
- Pericardial effusion
- Cardiac tamponade

Pericardial disease syndromes may present in isolation or as a complication of systemic illness.

Pericardium and Pericardial Fluid

There is usually a volume of 15–50 ml of pericardial fluid lubricating the space between the single layer of mesothelial cells, termed the visceral pericardium, and the parietal pericardium which consists of mainly collagen and elastin. These envelope the heart and fuse around the great vessels, forming a relatively inelastic capsule.

Pericarditis

Pericarditis is the most common form of pericardial disease and accounts for 0.1 per cent of hospital admissions. Pericarditis may be associated with pericardial effusion or severe illness (commonly sepsis or pneumonia). Although most cases of pericarditis follow a benign course, hospital admission is recommended for patients with high-risk features, including: fever >38°C, subacute onset and large pericardial effusion (diastolic echo-free space >20 mm), cardiac tamponade or failure to respond within 7 days to non-steroidal anti-inflammatory drugs (NSAIDs). Of patients admitted with pericarditis, the in-hospital mortality rate is 1.1 per cent, strongly associated with increasing age and severe co-infections such as pneumonia or septicaemia. Treatment is with anti-inflammatory drugs, NSAIDs and colchicine.

Pericardial Effusion

Clinical presentation is related to the speed of pericardial fluid accumulation. The viscoelastic properties of the pericardium allow it to stretch and accommodate large amounts of fluid if the effusion is chronic (up to 2000 ml). However, in the acute setting, even a small collection of fluid can cause severe haemodynamic compromise (as little as 150–250 ml in cases of bleeding associated with penetrating trauma or cardiac surgery). The pericardial pressure–volume curve behaves in a 'last drop' manner, whereby initial small increases in volume cause small increases in pericardial pressure until an upward inflection occurs at a critical volume. At this point, even very small increases in volume cause large increases in pressure (up to 20 mmHg), which, in turn, cause cardiac compression.

Treatment should be targeted towards the underlying aetiology. This is a known disease in around 60 per cent of cases. In the presence of inflammation, treatment is as for pericarditis. For large effusions, pericardiocentesis, pericardial window or pericardiectomy may be necessary. Small effusions are usually asymptomatic and do not require specific monitoring. Moderate to large idiopathic pericardial effusions may evolve to pericardial tamponade in up to one-third of cases and are followed more closely.

Constrictive Pericarditis

Thickened, fibrotic pericardium impairs ventricular diastolic function and can mimic tamponade, as it impairs cardiac filling and reduces cardiac output despite normal systolic function. Causes include viral pericarditis, cardiac surgery, collagen vascular disease, radiation and tuberculosis. In common with tamponade, it presents with augmented ventricular interdependence and respiratory variability. Pulsus paradoxus is possible but found less commonly. In cardiac tamponade, pressure is exerted on the myocardium throughout the cardiac cycle and haemodynamic effects are most prominent when intramyocardial pressures are low (right atrial and left atrial throughout cycle, right ventricular diastole). In contrast, with a constrictive pericardium, effects are not usually witnessed until mid- to late-diastole and atrial systole, when ventricles are unable to be filled further due to the constrictive effect of the pericardium.

Echocardiography typically shows a thickened pericardium with increased echogenicity if calcification is present (better seen on transoesophageal (TOE) than on transthoracic echocardiography (TTE)). Constrictive spectral Doppler studies reveal early diastolic flow dominance through the atrioventricular valves, with abrupt cessation of 'diastolic checking' as the limit of pericardial constriction is reached.

Cardiac Tamponade

This involves life-threatening compression of the heart due to pericardial accumulation of fluid, pus, blood, clots or gas. It is commonly due to pericarditis, tuberculosis, invasive cardiac procedures, trauma or neoplasms, or less commonly due to collagen vascular disease, radiation, post-myocardial infarction, uraemia, cardiac rupture, aortic dissection or bacterial infection. Whilst pericardial effusion is an anatomical diagnosis, cardiac tamponade is a physiological diagnosis in which the pericardial pressure exceeds the pressure in one or more cardiac chambers, leading to obstructive shock.

Signs of Cardiac Tamponade in the Spontaneously Ventilated Patient

Typical signs of cardiac tamponade relate to sympathetic-mediated compensatory mechanisms (tachycardia, tachypnoea, vasoconstriction, fluid retention, raised jugular venous pressure/right atrial pressure). Later in the process, signs of obstructive shock, including hypotension and oliguria, develop with more specific signs, including muffled heart sounds, pulsus paradoxus, low QRS voltages and electrical alterans on the electrocardiogram, and an enlarged cardiac silhouette on the chest X-ray (effusions of over 300 ml).

Echocardiography

Echocardiography is the most important diagnostic tool. It is used to identify the effusion and estimate its size (small <10 mm, moderate 10–20 mm, large >20 mm), location and degree of haemodynamic impact. It is also used to guide pericardiocentesis. Whilst computed tomography and cardiac magnetic resonance provide a larger field of view, patients with cardiac tamponade are usually too haemodynamically unstable to tolerate these imaging modalities.

Cardiac tamponade causes augmented ventricular interdependence, which can be demonstrated with echocardiography. During normal inspiration, negative intrathoracic pressure leads to increased venous return, right-sided filling and right-sided chamber size. The constrictive nature of tamponade fixes the overall cardiac chamber size, therefore compressing the left-sided chambers and leading to a drop in systolic arterial pressure in inspiration. This manifests clinically as pulsus paradoxus – an inspiratory systemic pressure drop of over 10 mmHg. The reverse happens in expiration. Echocardiographically, this phenomenon is seen as abnormal ventricular septal motion and respiratory variability in chamber size, pulmonary vein diastolic inflow, tricuspid and mitral inflow velocity and aortic outflow velocity.

Cardiac Tamponade in Post-operative Cardiac Surgical Patients

Tamponade is a common finding in hypotensive patients post-cardiac surgery. When it occurs in the first hours after cardiac surgery, it is usually due to haemorrhage and requires urgent surgical intervention to remove the compression and identify a source of bleeding.

Although tamponade is generally described as a clinical diagnosis, as opposed to an echocardiographic diagnosis, the usual clinical signs and haemodynamic variants may be absent, blunted or even reversed in positive pressure-ventilated, post-cardiac surgical patients. Common signs suggesting a low cardiac output state, including cool peripheries, oliguria, raised cardiac filling pressures and hypotension, may also be present, with primary myocardial dysfunction causing cardiogenic shock. When pericardial effusion and myocardial dysfunction occur together, the proportion attributed to the effusion may be difficult to determine, and the decision to reoperate involves assessing the size and speed of accumulation, ventricular function, filling status and degree of vasoplegia.

Confounding these difficulties, TTE windows in post-cardiac surgical patients are usually obstructed by chest tubes and hindered by supine positioning, positive pressure ventilation and valve surgery artefacts. Good visualisation of the haemopericardium (which may be fluid or solid blood clot) is difficult or, in some cases, impossible. The haemopericardium is often loculated and contained in far-field areas over the right atrial free wall, behind the left atrium and posterolateral to the right ventricle, compressing specific cardiac regions and causing regional tamponade. Furthermore, two-dimensional and Doppler findings consistent with large circumferential pericardial effusions are rarely found in this subset of intensive care patients. Typical findings representing pulsus paradoxus may be reversed with inspiration, impeding venous return in positive pressure-ventilated patients.

TTE in post-cardiac surgical patients has been found to miss pericardial tamponade in up to 20 per cent of cases. Diagnosis of tamponade in this subset of patients relies on demonstration of effusion with compression, impaired right heart filling (inferior vena cava plethora) and a left ventricle with reduced end-diastolic and systolic dimensions. Pseudohypertrophy is a common finding in which the ventricular cavity appears underfilled and wall thickness is increased.

A negative finding on TTE in this subset of patients with clinically suspected tamponade should be followed up with TOE.

Haemodynamic Goals

Maintaining venous return is critically important. Systemic venodilation should be minimised, and small fluid boluses may be beneficial if the patient is volume-depleted. However, excessive fluid risks worsening ventricular interdependence and reducing cardiac output. Positive pressure ventilation has the potential to drastically impair venous return. Increased end-expiratory intrathoracic pressures may impede venous return, even in expiration, and as such, use of positive end-expiratory pressure (PEEP) should be minimised and excessive inspiratory times avoided. Although afterload reduction is beneficial with respect to cardiac output, maintenance of systemic vascular resistance (SVR) is critically important for coronary perfusion pressure and, in turn, myocardial contractility. Vasopressor and/or inotropic support is often employed, although there is no consensus on ideal agents. Noradrenaline is used to maintain SVR, with no change in cardiac index. Some small studies on dogs suggest inotropic agents, such as dobutamine, isoprenaline and dopamine, can increase cardiac output but do so at the cost of increased metabolic requirements and decreased myocardial perfusion time. Vasopressors and inotropes need to be downtitrated rapidly when tamponade is relieved, as resulting high blood pressures may contribute to ongoing bleeding.

Pericardial Tamponade and Intubation

Extreme caution is required in the patient with pericardial tamponade who requires intubation. Indications may include a decreased level of consciousness, severe pulmonary oedema with left-sided compression or need for surgical intervention. It should only be attempted if strictly necessary, after instigation of invasive monitoring and ideally with the cardiothoracic surgical team ready to intervene. Maintenance of spontaneous ventilation until surgical drainage may be beneficial, but not always possible.

References and Further Reading

Adler Y, Charron P, Imazio M, *et al.* 2015 ESC Guidelines for the diagnosis and management of pericardial diseases: The Task Force for the Diagnosis and Management of Pericardial Diseases of the European Society of Cardiology (ESC) Endorsed by: The European

Association for Cardio-Thoracic Surgery (EACTS). *Eur Heart J* 2015;**36**:2921–64.

Bodson L, Bouferrache K, Vieillard-Baron A. Cardiac tamponade. *Curr Opin Crit Care* 2011;**17**:416–24.

Imazio M, Adler Y. Management of pericardial effusion. *Eur Heart J* 2013;**34**:1186–97.

Klein AL, Abbara S, Agler DA, *et al.* American Society of Echocardiography clinical recommendations for multimodality cardiovascular imaging of patients with pericardial disease: endorsed by the Society for Cardiovascular Magnetic Resonance and Society of Cardiovascular Computed Tomography. *J Am Soc Echocardiogr* 2013;**26**:965–1012 e15.

Keywords: cardiogenic shock, septic shock, oxygen delivery, shock trials

Introduction

Shock describes inadequate oxygen delivery to meet general end-organ demands leading to tissue hypoxia. Whilst respiratory disease can cause severe hypoxaemia and consequent generalised tissue hypoxia, shock relates more specifically to haemodynamic disturbances leading to this.

Oxygen Delivery

To understand shock in greater detail, it is essential to consider the constituents that make up oxygen delivery, such that they can be exploited during treatment (Box 3.1.11.1).

Box 3.1.11.1 Essential Equations Relevant to Oxygen Delivery (DO_2)

Oxygen delivery = cardiac output × oxygen content

Oxygen content = $[(Hb \times 1.34 \times SpO_2) + (PaO_2 \times 0.003)]$

Cardiac output = heart rate × stroke volume

The important drivers in oxygen delivery thus include cardiac output and oxygen content. Whilst oxygen content can be affected by haemoglobin concentration and SpO_2 (in the absence of hyperbaric therapy), not a great deal else can be directly manipulated until one considers the oxyhaemoglobin dissociation curve and how this can be manipulated. The vast majority of shock management therefore relates to the components of cardiac output – heart rate and stroke volume – which, in turn, are dependent on preload, contractility and afterload.

In practice, the clinical scenario usually involves an interaction between multiple physiological insults causing shock with a complex interplay between factors, but to illustrate the learning points more clearly, the isolated systems will be explained.

Role of Preload

Normal cardiac myofibril contraction will produce a predictable response to a given left ventricular end-diastolic volume (LVEDV) in the absence of inotropy or changes in afterload. The Frank–Starling mechanism describes how an increased preload increases myofibril stretching and subsequent force of contraction, increasing the stroke volume and therefore the cardiac output. The corollary of this is also true – that a fall in LVEDV will produce a lesser stroke volume. In a conceptually perfect left ventricle with maximal contractility, and hence the ability to overcome any amount of afterload, a lack of volume will lead to poor LVEDV, and when taken to an extreme, despite good contractility, the stroke volume (at an assumptive theoretical maximal heart rate), and ultimately the cardiac output, will fall. This is the archetypal physiology of the young trauma patient.

Requirement for Contractility

Inotropy describes the power of cardiac contraction for a given stretch or preload. When an exogenous inotropic drug is infused, the power of ventricular emptying increases, irrespective of the LVEDV, which leads to a greater stroke volume and a lower left ventricular end-systolic volume (LVESV). Conversely in the failing ventricle, reduced inotropy leads to a smaller stroke volume and a lower cardiac output. This classically reflects true heart failure.

Maintenance of Afterload

Afterload is the ventricular wall stress during ejection, and can be conceptualised as the aortic or pulmonary artery pressure against which the ventricle is trying to eject. As afterload increases, the stroke volume will fall (assuming there are no changes in the cardiac preload or contractility). The more common aetiologies of shock lead to vasodilation; thus, manipulation of afterload/systemic vascular resistance is the usual goal. The majority of clinical trials use mean arterial pressure (MAP) as a clinical target but use volume replacement as the means to achieve this, making the assumption that these patients are intravascularly deplete. Many large trials (see Table 3.1.11.2) endeavour to show benefits to various interventions.

Importance of Heart Rate

The natural physiological response to a low cardiac output state is to increase the stroke volume and heart rate. It is therefore important to acknowledge that a septic patient with relative bradyarrhythmia may need chronotropic assistance, either pharmacological or electrophysiological, to bridge ischaemic, infective or iatrogenic conduction abnormalities.

The above is obviously only a very simplistic way of summarising the factors influencing the cardiac output. However, it allows one to conceptualise the main components that can be manipulated during resuscitation of a shocked patient. Notably though, many pathologies lead to an upset of all cardiac output components directly, and treatment may further compound these imbalances. Take, for example, the septic diabetic patient:

- Preload may be low due to absolute volume depletion and vasodilation – often initially treated with boluses of intravenous crystalloid.
- Contractility may initially be considered adequate. However, in the setting of long-standing diabetes and atherosclerosis, oxygen supply may begin to be inadequate – particularly in a state of

increased demand such as sepsis. As myocardial demand starts to outstrip supply, the ensuing ischaemia may begin to compromise cardiac contractility (compounded by septic acidaemia). With impaired contractility, the LVESV begins to increase, leading to raised diastolic filling pressure, which further compromises diastolic perfusion and can lead to poor venous drainage of the lungs and consequent pulmonary oedema.

- Afterload may initially be low due to septic vasodilation. As myocardial contractility falls, a low afterload helps to augment left ventricular emptying, but as left ventricular perfusion is dependent on diastolic filling pressure, a low afterload will further hinder the ischaemic, septic myocardium.

Pressure versus Flow

The concept of shock invariably accompanies a description of hypotension. In the drive to resuscitate a patient, target blood pressures are thus often prescribed. However, in the oxygen delivery equation, blood pressure does not feature. Furthermore, generating an aortic root pressure through aggressive vasoconstriction may not necessarily improve tissue oxygen delivery, but rather may, in fact, reduce distal perfusion due to the arteriolar vasoconstriction required to achieve it. An alternative approach is to allow some vasodilation and instead target a hyperdynamic, low-pressure circulation. As always, in medicine, a middle ground is sought, and the SEPSISPAM trial comparing higher versus lower target MAP failed to show a benefit in mortality and ICU length of stay with a target MAP of 80–85 mmHg versus 65–70 mmHg, expanded upon by the 65 Trial.

Specific Management of Shock

Shock may be classified into:

1. Cardiogenic
2. Hypovolaemic
3. Distributive
4. Obstructive

Some specific causes and their treatment principles are outlined in Table 3.1.11.1.

Table 3.1.11.1 Specific causes and principles of treatment of shock

Classification	Specific causes	Treatment principles
Cardiogenic	Myocardial ischaemia	Cardiogenic shock may result through tachy-/brady-arrhythmias and/or embarrassment of ventricular function through the development of regional hypo-/akinesis. Treatment involves resuscitation and revascularisation. In the short term, nitrates can assist coronary dilation (but will cause aortic root dilation), whilst vasopressors will increase aortic root (and hence diastolic filling) pressure and potentially coronary artery perfusion pressure
	Valve dysfunction	Stenotic valve dysfunction is usually a slow-developing pathology. Valves may become acutely regurgitant (ischaemic, infective) and compromise forward blood flow. Management will ultimately require some form of surgical valve repair but, in the short term, can be aided by inodilators and reduction of afterload to help offload the heart Chronically stenotic valve pathology can become acutely crippling if there is sudden reduction in ventricular ability, e.g. in the setting of new ischaemia. In such circumstances, revascularisation is important, but techniques such as emergent balloon valvotomy may serve as a bridge to this in extremis
	Myocarditis	May present benignly or malignantly – in the latter form, cardiac dysfunction may take the form of brady-arrhythmias requiring temporary pacing wires, or tachy-arrhythmias requiring DCCV, with any degree of ventricular impairment. Due to the risk of precipitating severe tachy-arrhythmias, ventricular function should be augmented with as little in the way of catecholamines as possible, and mechanical circulatory support should be considered as a bridge to recovery or long-term device if appropriate
	Arrhythmias	In the event of brady-arrhythmias, pharmacological and/or electrophysiological assistance should be arranged. If thought to be secondary to ischaemia, revascularisation should be urgently considered In the event of tachyarrhythmias, advice may be taken from EP physicians for specific management, but ALS protocols should be followed in the first instance Implanted pacemakers or defibrillators may prove necessary after the emergent phase
	Drugs	Acute cardiogenic shock secondary to drugs normally only results after an overdose – in these cases, CVS support should be symptom- or cardiac output monitor-guided. In some refractory cases, haemodialysis may be able to augment removal of certain drugs. In the setting of beta-blocker or calcium channel blocker overdoses, techniques such as glucagon and high-dose insulin euglycaemic therapy may be considered
Hypovolaemic	Haemorrhage	Appropriate volume replacement, guided by local major haemorrhage protocols Early administration of anti-fibrinolytics is advocated Definitive surgery may be necessary if source does not stop Tourniquets, Sengstaken–Blakemore tubes, pelvic binders, REBOA and damage limitation surgery are the more invasive stabilising techniques
	Fluid loss (burns, GI losses, metabolic derangement)	Often leads to total body water deficit, and replenishment needs to take this into account Electrolyte abnormalities may be severe and should be anticipated and corrected
Distributive	Sepsis/toxin-mediated Anaphylaxis Neurogenic Drugs Fluid loss ('third-space', e.g. pancreatitis)	Use of targeted volume replacement Use of vasopressors Haemodialysis/filtration to remove drugs/toxins Specifically: antibiotics in sepsis; steroids/adrenaline in allergy; antidotes to certain drugs
Obstructive	Tension pneumothorax Pulmonary embolus Pericardial tamponade Intra-cardiac tumour SAM/LVOTO	Decompression of pneumothorax Lysing of thrombi Drainage of pericardial collections Surgical removal of intra-cardiac tumours Reduction of pressure gradient through aortic valve

Abbreviations: DCCV = direct current cardioversion; EP = electrophysiology; ALS = advanced life support; CVS = cardiovascular system; REBOA = resuscitative endovascular balloon occlusion of the aorta; GI = gastrointestinal; SAM = systolic anterior movement of the anterior mitral valve leaflet; LVOTO = left ventricular outflow tract obstruction.

Table 3.1.11.2 Prominent 'shock trials'

Intervention	Year	Known as	Cohort	Result
Protocols	2001	Rivers Trial	Septic shock ($n = 263$)	EGDT reduced in-hospital mortality from 46.5% to 30.5% (NNT = 6)
	2014	ProCESS	Septic shock ($n = 1341$)	Compared EGDT, a less invasive protocolised approach, and usual-therapy approach in emergency departments in the United States. No difference in primary endpoint (60-day in-hospital mortality) between any groups, but a much lower mortality rate seen than in the Rivers' EGDT trial
	2018	SMART	Shock in emergency department ($n = 15,802$)	Non-selected critically ill population in emergency department randomised to either 0.9% NaCl or balanced crystalloid as resuscitation fluid. Balanced crystalloids favoured an improvement in composite outcome of death and renal failure versus saline
	2020	65 Trial	Vasodilatory shock ($n = 2463$)	No difference between targeting MAP of 60 mmHg (permissive hypotension) versus normal care (presumed to be MAP >65 mmHg) in patients aged >65
Activated protein C	2014	PROWESS-SHOCK	Septic shock ($n = 1697$)	Use of drotrecogin alfa (activated protein C) showed no survival benefit, but increased side effects (particularly bleeding)
Blood products	2013	Transfusion Strategies for acute UGIB	Upper GI bleed ($n = 921$)	Use of transfusion trigger of <7 g/dl versus 9 g/dl was associated with reduced mortality (5% versus 9%) in patients undergoing endoscopy within 6 hours of presentation
	2014	TRISS	Septic shock ($n = 1005$)	No difference in 90-day mortality (43% versus 45%) when using a transfusion trigger of 7 g/dl or 9 g/dl
Steroids	2017	Cochrane Review	Septic shock ($n = 4268$)	Meta-analysis: low-quality evidence of mortality benefit in heterogeneous septic patients
	2018	ADRENAL	Septic shock ($n = 3658$)	Hydrocortisone infusion: no 90-day mortality benefit and increased adverse events in steroid group. Reduced time to resolution of shock in steroid group
Levosimendan	2017	CHEETAH	Cardiac surgery ($n = 506$)	Levosimendan administration conferred no mortality benefit versus placebo in a high-risk group of patients undergoing cardiac surgery
	2017	LeoPARDS	Septic shock ($n = 516$)	Levosimendan conferred no mortality benefit and did not improve organ dysfunction scores, compared to placebo, but had more adverse effects
IABP	2012	IABP-SHOCK II	Cardiogenic shock ($n = 600$)	No difference in 30-day mortality when comparing IABP to best medical therapy in cardiogenic shock post-MI

Abbreviations: EGDT = early goal-directed therapy; NaCl = sodium chloride; MAP = mean arterial pressure; GI = gastrointestinal; IABP = intra-aortic balloon pump; MI = myocardial infarction.

References and Further Reading

Gordon AC, Perkins GD, Singer M, *et al.* Levosimendan for the prevention of acute organ dysfunction in sepsis. *N Engl J Med* 2016;**375**:1638–48.

IABP-SHOCK II Trial Investigators. Intra-aortic balloon counterpulsation in acute myocardial infarction complicated by cardiogenic shock (IABP-SHOCK II): final 12 month results of a randomised, open-label trial. *N Engl J Med* 2012;**367**:1287–96.

Landoni G, Lomivorotov VV, Alvaro G, *et al.* Levosimendan for hemodynamic support after cardiac surgery. *N Engl J Med* 2017; **376**:2021–31.

Semler MW. Balanced crystalloids versus saline in critically ill adults. *N Engl J Med* 2018;**378**:829–39.

3.1.12

Aortic Dissection

Simon Mattison

Key Learning Points

1. Acute aortic dissection is a rare, but life-threatening disorder.
2. Presentation may be similar to that of an acute coronary syndrome and should always be considered as a differential diagnosis.
3. Immediate treatment should focus on analgesia and blood pressure control, followed by rapid referral to a specialist unit.
4. ECG-gated computed tomography is usually the imaging modality of choice.
5. Urgent surgery is usually required for type A dissections.

Keywords: acute aortic dissection, acute aortic syndrome

Pathophysiology

Acute aortic dissection (AAD) forms part of a range of acute aortic diseases which also include intramural haematoma, penetrating atherosclerotic ulcer, aortic pseudoaneurysm and traumatic aortic injury. These conditions can be collectively labelled as acute aortic syndrome (AAS). AAD (<14 days) is distinct from subacute (15–90 days) and chronic (>90 days) aortic dissection by virtue of their respective time frames.

Aortic dissections are severe, life-threatening conditions. The primary pathological feature is usually an intimal tear, followed by disruption and tracking of blood within the aortic media. There is subsequently either an aortic rupture or a second intimal tear allowing re-entry of blood into the lumen. This process can be either anterograde or retrograde.

Incidence

There are around six cases per 100,000 patient-years, with the average age of onset at 65 years and twice the incidence in men as in women.

Predisposing factors include systemic hypertension, previous cardiac surgery, aortic aneurysms, a family history of AAS and collagen disorders, including Marfan, Loeys–Dietz and Ehlers–Danlos syndromes.

Classification

There are two classification systems in common use. The DeBakey system, named after the cardiothoracic surgeon Michael E. DeBakey, is based on the site of the original intimal tear and also on the extent of the dissection. More frequently employed in clinical practice is the Stanford system. Stanford type A (proximal) involves the ascending aorta and/or the aortic arch but may extend to include the descending aorta. Stanford type B is limited to the descending aorta.

The distinction is important, as type A generally requires urgent surgical repair, whereas with type B, initial treatment is usually medical.

Presentation

AAD may present as the event itself, or with the consequences of it. The most common symptom is severe chest pain, which is abrupt in onset and may be sharp, ripping or tearing in character. Back and abdominal pain is also common. Other presenting features may include aortic regurgitation (AR), cardiac tamponade, heart failure, myocardial ischaemia (if the dissection involves the coronary arteries), syncope or neurological deficit (if the dissection involves the cerebral circulation) and signs of abdominal organ malperfusion, including renal failure and signs of shock.

The most important differential diagnosis is that of an acute coronary syndrome (ACS), as the administration of anti-platelet agents can make subsequent surgical management more challenging.

Diagnosis

Clinical Examination

Potential physical signs are diverse but may include some of the following features. Hypertension is common, either as a result of an acute catecholamine surge or due to underlying essential hypertension as a contributory factor. Shock may be present, and there may be signs of cardiac tamponade or a new diastolic murmur indicative of AR. If AR is acute and severe, there may be signs of left heart failure, including pulmonary oedema. A significant difference (>20 mmHg) in blood pressure between both arms is suggestive, but not diagnostic. Neurological deficits, which include a reduction in Glasgow Coma Score (GCS), altered mental state or focal deficits, may be present in up to 20 per cent of cases.

Investigations

Blood tests should include full blood count, renal and liver function, troponin, creatine kinase, blood gas, C-reactive protein and procalcitonin (if sepsis is being considered as an alternative diagnosis). A negative D-dimer may help to rule out the diagnosis in situations where there is low clinical suspicion.

An ECG may demonstrate evidence of myocardial ischaemia, and this either may be as a result of the dissection if it involves the coronary arteries or may point to an ACS as an alternative diagnosis.

Chest X-ray may show a widened mediastinum or left-sided pleural effusion. However, it is unreliable and cannot be relied upon to rule out the diagnosis. Clinical suspicion therefore mandates the use of a more sensitive imaging test.

Imaging

Transthoracic echocardiography (TTE) is quick, readily available and non-invasive. For type A dissections, the sensitivity is 77–80 per cent and specificity 93–96 per cent. Transoesophageal echocardiography (TOE) has a sensitivity of 99 per cent and a specificity of 89 per cent, albeit at the cost of being more invasive. Echocardiography is also useful for identifying and quantifying AR and pericardial effusions, and for localising the site of the intimal flap.

ECG-gated CT is the most commonly utilised imaging technique for the diagnosis and evaluation of AAD. It is quick (usually one breath-hold), widely available and highly accurate, with a sensitivity of >95 per cent. Information is also provided regarding the extent of the dissection and involvement of the various aortic side branches, e.g. carotid, coronary, renal or mesenteric circulations. Disadvantages include exposure to ionising radiation and the need for intravenous contrast.

MRI is the most accurate technique for diagnosis of aortic dissection, with a sensitivity and specificity of 98 per cent. It also provides excellent anatomical detail of the extent of the disease, including pericardial effusions and AR. Its usefulness in the acute setting, however, is limited by practical considerations.

The approach to the diagnostic workup for aortic dissection should initially be based on the pre-test probability of the diagnosis, followed by a stepwise progression based on the stability of the patient.

Negative imaging in the face of high clinical suspicion requires active monitoring followed by repeat imaging.

Treatment

Initial treatment in all patients should include pain relief and blood pressure control. Infusion of a short-acting beta-blocker, e.g. labetalol or esmolol, is often a first-line treatment if not contraindicated, followed by rapid referral to a specialist cardiothoracic centre.

Emergency surgery is the recommended treatment for acute type A aortic dissection. Surgery may involve the aortic valve, aortic root, ascending aorta and aortic arch. Decisions on whether to operate and the extent of surgery undertaken may best be made in specialist centres.

Uncomplicated type B aortic dissection in the absence of malperfusion or early disease progression is treated medically with analgesia and drugs to control the heart rate and blood pressure. This is usually followed by surveillance with either CT or MRI to identify signs of disease progression. If invasive treatment is required, this usually takes the form of thoracic endovascular aortic repair (TEVAR).

Outcomes

Surgery is high risk and perioperative mortality may be as high as 25 per cent, with a significant risk of neurological complications. Causes of early mortality include cardiogenic shock, cerebral ischaemia and haemorrhage. One significant factor influencing surgical outcome is the presence of visceral malperfusion at presentation, which may occur in up to 30 per cent of cases.

However, without surgery, mortality is 50 per cent within the first 48 hours, and surgery reduces 1-month mortality from 90 to 30 per cent. Of those treated medically, <10 per cent are alive after 1 year, and 10-year survival after surgery for type A aortic dissection is 50 per cent.

Of Historical Interest

Possibly the first record in the literature of an AAD describes the demise of King George II. It was described thus by Frank Nicholls in his autopsy report:

> On 25 October 1760 George II, then 76, rose at his normal hour of 6 am, called as usual for his chocolate, and repaired to the close-stool. The German valet de chambre heard a noise, memorably described as "louder than the royal wind," and then a groan; he ran in and found the King lying on the floor, having cut his face in falling. Mr Andrews, surgeon to the household, was called and bled His Majesty but in vain, as no sign of life was observed from the time of his fall. At necropsy the next day Dr Nicholls, physician to his late Majesty, found the pericardium distended with a pint of coagulated blood, probably from an orifice in the right ventricle, and a transverse fissure on the inner side of the ascending aorta 3.75 cm long, through which blood had recently passed in its external coat to form a raised ecchymosis, this appearance being interpreted as an incipient aneurysm of the aorta.
>
> Source: *British Medical Journal*, 1979, **2**, 260–262.

References and Further Reading

Chiappini B, Schepens M, Tan E, *et al*. Early and late outcomes of acute type A aortic dissection: analysis of risk factors in 487 consecutive patients. *Eur Heart J* 2005;**26**:180–6.

Erbel R, Aboyans V, Boileau C, *et al*. 2014 ESC Guidelines on the diagnosis and treatment of aortic diseases: Document covering acute and chronic aortic diseases of the thoracic and abdominal aorta of the adult. The Task Force for the Diagnosis and Treatment of Aortic Diseases of the European Society of Cardiology (ESC). *Eur Heart J* 2014;**35**:2873–926.

Erbel R, Engberding R, Daniel W, Roelandt J, Visser C, Rennollet H. Echocardiography in diagnosis of aortic dissection. *Lancet* 1989;**1**:457–61.

Hiratzka LF, Bakris GL, Beckman JA, *et al*. 2010 ACCF/AHA/AATS/ACR/ASA/SCA/SCAI/SIR/STS/SVM guidelines for the diagnosis and management of patients with thoracic aortic disease: a report of the American College of Cardiology Foundation/American Heart Association Task Force on Practice Guidelines, American Association for Thoracic Surgery, American College of Radiology, American Stroke Association, Society of Cardiovascular Anesthesiologists, Society for Cardiovascular Angiography and Interventions, Society of Interventional Radiology, Society of Thoracic Surgeons, and Society for Vascular Medicine. *Circulation* 2010;**121**:e266–369.

Iliceto S, Ettorre G, Francioso G, Antonelli G, Biasco G, Rizzon P. Diagnosis of aneurysm of the thoracic aorta. Comparison between two non-invasive techniques: two-dimensional echocardiography and computed tomography. *Eur Heart J* 1984;**5**:545–55.

Khandheria BK, Tajik AJ, Taylor CL, *et al*. Aortic dissection: review of value and limitations of two-dimensional echocardiography in a six-year experience. *J Am Soc Echocardiogr* 1989;**2**:17–24.

Mintz GS, Kotler MN, Segal BL, Parry WR. Two dimensional echocardiographic recognition of the descending thoracic aorta. *Am J Cardiol* 1979;**44**: 232–8.

Nienaber CA, von Kodolitsch Y, Nicolas V, *et al*. The diagnosis of thoracic aortic dissection by non-invasive imaging procedures. *N Engl J Med* 1993;**328**:1–9.

Novelline RA, Rhea JT, Rao PM, Stuk JL. Helical CT in emergency radiology. *Radiology* 1999;**213**:321–39.

Sommer T, Fehske W, Holzknecht N, *et al*. Aortic dissection: a comparative study of diagnosis with spiral CT, multiplanar transesophageal echocardiography, and MR imaging. *Radiology* 1996;**199**:347–52.

Trimarchi S, Nienaber CA, Rampoldi V, *et al*. Contemporary results of surgery in acute type A aortic dissection: The International Registry of Acute Aortic Dissection experience. *J Thorac Cardiovasc Surg* 2005;**129**:112–22.

Acute Kidney Injury

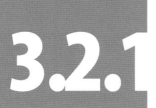

3.2.1

Nuttha Lumlertgul, Alistair Connell and Marlies Ostermann

Keywords: acute kidney injury, nephrotoxin, chronic kidney disease, renal failure

Key Learning Points

1. Acute kidney injury (AKI) is characterised by an acute decline in glomerular filtration rate, defined by an increase in serum creatinine and/or fall in urine output, according to the Kidney Disease: Improving Global Outcomes (KDIGO) criteria.

2. Clinical risk scores, biomarkers and stress tests have been developed for prediction and risk stratification in AKI. Combining risk scores with biomarkers or stress tests can increase accuracy in AKI prediction and prognostication.

3. Common causes of AKI in critically ill patients are hypovolaemia, sepsis, nephrotoxin exposure and haemodynamic instability, often in combination. Each cause has distinct and complex pathogenesis.

4. General principles of AKI management are optimisation of haemodynamic and fluid status with appropriate monitoring, serial measurement of creatinine and electrolytes, urine output monitoring, glucose control, avoidance of nephrotoxic drugs, treatment of the underlying cause, management of potential AKI-related complications and renal replacement therapy if indicated.

5. AKI is associated with short- and long-term complications, premature chronic kidney disease and end-stage renal disease and death. Monitoring of AKI survivors is essential.

Introduction

Acute kidney injury (AKI) is a syndrome characterised by a rapid deterioration of kidney function. It is common in ICUs and associated with increased morbidity, mortality and costs of care. AKI leads to accumulation of toxins and fluid, imbalances in electrolytes and dysfunction of non-renal organs. Long-term survivors also experience an increased risk of sequelae, including chronic kidney disease (CKD), end-stage renal disease (ESRD) and long-term morbidity and mortality. Although there are several therapies under ongoing investigation, there is currently no cure for AKI. Prevention, avoidance of risk factors, timely diagnosis and investigation for correctable causes, management of complications and renal replacement therapy (RRT) remain the cornerstones of therapy. This chapter aims to review the basic understanding of AKI diagnosis, causes, pathophysiology and diagnostic workup, and summarises the principles of AKI treatment in the critical care setting.

Diagnosis of AKI

AKI was previously defined by the Risk, Injury, Failure, Loss, End-stage kidney disease (RIFLE) criteria and later by the Acute Kidney Injury Network (AKIN) classification. In 2012, the Kidney Disease: Improving Global Outcomes (KDIGO) committee merged both definitions and established the KDIGO consensus criteria, consisting of an increase in serum creatinine (SCr) or a decline in urine output, or both. Based on the maximum rise in SCr and/or the degree of oliguria, there are three stages of AKI (Table 3.2.1.1). Higher AKI stages are associated with an increased risk of complications and mortality.

Table 3.2.1.1 AKI staging by the Kidney Disease: Improving Global Outcomes (KDIGO) criteria

AKI stage	Serum creatinine criteria	Urine output criteria
AKI stage 1	Increase by ≥0.3 mg/dl (≥26.4 µmol/l) Or Increase to 1.5–1.9 times from baseline	Urine output <0.5 ml/(kg hr) for 6–12 hours
AKI stage 2	Increase to 2.0–2.9 times from baseline	Urine output <0.5 ml/(kg hr) for ≥12 hours
AKI stage 3	Increase ≥3.0 times from baseline Or Increase to ≥4.0 mg/dl (≥354 µmol/l) Or Treatment with RRT Or In patients <18 years: decrease in estimated GFR to <35 ml/min per 1.73 m²	Urine output <0.3 ml/(kg hr) for ≥24 hours Or Anuria for ≥12 hours

Abbreviations: AKI = acute kidney injury; RRT = renal replacement therapy; GFR = glomerular filtration rate.

Limitations of Creatinine Criteria

Creatinine is a metabolite of creatine, which is synthesised from the amino acids glycine and arginine in the liver, pancreas and kidneys (Figure 3.2.1.1).

Creatine is transported via the bloodstream to skeletal muscle where it serves as an energy reservoir and is metabolised, through phosphorylation, to high-energy phosphocreatine. Creatine conversion to phosphocreatine is catalysed by creatine kinase (CK), leading to the formation of creatinine. Total creatinine production is determined by the productive capability of the liver, pancreas and kidneys and muscle function. In health, the production rate equals the renal excretion rate, as the molecular weight of creatinine is 113 Da and creatinine can be readily filtered through the glomeruli. In critical illness and sepsis, creatinine production is often impaired as a result of reduced function of the liver and skeletal muscle. In the case of decreased glomerular function, the half-life of SCr increases from 4 hours to 24–72 hours. Therefore, a detectable SCr increase may lag after an actual insult to the kidneys. Fluid overload may dilute SCr concentration further. Certain drugs may also compete with tubular creatinine secretion, such as trimethoprim or cimetidine, resulting in a SCr rise without any change in renal function. Finally, substances such as bilirubin or drugs may interfere with certain analytical techniques, namely Jaffe-based assays.

In addition, determination of baseline SCr is challenging as true baseline SCr values in steady state are not always available. Currently, it is recommended to use a historic SCr value from 7 to 365 days before admission as a baseline value. If no actual baseline

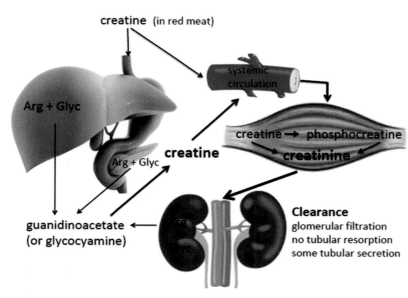

Figure 3.2.1.1 Generation and clearance of creatinine.

SCr is available, the first hospital admission SCr can be used. However, this method may not be reliable in community-acquired AKI with patients presenting with a high SCr on admission. Back calculation of the glomerular filtration rate (GFR) assuming an estimated glomerular filtration rate (eGFR) of 75 ml/min per 1.73 m² by the Modification of Diet in Renal Disease (MDRD) equation is also acceptable, although this method is likely to result in overestimation of the true GFR.

Daily variations in SCr may not reflect changes in the GFR. For example, an increase of SCr by 0.3 mg/dl in patients with underlying CKD might be insignificant, compared to a similar rise in patients with normal baseline renal function. Defining AKI stage 3 by RRT commencement is also problematic, as the timing of RRT initiation differs vastly in clinical practice. Lastly, the MDRD formula used to estimate the GFR is not valid in AKI due to an unsteady state, and should not be used to estimate the GFR during critical illness.

Limitations of Urine Criteria

Not all oliguric patients have AKI. Transient oliguria may be an appropriate physiological response of functioning kidneys during periods of prolonged fasting, hypovolaemia, after surgery and following stress, pain or trauma. The action of anti-diuretic hormone may concentrate the urine, with osmolarities of up to 1400 mOsm/l. The urine volume may physiologically decrease to 500 ml despite normal renal function. In obese patients, using actual weight instead of ideal body weight may mislead the AKI diagnosis. Therefore, ideal body weight is recommended for calculating the urine volume per kilogram per hour. Likewise, AKI can develop without any reduction in urine output – for instance, in acute interstitial nephritis where the kidneys may lose their concentrating ability.

Utilisation of AKI Biomarkers

Biomarkers with different functions have been developed to allow early diagnosis of renal dysfunction before SCr rises or urine output decreases. Various biomarkers have been discovered that reflect either glomerular or tubular damage (i.e. damage markers) or impairment of function (i.e. functional markers) (Figure 3.2.1.2).

Typically, they indicate different types of glomerular and/or tubular disorders, i.e. markers of glomerular filtration (cystatin C), glomerular integrity (albuminuria and proteinuria), tubular stress (insulin-like growth factor binding protein 7 (IGFBP-7), tissue inhibitor metalloproteinase 2 (TIMP2)), tubular damage (i.e. neutrophil gelatinase-associated lipocalin (NGAL), kidney injury molecule-1 (KIM-1), N-acetyl-β-D-glucosaminidase (NAG), liver fatty acid-binding protein (L-FAB)), and intrarenal inflammation (i.e. interleukin-18).

Patients with 'subclinical AKI', defined as those with positive damage biomarkers, but normal SCr and urine output, have increased risks of short- and long-term

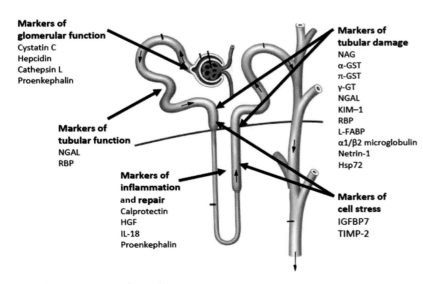

Markers of glomerular function
Cystatin C
Hepcidin
Cathepsin L
Proenkephalin

Markers of tubular function
NGAL
RBP

Markers of inflammation and repair
Calprotectin
HGF
IL-18
Proenkephalin

Markers of tubular damage
NAG
α-GST
π-GST
γ-GT
NGAL
KIM–1
RBP
L-FABP
α1/β2 microglobulin
Netrin-1
Hsp72

Markers of cell stress
IGFBP7
TIMP-2

Figure 3.2.1.2 New AKI biomarkers.

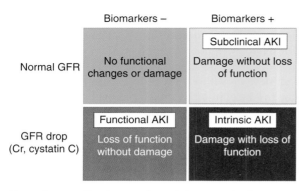

Figure 3.2.1.3 Classification of acute kidney injury by changes in function/damage. AKI = acute kidney injury; GFR = glomerular filtration rate; Cr = creatinine.
Source: Modified from Acute Disease Quality Initiative 23 (www.adqi .org) and used with permission.

complications, compared to those with negative biomarkers and SCr. In the future, these biomarkers might be incorporated into clinical practice to delineate patients into different spectra and might indicate a window for intervention in those with early damage, but without evident functional loss (Figure 3.2.1.3).

Differentiation between AKI, CKD and AKI on Top of CKD

CKD is defined as eGFR <60 ml/min per 1.73 m² or evidence of structural damage persisting for >3 months. Occasionally, patients may present to the ICU with high urea or SCr with no baseline creatinine available. Their symptoms might be attributed to AKI, CKD or AKI on top of CKD (AoCKD). Clues for CKD include medical history, history of repeated SCr measurements over time, presence of pre-morbid albuminuria, evidence of small-sized kidneys, cortical thinning, loss of corticomedullary differentiation and increased parenchymal echogenicity on renal ultrasonography. Metabolic complications from CKD, such as anaemia and mineral bone disorders (e.g. hyperphosphataemia, hyperparathyroidism), should be looked for. Urine microscopy might show evidence of broad casts, resulting from chronic tubular damage. Note that these features might be present in both AKI and CKD patients, and in some cases, it may not be possible to initially differentiate AKI and CKD. After hospital admission, a decrease in SCr might indicate resolving AKI. Note that AKI is on the same continuum as CKD, with a bidirectional relationship; AKI is a risk factor for CKD, and vice versa.

AKI Alerts

Computerised data systems can analyse online laboratory data and urine output for early diagnosis of AKI and readily notify physicians. They can also simultaneously flag risk factors such as nephrotoxin use and hypotension, and early management can be employed. Short- and long-term AKI outcomes can potentially be improved by combining electronic alerts with protocolised care bundles.

Common Causes of AKI in Intensive Care Units

Renal Hypoperfusion

Renal hypoperfusion can be caused by several factors, e.g. hypovolaemia, systemic vasodilation or increased vascular resistance. This activates adaptive mechanisms, such as autoregulation mechanisms, the sympathetic nervous system and the renin–angiotensin–aldosterone system (RAAS), to maintain the GFR. AKI frequently occurs in true hypovolaemic conditions such as haemorrhage or severe diarrhoea. When hypoperfusion is sustained and the adaptive response is inadequate, the GFR is initially decreased without parenchymal damage (functional AKI). If adequate renal perfusion is not restored, tubular injury follows. Some populations might have a higher risk of developing AKI following mild to moderate reductions in kidney perfusion due to the presence of co-morbidities, such as chronic hypertension or diabetes, and medications (e.g. non-steroidal anti-inflammatory drugs (NSAIDs), angiotensin-converting enzyme inhibitors (ACEIs), angiotensin receptor blockers (ARBs)). Hypervolaemia or volume overload can also be deleterious; venous congestion and intra-abdominal hypertension can increase intrarenal interstitial pressure, cause venous congestion and lower renal blood flow and subsequently GFR.

Sepsis-Associated AKI

Sepsis is defined as life-threatening organ dysfunction caused by dysregulated host response to infection. Sepsis-associated AKI (SA-AKI) occurs in 10–20 per cent of all sepsis patients and in 50–70 per cent of septic shock patients. In turn, AKI patients have increased risk of in-hospital and long-term sepsis due to suppressed immune function.

SA-AKI is not associated with hypoperfusion or ischaemic–reperfusion injury as previously thought.

Post-mortem histology has shown that renal histology is relatively well preserved without acute tubular necrosis. In fact, animal studies have shown normal, or even increased, renal blood flow in sepsis. Decreased GFR occurs due to efferent arteriolar vasodilation and intrarenal shunting, which leads to diversion of blood flow away from the medulla and subsequent medullary hypoxia. Septic cardiomyopathy may also contribute to renal hypoperfusion in SA-AKI. In addition, during sepsis, damage-associated molecular patterns (DAMPs) and pathogen-associated molecular patterns (PAMPs), such as lipopolysaccharide, enter the tubular lumen after being filtered and activate Toll-like receptors (TLRs) expressed on tubular and endothelial cells. Receptor activation triggers release of further pro-inflammatory mediators and recruitment of inflammatory cells. Lastly, microvascular dysfunction, inflammation and metabolic reprogramming contribute to SA-AKI.

Nephrotoxins

Exposure to nephrotoxins is a contributing factor in to up to 25 per cent of cases of AKI. Nephrotoxins can affect kidneys in different ways, including haemodynamic perturbations, direct cytotoxicity on renal tubular epithelial cells, interstitial inflammation, podocyte or endothelial cell damage leading to glomerular injury, and precipitation of metabolites or crystals or endothelial injury (Table 3.2.1.2).

Most cases are acute and non-oliguric, and resolve with discontinuation of the drugs. However, residual tubular dysfunction and CKD might persist after nephrotoxic AKI. Particular nephrotoxins of note include the following.

Contrast

Contrast-associated AKI is characterised by a decline in creatinine within days after iodinated contrast administration. Contrast agents are directly toxic to tubular epithelial cells, causing apoptosis, necrosis and tubular injury. They may also cause disturbances in intrarenal blood flow. Pre-existing CKD, high-osmolality contrast agent, use of contrast medium at a high volume (>350 ml or >4 ml/kg) or repeated administration within 72 hours and intra-arterial contrast administration are risk factors. Most patients recover, although a few patients eventually require RRT. Correction of intravascular hypovolaemia is recommended for prevention, although the optimal rate or timing of volume expansion has not been established. Risks may also be mitigated by minimising the infused volume of contrast and avoiding hyperosmolar contrast material.

An important differential diagnosis in patients with atherosclerosis undergoing coronary angiography or invasive intra-arterial procedures is renal atheroembolism. It manifests as a subacute decline in the GFR from weeks to months. Physical examination might reveal blue toes, livedo reticularis and evidence of cholesterol

Table 3.2.1.2 Mechanisms of drug-induced acute kidney injury

	Haemodynamic	Tubular	Interstitial	Glomerular	Crystal-induced tubular obstruction	Vascular injury
Type of injury	Haemodynamic alterations	Cytopathic or toxic injury	Inflammatory reactions	Nephritis, nephrotic syndrome	Intracellular deposition or intratubular obstruction	TMA
Mechanisms	Imbalances between afferent and efferent arteriolar tone	Mitochondrial damage	Hypersensitivity reaction	Podocyte or endothelial damage	Osmotic, obstructive or epithelial cell toxicity	Endothelial cell damage
Common agents	ACEIs ARBs IL-2 Ciclosporin NSAIDs Contrast	Aminoglycosides Cisplatin Contrast Vancomycin Amphotericin	Penicillin Proton pump inhibitors Allopurinol Aristolochic acid	Bisphosphonates Hydralazine Propylthiouracil	Phosphate, orlistat Indinavir Aciclovir Methotrexate	Calcineurin inhibitors Mitomycin C Clopidogrel Quinine

Abbreviations: TMA = thrombotic microangiopathy; ACEI = angiotensin-converting enzyme inhibitor; ARB = angiotensin receptor blocker; IL-2 = interleukin-2; NSAID = non-steroidal anti-inflammatory drug.

emboli in retinal arteries (Hollenhorst plaques). Laboratory investigations might show eosinophilia, increased lactate dehydrogenase and decreased complement levels (C3).

Proton Pump Inhibitors

Using proton pump inhibitors (PPIs) is associated with acute interstitial nephritis (AIN) and chronic tubulointerstitial nephritis. In most cases, recovery from AKI occurs after drug withdrawal; however, most patients are left with some level of residual renal dysfunction and incident CKD. Hyponatraemia and hypomagnesaemia are common electrolyte disorders following PPI use.

Antibiotics

Common antibiotics which potentially cause AKI are aminoglycosides, vancomycin, colistin or a combination of macrolide antibiotics with other inhibitors of cytochrome (CYP3A4) enzymes (e.g. statins or calcium channel blockers). Amphotericin B is a well-known anti-fungal drug which can cause AKI, nephrogenic diabetes insipidus and distal renal tubular acidosis.

Crystal Precipitation

Sulfadiazine, aciclovir, indinavir, triamterene, methotrexate, orlistat, oral sodium phosphate preparation, sulfamethoxazole and ciprofloxacin can cause AKI from crystal precipitation. Distinct crystal features can be found on urine microscopy. In addition, acute oxalate nephropathy can be caused by exogenous administration of ethylene glycol poisoning and diets, including nuts, rhubarb, vitamin C, starfruit, black tea, etc.

Drug-Induced Glomerular Injury

Intravenous bisphosphonates are associated with acute tubular injury and collapsing focal segmental glomerulosclerosis (FSGS). D-penicillamine, hydralazine, propylthiouracil and levamisole-adulterated cocaine are secondary causes of pauci-immune, rapidly progressive glomerulonephritis, which presents with a subacute decline in GFR, with urine sediments, proteinuria and hypertension.

Chemotherapy

Cisplatin, ifosfamide, pamidronate and zoledronic acid are well-known chemotherapy agents which are nephrotoxic. In the last few years, the field of oncology has advanced rapidly with the emergence of new therapies, of which some can cause AKI. Nivolumab and pembrolizumab are anti-programmed death-1 (PD-1) antibodies (sometimes referred to as checkpoint inhibitors) and associated with AIN and hyponatraemia. Bortezomib and carfilzomib are proteasome inhibitors used for the treatment of myeloma. These agents can cause AKI, ranging from pre-renal disease and tumour lysis-like phenomenon to thrombotic microangiopathy (TMA). The immunomodulatory drugs lenalidomide and pomalidomide used for treatment in myeloma and amyloidosis have also been associated with AKI. The B-rapidly accelerated fibrosarcoma (*BRAF*) oncogene inhibitors (e.g. vemurafenib and dabrafenib) are reported to be associated with AIN, acute tubular injury, subnephrotic-range proteinuria, hypokalaemia, hyponatraemia and hypophosphataemia.

Obstruction

Obstruction may occur at any point along the urinary tract, and is categorised into extrarenal (e.g. prostate hypertrophy, retroperitoneal fibrosis, lymph nodes, tumours) and intrarenal obstruction (e.g. nephrolithiasis, blood clots). Obstruction leads to an increase in intratubular pressure, impaired renal blood flow and triggering of inflammatory processes. Importantly, SCr may be normal in unilateral obstruction if the excretory function of the contralateral kidney is not impaired. Irreversible tubulointerstitial fibrosis will occur if the obstruction is not treated. Although several factors might contribute to the chance of full renal recovery (e.g. site of obstruction, severity, previous kidney function, the presence or absence of infection), the most important factor appears to be time to relief. Ultrasound and non-contrast spiral computed tomography remain the most commonly used forms of imaging in the acute stage.

After relief of obstruction, massive polyuria and natriuresis may occur. A number of factors are presumed to contribute to this, including osmotic effects of retained solutes, impaired ability to concentrate urine due to tubular damage and activation of natriuretic factors after volume expansion. Care should be taken that fluid is replaced without causing fluid overload. Multiple electrolyte abnormalities (e.g. hypokalaemia, hypomagnesaemia) may also occur and should be replaced.

Cardiac and Vascular Surgery-Associated AKI

Cardiac and vascular surgery-associated AKI (CVS-AKI) generally refers to AKI occurring within 2–7 days of cardiovascular surgery. The incidence is

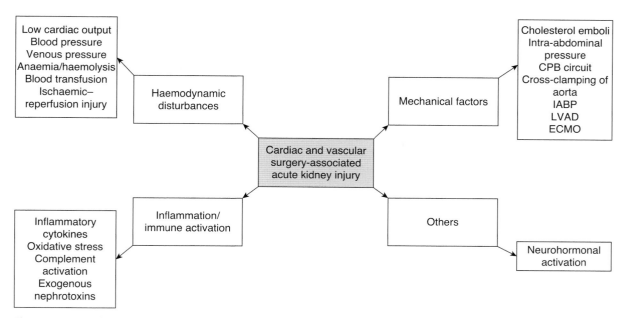

Figure 3.2.1.4 Pathogenesis of cardiac and vascular surgery-associated acute kidney injury. CPB = cardiopulmonary bypass; IABP = intra-aortic balloon pump; LVAD = left ventricular assist device; ECMO = extracorporeal membrane oxygenation.

approximately 20–30 per cent. Pre-surgical risk factors include CKD, diabetes, hypertension, heart disease, anaemia, proteinuria, emergency, cardiogenic shock, etc. The pathogenesis of CVS-AKI includes several processes (Figure 3.2.1.4).

Postulated mechanisms include renal hypoperfusion, neurohormonal activation, immunomodulation, inflammation and exposure to exogenous and endogenous nephrotoxins. Cardiac dysfunction is greater in cardiac surgery, and warm ischaemia–reperfusion injury to the kidneys and increased abdominal pressures are more prominent in vascular surgery. In cardiac surgery, bioincompatibility reaction from contact of blood and artificial surfaces of cardiopulmonary bypass (CPB) is a significant risk factor for AKI. CPB, cross-clamping of the aorta, high doses of exogenous vasopressors and blood product transfusion all enhance the risk of AKI. Associated tissue damage and reperfusion injury increase oxidative stress, inflammation and immune activation. The rewarming phase of CPB exacerbates medullary ischaemia because of the combination of high oxygen demand and low oxygen supply in the medulla. Furthermore, CPB leads to free haemoglobin liberation with the release of free iron, which is augmented by prolonged hypothermia (temperature as low as <18°C), and produces renal

vasoconstriction from scavenging of nitric oxide by free haemoglobin. Free haemoglobin and free ferrous iron then increase the production of reactive oxygen species and trigger further inflammation. Cholesterol embolisation is another cause of AKI during cardiovascular surgery and is caused by distal migration of cholesterol crystals when a cross-clamp is applied or released from the aorta, especially in patients with significant atherosclerosis. Intra-aortic balloon counterpulsation devices can increase the embolic load. Extracorporeal organ support (e.g. left ventricular assist device (LVAD) and extracorporeal membrane oxygenation (ECMO)) can also precipitate haemolysis and cause pigment-associated nephropathy.

Surgery-Associated AKI

Variable factors predict risks of surgery-associated AKI. Renal hypoperfusion may be caused by fluid depletion from blood losses, insensible losses, extravasation of fluid to the third space or systemic effects of anaesthetic drugs (e.g. peripheral vasodilation, myocardial depression). Intraoperative hypotension is an important determinant of AKI. In a similar manner to cardiac surgery, sustained pro-inflammatory and anti-inflammatory responses and immune responses can occur in response to tissue injury.

147

Hepatorenal Syndrome

Previously, hepatorenal syndrome was traditionally defined using an absolute cut-off of SCr $\geq$1.5 mg/dl (132 mmol/l); however, the recent definition incorporates the KDIGO criteria (Table 3.2.1.1).

Hepatorenal syndrome is described as volume-unresponsive kidney injury after exclusion of glomerular or structural causes and withdrawal of nephrotoxic drugs. It is a form of renal vasoconstriction with systemic and splanchnic vasodilation from increased nitric oxide. Activated sympathetic nervous system and RAAS, cirrhotic cardiomyopathy and abnormal renal autoregulation also play a role in the pathogenesis. Other causes of AKI in the setting of liver disease are intravascular hypovolaemia, large-volume paracentesis, intra-abdominal compartment syndrome from massive ascites, intrinsic renal disease and SA-AKI. Diagnostic workup in hepatorenal syndrome usually reveals very low urine sodium and fractional excretion of sodium (FE_{Na}).

Norfloxacin has been found to decrease the frequency of spontaneous bacterial peritonitis (SBP) and the rate of hepatorenal syndrome in patients with SCr $\geq$106 mmol/l (1.2 mg/dl), and improve survival. Rifaximin is a minimally absorbed broad-spectrum antibiotic with activity against Gram-negative, Gram-positive and anaerobic bacteria. It has been shown to treat hepatic encephalopathy, and decrease the risk of AKI, HRS and the requirement for RRT.

Cardio-renal Syndrome

There are five types of cardio-renal syndrome (CRS): type 1 – acute cardiac dysfunction leading to decreased kidney function; type 2 – chronic progressive disease due to chronic heart failure; type 3 – acute worsening of kidney function causing cardiac dysfunction; type 4 – chronic kidney disease leading to chronic cardiac dysfunction; and type 5 – systemic conditions, such as sepsis, causing simultaneous dysfunction of the heart and kidney. The pathogenesis of CRS is not simply based on decreased cardiac output but is also caused by increased venous congestion and increased intrarenal pressure, or both. Therefore, diuretic treatment to alleviate renal congestion is essential in the treatment of CRS. Other potential mechanisms involved are sympathetic nervous system and RAAS activation, chronic inflammation and imbalance in reactive oxygen species or nitric oxide production. There were no significant differences in symptom relief or renal outcomes

when furosemide was administered by bolus or continuous infusion. Continuous infusion of furosemide is associated with less ototoxicity, when compared with intermittent bolus dosing. Inotropes should be used in patients with low cardiac output state. Ultrafiltration (UF) should be reserved for those who are refractory to stepped diuretic therapy. Currently, there is insufficient evidence to recommend the routine use of UF as an alternative to diuretic therapy in acute decompensated heart failure.

Abdominal Compartment Syndrome

Normal intra-abdominal pressure (IAP) is 5–7 mmHg. Intra-abdominal hypertension (IAH) is defined as sustained elevation in IAP of $\geq$12 mmHg, and abdominal compartment syndrome (ACS) is defined as sustained IAP of >20 mmHg associated with new organ dysfunction. ACS can be caused by increased intra-abdominal content (mass, fluid or blood), interstitial oedema (fluid overload) or external compression (retroperitoneal bleeding). Risk factors include trauma, major burns, abdominal surgery, mechanical ventilation, obesity, ascites, haemoperitoneum, gastric or bowel distension, large-volume resuscitation and pancreatitis. IAH decreases perfusion of any abdominal organ, including the kidneys, and the effects can be transmitted to other compartments, leading to multiple organ failure, including decreased cardiac output, impaired ventilation and increased intracranial pressure. AKI from IAH is a result of both elevation in renal venous and parenchymal pressures and reduction of arterial inflow. Systemic inflammation from impaired visceral perfusion and increased cytokine levels also contribute to kidney damage. Furthermore, IAH has been implicated in the pathogenesis of both hepatorenal syndrome and CRS.

Rhabdomyolysis

Causes include trauma, exertion, muscle hypoxia, infection, severe electrolyte disturbances (e.g. hypokalaemia or hypophosphataemia), drugs (e.g. statin, alcohol, heroin, cocaine) and genetic defects. Pathogenesis includes hypovolaemia due to loss of fluid from muscle sequestration, renal vasoconstriction from decreased nitric oxide and increased thromboxane and endothelin, direct toxicity of myoglobin and generation of reactive oxygen species and intratubular obstruction from binding of myoglobin with Tamm–Horsfall proteins at distal tubules. Rhabdomyolysis is often seen in patients with CK levels of >5000 U/l. For prevention and treatment, hydration to maintain adequate urine output is the most important strategy. Urine output should be targeted at 2–3 ml/(kg hr). Electrolyte disturbances, including hyperkalaemia, hypocalcaemia and hyperphosphataemia, should be frequently checked. Urine alkalinisation with sodium bicarbonate to keep urine pH >6.5 might be ordered in selected patients. Finally, RRT should be started according to standard indications, e.g. hyperkalaemia refractory to medical treatment.

Tumour Lysis Syndrome

Tumour lysis syndrome results from the release of intracellular electrolytes and nucleic acids from malignant cells that were lysed spontaneously or by anticancer therapies. Nearly all haematological and solid organ cancers have been associated with tumour lysis syndrome, most commonly those with large tumour burden and high proliferation rates (e.g. Burkitt's lymphoma and acute lymphoblastic leukaemia). Tumour lysis syndrome is characterised by hyperuricaemia, hyperkalaemia, hyperphosphataemia and hypocalcaemia. The syndrome may be associated with AKI, cardiac arrhythmia, seizures or death. Cytokine release associated with acute tubular injury, acute uric acid nephropathy and acute nephrocalcinosis is an important factor in the development of AKI. Uric acid results from metabolism of purine nucleotides from cancer cells by xanthine oxidase into insoluble uric acid. High levels of uric acid may precipitate in renal tubules, causing intratubular obstruction, vasoconstriction and upregulation of inflammatory cytokines. In patients with hyperphosphataemia, calcium phosphate precipitation in renal tubules may also contribute to AKI, especially if the urine is alkaline. Prevention includes maintenance of an adequate volume status through intravenous hydration, aiming for a urine output of 2–3 ml/(kg hr) to be able to clear uric acid and potassium. However, urine alkalinisation is not recommended as it might enhance calcium phosphate precipitation in renal tubules. Prophylactic use of xanthine oxidase inhibitors, such as allopurinol or febuxostat, is recommended in patients who are at high risk of tumour lysis syndrome. Treatment with rasburicase, a recombinant urate oxidase, to convert uric acid to the more soluble allantoin, might be beneficial prior to chemotherapy in those with very high uric acid levels. However, rasburicase leads to the production of hydrogen peroxide, which can cause methaemoglobinaemia and haemolytic anaemia in patients with glucose-6-phosphate dehydrogenase (G6PD) deficiency. There is no role for prophylactic dialysis to prevent tumour lysis syndrome. Similarly, RRT should be initiated as per standard indications.

Intrinsic Causes of AKI

1. Diseases affecting the renal vasculature:
   a. Small-vessel vasculitides, e.g. thrombotic thrombocytopenia purpura and haemolytic uraemic syndrome, anti-phospholipid syndrome
   b. Diseases affecting larger vessels, e.g. systemic thromboembolism or acute renal vein thrombosis
2. Diseases affecting the glomeruli:
   a. *Acute glomerulonephritis* (onset days to weeks) or *rapidly progressive glomerulonephritis* (onset weeks to months) with active urinary sediment with dysmorphic red blood cells/cellular casts. Patients may also exhibit a variable degree of proteinuria. Systemic presentation may suggest the underlying cause. For example, pulmonary haemorrhage would suggest a diagnosis of pauci-immune glomerulonephritis or Goodpasture's syndrome; haematuria following a respiratory tract infection would suggest post-streptococcal glomerulonephritis; anaemia, rash, joint pain and serositis would suggest lupus glomerulonephritis
   b. *Diseases causing a nephrotic pattern of disease* may present with a spectrum of proteinuria, from subnephrotic (1–3 g proteinuria/day) to full nephrotic syndrome (>3.5 g proteinuria/day, with marked oedema and hyperlipidaemia). Causes of AKI in this category include primary renal diseases (e.g. minimal change disease, idiopathic membranous nephropathy, etc.) and a range of systemic disorders that affect the kidneys (lupus, cast nephropathy in myeloma). Hypovolaemic AKI may occur in patients with massive proteinuria causing leakage of fluid into the interstitium (nephrosarca) and resulting in ineffective intravascular volume. Renal vein thrombosis can develop in patients with massive proteinuria (>10 g/day) with risk factors such as hypercoagulable state and anti-phospholipid syndrome

149

3. Diseases affecting the tubules/interstitium:
   a. AIN is characterised by normal blood pressure and non-oliguric AKI due to impaired urine concentration. Maculopapular rash might be found in drug-induced AIN. Proteinuria and haematuria are most commonly found, followed by eosinophiluria/eosinophilia which are sometimes seen in drug-induced AIN
   b. Potential causes are antibiotics (penicillins, cephalosporins, quinolones), diuretics (thiazide, furosemide), analgesics (NSAIDs), anti-convulsants (phenytoin, carbamazepine, phenobarbitol), allopurinol, cimetidine and PPIs

Risk Stratification in AKI

Some patients might be at higher risk of AKI than others. There are different types of risk stratification. The goal is to identify high-risk patients before exposure, so that management can be guided to prevent the development of AKI.

Clinical Risk Scores

Several AKI risk scores have been developed (e.g. Cleveland Clinic Score, Dialysis Risk after Cardiac Surgery) to predict AKI with good accuracy. The renal anginal index (RAI) is based on a combination of clinically significant risk factors to identify high-risk patients for AKI development. Susceptibilities (advanced age, hypertension, diabetes, CKD) and exposures (volume depletion, nephrotoxins, sepsis) are used to categorise patients into moderate, high and very high risk. Then the clinical risk score is multiplied by the daily increase in SCr. The higher the RAI, the higher the risk of severe AKI within 3 days. More advanced techniques (e.g. Machine Learning) may utilise a larger volume of structured patient data to predict future AKI with improved accuracy. The output of risk scoring or prediction systems may be displayed in the electronic health record (EHR).

Other Risk Prediction Tools

1. **Biomarkers:** some novel biomarkers (TIMP2, IGFBP-7, NGAL and cystatin C) have been found to be predictive of adverse outcomes in high-risk patients (e.g. post-cardiac surgery, ICU, intubated and on vasopressors). Importantly, patients need to have high pre-test probability in order to achieve the best sensitivity and specificity. The

clinical settings and limitations of each biomarker should therefore be kept in mind with the interpretation of each test.

2. **Stress tests:** common stress tests are furosemide stress test (tubular stress test) and renal functional reserve (RFR) tests (glomerular stress test). The furosemide stress test constitutes of giving furosemide (1 mg/kg intravenously if furosemide-naïve, and 1.5 mg/kg if previously exposed to furosemide), in combination with intravenous fluid to avoid intravascular hypovolaemia. A urine output of <200 ml in 2 hours has been shown to have high accuracy for progression to AKI stage 3.

3. **Renal functional reserve (RFR) testing:** RFR testing aims to test the difference between 'resting GFR' and 'stress GFR' after an oral protein load, as an indicator of the RFR. Patients with low functional reserve have been shown to have a higher risk of AKI after cardiac surgery.

Clinical risk scores and biomarkers may be used together to improve early detection in high-risk patients. These tests should always be interpreted with the clinical context and combined with an action plan to prevent AKI.

Prevention

General principles of AKI prevention include management of risk factors, discontinuation/avoidance of nephrotoxic agents, avoidance of contrast media, proper renal dosing of all pharmacologic agents and optimisation of haemodynamics and fluid status. Adequate oxygenation and haemoglobin concentration (>70 g/l) should be maintained. A target mean arterial pressure (MAP) of at least 65 mmHg should be maintained in circulatory shock patients. Patients with chronic hypertension might benefit from a higher MAP (>80 mmHg). In older patients (≥65 years), MAP targets of 60–65 mmHg can be allowed, with no difference in mortality and kidney outcomes, compared with usual care.

Fluid should be administered judiciously, aiming to replenish the intravascular volume without causing fluid overload. Non-invasive and invasive monitoring, if necessary, should be employed to guide fluid management. Static measures (e.g. central venous pressure, central venous oxygen saturation ($ScVO_2$) or pulmonary wedge pressure) are not recommended; instead dynamic measures of volume responsiveness (e.g. pulse pressure variation, stroke volume variation, transthoracic or transoesophageal echocardiography Doppler, bioimpedance analysis and passive leg raising test) are recommended. If intravascular hypovolaemia has been corrected, but the patient remains hypotensive, vasopressors should be considered. Current guidelines recommend noradrenaline as the first-line vasopressor.

The choice of fluids is important. Hydroxyethyl starch is no longer advised, as it is associated with increased rates of AKI and RRT. Randomised controlled trials have not shown superiority of albumin over crystalloids. Saline 0.9% is associated with hyperchloraemic metabolic acidosis, which can lead to afferent renal vasoconstriction through the tubuloglomerular feedback system. Use of buffered solutions has been shown to decrease a composite endpoint of major adverse kidney events consisting of death, RRT and doubling of SCr at 30 days, compared with saline.

Contrast-associated AKI is becoming less common because of reduced toxicity of contrast and lesser amounts of contrast media used. *N*-acetylcysteine and bicarbonate have no role in preventing contrast-associated AKI.

Among patients undergoing cardiac surgery, off-pump coronary artery bypass grafting might attenuate AKI but should not be the sole reason for choosing this technique, as 5-year survival is lower with off-pump techniques, with no discernible differences in renal function. Moderate glucose control (7–10 mmol/l) is preferable to tight control (≤7 mmol/l) in patients undergoing coronary artery bypass grafting, with the most important factor being avoidance of glucose variability throughout the entire perioperative time frame. ACEIs and ARBs should be held before surgery.

Diagnostic Workup in AKI

AKI is a syndrome, and not a final diagnosis. Patients with AKI often encompass a variety of aetiologies and pathologies which are not as simple as pre-renal, renal and post-renal AKI as previously thought. After a diagnosis of AKI is made, investigation should focus on determining the underlying cause to allow prompt delivery of disease-specific interventions. Importantly, pre-renal AKI is not synonymous with 'hypovolaemic' AKI or 'transient' AKI and should not automatically trigger fluid administration. Tubular damage is commonly found in patients with pre-renal AKI and those with transient AKI. Recently, AKI has been more commonly categorised by its duration – 'transient' AKI, 'persistent or sustained' AKI and acute kidney disease.

Transient AKI is defined as total duration from AKI onset until recovery (SCr <1.5 times of baseline) of <48 hours. Persistent AKI is defined as total duration of >48 hours. Acute kidney disease is defined as AKI duration of >7 days, but not more than 90 days.

Some might prefer the differentiation between 'functional AKI' and 'damage AKI'. Functional AKI is defined by abnormal SCr due to loss of function without tubular or glomerular damage (for instance, ACEI-induced AKI). Examples of damage AKI are aminoglycoside-induced AKI or AIN.

The most common causes of AKI in intensive care are hypovolaemia, sepsis, CRS, major or cardiac surgery and nephrotoxic drugs. However, as many disease states cross such boundaries, it may make more sense to approach patients with an organised framework of specific syndromic diagnoses in mind (e.g. SA-AKI, CVS-AKI, nephrotoxic AKI, etc.).

Diagnostic Workup

- History and examination:
  - Are there any symptoms of AKI, e.g. oliguria, anuria, shortness of breath, orthopnoea, paroxysmal nocturnal dyspnoea?
  - Is there any indication of pre-existing renal disease or systemic disease with renal involvement, e.g. diabetes, chronic hypertension, liver disease, heart failure, connective tissue disease, vasculitis?
  - Is there any evidence of insult, e.g. sepsis, cardiac surgery, major surgery, nephrotoxic drugs?
  - Is there any history or evidence of trauma or obstruction to the genitourinary tract?

- Investigations:
  - **Blood urea and creatinine:** high urea-to-SCr ratio is suggestive of hypovolaemia. High SCr disproportionate to urea might suggest increased creatinine production (e.g. rhabdomyolysis)
  - **Blood and urine tests suggestive of pre-existing CKD:** such as chronic anaemia, hyperphosphataemia, hyperparathyroidism and broad casts
  - **Urinalysis:** urine sediments might give some clues to specific diagnoses. Urine white blood cells with or without eosinophiluria might suggest acute pyelonephritis or AIN. Urine red blood cells are found in catheterised

patients with trauma or glomerulonephritis patients. Haematuria and proteinuria are suggestive of glomerulonephritis. However, haematuria, leucocyturia or proteinuria are neither sensitive nor specific to a single cause of AKI. Interpretations should be made with the clinical history. Red supernatant urine with negative haem is from pigmenturia (e.g. beet, phenazopyridine, porphyria). Positive urine dipstick for haem without visible red blood cells or sediments on centrifugation is suggestive of rhabdomyolysis or haemolysis. Quantified proteinuria in the absence of albumin on dipstick signifies protein other than albumin (e.g. light chain – suggests myeloma)

○ **Urine microscopy:** urine sediments can be very useful with trained operators. For example, dysmorphic red blood cells with red cell casts are suggestive of glomerulonephritis. Urine crystals are unique to each type of crystalluria (e.g. calcium oxalate monohydrate, calcium oxalate dihydrate, triple phosphate crystals, uric acid crystal, drug crystals). Granular casts and epithelial cells are from acute tubular necrosis and can be used to predict progression of AKI

○ **Urine electrolytes:** a spot urine <20 mEq/l and FE_{Na} <1% may represent intact tubular function to reabsorb sodium in response to hypovolaemia. In contrast, spot urine >20 mEq/l and Fe_{Na} ≥2% may signify acute tubular necrosis. However, multiple factors can confound these findings and the results are not always indicative of the aetiologies. For instance, FE_{Na} <1% can be found with sepsis, acute obstruction, glomerulonephritis, rhabdomyolysis, radio-contrast agents, NSAID use and acute allograft rejection. Patients receiving diuretics or those with CKD might have FE_{Na} ≥1%. Alternatively, FE_{urea} <35% may represent low effective circulatory volume. The utility is lost with impaired proximal tubular function, such as in patients receiving acetazolamide, mannitol, glycosuria or high protein intake or those having cerebral salt wasting

○ **Renal ultrasonography:** it is very useful for evaluating pre-existing CKD and diagnosing obstruction of the urinary collecting system

○ **IAP:** this should be measured periodically in suspected ACS. IAP of >20 mmHg with organ dysfunction denotes ACS

• Additional investigations for specific causes:

○ **Autoimmune disease:** anti-nuclear antibody (ANA), anti-double-stranded deoxyribonucleic acid (anti-dsDNA), complement, antibodies to extractable nuclear antigens (anti-ENAs), anti-neutrophil cytoplasmic antibody (ANCA) profile and anti-glomerular basement membrane (anti-GBM) are commonly ordered when there is suspicion of immune-mediated, pauci-immune or anti-GBM glomerulonephritis. Further serologies may be sent for specific causes of glomerulonephritis (e.g. human immunodeficiency virus (HIV) antibody, hepatitis B antigen, anti-hepatitis C (HCV) antibody, cryoglobulin, rheumatoid factor, anti-streptolysin O (ASO), anti-DNAse B antibody)

○ **Myeloma:** serum or urine protein electrophoresis, immunofixation electrophoresis of blood or urine and serum free light chain should be sent to identify monoclonal proteins

○ **Anaemia, thrombocytopenia and increased lactate dehydrogenase:** these should be looked for in TMA

○ **Blood smear:** this should be reviewed to look for microangiopathic haemolytic anaemia (MAHA) blood picture in TMA

○ Reduced haptoglobin, Coombs' test, increased indirect bilirubin and increased reticulocyte counts are found in haemolysis

○ **CK** is increased in rhabdomyolysis

• **Kidney biopsy:** it is reserved for cases of suspected glomerular disease, interstitial nephritis or AKI with unclear aetiology. However, it is rarely done in ICUs due to high bleeding risks. Renal biopsy via the internal jugular vein is an alternative to the standard percutaneous route and is associated with a lower bleeding risk

Management of Complications

Traditionally, AKI was thought to be a single-organ process with complications. Traditional complications include hyperkalaemia, metabolic acidosis, hyper-phosphataemia, hypocalcaemia, volume overload and uraemic complications such as bleeding, pericarditis and altered mental status. Fluid overload, defined as accumulation of fluid of >10 per cent of baseline weight, has been proven to be associated with RRT, renal non-recovery and mortality in AKI. In view of increased RRT utilisation over the past few decades, death from AKI itself is rare. However, the concept of AKI has evolved over the past decade to AKI being a syndrome with interactions between organ systems, including the lung, heart, liver, brain and intestine. These non-traditional complications from 'organ–organ crosstalk' resulting in distant organ effects are the primary cause of high mortality in AKI. The leading cause of death in AKI is sepsis, which accounts for over 40 per cent of mortality, followed by cardiovascular complications.

Managing Complications in AKI

Volume Overload

Owing to an impaired ability to excrete salt and water, hypervolaemia may be evident on initial presentation or may develop after overzealous fluid administration. Diuretics can be of use as an initial treatment for hypervolaemia. An intravenous loop diuretic is usually used initially; depending on the clinical response to the initial treatment, increasing doses or addition of a thiazide may be necessary. Although RRT is the most efficient way of treating hypervolaemia, the clinical benefits of early RRT purely for volume management are unclear.

Hyperkalaemia

This is a common and potentially life-threatening complication of AKI. Broadly speaking, medical treatment for hyperkalaemia aims to achieve one of three things:

1. To ameliorate the effects of potassium on cell membranes (e.g. calcium gluconate)
2. To shift potassium into cells (e.g. insulin/dextrose infusions)
3. To remove potassium from the body (e.g. loop diuretics or dialysis)

Patients with serum potassium of >5.5 mmol/l, muscle weakness or cardiac conduction abnormalities should be treated as an emergency. Patients with potassium of >5.5 mmol/l who are oligo-anuric or where hyperkalaemia is refractory to medical treatment should be considered for RRT.

Metabolic Acidosis

Excretion of acid produced from normal cellular metabolism may be impaired in the setting of AKI. In addition, there may be increased production of ketoacids or lactic acid or increased bicarbonate loss (e.g. diarrhoea or renal tubular acidosis) in critical illness. Treatments for acidosis include RRT and administration of bicarbonate. Intravenous bicarbonate therapy to achieve pH >7.3 has shown a potential beneficial effect of avoiding RRT in severe AKI. However, adverse effects of bicarbonate administration may occur (i.e. hypernatraemia, volume overload, hypocalcaemia, intracellular acidosis, rebound metabolic alkalosis). RRT should be initiated in those with very severe metabolic acidosis (pH <7.1) or those who do not respond to bicarbonate administration.

Uraemia

Severe uraemia includes pericarditis, pleuritis, encephalopathy and bleeding. The latter is due to platelet dysfunction; circulating clotting factors and prothrombin/partial thromboplastin times are not deranged, unless there is coexisting coagulopathy. No absolute urea concentration should serve as an indication for initiation of RRT in AKI.

Hypocalcaemia

As eGFR falls, serum phosphate levels will increase, which can lead to hypocalcaemia. In the context of severe hyperphosphataemia, administration of calcium may lead to the deposition of calcium phosphate in tissue; dialysis against a high calcium dialysate may be required to normalise both calcium and phosphate in this setting. However, intravenous calcium gluconate should always be given where life-threatening symptoms or signs occur (e.g. tetany, paraesthesia, confusion, seizures or prolongation of the QT interval). Here, use of intravenous calcium gluconate will raise serum calcium for a few hours, allowing for dialysis to be arranged.

Hyperphosphataemia

Hyperphosphataemia may be treated with oral phosphate binders where it is severe, though the clinical benefits of treatment in the context of AKI are not clear. Alternatively, RRT may be used; this approach will reduce phosphate more quickly and prevent the precipitation of calcium and phosphate in tissues.

Principles of Management in AKI

Current management strategy of AKI should follow the KDIGO care bundle (Figure 3.2.1.5).

Treatment according to the underlying aetiology of AKI is advisable. For example, timely administration of antibiotics and source control are paramount

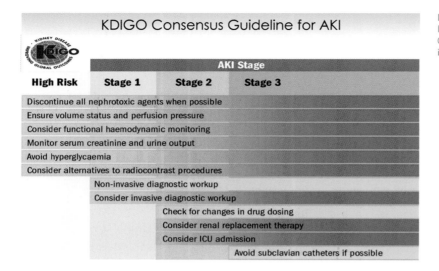

Figure 3.2.1.5 The Kidney Disease: Improving Global Outcomes (KDIGO) Consensus Guideline for acute kidney injury.

in sepsis. Fluid therapy should be provided to hypo-volaemic patients. Diuretics should be administered in acute CRS. Vasoconstrictors (e.g. terlipressin) plus albumin are recommended in hepatorenal syndrome. Correction of causes of ACS can alleviate IAP and restore renal perfusion.

Nutritional therapy should be encouraged, aiming for total energy intake of 20–30 kcal/(kg day) in any stage of AKI. Protein 0.8–1.0 g/kg should be targeted in non-dialysis, non-catabolic AKI patients, 1.0–1.5 g/kg in dialysis patients and >1.7 g/kg in patients receiving continuous RRT (CRRT). Haemoglobin target of >70 g/l should be met. Loop diuretics should be used only in patients with a hypervolaemic state and should not be used to prevent or hasten recovery in those without fluid overload. In patients who failed conservative measures in severe AKI, RRT should be offered. Principles of RRT in the ICU are discussed in detail in another chapter.

Drug Adjustment during AKI/RRT

Factors to consider when prescribing drugs in AKI include drug pharmacodynamics (glomerular and tubular kidney function; renal and non-renal drug metabolism) and pharmacokinetics as a result of decreased kidney function (volume of distribution, protein binding). Initiation and discontinuation of nephrotoxic drugs in high-risk or AKI patients should be considered, with alternative medications in mind. Each prescription should be reviewed during each phase of AKI (deterioration, maintenance,

RRT and recovery) for its appropriateness and correct dosing using evidence-based guidelines. Antibiotics have a concentration–effect relationship as time-dependent or concentration-dependent characteristics. Maintaining drug concentrations according to antibiotic characteristics and pharmacodynamics is crucial. If possible, drug levels should be monitored and adjusted to achieve target levels.

During RRT, drug clearance is dependent on molecular size, charge, volume of distribution, water solubility and protein binding. Non-ionised drugs with high fat solubility and large volume of distribution will not be cleared efficiently by dialysis. For intoxication, including methanol, lithium, metformin and salicylate, readers are referred to the 'EXtracorporeal TReatments In Poisoning' (EXTRIP) Workgroup guidelines. Regular reassessment should focus on medication indications, regimen and dosing, adverse events and duration of these medications, to minimise exposure as much as possible.

Palliative Care Nephrology

Palliative care is a multidisciplinary support system that assists patients and their surrogates with communication about their prognosis and advance care planning. It also provides emotional and spiritual support and focuses on symptom identification and management. Decision to initiate or discontinue RRT should incorporate palliative care into the decision-making. If overall prognosis is poor, providers should re-examine whether RRT is likely to provide any meaningful benefit. Given that prognostication in ICU patients is difficult, offering RRT may, at times, be appropriate. Time-limited trials are agreements between providers and a patient and/or surrogates to use certain medical therapies over a defined period to see if the patient improves or deteriorates according to agreed outcomes. Similarly, RRT can be offered using time-limited trials, with global factors such as shock resolution or extubation or tolerance of RRT, i.e. haemodynamic tolerance, as outcomes. If these outcomes are not met, withdrawal of therapy may be discussed to facilitate maximal comfort care.

Long-Term Effects of AKI and Post-AKI Care

AKI is associated with proteinuria, hypertension, CKD, end-stage renal disease (ESRD) and death. Moreover, non-renal complications include myocardial infarction, heart failure, stroke, infection, bleeding, malignancy and disability. The mechanisms are thought to be a maladaptive repair process involving transformation of tubular cells into fibroblasts, pro-inflammatory cytokines and vascular dropouts. Key elements in the natural history of AKI that determine prognosis include pre-existing CKD, timing of onset, severity of injury, duration of injury, number of episodes of AKI and recovery status. The KDIGO guideline recommends an initial 3-month follow-up of AKI survivors by measuring SCr and proteinuria and monitoring for CKD progression. There is currently no consensus regarding who should be reviewed, the frequency of follow-up, what targets should be monitored and what drugs are appropriate to prevent long-term complications.

Conclusion

As there is currently no pharmacologic breakthrough for AKI prevention and treatment, reduction in AKI morbidity and mortality comes from AKI recognition and rapid response. When AKI is established, causes should be delineated to determine treatable factors. Optimisation of haemodynamics, avoidance and withdrawal of nephrotoxic drugs and close monitoring are still principles in early AKI management. Complications of AKI should be treated conservatively; then referral for RRT should be considered in those who have failed conservative therapy. Palliative care should be addressed and discussed thoroughly with the patient and/or surrogates, with consideration of time-limited trials. Finally, AKI is associated with distant organ dysfunctions and worse long-term consequences. Therefore, AKI survivors should be monitored for long-term complications.

References and Further Reading

Griffin BR, Liu KD, Teixeira JP. Critical care nephrology: core curriculum 2020. *Am J Kidney Dis* 2020;**75**:435–52.

Khwaja A. KDIGO clinical practice guidelines for acute kidney injury. *Nephron Clin Pract* 2012;**120**:c179–84.

Koyner JL, Thakar CV. Acute kidney injury and critical care nephrology. *Nephrology Self-Assessment Program* 2017;**16**(2).

Moore PK, Hsu RK, Liu KD. Management of acute kidney injury: core curriculum 2018. *Am J Kidney Dis* 2018;**72**:136–48.

Ostermann N, Joannidis M. Acute kidney injury 2016: diagnosis and diagnostic workup. *Crit Care* 2016;**20**:299.

Ronco C, Bellomo R, Kellum JA. Acute kidney injury. *Lancet* 2019;**394**:1949–64.

3.3.1

Acute-on-Chronic Liver Failure

Michael Spiro and Jeremy Fabes

Key Learning Points

1. The acute-on-chronic liver failure (ACLF) syndrome describes acute decompensation of liver function in the context of chronic liver disease.
2. ACLF is associated with extra-hepatic organ failure and high mortality.
3. Underlying chronic liver disease reflects typical population prevalence; the acute precipitant is often alcohol toxicity, systemic sepsis or viral hepatitis, although up to half of cases have no discernible aetiology.
4. Systemic inflammation and bacterial translocation are major pathophysiological components.
5. At present, there are no evidence-based interventions for ACLF, other than supportive care in the intensive care unit and assessment for urgent liver transplantation.

Keywords: acute liver failure, chronic liver failure, decompensation, transplantation, liver support devices

Introduction

Acute-on-chronic liver failure (ACLF) describes a syndrome of rapid-onset deterioration in hepatic and extra-hepatic organ function from a range of causes on a background of chronic hepatic disease, with or without cirrhosis. This syndrome does not fit within the classic chronic compensated–decompensated liver disease model, and represents an alternative endpoint to decompensation in the evolution of chronic liver disease. ACLF is common – approximately 5 per cent of patients admitted to hospital with cirrhosis have ACLF – and is further differentiated from decompensated liver disease by the presence of high mortality.

Definition

A broad range of definitions of ACLF exists without consensus. The Asian Pacific Association for the Study of the Liver consensus definition describes ACLF as 'an acute hepatic insult manifesting as jaundice and coagulopathy complicated within four weeks by clinical ascites and/or encephalopathy in a patient with previously diagnosed or undiagnosed chronic liver disease/cirrhosis, and is associated with a high 28-day mortality'. The major difference between this definition and that put forward by other groups is the requirement for hepatic failure.

Diagnosis and Classification

There are no currently accepted or validated diagnostic criteria for ACLF, and various models have been put forward. Furthermore, there are no biomarkers for ACLF to differentiate it from more classical hepatic decompensation and acute liver failure.

The definition of ACLF in the majority of published data sets requires:

- Acute hepatic decompensation
- Extra-hepatic organ failure
- High short-term mortality

The World Gastroenterology Organisation Working Party classifies ACLF into three groups (Figure 3.3.1.1):

- Type A – in the context of chronic liver disease
- Type B – in the context of compensated cirrhosis
- Type C – in the context of decompensated cirrhosis

Aetiology

The underlying aetiology of chronic liver failure (CLF) in patients with ACLF mirrors that of the general CLF population, with alcoholic liver disease and viral hepatitis predominating, as well as more recently recognised metabolic conditions such as non-alcoholic fatty liver disease (NAFLD) and non-alcoholic

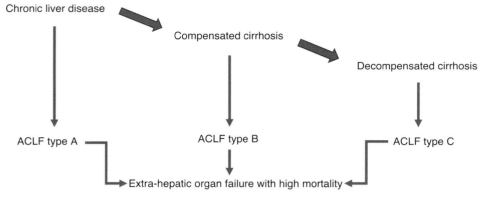

Figure 3.3.1.1 The World Gastroenterology Organisation Working Party classification of acute-on-chronic liver failure.

steatohepatitis (NASH). Precipitants for ACLF are also comparable to those of acute cirrhotic decompensation, including acute drug or alcohol toxicity, surgery, sepsis, transjugular intrahepatic portosystemic shunt (TIPSS) insertion, reactivation of hepatic viruses and gastrointestinal haemorrhage. However, ACLF patients are often younger and alcohol toxicity or bacterial infections are more common precipitants, when compared to those with acute cirrhotic decompensation. It should also be borne in mind that up to a third of ACLF episodes may have no clear precipitant.

Pathophysiology

Precipitants of ACLF are typically pro-inflammatory, including systemic or localised sepsis, such as spontaneous bacterial peritonitis (SBP), and acute alcohol toxicity. Evidence indicates a causative role for systemic inflammation and/or gastrointestinal bacterial translocation in the evolution of the ACLF syndrome. At-risk hepatocytes injured by the precipitating insult attract and activate inflammatory cells, leading to cytokine release and systemic inflammation. These physiological insults, combined with a reactive immunoparesis, lead to systemic sepsis, multi-organ failure and progressive liver dysfunction.

Acute organ failure in ACLF commonly affects the organs at risk in CLF. Encephalopathy and renal dysfunction, often requiring renal replacement therapy, occur in over 50 per cent of cases, with respiratory failure, coagulopathy and vasoplegia also common.

Prognosis

The CANONIC study (a prospective European observational study) reported high overall 28-day mortality of 33 per cent, in keeping with acute liver failure, with more severe ACLF at diagnosis, correlating with higher short-term mortality. ACLF-specific severity scores are still in genesis, with the CLIF-C ACLF score (based on the Sequential Organ Failure Assessment score) demonstrating good correlation with outcome. Simplified severity grading, based on the number of failing extra-hepatic organs, correlates well with mortality. Respiratory failure, or the presence of two or more other extra-hepatic organ failures, correlates with high mortality, whilst those with ACLF grade 3 (three or more extra-hepatic organ failures) have a 28-day mortality rate of 73 per cent.

Management

The relatively short time span of recognition of ACLF as a separate entity means that there are no disease-specific interventions – rather management is supportive, whilst concurrently identifying and treating the underlying precipitant and complications as they emerge. Patients should be managed in a specialist transplant centre intensive care unit.

Poor prognosis of ACLF and the lack of definitive interventions leave transplantation as a final option. Commonly, however, these patients are too unwell to undergo major surgery, despite being prioritised for organ allocation due to their Model for End-Stage Liver

Disease (MELD) scoring. At present, there are few data regarding outcome following transplantation for ACLF. However, the CANONIC study demonstrated a survival increase from 20 to 80 per cent in grade 2–3 ACLF. Decision-making regarding transplantation in ACLF must be expedited. Outcomes following liver transplantation performed early in disease progression appear to be comparable to those without ACLF, whilst transplantation following the onset of multi-organ failure is likely to be futile.

There is a potential role for extracorporeal liver support systems in bridging ACLF patients to transplantation or as additional organ support. A clinical trial of an albumin dialysis-based device (the RELIEF study) did not demonstrate a survival benefit at 28 days but did demonstrate some improvement in renal, hepatic and cardiovascular function in decompensated cirrhosis. Experimental interventions with some evidence base include the use of granulocyte colony-stimulating factor, erythropoietin and umbilical cord stem cells. However, there were limited patient numbers included in each trial.

References and Further Reading

Blasco-Algora S, Masegosa-Ataz J, Gutiérrez-García ML, et al. Acute-on-chronic liver failure: pathogenesis, prognostic factors and management. *World J Gastroenterol* 2015;**21**:12125–40.

Hernaez R, Solà E, Moreau R, et al. Acute-on-chronic liver failure: an update. *Gut* 2017;**66**:541–53.

Jalan R, Yurdaydin C, Bajaj JS, et al. Toward an improved definition of acute-on-chronic liver failure. *Gastroenterology* 2014;**147**:4–10.

Sarin SK, Kedarisetty CK, Abbas Z, et al. Acute-on-chronic liver failure: consensus recommendations of the Asian Pacific Association for the Study of the Liver (APASL). *Hepatol Int* 2014;**8**:453.

Jaundice

3.3.2

Michael Spiro and Jeremy Fabes

Key Learning Points

1. Jaundice is the clinical manifestation of high serum and tissue bilirubin levels.
2. Jaundice is usually benign in adults; however, it may cause significant encephalopathy and neurological damage in neonates.
3. High bilirubin levels may be from pre-hepatic, hepatic or post-hepatic causes.
4. Management is typically of the underlying cause, rather than of the jaundice itself.

Keywords: icterus, kernicterus, cholestasis, ERCP, bilirubin, haem metabolism

Introduction

Jaundice (icterus) describes yellow pigmentation of the skin and sclerae secondary to raised bilirubin levels. Whilst jaundice itself is usually benign, the aetiology may be trivial or carry high mortality. Normal total bilirubin levels are variably quoted as below 17 μM in serum, of which 5 per cent or less is conjugated. Typically, clinical evidence of hyperbilirubinaemia is not detectable until plasma levels are >35 μM, best seen on the oral mucosa and peripheral conjunctivae.

Haem Metabolism

Normal metabolism of the haem co-factor generates bilirubin, which is highly bound to serum proteins, predominantly albumin. Hepatic phase II metabolism via conjugation to glucuronic acid (by glucuronyl transferase) generates water-soluble bilirubin that is excreted into the bile ducts. Subsequent deconjugation of bilirubin by colonic bacteria generates urobilinogen which undergoes oxidation to stercobilin (and contributes to normal stool colour). Urobilinogen is reabsorbed in small amounts via the portal enterohepatic circulation and subsequently undergoes metabolism from this colourless form to yellow urobilin that is renally excreted (Figure 3.3.2.1).

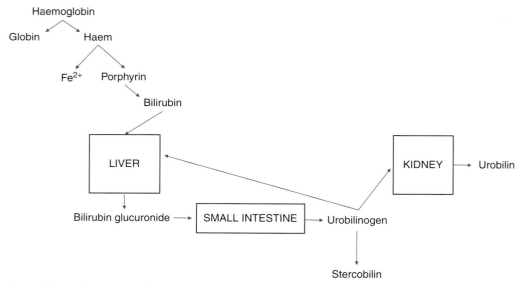

Figure 3.3.2.1 Haem metabolism.

Hepatic dysfunction or biliary obstruction can lead to displacement of conjugated bilirubin into the urine, leading to the classic dark urine of jaundice (with associated pale stools secondary to a reduction in faecal stercobilin). However, jaundice in the context of high haem metabolism generates excess unconjugated serum bilirubin, and this cannot enter the urine due to low water solubility. This excess bilirubin undergoes normal metabolism and enterohepatic circulation to generate excess urine urobilinogen.

Toxicity

Whilst adults are relatively resistant to cellular damage from hyperbilirubinaemia, higher permeability of the neonatal blood–brain barrier permits cerebral accumulation of unconjugated bilirubin. The basal nuclei are particularly sensitive, and bilirubin neural toxicity leads to irreversible sequelae, including ophthalmoplegia, seizures and abnormal reflexes known as kernicterus.

Classification of Jaundice

By Conjugation

Excess bilirubin may be conjugated to glucuronic acid or unconjugated, or a mixed picture may be present. Unconjugated hyperbilirubinaemia is typically driven by raised red blood cell (RBC) turnover, and impaired hepatic bilirubin uptake or conjugation. Jaundice due to a combination of conjugated and unconjugated bilirubin develops subsequent to hepatocellular disease, reduced biliary excretion or biliary tree obstruction.

By Aetiology

Jaundice may be classified according to the primary source of raised bilirubin:

- Pre-hepatic or haemolytic: due to intrinsic defects in RBCs or non-hepatic causes extrinsic to RBCs (see below)
- Hepatic: driven by parenchymal liver disease
- Post-hepatic or cholestatic: caused by obstruction of the biliary tree

Pre-hepatic Jaundice

Abnormal levels of RBC turnover, with resultant high levels of haem catabolism, generate excess unconjugated bilirubin. The liver's reserve capacity to process these breakdown products increases conjugated bilirubin levels and downstream end-products, and thereby excretion. For this reason, pre-hepatic jaundice is typically mild.

Investigations in the context of haemolysis will demonstrate reticulocytosis and low haptoglobin levels. Whilst urinary urobilinogen increases, free urinary bilirubin does not; hence, stool and urine colour remains unchanged. As the liver's capacity to conjugate bilirubin outweighs typical maximum rates of bilirubin generation, total serum bilirubin will remain below approximately four times the normal range (approximately 68 μmol/l), and conjugated bilirubin will remain below 5 per cent of the total. In patients with any degree of hepatic disease, bilirubin levels will rise substantially higher.

The aetiology of RBC breakdown may be intrinsic to the red cell itself or extrinsic (Table 3.3.2.1).

Iatrogenic precipitation of red cell crises in glucose-6-phosphate dehydrogenase (G6PD) deficiency may be due to a range of drugs, including antibiotics of the sulphonamide and quinolone families, nitrofurantoin, isoniazid, dapsone and methylene blue.

Hepatic Jaundice

Hepatocellular dysfunction or necrosis disrupts bilirubin metabolism and biliary excretion, leading to excessive serum conjugated and unconjugated bilirubin. Laboratory testing is likely to demonstrate transaminitis, with abnormal markers of hepatic synthetic function.

Hepatocellular aetiologies include:

- Acute or chronic hepatitis (viral, drug-induced)
- Hepatic cirrhosis
- Alcoholic liver disease

Table 3.3.2.1 Aetiology of red blood cell breakdown

Intrinsic aetiologies	Extrinsic aetiologies
- Haemoglobinopathy, e.g. sickle cell, thalassaemia - Red blood cell structure: hereditary spherocytosis and elliptocytosis - Red blood cell metabolism: glucose-6-phosphate dehydrogenase deficiency, pyruvate kinase deficiency	- Infectious: malaria, Gram-positive sepsis - Disseminated intravascular coagulation - Errors in bilirubin metabolism: Gilbert's syndrome, Crigler–Najjar syndrome - Autoimmune haemolysis, hypersplenism - Drug-induced, e.g. lead poisoning - Mechanical haemolysis: metallic heart valves, burns - HELLP syndrome of pregnancy - Haemolytic disease of the newborn

Abbreviations: HELLP = haemolysis, elevated liver enzymes and low platelets.

- Neonatal jaundice (due to immature bilirubin metabolic pathways)
- Infectious: leptospirosis
- Drug-induced hepatitis: paracetamol, cocaine, phenytoin, methyldopa, methotrexate, amiodarone, atorvastatin

Post-hepatic (Cholestatic) Jaundice

Cholestatic jaundice results from failure of biliary drainage of conjugated bilirubin and subsequent displacement to plasma. Disruption of normal bilirubin excretion leads to reduced stool stercobilin levels and increased urinary conjugated bilirubin levels, leading to the classic pale stools and dark urine. The site of cholestasis may be intra- or extra-hepatic (Table 3.3.2.2).

Post-operative Jaundice

In the post-operative setting, the precise aetiology of new-onset jaundice may not be apparent and is often multifactorial. Patients with pre-existing liver dysfunction, as well as acute or chronic renal failure, are at higher risk. Common causes include packed red cell transfusion, extracorporeal circuit haemolysis, sepsis and drugs precipitating haemolysis or liver dysfunction, as well as perioperative hypoxia or hypotension. Surgery to the liver or associated organs may be causative. Benign causes include Gilbert's syndrome in the context of a fasting patient.

Patients with jaundice are at increased risk of renal dysfunction post-operatively, and optimisation of fluid status, renal perfusion and urine output may reduce this risk.

Jaundice in the Transplant Recipient

The transplant recipient is at high risk of cholestatic jaundice due to pre-existing liver disease, significant surgical stress with intraoperative instability and exposure to a range of hepatotoxins. In patients undergoing liver transplantation, cholestatic jaundice may indicate a biliary leak, as well as acute or chronic organ rejection.

Investigations

Initial investigations to complement history and examination should include serum total, conjugated and unconjugated bilirubin, aspartate aminotransferase (AST), alanine aminotransferase (ALT), alkaline phosphatase (ALP), prothrombin time (PT) and albumin. Hepatocellular disease demonstrates greater transaminitis than ALP rise, whilst cholestatic disease typically shows the converse. Abnormal synthetic function may be present in both cases and the degree of conjugated versus unconjugated bilirubin may also not be informative.

Hypoalbuminaemia takes time to develop, implying a more chronic picture. A deranged PT that corrects with vitamin K indicates malabsorption secondary to cholestatic hyperbilirubinaemia, whilst failure to correct suggests hepatocellular injury. ALT is more specific than AST for hepatocellular injury, with an AST:ALT ratio of 2 or more, with raised gamma-glutamyl transferase (γGT) suggesting alcoholic liver disease.

Investigation of cholestatic disease includes hepatic imaging with ultrasound, magnetic resonance cholangiopancreatography (MRCP) or endoscopic retrograde cholangiopancreatography (ERCP) for obstruction or bile duct dilation. Where an obstructive pathology is unlikely, an abdominal CT may be an appropriate first investigation to exclude biliary pathology and assess for hepatocellular disease. In the context of predominant transaminitis, further investigations include serology for viral hepatitis, thyroid function, haemochromatosis, autoimmune hepatitis and primary biliary cirrhosis. Diagnosis may require liver biopsy.

Table 3.3.2.2 Site of cholestasis

Intrahepatic cholestasis	Extra-hepatic cholestasis
- Alcoholic hepatitis and non-alcoholic steatohepatitis - Primary biliary sclerosis and primary sclerosing cholangitis - Viral hepatitis - Thyrotoxicosis - Cholestasis of pregnancy - Infiltration: sarcoid, tuberculosis, lymphoma, amyloidosis - Vascular: Budd–Chiari syndrome - Drug-induced hepatitis: chlorpromazine, erythromycin, halothane, angiotensin-converting enzyme inhibitor, terbinafine, flucloxacillin - Autoimmune hepatitis - Total parenteral nutrition - Genetic: Dubin–Johnson syndrome, Rotor syndrome - Non-specific: sepsis, post-operative	- Cholelithiasis - Pancreatitis - Primary sclerosing cholangitis - Cystic fibrosis - Human immunodeficiency virus cholangiopathy - Biliary stricture - Malignancy: pancreatic and cholangiocarcinoma

Management and Prognosis

Neonatal jaundice may require phototherapy or exchange transfusion to reduce the risk of kernicterus. In adults, management of jaundice is predominantly medical – aimed at addressing the aetiology and sequelae, which may include prolonged international normalised ratio (INR) and fat-soluble vitamin malabsorption. Surgical and endoscopic intervention is reserved for reversible biliary tree obstruction. Prognosis is dependent on the underlying aetiology.

References and Further Reading

Anand AC, Garg HK. Approach to clinical syndrome of jaundice and encephalopathy in tropics. *J Clin Exp Hepatol* 2015;5(Suppl 1):S116–30.

Kruger D. The assessment of jaundice in adults: tests, imaging, differential diagnosis. *JAAPA* 2011;**24**:44–9.

3.3.3 Ascites

Michael Spiro and Jeremy Fabes

Key Learning Points

1. The most common cause of ascites in the UK is hepatic cirrhosis.
2. Diagnosis of the underlying aetiology is key for management and dependent on a robust history and examination, with appropriate tests on serum and paracentesis samples.
3. Whilst certain routine tests should be performed on all paracentesis samples, more specialist tests should be ordered, dependent on clinical findings.
4. Clinical suspicion of spontaneous bacterial peritonitis requires rapid diagnosis and management to prevent deterioration.
5. Ascites secondary to portal hypertension that is resistant to medical therapy is an indication for liver transplantation.

Keywords: ascites, paracentesis, spontaneous bacterial peritonitis, cirrhosis, SAAG, transudate, exudate

Pathophysiology

Ascites describes the accumulation of a broad range of fluids within the peritoneum. Ascitic fluid may be exudative or transudative in nature, and it is not uncommon for patients to have multiple concurrent aetiologies. Transudative fluid develops secondary to portal hypertension driving persistent passive fluid migration due to hydrostatic pressure within the splanchnic bed. Transudates typically contain low protein, white blood cell and lactate dehydrogenase (LDH) levels, with glucose and pH levels comparable to serum levels. Exudates accumulate as a result of active fluid secretion into the peritoneal cavity due to localised inflammation, and contain higher levels of protein, albumin and white blood cells; they may be acidic, low in glucose and high in LDH, depending on their aetiology.

Sequelae from the development of ascites include progressive abdominal tension and compression of intra-abdominal organs and vasculature, activation of the renin–angiotensin–aldosterone axis and upregulation of sympathetic tone. Consequent retention of sodium and free water leads to worsening ascites and oedema. Significant renal vasoconstriction, coupled with extrinsic compression from ascitic fluid, can lead to renal hypoperfusion and subsequent hepatorenal syndrome.

Clinical

Physical signs in ascites include lateral dullness to percussion, with shifting dullness on axial rotation of the patient, as well as a fluid thrill. Concurrent pleural effusions are common due to heart failure, hypoproteinaemia, malignancy or hepatic hydrothorax (transdiaphragmatic migration of ascites). In combination with progressive abdominal distension, this may cause respiratory decompensation.

As well as the symptoms and signs of ascites, patients may have clinical evidence of the underlying aetiology. In the context of cirrhotic ascites, the most common cause in the UK, patients will demonstrate signs of hepatic failure and decompensation.

Serum–Ascites Albumin Gradient

Previous classification of ascites by total protein concentration (exudative versus transudative) has now been superseded by the serum–ascites albumin gradient (SAAG) as a marker of the presence of portal hypertension, the major aetiology (Box 3.3.3.1). A high ascitic fluid total protein concentration (above 3 g/dl) can be classified as exudative, but below this threshold, the SAAG criteria are employed. The presence of a high SAAG does not help determine whether the underlying aetiology of portal hypertension is cirrhotic or non-cirrhotic, and further investigations are required.

Box 3.3.3.1 Serum–Ascites Albumin Gradient (SAAG)

SAAG = serum albumin concentration – ascitic fluid albumin concentration

The presence of a high SAAG (>1.1 g/dl) has a high sensitivity for the presence of portal hypertension, in keeping with transudative ascites. SAAG values below this threshold indicate an exudative pathology.

Classification by SAAG

Table 3.3.3.1 shows the classification of ascites by SAAG.

Aetiology

Table 3.3.3.2 shows the aetiology of ascites by system.

Table 3.3.3.1 Classification by serum–ascites albumin gradient

High SAAG/transudate	Low SAAG/exudate
• Hepatic cirrhosis and other hepatic aetiologies • Heart failure and constrictive pericarditis • Hypoalbuminaemia and malnutrition	• Malignancy • Infective • Pancreatitis • Bowel infarction or obstruction • Nephrotic syndrome

Table 3.3.3.2 Aetiology by system

Physiological system	Cause
Hepatic	• Cirrhosis[a] (75% of cases in the UK), including haemorrhagic ascites • Portal hypertension • Acute or chronic liver failure • Hepatitis (including alcohol-induced) • Budd–Chiari syndrome
Cardiogenic	• Heart failure[a] • Constrictive pericarditis
Oncological	• Malignant (including mesothelioma and multiple myeloma) • Leukaemia and lymphoma
Renal	• Nephrotic syndrome • Haemodialysis and peritoneal dialysis
Other	• Hypothyroidism • Crohn's disease • Bowel obstruction and infarction • Malnutrition, hypoalbuminaemia, protein-losing enteropathies • Endometriosis • Systemic lupus erythematosus, vasculitic disease • Pancreatitis • Amyloid • Infectious (including HIV-associated infections)
Anatomical and surgical	• Ureteric or bladder disruption • Haemoperitoneum • Pancreatic or biliary leak • Chylous and lymphatic injury • Ventriculoperitoneal shunt

[a] Common causes in the UK.

Investigations

Investigations, guided by clinical findings, are required to determine the nature and aetiology of the ascites and thereby direct management. Serum for full blood count, urea and electrolytes, liver function, albumin, clotting function and C-reactive protein (CRP) should be drawn routinely. Abdominal paracentesis is essential to determine the aetiology, as well as to exclude SBP which may be acutely life-threatening. Guidelines vary as to which patients undergo paracentesis, but typically any patient with new-onset ascites, a significant change to pre-existing ascitic burden, those being admitted or those in whom a novel pathology is being considered should undergo the procedure. Visual inspection of the ascitic fluid may give some clues to its nature (i.e. chylous, haemorrhagic, turbid) and direct subsequent laboratory investigations.

Abdominal ultrasound will provide information regarding the volume of ascites and hepatic and splenic pathology. Doppler studies will demonstrate the direction of portal venous flow, Budd–Chiari syndrome and portal vein thrombosis. Ultrasound may also be of use in draining anatomically difficult or loculated ascites. CT and MRI will also be diagnostic, as well as providing additional information on intra-abdominal pathology such as bowel perforation.

If no underlying aetiology is determined, then a diagnostic laparoscopy should be considered to rule out malignancy and infection.

Ascitic Fluid Investigations

Box 3.3.3.2 shows routine tests for investigation of ascitic fluid.

Box 3.3.3.2 Routine Tests for Ascitic Fluid Investigation

• Cell count and white cell differential
• Albumin and total protein (with calculation of SAAG)

Box 3.3.3.2 (cont.)

- **Secondary tests (guided by clinical findings and visual inspection of fluid):**
  - Microscopy, Gram stain, culture and sensitivity – with direct culture bottle inoculation at bedside (SBP or secondary infection from bowel rupture)
  - Lactate dehydrogenase (low in transudative aetiologies and high in the presence of exudates)
  - Glucose (decreased in secondary bacterial peritonitis, intra-peritoneal malignancy or infection)
  - Amylase (pancreatic aetiology or bowel perforation)
  - pH (bacterial infection generates a more acidic fluid)
  - Triglycerides (chylous ascites)
  - Tuberculosis-specific culture and local testing strategies
  - Bilirubin (perforation of bowel or biliary tree)
  - Cytology and carcinoembryonic antigen (malignancy)
  - Serum N-terminal pro-B-type natriuretic peptide (heart failure)

Management

Management is directed at the underlying cause, with ascitic drainage for symptomatic relief where appropriate. Mild and uncomplicated transudative ascites can be managed as outpatients with salt restriction, fluid restriction and diuretics (spironolactone and furosemide), whilst monitoring body weight and sodium and potassium balance. Patients with exudative aetiologies require management of the underlying aetiology, with repeated paracentesis to control the ascitic burden. Medically refractory ascites secondary to portal hypertension requires assessment for liver transplantation. Bridging therapy whilst awaiting transplantation may be performed using a transjugular intrahepatic porto-systemic shunt (TIPSS), although with the attendant risk of precipitating hepatic encephalopathy.

Patients with significant volume or tense ascites, respiratory or other organ decompensation or evidence of novel or significant underlying aetiology should be admitted for management and paracentesis. Paracentesis is diagnostic, as well as therapeutic, and may require albumin infusion to cover losses in drained ascitic fluid and subsequent redistribution from the vascular space to the peritoneum, with cardiovascular decompensation. Drainage of ascitic volumes of above 2 l should be covered using a human albumin solution (HAS) infusion. Excessively rapid ascitic fluid drainage, or failure to cover for consequent volume loss, can cause rapid hypovolaemia and hypotension.

Spontaneous Bacterial Peritonitis

Spontaneous bacterial peritonitis (SBP) describes non-surgical infection of ascites and occurs most commonly in hepatic cirrhosis. Ascitic fluid contains low levels of complement and other anti-microbial serum proteins; hence, dissemination of bacteria and other infectious agents from extra-peritoneal sites, or breakdown of gut integrity with bacterial translocation, can cause a sudden onset of intra-peritoneal infection without an obvious precipitant. Clinical indications include abdominal pain, signs of sepsis and delirium, but these may be absent and a low threshold for suspicion must be maintained.

Infective ascites leads to progressive clinical deterioration, morbidity and mortality. Paracentesis in these patients should be performed urgently, ideally prior to the administration of antibiotics, with a rapid cell differential analysis for a corrected neutrophil count. Diagnostic criteria include corrected neutrophil count of above $250/mm^3$, positive ascitic fluid culture results and exclusion of other causes of intra-abdominal infection. The diagnosis is supported by a low ascitic protein concentration (below 1 g/dl). Early identification, with guideline-defined antibiotics and consideration for HAS infusion, leads to improved outcomes.

The presence of infective ascites may be due to SBP or secondary to infection of ascitic fluid due to perforation of an abdominal viscus (secondary bacterial peritonitis). The latter requires surgical intervention, in addition to urgent antibiotics and management of sepsis. Differentiating these may be challenging but is essential for correct management. In those patients in whom the corrected neutrophil count meets the criteria, the presence of raised ascitic total protein (above 1 g/dl), raised LDH or low glucose (<2.8 mmol/l) supports the presence of intra-abdominal perforation. Gram staining may also be helpful; the presence of a single microbial species on Gram staining is in keeping with SBP, whilst multiple microbial species suggests a secondary cause of bacterial peritonitis and bowel or other visceral injury should be considered.

References and Further Reading

Runyon BA. Introduction to the revised American Association for the Study of Liver Diseases Practice Guideline management of adult patients with ascites due to cirrhosis 2012. *Hepatology* 2013;**57**:1651.

Runyon BA, Montano AA, Akriviadis EA, Antillon MR, Irving MA, McHutchison JG. The serum-ascites albumin gradient is superior to the exudate-transudate concept in the differential diagnosis of ascites. *Ann Intern Med* 1992;**117**:215–20.

Saab S, Nieto JM, Lewis SK, Runyon BA. TIPS versus paracentesis for cirrhotic patients with refractory ascites. *Cochrane Database Syst Rev* 2006;**4**:CD004889.

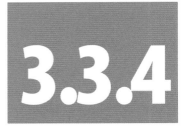

Portal Hypertension

Michael Spiro and Jeremy Fabes

Key Learning Points

1. Common causes include cirrhosis, venous obstruction and (worldwide) schistosomiasis.
2. High portal venous pressures may cause ascites and bleeding from variceal sites.
3. Management is of the underlying cause and complications of portal pressures.
4. Portal gastropathy is common but rarely causes acute haemorrhage.
5. Transjugular portosystemic shunting can decompress the portal system.

Keywords: transjugular portosystemic shunting, gastrointestinal bleeding, gastropathy

Introduction

Portal hypertension (PH) is a consequence of increased resistance to portal venous flow from a broad range of intra- and extra-hepatic causes. These structural changes are accompanied by activation of peri-sinusoidal stellate cells and myofibroblasts, brought about by changes in the balance of local and systemic vasoconstrictors and vasodilators, including nitric oxide.

Progression of PH leads to paracrine vasodilation of the splanchnic arteries, with subsequent increases in portal pressures due to enhanced portal blood flow. This also drives relative hypovolaemia, low systemic vascular resistance (SVR) and a high cardiac output state associated with liver disease. Systemic hypotension drives salt and free water retention through the renin–angiotensin and sympathetic nervous systems, leading to the development of ascites, hepatic hydrothorax and respiratory embarrassment. Splanchnic vasodilation leads to reflex renal vasoconstriction, with resultant renal hypoperfusion, reduced glomerular filtration rate (GFR) and increased sodium retention.

The increased portosystemic gradient leads to enhancement of collateral venous drainage, with the development of varices at the gastro-oesophageal junction and anorectum that are friable and prone to bleeding. The raised portal pressure also leads to increased splenic venous pressure, with resultant splenomegaly and thrombocytopenia.

Aetiology

1. Cirrhotic liver disease (the most common cause in Western countries)
2. Non-cirrhotic causes (<10 per cent of cases in Western countries)
   a. Pre-hepatic
      i. Increased portal blood flow (splenomegaly, arteriovenous fistulae)
      ii. Thrombosis of the splenic vein or portal vein
   b. Hepatic
      i. Chronic pancreatitis
      ii. Biliary disease (primary biliary cirrhosis, primary sclerosing cholangitis)
      iii. Schistosomiasis (most common cause worldwide)
      iv. Fatty liver disease, including non-alcoholic fatty liver disease
      v. Viral hepatitis
      vi. Infiltrative and granulomatous diseases of the liver
   c. Post-hepatic
      i. Venous obstruction (Budd–Chiari syndrome, hepatic vein thrombosis, inferior vena cava obstruction)
      ii. Cardiac disease (restrictive cardiomyopathy, constrictive pericarditis)

Clinical Findings

Early PH is usually asymptomatic and manifests through sequelae and complications. Classical signs and symptoms include:

- Ascites, hepatic hydrothorax and spontaneous bacterial peritonitis
- Splenomegaly with secondary thrombocytopenia
- Cirrhotic cardiomyopathy
- Consequences of collateral venous drainage with variceal disease of the oesophagus and anorectum (haemorrhoids), caput medusae and upper gastrointestinal haemorrhage

PH also plays a key role in pathogenesis of portopulmonary hypertension, portal hypertensive gastropathy and hepatorenal and hepatopulmonary syndromes.

Diagnosis

A clinical diagnosis of PH in patients with risk factors and signs of disease can be made without investigation. Ultrasound is not sufficiently sensitive for PH diagnosis but will demonstrate the presence of complications such as venous collateralisation and thrombosis, splenomegaly and ascites.

Transhepatic venous pressure gradient (using hepatic venous wedge pressure as a surrogate for portal pressure) is the gold standard for diagnosis and grading the severity of portal hypertensive disease. The technique involves balloon catheterisation of the hepatic vein via the internal jugular vein, and is typically performed at the same time as transjugular intrahepatic portosystemic shunt (TIPSS) insertion or liver biopsy.

Higher degrees of pressure gradient correlate with an increased risk of complications and mortality (Table 3.3.4.1).

A diagnosis of PH in the absence of risk factors necessitates workup to determine the presence of cirrhosis or other underlying aetiology.

Management

Treatment of the underlying cause of PH depends on the aetiology and is beyond the scope of this chapter. Further management is focused on complications of disease and is covered in additional detail in other chapters.

Prevention of bleeding from oesophageal variceal disease involves endoscopic screening for the presence of disease with banding, as well as medical therapy with non-specific beta-blockers to lower portal pressures and splanchnic vasoconstrictors such as terlipressin. Management of an acute variceal bleed, other than resuscitation, requires endoscopic therapy or transjugular portosystemic shunt insertion.

Management of ascites in PH includes salt restriction, diuresis (typically spironolactone), recurrent therapeutic paracentesis with albumin cover and TIPSS insertion. Caution must be applied to avoid hypovolaemia which may induce hepatorenal syndrome, pre-renal renal failure and encephalopathy.

PH itself may be addressed through insertion of a transjugular portosystemic shunt and this reduces the risk of variceal rebleeding.

Transjugular Intrahepatic Portosystemic Shunt

The TIPSS provides an anatomical communication between the hepatic and portal venous systems, with low flow resistance. TIPSS has found a role in management of bleeding from oesophageal varices and gastropathy, as well as refractory ascites and hepatorenal syndrome. Contraindications include significant systemic infection, hepatic encephalopathy, heart failure, severe pulmonary hypertension and tricuspid regurgitation.

The procedure can be performed under sedation and local anaesthesia. Percutaneous TIPSS deployment usually occurs through the right internal jugular vein under fluoroscopic guidance. A catheter is passed via the hepatic vein through the liver parenchyma into the intrahepatic portal vein. This vascular communication is then stented open.

Complications of TIPSS include those of vascular insertion and manipulation, thrombosis and stenosis of the stent or other vascular territories, portosystemic encephalopathy and precipitation of heart failure through increased preload.

Portal Hypertensive Gastropathy

Increased gastric blood flow in PH leads to changes in the gastric mucosa and the development of ectatic blood vessels that are prone to rupture and bleeding. Chronic mucosal ooze may lead to subclinical bleeding

Table 3.3.4.1 Complications associated with different pressure gradients

Transhepatic venous pressure gradient (mmHg)	Complications
≥6	Diagnosis of portal hypertension
≥10	Clinically significant with variceal disease
≥12	Complications, including ascites and variceal haemorrhage

169

and anaemia. Whilst gastropathy is common in PH, and probably present in most cases, clinically significant bleeding is rare and more commonly due to other causes of gastrointestinal bleeding associated with PH. That said, higher degrees of portal pressure are associated with more severe gastropathy and bleeding risk.

Diagnosis is endoscopic, with a classic mosaic patterning of the mucosa throughout the stomach and the presence of ectatic vessels on biopsy.

Medical management of asymptomatic disease or chronic low-grade bleeding includes reduction of portal pressure through beta-blockade. Acute gastrointestinal bleeding may respond to anti-fibrinolytics or splanchnic vasoconstrictors such as octreotide or terlipressin. A third-generation cephalosporin (or other) antibiotic should be prescribed as prophylaxis against spontaneous bacterial peritonitis. Endoscopic approaches include argon plasma coagulation and electrocautery but are of limited benefit in diffuse disease. Targeting the underlying PH through TIPSS or liver transplantation is effective in regressing portal gastropathy.

References and Further Reading

Buob S, Johnston AN, Webster CR. Portal hypertension: pathophysiology, diagnosis, and treatment. *J Vet Intern Med* 2011;**25**:169–86.

Iwakiri Y. Pathophysiology of portal hypertension. *Clin Liver Dis* 2014;**18**:281–91.

Leung JC, Loong TC, Pang J, Wei JL, Wong VW. Invasive and non-invasive assessment of portal hypertension. *Hepatol Int* 2018;**12**(Suppl 1):44–55.

Strunk H, Marinova M. Transjugular intrahepatic portosystemic shunt (TIPS): pathophysiologic basics, actual indications and results with review of the literature. *Rofo* 2018;**190**:701–11.

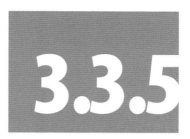

3.3.5 Hepatorenal Syndrome and Hepatopulmonary Syndrome

Michael Spiro and Jeremy Fabes

Key Learning Points

1. Hepatorenal syndrome (HRS) is the end result of progressive impairment of renal perfusion secondary to worsening hepatic failure.
2. HRS is a diagnosis of exclusion of acute kidney injury in chronic liver disease.
3. Both forms of HRS (types 1 and 2) have a poor prognosis, although HRS 1 typically leads to death within weeks.
4. Hepatopulmonary syndrome (HPS) develops from transpulmonary shunting, with resultant hypoxaemia.

Keywords: kidney injury, kidney failure, liver transplantation, liver cirrhosis, hepatorenal syndrome, hepatopulmonary syndrome

Hepatorenal Syndrome

Background

Hepatorenal syndrome (HRS) describes the development of renal dysfunction secondary to portal hypertension and ascites in chronic liver failure or, less commonly, fulminant hepatic failure. This usually occurs in the context of cirrhosis, severe alcoholic hepatitis or (less often) metastatic tumours. HRS represents the end-stage of progressive reductions in renal perfusion due to worsening hepatic injury. HRS is a diagnosis of exclusion and is associated with a poor prognosis.

HRS occurs in 40 per cent of patients with end-stage liver disease with cirrhosis and ascites. The risk of developing HRS if hospitalised with cirrhosis and ascites is 10 per cent or higher. HRS also occurs frequently in acute liver disease, particularly alcoholic hepatitis.

Presentation and Classification

Key components of the presentation include:
- Oliguria with a progressive rise in creatinine level
- Minimal proteinuria (<500 mg/day)
- Low urinary sodium excretion (<10 mEq/l)

Two forms of HRS are classically described, based on the rate of renal function decline:
- **Type 1** – twofold or greater increase in serum creatinine level to >221 μmol/l over 2 weeks or less
- **Type 2** – less severe renal failure; typically presenting with diuretic-resistant ascites

Aetiology

HRS may develop idiopathically or may be precipitated by a range of insults, including hepatic damage, gastrointestinal bleeding, acute hypovolaemia (i.e. paracentesis without volume replacement, although not diuresis) and infection. A quarter of spontaneous bacterial peritonitis (SBP) cases develop HRS 1 despite appropriate antibiotic use.

Risk factors for the development of HRS include mean arterial blood pressures below 80 mmHg with dilutional hyponatraemia, high plasma renin and secondary urinary sodium retention. However, advanced liver disease and deteriorating hepatic function do not increase the risk.

Pathophysiology

Splanchnic vasodilation secondary to portal hypertension in progressive liver disease leads to a high cardiac output and a low systemic vascular resistance (SVR) state, despite reflex constriction in renal and femoral circulations mediated by the renin–angiotensin and sympathetic nervous systems. HRS is a functional condition brought about by this progressive renal vasoconstriction, with resultant renal hypoperfusion, reduced glomerular filtration rate (GFR) and sodium retention.

Diagnosis

Patients with cirrhosis and acute kidney injury (AKI) are more likely to have another causative factor of HRS, e.g. pre-renal or sepsis-induced AKI. That said, it is important to differentiate HRS from other causes of AKI, due to significantly different prognoses and management.

Renal dysfunction in HRS can be significantly worse than indicated by serum urea and creatinine, due to synthetic liver disease, muscle wasting and poor oral intake. Urea levels may also be higher than expected due to renal sodium and water reabsorption.

HRS is a clinical diagnosis of exclusion without a specific test, but potential criteria for diagnosis include:

- Advanced hepatic failure with portal hypertension
- A rise in serum creatinine level (pre-existing renal failure does not exclude HRS)
- Absence of another cause

Prognosis

Whilst the kidneys are normal structurally and histologically, the development of HRS in liver failure significantly worsens prognosis. Prognosis without liver transplantation is poor, as this is the only intervention that robustly leads to reversal of renal dysfunction. The functional nature of the condition is apparent by rapid resolution of renal function following restoration of SVR and of renal haemodynamics following liver transplantation.

Whilst HRS 1 and 2 have comparable pathophysiology, their outcomes are very different:

- HRS 1 presents with rapidly progressive renal failure and median survival of 2 weeks
- HRS 2 causes a more steady progression of renal failure, with median survival of 3–6 months

Management

- Routine management of AKI, including avoidance of nephrotoxics
- Treatment of underlying precipitant – alcohol abstention for alcoholic hepatitis, antiviral treatment of decompensated hepatitis B or liver transplantation. Notably, antibiotics alone will not correct HRS in spontaneous bacterial peritonitis

- Medical management of renal hypoperfusion, using a range of interventions, depending on the setting, is generally required for two or more weeks:
  - Noradrenaline with albumin
  - Vasopressin
  - Terlipressin with albumin
  - Midodrine, octreotide and albumin

The renal response to medical therapy is proportional to the improvement in arterial pressure generated and, frequently, pressures above 80 mmHg are required. Alternative strategies, employed where the above are insufficient, include transjugular intrahepatic portosystemic shunting and renal replacement therapy, depending on patient suitability for liver transplantation.

Hepatopulmonary Syndrome

Aetiology and Pathophysiology

Hepatopulmonary syndrome (HPS) describes dyspnoea and hypoxaemia in the setting of chronic liver disease. Progressive imbalance in pre- and post-capillary vascular tone leads to the development of widespread intrapulmonary arteriovenous shunting. The aetiology is currently unclear, but a role for excessive nitric oxide in mediating capillary vasodilation is likely.

Clinical Examination

Other than classical signs of liver disease and those of clubbing, dyspnoea and hypoxaemia, patients with HPS may demonstrate platypnoea and orthodeoxia – where dyspnoea and oxygen saturations, respectively, improve in the supine position and worsen when erect or sitting.

Investigation

Other causes of hypoxaemia must be excluded, including acute or chronic lung disease, high-output heart failure of chronic liver disease, significant pleural effusion or collapse and compression atelectasis secondary to ascites. Arterial blood gases will demonstrate positional hypoxaemia with a raised alveolar–arterial gradient.

Diagnosis requires demonstration of intrapulmonary shunting, which can be achieved using technetium-Tc[99] scanning or bubble contrast echocardiography, in which late transitioning of bubbles from right to left heart (3–5 cardiac cycles) is evident. Pulmonary artery catheterisation can also assist with diagnosis, whilst pulmonary angiography can identify regions of disease that might be amenable to embolisation.

Management and Prognosis

Medical management of the underlying condition has not been demonstrated to be effective. Regional disease may be amenable to angiographic embolisation, but liver transplantation is typically required, without which mortality from chronic hypoxaemia is high.

HPS resolves slowly following transplantation, as the pulmonary microvasculature remodels, and three-quarters of transplant recipients survive to 5 years.

References and Further Reading

Grace JA, Angus PW. Hepatopulmonary syndrome: update on recent advances in pathophysiology, investigation, and treatment. *J Gastroenterol Hepatol* 2013;**28**:213–19.

Krowka MJ, Fallon MB, Kawut SM, *et al*. International Liver Transplant Society Practice Guidelines: diagnosis and management of hepatopulmonary syndrome and portopulmonary hypertension. *Transplantation* 2016;**100**:1440–52.

Salerno F, Gerbes A, Gines P, Wong F, Arroyo V. Diagnosis, prevention and treatment of hepatorenal syndrome in cirrhosis. *Gut* 2007;**56**:1310–18.

Wong F. The evolving concept of acute kidney injury in patients with cirrhosis. *Nat Rev Gastroenterol Hepatol* 2015;**12**:711–19.

3.3.6

Encephalopathy

Michael Spiro and Jeremy Fabes

Key Learning Points

1. Encephalopathy describes potentially reversible neuropsychiatric abnormalities that are common in those with liver failure.
2. A wide range of motor and cognitive defects are described in hepatic encephalopathy, with clinical grading by the West Haven classification.
3. Investigations are useful to determine the aetiology of encephalopathy and to exclude differentials.
4. Whilst there is a clear role for ammonia in the pathogenesis, raised ammonia levels are not necessary or sufficient for a diagnosis of hepatic encephalopathy.
5. Management is aimed at correcting the underlying precipitant, lowering systemic ammonia absorption, and managing symptoms and complications.

Keywords: hepatic encephalopathy, ammonia, transjugular intrahepatic portosystemic shunt, TIPSS

Introduction

Encephalopathy describes a syndrome of cerebral dysfunction with multiple aetiologies. It may be intracranial or systemic in derivation and permanent or reversible, and the onset may be gradual or abrupt. This chapter will focus predominantly on hepatic encephalopathy (HE), which is present at some point in up to half of cirrhotic patients and those with a transjugular intrahepatic portosystemic shunt (TIPSS).

Aetiology

Common encephalopathy aetiologies in the UK include:

- Metabolic
  - Uraemia
  - Alcohol toxicity and withdrawal
  - Electrolyte derangement (hyper- or hypocalcaemia and hyper-/hyponatraemia)
  - Hyper- or hypoglycaemia
  - Toxins (lead, mercury, ammonia)
  - Nutritional (Wernicke's encephalopathy)
- HE
- Infectious (including prion disease, HIV, hepatitis B virus (HBV), hepatitis C virus (HCV), meningitis)
- Brain injury
  - Traumatic
  - Hypoxic
  - Cerebral oedema
  - Raised intracranial pressure

Other aetiologies include:

- Mitochondrial
- Autoimmune (Hashimoto's)
- Lyme disease
- Spongiform

Pathogenesis

There are multiple contributory mechanisms of injury in HE that coexist and interact to produce the clinical syndrome. These include metabolic and electrolyte derangements, increased sensitivity to sedatives and analgesics, cerebral hypoperfusion, hypoxia and oedema (present in a high proportion of HE patients). Additionally, blood–brain barrier dysfunction, abnormal cerebral metabolism and neurotransmitter dysfunction or dysregulation play a role. Cerebral hypoperfusion may be driven by systemic hypotension compounded by failure of cerebral perfusion autoregulation.

Raised ammonia levels are a significant contributory factor, although neither necessary nor sufficient for a diagnosis of HE. Ammonia is generated by gastrointestinal metabolism of glutamine and synthesis by enteric commensal bacteria. Levels of ammonia are raised in liver dysfunction due to reduced hepatic clearance and collateral portal venous bypass, leading to systemic and cerebral exposure.

Ammonia brings about cerebral dysfunction through a range of mechanisms, including:

- Increased astrocyte osmolality, with cellular swelling and deranged function, without clinically detectable rises in intracranial pressure
- Abnormal neurotransmitter synthesis and neural firing
- Excessive reactive oxidative species and cellular oxidative stress
- Raised intracerebral glutamine driving astrocyte dysfunction

Precipitants of Hepatic Encephalopathy

Common precipitants include:

- Hypoxia
- Infection, including spontaneous bacterial peritonitis (SBP), urinary tract infection and lower respiratory tract infection
- Hypovolaemia from excessive diuresis, paracentesis or gastrointestinal bleeding
- Metabolic derangement, including hypoglycaemia, hyponatraemia and hypokalaemia
- Injudicious use of sedatives, narcotics and alcohol
- Onset of renal failure
- Constipation
- Excessive nitrogen loading (dietary, from gastrointestinal bleeding or renal failure and poor urea clearance)
- Surgery
- Acute-on-chronic liver injury (i.e. alcoholic or viral hepatitis)

Insertion of a TIPSS can precipitate HE in up to one-third of patients, due to ammonia-rich portal blood bypassing the liver and entering the systemic circulation. This may be refractory to therapy, thus requiring urgent liver transplantation.

Classification

The World Congress of Gastroenterology classification defines three HE subtypes, based on aetiology:

- Type A – acute, associated with acute liver failure, typically with cerebral oedema
- Type B – bypass, induced by portosystemic shunting
- Type C – cirrhotic

Clinical Manifestations

Pure signs of HE may overlap with those of the underlying cause of liver dysfunction, i.e. Wilson's disease or drug and alcohol abuse. Early neurological phenomena include abnormal sleep patterns and day–night reversal, change in mood, disorientation, confusion and drowsiness. Cognitive dysfunction presents as memory impairment and attention deficit. Neurological signs are classically cerebellar, including rigidity, bradykinesia, hyper-reflexia, ataxia, myoclonus and asterixis.

The West Haven classification is based on clinical criteria shown in Box 3.3.6.1.

Box 3.3.6.1 The West Haven Classification

Minimal – subclinical disease that can only be detected through neuropsychological testing

Grade I – orientated, but subtle confusion, altered behaviour or sleep, subtle asterixis, slurred speech

Grade II – disorientated in time, asterixis, personality change, lethargy

Grade III – disorientated to place, gross asterixis, somnolence, clonus, positive Babinski sign

Grade IV – unresponsive, seizures, death

Diagnosis and Investigation

The diagnosis of an encephalopathic syndrome is predominantly clinical. However, investigation into the underlying cause, and to exclude differentials, is key to management.

- Routine blood tests – liver function, electrolytes, full blood count, thyroid function
- Specific tests – ammonia, α-fetoprotein
- Blood glucose
- Toxin and alcohol screen
- Microbiology – blood and urine microscopy, culture and sensitivity
- Paracentesis (for SBP)
- Cerebrospinal fluid microscopy, culture and sensitivity
- Electroencephalography (usually normal in grade I and abnormal in higher grades)

- Computed tomography or magnetic resonance imaging head (cerebral oedema, space-occupying lesion)

Psychometric testing may pick up more subtle degrees of HE not apparent on simple history and examination.

Management

Admission to the intensive care unit is usually required for higher grades of encephalopathy where concerns exist about conscious level and maintenance of airway patency, as well as the need for intensive nursing and medical input. Management is of the underlying precipitant, correcting the pathophysiological processes driving the encephalopathy and managing symptoms and complications. Agitation or aggression typically resolves with management of HE, and pharmacological management should avoid benzodiazepines due to oversensitivity.

Ammonia is a key component of the pathophysiological process, and levels can be decreased in a number of ways. Absence of a raised ammonia level does not preclude these approaches:

- Lactulose – a non-absorbable disaccharide that decreases gastrointestinal absorption of ammonia; to generate 2–3 soft stools per day
- Rifaximin (as a second-line agent) – acts by reducing the gut bacterial load and/or altered metabolic function
- Neomycin and alternative antibiotics are third-line agents due to their higher side effect profile
- Probiotics may have some benefit

Nutritional management should be based on ideal body weight and encompasses approximately 40 kcal/kg and up to 1.5 g/kg protein per day. Branched-chain amino acid supplementation might also improve symptoms, but no mortality benefit has been demonstrated.

Other interventions such polyethylene glycol, flumazenil, ammonia scavengers, L-ornithine, L-aspartate and zinc do not have a robust evidence base as yet. Extracorporeal interventions, such as albumin dialysis with molecular adsorbent recirculating system (MARS), reduce levels of ammonia and bilirubin; however, evidence to date does not support their use in HE. Some units employ continuous veno-venous haemofiltration to lower ammonia levels, although with unproven benefit.

Prognosis

Following resolution of the acute HE episode, residual cognitive deficits are usually present and these are additive over time with further HE episodes. Over half of patients with higher-grade HE in the context of cirrhosis die within a year of onset. Those who receive a liver transplant have 70 per cent 5-year survival.

References and Further Reading

Felipo V. Hepatic encephalopathy: effects of liver failure on brain function. *Nat Rev Neurosci* 2013;**14**:851–8.

Suraweera D, Sundaram V, Saab S. Evaluation and management of hepatic encephalopathy: current status and future directions. *Gut Liver* 2016;10:509–19.

Wijdicks E. Hepatic encephalopathy. *N Engl J Med* 2016;**375**:1660–70.

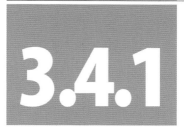

Decreased Consciousness

Chris Whitehead and Ian Tweedie

Key Learning Points

1. Initial resuscitation is key to improving outcome.
2. Breaking down the Glasgow Coma Score into sub-scores provides additional information to the total score.
3. Causes of impaired consciousness can be broadly divided into structural and diffuse aetiologies.
4. A structured approach can aid rapid assessment and confirmation of the diagnosis.
5. Accurate prognostication can take time and may require extensive investigation.

Keywords: consciousness disorders, Glasgow Coma Score, resuscitation

Introduction

Patients with impaired consciousness are at substantial risk of death and disability. Critical care staff are often required to become involved in the management of impaired consciousness, including: resuscitation, to prevent secondary neurological injury; diagnosis, including identification of easily remediable causes; and ongoing support and treatment of such patients. This can be achieved by using an organised and systematic approach (Figure 3.4.1.1).

Signs of brainstem dysfunction include those seen in Box 3.4.1.1.

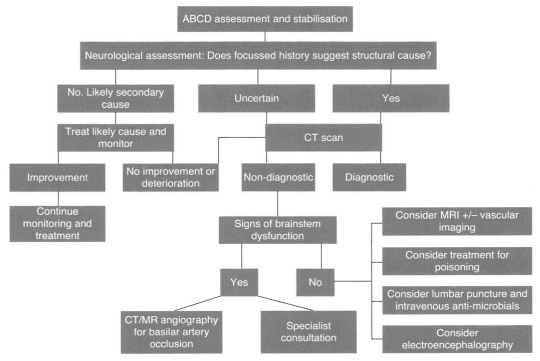

Figure 3.4.1.1 Algorithm for the diagnosis of impaired consciousness.

177

Box 3.4.1.1 Signs of Brainstem Dysfunction

- Vestibulo-ocular reflex (cold caloric testing) absent
- Abnormal motor response to supraorbital pressure
- Abnormal/absent respiration
- Gag and cough reflexes absent
- Corneal reflex absent
- Abnormal pupillary function (size, reactivity and symmetry)

Initial Resuscitation of the Unconscious Patient

Predictive outcome models indicate that secondary insults have a very significant influence on brain injury outcomes. It is possible that their prevention or elimination represents the area of early brain injury treatment with the greatest potential for improving outcome. Consequently, the fundamental requirement of initial resuscitation is to ensure satisfactory oxygen delivery. The patient's airway (including cervical spine stabilisation), breathing and circulation should be assessed and treated in sequence. The initial targets for immediate resuscitation and early (within the first hour) management are:

1. PaO_2 >13 kPa
2. $PaCO_2$ 4.5–5.0 kPa
3. Mean arterial blood pressure >80 mmHg
4. Exclusion and treatment of hypoglycaemia and opioid overdose
5. Serum biochemistry, arterial blood gas and urine toxicology screen
6. CT scan of the brain if structural or uncertain aetiology

Assessment of Level of Consciousness

The Glasgow Coma Score (GCS) (Table 3.4.1.1) is the most common tool for quantitative assessment of the level of consciousness. It is most useful in providing sequential examination responses in a particular

Table 3.4.1.1 Glasgow Coma Score

Criterion	Rating	Score
Eye opening		
Open before stimulus	Spontaneous	4
After spoken or shouted request	To sound	3
After fingertip stimulus	To pressure	2
No opening at any time, no interfering factor	None	1
Closed by local factor	Non-testable	NT
Verbal response		
Correctly gives name, place and date	Orientated	5
Not orientated, but communicating coherently	Confused	4
Intelligible single words	Words	3
Only moans/groans	Sounds	2
No audible response, no interfering factor	None	1
Factor interfering with communication	Non-testable	NT
Motor response		
Obey two-part request	Obeys commands	6
Brings hand above clavicle to stimulus on head/neck	Localising	5
Bends arm at elbow rapidly, but features not predominantly abnormal	Normal flexion	4
Bends arm at elbow, features clearly predominantly abnormal	Abnormal flexion	3
Extends arm at elbow	Extension	2
No movement in arms/legs, no interfering factor	None	1
Paralysed or other limiting factor	Non-testable	NT

patient. Identical overall scores can mask very different presentations because of the different combinations of eye, verbal and motor responses. Notably, brainstem function, hemiparesis and aphasia are not assessed by the GCS. Total and sub-scores should be recorded.

Causes of Impaired Consciousness

Causes of impaired consciousness can be classified into two groups (Table 3.4.1.2):

1. Primary (structural) brain disease
2. Secondary (diffuse) neuronal dysfunction

Information from the history often indicates the cause of impaired consciousness. Sudden onset suggests stroke, haemorrhage, seizure or a cardiac event causing impaired cerebral perfusion. A slower onset suggests metabolic or other secondary causes. Past medical and drug histories can provide important information about pre-existing conditions, as well as identifying potential overdose that may be contributing to impaired consciousness.

Further Investigations

Brain Imaging

Non-contrast CT scans can demonstrate structural causes of impaired consciousness, e.g. cerebral infarction, haemorrhage, brain masses, cerebral oedema and acute hydrocephalus. Contrast CT scans can evaluate abscesses, extra-axial fluid collections, haemorrhagic changes and infarctions – all of which are important to assess for prior to undertaking a lumbar puncture (LP) and cerebrospinal fluid (CSF) analysis.

CT angiography and perfusion scanning can help determine regional perfusion, vascular anatomy and patency in ischaemic stroke or subarachnoid haemorrhage.

MRI scanning may be superior to CT scanning in hyper-acute ischaemic stroke where the cause of impaired consciousness has not otherwise been identified and where subtle structural changes have caused new-onset, or changes in, seizure patterns.

Table 3.4.1.2 Causes of impaired consciousness

Structural brain disease	Diffuse neuronal dysfunction
Mass lesion (e.g. tumour, abscess)	Metabolic/endocrine disorders
Raised intracranial pressure	Hypoglycaemia
Subdural or extradural haematoma	Hyperglycaemia
Intracerebral haemorrhage	Hyponatraemia
Subarachnoid haemorrhage	Hypercalcaemia
Acute ischaemic stroke	Hypovolaemia/hypotension
Hydrocephalus	Hyperammonaemia/hepatic encephalopathy
Cerebral oedema resulting from stroke	Renal failure
Cerebellar oedema resulting from stroke	Thyroid disorders
Cerebral venous sinus thrombosis	Adrenal insufficiency
Intracranial sepsis/central nervous system infections	Hypopituitarism
Anoxic/hypoxic brain damage post-cardiac arrest	Wernicke's encephalopathy
Non-convulsive status epilepticus	Drugs/toxins: • Sedatives/hypnotics/opioids • Dissociative agents, e.g. ketamine • Cholinergic agents • Carbon monoxide • Cyanide • Asphyxiants • MDMA Neuroleptic malignant syndrome Serotonin syndrome
Autoimmune/neuroinflammatory disorders, e.g. vasculitis, NMDA encephalitis	

Abbreviations: MDMA = 3,4-methylenedioxymethamphetamine; NMDA = *N*-methyl-*D*-aspartate.

Unfortunately, however, the magnetic field and isolated environment of MRI scanners pose particular challenges for the safe care of critically ill patients.

Lumbar Puncture

An LP is indicated when raised intracranial pressure has been excluded and there is suspicion of:

- Central nervous system (CNS) infection
- Neuroinflammatory/autoimmune disease
- Subarachnoid haemorrhage not demonstrated on CT

Electroencephalography

An electroencephalogram (EEG) is needed to confirm the diagnosis of non-convulsive status epilepticus. This is suspected where there is a history of epilepsy or witnessed seizure. The only signs otherwise present may be fine twitching or tremor.

Prognosis

Prognosis for a patient with decreased consciousness can vary from death, through varying degrees of functional deficit, to complete recovery. The Glasgow Outcome Score (GOS) is the most commonly used objective measure of outcome. Prognostication of coma can be guided by consideration of the aetiology, clinical signs, electrophysiological and biochemical tests and neuroimaging. Subsequent results can, in turn, help guide decision-making in the ICU, e.g. about the intensity of ongoing treatment, withdrawal of life support and the potential for rehabilitation. There is a growing body of evidence that even in the most severe cases, it may be necessary to continue active management for at least 72 hours from the time of brain injury, before such decisions can be taken. In many cases, it may take much longer.

Ongoing Critical Care Management

In addition to treating the underlying cause, unconscious patients needing critical care need careful multidisciplinary management to prevent the huge array of possible complications – venous thromboembolism (deep vein thrombosis), ventilator-associated pneumonias and development of contractures, to name but a few.

References and Further Reading

Cadena R, Sarwal A. Emergency neurological life support: approach to the patient with coma. *Neurocrit Care* 2017;**27**(Suppl 1):74–81.

Edlow JA, Rabenstien A, Traub SJ, Wijdicks EFM. Diagnosis of reversible causes of coma. *Lancet* 2014;**384**:2064–76.

Farling P, Andrews PJD, Cruickshank S, *et al*. Recommendations for the safe transfer of patients with brain injury. London: Association of Anaesthetists of Great Britain & Ireland; 2006.

Royal College of Physicians and Surgeons of Glasgow. The Glasgow structured approach to assessment of the Glasgow Coma Scale. www.glasgowcomascale.org

Souter MJ, Blissitt PA, Blosser S, *et al*. Recommendations for the critical care management of devastating brain injury: prognostication, psychosocial, and ethical management. *Neurocrit Care* 2015;**23**:4–13.

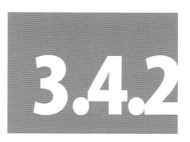

3.4.2 Seizures and Status Epilepticus

Chris Whitehead

Key Learning Points

1. Over a lifetime, many people will suffer seizures, but only a small proportion of these develop into epilepsy.
2. Acute symptomatic seizures may be classified into those with a primary cerebral cause and those of a secondary cause, e.g. drug intoxication or hypoglycaemia.
3. If seizures are prolonged, they may become resistant to pharmacological control and mortality is high. Early termination of seizures is thus a priority.
4. A stepwise approach to seizure management is recommended until electrographic seizures are stopped.
5. Critical care treatment and monitoring should be started in conjunction with initial therapy. It should then be continued until therapy is considered successful or futile.

Keywords: seizures, epilepsy, status epilepticus

Introduction

A seizure is a sudden change in behaviour caused by electrical hypersynchronisation of neuronal networks in the cerebral cortex. They are estimated to affect 8–10 per cent of the population over a lifetime.

Acute Symptomatic Seizure

Acute symptomatic seizures refer to seizures that occur at the time of a systemic insult or in close temporal association with a documented brain insult. They may be thought of as primary or secondary (Table 3.4.2.1).

Unprovoked Seizure

An unprovoked seizure refers to a seizure of unknown aetiology, as well as one that occurs in relation to a pre-existing brain lesion or a progressive nervous system disorder. They carry a higher risk of future epilepsy, compared with acute symptomatic seizures.

Epilepsy

Epilepsy is defined when any of the following exists:

1. At least two unprovoked (or reflex) seizures occurring >24 hours apart
2. One unprovoked (or reflex) seizure, and a probability of further seizures similar to the general recurrence risk after two unprovoked seizures (e.g. ≥60 per cent), occurring over the next 10 years. This may be the case with remote structural lesions such as stroke, central nervous system infection or certain types of traumatic brain injury
3. Diagnosis of an epilepsy syndrome

Seizures are further categorised as either focal or generalised, depending on whether the abnormal electrical activity involves a focal region of the brain or the entire cortex. Clinical manifestations of seizures vary, based both upon the location of the seizure in the brain and on the amount of cortex that is involved. They are classified in numerous different ways, one of which is seen in Figure 3.4.2.1.

Table 3.4.2.1 Acute symptomatic seizures

Primary cerebral causes	Secondary causes
• Acute ischaemic or haemorrhagic stroke, particularly lobar haemorrhage • Subdural haematoma/contusion • Subarachnoid haematoma • Hypoxic brain injury • Meningitis/encephalitis • Brain abscess • Post-neurosurgery	• Hypo-/hyperglycaemia • Hyponatraemia • Hypocalcaemia • Hypomagnesaemia • Uraemia • Hyperthyroidism • Withdrawal states • Drug intoxication, poisoning and overdose • Disorders of porphyrin metabolism

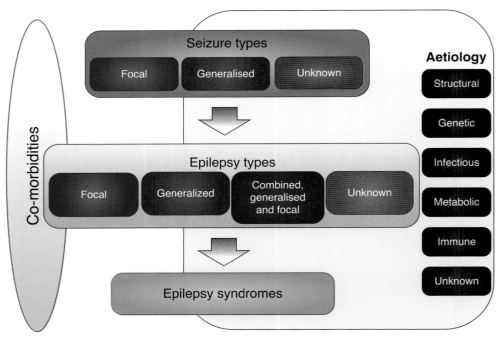

Figure 3.4.2.1 International League Against Epilepsy classification of epilepsies.
Source: Position paper of the ILAE Commission for Classification and Terminology.

Early Post-seizure Management

Most seizures stop spontaneously within 2 minutes, and rapid administration of a benzodiazepine (lorazepam or diazepam) or an anti-epileptic drug (AED) is not needed.

Acute symptomatic seizures should be managed by identifying and treating any underlying metabolic disturbances or infectious aetiologies. If present, severe hyponatraemia should be corrected slowly to avoid the risk of central pontine myelinolysis.

Differential Diagnosis

In adults, the primary conditions to consider in patients presenting with transient or paroxysmal neurological events are:

- Syncope
- Transient ischaemic attack (particularly in older adults)
- Migraine
- Panic attack and anxiety
- Psychogenic non-epileptic seizure
- Transient global amnesia (rare before the age of 50 years)
- Narcolepsy with cataplexy
- Paroxysmal movement disorders

The diagnosis of seizure is largely clinical, determined by a diagnosis based on the history, physical and neurological examinations and selected additional investigations to identify an underlying cause. The history should focus on obtaining a detailed description of events before the seizure, what happened during the event and the post-ictal condition of the patient. A history of similar previous events should be elicited in the past medical history, and a full physical and neurological examination should be performed.

Investigations

Initial investigations should include laboratory studies (electrolytes, glucose, calcium, magnesium, full blood count, renal function tests, liver function tests, urinalysis and toxicology screens) and AED drug levels. Further investigations may include electrocardiography, electroencephalography (EEG) (urgently when impaired sensorium is persistent), neuroimaging studies and a lumbar puncture, depending on the clinical circumstances.

Status Epilepticus

Status epilepticus is currently defined as an epileptic seizure that continues for >5 minutes or when seizures occur without recovery between the seizures. Overall mortality reaches almost 20 per cent. Initial management is focused on ABCDE assessment and stabilisation with rapid termination of seizure activity to reduce the risk of systemic dysfunction, neurological injury and pharmacological resistance – the latter of which increases with the duration of the seizure. Input from critical care is required if the patient does not respond to initial attempts to control the seizures (Table 3.4.2.2).

It has been demonstrated that benzodiazepine-refractory convulsive status epilepticus may be controlled in about 50 per cent of patients by administration

Table 3.4.2.2 Management of status epilepticus

0 minute	10 minutes	30 minutes	60 minutes	90 minutes

First stage (0–10 minutes)
Early status

- Secure airway and resuscitate
- Administer oxygen
- Assess cardiorespiratory function
- Establish intravenous access

Drug treatment

- Lorazepam (intravenous) 0.1 mg/kg (usually a 4-mg bolus, repeated once after 10–20 minutes; rate not critical)
- Give usual AED medication if already on treatment
- For sustained control or if seizures continue, treat as below

Second stage (0–30 minutes)

- Institute regular monitoring
- Consider the possibility of non-epileptic status
- Emergency AED therapy
- Emergency investigations
- Administer glucose (50 ml of 50% solution) and/or intravenous thiamine (250 mg) as high-potency intravenous Pabrinex® if any suggestion of alcohol abuse or impaired nutrition
- Treat acidosis if severe

Third stage (0–60 minutes)
Established status

- Establish aetiology
- Alert anaesthetist and intensive care
- Identify and treat medical complications
- Pressor therapy when appropriate

Drug treatment

Phenytoin infusion at a dose of 15–18 mg/kg at a rate of 50 mg/min
Or
Fosphenytoin infusion at a dose of 15–20 mg phenytoin equivalents (PE)/kg at a rate of 50–100 mg PE/minute
And/or
Phenobarbital bolus of 10–15 mg/kg at a rate of 100 mg/min

Fourth stage (30–90 minutes)
Refractory status

- Transfer to intensive care
- Establish intensive care and EEG monitoring
- Initiate intracranial pressure monitoring where appropriate
- Initiate long-term maintenance AED therapy

Drug treatment

General anaesthesia, with one of:

- Propofol (1–2 mg/kg bolus, then 2–10 mg/(kg hr)) titrated to effect
- Midazolam (0.1–0.2 mg/kg bolus, then 0.05–0.5 mg/(kg hr)) titrated to effect
- Thiopental sodium (3–5 mg/kg bolus, then 3–5 mg/(kg hr)) titrated to effect; after 2–3 days, infusion rate needs reduction as fat stores are saturated

Anaesthetic should be continued for 12–24 hours after the last clinical or electrographic seizure, then dose tapered

Abbreviations: AED = anti-epileptic drug; EEG = electroencephalogram.

of levetiracetam, fosphenytoin or sodium valproate, leading to seizure cessation and improved alertness by 60 minutes. The three drugs were associated with similar incidences of adverse events.

References and Further Reading

Betjemann JP, Lowenstein DH. Status epilepticus in adults. *Lancet Neurol* 2015;**14**:615–24.

Brophy GM, Bell R, Claassen J, *et al.* Guidelines for the evaluation and management of status epilepticus. *Neurocrit Care* 2012;**17**:3–23.

Claassen J, Goldstein JN. Emergency neurological life support: status epilepticus. *Neurocrit Care* 2017;**27**(Suppl 1):S152–8.

Kapur J, Elm J, Chamberlain JM, *et al.* Randomized trial of three anticonvulsant medications for status epilepticus. *N Engl J Med* 2019;**381**:2103–13.

National Institute for Health and Care Excellence. 2004. Appendix F: Protocols for treating convulsive status epilepticus in adults and children. www.nice.org.uk/guidance/cg137/chapter/appendix-f-protocols-for-treating-convulsive-status-epilepticus-in-adults-and-children-adults#treating-convulsive-status-epilepticus-in-adults-published-in-2004

Scheffer IE, Berkovic S, Capovilla G, *et al.* ILAE classification of the epilepsies: position paper of the ILAE Commission for classification and terminology. *Epilepsia* 2017;**58**:512–21.

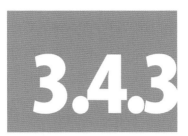

Acute Cerebrovascular Accident and Its Complications

Chris Whitehead

Key Learning Points

1. Best outcomes for stroke patients are achieved in well-organised stroke systems which involve pre-hospital care, emergency departments, a stroke service, diagnostic and interventional radiology, critical care, anaesthesia and neurosurgery.
2. Success of interventions aimed at reducing morbidity and mortality is time-dependent.
3. Patients may need close monitoring and prompt intervention, particularly for blood pressure control and for neurological deterioration.
4. Some patients need neurosurgical intervention and may need critical care post-operatively.
5. Uncertainty remains about patient and treatment selection for intervention, and this is an area of intensive ongoing research.

Keywords: stroke, thrombolytic therapy, thrombectomy, intracranial haemorrhages

Introduction

Stroke is defined by the World Health Organization as: 'a clinical syndrome consisting of rapidly developing clinical signs of focal (at times global) disturbance of cerebral function, lasting more than 24 hours, or leading to death, with no apparent cause other than that of vascular origin'. Worldwide, 6.3 million deaths per annum are caused by stroke. The morbidity and mortality associated with stroke can be reduced by effective systems of care. In the UK, the FAST (Face, Arm, Speech, Time) campaign is used to educate the public about the importance of early recognition and hospitalisation in suspected stroke.

Initial Assessment

The most important part of initial assessment is time of symptom onset. This is defined as the last time the patient was known to be 'normal' or awake and symptom-free. This is because the likelihood of success of further interventions intended to improve outcome (e.g. thrombolysis or mechanical thrombectomy) is time-dependent. Enquiry should also be made about any history of seizure, trauma, infection or pregnancy, risk factors for atherosclerosis and cardiovascular disease and a detailed drug history – particularly those that may alter clotting.

After an initial ABCDE assessment, general examination should focus not only on neurological signs and deficits, but also on potential causes of a stroke and identification of any co-morbidities, e.g. carotid bruits, irregular pulse, stigmata of coagulopathies, signs of embolism.

Unlike in many acute situations, high-flow oxygen should not be routinely given to suspected stroke patients. Hyperoxia may, in fact, be harmful in the acute setting and there is no evidence to support the need for supplemental oxygen if an SaO_2 ≥94 per cent can be achieved.

Recommendations concerning blood pressure control in ischaemic stroke vary slightly between the United States and the UK. The National Institute for Health and Care Excellence (NICE) recommends blood pressure is lowered in the presence of:

- Hypertensive encephalopathy
- Hypertensive nephropathy
- Hypertensive cardiac failure/myocardial infarction
- Aortic dissection
- Pre-eclampsia/eclampsia
- Intracerebral haemorrhage with systolic blood pressure >200 mmHg

In the United States, guidelines recommend blood pressures above 220/120 mmHg should be lowered.

If thrombolysis is indicated, the blood pressure target for initiation of therapy is <185/110 mmHg, and this should be lowered to <180/105 mmHg for the first 24 hours after completion of thrombolysis. Short-acting intravenous anti-hypertensive agents, such as labetalol, hydralazine and nicardipine, allow careful lowering of blood pressure. Blood pressures above these thresholds increase the likelihood of intracranial haemorrhage.

Neurological assessment using a validated stroke severity score (e.g. National Institute for Health Stroke Scale (NIHSS)) improves communication, quantifies the extent of neurological injury, assists in assessing prognosis and helps predict the risk of complications. The score can range from zero (no neurological deficit) to 42. As with the Glasgow Coma Score (GCS), it is of limited value in determining brainstem injury.

After initial assessment, in either the community or the emergency department, all people with suspected stroke should be admitted directly to an acute stroke unit. Brain imaging should be performed immediately in the presence of:

1. Indications for thrombolysis or early anticoagulant treatment
2. Already on anticoagulant treatment
3. A known bleeding tendency
4. GCS <13
5. Unexplained progressive or fluctuant symptoms
6. Papilloedema, neck stiffness or fever
7. Severe headache at onset of stroke symptoms

Thrombolysis

Consideration for thrombolysis with alteplase is recommended if all the following apply:

- Acute ischaemic stroke with a measurable deficit
- Within 4.5 hours of symptom onset
- If intracranial haemorrhage has been excluded radiologically
- In patients aged >18 years

If administered within 3 hours, the risk of both death and disability is reduced. If administered between 3 and 4.5 hours, a reduction in mortality has not been demonstrated; however, disability is reduced. Alteplase can be administered by emergency department staff trained in its administration and supported by appropriate stroke and neuroradiological services.

Currently, the best performing stroke services aim to start fibrinolysis in 80 per cent of eligible patients within 60 minutes of arrival at hospital, as minimising the ischaemic time is fundamental to improving outcome. Absolute and relative exclusion criteria include recent trauma or surgery, intracranial pathology at risk of bleeding, active bleeding at other sites, recent myocardial infarction and untreated hypoglycaemia. Exclusion criteria for treatment between 3 and 4.5 hours include age >80 years, oral anticoagulation regardless of the international normalised ratio (INR), baseline NIHSS score >25, history of stroke and diabetes and evidence of extensive middle cerebral artery territory infarction.

Endovascular Interventions

Successful recanalisation is the best predictor for good outcome, and although thrombolysis is effective, its benefit is reduced when large-vessel occlusion occurs. Both European guidelines and guidelines in the United States now recommend endovascular intervention within 6 hours when there has been no improvement after thrombolysis. Current evidence supports the use of stent retrievers and bridging thrombolysis. Uncertainty, however, remains, with regard to thresholds for patient selection, treatment time limits, the range of thrombectomy devices and the exact benefit of intravenous tissue plasminogen activator (tPA), in addition to endovascular thrombectomy.

There is also recent controversy as to whether mechanical thrombectomy should be performed under general anaesthesia or with local anaesthesia ± sedation. Initial trials (with major limitations) suggested worse outcomes with general anaesthesia. However, more recently published higher-quality evidence has demonstrated no difference in outcomes.

Neurosurgery

Indications for neurosurgery in the presence of intracranial haemorrhages are contentious. There is some evidence to support craniotomy for superficial haemorrhages (<1 cm from the cortical surface), but it is not recommended for small, deep haemorrhages, lobar haemorrhage without neurological deterioration, large haemorrhage with significant co-morbidities and GCS <8 in the absence of hydrocephalus or posterior fossa haemorrhage.

Insertion of external ventricular drains may be beneficial for symptomatic hydrocephalus, and decompressive craniectomy should be considered for middle cerebral artery infarction in patients aged <60 years with an NIHSS >15 and with an infarct size >50 per cent of the middle cerebral artery territory on CT scan.

Other General Measures

- Anticoagulation and thromboprophylaxis are not recommended because of an increased risk of intracranial haemorrhage.
- Blood glucose should be maintained between 4 and 11 mmol/l, using intravenous insulin and glucose where necessary. High levels are associated with increased mortality.
- A swallowing assessment should be made on admission before food, fluids or medication are administered orally. If swallowing is inadequate, food and fluids should be given in a form that can be swallowed without the risk of pulmonary aspiration, and may involve nasogastric feeding.

- Early sitting up and mobilisation are key elements in the prevention of pneumonia and are a key part of the active management plan in acute stroke units.

References and Further Reading

Gross H, Grose N. Emergency neurological life support: acute ischaemic stroke. *Neurocrit Care* 2017;**27**(Suppl 1):S102–15.

National Institute for Health and Care Excellence. Stroke and transient ischaemic attack in over 16s: diagnosis and initial management. London: National Institute for Health and Care Excellence; 2008.

Powers WJ, Rabinstein AA, Ackerson T, *et al.* 2018 guidelines for the early management of patients with acute stroke: a guideline for healthcare professionals from the American Heart Association/American Stroke Association. *Stroke* 2018;**49**:e46–110.

Steiner T, Al-Shahi Salman R, Beer R, *et al.* European Stroke Organisation (ESO) guidelines for the management of spontaneous intracerebral hemorrhage. *Int J Stroke* 2014;**9**:840–55.

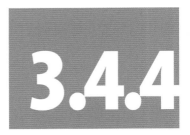

Meningitis

Arun Krishnamurthy

Key Learning Points

1. Bacterial meningitis is more often fatal than other forms of meningitis.
2. Viral meningitis is usually self-limiting.
3. Immunocompromised patients are susceptible to tuberculosis and fungal infections.
4. If you suspect bacterial meningitis, antibiotics should be administered immediately.
5. Use of corticosteroids in the management of meningitis is still debatable. Evidence shows that use does not reduce mortality; however, it does show a reduction in neurological complications, especially hearing loss.

Keywords: meningitis, immunocompromised, corticosteroids, antibiotics

Definition

Meningitis is a life-threatening illness that involves acute inflammation of the meninges. Inflammation of the brain itself is known as encephalitis.

Causes

Meningitis is typically caused by an infection, the most common causes being viral and then bacterial. Other causes include fungal and a variety of non-infectious causes. Transmission occurs mainly through close contact and droplet spread, though some pathogens such as *Listeria monocytogenes* and *Escherichia coli* may be spread via food. Identifying the cause of meningitis is important, as the bacterial form can be rapidly fatal.

Bacterial Meningitis

The most common causes of bacterial meningitis are seen in Box 3.4.4.1. Immunocompromised patients may also be susceptible to tuberculosis and fungal infections.

Box 3.4.4.1 Common Causes of Bacterial Meningitis

- *Streptococcus pneumoniae*
- *Neisseria meningitidis* (meningococcal meningitis) – highly contagious infection and common in young adults
- *Haemophilus influenzae* type b
- *Listeria monocytogenes* (listeria) – common in patients who have some form of immunocompromise, including pregnant women, newborns and older adults
- Group B *Streptococcus*
- Gram-negative bacilli

Viral Meningitis

This is more common than the bacterial form and generally less serious. Symptoms may be mild, and generally people with this form of the disease will recover without any treatment. Common causes of viral meningitis are seen in Box 3.4.4.2.

Box 3.4.4.2 Common Causes of Viral Meningitis

- Enteroviruses (most common pathogen)
- Herpes simplex virus (generally type II)
- Varicella-zoster virus
- Mumps
- Human immunodeficiency virus

Other Causes

There are a number of non-infectious causes which can lead to meningitis. Disorders such as sarcoidosis, systemic lupus erythematosus and spread of cancer to the meninges are all possible causes.

Risk Factors

Certain groups of people are at an increased risk of developing meningitis (Box 3.4.4.3).

Box 3.4.4.3 Risk Factors for Infective Meningitis

- Extremes of age
- Immunocompromised patients
- Diabetes mellitus, chronic renal failure, adrenal insufficiency, alcoholism and cirrhosis
- Head injury
- Neurosurgery
- Ear/sinus infection
- Crowding, areas such as schools and university where large groups of people gather together
- Travel

Presentation

The classic presentation is a triad of fever, headache and neck stiffness. That said, less than half of adults will present with this and instead often have other signs and symptoms such as non-blanching rash, lethargy, altered conscious level, photophobia, confusion, seizures and nausea and vomiting. There may also be signs of systemic infection such as tachypnoea, tachycardia and associated hypotension.

Symptoms may develop acutely or may occur over several days. It can often be preceded by a prodromal illness, with lethargy and lack of appetite. This is especially true in patients with viral meningitis.

Differential Diagnosis

This could include any other causes of severe headache such as those seen in Box 3.4.4.4.

Box 3.4.4.4 Common Causes of a Severe Headache

- Subarachnoid haemorrhage
- Migraine
- Non-infectious meningitis
- Stroke
- Central nervous system vasculitis
- Encephalitis
- Other causes of raised intracranial pressure

Diagnosis

The history and examination should lead to a high index of suspicion of meningitis.

Blood Tests

- Full blood count and C-reactive protein (CRP) – looking at markers of inflammation

- Coagulation profile
- Blood cultures
- Whole-blood polymerase chain reaction (PCR) for *N. meningitidis*
- Blood glucose, which is compared to cerebrospinal fluid (CSF) glucose

Imaging

- Head CT or MRI to exclude other causes of raised intracranial pressure
- If there is evidence of raised intracranial pressure, do not perform a lumbar puncture
- Do not delay treatment in order to perform a CT scan

Lumbar Puncture

Unless this is contraindicated, this is the diagnostic test of choice.

The CSF sample is examined for the presence and types of white blood cells, red blood cells, protein content and glucose level (Table 3.4.4.1). Gram staining of the sample may demonstrate bacteria in bacterial meningitis. However, absence of bacteria does not exclude bacterial meningitis, as they are only seen in 60 per cent of cases.

Management

Management is aimed at early recognition. If you suspect bacterial meningitis, antibiotics should be administered immediately.

Table 3.4.4.1 Typical cerebrospinal fluid findings

	Appearance	White blood cells	Protein	Glucose
Normal	Clear	0–5 cells/mm^3	0.15–0.45 g/dl	2.8–4.2 mmol/l >60% serum glucose
Bacterial meningitis	Clear/cloudy/purulent	>1000 cells/mm^3	Elevated	Low <40% glucose
Viral meningitis	Clear	10–1000 cells/mm^3	Elevated	Elevated >60% glucose
Fungal meningitis	Clear/cloudy	10–500 cells/mm^3	Elevated	Low

Immediate Management

Airway

- Administer 100% oxygen.
- Assess the airway and consider intubation if there is:
  - A reduction in Glasgow Coma Score (GCS)
  - Evidence of respiratory failure

Breathing

- Ensure breathing/ventilation is adequate.

Circulation

- Secure intravenous access; take blood tests (including blood cultures) and start fluid resuscitation.
- You may need to consider inotropic support.

Disability

Assess neurological status, looking for:
- Conscious level
- Signs of meningeal irritation
- Focal neurological signs
- Papilloedema
- Signs of raised intracranial pressure

Specific Management

- Treat suspected bacterial meningitis with antibiotics according to local policies.
- May need to perform a CT scan to exclude evidence of raised intracranial pressure.
- Perform a lumbar puncture if no contraindications.
- Take samples of CSF and send for Gram staining, microscopy, culture, protein, glucose and PCR (particularly important for herpes encephalitis).
- Take paired blood samples for blood glucose.
- Review the antibiotic regime after results of Gram staining.
- Use of corticosteroids in the management of meningitis is still debatable. Evidence shows that corticosteroids do not reduce mortality; however, it does show a reduction in neurological complications, especially hearing loss.

Although some patients require imaging prior to lumbar puncture, antibiotics should not be delayed, as this is associated with poor outcomes, including chronic neurological deficits and death.

Further Management

Treat immediate complications:
- Septic shock
- Disseminated intravascular coagulation
- Coma
- Seizures
- Cerebral oedema
- Electrolyte disturbances: hypoglycaemia, hypokalaemia, acidosis

Long-Term Sequelae

These include:
- Hearing loss or deafness
- Blindness
- Seizures
- Cranial nerve dysfunction
- Hydrocephalus
- Ataxia

Prognosis

In patients with viral meningitis, the prognosis is generally favourable, with a mortality rate of <1 per cent. Those at extremes of age and those who are immunocompromised or have significant co-morbidities may have a worse prognosis.

Bacterial meningitis has a higher mortality rate, varying from 3 to 30 per cent, depending on the organism involved, the age of the patient and the underlying cause. *S. pneumoniae* has the highest mortality – up to 30 per cent. Meningococcal meningitis has low mortality. However, if there is associated meningococcal septicaemia, this goes up to 20–30 per cent. Disease caused by *H. influenzae* has a good prognosis, with a mortality rate of 3–5 per cent.

References and Further Reading

Brouwer MC, McIntyre P, Prasad K, Van de Beek D. Corticosteroids for acute bacterial meningitis. *Cochrane Database Syst Rev* 2015;**9**:CD004405.

Van de Beek D, de Gans J, Spanjaard L, Weisfelt M, Reitsma J, Vermeulen M. Clinical features and prognostic factors in adults with bacterial meningitis. *N Engl J Med* 2004;**351**:1849–59.

Van de Beek D, de Gans J, Tunkel AR, Wijdicks EF. Community-acquired bacterial meningitis in adults. *N Engl J Med* 2006;**354**:44–53.

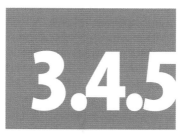

3.4.5

Tetanus

Sachin Mehta and Manpreet Bahra

Key Learning Points

1. Tetanus is a potentially lethal condition that must be considered in patients with muscle spasms and inadequate immunisation.
2. Initial management focuses on administration of human tetanus immunoglobulin, followed by wound cleaning and debridement.
3. Patients with shorter incubation periods have increased disease severity and mortality.
4. Supportive care is the mainstay of management to avoid complications such as fractures, rhabdomyolysis and respiratory failure.
5. Autonomic instability indicates severe disease and is the most common cause of death.

Keywords: tetanus, *Clostridium tetani*, tetanospasmin, tetanus toxoid

Pathophysiology

Clostridium tetani is an anaerobic, spore-forming, Gram-positive bacillus that produces the exotoxin tetanospasmin. It can be found in soil, saliva and manure, and enters the body through breaks in the skin caused by cuts, bites or penetrating trauma. Drug users, particularly those that inject subcutaneously, are also at risk of contracting tetanus. Once in the body, tetanospasmin ascends via the axons of motor and autonomic neurones and prevents the release of inhibitory neurotransmitters. This leads to uncontrolled muscle spasms and the autonomic features seen in more severe cases. Previous immunisation confers some protection, such that milder or localised symptoms may be experienced in a sensitised individual.

Signs and Symptoms

There are four distinct clinical patterns of tetanus:

1. Generalised – the most common form as detailed in this chapter
2. Local – muscle contractions occur in one extremity or body region (a rare form)
3. Cephalic – may present after head injuries and initially involves one cranial nerve
4. Neonatal – occurs from failure of aseptic techniques in managing the umbilical stump

The incubation period (i.e. time from injury to first symptoms) is usually between 3 and 14 days. The onset time (i.e. time from first symptom to first spasm) is 1–7 days. The hallmark features are gradual-onset muscle pain and stiffness, hypertonia, rigidity, spasm and dysphagia. Dysphagia is often followed by laryngospasm, which is easily provoked (e.g. by swallowing) like the other types of spasm seen. Classically, these spasms begin in the jaw and spread to the rest of the body. They usually last a few minutes at a time and occur frequently during the course of the disease. Other symptoms may include headache, pyrexia, diaphoresis, drooling, incontinence and autonomic instability (arrhythmias, myocardial ischaemia, hypertension with tachycardia and later hypotension with bradycardia).

Initial Management

The wound should be cleaned, and non-viable tissue debrided. Patients with a significant wound and no or incomplete vaccination should receive 3000–6000 units of human tetanus immunoglobulin intramuscularly prior to surgical debridement (with part of the dose infiltrated around the wound). All patients should also receive three doses of tetanus toxoid spaced at least 2 weeks apart for active immunity (in a different site to the immunoglobulin administration). Appropriate initial antibiotics include intravenous metronidazole (500 mg 8-hourly) or benzylpenicillin (1.2 g 6-hourly) for 7–10 days. There is some evidence to favour metronidazole. This should be tailored to the type of bite/injury, other potential contaminants and local anti-microbial policies. Wounds with a greater risk of tetanus contamination include those with significant amounts of non-viable tissue, those which have come into contact with soil/manure, puncture wounds and wounds that occurred >6 hours before surgical debridement or have evidence of established infection.

Investigations

The diagnosis is clinical and based on the triad of rigidity, muscle spasms and autonomic dysfunction (in severe cases). There are currently no serological tests for diagnosing tetanus. *C. tetani* is isolated from wounds of affected patients in only 30 per cent of cases. It can be isolated from patients without tetanus.

A 'spatula test' is a clinical test for tetanus that involves touching the posterior pharynx with a spatula and observing the effect. Reflex contraction of the jaw (biting the spatula) indicates a positive test, whereas a normal gag reflex indicates a negative test. Arterial blood gases may herald the development of respiratory failure, and creatine kinase monitoring should be undertaken to identify rhabdomyolysis.

Other investigations can be used to help exclude differential diagnoses, such as strychnine poisoning, hypocalcaemic tetany, trismus due to oro-facial infection, seizure disorder and meningism. Malignant neuroleptic syndrome and acute dystonia should also be considered, as well as stroke (in the context of cephalic tetanus).

Severity

Onset of symptoms within 5 days signifies a substantial toxin load and severe disease. Autonomic instability is also a sign of severe disease. Approximately 50 per cent of patients die without treatment, and 10–25 per cent of patients die despite intensive care. Autonomic failure is the most common cause of death. The mortality rate is higher in patients without prior immunisation and those over the age of 60 years. Neonatal tetanus accounts for half of tetanus deaths worldwide.

Management

Mild tetanus is defined by the presence of mild symptoms with delayed onset and no respiratory embarrassment. These patients should be managed in a quiet environment after the initial management described above. Light sedation, e.g. oral diazepam, is administered to prevent spasms.

Severe tetanus should be treated expectantly in the ICU. Prolonged respiratory muscle spasm can lead to respiratory failure requiring intubation and ventilation. Intravenous benzodiazepines are the sedative of choice. A high requirement of sedatives in itself may necessitate intubation. Early tracheostomy is often needed, as oral endotracheal tubes can precipitate further spasms. Bronchial secretions are copious and require frequent suctioning. Sedation and mechanical ventilation are often necessary for 2–3 weeks until spasms cease. Ongoing muscle rigidity is treated with intravenous magnesium sulphate (20 mmol/hr). Refractory cases may require the addition of non-depolarising muscle relaxants. Intrathecal baclofen has been used successfully. Spasms may be so severe that bone fractures can result.

Autonomic instability is minimised by sedation or general anaesthesia. Haemodynamics should be supported with intravenous fluid and short-acting agents due to lability of cardiovascular fluctuations. Such agents include intravenous atropine (1–20 mg/hr), labetalol (15–120 mg/hr) and magnesium sulphate (20 mmol/hr). Beta-blockade without concomitant alpha-blockade should be avoided.

Nutritional support is necessary in the face of significantly increased muscle activity. A high-calorie and protein supplementation regime should be instituted and maintained throughout the course of the disease. Gastric stasis and ileus are common and may necessitate instigation of parenteral nutrition. Close attention should be paid to preventing pressure sores, stress ulcers and venous thromboembolism.

Complete recovery takes 4–6 weeks, as destroyed nerve axon terminals must regenerate. Exposure to the disease does not provide lifelong immunity; therefore, prophylaxis is mandatory prior to hospital discharge and every 10 years thereafter.

References and Further Reading

Ahmadsyah I, Salim A. Treatment of tetanus: an open study to compare the efficacy of procaine penicillin and metronidazole. *Br Med J (Clin Res Ed)* 1985;**291**:648.

Rushdy AA, White JM, Ramsay ME, Crowcroft NS. Tetanus in England and Wales, 1984–2000. *Epidemiol Infect* 2003;**130**:71.

Santos ML, Mota-Miranda A, Alves-Pereira A, *et al.* Intrathecal baclofen for the treatment of tetanus. *Clin Infect Dis* 2004;**38**:321.

Thwaites CL, Farrar JJ. Preventing and treating tetanus. *BMJ* 2003;**326**:117.

Thwaites CL, Yen LM, Loan HT, *et al.* Magnesium sulphate for treatment of severe tetanus: a randomised controlled trial. *Lancet* 2006;**368**:1436.

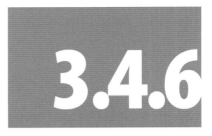

Delirium

Tamas Bakonyi and Valerie Page

Key Learning Points

1. Delirium is an independent predictor of poor patient outcomes.
2. Routine daily screening for delirium is essential.
3. Daily targeted light sedation reduces the risk of delirium.
4. Early mobilisation needs to be a priority.
5. Only use anti-psychotics to reduce symptoms of agitation.

Keywords: delirium, anti-psychotics, CAM-ICU, disorientation

Introduction

Delirium is associated with increased mortality, prolonged ICU and hospital length of stay and development of long-term cognitive impairment in adult ICU patients. The longer delirium persists, the worse the outcomes for the patient.

Definition and Presentation

Delirium is an acute, transient mental dysfunction with inattention, altered level of 'awakeness' and cognitive changes, i.e. disorientation, memory deficit, language disturbances and perceptual abnormalities (illusions and hallucinations). It is typical for symptoms to fluctuate in modality and intensity. Patients will always have inattention, i.e. inability to focus, maintain and shift attention; however, perceptual disturbances are not necessary for a diagnosis of delirium.

Delirium is categorised into three motoric subtypes, according to the presenting psychomotor activity of the patient. The most common subtype is the hypoactive patient presenting with lethargy and reduced level of consciousness, often difficult to diagnose since the patient is quiet and compliant. In hyperactive delirium, the patient is restless and agitated, sometimes combative. In the mixed subtype, symptoms vary and fluctuate with time, even within a few hours.

Risk Factors

Delirium is precipitated by a medical condition and/or drugs, administration or withdrawal. Delirium may be the first symptom of acute disease and it will continue until the cause(s) are managed.

Predisposing Factors

Baseline factors making patients more prone to developing delirium are age, chronic medical conditions, hypertension, cognitive impairment, especially dementia, alcohol or illicit drug abuse and high severity of illness. Aggravating factors include visual and hearing impairment, immobility and disturbances in the circadian rhythm.

Precipitating Factors

Treatment-associated causes include medical interventions (surgical interventions, mechanical ventilation, use of bladder catheter), depth and duration of sedation and use of anti-cholinergic drugs or benzodiazepines and other psychotropic drugs.

Common medical causes are infections, metabolic disorders (hypoglycaemia, acid–base imbalance, electrolyte disturbances, hepatic or renal failure), hypoperfusion states, primary brain pathologies, vitamin deficiencies, abnormal thyroid function and/or uncontrolled pain.

Recognition

Delirium is an independent risk predictor of negative clinical outcomes. Because hypoactive delirium is often missed, to detect delirium in critically ill patients, clinicians need to routinely use a screening tool. Two screening tools are validated for use in intubated patients on sedative drugs – Confusion Assessment

Method-ICU (CAM-ICU) and the Intensive Care Delirium Screening Checklist (ICDSC). They are usually undertaken by the bedside nurse.

CAM-ICU

This assesses four items:

1. Change in mental status
2. Inattention (can the patient squeeze the assessor's hand on the 'A's in a sequence of letters?)
3. Level of consciousness other than awake and aware
4. Disorganised thinking (four yes/no questions and a simple command)

If the patient has >2 mistakes during looking for inattention and has an altered level of consciousness and/or disorganised thinking, they are assessed as positive for delirium.

ICDSC

This consists of eight items that can be observed throughout an ICU shift: level of consciousness, inattention, disorientation, hallucination/delusion/psychosis, psychomotor agitation or retardation, inappropriate speech or mood, sleep/wake disturbance and fluctuation of symptoms. If there are four or more present, the patient is assessed as positive for delirium.

The CAM-ICU and ICDSC are not particularly sensitive in acute medical patients. In patients who are not intubated, a useful screen for inattention is asking the patient to say the months of the year going backwards, normally achieved without mistakes.

(ICU delirium assessment tool implementation and training resources are available at www.icudelirium.org)

Management

The cornerstone of managing delirium in patients is to treat any, and all, modifiable causes.

Non-pharmacological

A 'delirium bundle' has proved to be useful in other patient populations. The interventions are designed to achieve an optimal caring environment to reduce delirium. It includes regular orientation, avoiding constipation and dehydration and providing hearing and visual aids if needed. Promoting a normal sleep–wake cycle by decreasing activities and stimuli at night, i.e. controlling noise and light, removing unnecessary lines/catheters and monitoring devices. Early mobilisation has been shown to decrease delirium in the critically ill population and needs to be a priority. Involving the ICU pharmacist is key – a large number of drugs in common use have the potential to precipitate or aggravate delirium, e.g. steroids, drugs with anti-cholinergic properties.

National and international guidelines recommend mechanically ventilated patients in the ICU are kept pain-free and comfortable, whilst being awake or easily aroused. Deep sedation, even within the first 48 hours, is associated with worse outcomes. Daily sedation monitoring with a targeted sedation level is not only good clinical practice – it is essential to reduce the risk of delirium in this vulnerable patient group.

An effective sedation protocol needs to be user-friendly and analgesia-based, include clinical indications for deep sedation, e.g. proning, and facilitate dynamic management of sedation by nurses. This includes appropriate use of supplementary analgesia, anti-psychotics and alpha-agonists, as needed for agitation. If each patient is to be optimally sedated, doctors need to take an ongoing and active interest supporting the bedside nurse. Benzodiazepines are well-known risk factors for delirium. However, their use is recommended for patients with severe alcohol withdrawal.

Pharmacological Management

There is no evidence to support the use of drugs to prevent or treat ICU delirium. The goal of drug use in delirium is to control agitation.

Haloperidol is the most commonly used anti-psychotic in the ICU, and it can be given intravenously. It can prolong the QT interval, potentially leading to torsades de pointes; thus, its administration is contraindicated in patients with prolonged QTc. Olanzapine is currently the only other drug that can be given parenterally or as an intramuscular injection. Quetiapine and risperidone (orally) are useful adjuncts and have fewer side effects.

Alpha-agonists, clonidine and the newer, more selective drug dexmedetomidine may also be used. However, they are not always effective and currently there is limited evidence for their use in delirium.

Patients and Families

Delirium is often a distressing experience for patients, and for families to witness. Families want to know about the risk of delirium and the steps being taken to manage it. Written information, as provided by www.icusteps.org, is useful and free to download. Once patients have recovered, they usually find it helpful and reassuring to talk about and understand their delirious experience as part of their illness.

References and Further Reading

Barr J, Fraser GL, Puntillo K, *et al.*; American College of Critical Care Medicine. Clinical practice guidelines for the management of pain, agitation, and delirium in adult patients in the intensive care unit. *Crit Care Med* 2013;**41**:263–306.

Cerejeira J, Nogueira V, Luís P, Vaz-Serra A, Mukaetova-Ladinska EB. The cholinergic system and inflammation: common pathways in delirium pathophysiology. *J Am Geriatr Soc* 2012;**60**:669–75.

Gusmao-Flores D, Salluh JI, Chalhub RA, Quarantini LC. The Confusion Assessment Method for the Intensive Care Unit (CAM-ICU) and Intensive Care Delirium Screening Checklist (ICDSC) for the diagnosis of delirium: a systematic review and meta-analysis of clinical studies. *Crit Care* 2012;**16**:R115.

Mehta S, Cook D, Devlin JW, *et al.* Prevalence, risk factors, and outcomes of delirium in mechanically ventilated adults. *Crit Care Med* 2015;**43**:557–66.

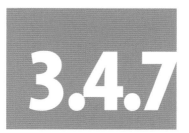

Neuromuscular Disorders

3.4.7

Sachin Mehta and Manpreet Bahra

Key Learning Points

1. Several conditions exist that may lead to profound muscle weakness and death.
2. The most common conditions leading to admission to the ICU are Guillain–Barré syndrome and myasthenia gravis.
3. Early identification and supportive care can be lifesaving.
4. Specific therapies initiated in a timely manner can improve the prognosis significantly.
5. ICU-acquired weakness should be considered in ICU patients with flaccid, generalised weakness or weaning difficulties.

Keywords: neuromuscular disorders, myasthenia, Guillain–Barré, myopathy, polyneuropathy

Introduction

Neuromuscular disorders lead to voluntary muscle weakness via disruption of their innervation, motor end-plate unit or intrinsic muscle function. Muscle weakness can develop during the course of several conditions, both acute and chronic. The mechanisms through which acute organ failures occur are the same, however – respiratory muscle weakness can lead to respiratory failure and coma, and bulbar dysfunction can lead to aspiration and respiratory failure. Death and disability can also occur from sequelae specific to these conditions, e.g. cardiac arrhythmias.

The most common neuromuscular disorders leading to admission to the ICU are metabolic myopathies, pontine cerebrovascular accident (CVA), multiple sclerosis, myasthenia gravis (MG) and Guillain–Barré syndrome (GBS). Poisoning with benzene-containing compounds can also cause neuromuscular weakness. ICU-acquired weakness (ICU-AW) can mimic these disorders but occurs as a result of critical illness in patients already admitted to the ICU.

Initial management of patients with significant neuromuscular weakness involves assessment/support of the airway and respiratory and cardiovascular systems. Efforts to identify the underlying diagnosis should be undertaken simultaneously to allow timely preparation of definitive treatments. Specific management of myasthenia gravis, GBS and ICU-AW is described in further detail below.

Myasthenia Gravis

MG, although relatively rare, is the most common disorder of neuromuscular transmission. Weakness is caused by autoantibodies directed against nicotinic acetylcholine receptors on the post-synaptic membrane of the neuromuscular junction. Ten to 15 per cent of patients have an associated thymoma where these antibodies arise, and thymectomy may provide remission. It is characterised by fluctuating weakness in limb, bulbar, ocular and respiratory muscles. The weakness is *not* associated with pain or loss of tendon reflexes. Weakness deteriorates after exertion, infection, stress, trauma or certain drugs (see below) and recovers following rest. Respiratory muscle involvement can be fatal and is termed 'myasthenic crisis'. Age of onset demonstrates a bimodal distribution. The first peak occurs in the second and third decades, with a female predominance. The second peak occurs in the sixth to eighth decades, with a male predominance.

Lambert–Eaton myasthenia syndrome is a rare variant of MG, in which pre-synaptic voltage-gated calcium channels are the subject of autoantibody disruption. It can be distinguished clinically from MG by demonstrating predominant leg weakness, temporary improvement of weakness after exertion and relative absence of eye involvement. Sixty per cent of cases are paraneoplastic, and treatment is directed at the underlying malignancy. In the remaining cases, immuno-modulation treatments are used as for MG, but are not as effective.

The diagnosis of MG can be established through clinical and serological testing. The edrophonium, or 'Tensilon®', test, is used in patients with obvious ptosis or ophthalmoparesis where improvement after administration of this short-acting anti-cholinesterase can be easily observed. In known myasthenic patients, the test can distinguish a myasthenic from a cholinergic crisis (see below). The diagnosis is confirmed by detecting the presence of antibodies against acetylcholine receptors or muscle-specific tyrosine kinase. Electrophysiological testing may be used to confirm the disease in seronegative cases. Chest CT/MRI scan should then be undertaken to identify possible thymoma. Studies to exclude other diseases such as thyrotoxicosis, meningitis or associated rheumatological conditions should be considered in selected patients.

MG is treated with four therapeutic options. Anti-cholinesterase drugs, such as pyridostigmine, provide the mainstay of symptomatic treatments. Remission can be induced with chronic (corticosteroids or other immunomodulating agents) or rapid immunotherapies (plasma exchange or intravenous immunoglobulin). Finally, thymectomy may offer remission in some cases. Treatment strategies are determined by patient age, disease severity and rate of progression.

Myasthenic crisis is a potentially life-threatening condition characterised by acute respiratory failure. It may be precipitated by events such as surgery, infection and immunosuppressant withdrawal, but may also occur spontaneously. Rarely, a myasthenic crisis can be the first presenting feature of the disease. Several drugs can worsen weakness in MG and may also precipitate a crisis. Drugs commonly encountered in the ICU that should be used with caution in MG include those seen in Box 3.4.7.1.

Box 3.4.7.1 Drugs Commonly Encountered in ICU that Should Be Used with Caution in Myasthenia Gravis

- Vancomycin
- Clindamycin
- Aminoglycosides
- Ketolides (contraindicated)
- Fluoroquinolones
- Local anaesthetics
- Opiates
- Muscle relaxants
- Magnesium sulphate
- Beta-blockers

Admission to the ICU is recommended for patients with moderate/severe exacerbations of MG who are deteriorating. Close monitoring, including regular vital capacity (VC) and/or maximal inspiratory pressure (MIP) measurements (up to 2-hourly in some cases), should be undertaken. Intubation is indicated when VC drops below 15–20 ml/kg body weight, the MIP measurement becomes less negative than −30 cmH_2O or respiratory distress is clinically evident. Once intubated, anti-cholinesterase medication can be stopped to reduce airway secretions. Rapid therapy with plasma exchange (PLEX) or intravenous immunoglobulins (IVIGs) is initiated, alongside chronic immunomodulatory medication, to maintain the transient benefit of these therapies. Spontaneous breathing trials can be attempted once rapid therapies have been instituted and signs of improving respiratory function are seen.

Cholinergic crisis describes a state of overstimulation at the neuromuscular junction due to excess acetylcholine. Typical cholinergic features, such as sweating, confusion, miosis, arrhythmias and seizures, will be present. Muscles subsequently stop responding to excess acetylcholine, which leads to flaccid paralysis and respiratory failure. Mechanical ventilation is indicated as for myasthenic crisis, and atropine may need to be administered. Repeat edrophonium tests are undertaken once the patient is stable, and anti-cholinesterase drugs reinitiated once positive.

Guillain–Barré Syndrome

GBS is an acute condition characterised by rapidly progressive polyneuropathy with muscle weakness or paralysis. It is an immunologically mediated demyelinating polyradiculopathy, commonly precipitated by viruses and immunisations. Weakness is largely symmetrical and accompanied by decreased or absent tendon reflexes. Progression is typically over a 2-week period. Weakness ranges in severity, from mild difficulty in walking to almost complete paralysis of voluntary muscles. Approximately 30 per cent of affected patients require ventilatory support, and 20 per cent will develop severe autonomic dysfunction warranting ICU admission.

GBS has various clinical patterns. Acute inflammatory demyelinating polyneuropathy is the most prevalent in the Western world. Miller Fisher syndrome is a variant of GBS, featuring ophthalmoplegia and ataxia. Diagnosis is clinical and supported by cerebrospinal fluid (CSF) findings of increased protein and normal white cell count, known as the 'albumi-nocytological dissociation'. Nerve conduction studies can also aid confirmation, as well as demonstrate the type of GBS variant present. The presence of serum immunoglobulin G (IgG) antibodies to GQ1b may also be useful for diagnostic purposes where available. Further investigations are targeted at excluding differentials such as neuromuscular disorders and other polyneuropathies.

Similar measures for close monitoring, as described above for MG, should be undertaken. Additionally, closer monitoring of cardiovascular status is necessary, given the frequency of autonomic dysfunction encountered. Baseline VC and MIP measurements must be taken on admission, and repeated frequently whilst weakness is progressing. Intubation is indicated when VC drops below 20 ml/kg, or MIP is less negative than $-30 \text{ cmH}_2\text{O}$. Suxamethonium is contraindicated as it is likely to precipitate arrhythmias, hyperkalaemia and cardiac arrest. Early tracheostomy is useful, as ventilation is often prolonged, and may also be warranted in self-ventilating patients with bulbar dysfunction. Physiotherapy and rehabilitation should be initiated early, along with the provision of psychological support. Pain occurs in approximately two-thirds of patients. It is often severe and prolonged, and must be sought and treated appropriately. Paralytic ileus may develop; therefore, daily abdominal examination is required. Parenteral nutrition is often necessary if ileus is present.

Treatment with PLEX or IVIG is effective if initiated within 2 weeks of symptom onset, though they can be used up to within 4 weeks. Outcomes are equivalent with either treatment, and selection is largely determined by local availability/expertise, patient preference and contraindications. Corticosteroid treatment is not recommended in adult patients. 'Treatment-related fluctuations' refer to deteriorations after initial improvement/stabilisation following PLEX or IVIG. They occur in approximately 10 per cent of cases and usually occur within the first 2 months of treatment. Repeated treatment with IVIG is indicated in such cases. Prevention of venous thromboembolism and pressure sores is important due to prolonged immobility.

The typical course of GBS is progressive weakness for 2 weeks, followed by a plateau between 2 and 4 weeks, followed by gradual improvement in muscle strength thereafter. At 1 year following treatment, approximately 60 per cent of patients have full recovery of muscle strength, and 14 per cent have persistent, severe weakness. Approximately 5 per cent of patients will die in spite of ICU care.

ICU-Acquired Weakness

Critically ill patients who develop flaccid, generalised weakness or failure to wean from mechanical ventilation should be assessed for the presence of ICU-AW. ICU-AW includes critical illness myopathy (CIM) and critical illness polyneuropathy (CIP), or a combination of the two. ICU-AW is very common in critically ill patients, with an incidence of 25–60 per cent seen in patients who are mechanically ventilated for >7 days. It can lead to poor quality of life and weakness that persists long after ICU discharge.

The pathophysiology is multifactorial and likely to involve axonopathy, ischaemia, mitochondrial dysfunction, catabolism and immobility. Several risk factors exist, including pre-morbid nutritional status, female sex, sepsis/inflammation, poor glycaemic control, corticosteroids (controversial) and neuromuscular-blocking agents.

Onset is typically 1 week into critical illness. Diagnosis is clinical and based on the typical pattern of symmetrical, mostly proximal weakness, preserved, but diminished, reflexes and intact cranial nerve and autonomic function. Objective assessment of muscle strength using the Medical Research Council (MRC) sum score can be diagnostic where a patient scores <48 (indicating that average strength is limited to movement against gravity and partial resistance). Investigations to support the diagnosis are normal CSF studies, raised creatine kinase (CK) in CIM and nerve conduction studies displaying normal conduction velocities with decreased compound muscle action potentials. Investigations are often unnecessary but may aid exclusion of differential diagnoses. These include residual paralysis or sedation, rhabdomyolysis, acute myopathy, cachectic myopathy, neuromuscular junction disorders, spinal cord or brainstem lesions and GBS.

Management is aimed at aggressively treating medical conditions and minimising sedatives, neuromuscular-blocking agents and corticosteroids. Close attention should be paid to glycaemic control and electrolyte and nutritional optimisation. Rehabilitation is attempted through physiotherapy, electrical muscle stimulation and ventilator weaning.

ICU-AW is usually reversible over weeks to months; however, it leads to prolonged ventilation and ICU and

199

hospital stay. In CIP, residual functional deficits are relatively common. In general, most patients recover to be able to walk independently. Approximately 30 per cent of patients will, however, be left with severe quadriparesis, quadriplegia or paraplegia.

References and Further Reading

De Jonghe B, Sharshar T, Lefaucheur J-P, *et al.* Paresis acquired in the intensive care unit: a prospective multicenter study. *JAMA* 2002;**288**:2859.

Hough CL, Lieu BK, Caldwell ES. Manual muscle strength testing of critically ill patients: feasibility and interobserver agreement. *Crit Care* 2011;**15**:R43.

Hughes R, Cornblath D. Guillain-Barré syndrome. *Lancet* 2005;**366**:1653–66.

Sanders DB, Wolfe GI, Benatar M, *et al.* International consensus guidance for management of myasthenia gravis: executive summary. *Neurology* 2016;**87**:419.

Yuki N, Hartung HP. Guillain–Barré syndrome. *N Engl J Med* 2012;**366**:2294.

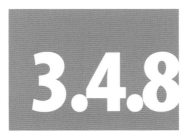

3.4.8 Non-traumatic Spinal Cord Injury

Manpreet Bahra and Sachin Mehta

Key Learning Points

1. Non-traumatic spinal cord injury (NTSCI) describes a heterogeneous group of diseases which cause myelopathy by mechanisms other than trauma.
2. The International Spinal Cord Society (ISCoS) have developed a useful classification system for the diverse range of aetiologies causing NTSCI.
3. Presentation of NTSCI may be highly variable, and prompt identification of cord syndromes is therefore important to prevent diagnostic delay.
4. Management should focus on timely resuscitation and supportive treatment, whilst seeking specialist assessment.
5. Prognosis depends on the neurological level and completeness of injury – those with higher or complete injuries suffer worse outcomes.

Keywords: non-traumatic, spinal cord injury

Introduction

Acute spinal cord injuries (ASCIs) include both traumatic and non-traumatic causes of damage to the spinal cord, resulting in temporary or permanent neurological deficit. Traumatic spinal cord injury (TSCI) is covered in depth in a separate chapter. Non-traumatic spinal cord injury (NTSCI) is an umbrella term for a heterogeneous group of diseases which cause myelopathy by mechanisms other than trauma. The breadth and depth of this topic are beyond the scope of this book. This chapter will therefore focus on common presentations of NTSCI and their implications in the critical care setting.

Epidemiology

In recent years, the epidemiology of ASCI has dramatically changed owing significantly to an ageing population. NTSCI can occur at any age (see below) and has a relatively equal gender distribution. Recent data have suggested equivalent, and occasionally higher, incidence of NTSCI, compared to TSCI, particularly in developed countries. This emerging pattern of higher incidence is predicted to continue to rise in the coming decades.

Classification

It is well recognised that NTSCI occurs as a result of a variety of aetiologies and pathophysiological processes. Leading causes in developed countries are degenerative disorders of the vertebral column, tumours, infection, vascular disorders and inflammatory and autoimmune diseases. The International Spinal Cord Society (ISCoS) classifies the aetiology of NTSCI by cause, time frame of onset and presence of iatrogenicity. In essence, this system subdivides aetiology into congenital diseases (spinal dysraphism, Arnold–Chiari malformation and skeletal malformations), genetic disorders (hereditary spastic paraplegia, spino-cerebellar ataxias, adreno-myeloneuropathies, other leukodystrophies and spinal muscular atrophies) and acquired abnormalities (vertebral column degeneration, metabolic and vascular disorders, inflammatory and autoimmune diseases, toxic, neoplastic, infectious and radiation-related injury).

Clinical Features

Irrespective of the underlying pathology, it is vital to consider time-critical diagnoses in any patient presenting with the following cord syndromes:

- **Anterior cord syndrome:** occurs due to interruption of the anterior spinal cord blood supply. Results in paralysis, loss of pain and temperature sensation and autonomic dysfunction below the level of the lesion. Vibration sensation and proprioception are preserved due to dorsal column sparing

- **Brown-Séquard syndrome:** hemi-section of the spinal cord (possibly due to inflammatory disease, e.g. multiple sclerosis; compression, e.g. spinal cord tumour; or infection, e.g. tuberculosis) which causes ipsilateral motor weakness, loss of fine touch, proprioception and vibration sensation and contralateral loss of pain and temperature sensation, below the level of the lesion
- **Cauda equina syndrome:** caused by lesions at or below the level of L2. Associated with leg weakness, saddle anaesthesia and autonomic dysfunction (urinary retention is almost always present). This is a neurosurgical emergency – immediate recognition and management may prevent permanent neurological damage
- **Central cord syndrome:** commonly resulting from hyperextension of the neck, typically in elderly patients with cervical spondylosis. Causes weakness and sensory loss, greater in the upper limbs, and autonomic dysfunction (particularly bladder)

Diagnosis

Where a high index of suspicion exists for NTSCI, a targeted history and examination form the basis for prompt diagnosis. Key features to ascertain from the history are the presence of:

- **Risk factors:** history of malignancy, previous radiotherapy, increasing age, corticosteroid use, degenerative conditions (e.g. osteoarthritis, osteoporosis, Paget's disease), intravenous drug use, immunosuppression, nutritional deficiencies (vitamin B12, folate, copper), exposure to toxic substances (organophosphates, nitric oxide), coagulopathies
- **Neurological symptoms:** paraesthesia or loss of sensation, muscle weakness/wasting or paralysis, autonomic dysfunction, altered reflexes, altered tone, claudication, relapsing and remitting symptoms
- **Infective symptoms:** fever, other recent infections
- **Red flag symptoms:** unexplained weight loss, neck or back pain

A thorough neurological examination in accordance with the American Spinal Injury Association (ASIA) Impairment Scale allows the level and completeness of spinal cord injury to be deduced. It is important to remain mindful of the various aetiologies and differential diagnoses which cause NTSCI when conducting a general examination. Certain features may indicate specific pathologies, e.g. signs of sepsis pointing towards an infective process.

Imaging plays a critical role in evaluation of NTSCI, specifically for determining the location and extent of injury. MRI is the imaging modality of choice; it is more sensitive and provides superior images of the spinal cord, spinal ligaments, intervertebral discs and paraspinal soft tissues, when compared to plain CT. Conventional T1- and T2-weighted fast spin-echo images are useful for diagnosis of degenerative disc disease. Gadolinium-enhanced MRI is effective for infectious causes (e.g. epidural abscess, osteomyelitis). CT myelography may be used where MRI is contraindicated. Laboratory studies such as blood tests and cerebrospinal fluid analysis are often non-specific; however, they may aid diagnosis and exclude certain pathologies.

Management

The role of the intensive care physician is to identify NTSCI, implement timely resuscitation, investigate the likely causes and provide supportive management, whilst seeking specialist assessment. Individuals with high thoracic and cervical spine injuries are at risk of cardiovascular and respiratory compromise. Resuscitation for unstable patients is therefore in accordance with the advanced life support (ALS) algorithm using an ABC approach.

Supportive management involves optimisation of physiological parameters, as well as instigation of general principles of intensive care (risk-assessed venous thromboembolism prophylaxis, stress ulcer prophylaxis, ventilator-associated pneumonia prevention, nutritional support, aperients and adequate sedation and analgesia), as described in Chapter 3.13.4, Traumatic Spinal Cord Injuries.

Treatment of the underlying cause of NTSCI should ideally be undertaken in a specialist spinal injury unit. Urgent surgical decompression for progressive neurological deterioration is indicated in intervertebral disc compression (cauda equina syndrome), spinal stenosis, malignant spinal cord compression and epidural abscess or haematoma. Specific treatments include anti-microbial therapy for infectious causes, targeted chemotherapy, radiotherapy and/or corticosteroids for spinal tumours (depending on the type and location) and immunomodulatory drugs and/or corticosteroids for inflammatory or autoimmune diseases (e.g. multiple sclerosis, sarcoidosis, transverse myelitis).

Prognosis

Recovery from NTSCI can be a lengthy process, best managed in a specialist spinal injury centre where optimal rehabilitation facilities are available. Prognosis depends on the level and completeness of neurological injury. Like TSCI, those with higher or complete injuries suffer worse outcomes.

References and Further Reading

Bonner S, Smith C. Initial management of acute spinal cord injury. *Contin Educ Anaesth Crit Care Pain* 2013;**13**:224–31.

New PW, Marshall R. International spinal cord injury data sets for non-traumatic spinal cord injury. *Spinal Cord* 2014;**52**:123–32.

New PW, Reeves RK, Smith E, *et al*. International retrospective comparison of inpatient rehabilitation for patients with spinal cord dysfunction: epidemiology and clinical outcomes. *Arch Phys Med Rehabil* 2015;**96**:1080–7.

van den Berg MEL, Castellote JM, Mahillo-Fernandez I, de Pedro-Cuesta J. Incidence of spinal cord injury worldwide: a systematic review. *Neuroepidemiology* 2010;**34**:184–92.

Gastrointestinal Haemorrhage

3.5.1

Megan Fahy and Liza Keating

Key Learning Points

1. In suspected variceal bleeding, terlipressin and prophylactic antibiotics should be administered at presentation.
2. In upper gastrointestinal bleeding, a restrictive approach to blood transfusion reduces rebleeding rates and mortality.
3. Following a non-variceal upper gastrointestinal bleed in those taking aspirin for secondary prevention of vascular events, aspirin should be restarted when haemostasis is achieved.
4. Haematochezia is caused by an upper gastrointestinal bleed in approximately 10 per cent of presentations.
5. Early initiation of enteral feeding is effective in preventing bleeding from stress ulcer in critically unwell adults.

Keywords: terlipressin, transfusion, variceal bleeding, haematochezia, haemostasis

Upper Gastrointestinal Bleeding

Acute upper gastrointestinal bleeding (UGIB) is a common medical emergency which is associated with a 7 per cent mortality rate in those presenting to hospital, and a 26 per cent mortality rate for those who develop a bleed whilst an inpatient. The principal causes of UGIB are peptic ulceration (26 per cent), oesophagitis (17 per cent), gastritis or gastric erosions (16 per cent), duodenitis (9 per cent), varices (8 per cent), Mallory–Weiss tear (3 per cent), portal hypertensive gastropathy (4 per cent), malignancy (3 per cent) and vascular ectasia (2 per cent), with no cause identified in 12 per cent of cases.

Clinical Presentation

The most common presenting signs of an UGIB are haematemesis (fresh blood or altered blood with a coffee ground appearance), melaena, fresh blood per rectum (if the bleed is particularly brisk) or an unexplained fall in haemoglobin level. A focused patient history should be taken for anticoagulant/anti-platelet medication, non-steroidal anti-inflammatory drug (NSAID) use, alcohol excess or liver disease, weight loss and previous peptic ulcer disease.

Investigations and Management

Immediate management is assessment of haemodynamic stability and resuscitation as appropriate. Airway compromise is possible from either massive haematemesis or a reduced level of consciousness, e.g. in hepatic encephalopathy.

Blood products may be required in resuscitation. In haemodynamically stable patients, a restrictive approach to blood transfusion has been shown in randomised controlled trials to be beneficial over more liberal transfusion practices. A target haemoglobin of 70–90 g/l is associated with lower rebleeding rates, adverse events and mortality at 6 weeks. In variceal bleeds, more liberal transfusion practices may increase portal pressures.

In patients actively bleeding, platelet transfusion is appropriate only in those with platelet counts of $<50 \times 10^9/l$. Fresh frozen plasma (FFP) should be given to those with a prothrombin time or an activated partial thromboplastin time >1.5 times the normal range. If the fibrinogen level is <1.5 g/l, the first-line treatment is FFP, followed by cryoprecipitate. In patients taking warfarin, normalise the international normalised ratio (INR) with prothrombin complex concentrate and vitamin K (phytomenadione). The INR needs to be <2.5 for endoscopy to be performed. The HALT-IT trial on the use of tranexamic acid in gastrointestinal bleeding closed in 2019 and results are eagerly anticipated.

Endoscopy is the investigation of choice in UGIB, as it both provides a diagnosis and allows therapeutic intervention to be delivered. In an unstable patient, endoscopy should be performed immediately following resuscitation, and in stable patients within 24 hours.

Assessment of severity and prediction of clinical outcomes are facilitated using validated scoring systems – the Glasgow–Blatchford score can be used as a triaging tool prior to endoscopy, and the Rockall score is used pre- and post-endoscopy.

Non-variceal Bleeding

For practical purposes, UGIB is divided into variceal and non-variceal bleeds, and there are important differences in their management. In non-variceal bleeds, opinions are divided regarding the use of proton pump inhibitors (PPIs) prior to endoscopy. Concerns exist that they may reduce the stigmata of recent haemorrhage on endoscopy, and thus may mask the need for endoscopic therapy. This, however, has not been shown to increase the risk of rebleeding or mortality. Following endoscopy, if stigmata of current or recent bleeding are identified, a PPI should be initiated. High-risk findings on endoscopy include active bleeding, adherent clot and a non-bleeding visible vessel. Endoscopic treatments aim to provide definitive haemostasis. In those who rebleed following endoscopy, repeat endoscopy or interventional radiology input for CT angiography and transcatheter arterial embolisation are indicated.

Patients requiring aspirin for secondary prophylaxis of vascular disease who develop UGIB should have aspirin restarted as soon as haemostasis is achieved. Randomised controlled trials show this approach reduces all-cause mortality at 8 weeks.

Variceal Bleeding

If a variceal bleed is suspected on presentation, prophylactic antibiotics should be administered. Bacterial infection is strongly associated with a risk of rebleeding and mortality, and a fluoroquinolone or third-generation cephalosporin is recommended. A vasopressin analogue such as terlipressin should also be commenced, and this should be continued either until definitive treatment of the bleeding source or for a total of 5 days. Terlipressin has been shown to produce haemostasis in 75–80 per cent of variceal bleeds by reducing portal pressures. Contraindications to its use include vascular disease, QT prolongation, heart failure and hyponatraemia.

At endoscopy, oesophageal varices are most successfully treated with band ligation, whilst in gastric varices, injection of cyanoacrylate is advised. In oesophageal and some gastric varices, balloon tamponade with devices such as a Sengstaken–Blakemore tube is an option if initial strategies are unsuccessful. Patients are likely to need admission to the ICU for sedation whilst the device is *in situ*, and rebleeding rates are high following balloon deflation. If these methods fail, insertion of a transjugular intrahepatic portosystemic shunt (TIPSS) should be considered.

Acute Severe Lower Gastrointestinal Bleeding

Up to 10 per cent of patients who present with haematochezia (passage of fresh red blood per rectum) have a UGIB source, and if suspected, an endoscopy should be the first-line investigation. Lower gastrointestinal causes include diverticular disease, ischaemic bowel, complications of inflammatory bowel disease, malignancy, angiodysplasia and rarely aorto-enteric fistula. Spontaneous resolution of haemorrhage can be expected in 80–85 per cent of cases, and outcomes are considered more favourable than in UGIB. However, much depends on patient co-morbidities.

In a presumed lower gastrointestinal bleed, the first-line investigation is CT angiography, followed by embolisation if active bleeding is detected. Embolisation has up to a 90 per cent success rate. If active bleeding is not detected, a prepared colonoscopy should be performed, with the aim of definitive endoscopic haemostasis. Surgical input is appropriate in the event of failure of the above interventions or in the instance of rebleeding. If the bleeding source has not been identified, examination of the small bowel should be considered.

Prevention of Upper Gastrointestinal Bleeding in Critical Care

The proportion of intensive care admissions experiencing a significant gastrointestinal bleed related to stress ulceration is estimated to be 1.5–8.5 per cent.

Gastric and oesophageal stress ulceration results from an imbalance between gastric acid secretion and maintenance of the protective mucosal barrier. Reduced mucosal protection is likely multifactorial, with poor gut perfusion often contributing. Significant risk factors for developing stress ulceration and bleeding include previous peptic ulcer disease, mechanical ventilation for >48 hours, absence of enteral feeding, chronic liver disease and coagulopathy. Minor risk factors include renal failure, glucocorticoid therapy and anti-platelet medication.

Medications that have been shown to be effective in reducing stress ulcer development and bleeding are PPIs and histamine-2 receptor blockers (H2RBs). Both, however, have been associated with increased rates of nosocomial pneumonia in the critically ill patient. The recent PEPTIC randomised controlled trial directly compared the use of PPI versus H2RBs for stress ulcer prophylaxis in mechanically ventilated patients and identified no statistically significant difference in mortality between the treatment groups.

Enteral feeding when initiated early is effective in preventing stress ulcer bleeding, and patients who are mechanically ventilated and enterally fed are unlikely to benefit from prophylaxis in the absence of other risk factors. Stress ulcer prophylaxis medication is beneficial in reducing gastrointestinal bleeding for patients with significant risk factors. For those without risk factors, the benefit of prophylaxis is not proven. Also, this reduction of gastrointestinal bleeding has not been shown by a recent meta-analysis to lead to a reduced length of ICU stay or mortality.

References and Further Reading

Gralnek I, Dumonceau JM, Kuipers E, *et al*. Diagnosis and management of nonvariceal upper gastrointestinal haemorrhage: European Society of Gastrointestinal Endoscopy (ESGE) Guidelines. *Endoscopy* 2015;**47**:1–46.

National Institute for Health and Care Excellence. 2012. Acute upper gastrointestinal bleeding in over 16s: management. Clinical guideline [CG141]. www.nice.org.uk/guidance/cg141

Osman D, Djibre M, Da Silva D, Goulenok C. Management by the intensivist of gastrointestinal bleeding in adults and children. *Ann Intensive Care* 2012;**2**:46.

PEPTIC Investigators for the Australian and New Zealand Intensive Care Society Clinical Trials Group, Alberta Health Services Critical Care Strategic Clinical Network, the Irish Critical Care Trials Group; Young PJ, Bagshaw SM, Forbes AB, *et al*. Effect of stress ulcer prophylaxis with proton pump inhibitors vs histamine-2 receptor blockers on in-hospital mortality among ICU patients receiving invasive mechanical ventilation: the PEPTIC randomized clinical trial. *JAMA* 2020;**323**:616–26.

Siau K, Chapman W, Sharma N, *et al*. Management of acute upper gastrointestinal bleeding: an update for the general physician. *J R Coll Physicians Edinb* 2017;**47**:218–30.

Tripathi D, Stanley AJ, Hayes PC, *et al*. UK guidelines on the management of variceal haemorrhage in cirrhotic patients. *Gut* 2015;**64**:1680–704.

Wang Y, Ye Z, Ge L, *et al*. Efficacy and safety of gastrointestinal bleeding prophylaxis in critically ill patients: systematic review and network meta-analysis. *BMJ* 2019;**367**:l16744.

3.5.2

Acute Pancreatitis

Mike Peters and Liza Keating

Key Learning Points

1. Diagnosis requires two of the following criteria: abdominal pain consistent with acute pancreatitis, serum amylase/lipase over three times the reference range or findings suggestive of acute pancreatitis on cross-sectional imaging.
2. Severe acute pancreatitis is characterised by organ failure persisting for over 48 hours, and carries a mortality risk of 15–20 per cent.
3. Management is predominantly supportive. Operative intervention has a role only in the later stages of the disease.
4. Prophylactic antibiotics are not recommended; however, they may be indicated in the event of a secondary infection.
5. Enteral nutrition can be given via nasogastric or nasojejunal routes, and is preferred to parenteral nutrition.

Keywords: pancreatitis, multi-organ failure, necrotising, surgery

Introduction

Acute pancreatitis is an inflammatory condition of the pancreas which causes severe abdominal pain and an elevation of serum levels of pancreatic enzymes. As a clinical entity, it ranges from a mild, self-limiting disease, with minimal sequelae, to massive pancreatic necrosis associated with multi-organ failure and a mortality rate of up to 20 per cent.

Aetiology and Pathogenesis

Gallstones are the most common cause of acute pancreatitis (40 per cent), followed by alcohol (30 per cent) and hypertriglyceridaemia (2–5 per cent). Less common causes include drugs, infection, autoimmune disease, injury during endoscopic retrograde cholangiopancreatography (ERCP) and trauma. In the case of alcohol, prolonged use (4–5 drinks daily for at least 5 years) is required to cause pancreatitis, and the presentation with acute pancreatitis in this context may be an acute flare of underlying chronic disease. Multiple drugs (azathioprine, 6-mercaptopurine, valproate, angiotensin-converting enzyme (ACE) inhibitors, mesalazine) have been implicated, but it may be difficult to determine if a drug is responsible in individual cases. Drug-induced pancreatitis is usually mild.

The exact pathophysiology of acute pancreatitis remains incompletely understood. The initial mechanism of pancreatic injury depends on the cause, but a similar progression is thought to occur in all cases. Active pancreatic enzymes are released into the duct system, causing auto-digestion and injury to the pancreas and surrounding tissue. Micro-circulatory changes, and possibly ischaemia–reperfusion injury, lead to altered vascular permeability and localised oedema. In severe cases, systemic inflammatory response is thought to be initiated by both activated pancreatic enzymes (trypsin, elastase, phospholipase) and pro-inflammatory cytokines (tumour necrosis factor (TNF) alpha, platelet-activating factor), which are released into the peripheral circulation following the initial insult. In 15–20 per cent of cases, gland necrosis occurs, resulting in necrotic fluid collections which eventually become walled off and are at risk of secondary infection in the subacute phase of the illness. Inflammatory changes may result in compromise of gut wall integrity, and this lends itself to an increased risk of bacterial translocation and secondary infection.

Clinical Presentation, Investigation and Diagnosis

Presentation is typically with acute, severe epigastric pain, accompanied by nausea and vomiting that persists for several hours. Classical signs such as

Grey-Turner's (bruising of the flanks) and Cullen's (superficial oedema and bruising in the subcutaneous fatty tissue around the umbilicus) signs occur in severe disease and are rare, but patients may have pyrexia, tachypnoea, tachycardia and hypotension, in keeping with a massive systemic inflammatory response.

Serum amylase rises within 6–12 hours of onset of pancreatitis and falls within 3–5 days. Serum lipase rises within 4–8 hours and falls within 8–14 days. Lipase may therefore be more useful in patients presenting several days after the initial onset of symptoms. Levels are useful in diagnosis, but neither marker is a useful predictor of severity or prognosis.

Ultrasound imaging should be considered early to assess for the presence of gallstones in the common bile duct, as this may be an indication for early ERCP. CT imaging at presentation provides little information, unless the diagnosis is in question; however, a CT scan later in the disease course may be useful to guide management of complications.

The 2012 Revised Atlanta consensus on the definition and classification of acute pancreatitis stipulates that diagnosis requires two of the following features:

- Abdominal pain consistent with acute pancreatitis (severe, epigastric, may radiate to the back)
- Elevation of serum amylase or lipase activity of at least three times the normal limit
- Characteristic findings of acute pancreatitis on contrast CT, MRI or transabdominal ultrasonography

It divides pancreatitis into two broad categories:

- Acute interstitial pancreatitis: acute inflammation of the pancreas and peri-pancreatic parenchyma without necrosis (80–85 per cent)
- Acute necrotising pancreatitis: inflammation with pancreatic parenchymal or peri-pancreatic necrosis (15–20 per cent)

It also suggests classification of severity according to the following:

- Mild pancreatitis: no local complications or organ failure. Usually resolves within a week
- Moderately severe acute pancreatitis: transient organ failure (lasting <48 hours) and/or local complications
- Severe acute pancreatitis: persistent organ failure (lasting >48 hours)

The above classification provides useful standardised definitions but is not suitable for prospective risk stratification. Multiple scoring systems have been developed for this purpose, incorporating a variety of clinical, laboratory and radiological parameters. These include the Glasgow score, the Ranson Criteria, the Harmless Acute Pancreatitis Score (HAPS), the Bedside Index for Severity in Acute Pancreatitis (BISAP) and the Balthazar CT severity index. None of these, however, has a high specificity for predicting acute pancreatitis in the individual patient, but they may have a role in triggering early consideration for escalation of care.

Specific clinical features which tend to correlate with severity include advanced age, level of co-morbidity, a rising urea or haematocrit at 48 hours and persistence of systemic inflammatory response syndrome (SIRS) features after initial resuscitation.

Management

Management focuses on supportive care in the early phases. Aggressive fluid resuscitation with a balanced crystalloid (5–10 ml/(kg hr)) has previously been advocated in the first 12–24 hours, although there is a paucity of trial evidence in this area. The aim is to restore intravascular volume, which is normally low due to excessive third space fluid loss, but the risk of fluid overload resulting from over-resuscitation should also be considered. Early referral to the ICU for inotropes should be considered.

Patients with pancreatitis severe enough to warrant ICU admission are likely to require nutritional support. Evidence shows enteral nutrition is safer and more effective than parenteral nutrition. Randomised trials and meta-analyses have also shown that nasogastric or nasoduodenal feeding is clinically equivalent to nasojejunal feeding. Parenteral nutrition should be used in cases where enteral feeding is not tolerated. Current guidance from several international working groups advises early initiation of enteral feeding (within 24–48 hours) to preserve gut integrity and reduce the risk of bacterial translocation.

Multiple trials and meta-analyses have shown no benefit of prophylactic antibiotics in acute pancreatitis. Antibiotics may be indicated later in the disease course if infection of a necrotic collection is suspected.

Early ERPC should be performed in cases of pancreatitis with concurrent cholangitis, and considered where there is common bile duct obstruction on imaging.

Management of Complications

Acute peri-pancreatic fluid collections should not be drained. Walled-off collections occurring in the weeks following the initial event are at risk of secondary infection. If this occurs, invasive intervention should be delayed, if possible, to allow the collection to become fully demarcated (usually at least 4 weeks). Minimally invasive debridement techniques (e.g. endoscopy, laparoscopy) are usually preferred to open necrosectomy. Patients with extensive necrosis or other complications should be referred to a specialist unit.

Patients with severe pancreatitis are at risk of abdominal compartment syndrome, and this diagnosis should be considered in the event of new, or worsening, organ failure.

References and Further Reading

Banks PA, Bollen TL, Dervenis C, *et al*. Classification of acute pancreatitis–2012: revision of the Atlanta classification and definitions by international consensus. *Gut* 2013;**62**:102.

Forsmark C, Vege SS, Wilcox CM. Acute pancreatitis. *N Engl J Med* 2016;**375**:1972–81.

Meier R, Ockenga J, Pertkiewicz M, *et al*. ESPEN Guidelines on enteral nutrition: pancreas. *Clin Nutr* 2006;**25**:275–84.

Mirtallo JM, Forbes A, McClave SA, *et al*. International consensus guidelines for nutrition therapy in pancreatitis. *JPEN J Parenter Enteral Nutr* 2012;**36**:284–91.

Sah R, Dawra RK, Saluja AK. New insights into the pathogenesis of pancreatitis. *Curr Opin Gastroenterol* 2013;**29**:523–30.

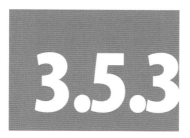

Peritonitis and the Acute Abdomen

Shona Johnson and Liza Keating

Key Learning Points

1. The acute abdomen requires prompt diagnosis and management to improve patient outcomes.
2. In the critically ill adult, causes of an acute abdomen can be broadly divided into mechanical, inflammatory and vascular.
3. Peritonitis is due to infection in most cases. It may be generalised or localised, and is further divided into primary, secondary and tertiary infection.
4. Acute mesenteric ischaemia is an uncommon vascular cause of the acute abdomen but is associated with high mortality.
5. Radiological findings are useful, although the diagnosis is mainly clinical.

Keywords: acute abdomen, peritonitis, intra-abdominal infection, acute mesenteric ischaemia

Introduction

The 'acute abdomen' refers to the rapid onset of symptoms requiring urgent surgical intervention. The underlying pathology needs prompt diagnosis and management, as frequently it has a steadily worsening prognosis. Pain is the predominant feature for the majority of patients; however, a pain-free acute abdomen can occur in the elderly, the immunocompromised, children and pregnant women. Causes of an acute abdomen in the critically ill adult can be broadly divided into inflammatory, vascular and mechanical.

Causes

Inflammatory

Peritonitis

The peritoneum is normally a sterile environment. Peritonitis is inflammation of the serosal lining of the abdominal wall and viscera. It occurs in response to an inflammatory pathological stimulus causing an infectious or sterile peritonitis, depending on the underlying cause.

Bacterial invasion may occur in four ways:

1. Introduced: during laparotomy or in a penetrating wound
2. From intra-abdominal viscera:

a. Gangrene, i.e. acute appendicitis
b. Perforation, i.e. perforated duodenal ulcer
c. Iatrogenic, i.e. anastomotic leak

3. Haematogenous spread
4. Direct spread from the female genital tract

Intra-abdominal infections may be further classified as either localised or generalised. Furthermore, they can be divided into primary, secondary or tertiary:

- **Primary:** spontaneous bacterial peritonitis (SBP) is defined as an infection of ascitic fluid without an obvious surgically treatable source. In adults, it almost always occurs in those with cirrhosis and ascites, and usually a single organism is responsible. Early initiation of appropriate anti-microbials is associated with improved outcomes. In one retrospective study of patients with SBP who developed septic shock, mortality was 82 per cent and the adjusted odds ratio for mortality was 1.9 for every hour delay in administering anti-microbials.

- **Secondary:** a localised or generalised process in a visceral organ that may be further divided by their management into:
  - *Operative:* intestinal perforation, biliary obstruction, appendicitis, refractory inflammatory bowel disease, diverticulitis
  - *Supportive:* pancreatitis, infectious colitis, hepatic abscess
- **Tertiary:** persistent or recurrent infection despite initial treatment, e.g. formation of a post-operative collection. This is more common in immunocompromised patients.

Perforation

Peritoneal contamination of faecal fluid will result in intra-abdominal sepsis. Contamination by gastric contents and bile is more likely to cause chemical peritonitis, although it can be complicated by secondary bacterial infection. Consequently, upper gastrointestinal (GI) events (stomach and duodenum) have lower morbidity and mortality than lower GI events.

Vascular

Ischaemia

Mesenteric ischaemia is an uncommon, but life-threatening, condition in which splanchnic hypo-perfusion leads to inflammation and eventually bowel necrosis. The onset can be acute or chronic. Acute mesenteric ischaemia (AMI) is arterial or venous in aetiology. The underlying process may be thrombotic or non-occlusive, with the extent of bowel damage proportional to the decrease in blood flow.

1. **Arterial embolism:** make up to 50 per cent of acute ischaemic conditions. The superior mesenteric artery is most susceptible due to its higher flow and acute angle at the aorta. Typical causes of emboli include mural thrombi following acute myocardial infarction, thrombi from atrial fibrillation or septic emboli from endocarditis.
2. **Arterial thrombus:** typically occurs at the origin of the mesenteric arteries, causing extensive infarcts. Usually a complication of pre-existing atherosclerotic disease, in which an acute decrease of the already compromised blood flow occurs.
3. **Venous thrombosis:** these make up approximately 10 per cent of cases of AMI. Local factors (e.g. pancreatitis) are associated with large-vessel thrombosis with systemic hypercoagulable states,

leading to thrombus in smaller vessels. Superior mesenteric venous occlusion occurs at the ileum in the majority of cases.

4. **Non-occlusive mesenteric ischaemia (NOMI):** usually a result of severe and prolonged visceral vasoconstriction – this can occur with all forms of shock. It may also arise as a result of raised intra-abdominal pressure caused by tumours, or abdominal compartment syndrome.

Haemorrhage

Blood is an irritant to the peritoneum and will produce an acute abdomen, e.g. in the context of a leaking aortic aneurysm. GI bleeding will be discussed elsewhere.

Clinical Features

The underlying pathology may have definite clinical features, e.g. migratory right iliac fossa pain in appendicitis. The patient will usually lie very still. The classical signs of peritonitis are: rigid 'washboard' abdomen, involuntary guarding, percussion and rebound tenderness.

Other signs include fever, tachycardia, hypotension and abnormal or absent bowel sounds suggesting ileus or obstruction.

Investigations

Laboratory tests are often non-specific, but the following can be used to support clinical findings:

- Full blood count: leucocytosis is often present
- Urea and electrolytes: hypochloraemia and hypokalaemia occur late in obstruction, elevated glucose in pancreatitis
- Liver function tests: high amylase, often indicative of pancreatitis
- Clotting: may indicate sepsis-related disseminated intravascular coagulation or hypercoagulable state in AMI
- Venous blood gas: metabolic acidosis is common, but non-specific in AMI

Imaging views will be guided by suspected pathology:

- Plain X-ray is of some benefit in intra-peritoneal perforation: subdiaphragmatic free air may be seen on an erect chest X-ray, and a ruptured oesophagus may result in pneumomediastinum
- Ultrasound is useful if venous thrombosis is suspected or paracentesis required

- CT abdomen is useful in evaluating many causes of the acute abdomen; however, it is important to remember that imaging will delay time to laparotomy
- CT angiography may be used to assess occlusive disease in AMI; however, CT findings are non-specific in NOMI

Prompt surgical assessment of the ICU patient is advised, owing to difficulties in diagnosing acute abdominal issues in the unconscious and ventilated patient.

Management

General principles of treatment are:
- Source control:
  - Conservative: removal of indwelling catheters or CT-guided drain of localised abscesses in sepsis
  - Operative: laparotomy to repair a perforation or resect infarcted bowel
  - Laparostomy in cases of intra-abdominal sepsis causing abdominal compartment syndrome
- Systemic antibiotics in peritonitis
- Supportive therapy: fluid and electrolyte replacement, blood products or inotropes

- Pain relief
- Gastric decompression with nasogastric tube to reduce risk of aspiration

References and Further Reading

Doherty GM. The acute abdomen. MS Loeb, K Davis (eds). *Current Diagnosis and Treatment: Surgery*, 13th edn. New York, NY: McGraw-Hill; 2010. pp. 451–63.

Ellis H, Calne R, Watson C. Peritonitis. In: H Ellis, R Calne, C Watson (eds). *Lecture Notes: General Surgery*, 11th edn. Malden, MA: Blackwell Publishing; 2006. pp. 231–6.

Karvellas CJ, Abraldes JG, Arabi YM, *et al.*; Cooperative Antimicrobial Therapy of Septic Shock (CATSS) Database Research Group. Appropriate and timely antimicrobial therapy in cirrhotic patients with spontaneous bacterial peritonitis-associated septic shock: a retrospective cohort study. *Aliment Pharmacol Ther* 2015;**41**:747–57.

Mastoraki A, Mastoraki S, Tziava E, *et al.* Mesenteric ischemia: pathogenesis and challenging diagnostic and therapeutic modalities. *World J Gastrointest Pathophysiol* 2016;**7**:125–30.

Strachan S, Soni N. Intra-abdominal sepsis. In: C Waldmann, N Soni, A Rhodes (eds). *Oxford Desk Reference: Critical Care*. New York, NY: Oxford University Press; 2008. p. 336.

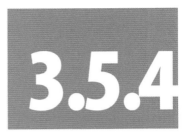

Ileus and Bowel Obstruction

Charles Rich and Liza Keating

Key Learning Points

1. Ileus is the absence of bowel motility and is common in intensive care patients.
2. Ensure early surgical input to all cases of mechanical bowel obstruction.
3. In adults, large bowel obstruction is most commonly caused by cancer.
4. Resuscitation and correction of electrolyte disturbance are required in all cases.
5. Untreated bowel obstruction leads to dilation and increases the risks of perforation and ischaemia.

Keywords: ileus, bowel obstruction, paralytic ileus

Introduction

Bowel obstruction is a common indication for emergency laparotomy. Over 3 million cases of bowel obstruction are diagnosed globally each year, with >10 per cent mortality. This condition affects males and females equally and can occur at any age.

Adhesions are implicated in up to 80 per cent of all cases of small bowel obstruction (SBO). Therefore, it is far more common in patients who have previously had abdominal surgery. Most cases of large bowel obstruction (LBO) are due to colonic malignancy, and it is often the first presentation of the disease. Causes of bowel obstruction can be overall classed as intrinsic (e.g. Crohn's disease, cancer, vascular causes, intussusception, volvulus, diverticulosis), extrinsic (e.g. adhesions, hernias, endometriosis, abscess) or intraluminal (e.g. faeces, bezoar, foreign body). SBO accounts for 80 per cent of cases of mechanical bowel obstruction.

Paralytic ileus is common in intensive care patients and constipation is related to longer stays in the ICU and worse outcomes. Enteric neuropathy associated with critical illness and major surgery affects the peristaltic propulsion of intestinal contents through the digestive tract and results in colonic dilation (Ogilvie's syndrome) and failure to pass flatus or faeces. This condition is commonly exacerbated by drugs that slow intestinal motility such as opiates.

Symptoms and Signs

Abdominal pain and tenderness, abdominal distension and intolerance of enteral feeding are common features of both mechanical and functional intestinal obstructions. Vomiting is an earlier and more prominent feature of SBO, whereas constipation is an earlier and more prominent feature of LBO. The distended abdomen can cause diaphragmatic splinting, with subsequent ventilatory compromise. Excessive vomiting risks dehydration and electrolyte depletion. Prolonged or severe obstruction risks ischaemia and perforation if untreated. Spasmodic cramps caused by SBO are often felt in the peri-umbilical region and typically last a few minutes. LBO typically causes longer spasms of pain felt lower down in the abdomen. Mechanical bowel obstruction is associated with high-pitched, 'tinkling' bowel sounds on auscultation, whereas patients with ileus will often have absent bowel sounds.

Diagnosis

Diagnosis is made on plain abdominal X-ray (AXR) in 50–60 per cent of cases. Radiographic signs include >5 fluid levels on erect AXR or dilated loops of bowel. Small bowel diameter of >3.5 cm or large bowel diameter of >5 cm are usually pathological. Ultrasound can be useful where dilated loops of the small bowel are filled with fluid; however, most adhesional obstruction features gas-filled loops which will rarely allow the sonographic diagnosis of SBO. CT is a commonly used modality that has a high sensitivity for high-grade SBO, and confers detail about the location, extent, type and cause of obstruction. CT is diagnostic of SBO where small bowel loops proximal to a transition point have a diameter of >2.5 cm and normal or reduced diameter distal to the transition point.

Where radiological diagnosis of SBO remains equivocal, contrast follow-through or enemas, enteroclysis or CT enteroclysis can provide more detailed images of the extent and location of the obstruction. When imaging is performed 3 hours after the administration of an enteral contrast agent, obstruction is considered total if no contrast is seen past the transition point, high-grade if movement of contrast is delayed and low-grade if passage of contrast is sufficient. The difference in calibre between the diameter of the bowel proximal and distal to the transition point is also helpful in differentiating whether obstruction is high-grade or low-grade. Closed-loop obstructions, where a bowel loop is occluded at two points along its length, have a higher rate of strangulation leading to ischaemia and carry higher mortality.

Management

Conservative management involves intestinal decompression via a nasogastric tube, reduction in enteral feeding (now preferred to complete cessation of feeding), intravenous fluids, electrolyte replacement (particularly potassium and magnesium), anti-emetics and analgesia. All potentially causative contributory drugs must be stopped where possible, and underlying causes otherwise addressed. Parenteral nutrition may be required to maintain calorie intake during episodes of significant enteral failure. Where conservative approaches are taken, serial examination and X-ray ensure that critical deterioration is detected early and appropriate management can be instituted.

Motility stimulants, such as metoclopramide and erythromycin, as well as peripherally acting μ-opiate receptor antagonists, are helpful in cases of ileus, and neostigmine or colonoscopy can be used to help acutely decompress the colon.

Surgery is needed to treat or prevent sepsis, ischaemia or intestinal perforation in cases of mechanical obstruction, and where spontaneous resolution of the underlying cause is unlikely. It may also be needed in cases of ileus in the context of abdominal compartment syndrome.

References and Further Reading

Bauer A, Schwarz NT, Moore B, Türler A, Kalff JC. Ileus in critical illness: mechanisms and management. *Curr Opin Crit Care* 2002;**8**;152–7.

Garden OJ, Parks RW. *Principles and Practice of Surgery*, 7th edn. Edinburgh: Elsevier; 2018.

Martindale RG, McClave SA, Vanek VW, *et al.*; American College of Critical Care Medicine; ASPEN Board of Directors. 2009 Guidelines for the provision and assessment of nutrition support therapy in the adult critically ill patient: Society of Critical Care Medicine and American Society for Parenteral and Enteral Nutrition: executive summary. *Crit Care Med* 2009;**37**:1757–61.

Paulson EK, Thompson WM. Review of small-bowel obstruction: the diagnosis and when to worry. *Radiology* 2015;**275**;332–42.

Stevens P, Dark P. Ileus and obstruction in the critically ill. In: A Webb, D Angus, S Finfer, L Gattinoni, M Singer (eds). *Oxford Textbook of Critical Care*, 2nd edn. Oxford: Oxford University Press; 2016. pp. 856–9.

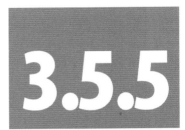

3.5.5 Intra-abdominal Hypertension and Abdominal Compartment Syndrome

Dominic Moor, Katie Wimble and Ravi Kumar

Key Learning Points

1. Although intra-abdominal hypertension and abdominal compartment syndrome (ACS) form part of a scale in clinical practice, they are different entities as the former may be chronic, but the latter involves acute organ failure.
2. The prevalence of ACS in the intensive care unit has been reported as 8.2 per cent, with a higher prevalence in medical patients (10.5 per cent), compared to the surgical cohort (5 per cent).
3. Palpation of the abdomen is highly unreliable as a method of detection.
4. A standardised measurement protocol is important to avoid significant inter-individual variability.
5. Management of these syndromes should be protocol-based and multi-modal.

Keywords: intra-abdominal hypertension, abdominal compartment syndrome, pressure, WSACS

Definitions

The World Society of the Abdominal Compartment Syndrome (WSACS) has set out clear definitions.

- Intra-abdominal hypertension (IAH) is defined as a measured intra-abdominal pressure in excess of 12 mmHg.
- Abdominal compartment syndrome (ACS) is a distinct entity that should not be thought of as being synonymous with IAH. It is defined as an intra-abdominal pressure (IAP) of >20 mmHg, with signs of new organ dysfunction or failure.

In clinical practice, both IAH and ACS form part of a scale. Raised IAP by itself may be a chronic state, e.g.

Table 3.5.5.1 Grades of raised intra-abdominal pressure

Grade	Intra-abdominal pressure (mmHg)
I	12–15
II	16–20
III	21–25
IV	>25

in the morbidly obese or in those with various types of chronic abdominal pathology. ACS, however, is by definition an acute condition. For research purposes, a classification exists that grades raised IAP (Table 3.5.5.1).

Risk Factors

IAH has a prevalence of up to 50 per cent in the intensive care environment. Perhaps surprisingly, ACS is actually more common in the medical, rather than surgical, population in the ICU. This may, in part, be due to the higher threshold for measuring IAP in the medical population, and therefore, the pathology has progressed to an advanced stage by the time the possibility is considered. A single cause is often hard to ascertain. However, risk factors can be thought of in the following categories:

1. Increased intraluminal contents:
   a. Bowel obstruction
   b. Ileus
2. Increased intra-abdominal contents:
   a. Haemoperitoneum/pneumoperitoneum
   b. Ascites
   c. Abdominal collections
3. Reduced abdominal wall compliance:
   a. Mechanical ventilation
   b. Recent abdominal surgery
   c. Trauma/burns
   d. Body mass index >30 kg/m^2

4. Capillary leak and oedema:
   a. Sepsis
   b. Non-infective inflammatory response (e.g. burns, trauma, pancreatitis)
   c. Large-volume blood or fluid resuscitation

There is also a considerable secondary wind-up effect from impaired perfusion, whereby free radical formation and subsequent capillary leak, oedema and gut translocation amplify impending organ failure.

Measurement of Intra-abdominal Pressure

Whilst many different techniques have been evaluated for the measurement of IAP, including intra-gastric and inferior vena cava (IVC) pressure monitoring, the WSACS recommends the use of a modified Kron technique using urinary bladder pressure measurement. This technique has shown the least variability amongst users. Importantly, palpation of the abdomen has only been shown to have a 50 per cent rate of successful detection of IAH.

Modified Kron Technique for Measurement of Intra-abdominal Pressure

This is achieved by instilling up to 25 ml of saline into the bladder, clamping the catheter tubing and waiting 1 minute to account for detrusor muscle resistance. The patient should be supine and the abdominal muscles should be relaxed, although paralysis is not mandatory. Measurement should be taken at the end of expiration, with the transducer at the level of the mid-axillary line. Pressure should be measured within the lumen of the urinary catheter, with either a specially intended measurement device or a needle connected to a transducer that is inserted into a side port of the clamped catheter.

Limitations of measurement techniques include:
- Equipment failure
- Abdominal muscle contraction
- Bladder pathology (e.g. neuropathic bladder)
- Urinary catheter obstruction

Clinical Impact

Clearly, the impact of pathologically raised IAP is potentially devastating on several different organ systems.

Abdominal Organs

Raised pressure may impact the abdominal viscera in a number of different ways:
- Impaired arterial perfusion: the concept of abdominal perfusion pressure (= mean arterial pressure – IAP) is broadly analogous to that of cerebral perfusion pressure, albeit without the constraints of the rigid cranial vault
- Impaired venous drainage: either through direct venous compression or through the subsequent effect of venous stasis on the incidence of thromboembolic complications
- Impaired biliary drainage and reduced gut transit time

Clearly, all abdominal organs, both visceral and retroperitoneal organs, can be affected. However, evidence suggests that hepatic and renal perfusion are compromised before that of the gut – which, in turn, seems to be affected prior to a significant reduction in cardiac output.

Extra-abdominal Organ Systems

- Respiratory: impaired diaphragmatic excursion, with increased work of breathing and reduced tidal volumes
- Cardiovascular: impaired IVC flow reduces the appearance of an intravascularly depleted state
- Neurological: in patients with compromised cerebral perfusion, there is evidence to suggest that raised IAPs can cause deleterious secondary effects on intracranial pressure (ICP). Some centres employ rescue decompressive laparotomy as a mode of treatment for raised ICP
- Lower limbs: venous return is compromised, and in a subsection of patients, there may also be a significant impact on arterial perfusion

Treatment

Treatment of ACS may be thought of in five domains:

1. Reducing intraluminal contents:
   a. This includes evacuation of the gastrointestinal tract with use of gastric tubes, rectal tubes, laxatives/prokinetics, enemas and endoscopic decompression, as well as limiting or discontinuing enteral nutrition

2. Evacuation of intra-abdominal space-occupying lesions:

   a. CT- or ultrasound-based surveys of the abdomen and pelvis allow identification of collections or masses that may be removed. This is increasingly being achieved using interventional radiology; however, open surgical intervention continues to be a last resort

3. Optimising abdominal wall compliance:

   a. Consider intubation and ventilation; optimise sedation and analgesia; consider abdominal escharotomy in burns patients; consider reverse Trendelenburg position, and as a last resort, neuromuscular blockade may be appropriate

4. Optimise fluid status:

   a. Avoid excessive fluid resuscitation: set daily neutral to negative fluid balance targets, using judicious diuresis where possible. Consider renal replacement therapy

5. Optimise systemic/regional perfusion:

   a. Goal-directed haemodynamic optimisation

Prognosis/Outcomes

Evidence suggests there is increased mortality associated with raised IAP in both the medical and surgical ICU populations. However, given the huge number of risk factors, heterogeneity of patients and the difficulty involved with screening patients, effective studies are difficult to run.

More reliable evidence exists in the surgical population, with studies reporting improved mortality in abdominal hypertension after damage control laparotomy of patients with the abdomen initially left open versus patients who underwent primary closure (10 per cent versus 39 per cent, respectively).

References and Further Reading

Berry N, Fletcher S. Abdominal compartment syndrome. *Contin Educ Anaesth Crit Care Pain* 2012;**12**:110–17.

Hunt L, Frost SA, Hillman K, Newton PJ, Davidson PM. Management of intra-abdominal hypertension and abdominal compartment syndrome: a review. *J Trauma Manag Outcomes* 2014;**8**:2.

Kirkpatrick AW, Roberts DJ, De Waele J, *et al*. Intra-abdominal hypertension and the abdominal compartment syndrome: updated consensus definitions and clinical practice guidelines from the World Society of the Abdominal Compartment Syndrome. *Intensive Care Med* 2013;**39**:1190–206.

Santa-Teresa P, Muñoz J, Montero I, *et al*. Incidence and prognosis of intra-abdominal hypertension in critically ill medical patients: a prospective epidemiological study. *Ann Intensive Care* 2012;**2**:S3.

3.6.1 Pulmonary Embolism

Benjamin Post

Key Learning Points

1. The critical care population is at high risk of venous thromboembolism.
2. Classification of pulmonary embolism is based on mortality risk.
3. The clinical presentation of pulmonary embolism in the critical care environment is atypical and diagnosis remains difficult.
4. Computed tomography pulmonary angiography is the investigation of choice for pulmonary embolism.
5. Anticoagulation is the mainstay of acute treatment, with thrombolysis being reserved for high-risk pulmonary embolism.

Keywords: pulmonary embolism, PE, venous thromboembolism, VTE, deep vein thrombosis, DVT

Definition

Pulmonary embolism (PE) occurs when a thrombus forms in the venous system (deep vein thrombosis (DVT)) or the right heart, and travels to the pulmonary arterial system, resulting in obstruction. Venous thromboembolism (VTE) collectively refers to both PE and DVT. This may occur in association with a known risk factor – *provoked* – or in the absence of any observed risk factors – *unprovoked*.

Epidemiology

The annual incidence of PE in the general population is approximately 0.21–0.31 per 1000. The intensive care population is at high risk of DVT, with rates of 22–80 per cent, with PE being identified in 1.9 per cent of patients. Mortality is variable but may exceed 50 per cent when circulatory shock is present.

Aetiology

Virchow's triad describes the conditions required for thrombus to form in the venous system: venous stasis, trauma and hypercoagulability. Risk factors for VTE are shown in Table 3.6.1.1.

Classification

Classification is based on 30-day mortality risk:

- High (>15 per cent mortality): shock or hypotension present

Table 3.6.1.1 Risk factors for venous thromboembolism

Acquired hypercoagulable states
• Surgery
• Trauma
• Immobility (>5 days)
• Catheters/foreign bodies in the venous system
• Burns
• Recent myocardial infarction
• Sepsis
• Recent blood transfusion
• Malignancy
• Pregnancy
• Obesity
• Chronic obstructive pulmonary disease
• Smoking
• Oestrogen-containing oral contraceptive and hormone replacement therapy
• Limb paralysis
• Heart failure
• Recent air travel
Primary and non-modifiable risk factors
• Increasing age
• History or family history of venous thromboembolism
• History of spontaneous abortion/miscarriage
• Anti-thrombin III deficiency
• Protein C deficiency
• Prothrombin gene mutation
• Protein S deficiency
• Factor V Leiden mutation
• Hyperhomocysteinaemia and Behçet's disease
• Lupus anticoagulant (anti-phospholipid antibody)

- Intermediate to high: signs of right ventricular (RV) dysfunction *and* biochemical evidence of myocardial injury
- Intermediate to low: signs of RV dysfunction *or* biochemical evidence of myocardial injury
- Low (<1 per cent mortality): none of the above present

Presentation and Diagnosis

PE has a broad range of clinical presentations and requires a high level of clinical suspicion. The most common presenting symptoms are non-specific: dyspnoea, chest pain and cough. Diagnosis in the intensive care unit is challenging as patients may not communicate symptoms and investigations are confounded by concomitant pathological processes.

The use of scoring systems can aid the diagnosis of PE. The Wells score and the Revised Geneva Score both assign 'points' to salient features from the clinical history (e.g. previous PE or DVT, recent surgery or immobilisation, active cancer) and physical examination (heart rate, clinical signs of DVT) to determine a *low* (10 per cent), *intermediate* (30 per cent) or *high* (65 per cent) probability of PE.

Investigations

- **Arterial blood gas analysis:** hypoxaemia and hypocapnia
- **Chest radiograph:** often normal, but signs may include atelectasis, effusion, peripheral oligaemia, elevated hemidiaphragm and wedge-shaped infarctions
- **ECG:** tachycardia (the most common finding – may be the only anomaly in 40 per cent of patients with a small PE), atrial arrhythmias, non-specific ST depression/T wave inversion or, in larger PEs, signs of RV strain (anterior T wave inversion, right bundle branch block, right axis deviation or the classic S1, Q3, T3 pattern).
- **D-dimer:** levels are elevated due to clot breakdown (fibrinolysis). This test has a high negative predictive value, but a low positive predictive value, so it is most useful when used for patients with a low or moderate clinical probability score. Its use in the context of critical illness may be limited
- **Computed tomography pulmonary angiography (CTPA):** the imaging study of choice, with the best diagnostic accuracy of all non-invasive imaging methods. Thrombus can be reliably visualised at least down to the segmental level. Its accuracy is dependent on clinical probability, and a high index of suspicion in the context of negative result should prompt further imaging. The increasing quality of CT images may lead to the identification of small sub-segmental PEs – the significance of these findings is not always clear
- **Ventilation/perfusion (V/Q) scintigraphy:** largely superseded by CTPA, but used when CTPA is contraindicated (e.g. contrast allergy, moderate to severe renal failure). The test is based on intravenous injection of technetium (Tc)-99m-labelled albumin particles. This can be combined with a ventilation scan (commonly xenon-133) to improve specificity. Its role in pregnancy is a point of debate, as it may reduce radiation dose to the mother but increases fetal exposure, when compared to CTPA
- **Pulmonary angiography:** previously considered the 'gold standard'; however, CT angiography now offers comparable accuracy. Its use in current practice is mainly to facilitate catheter-directed PE treatment. Risk of death from pulmonary angiography is approximately 0.5 per cent
- **Echocardiography:** acutely, its use is confined to the investigation of high-risk PE, to identify RV dysfunction or mobile right heart thrombi. The absence of these findings in the haemodynamically unstable patient practically excludes PE as the cause
- **Compression venous ultrasonography:** the finding of a proximal DVT in a patient suspected of having a PE obviates the need for further investigation

Treatment

Resuscitation

In high-risk PE, acute RV failure is the main cause of death. Aggressive volume resuscitation is likely harmful and a targeted bolus approach is preferable. Vasoactive substances may be required to support RV function – adrenaline and noradrenaline are suitable first-line agents (positive inotropic effect and improved coronary perfusion by peripheral vasoconstriction). If mechanical ventilation is required, a low tidal volume strategy should be implemented.

Anticoagulation

Anticoagulation prevents recurrence and reduces mortality from PE; unfractionated heparin (UFH), low-molecular-weight heparin (LMWH) and fondaparinux have all been used successfully. Compared with LMWH, UFH has a higher risk of major bleeding and heparin-induced thrombocytopenia, but may be more appropriate in renal failure.

Thrombolysis

Thrombolysis is indicated in haemodynamic compromise or RV dysfunction associated with PE. Over 90 per cent of patients respond favourably to treatment. Catheter-directed approaches, to reduce the total dose of thrombolytic agent, do not offer any advantage over systemic treatment. Thrombolysis in non-high-risk PE does not seem to improve long-term survival and morbidity.

Surgical Embolectomy

Surgical embolectomy should be considered in patients with high-risk PE, in whom thrombolysis is contraindicated. Catheter-based embolectomy techniques are also available, e.g. suction thrombectomy.

Venous Filters

Venous filters are (generally) placed in the infrarenal inferior vena cava (IVC), and indicated in patients with absolute contraindications to anticoagulation and a high risk of VTE recurrence. They have a significant complication rate and should be removed as soon as anticoagulation can be implemented.

Long-Term Anticoagulation

The aim of anticoagulation in VTE is to prevent recurrence (rates are similar between PE and DVT). Vitamin K antagonists (VKAs) (e.g. warfarin), LMWH and the newer novel oral anticoagulants (NOACs) are all valid options. Anticoagulation should be continued for a minimum of 3 months, but haematology guidance is often warranted.

Pulmonary Hypertension

Chronic thromboembolic pulmonary hypertension is a debilitating long-term complication of PE that may be related to increasing thrombus mass and inadequate anticoagulation. Prognosis is poor without surgical intervention.

References and Further Reading

Attia J, Ray JG, Cook DJ, Douketis J, Ginsberg JS, Geerts WH. Deep vein thrombosis and its prevention in critically ill adults. *Arch Intern Med* 2001;**161**: 1268–79.

Konstantinides SV, Torbicki A, Agnelli G, *et al.* 2014 ESC Guidelines on the diagnosis and management of acute pulmonary embolism. *Eur Heart J* 2014;**35**:3033–80.

Konstantinides SV, Vicaut E, Danays T, *et al.* Impact of thrombolytic therapy on the long-term outcome of intermediate-risk pulmonary embolism. *J Am Coll Cardiol* 2017;**69**:1536–44.

Meyer G, Vieillard-Baron A, Planquette B. Recent advances in the management of pulmonary embolism: focus on the critically ill patients. *Ann Intensive Care* 2016;**6**:19.

Pollack CV, Schreiber D, Goldhaber SZ, *et al.* Clinical characteristics, management, and outcomes of patients diagnosed with acute pulmonary embolism in the emergency department: initial report of EMPEROR (Multicenter Emergency Medicine Pulmonary Embolism in the Real World Registry). *J Am Coll Cardiol* 2011;**57**:700–6.

3.6.2

Asthma

Leon Cloherty and Gary Masterson

Key Learning Points

1. Asthma is difficult to diagnose and may coexist with chronic obstructive pulmonary disease.
2. Be aware of the markers of life-threatening asthma.
3. Administer steroids quickly.
4. Give high-dose oxygen.
5. Antibiotics are rarely indicated in acute asthma.

Keywords: asthma, ICU, critical care, permissive hypercapnia

Introduction

Asthma is a common chronic respiratory condition. The UK has the highest prevalence of asthma in Europe at 10 per cent, almost double that of the European Union (EU) (average 6.1 per cent). The total financial burden of asthma in the EU is estimated to be €72 billion per annum.

Despite advances in care, deaths from asthma in the UK have remained static since 2001, with over 1000 deaths per year. Most of these deaths occur before the patient reaches hospital.

Over a 10-year period, there were 11,948 asthma admissions (1.4 per cent of total) to adult critical care units in England and Wales. Median length of stay in the critical care unit was 1.8 days, with a median overall hospital stay of 7 days. Of note, nearly half of these patients were invasively ventilated. However, critical care unit survival rate was 95.5 per cent, with a rate of survival to hospital discharge of 93.3 per cent.

This chapter aims to aid the identification of the small subset of patients who are at risk of fatal asthma, and describes the strategies which can be employed to treat them once admitted to critical care.

Pathophysiology

Busse and Horwitz *et al.* have defined asthma as 'airway inflammation, intermittent airflow obstruction, and bronchial hyper-responsiveness'. The mechanism of inflammation in asthma may be acute, subacute or chronic, and the presence of airway oedema and mucus secretion also contribute to airflow obstruction. Varying degrees of mononuclear and eosinophil cellular infiltration, mucus hypersecretion, desquamation of the epithelium, smooth muscle hyperplasia and airway remodelling are present.

Signs and Symptoms

Typically, recurrent episodes of symptoms include wheeze, dyspnoea, chest tightness and cough, which vary over time in the absence of an alternative diagnosis. These symptoms may be chronic, subacute or acute. Asthma may coexist with atopic conditions, including atopic eczema/dermatitis and allergic rhinitis.

Investigations

Spirometry is the investigation of choice for asthma. The British Thoracic Society (BTS)/Scottish Intercollegiate Guidelines Network (SIGN) guideline states that 'confirmation of an asthma diagnosis hinges on the demonstration of airflow variability over short periods of time'. However, both signs and symptoms, as well as objective tests, have significant false positive and false negative rates. A normal spirogram obtained when the patient is asymptomatic does not, therefore, exclude the diagnosis of asthma. In a population of adults presenting to primary care with new respiratory symptoms, only a third of those with obstructive spirometry had asthma, and almost two thirds had COPD.

Grading of Severity

Assessment of the asthma patient and subsequent decision to admit to critical care can be difficult. Most patients will improve with medical management alone.

Critical care involvement often occurs at an early stage when optimum therapy has not been achieved, and a 'watch and wait' strategy can be employed. Repeated assessment is mandatory.

Objective measures have been described to help assess clinical severity. The presence of any of the features described below should prompt consideration of admission to the ICU and potential invasive ventilation.

Life-threatening features include:

1. Peak expiratory flow (PEF) <33 per cent (not particularly useful)
2. SpO_2 <92 per cent
3. Silent chest, cyanosis or feeble respiratory effort
4. Arrhythmia or hypotension
5. Exhaustion or altered conscious level

If any of these exist, then an arterial blood gas (ABG) is recommended. However, valuable time should not be wasted attempting arterial puncture if the patient is clearly peri-arrest.

Blood gas markers of a life-threatening attack include:

1. Normal or high $PaCO_2$ >4.6 kPa
2. Severe hypoxia: PaO_2 <8 kPa
3. Low pH

The UK-wide National Review of Asthma Deaths and previous Confidential Enquiries into asthma deaths have established other risk factors which should highlight a patient at risk of developing near-fatal or fatal asthma (Table 3.6.2.1).

Admission to ICU and Management

Drug Therapy

By the time the sick asthmatic reaches the ICU, drug therapy will usually have reached the intravenous phase and second-line therapies will be in consideration. Below is an overview of common and evidence-based therapies.

Oxygen

Give it in high concentration.

Do not use Heliox® – as whilst this decreases the density (and thus aids flow), it dilutes the administered oxygen.

Beta-2 Agonists

Use high-dose inhaled beta-2 agonists as first-line agents in patients with acute asthma, and administer as early as possible. Repeat nebulised dose every 15–30 minutes. Reserve intravenous beta-2 agonists for those patients in whom inhaled therapy cannot be used reliably.

Intravenous salbutamol may be administered as a bolus of 250 µg and repeated as necessary. This is diluted to a concentration of 50 µg/ml.

Alternatively, an infusion may be commenced at a rate of 5 µg/min, and adjusted to response and heart rate. The usual dose range is 3–20 µg/min, although higher doses may be required. Consider monitoring serum lactate for toxicity if intravenous beta-2 agonists are used.

Steroids

Give steroids (prednisolone (40–50 mg daily) or parenteral hydrocortisone (100 mg 6-hourly)) promptly to all patients with an acute attack, and continue for at least 5 days or until recovery. They can be stopped abruptly, provided the patient continues on an inhaled corticosteroid.

Ipratropium Bromide

Use nebulised ipratropium bromide (0.5 mg 4- to 6-hourly).

Table 3.6.2.1 Risk factors highlighting a patient at risk of developing near-fatal or fatal asthma

A combination of severe asthma, recognised by one or more of:
• Previous near-fatal asthma, e.g. previous ventilation or respiratory acidosis and previous admission for asthma, especially if in the last year • Requiring three or more classes of asthma medication • Heavy use of beta-2 agonist • Repeated attendances at emergency department for asthma care, especially if in the last year
AND adverse behavioural or psychosocial features, recognised by one or more of:
• Non-adherence with treatment or monitoring, failure to attend appointments • Fewer general practitioner contacts • Frequent home visits • Self-discharge from hospital • Psychosis, depression, other psychiatric illness or deliberate self-harm • Current or recent major tranquilliser use • Denial • Alcohol or drug abuse • Obesity • Learning difficulties • Employment problems • Income problems • Social isolation • Childhood abuse • Severe domestic, marital or legal stress

Magnesium Sulphate

Magnesium has bronchodilator effects and is used extensively in paediatric practice. Up to 2 g can be infused intravenously over 20 minutes. The safety and efficacy of repeated intravenous doses of magnesium sulphate have not been assessed. Repeated doses could cause hypermagnesaemia, with resultant muscle weakness and respiratory fatigue. Nebulised magnesium is not recommended.

Aminophylline

Aminophylline may be used as a second-line agent. Intravenous aminophylline is administered as a 5 mg/kg loading dose over 20 minutes (unless on maintenance oral therapy), followed by an infusion of 0.5–0.7 mg/(kg hr). Side effects are common and include nausea and cardiac arrhythmias. Levels should be checked at least daily.

Antibiotics

Infectious exacerbations of asthma are usually viral in nature and, therefore, antibiotics should not be routinely prescribed.

Other Therapies

Use of leukotriene receptor antagonists, recombinant human deoxyribonuclease and nebulised furosemide are not supported by current evidence.

Both ketamine and volatile anaesthesia are potent bronchodilators and are occasionally used when standard therapies have failed. Again, there is a lack of good-quality evidence.

Ventilatory Management

Non-invasive Ventilation

There is a lack of evidence to support non-invasive ventilation (NIV), although it is widely used in clinical practice.

Invasive Ventilation

The decision to invasively ventilate should be made when it is clear that medical management has failed. Intubation is difficult in these patients and should occur semi-electively in controlled conditions. The risks involved during induction of anaesthesia and the subsequent difficulties in ventilation should ensure a senior clinician is involved at an early stage. Hypotension is common on induction, primarily due to sedation, hypovolaemia and lung hyperinflation.

Instigation of positive pressure ventilation further worsens dynamic hyperinflation, and appropriate ventilator settings are of utmost importance.

Correction of hypoxia is the initial priority and this can usually be achieved with minimal addition of oxygen (FiO_2 of up to 0.5). Higher oxygen requirements indicate the possibility of a complication such as pneumonia, mucus plugging or pneumothorax. A chest X-ray is useful once stability is achieved.

Lung-protective strategies with permissive hypercapnia form the mainstay of ventilatory management. A prolonged expiratory phase will initially be required, and occasionally removal from the ventilator with manual compression of the thorax will help prevent breath stacking. The addition of extrinsic positive end-expiratory pressure (PEEP) in this context is controversial. Theoretically, work of breathing and gas trapping may be reduced, and PEEP has been demonstrated to reduce ventilator-associated lung injury. However, auto-PEEP may worsen gas trapping with a corresponding increase in ventilatory pressures. Careful titration and clinical observation are required.

Adequate sedation is mandatory and, in the authors' experience, muscle paralysis can be lifesaving.

The vast majority of ventilated patients will improve over a number of days, enabling a steady wean from the ventilator. There are, however, a small subsection of patients who, despite maximal therapy, fail to wean or deteriorate. Early discussion with regional extracorporeal membrane oxygenation (ECMO) providers is recommended when this becomes apparent.

References and Further Reading

British Thoracic Society. 2021. BTS/SIGN British guideline on the management of asthma. www.brit-thoracic.org .uk/quality-improvement/guidelines/asthma/

Busse WW, Calhoun WF, Sedgwick JD. Mechanism of airway inflammation in asthma. *Am Rev Respir Dis* 1993;**147**(6 Pt 2):S20–4.

European Respiratory Society. *EUROPEAN LUNG white book*. www.erswhitebook.org

Gibbison B, Griggs K, Mukherjee M, *et al.* Ten years of asthma admissions to adult critical care units in England and Wales. *BMJ Open* 2013;**3**:e003420.

Horwitz RJ, Busse WW. Inflammation and asthma. *Clin Chest Med* 1995;**16**:583–602.

Lim WJ, Akram RM, Carson KV, *et al.* Non-invasive positive pressure ventilation for treatment of respiratory failure due to severe acute exacerbations of asthma. *Cochrane Database Syst Rev* 2012;**12**:CD004360.

OECD and European Union. *Health at a Glance: Europe 2016. State of Health in the EU Cycle*. Paris: OECD Publishing; 2016. www.oecd-ilibrary.org/social-issues-migration-health/health-at-a-glance-europe-2016_9789264265592-en

Office for National Statistics. 2016. Asthma deaths in England and Wales, 2001 to 2015 occurrences. www.ons.gov.uk/peoplepopulationandcommunity/births deathsandmarriages/deaths/adhocs/005955 asthmadeathsinenglandandwales2001to2015 occurrences

Royal College of Physicians. 2015. Why asthma still kills. National Review of Asthma Deaths. www.rcplondon.ac.uk/projects/outputs/why-asthma-still-kills

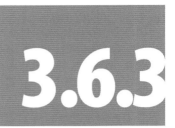

3.6.3 Chronic Obstructive Pulmonary Disease

Lee Poole and Gary Masterson

Key Learning Points

1. Chronic obstructive pulmonary disease (COPD) is the preferred term for the conditions in patients with airflow obstruction who were previously diagnosed as having chronic bronchitis or emphysema.
2. A diagnosis of COPD should be considered in patients over the age of 35 who have a risk factor (generally smoking) and who present with exertional breathlessness, chronic cough, regular sputum production, frequent winter 'bronchitis' or wheeze.
3. There is no single diagnostic test for COPD.
4. Co-morbidities are common in COPD and should be actively identified.
5. Clinicians should be aware that they are likely to underestimate survival in an acute exacerbation of COPD treated by invasive mechanical ventilation.

Keywords: chronic obstructive pulmonary disease, COPD, bronchitis, emphysema, MRC dyspnoea scale

Introduction

An estimated 3 million people have chronic obstructive pulmonary disease (COPD) in the UK. About 900,000 have diagnosed COPD, and an estimated 2 million people have COPD which remains undiagnosed. A diagnosis of COPD should be considered in patients over the age of 35 who have a risk factor (generally smoking) and who present with exertional breathlessness, chronic cough, regular sputum production, frequent winter 'bronchitis' or wheeze.

COPD is characterised by airflow obstruction that is not fully reversible. The airflow obstruction does not change markedly over several months and is usually progressive in the long term. The presence of airflow obstruction should be confirmed by performing post-bronchodilator spirometry.

The following are used as a definition of COPD:

- Airflow obstruction is defined as a reduced FEV_1/FVC ratio (where FEV_1 is forced expiratory volume in 1 second and FVC is forced vital capacity), such that FEV_1/FVC is <0.7.
- If FEV_1 is $\geq$80 per cent predicted, a diagnosis of COPD should only be made in the presence of respiratory symptoms, e.g. breathlessness or cough.

Airflow obstruction is present because of a combination of airway and parenchymal damage. The damage is the result of chronic inflammation which differs from that seen in asthma and which is usually the result of tobacco smoke. Significant airflow obstruction may be present before the person is aware of it.

Grading of COPD

There are a number of grading systems that can be used to classify the severity of COPD. The Medical Research Council (MRC) dyspnoea scale utilises symptoms to classify patients (Table 3.6.3.1).

The GOLD (Global Initiative for Chronic Obstructive Lung Disease) guide classifies the disease according to spirometry and FEV_1 (Table 3.6.3.2).

Table 3.6.3.1 MRC dyspnoea scale for COPD patients

Grade	Impact
1	Not troubled by breathlessness, except on vigorous exertion
2	Short of breath when hurrying or walking up inclines
3	Walks more slowly than contemporaries because of breathlessness or has to stop for breath when walking at own pace
4	Stops for breath after walking about 100 m or stops after a few minutes walking on the level
5	Too breathless to leave the house or breathless on dressing or undressing

Table 3.6.3.2 The GOLD classification of COPD

Spirometric classification of COPD severity based on post-bronchodilator FEV_1		
Stage I	Mild	$FEV_1/FVC <0.70$ $FEV_1 >80\%$ predicted
Stage II	Moderate	$FEV_1/FVC <0.70$ $50\% < FEV_1 <80\%$ predicted
Stage III	Severe	$FEV_1/FVC <0.70$ $30\% < FEV_1 <50\%$ predicted
Stage IV	Very severe	$FEV_1/FVC <0.70$ $FEV_1 <30\%$ predicted or $FEV_1 <50\%$ predicted plus chronic respiratory failure

Abbreviations: COPD = chronic obstructive pulmonary disease; FEV_1 = forced expiratory volume in 1 second; FVC = forced vital capacity.
Source: GOLD COPD.

Investigations

There is no single diagnostic test for COPD. Making a diagnosis therefore relies on clinical judgement based on a combination of history, physical examination and confirmation of the presence of airflow obstruction using spirometry.

At the time of a patient's initial diagnostic evaluation, in addition to spirometry, all patients should have:

- A chest radiograph to exclude other pathologies
- A full blood count to identify anaemia or polycythaemia
- Body mass index (BMI) calculated

Additional tests may be required in certain circumstances to exclude other diagnoses (e.g. alpha-1-anti-trypsin or heart failure), and an alternative diagnosis should be considered in:

- Older people without typical symptoms of COPD where the FEV_1/FVC ratio is <0.7
- Younger people with symptoms of COPD where the FEV_1/FVC ratio is ≥0.7

General Management

All COPD patients still smoking, regardless of age, should be encouraged to stop (and offered help to do so) at every opportunity. In the community, inhalers are the mainstay of treatment, and in those with stable COPD who remain breathless or have exacerbations despite use of short-acting bronchodilators as required, the following may be used as maintenance therapy:

- If FEV_1 ≥50 per cent predicted: either long-acting beta-2 agonist (LABA) or long-acting muscarinic antagonist (LAMA)
- If FEV_1 <50 per cent predicted: either LABA with an inhaled corticosteroid (ICS) in a combination inhaler, or LAMA
- Offer LAMA, in addition to LABA + ICS, to people with COPD who remain breathless or have exacerbations despite taking LABA + ICS, irrespective of their FEV_1

Long-Term Oxygen Therapy

Long-term oxygen therapy (LTOT) is indicated in patients with COPD who have:

- PaO_2 <7.3 kPa when stable, or
- PaO_2 between 7.3 and 8 kPa when stable and one of:
  - Secondary polycythaemia
  - Nocturnal hypoxaemia (SaO_2 <90 per cent for >30 per cent of the time)
  - Peripheral oedema
  - Pulmonary hypertension

To benefit from LTOT, patients should breathe supplemental oxygen for at least 15 hours per day. Even greater benefits are seen in patients receiving oxygen for 20 hours per day.

Acute Exacerbations of COPD

This is defined as an acute change in baseline status (dyspnoea, cough and/or sputum) beyond day-to-day variability, sufficient to warrant an alteration in therapy. This can be infective or non-infective. Prognosis is worse in those patients requiring three or more admissions to hospital for acute exacerbations of COPD (AECOPD) treatment.

COPD and Critical Care

Patients with exacerbations of COPD should be considered for intensive care unit admission, including for invasive ventilation when this is thought to be necessary.

When assessing suitability for intubation and ventilation during exacerbations of COPD, it is essential to gather information regarding the patient's functional status, BMI, requirement for oxygen when stable, co-morbidities, previous admissions to intensive care units and FEV_1. The latter, however, along with age, should not be used in isolation when assessing suitability.

Non-invasive Ventilation

Non-invasive ventilation (NIV) should be used as the treatment of choice for persistent hypercapnic ventilatory failure during acute exacerbations not responding to medical therapy. Staff trained in its application, experienced in its use and aware of its limitations should deliver it.

Adequately treated patients with chronic hypercapnic respiratory failure who have required assisted ventilation (whether invasive or non-invasive) during an exacerbation, or who are hypercapnic or acidotic on LTOT, should be referred to a specialist centre for consideration of long-term NIV.

In all instances, when patients are started on NIV, there should be a clear plan covering what to do in the event of deterioration, and ceilings of therapy should be agreed.

Invasive Ventilation

When considering the appropriateness of invasive mechanical ventilation (IMV) for a patient (and the subsequent prognosis), a number of prognostic scoring systems exist. These include the BODE and DECAF score (which are designed for use in the more stable setting), and the APACHE 2 and CAPS Score (in the more acute setting). The scoring systems are, however, poorly predictive for individual patient use, and clinicians should be aware that they are likely to underestimate survival in an AECOPD patient treated with IMV.

General principles of invasive ventilation that apply to acute hypercapnic ventilatory failure (AHVF) due to COPD include the following:

- A low tidal volume strategy improves survival.
- Dynamic hyperinflation due to airflow obstruction should be minimised by prolonging the expiratory time (I:E ratio 1:3 or greater) and setting a low ventilatory frequency (10–15 breaths/min).
- Applied extrinsic positive end-expiratory pressure (ePEEP) should not normally exceed 12 cmH$_2$O.
- Permissive hypercapnia (aiming for pH 7.2–7.25) may be required to avoid high airway pressures when airflow obstruction is severe.
- NIV-supported extubation should be employed, in preference to inserting a tracheostomy.

It is also important that following an episode requiring IMV, clinicians should discuss the management of possible future episodes of AHVF with patients, because there is a high risk of recurrence.

References and Further Reading

Davidson AC, Banham S, Elliott M, *et al.* BTS/ICS guideline for the ventilatory management of acute hypercapnic respiratory failure in adults. *Thorax* 2016;**71**:ii1–ii35.

Global Initiative for Chronic Obstructive Lung Disease. goldcopd.org

National Institute for Health and Care Excellence. 2010. Chronic obstructive pulmonary disease in over 16s: diagnosis and management. Clinical guideline [CG101]. www.nice.org.uk/guidance/cg101

Soler-Cataluña JJ, Martínez-García MA, Román Sánchez P, Salcedo E, Navarro M, Ochando R. Severe acute exacerbations and mortality in patients with chronic obstructive pulmonary disease. *Thorax* 2005; **60**: 925–31.

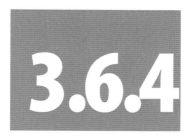

Pneumonia

Mahmoud Wagih

Key Learning Points

1. Diagnosis and treatment of pneumonia should be based on the clinical picture.
2. The CURB-65 score is a clinical prediction tool that has been validated for predicting mortality in community-acquired pneumonia, and it is recommended by the British Thoracic Society for assessment of the severity of pneumonia.
3. Chest radiographs have historically been perceived as a reliable tool for diagnosing pneumonia; however, despite their availability and widespread use, they have their limitations.
4. Antibiotics should be used early.
5. Nationally accepted protocols and the local antibiogram should be utilised when treating pneumonia.

Keywords: pneumonia, CURB-65, British Thoracic Society, CXR

Introduction

Pneumonia is an acute infection of the lung parenchyma, usually caused by one or multiple co-infecting pathogens. It excludes the well-defined condition of bronchiolitis, the primary cause of which is almost always a viral agent.

Classification

Attempts have been made to classify pneumonia according to its causative pathogen, the clinical presentation or the patient's background. These classifications failed to guide treatment or support the research methodology, due to the heterogeneity of pathogens involved. A widely acceptable clinical classification has been adopted by the National Heart, Lung and Blood Institute where pneumonia is classified as:

1. **Community-acquired pneumonia (CAP):** pneumonia that is acquired outside hospital (pneumonia that develops in a nursing home resident is included in this definition)
2. **Hospital-acquired pneumonia (HAP):** pneumonia that develops 48 hours or more after hospital admission and was not incubating at hospital admission. When managed in hospital, the diagnosis is usually confirmed by chest X-ray. Pneumonia that develops in hospital after intubation (ventilator-associated pneumonia) is excluded from this definition
3. Ventilator-associated pneumonia (VAP)
4. Atypical pneumonia
5. Aspiration pneumonia

Note lower respiratory tract infections are an acute illness (present for 21 days or less), usually with cough as the main symptom and with at least one other lower respiratory tract symptom (such as fever, sputum production, breathlessness, wheeze or chest discomfort or pain) and no alternative explanation (such as sinusitis or asthma). Pneumonia, acute bronchitis and exacerbation of chronic obstructive airways disease are included in this definition.

Common Causative Organisms

Common causative organisms and their specific features are shown in Table 3.6.4.1.

The Clinical Picture

History

Exposure/co-morbidities may indicate the potential causative organism, such as those seen in Table 3.6.4.2.

Presentation

In addition to the generic symptoms associated with infection (e.g. fever, rigours, altered mental status), attempts have been made to link some symptoms,

Table 3.6.4.1 Common causative organisms and their specific features

Organism	Specific features
Bacterium	
Streptococcus pneumoniae	Most common bacterial cause
Staphylococcus aureus pneumonia	One of the most common causes of ventilator-associated pneumonia and hospital-acquired pneumonia
Legionella pneumophila	Atypical pneumonia. It is sometimes called legionnaire's disease and has caused serious outbreaks which are usually linked to contaminated water/humidity sources
Mycoplasma pneumoniae	Atypical pneumonia which affects younger sections of the population (schools, prisons). Usually mild and can be associated with skin rash and haemolysis
Chlamydia pneumoniae	Atypical pneumonia which is non-seasonal and affects an older age group
Viral	
Influenza or flu virus	Most common causative virus in adults
Respiratory syncytial virus	Most common cause of viral pneumonia in children younger than 1 year old
Rhinovirus, human parainfluenza virus and human metapneumovirus	Common causes for common cold
Fungal	
Pneumocystis jirovecii	Causes pneumocystis pneumonia in immunocompromised patients
Coccidioidomycosis	Causes valley fever
Histoplasmosis	Organism usually found in the soil
Cryptococcus	Organism usually found in bird droppings

Table 3.6.4.2 Examples of causative organisms and their associations

Background	Aetiological associations
Recent travel, contaminated air conditioning or water system	*Legionella*
Overcrowded institutions	*S. pneumoniae*, mycobacteria, *Mycoplasma*, *Chlamydophila*
Farm animals	*Coxiella burnetii, Bacillus anthracis, Yersinia pestis*
Altered mental status, anatomical anomalies, seizures	Aspiration
Asthma, chronic obstructive pulmonary disease, smoking	*Haemophilus influenzae*
Systemic lupus erythematosus	Lupus pneumonitis

particularly sputum characteristics, to specific causative agents. Examples include:

- *S. pneumoniae* – rust-coloured sputum
- *Pseudomonas* and *H. influenzae* – green sputum
- *Klebsiella* – redcurrant jelly sputum
- Anaerobic infections – foul-smelling sputum
- *L. pneumophila* – gastrointestinal symptoms

Notably, these clinical features should not be utilised alone to tailor anti-microbial therapy, as they are both subjective and non-specific.

Severity Evaluation

The CURB-65 score is a clinical prediction tool that has been validated for predicting mortality in CAP, and it is recommended by the British Thoracic Society for assessment of the severity of pneumonia.

The score is an acronym for each of the risk factors measured (Box 3.6.4.1), and each risk factor scores 1 point, with a maximum score of 5 attainable.

> **Box 3.6.4.1 CURB-65 Score**
>
> - **C**onfusion of new onset (defined as an Abbreviated Mental Test Score of 8 or lower)
> - Blood **U**rea nitrogen >7 mmol/l (19 mg/dl)
> - **R**espiratory rate of 30 breaths per minute or greater
> - **B**lood pressure <90 mmHg systolic or 60 mmHg or less diastolic
> - Age **65** or older

Table 3.6.4.3 Mortality risk and management of different CURB-65 scores

CURB-65 score	Mortality risk (%)	Management
0–1	1.5	Outpatient care
2	9.2	Inpatient care or close observation as outpatient
>3	22	Inpatient admission, with consideration for admission to the intensive care unit with a score of 4 or 5

As the score increases, so does the patient's mortality risk. As such, clinical management decisions can be based on the score (Table 3.6.4.3).

Other scoring systems for classifying the severity of pneumonia include the Japanese Respiratory Society's Severity Rating System, the Pneumonia Severity Index (PSI) and the Acute Physiology And Chronic Health Evaluation (APACHE) score.

Diagnostic Approach to Pneumonia

This includes laboratory tests, which may be specific or non-specific, microbiological assessment and radiological evaluation.

Laboratory Tests

Non-specific
- C-reactive protein (CRP) and white cell count (WCC)
- Procalcitonin (PCT)
- Venous blood gases (and serum lactate), serum cortisol, kidney function tests, coagulation studies
- Hyponatraemia (sodium level <130 mEq/l) and microhaematuria – which may be associated with *Legionella* pneumonia

Specific
- *Legionella*-specific fluorescent antibody can be sought in the sputum; however, the technique has a high false negative rate.
- Urinary antigen testing for *Legionella* serogroup 1 organisms is accurate; however, up to 30 per cent of infections are not caused by serogroup 1 organisms.
- A *Legionella* serum antibody titre of 1:128 or more is indicative of active infection.
- Pneumococcal antigen tests for serum, urine and saliva samples are available.

Notably, the American Thoracic Society (ATS) guidelines advise that clinical criteria alone are superior to biomarkers as an indication to start anti-microbial therapy in HAP/VAP.

Microbiological Assessment

Blood Cultures

Blood cultures show poor sensitivity in pneumonia, and findings are positive in only approximately 40 per cent of cases of HAP (6–9 per cent in CAP). The chances of a positive test result are higher in the more severe forms of the disease; however, even in pneumococcal pneumonia, the results are often negative. Recommendations have thus changed to eliminate taking blood cultures routinely in CAP (unless of a certain severity or previous failed treatment), as their outcome rarely impacts the choice of the empirical antibiotic regime.

Pulmonary/Bronchial Sampling

Invasive (e.g. broncho-alveolar lavage) and non-invasive (e.g. endotracheal aspiration) methods may be used to obtain samples. However, a recent Cochrane review has demonstrated that invasive sampling rarely offers any advantage over non-invasive sampling in pneumonia. Clinicians might opt to use invasive sampling in complicated VAP or if failed treatment despite multiple anti-microbial regimes.

All samples obtained through these tests can be assessed quantitatively or semi-quantitatively. Semi-quantitative sampling is as effective as quantitative, and remains the recommended method of testing. For patients with suspected VAP whose invasive quantitative culture results are below the diagnostic threshold (e.g. colony counts) for VAP, it is suggested that antibiotics be withheld rather than continued.

Radiological Evaluation

Chest Radiographs

Chest radiographs have historically been perceived as a reliable tool for diagnosing pneumonia. Despite their availability and widespread use, they have their limitations such as:
- **Time to develop changes:** this can be affected by the immunological status of the patient (slow/non-specific changes in immunocompromised patients). Chest X-ray signs usually develop within 12 hours of symptom appearance. This might be adequate in CAP, but in a hospital setting, early

radiographs might lead to false reassurance and under-diagnosis

- **Time to resolution of radiological changes:** radiological changes can worsen initially despite clinical improvement after initiation of treatment. X-rays are also limited in terms of differentiating between pneumonia and other chest pathologies (e.g. pulmonary embolism, pulmonary fibrosis, malignancies)

Lobar pneumonia radiographically appears as homogeneous consolidation involving one (or rarely more) lobe. Patent larger bronchi create the characteristic air bronchogram. *S. pneumoniae* is known to cause lobar pneumonia which occasionally takes a round form, i.e. round pneumonia. Radiographic findings in aspiration pneumonia depend on the position of the patient at the time of aspiration. The right lung is twice as likely to be affected, but in recumbent patients, the posterior segments of the upper lobes are more commonly affected. *Klebsiella pneumoniae* shows tendency towards lobar expansion. Upper lobe involvement and cavitation are also commonly associated with this infection. *Legionella* affects the lower lung zones with a protracted radiological recovery course (10–12 weeks).

Bronchopneumonia presents as peribronchial thickening and patchy areas of consolidation involving the terminal and respiratory bronchioles. These can coalesce to create a lobular or lobar pattern late in the course of the disease. Air bronchograms are typically absent. They are associated with more destructive organisms such as *S. aureus*, *H. influenzae*, *Pseudomonas aeruginosa*, *Escherichia coli*, *K. pneumoniae* and *Proteus* species.

Importantly, chest radiographs are normal in 10–15 per cent of symptomatic patients with proven infiltrative lung disease, in up to 30 per cent of those with bronchiectasis and in close to 60 per cent of patients with emphysema.

Lung Ultrasound

A recent review has confirmed that lung ultrasound (LUS) has superior sensitivity and specificity for the diagnosis of pneumonia, compared to chest radiographs. Due to its availability, low radiation exposure and its ability to identify other lung pathologies (e.g. pleural effusion), LUS is being increasingly used to diagnose pneumonia. Issues related to training and logistical feasibility of use are unfortunately slowing down the uptake of this technique by clinicians.

Computed Tomography

CT scans are rarely used as a first-line imaging technique for pneumonia, but they have their uses, which include:

- X-ray-negative pneumonia with dominant clinical features and equivocal chest X-ray
- Investigation of non-resolving lesions
- Evaluation of complications (e.g. pneumothorax, empyema)
- Failed weaning from mechanical ventilation
- Considering alternative/underlying diagnosis (e.g. pulmonary fibrosis)

Logistical challenges associated with CT scans, alongside their related cost and high radiation exposure, limit their routine use.

Treatment: General Approach to Anti-microbial Therapy

Community-Acquired Pneumonia

The National Institute for Health and Care Excellence (NICE) offers advice to support the diagnosis and subsequent anti-microbial therapy for CAP. It follows these broad lines:

- Do not routinely offer microbiological tests to patients with low-severity CAP.
- For patients with moderate- or high-severity CAP:
  - Blood and sputum cultures should be obtained
  - Pneumococcal and *Legionella* urinary antigen tests should be considered.

Low-Severity Community-Acquired Pneumonia

The patient should be offered a 5-day course of a single antibiotic (longer with poor initial response). Amoxicillin should be considered in preference to a macrolide or a tetracycline, unless the patient is allergic to penicillin.

Moderate- and High-Severity Community-Acquired Pneumonia

Dual antibiotic therapy with amoxicillin and a macrolide is recommended. Beta-lactam antibiotics (e.g. co-amoxiclav, cephalosporins and piperacillin with tazobactam) and a macrolide are an acceptable alternative. Glucocorticoid treatment should not be used routinely.

Consider measuring a baseline CRP concentration in patients with CAP on admission to hospital, and repeat the test if clinical progress is uncertain after 48–72 hours.

Hospital-Acquired Pneumonia

All hospitals should regularly generate and disseminate a local antibiogram – ideally one that is specific to their intensive care population(s), if possible.

Antibiotic therapy should be started within 4 hours of diagnosis, according to the local hospital policy (antibiogram), and continued for 5–10 days.

The diagnosis of HAP is mainly clinical, with a minimal role for biomarkers (e.g. CRP, PCT, broncho-alveolar lavage fluid) or severity scoring systems, according to ATS guidelines.

Ventilator-Associated Pneumonia

Empirical anti-microbial therapy in VAP according to the Infectious Diseases Society of America (IDSA)/ATS should be planned as follows:

- In suspected VAP, coverage for *S. aureus*, *P. aeruginosa* and other Gram-negative bacilli should be included in all empirical regimens.
- Meticillin-resistant *S. aureus* (MRSA) cover should be included only in patients with any of the following:
  - Risk factors for anti-microbial resistance (Box 3.6.4.2)
  - Patients being treated in units where >10–20 per cent of *S. aureus* isolates are meticillin-resistant
  - Patients in units where the prevalence of MRSA is not known

---

Box 3.6.4.2 Risk Factors for Anti-microbial Resistance

- Prior intravenous antibiotic use within the last 90 days
- Septic shock at the time of ventilator-associated pneumonia
- Acute respiratory distress syndrome preceding ventilator-associated pneumonia
- >5 days of hospitalisation prior to ventilator-associated pneumonia
- Acute renal replacement therapy prior to ventilator-associated pneumonia

---

An agent active against meticillin-sensitive *S. aureus* (MSSA) (and not MRSA) should be used for empirical treatment of suspected VAP in patients without risk factors for anti-microbial resistance who are being treated in ICUs where <10–20 per cent of *S. aureus* isolates are meticillin-resistant.

Two anti-pseudomonal antibiotics from different classes should be used for empirical treatment of suspected VAP only in patients with any of the following:

1. A risk factor for anti-microbial resistance (Box 3.6.4.2)
2. Patients in units where >10 per cent of Gram-negative isolates are resistant to an agent being considered for monotherapy
3. Patients in an ICU where local anti-microbial susceptibility rates are not available

Other factors which may affect the decision to continue/discontinue antibiotics in VAP include:

- The likelihood of an alternative source of infection
- Prior anti-microbial therapy at the time of culture
- Degree of clinical suspicion
- Signs of severe sepsis
- Evidence of clinical improvement

References and Further Reading

Kalil AC, Metersky ML, Klompas M, *et al*. Management of adults with hospital-acquired and ventilator-associated pneumonia: 2016 clinical practice guidelines by the Infectious Diseases Society of America and the American Thoracic Society. *Clin Infect Dis* 2016;**63**:e61–111.

Kohno S, Seki M, Takehara K, *et al*. Prediction of requirement for mechanical ventilation in community-acquired pneumonia with acute respiratory failure: a multicenter prospective study. *Respiration* 2013;**85**:27–35.

Mackenzie G. The definition and classification of pneumonia. *Pneumonia (Nathan)* 2016;**8**:14.

Metlay JP, Fine MJ. Testing strategies in the initial management of patients with community-acquired pneumonia. *Ann Intern Med* 2003;**138**:109–18.

World Health Organization. 2016. ICD-10 Version: 2016. apps.who.int/classifications/icd10/browse/2016/en

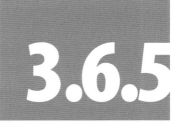

Acute Respiratory Distress Syndrome

Mahmoud Wagih

Key Learning Points

1. Due to the diverse heterogeneity in its aetiology, acute respiratory distress syndrome (ARDS) has been described as a symptom, rather than a distinct pathology in its own right.
2. Conventionally, ARDS can be categorised as either pulmonary or non-pulmonary in origin.
3. The Berlin definition has redefined the diagnostic criteria.
4. The ARDS Network trial has helped to understand the condition and identified a modifiable approach to change the outcome.
5. Key to its management is adherence to volume- and pressure-limited lung-protective ventilation to minimise ventilator-associated lung injury.

Keywords: acute respiratory distress syndrome, ARDS, Berlin definition, ARDSNet

Definition

Acute respiratory distress syndrome (ARDS) is a form of acute lung injury characterised by inflammation and increased endothelial and epithelial permeability. Pathological findings include lung oedema, inflammation and haemorrhage and alveolar epithelial cell injury.

History

Ashbaugh and colleagues were the first to use the term ARDS in 1967. The nomenclature has changed several times until more formerly defined in 1994 by the American European Consensus Conference (AECC), whereby a degree of standardisation was achieved. This was crystallised further in the most recent Berlin definition (2012) where the oxygenation standards and mutually exclusive PaO_2/FiO_2 thresholds were agreed to define the severity of ARDS, the diagnostic thresholds were broadened and the term acute lung injury (ALI) was discouraged.

Incidence

The incidence of ARDS ranges from 1.5 to 79 cases per 100,000. This variation reflects the heterogeneity in its definition, diagnosis and the population scanned. According to the LUNG SAFE study, ARDS represents 10.3 per cent of admissions to the ICU, and 23 per cent of these patients require mechanical ventilation.

Causes

Due to the diverse heterogeneity in its aetiology, ARDS has been described as a symptom, rather than as a distinct pathology in its own right. Causes have been classified as either pulmonary or extra-pulmonary (Table 3.6.5.1).

Risk Factors

In a survey of 19,003 patients in the United States, the following were identified as risk factors for ARDS:

- Sepsis
- Cirrhosis
- Surgical/medical mishaps
- Smoking
- Increased body mass index (BMI)
- Recent chemotherapy

Table 3.6.5.1 Causes of acute respiratory distress syndrome

Pulmonary causes	Non-pulmonary causes
Pneumonia	Sepsis
Aspiration	Trauma
Inhalation injury	Pancreatitis
Near drowning	Burns
Pulmonary contusion	Fat embolism

Interestingly, patients with chronic lung disease were found to be less likely to develop ARDS secondary to pneumonia.

Clinical Presentation

Patients initially develop dyspnoea on exertion, which progresses to severe dyspnoea at rest, tachypnoea, anxiety, agitation and increased work of breathing and oxygen requirements. Symptoms typically present within 12–48 hours of an inciting event but may occasionally take longer. On assessment, manifestations of any underlying aetiology should be sought out (e.g. burns or surgical wounds), and local examination of the chest may reveal bibasal or widespread crepitations. Clinical assessment should also focus on manifestation of acute-on-chronic cardiac failure (e.g. jugular venous distension, cardiac murmurs and gallops, hepatomegaly and peripheral oedema), as it is important to rule out cardiogenic pulmonary oedema as the cause.

Diagnostic Criteria

The Berlin definition (Table 3.6.5.2) has simplified the diagnosis by including the following as essential.

Bilateral Lung Infiltrates

These can be detected on chest X-ray or CT scan. They should not be secondary to malignancy, lung collapse or pleural effusion.

PO_2/FiO_2 Ratio

The thresholds agreed are 300–200 mmHg (mild), 200–100 mmHg (moderate) and <100 mmHg (severe).

Table 3.6.5.2 Berlin definition of acute respiratory distress syndrome

Timing	Within 1 week of a known clinical insult or new worsening respiratory symptoms
Chest imaging	Bilateral opacities – not fully explained by effusion, lobar/lung collapse or nodules
Origin of oedema	Respiratory failure not fully explained by cardiac failure or fluid overload. Objective assessment needed (e.g. Echo) to exclude hydrostatic oedema if no risk factor present
Oxygenation (with PEEP or CPAP ≥5 cmH₂O)	• Mild 200–300 mmHg (<39.9 kPa) • Moderate 100–200 mmHg (<26.6 kPa) • Severe ≤100 mmHg (13.3 kPa)

Abbreviations: Echo = echocardiography; PEEP = positive end-expiratory pressure; CPAP = continuous positive airway pressure.

(To obtain the equivalent in kilopascals, divide these figures by 7.5.) Importantly, all these numbers are obtained on positive end-expiratory pressure (PEEP) of 5 cmH₂O.

Duration

The clinical picture of ARDS should present <1 week after the causative event. Most cases develop within 72 hours.

Cardiogenic Pulmonary Oedema

The Berlin definition does not require rigid exclusion of cardiogenic pulmonary oedema (CPO). It states that the respiratory failure is not 'fully explained' by cardiac failure or fluid overload. This exclusion can be achieved clinically or, if feasible, through any form of cardiac output measurement. Notably, this is contrary to the previous definition, which was based on a direct pulmonary artery pressure measurement criterion.

Investigations (Laboratory/Radiological)

1. Investigation of the cause (Table 3.6.5.3)
2. Laboratory
3. Arterial blood gases (ABGs) are used to diagnose and assess the severity of ARDS (PO_2/FiO_2 ratio)
4. Radiological – chest X-ray or CT scan

Table 3.6.5.3 Investigating the cause

Aetiology	Investigation
Pulmonary (direct)	
Pneumonia	Sputum culture, urinary antigens, CRP, procalcitonin, CXR
Aspiration	CXR
Inhalation injury	History, direct and indirect airway examination
Near drowning	History, serum electrolytes
Non-pulmonary (indirect)	
Sepsis	History, CRP, procalcitonin, radiology
Trauma	History, CK, urine/serum myoglobin
Pancreatitis	Lipase, amylase, CRP
Burns	History, albumin, CRP, procalcitonin
Fat embolism	History, CT or CXR

Abbreviations: CRP = C-reactive protein; CXR = chest X-ray; CK = creatine kinase.

Management

Treatment of Underlying Cause

The severity or chronicity of ARDS depends on the amount of aetiological substances and the corresponding immune reactions. No effective measures have been identified to modulate the immune reaction. However, a sensible initial step would be to address the aetiological factors (e.g. sepsis or pneumonia).

Ventilatory Strategies

The ARDS guidelines promote volume- and pressure-limited lung-protective ventilation to minimise ventilator-associated lung injury (VALI).

The lungs of ARDS patients are affected heterogeneously, i.e. parts of the lungs are oedematous and inflamed and have limited elasticity, whilst other parts demonstrate near-normal elasticity. Overall, a markedly reduced volume of the lung tissue is available for ventilation, and as such, mechanical ventilation can result in lung injury when volumes and pressures meant for the entire lung are forced into only a small portion of healthy pulmonary tissue.

VALI occurs via numerous mechanisms, including exposure to high inflation pressures or overdistension (barotrauma or volutrauma), repetitive opening and closing of alveoli (atelectrauma) and mechanotransduction resulting in upregulated cytokine release and a systemic inflammatory response (biotrauma).

According to the ARDS Network trial, protective/open lung ventilation reduces mortality by nearly 10 per cent.

The parameters recommended by the ARDS Network include tidal volume (Vt) of 6 ml/kg of ideal body weight (with a range of 4–8 ml/kg, depending on plateau pressure and pH) and reduced plateau pressure (measured after a 0.5-second end-inspiratory pause) of ≤30 cmH$_2$O.

Permissive hypercapnia is accepted and refers to acceptance of a rise in carbon dioxide (CO_2) as a consequence of low Vt. There is no well-identified limit for an acceptable rise in CO_2. However, evidence suggests that it is well tolerated. Measures recommended by the ARDS Network include considering increasing the respiratory rate to up to 35 breaths/min, use of a bicarbonate buffer and increasing the Vt for management of acidosis.

Fluid Management

The ARDS Network trial, which compared liberal versus conservative fluid management strategies, showed no effect on overall mortality between cohorts. However, the conservative fluid group demonstrated an improved oxygenation index and lung injury score, as well as an increase in ventilator-free days, without an increase in non-pulmonary organ failures. On this occasion, the conservative group had a neutral, rather than a negative, fluid balance and this is thought to explain why other studies demonstrated more favourable mortality outcomes with conservative fluid management.

Use of Muscle Relaxants

In 2010, a study concluded that early (first 48 hours) administration of a neuromuscular-blocking agent improved the adjusted 90-day survival and increased the time off the ventilator in patients with severe ARDS, without increasing muscle weakness.

Nutrition in Acute Respiratory Distress Syndrome

- Enteral versus parenteral: a meta-analysis of studies comparing both approaches found no difference in survival; however, enteral nutrition was associated with a lower incidence of infectious complications. This has traditionally been ascribed to the trophic effect enteral nutrition has on the gut mucosa which reduces the chance of translocation
- Early versus late initiation of nutritional support: early introduction of nutrition (48 hours) was associated with a reduction in both mortality and infectious complications
- Caloric prescription: to settle the long-standing debate of whether restrictive (trophic) feeding has survival benefit over full feeding, the National Heart, Lung and Blood Institute's ARDS Network recently published a large randomised controlled trial of trophic enteral feeding versus full enteral feeding. No differences were observed in the number of ventilator-free days, mortality at 60 days, organ failure-free days or infectious complications

Management of Severe Hypoxia

Proning

Guérin *et al.* in 2013 demonstrated that in severe ARDS, early proning for prolonged periods (16 hours) reduced the 28- and 90-day mortality. This outcome negated the well-held notion that proning is a mere rescue measure in refractory hypoxaemia. There is, however, no universal approach to proning (i.e. timing, threshold, technique and duration), so different institutes have devised their own protocols for the process.

Extracorporeal Membrane Oxygenation

After the first successful use of extracorporeal membrane oxygenation (ECMO) in an adult respiratory failure patient was reported in 1972, a number of studies throughout the eighties subsequently reported no difference in outcomes for patients randomised to, or not to, receiving ECMO. Since then, the CESAR trial demonstrated favourable outcomes in patients who underwent ECMO and this has been supported by other studies during the 2009 influenza pandemic.

Proposed criteria for initiating veno-venous ECMO include:

- Acute reversible lung disease when conventional therapy cannot sustain life
- Severe hypoxaemia (PaO_2/FiO_2 ratio <80 mmHg) and/or
- Uncompensated hypercapnia (pH <7.20)

Contraindications include advanced cancer, chronic lung disease, pulmonary fibrosis and ARDS associated with bone marrow transplantation.

Prognosis

Hospital mortality has been reported to be as high as 34.9 per cent for those with mild ARDS, 40.3 per cent for those with moderate ARDS and 46.1 per cent for those with severe ARDS. However, due to the heterogeneity in the underlying pathology and aetiology behind ARDS, huge variations exist.

References and Further Reading

Acute Respiratory Distress Syndrome Network; Brower RG, Matthay MA, Morris A, *et al.* Ventilation with lower tidal volumes as compared with traditional tidal volumes for acute lung injury and the acute respiratory distress syndrome. *N Engl J Med* 2000;**342**:1301–8.

Baig S, Ahmad S, Devogel N, *et al.* Risk factors for the development of acute respiratory distress syndrome (ARDS) in patients with pneumonia, a nationwide retrospective study using the Nationwide Inpatient Sample (NIS) Database from year 2002–2012. *Am J Respir Crit Care Med* 2016;**193**:A1826.

Bellani G, Laffey JG, Pham T, *et al.* Epidemiology, patterns of care, and mortality for patients with acute respiratory distress syndrome in intensive care units in 50 countries. *JAMA* 2016;**315**:788–800.

Guérin C, Reignier J, Richard J-C, *et al.* Prone positioning in severe acute respiratory distress syndrome (ARDS). *N Engl J Med* 2013;**368**:2159–68.

National Heart, Lung, and Blood Institute Acute Respiratory Distress Syndrome (ARDS) Clinical Trials Network; Wiedemann HP, Wheeler AP, Bernard GR, *et al.* Comparison of two fluid-management strategies in acute lung injury. *N Engl J Med* 2006;**354**:2564–75.

Papazian L, Forel JM, Gacouin A, *et al.* Neuromuscular blockers in early acute respiratory distress syndrome. *N Engl J Med* 2010;**363**:1107–16.

Ranieri VM, Rubenfeld GD, Thompson BT, *et al.* Acute respiratory distress syndrome: the Berlin definition. *JAMA* 2012;**307**:2526–33.

Retamal J, Libuy J, Jiménez M, *et al.* Preliminary study of ventilation with 4 ml/kg tidal volume in acute respiratory distress syndrome: feasibility and effects on cyclic recruitment – derecruitment and hyperinflation. *Crit Care* 2013;**17**:R16.

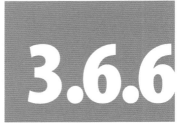

Pulmonary Oedema

3.6.6

Marc Zentar and Kate Tatham

Keywords: pulmonary oedema, cardiogenic pulmonary oedema, non-cardiogenic pulmonary oedema

Definition and Pathophysiology

Pulmonary oedema is a common and potentially fatal cause of acute respiratory failure caused by excess fluid influx into the alveolar space. This occurs owing to alterations in the 'Starling forces' which determine fluid balance between the pulmonary microvasculature and the interstitium, as detailed by the equation in Box 3.6.6.1, for filtration across semi-permeable membranes. Disproportionate changes in hydrostatic pressure or permeability across the membrane can result in flooding of the interstitial and alveolar spaces. Untreated, this may result in significantly impaired gas exchange, hypoxaemia, impaired tissue oxygenation, organ failure and death. However, these changes in net filtration seldom occur in isolation, and it may be more informative, when determining the best management strategy, to define pulmonary oedema as either cardiogenic or non-cardiogenic in origin.

Box 3.6.6.1 Starling's Equation

Net filtration $= k_f [(P_c - P_i) - \sigma(\Pi_c - \Pi_i)]$

Where $k_f =$ filtration coefficient (a product of capillary 'porosity' or permeability and surface area)

P_c and $P_i =$ capillary and interstitial fluid hydrostatic pressures, respectively

Π_c and $\Pi_i =$ capillary and interstitial fluid oncotic pressures, respectively

$\sigma =$ reflection coefficient of proteins across the capillary wall (with values ranging from 0, if completely permeable, to 1 if completely impermeable)

Cardiogenic Pulmonary Oedema

Increases in left ventricular and atrial filling pressures result in a corresponding rise in pulmonary venous and capillary pressures, thus driving protein-poor fluid into the pulmonary interstitium. This increased interstitial pressure drives fluid across the visceral pleura causing pleural effusions, and across the alveolar membrane resulting in alveolar flooding and impaired gas exchange. Compensatory mechanisms to remove fluid from the alveoli, utilising active transport of sodium and chloride ions by type 2 epithelial cells, with water following via aquaporin receptors on type 1 epithelial cells, and increased lymphatic clearance from the interstitium, are unable to compensate for such acute rises in hydrostatic pressure.

Although it is widely recognised that increased hydrostatic pressure represents the primary driving force in cardiogenic pulmonary oedema, it is likely that inability of the pulmonary capillaries to respond to such stressors ('stress failure') also plays a role. This results in permeability changes across the membrane which exacerbates the situation. Furthermore, activation of the renin–angiotensin and sympathetic nervous systems results in tachycardia-mediated shortening of diastolic filling time and increased afterload, which increases myocardial oxygen demand and worsens cardiac ischaemia.

Non-cardiogenic Pulmonary Oedema

Non-cardiogenic pulmonary oedema encompasses a diverse group of conditions, including those driven primarily by increased pulmonary capillary permeability or by alterations in hydrostatic pressures, in the absence of cardiac dysfunction.

Systemic inflammatory states, such as those seen in sepsis or following trauma, may cause direct or indirect lung injury, which impairs pulmonary microvascular permeability. Irrespective of the underlying cause, mediator release (e.g. the cytokines interleukin-1, interleukin-8 and tumour necrosis factor) recruits pro-inflammatory leucocytes to pulmonary microcirculation, contributing to endothelial dysfunction, and thus diffusion of protein-rich fluid into the interstitium. The degree of alveolar flooding depends upon the capacity of the epithelial cells and lymphatic system to remove the fluid, mechanisms that are significantly impaired in acute lung injury.

In other forms of non-cardiogenic pulmonary oedema, increased hydrostatic pressure, in the absence of raised cardiac pressures, results in alveolar flooding and pulmonary capillary stress failure. The most common example of this is neurogenic pulmonary oedema, in which brain injury causes profound sympathetic activation, resulting in pulmonary vasoconstriction and raised capillary pressures. The altered permeability is thought to occur via both direct stress failure and cytokine release, further highlighting the degree of interaction between hydrostatic and permeability changes in these conditions.

Common Causes

Cardiogenic Pulmonary Oedema

- Heart failure with left ventricular systolic dysfunction, in either the presence or absence of other cardiac pathology, e.g. myocardial ischaemia, malignant hypertension or valvular pathology
- Heart failure with diastolic dysfunction, either in the presence or absence of other cardiac pathology, e.g. myocardial ischaemia, malignant hypertension, valvular pathology
- Transfusion-associated circulatory overload (TACO)
- Renal artery stenosis and/or severe renal disease

'Flash' pulmonary oedema is an extension of cardiogenic pulmonary oedema, in which the same pathological processes are in effect, but the progression to severe pulmonary oedema and hypoxia requires rapid treatment and assessment of the underlying pathology. This is typically associated with acute myocardial ischaemic events, acute valvular obstruction, hypertensive crisis or tachy-arrhythmias.

Non-cardiogenic Pulmonary Oedema

- Acute respiratory distress syndrome (ARDS)
- Neurogenic pulmonary oedema
- High-altitude pulmonary oedema
- Opiate toxicity
- Pulmonary embolism (PE) and reperfusion pulmonary oedema (following removal of pulmonary thromboembolic obstruction)
- Re-expansion pulmonary oedema (following rapid re-expansion of a collapsed lung)
- Eclampsia
- Transfusion-related acute lung injury (TRALI)

Assessment and Investigations

History of Presenting Complaint

Presenting clinical features of both cardiogenic and non-cardiogenic pulmonary oedema are similar. Dyspnoea and tachypnoea are often accompanied by hypertension and tachycardia.

The history should focus on typical features of cardiogenic and non-cardiogenic pulmonary oedema:

- For cardiogenic oedema, acute symptoms may include a typical history of myocardial ischaemia (e.g. central crushing chest pain), tachy-arrhythmias (e.g. palpitations) or valvular pathology (e.g. symptoms/signs of bacterial endocarditis). Decompensated chronic heart failure might present with findings of paroxysmal nocturnal dyspnoea, orthopnoea, reduced exercise tolerance and increased peripheral oedema.

239

- Non-cardiogenic oedema features include signs and symptoms of infection, decreased level of consciousness possibly associated with vomiting or seizure activity, trauma, current pregnancy and drug or transfusion history.

Examination Findings

- Examination findings of pulmonary oedema typically include bilateral inspiratory crepitations and rhonchi, with or without signs of pleural effusions.
- On examination, patients with left ventricular systolic dysfunction may have signs of elevated left ventricular end-diastolic volume with an S3 gallop, which is a sensitive, but not specific, sign for cardiogenic pulmonary oedema.
- Patients with valvular pathology may have audible murmurs on auscultation.
- Patients with volume overload and chronic decompensated heart failure resulting in cardiogenic pulmonary oedema will have typical findings such as elevated jugular venous pressure, peripheral oedema and a tender and/or enlarged liver edge.

Investigations

- **Troponin:** measurement is recommended in the 2016 European Society of Cardiology acute heart failure guidelines, and a dynamic and significant rise is suggestive of acute coronary syndrome, especially in the context of corresponding ECG changes or typical cardiac chest pain. Caution should be taken in the absence of these features in critically unwell patients, as troponin may also be raised in other conditions such as sepsis and renal impairment.
- **B-type natriuretic peptide (BNP):** measurement is also recommended in the European Society of Cardiology acute heart failure guidelines. Raised levels correlate well with raised left ventricular end-diastolic pressures; however, in critically unwell patients, positive or intermediate levels should be interpreted with caution. Values of <35 pg/ml (or N-terminal pro-BNP (NT-pro-BNP) <125 pg/ml) have a good negative predictive value.
- **Toxin screen:** may reveal unsuspected ingestion and/or overdose, and should be performed in obtunded patients with pulmonary oedema.
- **Serum amylase/lipase:** should also be performed in obtunded patients with pulmonary oedema where intra-abdominal pathology is being considered.
- **Other blood tests** recommended include renal and liver function tests, electrolytes, thyroid function tests, glucose, full blood count, D-dimer, lactate and **arterial blood gas** analysis.
- **Chest X-ray:** typical cardiogenic pulmonary oedema appearances include cardiomegaly, increased width of the vascular pedicle, central distribution of oedema ('bat-wing' appearance), pleural effusion, septal (Kerley B) lines and peribronchial cuffing. Absence of these findings, with or without a more patchy or uneven distribution of oedema, and air bronchograms are suggestive of non-cardiogenic pulmonary oedema.
- **ECG:** to elicit evidence of, for example, acute cardiac ischaemia, tachy-arrhythmias, left axis deviation or PE.
- **Echocardiography:** two-dimensional transthoracic bedside scans can reliably identify myocardial and valvular pathology, showing raised left ventricular end-diastolic pressures, left ventricular systolic dysfunction, valvular pathology, regional wall movement abnormalities and raised right-sided/pulmonary pressures. Although studies are more challenging in critically unwell patients, they have nevertheless been shown to agree with pulmonary artery catheter measurements.
- **Pulmonary wedge/occlusion pressure measurement:** direct measurements can be done with a pulmonary artery catheter. This allows continuous monitoring of cardiac filling pressures, cardiac output and systemic vascular resistance during treatment (a pulmonary artery wedge pressure of, for example, ≤18 mmHg indicates a non-cardiogenic cause). Although echocardiography has largely replaced pulmonary artery catheter use in evaluating the causes of pulmonary oedema/heart failure, it remains a useful tool if there is diagnostic uncertainty or for continual monitoring in cases with hypotension and hypoperfusion, most commonly in cardio-thoracic intensive care.

Management

Recognition and treatment of the underlying pathology are paramount, and specific management is covered in the respective sections of this textbook. Initial general measures include admission to the high dependency unit, with invasive monitoring and other supportive measures such as oxygen therapy. Early consideration of non-invasive ventilation (NIV) with continuous positive airway pressure (CPAP) or endotracheal intubation and mechanical ventilation is recommended.

In cardiogenic oedema, it is recognised that patients presenting with acute heart failure and hypertension are often euvolaemic or hypovolaemic, due to fluid redistribution. Use of diuretics, over vasodilators, in these patients is associated with increased mortality, the need for mechanical ventilation and myocardial infarction. Pharmacological or mechanical circulatory support may be indicated in severe cases. Patients who remain significantly hypoxic, despite oxygen therapy, should be considered for NIV, as studies suggest prompt CPAP use may reduce mortality, the need for endotracheal intubation and length of critical care stay. For patients with a chronic history of decompensated heart failure, with volume overload, intravenous diuresis should be initiated and targeted against the patient's clinical condition, urine sodium excretion and/or daily weight.

In patients with non-cardiogenic pulmonary oedema who have failed standard oxygen therapy, NIV may be considered; however, there are conflicting data regarding its efficacy and endotracheal intubation should be strongly considered in most cases. In ARDS, the high positive end-expiratory pressure (PEEP) often required for adequate oxygenation may be associated with patient discomfort, and face mask leakage when using NIV. Recent data have suggested that delivery of NIV via a helmet may be an effective alternative, reducing the need for endotracheal intubation and 90-day mortality. In patients who do progress to mechanical ventilation, lung-protective ventilation measures are recommended, as described in the 2018 Intensive Care Society 'Guidelines for management of acute respiratory distress syndrome'.

References and Further Reading

Gandhi SK, Powers JC, Nomeir AM, *et al.* The pathogenesis of acute pulmonary oedema associated with hypertension. *N Engl J Med* 2001;**344**:17–22.

Griffiths MJD, McAuley DF, Perkins GD, *et al.* Guidelines on the management of acute respiratory distress syndrome. *BMJ Open Respir Res* 2019;**6**:e000420.

Patel BK, Wolfe KS, Pohlman AS, Hall JB, Kress JP. Effect of non-invasive ventilation delivered by helmet vs facemask on the rate of endotracheal intubation in patients with acute respiratory distress syndrome: a randomised clinical trial. *JAMA* 2016;**14**:2435–41.

Ponikowski P, Voors AA, Ankers SD, *et al.* 2016 ESC Guidelines for the diagnosis and treatment of acute and chronic heart failure: The Task Force for the diagnosis and treatment of acute and chronic heart failure of the European Society of Cardiology (ESC). Developed with the special contribution of the Heart Failure Association (HFA) of the ESC. *Eur Heart J* 2016;**37**;2129–200.

Vital FMR, Ladeira MT, Atallah AN. Non-invasive positive pressure ventilation (CPAP or bilevel NPPV) for cardiogenic pulmonary oedema). *Cochrane Database Syst Rev* 2013;**5**:CD005351.

Ware LB, Matthay MA. Acute pulmonary oedema. *N Engl J Med* 2005;**353**:2788–96.

3.6.7

Pulmonary Hypertension

Raj Saha

Key Learning Points

1. Pulmonary hypertension (PH) is present when the mean pulmonary arterial pressure is ≥25 mmHg at rest.
2. The World Health Organization classifies PH into five groups.
3. Clinical features of PH may be non-specific, and thus challenging to recognise.
4. Identification and treatment of any potential reversible causes are fundamental to the management of PH.
5. PH is progressive and can be fatal if untreated.

Keywords: pulmonary hypertension, WHO classification, pulmonary arterial hypertension, echocardiography, right heart catheterisation

Introduction

Critical care healthcare professionals may encounter pulmonary hypertension (PH) in an array of different settings. Such settings may involve the management of patients:

- For an acute illness unrelated to their PH
- For an acute illness related to their PH
- With known PH following elective or emergency surgery
- With circulatory collapse after induction of anaesthesia or mechanical ventilation

Critical care management of patients with PH benefits from knowledge of the classification, pathogenesis, clinical features, diagnostic investigations, treatment and prognosis for the condition, as outcome is dependent on these variables.

Classification

PH is present when the mean pulmonary arterial pressure is ≥25 mmHg at rest. The World Health Organization (WHO) classifies PH into the following five groups:

- Group 1: pulmonary arterial hypertension (Box 3.6.7.1)
- Group 2: PH secondary to left heart disease
- Group 3: PH secondary to chronic lung disease and/or hypoxaemia
- Group 4: PH secondary to chronic thromboembolic pulmonary hypertension
- Group 5: PH secondary to unclear multifactorial mechanisms

Causes of Group 1 pulmonary arterial hypertension include those in Box 3.6.7.1.

> **Box 3.6.7.1 Causes of Group 1 Pulmonary Arterial Hypertension**
>
> - Idiopathic pulmonary arterial hypertension
> - Heritable pulmonary arterial hypertension
> - Congenital heart disease (atrial, ventricular and great artery defects)
> - Drugs
> - Toxins
> - Connective tissue diseases (systemic sclerosis, rheumatoid arthritis, systemic lupus erythematosus, Raynaud's disease, mixed connective tissue diseases)
> - Portal hypertension
> - Human immunodeficiency virus
> - Schistosomiasis

Pathogenesis of Pulmonary Hypertension

PH can be categorised by the anatomical location that is affected. These include:

- Pre-capillary pulmonary arteries and arterioles
- Alveoli and capillaries
- Post-capillary pulmonary veins and venules

Idiopathic pulmonary arterial hypertension results from increased vasoconstriction, pulmonary vascular remodelling and thrombosis. Group 3 PH may be caused by vascular destruction and alveolar hypoxaemia. Left ventricular diastolic dysfunction, valvular heart disease and pulmonary venous disorders may lead to pulmonary venous hypertension. PH may be associated with impaired nitric oxide (NO) and prostacyclin production, with resultant impairment of vascular dilation.

Increased pulmonary vascular resistance results from these abnormal molecular and cellular pathways. The resultant impedance to flow leads to right ventricular strain and eventually right ventricular volume and pressure overload.

Clinical Features

These may be non-specific, and thus challenging to recognise. Initial symptoms of PH may result from the inability to adequately increase cardiac output during exercise. Presentation may be with exertional dyspnoea and fatigue. Acute decompensation may occur with cardio-respiratory deterioration upon a background of progressive decline. Patients may present with other concomitant conditions. Pre-operative assessment of patients scheduled for surgery may reveal previously undiagnosed PH. Alternatively, in patients with previously undiagnosed PH, presentation may follow circulatory collapse after induction of mechanical ventilation or anaesthesia. Once severe PH has developed, features of right ventricular failure, such as exertional chest pain, syncope, peripheral oedema, ascites and pleural effusion, may become evident. Physical signs of PH may include those seen in Box 3.6.7.2.

> **Box 3.6.7.2** Physical Signs of Pulmonary Hypertension
>
> - Loud pulmonary component of second heart sound
> - Prominent *a* wave in the central venous pressure
> - Fourth heart sound
> - Left parasternal heave
> - Right bundle branch block
> - Systolic tricuspid regurgitation murmur
> - Systolic ejection murmur
> - Diastolic pulmonary regurgitation murmur

Diagnostic Investigations

Specific diagnostic investigations include:
- Echocardiography
- Right heart catheterisation

With respect to echocardiography in patients with PH, it can be challenging to interpret the asymmetrical shape of the right ventricle, and thus its resultant function. The degree of septal bowing on echocardiography can be quantified by the deformity index, which assesses the degree of right ventricular influence on the left ventricle.

Use of pulmonary artery catheters in patients with severe pulmonary hypertension and right ventricular failure facilitates measurement of atrial pressures, cardiac output and mixed venous oxygen saturations (SvO_2).

The diagnosis of pulmonary arterial hypertension requires right heart catheterisation and the following criteria to be met:
- Mean arterial pressure $\geq$25 mmHg at rest
- Mean pulmonary capillary wedge pressure <15 mmHg
- Absence of chronic lung diseases and other causes of hypoxaemia
- Absence of venous thromboembolic disease

Treatment

The aims of management of PH in the critical care setting include:

1. Treatment of any potential reversible causes and organ support – importantly, interventions used in the critical care setting, such as volume resuscitation, mechanical ventilation and anaesthesia, may worsen haemodynamics in patients with PH

2. Monitoring the response to interventions – the aims of monitoring the response to interventions include evaluation of cardiac function and evaluation of end-organ function

3. Management of right ventricular failure – management of patients with right ventricular failure due to pulmonary arterial hypertension may be complex and may benefit from specialised expertise. In this instance, early referral and transfer to an appropriate tertiary centre should be considered. Any potential reversible cause of right ventricular decompensation should be treated appropriately, and strategies used to improve right ventricular function include optimisation of right ventricular preload, contractility and afterload. The beta-1 receptor agonist dobutamine augments myocardial contractility and reduces right and left ventricular afterload. It may

offer benefit for patients with right ventricular failure. Phosphodiesterase-3 inhibitors, which lack chronotropic properties, may benefit some patients. This may be partly due to the absence of adverse effects of a reduced diastolic filling time secondary to tachycardia

Regarding longer-term management, prostanoid, endothelin receptor antagonists and phosphodiesterase-5 inhibitors may improve survival. This survival benefit, however, may not occur in all subgroups.

Prognosis

PH is progressive and can be fatal if untreated. Prognosis is variable and depends on the aetiology and severity. In general, Group 1 pulmonary arterial hypertension has worse survival than Groups 2 to 5. Severe PH (mean pulmonary arterial pressure ≥35 mmHg and/or right heart failure) has a poor prognosis.

Critical care healthcare practitioners may encounter patients with PH whose reduced cardiac function predisposes them to organ dysfunction or failure. This may include decreased bowel perfusion, loss of intestinal barrier function and bacterial translocation. Poor cardiac function may also lead to kidney or liver dysfunction.

Factors associated with poor prognosis include those seen in Box 3.6.7.3.

Box 3.6.7.3 Factors Associated with Poor Prognosis

- Age >50 years
- Male gender
- World Health Organization functional class 3 or 4
- Failure to improve World Health Organization functional class during treatment
- Right ventricular dysfunction
- Decreased pulmonary arterial capacitance
- Hypocapnia
- Chronic obstructive pulmonary disease

- Diabetes mellitus
- Pulmonary arterial hypertension associated with connective tissue diseases
- Selective serotonin reuptake inhibitors
- Low von Willebrand factor levels
- Bone morphogenetic protein receptor type 2 mutations

Death in patients with pulmonary arterial hypertension is commonly secondary to right heart failure with resultant circulatory collapse and respiratory failure. Circulatory collapse is a risk when mechanical ventilation or anaesthesia is instigated in these patients. Cardiopulmonary resuscitation is rarely successful in patients with pulmonary arterial hypertension.

References and Further Reading

Hoeper MM, Galie N, Murali S, *et al.* Outcome after cardiopulmonary resuscitation in patients with pulmonary arterial hypertension. *Am J Respir Crit Care Med* 2002;**165**:341–4.

Hoeper MM, Granton J. Intensive care unit management of patients with severe pulmonary hypertension and right heart failure. *Am J Respir Crit Care Med* 2011;**184**:1114–24.

Ishikawa S, Miyauchi T, Sakai S, *et al.* Elevated levels of plasma endothelin-1 in young patients with pulmonary hypertension caused by congenital heart disease are decreased after successful surgical repair. *J Thorac Cardiovasc Surg* 1995;**110**:271–3.

Rubin LJ, Hopkins W. Clinical features and diagnosis of pulmonary hypertension of unclear etiology in adults. UpToDate. Waltham, MA: Wolters Kluwer Health. www.uptodate.com/contents/8249

Simonneau G, Gatzoulis MA, Adatia I, *et al.* Updated clinical classification of pulmonary hypertension. *J Am Coll Cardiol* 2013;**62**(25 Suppl):D34–41.

Zamanian RT, Haddad F, Doyle RL, Weinacker AB. Management strategies for patients with pulmonary hypertension in the intensive care unit. *Crit Care Med* 2007;**35**:2037–50.

Anaphylaxis

3.7.1

Claire McCann

Keywords: anaphylaxis, hypersensitivity reactions, tryptase

Key Learning Points

1. Anaphylaxis is an immune-mediated hypersensitivity reaction. 'Non-immune anaphylaxis', previously termed 'anaphylactoid' reactions, can be clinically identical but do not involve sensitisation and immunoglobulin E (IgE) antibody production.
2. Inflammatory mediators released cause vasodilation, increased capillary permeability and smooth muscle contraction.
3. Risk factors exist for particularly severe or fatal reactions.
4. The recommended route for administration of adrenaline is intramuscular.
5. A negative mast cell tryptase result does not exclude anaphylaxis as the diagnosis.

Introduction

Anaphylaxis is a serious, life-threatening generalised or systemic hypersensitivity reaction. Hypersensitivity reactions are immune responses which result in tissue or organ damage. There are five types.

Type 1: Anaphylactic or Immediate

- At sensitisation, B cells are stimulated to produce immunoglobulin E (IgE) antibodies specific to an antigen.
- IgE antibodies bind to receptors on the surface of tissue mast cells and blood basophils.
- On a second exposure, the antigen binds to IgE on mast cell surfaces, triggering degranulation and the release of vasoactive substances, e.g. acute drug reactions, atopy.

Type 2: Antibody-Dependent

- Circulating immunoglobulin G (IgG) or immunoglobulin M (IgM) antibodies bind to antigens on cells, causing activation of complement and phagocytosis, e.g. Goodpasture's syndrome.

Type 3: Immune Complex-Mediated

- Circulating antibodies bind to free antigens to create complexes that activate complement and cause inflammation, e.g. pigeon fancier's lung.

Type 4: Cell-Mediated

- T cells bind to antigens, e.g. graft-versus-host disease.

Type 5: Stimulatory

- Autoantibody binds to a cell surface receptor and stimulates it, e.g. Graves' disease.

'Anaphylactoid reactions' are now termed 'non-immune anaphylaxis' and describe a similar or identical reaction to that of anaphylaxis, but the mechanism does not involve immune activation. They may be caused by drugs that directly cause histamine release (e.g. opioids) or by other mechanisms (e.g. X-ray contrast may activate the complement system).

Mediators and Their Actions

Inflammatory mediators released in an anaphylactic reaction include histamine, tryptase, chemokines, cytokines and those derived from phospholipids (e.g. prostaglandins, leukotrienes, thromboxane A2, platelet-activating factor). The principal effects are vasodilation, increased capillary permeability, increased glandular secretion and smooth muscle contraction.

Aetiology and Risk Factors for Severe or Fatal Episodes

Common causes of anaphylaxis include food products and insect stings – especially in children and young adults. Idiopathic anaphylaxis and reactions to medications become more common in adults. In hospital, triggers commonly include drugs (e.g. antibiotics, anaesthetic agents, chemotherapy agents), blood products, colloids, contrast media and latex. In addition, there are several patient risk factors that predispose to a more severe or fatal reaction, e.g. young or old age, chronic respiratory or cardiovascular disease, mastocytosis, severe atopy, concurrent use of medications such as beta-blockers and angiotensin-converting enzyme inhibitors. Acute intercurrent infections, fever, use of alcohol or non-steroidal drugs and exercise are co-factors that can augment an anaphylactic reaction.

Clinical Features

Presentation of an anaphylactic reaction is variable, but the main features are cutaneous, with skin signs present in over 80 per cent of cases, according to the World Allergy Organization. Additionally, 70 per cent have respiratory involvement and 45 per cent have cardiovascular and gastrointestinal features. The signs and symptoms are detailed in Table 3.7.1.1, according to organ system.

A history of allergy or exposure to a novel antigen will point towards the diagnosis, but in the absence of cutaneous signs on examination, anaphylaxis can be harder to diagnose. The differential diagnosis includes asthma attack or bronchospasm of any cause, ingestion of vasoactive substance, primary cardiac arrhythmia, myocardial infarction, pulmonary embolism, sepsis or, more rarely, hereditary angio-oedema or phaeochromocytoma.

Management

Anaphylaxis is a medical emergency, for which treatment guidelines exist. All possible triggers should be stopped, and the patient should be resuscitated in a systematic ABCDE manner.

First-Line Treatment

Specific treatment with adrenaline should be given as early as possible, at an initial dose of 50 µg intravenously (IV) or 0.5 mg intramuscularly (IM). As IM adrenaline rapidly reaches the central circulation and is associated with easier administration in a non-specialist environment, it is the route of choice for initial administration.

The effects of adrenaline include:

- Alpha-1 receptors: vasoconstriction, restoration of perfusion pressure, decreased airway oedema and improved upper airway obstruction
- Beta-1 receptors: chronotropy and inotropy
- Beta-2 receptors: inhibiting further release of histamine from mast cells and stabilising cell membranes, decreasing urticaria and angio-oedema, bronchodilation

Adverse effects of adrenaline administration are seen with an overdose, and include hypertensive crisis, pulmonary oedema, cardiac arrhythmias and coronary artery spasm.

Second-Line Treatment

There is limited evidence to support the use of other specific treatments for anaphylaxis. This is largely because there are no randomised controlled trials due to the nature of the condition, and recommendations are thus largely based on historical practice and extrapolation from treatment of similar conditions such as asthma. Other medications utilised include the following.

Anti-histamines

These drugs relieve cutaneous symptoms but have no significant effect on life-threatening cardio-respiratory features.

Glucocorticoids

Steroids are given to prevent biphasic anaphylactic reactions and have no benefit during resuscitation.

Table 3.7.1.1 Features of an anaphylactic reaction

System	Features
Cardiovascular	Chest pain, tachy- or bradycardia, arrhythmias, hypotension, cardiac arrest
Respiratory	Bronchospasm, stridor, rhinitis
Cutaneous	Urticaria, flushing, itching, sweating, angio-oedema, oedema, conjunctival injection
Gastrointestinal	Abdominal pain, diarrhoea, nausea and vomiting
Neurological	Feeling of impending doom, loss of consciousness
Other	Metallic taste

Beta-2 Adrenergic Agonists and Phosphodiesterase Inhibitors

On the basis of their usual role in the management of asthma, both classes of drug are useful adjuncts in the treatment of bronchospasm.

Investigation and Follow-Up

Blood levels of mast cell tryptase, and less commonly histamine or antigen-specific IgE, can be measured. Mast cell tryptase levels rise in the first hour after the reaction and stay elevated for up to 4 hours, so clotted blood samples should be taken as soon as is feasible at presentation, at the first hour and then at 24 hours (or in the follow-up allergy clinic) to obtain a baseline measurement. Notably, however, a negative mast cell tryptase result does not exclude anaphylaxis, and all patients should be referred to a specialist clinic for further investigation which may involve skin prick testing or intradermal tests.

Once specific triggers have been identified, long-term management involves strict avoidance of precipitating factors and training in use of an emergency adrenaline injector, i.e. an EpiPen® (= 300 μg adrenaline). For anaphylaxis caused by stinging insects, subcutaneous immunotherapy can hyposensitise the patient to the antigen and protect from subsequent attacks.

References and Further Reading

Harper NJN, Dixon T, Dugué P, *et al.*; Working Party of the Association of Anaesthetists of Great Britain and Ireland. Suspected anaphylactic reactions associated with anaesthesia. *Anaesthesia* 2009;**64**:199–211.

Muñoz-Cano R, Pascal M, Araujo G, *et al.* Mechanisms, cofactors, and augmenting factors involved in anaphylaxis. *Front Immunol* 2017;**26**:1193.

Resuscitation Council UK. 2021. Emergency treatment of anaphylactic reactions: guidelines for healthcare providers. www.resus.org.uk/library/additional-guidance/guidance-anaphylaxis/emergency-treatment

Simons FE, Ardusso LR, Bilo MB, *et al.* World Allergy Organization guidelines for the assessment and management of anaphylaxis. *World Allergy Organ J* 2011;**4**:13–37.

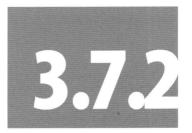

3.7.2 Host Defence Mechanisms and Immunodeficiency Disorders

Claire McCann

Key Learning Points

1. The innate immune system is immediate and non-specific, whilst the adaptive immune system mounts a slower, specific response to pathogens.
2. The complement system can be activated by either the innate or the adaptive immune system.
3. There are five classes of antibody, with variable roles.
4. Primary immunodeficiency disorders are genetic or congenital in origin, are present early in life and are rare.
5. Secondary acquired immunodeficiency is more common and linked to drug treatment, haematological disease, human immunodeficiency virus infection and critical illness.

Keywords: complement, antibodies, innate immunity, adaptive immunity

Introduction

In defence against invading pathogens, the immune system must identify and destroy a wide spectrum of microorganisms quickly, and at the same time avoid causing damage to the host tissues. In order to achieve this, the immune system is composed of both an innate immune response, which provides an immediate reaction to infection (based on pre-programmed recognition of microbe molecular patterns which differ from those of humans), and an adaptive immune response that can respond to specific antigens and retain immunological 'memory'. These two systems are synergistic and complementary, and both are required to be intact to achieve complete host defence. Unfortunately, any element of either of these immune systems may suffer a primary or acquired deficiency, thus leading to one of several immunodeficiency disorders.

The Innate Immune System

The innate immune system is non-specific and consists of anatomical, chemical and cell-based mechanisms (e.g. epithelial barriers, mucociliary escalators, gastric acid, complement proteins in secretions). Cells involved in the innate system are phagocytes such as macrophages, dendritic cells, neutrophils and natural killer cells – all of which are constitutionally present in tissues. When tissues are damaged by infection or trauma, these cells and others release cytokines (e.g. tumour necrosis factor-α and interleukin-1) and chemokines to attract inflammatory mediators and activate the adaptive immune response.

Complement

The complement system consists of a cascade of plasma proteins which result in the production of proteins with specific roles in host defence. It includes:

- C3b – responsible for opsonisation of targets for phagocytosis
- C3a and C5a – mediate chemotaxis and inflammation
- C5–C9 – form the membrane attack complex responsible for lysis of target cells

The cascade can be activated by the presence of bacterial cell wall components, e.g. polysaccharides (in the alternative pathway) or mannose (in the lectin-binding pathway), and this is part of the innate immune response. Alternatively, the classical pathway of complement activation may be initiated by antigen–antibody complexes and this is part of the adaptive immune system.

The Adaptive Immune System

The main functions of the adaptive immune system involve recognition of foreign antigens from 'self', mounting a specific response against those antigens and then retaining memory immune cells. The main component is the lymphocyte, of which there are T and B cell lymphocytes.

T cell lymphocytes are produced in the bone marrow and then travel to the thymus to mature whereby they differentiate into CD8 or CD4 T cells. CD8 T cells are cytotoxic and kill cells infected with microorganisms, and CD4 T cells consist of two types – T-helper 1 and T-helper 2 cells. T-helper 1 cells support cell-mediated immunity, whilst T-helper 2 cells support B cell lymphocytes and antibody production.

T cell lymphocytes are activated when antigen-presenting cells present antigens to them in one of several ways.

- Phagocytic cells in the innate immune system take up and digest exogenous antigens, then migrate to lymph nodes and interact with T cells.
- Infected endogenous cells break down proteins from infecting microorganisms and present them on their surfaces to reveal an infection.

In both cases, the mechanism of antigen presentation is via a cell surface glycoprotein called the major histocompatibility complex (MHC) – also known as human leucocyte antigen (HLA). Exogenous antigens are presented via MHC class II, and endogenous antigens via MHC class I.

B cell lymphocytes form in the bone marrow and migrate to the spleen and lymph nodes to mature. They are activated by contact with either antigen-presenting cells and/or T-helper 2 cells. Some antigens (e.g. toxic shock syndrome toxin-1, lipopolysaccharide) are known as 'superantigens', and these can activate large numbers of lymphocytes directly, causing a massive inflammatory response (e.g. toxic shock syndrome).

Antibodies

Once activated, B cell lymphocytes differentiate into plasma cells and these undergo clonal expansion and secrete antibodies. There are five types:

- Immunoglobulin A (IgA) – produced mainly in mucosa-associated lymphoid tissue (MALT) and prevents colonisation by microbes
- Immunoglobulin D (IgD) – activates basophils and mast cells
- IgM – responsible for acute elimination of microorganisms
- IgG – the major antibody acting against pathogens
- IgE – triggers mast cell degranulation

Antibodies have the following functions:

- Activation of complement via the classical pathway
- Opsonisation and agglutination of antigen for phagocytosis
- Neutralisation of toxins

Immunodeficiency Disorders

Immunodeficiency disorders can be primary genetic disorders or acquired syndromes secondary to another condition. They result not only in susceptibility to certain types of infection, but also to neoplasms, atopy and autoimmunity. Causes of acquired immunodeficiency include:

- B cell deficit or immunoglobulin deficiency due to: drugs (phenytoin, gold), haematological malignancy or protein loss (nephrotic syndrome)
- Cellular deficiency due to: drugs (steroids, immunosuppressants), haematological malignancy or human immunodeficiency virus (HIV) infection
- Combined immunodeficiency due to: haematopoietic stem cell transplant, critical illness, previous splenectomy or hyposplenism (e.g. in sickle cell disease)

Common causes of immunodeficiency and their sequelae can be seen in Table 3.7.2.1.

Table 3.7.2.1 Common causes of immunodeficiency and their sequelae

Immune system deficit	Effect
Complement deficiency: • Congenital C3 deficiency • Acquired persistent activation depletes components, e.g. SLE, chronic infection	• C3 deficiency impairs elimination of encapsulated organisms, e.g. pneumococci • MAC deficiency impairs response to *Neisseria* infection • SLE-like syndrome
B cell disorders: • Common variable immunodeficiency • IgA deficiency • Bruton's X-linked agammaglobulinaemia	• Recurrent bacterial infection, particularly with encapsulated organisms, e.g. *Streptococcus*, *Neisseria*, *Haemophilus*
T cell disorders: • di George syndrome	• Increased susceptibility to intracellular pathogens, e.g. viruses, protozoa, fungi, mycobacteria • Increased incidence of neoplasia
Combined B and T cell disorders: • Severe combined immunodeficiency	• Combined effect of lack of humoral and cell-mediated immunity • Fatal if untreated

249

Table 3.7.2.1 (cont.)

Immune system deficit	Effect
Phagocyte/neutrophil disorders: • Chronic granulomatous disease	• Recurrent pyogenic bacterial infection
Disorders of innate immunity: • Natural killer cell deficiency	• Increased viral and fungal infections

Abbreviations: SLE = systemic lupus erythematosus; MAC = membrane attack complex; IgA = immunoglobulin A.

References and Further Reading

Chaplin D. Overview of the human immune response. *J Allergy Clin Immunol* 2006;**117**:S430–5.

McGoughlin S, Padiglione AA. Host defence mechanisms and immunodeficiency disorders. In: A Bersten, N Soni (eds). *Oh's Intensive Care Manual*, 7th edn. Oxford: Butterworth Heinemann; 2014. pp. 703–9.

Nikita R, Dinakar C. Overview of immunodeficiency disorders. *Immunol Allergy Clin North Am* 2015;**35**:599–623.

3.7.3

HIV and AIDS

Claire McCann

Key Learning Points

1. There are four stages of human immunodeficiency virus (HIV) infection: primary HIV infection with a CD4 count of >500, chronic asymptomatic infection with a CD4 count of >350, symptomatic infections with a CD4 count of <350 and acquired immune deficiency syndrome (AIDS) accompanied by a CD4 count of <200.
2. CD4 T-helper cell lymphocytes are responsible for both adaptive and cell-based immunity, and are active against both infectious disease and neoplasms.
3. There are 27 AIDS-defining clinical conditions specified by the Centers for Disease Control and Prevention.
4. Recent evidence suggests improved outcomes for intensive care patients treated with highly active anti-retroviral therapy (HAART).
5. Intensive care patients not already treated with HAART, with a low CD4 count and an opportunistic infection, are at high risk of immune reconstitution inflammatory syndrome.

Keywords: HIV, AIDS, HAART, immune reconstitution inflammatory syndrome

Aetiology

The human immunodeficiency virus (HIV) is an RNA retrovirus and a member of the subgroup of lentiviruses which cause serious chronic disease characterised by a long ('lenti' meaning 'slow') incubation period. HIV-1 and HIV-2 are two distinct viruses which each have a number of subgroups. HIV-1 is responsible for 95 per cent of global infections, whilst HIV-2 is mainly found in West Africa and is less infectious and associated

with slower disease progression. In 2018, 37.9 million people were living with HIV and there were 1.7 million new infections and 770,000 deaths.

Infection and Natural History

HIV is transmitted via contact with infected blood, semen and pre-seminal, rectal and vaginal fluids. Vertical transmission describes transmission from mother to child, either *in utero*, at delivery or via breast milk. There are four stages of HIV infection, according to the World Health Organization (WHO) classification 2007:

1. Primary HIV infection from 2 to 4 weeks post-exposure, up to 6 months. This may be asymptomatic or associated with acute seroconversion illness. The CD4 count is >500 cells/mm^3 (normal range 500–16,000 cells/mm^3)
2. Chronic asymptomatic infection with a CD4 count of <500 cells/mm^3
3. Symptomatic infections (and opportunistic diseases such as pulmonary tuberculosis), accompanied by symptoms such as persistent generalised lymphadenopathy and chronic diarrhoea. The CD4 count drops to <350 cells/mm^3
4. Development of acquired immune deficiency syndrome (AIDS) with a CD4 count of <200 cells/mm^3

The main target of HIV is the CD4 T-helper cell, to which it binds, enters and then reverse-transcribes its own RNA into DNA in order to use the cell's machinery to replicate and further disperse, thus destroying the CD4 cell in the process. T-helper cells constitute 60 per cent of the body's T cells, and are responsible for helping B cell differentiation in adaptive immunity and cell-mediated immunity alongside macrophages. 'CD4' is a glycoprotein on the cell surface that recognises antigens on antigen-presenting cells, and depletion of CD4 T cell lymphocytes leaves the patient vulnerable to infections and neoplasm.

Acquired Immune Deficiency Syndrome

The diagnosis requires a CD4 count of <200 cells/mm^3 or the presence of one of several 'AIDS-defining clinical conditions' – severe opportunistic infections that reflect the degree to which the immune system has become impaired (Box 3.7.3.1).

Box 3.7.3.1 Centers for Disease Control and Prevention List of AIDS-Defining Clinical Conditions

- Bacterial infections – multiple or recurrent
- Candidiasis of the bronchi, trachea or lungs
- Candidiasis of the oesophagus
- Cervical cancer – invasive
- Coccidioidomycosis – disseminated or extra-pulmonary
- Cryptococcosis – extra-pulmonary
- Cryptosporidiosis – chronic intestinal (>1 month's duration)
- Cytomegalovirus disease (other than the liver, spleen or nodes)
- Cytomegalovirus retinitis (with loss of vision)
- Encephalopathy – HIV-related
- Herpes simplex – chronic ulcers (>1 month's duration) or bronchitis, pneumonitis or oesophagitis
- Histoplasmosis – disseminated or extra-pulmonary
- Isosporiasis – chronic intestinal (>1 month's duration)
- Kaposi's sarcoma
- Lymphoid interstitial pneumonia or pulmonary lymphoid hyperplasia complex
- Lymphoma – Burkitt's
- Lymphoma – immunoblastic
- Lymphoma – primary, of the brain
- *Mycobacterium avium* complex or *Mycobacterium kansasii* – disseminated or extra-pulmonary
- *Mycobacterium tuberculosis* of any site – pulmonary, disseminated or extra-pulmonary
- *Mycobacterium*, other species or unidentified species – disseminated or extra-pulmonary
- *Pneumocystis jirovecii* pneumonia
- Pneumonia – recurrent
- Progressive multifocal leukoencephalopathy
- *Salmonella* septicaemia, recurrent
- Toxoplasmosis of the brain
- Wasting syndrome attributed to HIV

HIV and ICU

HIV patients may be encountered in the ICU either after their first presentation of HIV – classically with critical AIDS-defining illness – or incidentally whilst admitted with other unrelated pathology. Considerations in managing these patients in the ICU include timing and administration of highly active anti-retroviral therapy (HAART) and immune reconstitution inflammatory syndrome (IRIS).

Highly Active Anti-retroviral Therapy

There are six classes of drugs used against HIV, and each targets a step in the viral life cycle. They are:
- Entry inhibitors (e.g. enfuvirtide)
- Fusion inhibitors (e.g. enfuvirtide)
- Nucleoside and nucleotide reverse transcriptase inhibitors (e.g. emtricitabine, lamivudine, tenofovir, zidovudine)
- Non-nucleoside reverse transcriptase inhibitors (e.g. efavirenz, nevirapine)
- Integrase inhibitors (e.g. raltegravir)
- Protease inhibitors (e.g. indinavir, darunavir)

Treatment consists of a combination of three drugs from two or more classes, e.g. Atripla® (= efavirenz, tenofovir and emtricitabine). The goals of treatment are threefold – to suppress plasma HIV viral load, to restore immune function and to reduce transmission. Timing of treatment initiation is debated, but there is recent evidence of improved survival rates in ICU patients treated early on with HAART. Current WHO guidelines state HAART should be initiated in all adults living with HIV, regardless of their CD4 count or stage of disease and, once initiated, treatment should be continued. HAART drugs are generally only available via the enteral route, and this may prove problematic in some ICU patients if they do not have a functioning gastrointestinal tract and absorption. Additionally, medications require dose adjustment in hepatic and renal impairment and they may interact with many commonly used drugs in the ICU. Examples include non-nucleoside reverse transcriptase inhibitors increasing the plasma level of midazolam and protease inhibitors interacting with amiodarone, proton pump inhibitors and histamine 2 receptor antagonists. Serious side effects and toxicity related to HAART include renal impairment (acute and chronic), hepatotoxicity, pancreatitis, lactic acidosis, Stevens–Johnson syndrome and insulin resistance and hyperlipidaemia leading to ischaemic heart disease in the longer term.

Immune Reconstitution Inflammatory Syndrome

IRIS may occur days to weeks after initiation of HAART and recovery of immune function. Upon recovery, the immune system has the ability to respond to previously acquired opportunistic infections, and initiates an inflammatory response to the antigens. Consequently, IRIS may unmask an untreated infection or a previously treated infection may relapse. Examples include *Pneumocystis jirovecii* pneumonia (PJP), tuberculosis (TB) and cytomegalovirus (CMV) infection. IRIS and symptoms of the underlying pathology can be life-threatening, and risk factors include a low CD4 count, the presence of any opportunistic infections and a good response to HAART. The latter is of particular concern, as it means initiating treatment for opportunistic infection in critically ill ICU patients puts them at high risk of IRIS. Management predominantly involves titration of HAART, although steroids may be useful, and this should be guided by an HIV specialist.

Specific Conditions Related to HIV

Pneumocystis jirovecii Pneumonia

Since the advent of HAART, respiratory failure requiring ICU admission is more likely to be secondary to bacterial pneumonia, rather than to PJP. PJP more commonly presents in patients with a CD4 count of <200 cells/mm³, with symptoms of cough, dyspnoea and hypoxia out of proportion to chest X-ray changes. Pneumothoraces are a common feature, and the differential diagnosis of diffuse bilateral infiltrates in HIV infection includes non-infective (pulmonary oedema, pulmonary haemorrhage), infective (typical and atypical bacteria, TB; viral: CMV, influenza; protozoan and fungal) and neoplastic (Kaposi's sarcoma) causes. Diagnosis is via polymerase chain reaction (PCR) of induced sputum or a broncho-alveolar lavage (BAL) sample, and beta *D*-glucan level is raised. First-line treatment is with steroids and co-trimoxazole (Septrin®), and primaquine is second line.

Tuberculosis

TB co-infection with HIV exacerbates and accelerates both diseases. Primary pulmonary infection may present classically with a cough and sputum for >3 weeks, dyspnoea and haemoptysis, or it may be subclinical with few symptoms, thus delaying the diagnosis. Patients with HIV are more likely to have extra-pulmonary TB and are more susceptible to secondary disease due to reactivation or re-infection. Presentations requiring ICU admission may include massive haemoptysis, respiratory failure, pericardial effusions, TB meningitis, small bowel obstruction secondary to tuberculoma and multi-organ failure.

Cryptococcal Meningitis

Cryptococcal meningitis is seen in patients whose CD4 count is <200 cells/mm³. It presents with symptoms of headache, and deterioration in the Glasgow Coma Score (GCS) is secondary to fungal invasion of the meninges. There are no specific signs on CT head imaging, and diagnosis is made on cerebrospinal fluid (CSF) sampling which demonstrates a low white cell count (WCC), low glucose level and moderately raised protein level. A positive India ink stain is associated with *Cryptococcus*, and culture from the CSF confirms the diagnosis. Treatment is with amphotericin B and then fluconazole.

Toxoplasma gondii

Toxoplasma gondii is a protozoan causing infection when the CD4 count is <100 cells/mm³. It presents with symptoms of headache, confusion and reduced GCS. Ring-enhancing lesions are classically seen on CT head imaging, and a plasma sample will be positive for *T. gondii* IgG antibody. Treatment is with pyrimethamine, with dexamethasone added if there are signs of raised intracranial pressure. Notably, the differential diagnosis of intracranial mass lesions in HIV includes primary cerebral lymphoma, tuberculoma or cerebral abscess.

References and Further Reading

Andrade HB, Shinotsuka CR, da Silva IRF, *et al.* Highly active antiretroviral therapy for critically ill HIV patients: a systematic review and meta-analysis. *PLoS One* 2017;**12**:e0186968.

Centers for Disease Control and Prevention. HIV basics. www.cdc.gov/hiv/basics/index.html

HIVinfo.NIH.gov. Clinical guidelines [guidelines on use of anti-retroviral agents in adults and adolescents living with HIV]. aidsinfo.nih.gov/guidelines

Huang L, Quartin A, Jones D, *et al.* Intensive care of patients with HIV infection. *N Engl J Med* 2006;**355**:173–81.

Joint United Nations Programme on HIV/AIDS (UNAIDS). 2019. UNAIDS data 2019. www.unaids.org/sites/default/files/media_asset/2019-UNAIDS-data_en.pdf

3.7.4

Sepsis and Septic Shock

Ravi Bhatia

Key Learning Points

1. Sepsis is defined as life-threatening organ dysfunction caused by a dysregulated host response to infection.
2. A change in the Sequential Organ Failure Assessment (SOFA) score post-infection of 2 or above is taken as a diagnosis of sepsis.
3. Once the diagnosis is made, treatment should be immediate and should involve source control, blood cultures, broad-spectrum antibiotics, 30 ml/kg crystalloid and vasopressors to achieve a mean arterial pressure of >65 and a lactate level of <2.
4. A quick SOFA (qSOFA) score of 2 or more is a bedside test designed to identify those suspected infective patients with higher morbidity and mortality, and should not be used as a diagnostic test for sepsis.
5. A SOFA score change of 2 or more represents an overall mortality risk of approximately 10 per cent.

Keywords: infection, immune response, scoring systems in critical care

Definition

Sepsis is defined as life-threatening organ dysfunction caused by a dysregulated host response to infection. Organ dysfunction is characterised by an increase in the Sequential (Sepsis-related) Organ Failure Assessment (SOFA) score of 2 and above (Table 3.7.4.1), which is associated with in-hospital mortality of >10 per cent.

Severe sepsis is a term previously used to grade severity of illness on a spectrum between systemic inflammatory response syndrome (SIRS) (Box 3.7.4.1) and septic shock. Severe sepsis was consequently defined as an insult due to infection resulting in SIRS and additionally cellular and metabolic dysfunction, hypoperfusion or hypotension. Hypoperfusion and perfusion abnormalities included lactic acidosis, oliguria or an acute alteration in mental state. Increase in severity of cellular organ dysfunction between sepsis, severe sepsis and septic shock, respectively, corresponded to increased mortality.

Pathophysiology

Sepsis is a multifaceted host response to an infecting pathogen that may be significantly amplified by endogenous factors. The specific response is greatly influenced by the causative pathogen (load and virulence) and the host (age, sex, ethnicity, genetics and coexisting illnesses). It is a dysregulated host response and organ dysfunction that differentiate sepsis from infection. The molecular interplay between the exogenous pathogens that results in the host response involves early activation of both pro- and anti-inflammatory responses. Pro-inflammatory reactions (directed at eliminating invading pathogens) are thought to be responsible for collateral tissue damage in severe sepsis. Immune pathways include recognition of pathogen-associated molecular patterns (PAMPs), including microbial cell wall components (e.g. endotoxin) and/or exotoxins (antigenic proteins produced by bacteria). Interaction between these and host immune system leucocytes promotes the production of a wide variety of pro-inflammatory cytokines and endothelium-derived vasoactive mediators. Although beneficial when targeted against local areas of infection or necrotic tissue, dissemination of this 'innate immune' response can produce shock and widespread tissue damage. Anti-inflammatory responses (important for limiting local and systemic tissue injury) are implicated in heightened susceptibility to secondary infections.

These immune responses also result in modifications in cardiovascular, neuronal, autonomic, hormonal, mitochondrial, metabolic and coagulation pathways. For example, initial activation of the coagulation cascade instigates platelet aggregation and widespread microvascular thrombosis and this leads to inadequate tissue perfusion. Additionally, in sepsis, there is a primary defect of cellular oxygen utilisation caused by mitochondrial dysfunction which further worsens this tissue hypoxia. Once clotting factors and platelets are consumed, they are unavailable for haemostasis elsewhere and a coagulation defect results. This heralds the development of disseminated intravascular coagulation (DIC) which often precedes multiple organ failure.

Similar biological responses may be triggered by non-infective pathology, e.g. major surgery and pancreatitis. SIRS is the clinical syndrome that describes this disseminated inflammation.

Clinical Features and Diagnosis

There is currently no single laboratory test or imaging modality that will identify a septic patient. Clinical findings may initially vary, depending on the source of infection. General initial symptoms may be subtle and non-specific, and are easily missed in the elderly and children. They include pyrexia or hypothermia,

nausea and confusion. Signs may include peripheral vasodilation, reduced conscious level, oliguria and hypotension. Bleeding from puncture sites (due to DIC), jaundice, rash, meningism and stupor may indicate more severe sepsis.

SIRS has previously been used to help diagnose sepsis. However, its lack of specificity means it is now being replaced by the SOFA score (Table 3.7.4.1) as a more discriminant marker of organ failure. A SOFA score change post-infection of 2 and above is taken as a diagnosis of sepsis. Those with no previous organ dysfunction have a baseline score of 0. Patients with septic shock can be identified by making a diagnosis of sepsis together with noting persisting hypotension requiring vasopressors to maintain a mean arterial pressure (MAP) of >65 mmHg and having a serum lactate level of >2 mmol/l despite adequate volume resuscitation.

Patients with suspected infection who are likely to have higher morbidity and mortality can be promptly identified at the bedside with a quick SOFA (qSOFA) score of 2 or more (Box 3.7.4.2). A positive qSOFA should lead on to a calculation of the SOFA score to confirm the diagnosis of sepsis. A negative qSOFA score can be easily repeated, should there be a change in the patient's clinical status.

Table 3.7.4.1 Sequential (Sepsis-Related) Organ Failure Assessment score

System	Criteria			Score		
		0	**1**	**2**	**3**	**4**
Respiration	PaO$_2$/FiO$_2$, mmHg (kPa)	≥400 (53.3)	<400 (53.3)	<300 (40)	<200 (26.7) with respiratory support	<100 (13.3) with respiratory support
Coagulation	Platelets, × 10^3/μl	≥150	<150	<100	<50	<20
Liver	Bilirubin, mg/dl (μmol/l)	<1.2 (20)	1.2–1.9 (20–32)	2.0–5.9 (33–101)	6.0–11.9 (102–204)	≥12 (204)
Cardiovascular		MAP ≥70 mmHg	MAP <70 mmHg	Dopamine <5 or dobutamine (any dose)	Dopamine 5.1–15 or adrenaline ≤0.1 or noradrenaline 0.1	Dopamine >15 or adrenaline >0.1 or noradrenabline >0.1
CNS	Glasgow Coma Score	15	13–14	10–12	6–9	<6
Renal	Creatinine, mg/dl (μmol/l)	<1.2 (110)	1.2–1/9 (110–170)	2.0–3.4 (171–299)	3.5–4.9 (300–440)	>5.0 (>400)
	Urine output (μl/day)				<500	<200

Catecholamine doses in micrograms per kilogram per minute.
Abbreviations: PaO$_2$ = partial pressure of oxygen; FiO$_2$ = fraction of inspired oxygen; MAP = mean arterial pressure; CNS = central nervous system.

Box 3.7.4.1 SIRS Features

- Temperature >38°C or <36°C
- Heart rate >90 bpm
- Respiratory rate >20 breaths/min or $PaCO_2$ <4.3 kPa
- White cell count >12 × 10^9/l, <4 × 10^9/l or >10 per cent immature forms

Box 3.7.4.2 qSOFA Criteria

- Respiratory rate >22 breaths/min
- Altered mentation
- Systolic blood pressure <100 mmHg

Investigations and Management

A diagnosis of sepsis is a medical emergency which requires immediate resuscitation and treatment. Although goal-directed protocoled management targeting an MAP of >65 mmHg, central venous pressure (CVP) of 8–12 mmHg (>12 mmHg if mechanically ventilated), urine output of >0.5 ml/(kg hr) and central venous oxygen saturation ($ScvO_2$) ≥70 per cent was previously advocated, recent evidence has demonstrated no mortality benefit to this. This may be because standard care has improved significantly since these were first advocated and their use, alongside the 'Septic Six' (Box 3.7.4.3), should still be considered if thought necessary.

Source control should be implemented as soon as logistically possible. Empirical broad-spectrum antibiotics, aiming at the most likely suspected pathogens, should be delivered as soon as possible, preferably within an hour of diagnosis and ideally after blood (and other relevant) samples have been sent for culture. (Notably, the timing of antibiotic delivery is a matter of recent debate.) Combination therapy using antibiotics of two different classes should be considered,

Box 3.7.4.3 The Septic Six 'Give and Take'

- Give oxygen
- Give intravenous fluids
- Give empirical antibiotics
- Take blood cultures
- Take (measure) serum lactate levels
- Take (measure) urine output

especially for neutropenic sepsis; 30 ml/kg of crystalloid should be given initially to correct hypoperfusion, and further fluid guided by frequent reassessment of the haemodynamic status, including dynamic signs such as response to passive leg raise. Should excessive fluid be required, albumin could be considered as an alternative.

Once a central venous catheter (CVC) line has been placed, CVP and mixed venous oxygen saturation (SvO_2) can be used to guide resuscitation. Noradrenaline should be used as first-line vasopressor, and either vasopressin or adrenaline as second-line agents. Targets for resuscitation include an MAP of >65 mmHg and normalisation of lactate levels. If shock does not resolve quickly, then assessment of cardiac function should be made to determine the aetiology of shock. Hydrocortisone 200 mg daily may reduce vasopressor requirement in refractory septic shock, but it may not affect overall mortality. Antibiotics should be reviewed daily and tailored to the results of cultures and investigations. Glucose management should be protocoled with a target of <10 mmol/l. Renal replacement therapy should not be instated specifically for sepsis.

Outcome

A SOFA score change of 2 or more reflects an overall mortality risk of approximately 10 per cent in a general hospital population with suspected infection. Those diagnosed with septic shock can have a hospital mortality rate in excess of 40 per cent. These figures underline the significance of the condition and the urgency with which treatment should be administered.

References and Further Reading

Angus D, van der Poll T. Severe sepsis and septic shock. *N Engl J Med* 2013;**369**:840–51.

Gyawali B, Ramakrishna K, Dhamoon AS. Sepsis: the evolution in definition, pathophysiology, and management. *SAGE Open Med* 2019;7:1–13.

Howell MD, Davis AM. Management of sepsis and septic shock. *JAMA* 2017;**317**:847–8.

Opal SM, Wittebole X. Biomarkers of infection and sepsis. *Crit Care Clin* 2020;**36**:11–22.

Singer M, Deutschman CS, Seymour CW, *et al.* The Third International consensus definitions for sepsis and septic shock (Sepsis-3). *JAMA* 2016;**315**:801–10.

3.7.5 Multiple Organ Dysfunction Syndrome

Ravi Bhatia

Key Learning Points

1. Multiple organ dysfunction syndrome (MODS) is a complex biological process in which an acute injury leads to sequential organ dysfunction.
2. The pathogenesis of MODS is still poorly understood but thought to be due to a dysregulated pro- and anti-inflammatory response to illness.
3. The clinical features of MODS comprise systemic inflammatory response syndrome plus sequential organ failure over hours or days.
4. To date, no clinical treatments have been shown to be beneficial in specifically treating MODS.
5. Evidence-based supportive care, alongside management of the underlying illness, is the current mainstay of treatment.

Keywords: inflammatory response, sepsis, organ failure, immune dysregulation

Definition

Multiple organ dysfunction syndrome (MODS) is a complex biological process in which an acute disease or injury provokes deterioration and deranged function in a number of organ systems. The term arose after it was noted that pathological specimens from critically ill patients examined post-mortem were similar, irrespective of their admission diagnosis (e.g. demonstrating microvascular thrombi, hepatic necrosis, gastric ulcers, etc.). MODS therefore describes these unifying pathological processes, all of which may lead to organ failure and death.

Pathophysiology

MODS is thought to have an underlying immune basis, with a dysregulated pro- and anti-inflammatory response to illness or injury. Upon injury, there is release of pro-inflammatory mediators, such as interleukin-6 and -8 and tumour necrosis factor (TNF), which gives rise to the systemic inflammatory response syndrome (SIRS) often associated with MODS (Box 3.7.5.1).

Compensatory anti-inflammatory cytokines (e.g. interleukin-4 and -10) are also released to regulate the immune response, and it is thought the disordered interplay between pro- and anti-inflammatory responses leads to either hyper-stimulation of the immune system or immunosuppression.

Immune activation triggers coagulation and neurohumoral and macro- and microcirculatory changes – all of which contribute to functional tissue hypoxia. Activation of the coagulation system, with upregulation of pro-thrombotic factors, promotes microvascular thrombosis. Stress hormones, such as cortisol, may be released, but relative glucocorticoid resistance contributes to blunting of their effect. There is an increased production of the biologically inactive reverse T3, which gives rise to the 'sick euthyroid' condition. Release of vasoactive substances, such as nitric oxide, reduces flow to organs and increases microvascular shunting. Relative capillary endothelial disruption leads to oedema, which compresses capillaries

---

Box 3.7.5.1 Features of Systemic Inflammatory Response Syndrome

- Temperature >38°C or <36°C
- Heart rate >90 bpm
- Respiratory rate >20 breaths/min or $PaCO_2$ <4.3 kPa
- White cell count >12 × 10^9/l, <4 × 10^9/l or >10 per cent immature forms

and further restricts tissue blood flow and oxygen delivery to mitochondria. Whilst beneficial when targeted against local areas of infection or necrotic tissue, this widespread, unchecked immune response produces extensive tissue damage, ultimately progressing to MODS, sequential organ failure and eventually death.

Clinical Features

The main features of MODS include the SIRS criteria, together with a variable course progressing to multi-organ failure over hours or days. Organ failure is usually measured using scoring systems such as the Sequential (Sepsis-Related) Organ Failure Assessment (SOFA) score or the Multiple Organ Dysfunction Score. The latter is based upon specific descriptors in six organ systems (respiratory, renal, neurological, haematological, cardiovascular and hepatic). Each system is scored, and the total score used to predict mortality (Table 3.7.5.1).

Therapies

There are currently no specific therapies that either prevent MODS or modulate its course. The focus of treatment is thus to identify and treat the precipitating condition, thereby preventing

further organ dysfunction with supportive therapy. Immunomodulation has been utilised as potential therapy, since the pro-inflammatory nature of SIRS is an attractive target to modulate MODS. However, when trialled, use of anti-TNF agents in MODS actually led to increased mortality. In a similar manner, endotoxin antibody, non-steroidal anti-inflammatories, interleukin-1 receptor antagonists, platelet-activating factor (PAF) antagonists, bradykinin antagonists, interferon-γ, nitric oxide (NO) synthase inhibition, NO antagonists, anti-thrombin III concentrate and activated protein C have not shown any benefit. This may be because MODS is thought to be due to a dysregulated immune balance, rather than a hyper-stimulated immune response per se.

Outcomes

Whilst no specific treatments have been shown to be beneficial in treating MODS, outcomes seemed to have improved over time, despite an increasingly complex, older cohort of patients navigating through critical care. This may represent a better understanding and treatment of the underlying conditions that lead to the syndrome, or better application of evidence-based supportive care in critical care itself (e.g. using lower tidal volumes to prevent pro-inflammatory cytokine release in ventilated lungs).

References and Further Reading

Marshall JC. Measuring organ dysfunction. *Med Klin Intensivmed Notfmed* 2020;**115**(Suppl 1):15–20.

Ramírez M. Multiple organ dysfunction syndrome. *Curr Probl Pediatr Adolesc Health Care* 2013;**43**:273–7.

Singer M. The role of mitochondrial dysfunction in sepsis-induced multi-organ failure. *Virulence* 2014;**5**:66–72.

Varela ML, Mogildea M, Moreno I, *et al.* Acute inflammation and metabolism. *Inflammation* 2018;**41**:1115–27.

Table 3.7.5.1 Mortality associated with different Multiple Organ Dysfunction Scores

MODS score (points)	Mortality risk (%)
9–12	25
13–16	50
17–20	75
>20	100

Nosocomial Infections

3.7.6

Ravi Bhatia

Key Learning Points

1. Nosocomial infections are acquired during an encounter in a healthcare facility and were not present at the time of admission.
2. Nosocomial infections have significant associated morbidity, mortality and financial costs.
3. The combination of certain patient, organisational and microbial factors encountered in critical care makes it a potential focus for nosocomial infections.
4. The most common nosocomial infections encountered in critical care include ventilator-associated pneumonias, surgical site infections and catheter-associated bloodstream infections.
5. Meticulous hand hygiene, aseptic non-touch techniques and cleanliness are the pillars of preventing nosocomial infections.

Keywords: hospital-acquired infection, iatrogenic patient harm, asepsis, hand hygiene

Definition

A nosocomial infection may be defined as an '[i]nfection acquired during an encounter in a healthcare facility, which was not present or incubating at time of admission'.

Epidemiology

The prevalence of nosocomial infections varies with the institution, ward and patient case-mix. Rates have been reported to be as high as 10 per cent of inpatients in recent times, although the incidence of certain infections is decreasing with rising awareness. Mortality data suggest that nosocomial infections contribute directly to 5000 deaths in the UK every year, and another 15,000 per year indirectly. This does not take into account associated patient morbidity and financial cost to the NHS which is estimated to be approximately £1 billion per year.

In critical care, the most common nosocomial infections encountered include surgical site infections (SSIs), ventilator-associated pneumonias (VAPs) and intravenous catheter-associated bloodstream infection (CABSI). These result in 12, 13 and 14 attributable extra hospital days, respectively.

Risk Factors

Critical care combines certain patient, organisational and microbial qualities, to make it a cauldron for nosocomial infections.

Patients in critical care are often severely ill with multiple pathologies and are relatively nutritionally deplete. They are frequently immunosuppressed, both from the underlying critical illness and also from their administered treatments which may include steroids and blood transfusions. They may have undergone numerous surgical procedures, often necessitating lines, catheters, tubes and drains to be placed into various orifices, and can even be left with open wounds. Their stay may be/have been prolonged, and they may have received multiple courses of potent broad-spectrum antibiotics – all of which allow resistant bacteria to breach the natural defences of the body and subsequently cause nosocomial infections.

In terms of environmental factors which can exacerbate the risk of nosocomial infection, lack of isolation rooms, poor aseptic techniques and cleanliness and workforce shortages can all contribute to the spread of infection.

Microbial Pathogens

The common pathogens implicated in nosocomial critical care infections are shown in Box 3.7.6.1. However, it is known that there will be local variation. There is also dynamism in common organisms affecting a

- Meticillin-resistant *Staphylococcus aureus* (MRSA)
- Coagulase-negative *Staphylococcus*
- *Enterococcus* species
- *Pseudomonas aeruginosa*
- *Acinetobacter baumanii*
- *Stenotrophomonas maltophilia*
- *Enterobacter* species
- *Klebsiella* species
- *Escherichia coli*
- *Serratia marcescens*
- *Proteus* species
- *Candida* species (*C. albicans, C. glabrata, C. krusei*)

particular institution, as this is influenced by both the surgical environment and the patient cohort. In severely immunocompromised patients (e.g. haematological malignancy, HIV), other organisms may be prominent.

Many of the organisms that cause nosocomial infections in critical care are characterised by microbial resistance, and this may have been acquired in one or more of the following ways:

- Enzymatic inactivation of anti-microbials (e.g. β-lactamases)
- Altered drug-binding site (penicillin-binding protein in *Streptococcus pneumoniae* leading to acquired resistance)
- Decreased uptake of drug, either by decreased permeability or upregulated efflux pumps (e.g. penicillins in Gram-negative bacteria)
- Development of novel metabolic bypass pathways
- Overproduction of target site

Specific Infections Seen in Critical Care

Surgical Site Infections

These represent approximately 20 per cent of all nosocomial infections. Prevalence varies from 15 per cent in potentially 'contaminated' surgery (e.g. bowel resection) to up to 40 per cent in surgery where infection already exists.

Preventative measures include:

- Meticulous asepsis, cleanliness and hand hygiene by all perioperative healthcare professionals
- Good surgical technique

- Use of antibiotic prophylaxis – which should be given 1 hour prior to surgical incision to give time for it to reach peak dosage at the time of surgery. A single dose should suffice unless there is prolonged surgery or significant blood loss

Ventilator-Associated Pneumonia

The incidence of VAP is 15–30 per cent in critically ill ventilated patients. VAP is defined as occurring 48 hours post-intubation or within 24 hours of extubation. It may be due to haematogenous spread and/or aspiration. Intubated patients have a higher rate of nosocomial infection than patients receiving non-invasive ventilation, due to bypassing of the natural defences provided by the upper respiratory tract. Factors predisposing specifically to VAP include chronic lung disease, recent surgery to the thorax or abdomen, endotracheal intubation with frequent changes of ventilator tubing, use of nasogastric tubes and bronchoscopy. The relationship between VAP and neutralisation of gastric acid by H_2 receptor antagonists and proton pump inhibitors is still debated.

Causative microbes include Gram-negative organisms such as *Klebsiella* species, *Escherichia coli* and *Pseudomonas* species. In more immunocompromised patients or in those with a delayed onset of VAP (5–7 days post-intubation), meticillin-resistant *Staphylococcus aureus* (MRSA), *Pseudomonas aeruginosa*, *Acinetobacter baumannii* and *Stenotrophomonas maltophilia* are more commonly found.

VAP prevention is often protocolised and involves the principles seen in Table 3.7.6.1.

Treatment involves the combination of broad-spectrum antibiotics against the most likely pathogens – usually with a β-lactam and an aminoglycoside. Given increasing concerns over antibiotic resistance, shorter courses of antibiotics are being advocated (except for specific pathogens, e.g. MRSA or pseudomonal pneumonia).

Catheter-Associated Bloodstream Infection

Fifteen per cent of all nosocomial infections are CABSIs. Central venous catheters (CVCs) have the highest rates of infection. However, all catheters and tubes which breach the patient's skin barrier are an infection risk, and this is proportionate to the length of their use. Specific prevention measures include:

- Meticulous handwashing and aseptic non-touch techniques (ANTTs) during insertion and line use
- Minimising access to lines

Table 3.7.6.1 Principles of ventilator-associated pneumonia prevention

Principle	Involves
To reduce aspiration	• Positioning the patient to 30–45° head up • Regular subglottic suctioning
To diminish contamination of respiratory devices and lower respiratory tract	• Use of closed-loop tracheal suctioning • Changing ventilator circuits at longer intervals • Non-invasive, rather than invasive, ventilation • Orotracheal, rather than nasotracheal, intubation • Heat and moisture exchange filter
To decrease the duration of ventilation	• Sedation holidays • Use of short-acting agents for sedation
To reduce bacterial load	• Selective decontamination of oral or digestive tract[a]

[a] Although shown to help reduce the prevalence of VAP, this may encourage anti-microbial resistance.

- Local antiseptic and sterile dressings
- Frequent inspection of line sites, aided by use of a clear, transparent dressings
- Use of bonded CVCs

Colonisation of intravenous catheters is a common problem and represents a precursor of infection – especially in tunnelled catheters. Organisms implicated include coagulase-negative staphylococci, *Staphylococcus aureus*, *Candida*, Gram-negative pathogens and *Pseudomonas*. The organisms form an extracellular biofilm on the prosthetic material of the catheter, which can be extremely resistant to eradication with antibiotics. Device removal is therefore mandated, with administration of required antibiotics via a new intravenous catheter.

Infection Prevention and Control

Critical care has a crucial role within an institution, to advocate and educate staff on rigorous hand hygiene and ANTT. Effective screening of patients prior to admission, isolation of infectious patients and responsible antibiotic stewardship all assist in reducing the burden of nosocomial infections. In turn, this helps reduce antibiotic use and length of stay, and prevent antibiotic resistance.

References and Further Reading

Centers for Disease Control and Prevention. Healthcare-associated infections (HAIs). www.cdc.gov/hai/index.html

Khan HA, Baig FK, Mehboob R. Nosocomial infections: epidemiology, prevention, control and surveillance. *Asian Pac J Trop Biomed* 2017;7:478–82.

Lyons PG, Kollef MH. Prevention of hospital-acquired pneumonia. *Curr Opin Crit Care* 2018;24:370–8.

Rigby R, Pegram A, Woodward S. Hand decontamination in clinical practice: a review of the evidence. *Br J Nurs* 2017;26:448–51.

Severe Soft Tissue Disorders

3.7.7

Elizabeth Potter, Gabor Dudas and Alexander Fletcher

Key Learning Points

1. Many soft tissue disorders carry high morbidity and mortality.
2. Early diagnosis and rapid definitive management are crucial for a successful outcome.
3. Multidisciplinary working is essential.
4. Consider using isolation rooms to prevent infection if there is significant loss of the skin barrier.
5. In severe cases, admission to the intensive care unit can be beneficial.

Keywords: soft tissue disorders, pressure ulcers, toxic shock syndrome, cellulitis, necrotising fasciitis, toxic epidermal necrolysis, compartment syndrome

Pressure Ulcers

Pressure ulcers are not a severe tissue disorder. However, they are an important cause of largely preventable morbidity in critical care and are estimated to cost the NHS £1.4–2.1 billion annually. A pressure ulcer (or sore) involves the localised destruction of the epidermis, often caused by necrosis secondary to hypoperfusion of the skin overlying a bony prominence. All patients admitted to the ICU should be initially risk-assessed for the presence of pressure ulcers, and subsequently pressure ulcers should be actively sought for on a daily basis during routine examination of patients. Pressure sores can be graded, according to the international National Pressure Ulcer Advisory Panel (NPUAP) and European Pressure Ulcer Advisory Panel (EPUAP) pressure ulcer staging, as seen in Table 3.7.7.1.

Prevention is better than cure, and preventative measures consist of use of an appropriate mattress, regular repositioning, regular skin cleansing, optimisation of nutrition and appropriate incontinence management. Should a pressure ulcer be identified, management should be guided by tissue viability specialist nurses with local knowledge of specialist equipment and facilities. There are numerous different specialised dressings on the market with bacteriostatic properties which serve to promote healing, and sometimes surgical debridement is required. Other techniques of debridement are available, including wet-to-dry gauze application and maggot therapy, and other management options include skin grafts and hyperbaric oxygen.

Table 3.7.7.1 The National Pressure Ulcer Advisory Panel (NPUAP) and European Pressure Ulcer Advisory Panel (EPUAP) staging score for pressure ulcers

Stage	Description
I	Non-blanching erythema
II	Partial thickness
III	Full-thickness skin loss – involving subcutaneous tissue (underlying fascia is intact)
IV	Full-thickness tissue loss – involving underlying bone, tendon, muscle or cartilage

Skin and Soft Tissue Infections

Skin and soft tissue infections (SSTIs) are common and potentially life-threatening. Table 3.7.7.2 outlines a number of these – their causative organisms, key features and management.

Generally, management requires rapid recognition, followed by anti-microbial administration, surgical input and supportive care. Early critical care admission for management of associated shock (and potential multi-organ failure) should be considered, and assistance from microbiology colleagues is essential as there are regional variations in causative organisms and resistances.

Table 3.7.2 Skin and soft tissue infections

Infection type	Predominant pathogens	Characteristic features	Treatment
Impetigo	*Staphylococcus aureus, Streptococcus pyogenes*	Honey-crusted lesions. Less common bullous variant	PO penicillins, first-generation cephalosporins or clindamycin
Ecthyma	*S. aureus, S. pyogenes*	Dry, crusted lesions that involve the dermis and lead to scarring. Predilection for lower extremities	PO penicillins, first-generation cephalosporins or clindamycin. If MRSA suspected, doxycycline, TMP-SMX or clindamycin
Ecthyma gangrenosum	*Pseudomonas aeruginosa, S. aureus, S. pyogenes*; less commonly, other Gram-negative rods, fungi and mould	Cutaneous vasculitis, typically seen between the umbilicus and the knees, and has the potential for rapid increases in size. Erythematous nodules that evolve into necrotic ulcers with eschar	Broad-spectrum antibiotics. Pathogen-directed therapy when culture results available
Purulent skin and soft tissue infections – abscesses, furuncles, carbuncles	*S. aureus*	Pustules surrounded by erythema. Furuncles and carbuncles centred on hair follicles. May exhibit the five cardinal signs of infection – calor, rubor, dolor, tumour and fluor	Incision and drainage. Antibiotic therapy for MRSA in patients meeting SIRS criteria or who are immunocompromised
Cellulitis	Beta-haemolytic staphylococci, *S. aureus*	Diffuse, superficial spreading erythema. May be associated with lymphangitis	**Mild:** PO therapy directed against MSSA and streptococci **Moderate:** as above, consider IV route **Severe:** surgical input. Broad-spectrum antibiotics directed against MRSA, *Pseudomonas* and anaerobes
Pyomyositis	*S. aureus*	Localised pain in a single muscle group with associated fever. Overlying skin may have a 'woody' feel	Surgical input. Vancomycin. Addition of Gram-negative agents if immunocompromised or penetrating trauma
Surgical site infections	Dependent on surgical site	Wound drainage, local inflammation	Surgical input. Anti-microbials dependent on surgical site and severity of illness
Toxic shock syndrome	*S. aureus, S. pyogenes*; rarely, other streptococci	Staphylococcal disease: erythroderma that starts on the trunk and spreads to the extremities (including palms and soles). Streptococcal disease: scarlatiniform rash may be seen	Vancomycin PLUS clindamycin for toxin production OR linezolid monotherapy (limited studies)
Gas gangrene/myonecrosis	*Clostridium* species: *C. perfringens* – trauma-related, *C. septicum* – non-traumatic	Bullae, crepitus	Immediate surgical input. Broad-spectrum agents – vancomycin PLUS piperacillin/tazobactam, an anti-pseudomonal carbapenem OR cefepime PLUS metronidazole
Necrotising fasciitis	Polymicrobial aerobes and anaerobes (type 1), group A *Streptococcus* or *S. aureus* (type II)	Classic finding of pain which is out of proportion to examination. Spectrum from normal external appearance to woody feel of subcutaneous tissues with obliterated fascial planes/muscle groupings	Immediate surgical input. Vancomycin OR linezolid PLUS cefotaxime and metronidazole OR piperacillin/tazobactam

Abbreviations: PO = oral; MRSA = meticillin-resistant *Staphylococcus aureus*; TMP-SMX = trimethoprim/sulfamethoxazole; SIRS = systemic inflammatory response syndrome; MSSA = meticillin-sensitive *Staphylococcus aureus*; IV = intravenous.

Source: Burnham JP, Kirby JP, Kollef MH. Diagnosis and management of skin and soft tissue infections in the intensive care unit: a review. *Intensive Care Med.* 2016;**42**: 1899–1911.

Cellulitis

The most common causative organisms found in cellulitic patients requiring ICU admission are *Staphylococcus aureus*, *Streptococcus pyogenes* and *Escherichia coli*. Patients with cellulitis necessitating admission to intensive care tend to have more co-morbidities, when compared to patients with necrotising fasciitis (NF), and lower Sequential Organ Failure Assessment (SOFA) scores, with a decreased incidence of shock. Interestingly, however, once in intensive care, short- and long-term mortality rates are very similar in cellulitic and NF patients.

Toxic Shock Syndrome

Toxic shock syndrome (TSS) is a fulminant Gram-positive infection, usually secondary to *S. aureus* (SaTSS) or *S. pyogenes* (SpTSS). The annual incidence of SaTSS and SpTSS is 0.5/100,000 and 0.4/100,000, respectively, with mortality rates of <0.5/100,000 for menstrual SaTSS, 5–22 per cent for non-menstrual SaTSS and 30–70 per cent for SpTSS. When treating TSS, it is essential to provide antibiotic cover for resistant organisms. It should be noted that when nafcillin or oxacillin are used as single agents, they can actually increase toxin production, and thus must be used in combination with clindamycin. Clindamycin and linezolid both decrease superantigen production. Intravenous immunoglobulin (IVIG) has been used in treatment and is thought to bind non-specifically to, and then inactivate, super-antigens, thus limiting the cytokine storm. However, the clinical benefits remain disputed.

Necrotising Fasciitis

NF is an aggressive soft tissue injury involving the deep fascial planes, with reported mortality rates of as high as 40 per cent. Traditionally, NF has been split into types 1 and 2 – type 1 signifying infection in an immunocompromised individual (caused by a range of pathogens) and type 2 infections occurring secondary to *S. pyogenes* in otherwise healthy individuals. The differentiation is, however, largely academic as management remains the same.

The 'Laboratory Risk Indicator for Necrotising Fasciitis' (LRINEC) (Table 3.7.7.3) is a scoring system devised to enable early identification of NF and further aids in differentiating NF from simple cellulitis.

Although there have been some studies which have questioned its applicability, a meta-analysis of 16

Table 3.7.7.3 Laboratory Risk Indicator for Necrotising Fasciitis (LRINEC)

Parameter	Range	Score
Hb (g/dl)	>13.5	0
	11–13.5	1
	<11	2
White blood cells (10,000/µl)	<15	0
	15–25	1
	>25	2
Sodium (mmol/l)	<135	2
Creatinine (µmol/l)	>141	2
Glucose (mmol/l)	>10	1
C-reactive protein (mg/l)	>150	4

Source: Bechar J, Sepehripour S, Hardwicke J, Filobbos G. Laboratory risk indicator for necrotising fasciitis (LRINEC) score for the assessment of early necrotising fasciitis: a systematic review of the literature. *Ann R Coll Surg Engl*. 2017;**99**:341–346 and Wong CH, Khin LW, Heng KS, Tan KC, Low CO. The LRINEC (Laboratory Risk Indicator for Necrotizing Fasciitis) score: a tool for distinguishing necrotizing fasciitis from other soft tissue infections. *Crit Care Med*. 2004;**32**:1535–1541.

studies confirmed a statistically significant correlation between the LRINEC score and a true diagnosis of NF. Clinical features include rapidly progressive necrotic soft tissue infection, bullae, pain out of proportion to that expected, tenderness extending beyond the margin of erythema, crepitus, dusky appearance of the skin, cutaneous anaesthesia, shock, lactic acidosis and renal failure. Radiological features include gas visible in soft tissue on plain film and enhancement of deep tissues and inflammation on MRI.

Notably, when NF involves the external genitalia and/or the perineum, it is termed 'Fournier's gangrene' and this is more commonly seen in diabetics, alcoholics or immunocompromised patients.

NF is a surgical emergency, and early source control can be a key determinant of outcome. Anti-microbials (vancomycin or linezolid PLUS cefotaxime and metronidazole OR piperacillin/tazobactam) and supportive care are important. However, rapid debridement is essential to prevent further spread. It is common to return to theatre every 24–48 hours for repeat examination and further debridement, though any clinical deterioration, such as an increase in vasopressor requirement, should expedite this. Hyperbaric oxygen therapy has been used in the management of necrotising soft tissue infections, and has been associated with a statistically significant decrease in mortality in a single-centre observational study when adjusted for other risk factors.

Gas Gangrene/Myonecrosis

Gas gangrene or myonecrosis is caused by the *Clostridium* species. *Clostridium perfringens* is associated with traumatic injuries, *Clostridium septicum* with gastrointestinal malignancies and immunocompromised patients, *Clostridium sordellii* with obstetric cases and *Clostridium perfringens*, *Clostridium novyi* and *Clostridium sordellii* with drug users who 'skin-pop'. Gas gangrene is another surgical emergency and necessitates early surgical consult and debridement, anti-microbials and supportive management. Antibiotic regimes include vancomycin with piperacillin/tazobactam or anti-pseudomonal carbapenem or cefotaxime with metronidazole.

Toxic Epidermal Necrolysis

Toxic epidermal necrolysis (TEN) is a rare, but severe, predominantly drug-induced immune reaction (Table 3.7.7.4), mediated by cytotoxic T cells, leading to keratinocyte apoptosis.

It is characterised by blistering and exfoliation of the epidermis, and in most cases, there is mucosal and ocular involvement. A prodrome of fever, malaise and respiratory symptoms normally precedes eruptions of purpuric macules, which, in time, become confluent, after which blisters appear and leave denuded areas as the epidermis exfoliates. Nikolsky's sign can be demonstrated, whereby the epidermis is easily detached on gentle lateral pressure.

Table 3.7.7.4 Drugs associated with toxic epidermal necrolysis

Category	Therapeutic agents
Anti-epileptics	Carbamazepine Lamotrigine Phenobarbital Phenytoin
Anti-inflammatory agents	Sulfasalazine Non-steroidal anti-inflammatory drugs – oxicam
Anti-microbials	Sulfamethoxazole
Others	Allopurinol

Source: Creamer D, Walsh SA, Dziewulski P, Exton LS, Lee HY, Dart JK, *et al*. U.K. guidelines for the management of Stevens–Johnson syndrome/toxic epidermal necrolysis in adults 2016. *Br J Dermatol*. 2016;**174**:1194–1227.

Table 3.7.7.5 SCORTEN severity scoring tool for toxic epidermal necrolysis

Category	Value	Score
Age (years)	>40	1
Malignancy	Presence of malignancy	1
Heart rate (bpm)	>120	1
Epidermal detachment (%)	>10 (at admission)	1
Serum urea (mmol/l)	>10	1
Serum glucose (mmol/l)	>14	1
Serum bicarbonate (mmol/l)	<20	1

Source: Creamer D, Walsh SA, Dziewulski P, Exton LS, Lee HY, Dart JK, *et al*. U.K. guidelines for the management of Stevens–Johnson syndrome/toxic epidermal necrolysis in adults 2016. *Br J Dermatol*. 2016;**174**:1194–1227.

It may be thought of as a continuum of Stevens–Johnson syndrome (SJS), with SJS involving <10 per cent of the body surface area (BSA), and TEN >10 per cent BSA and epidermal detachment. The overall incidence of SJS/TEN is 1–2 per million per year, with associated mortality rates of <10 per cent for SJS and up to >30 per cent for TEN.

When diagnosing TEN, it is important to take a thorough drug history and to calculate the SCORe of Toxic Epidermal Necrosis (SCORTEN) severity score which enables an estimation of mortality (Table 3.7.7.5). (Increased mortality is seen with each point scored.)

Epidermal loss exceeding 10 per cent BSA requires ICU admission as these cases can quickly progress to multi-organ failure and carry high morbidity and mortality, and isolation is mandatory due to high risk of infection as the skin barrier is lost. Management is generally supportive, with careful fluid balance, analgesia, stress ulcer prophylaxis and electrolyte replacement. A nasogastric tube should be passed, and enteral feeding commenced early. The tumour necrosis factor (TNF)-α antagonist etanercept improved clinical outcome in one randomised controlled trial, compared with the predicted SCORTEN mortality, though the accuracy of the predicted mortality using the SCORTEN model is debated.

Compartment Syndrome

Compartment syndrome classically occurs in the extremities such as the limbs, feet and hands. However, it can occur anywhere in the body where there is a

Table 3.7.7.6 Aetiology of compartment syndrome

	Volume expansion	Expansion limiting
Bones and fractures	Tibial diaphyseal	Casts and occlusive dressings
	Distal radius	Prolonged tourniquet time
	Crush syndrome	Burns
	Forearm diaphyseal	Fluid extravasation
	Femoral diaphyseal	Iatrogenic positioning, e.g. prolonged lithotomy
Vascular and bleeding	Vascular injury	Limb compression
	Coagulopathy/ anticoagulation	
	Ischaemia	
	Reperfusion injury	
	Venous obstruction	
Soft tissue injury	Bites, e.g. snake, insect	
	Drug abuse	
	Penetrating trauma	
Muscular injury	Tetany	
	Prolonged exercise	
	Seizure	
Drugs	Serotonin syndrome	
	Neuroleptic malignant syndrome	

compartment contained by fascial planes. The most common cause involves high-energy fractures; however, multiple other causes exist (Table 3.7.7.6).

Pathophysiologically, localised oedema increases interstitial pressure, which subsequently results in decreased venous drainage, further oedema, neural damage and eventual compromise of the arterial vasculature, thus causing widespread ischaemia and necrosis. Diagnosis is primarily clinical, and symptoms include pain out of proportion to the injury, pain on passive stretching, paraesthesia, prolonged capillary refill time distally and eventually ischaemia with loss of palpable pulses, skin mottling, pallor and myonecrosis. Blood tests demonstrate elevated serum creatinine kinase and lactate levels, and secondary rhabdomyolysis and acute kidney injury can occur.

Compartment syndrome is a limb-threatening condition, and surgical management (fasciotomies) is often required and may be guided by assessment of fascial compartment pressures (obtained using a manometer). As perfusion pressure may be considered as the diastolic blood pressure minus the compartmental pressure, a perfusion pressure of <20 mmHg is an indication for emergency fasciotomy, and <30 mmHg is a relative indication. Non-surgical management is otherwise supportive, involving maintenance of adequate oxygenation, hydration and perfusion pressures, and avoidance of other sequelae.

References and Further Reading

Bechar J, Sepehripour S, Hardwicke J, Filobbos G. Laboratory risk indicator for necrotising fasciitis (LRINEC) score for the assessment of early necrotising fasciitis: a systematic review of the literature. *Ann R Coll Surg Engl* 2017;**99**:341–6.

Burnham JP, Kirby JP, Kollef MH. Diagnosis and management of skin and soft tissue infections in the intensive care unit: a review. *Intensive Care Med* 2016;**42**:1899–911.

Burnham JP, Kollef MH. Understanding toxic shock syndrome. *Intensive Care Med* 2015;**41**:1707–10.

Cranendonk DR, van Vught LA, Wiewel MA, *et al.* Clinical characteristics and outcomes of patients with cellulitis requiring intensive care. *JAMA Dermatol* 2017;**153**:578–82.

Creamer D, Walsh SA, Dziewulski P, *et al.* UK guidelines for the management of Stevens–Johnson syndrome/ toxic epidermal necrolysis in adults 2016. *Br J Dermatol* 2016;**174**:1194–227.

Medical Advisory Secretariat. Pressure ulcer prevention: an evidence-based analysis. *Ont Health Technol Assess Ser* 2009;**9**:1–104.

National Pressure Ulcer Advisory Panel, European Pressure Ulcer Advisory Panel, Pan Pacific Pressure Injury Alliance. 2014. Prevention and treatment of pressure ulcers: quick reference guide. www.epuap.org/ wp-content/uploads/2016/10/quick-reference-guide-digital-npuap-epuap-pppia-jan2016.pdf

Wong CH, Khin LW, Heng KS, Tan KC, Low CO. The LRINEC (Laboratory Risk Indicator for Necrotizing Fasciitis) score: a tool for distinguishing necrotizing fasciitis from other soft tissue infections. *Crit Care Med* 2004;**32**:1535–41.

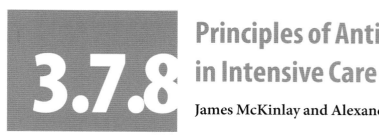

3.7.8 Principles of Antibiotic Use in Intensive Care

James McKinlay and Alexander Fletcher

Key Learning Points

1. Take samples; 'start smart' antibiotics based on the likely organism, then focused cover.
2. If no improvement, consider changing/stopping antibiotics or fungal/viral infection.
3. Short courses are usually sufficient (3–8 days).
4. Infective source control is vital, including potential removal of indwelling lines.
5. Poor use of antibiotics encourages resistant organisms and worsens patient outcomes.

Keywords: antibiotic, pathogens, Gram stain, sepsis, culture

Introduction

Anti-microbials may be anti-bacterial, antiviral, antifungal or anti-parasitic, all of which are covered by the umbrella term 'antibiotics', though generally (and in this chapter), this refers to low-molecular-weight organic solid drugs which kill or slow the growth of bacteria and which originally were derived from microbial metabolites. Antibiotic use is highly prevalent in the ICU, with as many as 71 per cent of ICU patients receiving antibiotics at any given time and around three times as many daily doses per hospital day as an average hospital patient. Selection pressure is high in ICUs, encouraging resistant strains of many organisms. Variability in prescribing practices and changing local microbial populations can contribute to antibiotic resistance. Furthermore, marked pharmacokinetic variability in ICU patients may lead to over- or under-dosing (exacerbating resistance). Sepsis likely affects around 31.5 million people each year globally

and kills around one in four severely septic patients. Appropriate and rational use of antibiotics is therefore critically important.

General Principles of Antibiotic Use in Intensive Care

Prevention of infection and its spread is ideal. Risk factors and reservoirs for infection should be reduced and fastidious hand hygiene remains the key to reducing transmission. Upon suspicion of infection, the following should occur:

- Careful history and examination to identify the likely source, severity and allergy status
- Two sets of peripheral blood cultures and any relevant body fluid specimens should be sent for urgent Gram staining, microscopy and culture and sensitivities. This should ideally be prior to antibiotic administration (otherwise culture sterilisation can occur rapidly) but should not delay lifesaving treatment. Samples should be incubated within 4 hours
- If treatment is deemed necessary, an appropriate empirical antibiotic should be started at an appropriate dose as soon as possible (within 1 hour for sepsis and septic shock). Gram staining may help direct therapy, and local guidelines should be followed
- Source control is vital and should occur as soon as possible (e.g. catheter removal or surgery)
- Other investigations may include appropriate imaging and standard haematology/biochemistry tests, including lactate and inflammatory markers (C-reactive protein (CRP)/procalcitonin) if locally available
- Consider atypical pathogen screening or polymerase chain reaction (PCR) tests for specific pathogens if appropriate

Table 3.7.8.1 Factors to consider when choosing empirical antibiotic therapy

Patient factors	Environmental factors	Organism factors	Drug factors
Likely site of infection	Length of stay >48 hours (HAI risk)	Body site (e.g. blood/tissue/abscess)	Spectrum of activity
Illness severity	Drug-resistant pathogens on unit	Prevalence of local pathogens	Tissue penetration
Co-morbidities	Long-term care resident	Susceptibility	Bactericidal/bacteriostatic
Mechanical ventilation	Recent antibiotics	Local resistance patterns	Side effect profile
Implants/lines/recent surgery	Prior MDR infection	Pathogenicity	Bioavailability (if not intravenous)
Organ dysfunction		Virulence	Pharmacokinetics and dose
Allergy		Intra-/extracellular organism	Monitoring requirement
Immune[a]/nutrition status		Local protocols	Drug–drug interactions

[a] Immune defects include: neutropenia, splenectomy, poorly controlled human immunodeficiency virus, immunoglobulin and complement or leucocyte function or production deficits. All above environmental factors and high illness severity are risk factors for MDR infections.
Abbreviations: HAI = healthcare-associated infection; MDR = multidrug-resistant.

How to Choose an Appropriate Antibiotic

The aim is to give the right antibiotic at the right dose, at the right time and for the right duration. The Department of Health and Public Health England suggest a 'Start smart, then focus' approach under their stewardship programme (see Chapter 4.2, Antibiotic Management and Monitoring). There are many factors to consider when commencing empirical antibiotics (Table 3.7.8.1). Not all the desired information may be available.

Body Site/Likely Pathogens

Pathogenic bacteria may be resident body flora in abnormal environments (e.g. bowel perforation) or they may be acquired (e.g. through exposure to hospital-acquired microbes), especially if immuno-compromised. In the absence of pathognomonic features suggesting specific organisms (e.g. infection with *Clostridium tetani*), appropriate specimen collection and organism definition are the key, though knowledge of common bacteria may be helpful in choosing an appropriate initial antibiotic. Gram-negative infections are more prevalent than Gram-positives (59 versus 49 per cent) in western European ICUs, the five most common organisms being *Escherichia coli*, *Pseudomonas aeruginosa*, *Staphylococcus aureus*, *Staphylococcus epidermidis* and *Klebsiella pneumoniae*. Figure 3.7.8.1 shows some of the more common bacteria found in patients, listing hospital-acquired bacteria where relevant. There is, of course, marked variation and many bacteria are not included. Table 3.7.8.2 lists several genera of bacteria divided by commonly used classification systems, including Gram staining. Table 3.7.8.3 shows commonly used antibiotics, classified according to the site of action and general spectrum of activity.

Rationalising Treatment

Having reviewed available investigations and considered the likely organism (Figure 3.7.8.1), appropriate broad-spectrum therapy should be started (following local protocols or antibiograms) until causative organisms are found and sensitivities performed, upon which therapy can be narrowed or 'de-escalated' accordingly. This may help to minimise 'collateral' damage, i.e. resistance, *Clostridium difficile* infection, side effects and drug interactions. This should be done in close liaison with microbiology/infectious diseases teams and ICU pharmacists. In the absence of positive cultures, continuing broad-spectrum cover for a planned duration may be a reasonable option. Most evidence has found increased mortality if (subsequently proven) inappropriate empirical therapy is started. In haemodynamically stable patients with suspected infection in the ICU, it may be beneficial to have objective evidence of infection prior to commencing antibiotics.

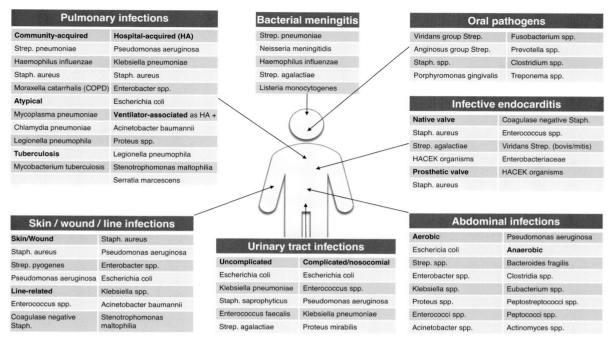

Figure 3.7.8.1 Common potential bacterial pathogens (genera or species) by body site. Viridans streptococci may include: anginosus, bovis, mitis, mutans, salivarius and sanguinis groups. The HACEK organisms are *Haemophilus influenzae, Aggregatibacter actinomycetemcomitans, Cardiobacterium hominis, Eikenella corrodens* and *Kingella kingae*, and account for around 5–10 per cent of non-intravenous drug use-related endocarditis infections. Coagulase-negative staphylococci include: epidermidis, haemolyticus, lugdunensis and saprophyticus. *Enterobacteriaceae* include: *Citrobacter, Enterobacter, Escherichia, Klebsiella, Morganella, Proteus, Salmonella, Serratia, Shigella* and *Yersinia*. Note that fungi may be responsible for infections in any of the above sites. spp. = species; Strep. = *Streptococcus*; Staph. = *Staphylococcus*.

Table 3.7.8.2 Classification of common genera of bacteria by Gram staining, morphology and oxygen requirements

	Morphology	Gram-positive	Gram-negative		
Aerobic/facultative anaerobes	**Bacilli**	***Bacillus*** *Corynebacterium* *Erysipelothrix* *Listeria* ***Nocardia***	*Burkholderia* *Campylobacter* *Citrobacter* *Eikenella* *Enterobacter* *Escherichia* *Helicobacter*	*Klebsiella* ***Legionella*** *Morganella* *Proteus* ***Pseudomonas*** *Rickettsia* *Salmonella*	*Serratia* *Shigella* ***Stenotrophomonas*** *Vibrio* *Yersinia*
	Coccobacilli		*Acinetobacter* *Aggregatibacter* *Bordetella*	*Brucella* *Chlamydia*[a] *Coxiella*	*Haemophilus* *Kingella*
	Cocci	*Enterococcus* *Staphylococcus* *Streptococcus*	*Moraxella* *Mycoplasma*[a] ***Neisseria***		
	Spirochaetes		*Borrelia*[a]	*Leptospira*[a]	*Treponema*[a]
Anaerobic	**Bacilli**	***Actinomyces*** ***Clostridium*** *Eubacterium* *Lactobacillus*	***Bacteroides*** ***Fusobacterium*** ***Porphyromonas*** ***Prevotella***		

Table 3.7.8.2 (cont.)

Morphology	Gram-positive	Gram-negative
Cocci	*Anaerococcus* **Peptostreptococcus**	*Acidaminococcus* *Megasphaera* **Veillonella**

[a] These organisms are difficult to, or do not, Gram-stain but are generally classified as Gram-negative. Organisms in bold are obligate aerobes/anaerobes. The list is generalised and not exhaustive. There is also some overlap; for example, *Streptococcus* species may be aerobic, facultative anaerobes or strict anaerobes and rickettsiae are pleomorphic. Mycobacteria are aerobic (or facultative anaerobes) but do not Gram-stain, though they have similarities to both groups. *Aggregatibacter, Campylobacter, Eikenella, Haemophilus* and *Neisseria* species may be capnophilic (increased growth in the presence of 5% carbon dioxide). *Chlamydia, Coxiella* and *Rickettsia* species are obligate intracellular pathogens.

Table 3.7.8.3 Commonly used antibiotics, general spectrum of activity and site of action

Spectrum	Gram activity	Site of antibiotic action				
		Cell wall	Protein synthesis	Nucleic acid synthesis	Folate synthesis	Cell membrane
Broad	**Both**	**Cefuroxime** **Amoxicillin** **Cefepime**[a] **Meropenem**[a] **Ertapenem** **Ceftriaxone** **Ceftazidime**[a] **Piperacillin**[a] **Nitrofurantoin**	Linezolid Clarithromycin Azithromycin Doxycycline Tigecycline **Gentamicin**[a] **Amikacin**[a] **Tobramycin**[a] Chloramphenicol	**Rifampicin** **Moxifloxacin** **Ciprofloxacin**[a] **Levofloxacin**[a] Nitrofurantoin	Sulfamethoxazole	
Narrow	**Positive**	**Flucloxacillin** **Meticillin** **Vancomycin** **Teicoplanin**	**Virginiamycin** **Quinupristin**	Fusidic acid		**Daptomycin**
	Both	**Penicillin G/V** **Cefalexin**	Clindamycin **Streptomycin**	**Metronidazole**	Trimethroprim	
	Negative	**Aztreonam**[a] **Temocillin** **Clavulanic acid** **Tazobactam**[b]				**Polymyxin B**[a] **Polymyxin E**[a] **(colistin)**

The broad/narrow classification is largely arbitrary, but conceptually useful. The position of an antibiotic in the 'both' rows relates loosely to a relatively greater degree of Gram-positive or negative cover. Antibiotics in bold are bactericidal, as opposed to bacteriostatic, though some bacteriostatic drugs may be bactericidal in some settings/doses (e.g. chloramphenicol, clindamycin, nitrofurantoin, linezolid). Choosing bactericidal drugs is more important in neutropenic/aplastic patients and in infective endocarditis.

[a] These antibiotics can be anti-pseudomonal, though resistance is possible.

[b] Clavulanic acid, sulbactam and tazobactam have weak intrinsic activity and are used in combination as β-lactamase inhibitors. Anti-tuberculous drugs (isoniazid, ethambutol, pyrazinamide) are specific to mycobacteria and are variably bacteriostatic or bactericidal. This is a rough guide only and local protocols should be followed.

A Note on Blood Cultures

Blood culture positivity rates are generally low at around 10 per cent (varying with infection locus), rising to 30–40 per cent in septic shock (the positivity rate of all microbiological samples is higher). Around 20–56 per cent of positive results may be contaminants. Early and repeated positivity of cultures is suggestive of true infection. Blood cultures taken from central lines at insertion have been shown to have higher contamination rates (8 per cent) than arterial line (at insertion) (3 per cent) and peripheral cultures (4 per cent), possibly due to skin flakes/dermal contamination. However, true pathogens were identified in 12 per cent of central line cultures versus 10 per cent for arterial line cultures and 8 per cent for peripheral cultures, which may be related to the volume taken for samples. For suspected line infections, cultures should be drawn both from the line and peripherally and demonstrate the same pathogen (e.g. with differing times to positivity) for confirmation. The timing of blood cultures is debated. A temperature 'spike' may be a marker of infection and trigger investigations for infection. However, temperature 'spikes' typically follow 1–2 hours after bacteraemia and there are many other potential causes for pyrexia (and some patients may not mount pyrexia). It would thus appear unnecessary to restrict culture sampling to times of raised temperature. The technique, number of cultures and volume of blood are likely more important factors in detecting bacteraemia.

Dose

Choosing the appropriate dose of antibiotics in critically ill patients is not straightforward. It is likely that many patients are under- and/or overdosed due to inherent and acquired variability in drug pharmacokinetics in this population. Local protocols and critical care microbiologists/pharmacists can aid decisions. Dosing and pharmacokinetics are covered in more detail in Chapter 3.7.9, Mechanism of Action and Activity of Commonly Used Antibiotics. Intravenous to oral 'switch' may occur if the patient is improving, the enteral route is available, oral bioavailability of the drug is high (e.g. clindamycin, linezolid, ciprofloxacin, metronidazole, rifampicin, clarithromycin) or there is a suitable alternative.

Timing and Duration

Early commencement of antibiotics is recommended, especially in sepsis and septic shock. Retrospective evidence suggested a 7.6 per cent survival decrease for each hour's delay in antibiotics in septic shock. However, as long as therapy for sepsis is given within 6 hours, the optimal time is not yet clear, nor is the point at which the 'clock' starts. Antibiotic course duration should generally be short (e.g. 3–8 days), depending on the clinical situation and response to therapy (see Chapter 3.7.9, Mechanism of Action and Activity of Commonly Used Antibiotics), except in specific circumstances, e.g. spontaneous bacterial endocarditis, osteomyelitis, necrotising fasciitis, tuberculosis, lung/brain/liver abscess, bacteraemia with *S. aureus*,

undrainable infection loci and possibly ventilator-associated pneumonia caused by non-lactose-fermenting Gram-negative bacilli (e.g. *Pseudomonas*, *Serratia*, *Stenotrophomonas*). Biomarkers such as macrophage-secreted procalcitonin (e.g. using a cut-off of <0.5 ng/ml in ICU patients and ≤0.25 ng/ml for respiratory infections) may be helpful in aiding antibiotic stop decisions, reducing the course duration. A recent Cochrane review found evidence to be of low to moderate quality and did not clearly support this approach, though it appears safe and likely cost-effective.

Reasons for Failure of Antibiotic Therapy

Treatment success may be difficult to determine, e.g. in patients with ongoing inflammatory states (e.g. pancreatitis or burns). Treatment may only appear to have failed in some cases (e.g. with drug-induced or centrally mediated pyrexia) or may, in fact, have failed (i.e. unresponsive infections). Failure may be multifactorial in origin and reasons include:

- Organism is susceptible to an antibiotic in vitro, but antibiotic is ineffective in vivo
- Inadequate spectrum of activity of antibiotic therapy
- Antibiotic resistance
- Inadequate target site drug levels
- Inadequate tissue/target site penetration
  - For example, cerebrospinal fluid, bone, prostate, ocular, biofilms on invasive lines
  - Reduced blood supply, e.g. osteomyelitis
  - Inactivation in tissues, e.g. daptomycin in the lung
- Drug–drug interactions (especially with drugs metabolised by cytochrome P450 system)
- Infected foreign bodies not removed or source control not achieved
- Non-infectious cause of fever, e.g. drug-induced, systemic lupus erythematosus
- Viral or fungal cause of infection

Monotherapy/Combination Antibiotic Therapy

There is debate over the use of monotherapy or combination therapy. Combination therapy may be appropriate:

- If agents exhibit synergistic activity against an organism:
  - For example, penicillin and gentamicin for *Enterococcus*-related infective endocarditis
  - Be aware of the risk of increased toxicity potential (e.g. penicillin and gentamicin)
- To extend the spectrum for likely/proven polymicrobial infections:
  - For example, cephalosporin and metronidazole for abdominal infections
- As empirical therapy in septic shock (until shock resolves)

In general, however, monotherapy is preferable and leads to reduced cost, fewer prescription/administration errors, fewer drug interactions and lower risk of antibiotic antagonism (e.g. penicillins and tetracyclines). It may help to reduce resistance, though in cases of multidrug-resistant (MDR) organisms (e.g. MDR tuberculosis), combinations may limit selection of resistant strains.

Acknowledgements

The authors would like to thank James Clayton, Consultant Microbiologist, for all his help with this chapter.

References and Further Reading

Covington EW, Roberts MZ, Dong J. Procalcitonin monitoring as a guide for antimicrobial therapy: a review of current literature. *Pharmacotherapy* 2018;**38**:569–81.

Cunha B, Hage J, Schoch P, Cunha C, Bottone E, Torres D. Overview of antimicrobial therapy. In: CB Cunha, BA Cunha (eds). *Antibiotic Essentials*, 11th edn. Sudbury, MA: Jones & Bartlett; 2012. pp. 2–15.

Lamy B, Dargère S, Arendrup MC, Parienti J-J, Tattevin P. How to optimize the use of blood cultures for the diagnosis of bloodstream infections? A state-of-the-art. *Front Microbiol* 2016;**7**:697.

Leekha S, Terrell CL, Edson RS. General principles of antimicrobial therapy. *Mayo Clin Proc* 2011;**86**:156–67.

Vincent J-L, Rello J, Marshall J, *et al.* International study of the prevalence and outcomes of infection in intensive care units. *JAMA* 2009;**302**:2323.

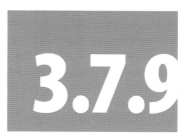

3.7.9 Mechanism of Action and Activity of Commonly Used Antibiotics

James McKinlay, Alexander Fletcher and Armine Sefton

Key Learning Points

1. Different antibiotics work through different mechanisms.
2. Resistance to antibiotics is of great concern.
3. Selecting the right antibiotics to target the identified organism is the primary goal.
4. The majority of available antibiotics work by inhibiting either cell wall formation or nucleic acid (DNA/RNA) synthesis of the organism.
5. Cross-reactivity in penicillin-allergic patients to carbapenems is around 1 per cent.

Keywords: selective toxicity, mechanism of action, spectrum, antibiotic resistance

Introduction

Antibiotics should destroy or inhibit bacterial cells, leaving host cells intact, i.e. they should exhibit selective toxicity. Bacteria have a number of features which can be targeted by antibiotics to kill or inhibit the growth of specific bacteria. All bacteria, except *Mycoplasma*, have a peptidoglycan cell wall – a feature missing from mammalian cells. This is used in Gram staining, named after Hans Christian Gram, for classifying bacteria. Gram-positive bacteria have a higher peptidoglycan and a lower lipid content in their cell wall and retain the purple stain. Gram-negative bacteria have a thinner cell wall, but an additional outer membrane consisting of lipopolysaccharide and proteins, which gives further protection against antibiotic entry, but the presence of porins allows a route in for some (small, hydrophilic) drugs. Aerobic or facultative anaerobic organisms possess enzymes capable of breaking down toxic products of oxygen metabolism, e.g. superoxide or hydrogen peroxide. Anaerobic organisms lack these enzymes and do not grow/perish in the presence of oxygen.

Antibiotics can be classified by structure, mechanism of action or spectrum of activity. The majority of antibiotics act by inhibiting either the bacterial cell wall or protein or nucleic acid synthesis. Some specific antibiotics, classified by chemical structure, are discussed in more detail below. Pharmacokinetic notes are provided below each section.

Cell Wall Inhibitors

Beta-Lactams (Penicillins, Cephalosporins, Carbapenems, Monobactams)

These compounds all contain a four-membered cyclic amide ring. They bind to various penicillin-binding proteins (PBPs) on bacteria, inhibiting cell wall peptidoglycan cross-linking. Beta-lactamases, which differ between Gram-positive and -negative bacteria, may inactivate the ring through hydrolysis.

Penicillins

- Contain a β-lactam/thiazolidine ring structure and one modifiable side-chain
- Often used with a β-lactamase inhibitor (e.g. clavulanic acid or tazobactam) to extend the spectrum of activity
- Benzylpenicillin is active against streptococci, *Neisseria* species and spirochaetes
- Flucloxacillin is mainly anti-staphylococcal but is also effective in high doses against beta-haemolytic streptococci
- Amoxicillin is active against streptococci, *Enterococcus faecalis* and some Gram-negative bacteria. Its spectrum of activity is improved by the addition of a β-lactamase inhibitor which gives it anti-staphylococcal activity and activity against the majority of β-lactamase-producing coliforms and most anaerobes
- Piperacillin is active against both Gram-positive and Gram-negative bacteria, including *Pseudomonas* species, but is inactivated by

273

β-lactamases unless combined with a β-lactamase inhibitor such as tazobactam which increases its activity against coliforms, staphylococci and anaerobes

- Temocillin is stable to most β-lactamases, but only active against Gram-negative bacteria
- Allergy is reported in 10 per cent of patients; however, approximately 90 per cent of these patients do not have immunoglobulin E (IgE) antibodies on testing

Pharmacokinetic Notes. Plasma half-lives are generally short. Protein binding is very variable. Tissue penetration is good – inflammation increases bone/blood–brain barrier penetration.

Cephalosporins

- Contain a β-lactam/dihydrothiazine ring structure and two modifiable side-chains
- Generally broader spectrum than penicillins (unless these are combined with β-lactamase inhibitors), but all lack enterococcal activity
- Improved Gram-negative, but generally less Gram-positive cover with increasing generations (1–3); for example, ceftazidime is highly active against most Gram-negative bacteria, including *Pseudomonas* species, but has minimal activity against streptococci and staphylococci
- Most cephalosporins have good activity against *Enterobacteriaceae* species, excluding extended-spectrum β-lactamase (ESBL)-producing coliforms. Cefuroxime, cefotaxime and ceftriaxone also have good activity against streptococci and staphylococci but are inactive against *Pseudomonas* species
- Cross-reactivity in skin prick-positive, penicillin-allergic patients is around 2–3% per cent
- May predispose to *Clostridium difficile*/vancomycin-resistant enterococci (VRE) infection

Pharmacokinetic Notes. Plasma half-lives generally short, except ceftriaxone which can be used once a day. Cefotaxime, ceftriaxone and ceftazidime penetrate the cerebrospinal fluid (CSF) well. Protein binding variable.

Carbapenems/Monobactams (Meropenem, Imipenem, Ertapenem/Aztreonam)

Carbapenems are very broad-spectrum. They are active against streptococci, staphylococci, most Gram-negative bacteria, including Ambler class C (AmpC) and ESBL producers, and anaerobes. Imipenem and meropenem both have reasonable activity against *Pseudomonas aeruginosa*, but ertapenem does not.

- Inactive against *Chlamydia*, *Legionella* and *Mycoplasma* species, meticillin-resistant *Staphylococcus aureus* (MRSA), *Stenotrophomonas maltophilia* and *Enterococcus faecium*. Moderate activity against *Enterococcus faecalis*
- Imipenem may cause seizures in seizure-prone patients
- Aztreonam has anti-Gram-negative activity only, including against *Pseudomonas* species, and is generally thought safe in penicillin allergy
- Cross-reactivity in penicillin-allergic patients to carbapenems is about 1 per cent.

Pharmacokinetic Notes. Renally cleared. Time-dependent killing. Minimally protein-bound.

Glycopeptides (Vancomycin, Teicoplanin)

These are naturally occurring large heterocyclic molecules. They bind to acyl-*D*-alanyl-*D*-alanine in peptidoglycan, preventing cell wall growth. They are given intravenously (IV) (except when oral vancomycin is used to treat pseudomembranous colitis). Vancomycin has to be given by slow IV infusion to prevent histamine release and 'red man syndrome', whereas teicoplanin can be given by slow IV injection.

- Active against streptococci and staphylococci, including MRSA. No activity against Gram-negative bacteria
- Excessive use of glycopeptides predisposes patients to VRE
- Some coagulase-negative staphylococci are less susceptible to teicoplanin than to vancomycin. Some VRE may be susceptible to teicoplanin

Pharmacokinetic Notes. Blood level monitoring needed to ensure adequate clearance/therapeutic levels.

Inhibitors of Protein Synthesis

Both mammalian and bacterial cells use ribosomes for protein synthesis. However, there exist sufficient differences between ribosomal structure and access to various targets to allow the use of antibiotics which may otherwise affect mammalian cells. Animals and fungi have 80S (Svedberg units of sedimentation rate) ribosomes, consisting of 60S and 40S subunits, whereas bacteria have 70S ribosomes, with 30S and 50S subunits, both of which may be targets for antibiotics.

Aminoglycosides (Gentamicin, Amikacin, Tobramycin, Streptomycin)

Aminoglycosides bind to the 30S subunit, blocking transfer ribonucleic acid (tRNA) attachment. Derived from either *Micromonospora* or *Streptomyces* species, these are large polar, linked rings of amino sugars and amino-substituted cyclic polyalcohols.

- Active against most Gram-negative bacteria, including *Pseudomonas* species and most staphylococci, but very limited activity against streptococci/enterococci unless used in combination with a β-lactam or a glycopeptide when they act synergistically
- Resistance is usually mediated through aminoglycoside-modifying enzymes
- Active transport into cells is required and is inhibited by calcium and magnesium ions, acidosis and hypoxia
- Nephrotoxicity is usually reversible and related to age. Ototoxicity is usually permanent
- Can increase the potency of non-depolarising muscle relaxants

Pharmacokinetic Notes. Low lipid solubility. Not absorbed orally. Concentration-dependent killing. Low protein binding. Poor cell/CSF/sputum concentrations. Excreted unchanged in the urine. Levels needed due to narrow therapeutic index.

Tetracyclines/Glycyclines (Doxycycline, Minocycline/Tigecycline)

These are polycyclic aromatic hydrocarbons, originally derived from *Streptomyces aureofaciens*. They bind to the 30S ribosomal subunit, blocking tRNA to messenger ribonucleic acid (mRNA) binding. Broad anti-Gram-positive (including MRSA) and negative activity (except against *Proteus* and *Pseudomonas* species). Also active against spirochaetes, some anaerobes and *Rickettsia*, *Chlamydia*, *Mycoplasma* and *Legionella* species.

- Resistant strains of *Enterobacteriaceae* species and streptococci increasing
- Tigecycline is IV only. It is sometimes used for treating hospital-acquired pneumonia, and multi-resistant and complicated skin/abdominal infections

Pharmacokinetic Notes. Tigecycline has poor plasma levels and is not normally recommended as monotherapy for bacteraemia.

Macrolides/Azalides (Clarithromycin, Erythromycin/Azithromycin)

These are 14- to 16-membered large lactone ring structures with various substitutions and attached sugars. They bind to the 50S ribosomal subunit, stimulating the dissociation of the peptide chain from the ribosome during elongation. Macrolides/azalides, lincosamides and the streptogramin B group of antibiotics (MLSB) are related in mechanism, and cross-resistance is likely.

- Have good anti-staphylococcal and anti-streptococcal activity. Often used in penicillin-allergic patients. Resistance is common in staphylococci and increasing in streptococci
- Also active against 'atypical' and intracellular bacteria (*Mycoplasma pneumoniae*, *Chlamydia* and *Legionella* species), some mycobacteria and *Campylobacter* species
- Azithromycin has improved Gram-negative cover over erythromycin/clarithromycin and can be used for treating typhoid
- Useful for respiratory tract and soft tissue infections
- Risk of prolonged QT interval; greatest with erythromycin and lowest with azithromycin

Pharmacokinetic Notes. Good tissue penetration. Azithromycin has a long half-life.

Lincosamides (Clindamycin)

Derived from *Streptomyces* species. It binds the 50S ribosomal subunit, preventing translocation and peptide elongation.

- Active against most Gram-positive aerobic cocci, except enterococci
- Effective against many Gram-positive and negative anaerobes
- May cause *C. difficile* toxin-induced diarrhoea
- Reduces the toxin-producing effects of *S. aureus* and *Streptococcus pyogenes*

Pharmacokinetic Notes. CSF penetration is poor. Bone/joint penetration is good. Highly protein-bound, widely distributed.

Streptogramins A/B (Dalfopristin/Quinupristin)

- Consisting of an unsaturated lactone peptide ring structure and a cyclic depsipeptide, they are only effective in combination. They alter the tRNA binding site and the peptide extrusion site, blocking protein synthesis. Used widely in Europe – not in the UK
- Active against aerobic Gram-positive organisms, including resistant staphylococci (MRSA) and *E. faecium* (*E. faecalis* is resistant)
- Limited degree of anaerobic cover

Nitrobenzenes (Chloramphenicol)

A peptidyl transferase inhibitor which reversibly binds to the 50S ribosomal subunit to prevent peptide bond formation and protein elongation.

- Active against many Gram-positive and -negative bacteria, including *Streptococcus pneumoniae*, *Neisseria meningitidis*, *Haemophilus influenzae* and anaerobes
- Useful for treating brain abscesses. Not useful for hepato-biliary (inactive metabolite in bile) or urine infections (low concentrations)
- Resistance is increasing
- Used mainly for treating serious infections where other agents are not appropriate due to side effects of bone marrow suppression (either dose-related and reversible or idiosyncratic and irreversible)

Pharmacokinetic Notes. Excellent CSF penetration. Excreted in bile as inactive metabolite.

Oxazolidinones (Linezolid)

These are heterocyclic molecules with oxygen and nitrogen in a five-membered oxazolidinone ring bridged by a carbonyl group. They have a unique mechanism of action. Linezolid binds to the 50S ribosomal subunit, preventing the formation of a 70S initiation complex and subsequent translation.

- Covers Gram-positive aerobes (including *Nocardia* and *Listeria* species) and some anaerobes, including *C. difficile* and *Bacteroides fragilis*
- Useful against VRE, MRSA and penicillin-resistant *S. pneumoniae* (PRSP)
- Reduces the toxin production of *S. aureus* and *S. pyogenes*
- Resistance low

- Cross-resistance with other protein synthesis inhibitors does not appear to occur
- Reversible bone marrow suppression may occur, especially if used for over 2 weeks. It has monoamine oxidase inhibitor effects and increases the risk of serotonin syndrome

Pharmacokinetic Notes. Well absorbed orally. Hepatic elimination – no renal dose adjustment. Can be used for central nervous system (CNS) infections. Good lung penetration.

Inhibitors of Nucleic Acid Synthesis

Fluoroquinolones (Ciprofloxacin, Levofloxacin, Ofloxacin, Moxifloxacin)

These are heterocyclic molecules with a four-quinolone core and various substituents, including fluorine at C-6. They are not derived from bacteria. They bind either to DNA gyrase and/or topoisomerase IV (required for DNA supercoiling) and result in cell death due to inhibition of DNA replication and repair.

- Broad anti-Gram-negative activity, including enteric pathogens, chlamydiae and meningococci. Also active against *Mycoplasma* species. Have some anti-Gram-positive activity. The only oral anti-microbials active against *Pseudomonas* species
- 'Respiratory quinolones' – levofloxacin and moxifloxacin – have excellent bioavailability and improved activity against *S. pneumoniae*/*S. aureus*, compared to ciprofloxacin, but are somewhat less active against Gram-negative bacteria, including *Pseudomonas* species
- Ciprofloxacin may reduce the seizure threshold

Pharmacokinetic Notes. Usually renal excretion. Excellent tissue penetration.

Nitroimidazoles (Metronidazole)

The 5-nitroimidazole group of imidazoles are ring structures with anti-bacterial and anti-protozoal activity. The mechanism is unclear but targets anaerobes as unionised metronidazole is taken up by anaerobic organisms, forming an active, charged reduction product, which induces DNA strand breakage, inhibiting DNA synthesis and repair and causing cell death.

- Covers most common anaerobes and protozoa (which exhibit anaerobic metabolism)
- Covers some Gram-negative micro-aerophiles, including *Helicobacter* species

- Metronidazole is an alternative to oral vancomycin for *C. difficile*-related colitis

Pharmacokinetic Notes. Hepatic elimination, but needs dose adjustment in renal failure. Does not bind to plasma proteins. Distributes widely in the brain, prostate, pleural fluid and cerebral abscesses.

Folic Acid Synthesis Inhibitors

Sulphonamides/Diaminopyrimidines (Sulfamethoxazole/Trimethoprim (Co-trimoxazole))

Bacteria use para-aminobenzoic acid (PABA) to synthesise folate. Sulphonamides, consisting of a sulphonyl and amine group, liberate sulphanilamide, a PABA analogue which competes for dihydropteroate synthase, inhibiting the synthesis of folate. Diaminopyrimidines, consisting of a pyrimidine ring structure with two amine groups, inhibit dihydrofolate reductase, which would otherwise aid the synthesis of tetrahydrofolate from dihydrofolate. The two agents act synergistically, lowering the required concentrations of each to inhibit bacterial growth.

Co-trimoxazole has activity against staphylococci, some streptococci, *Listeria* and *Nocardia* species and Gram-negative bacilli, including *Escherichia coli*, *Klebsiella*, *Proteus*, *Serratia* and *Stenotrophomonas* species, but is inactive against *Pseudomonas* species and anaerobes.

- Co-trimoxazole is used for the treatment and prophylaxis of *Pneumocystis jirovecii* pneumonia
- Trimethoprim is used on its own for treating lower urinary tract infections
- The sulphonamide component is usually responsible for any allergy/side effects

Pharmacokinetic Notes. Good tissue/CNS penetration. Excellent bioavailability.

Inhibitors of Membrane Function

Cyclic Lipopeptides (Daptomycin)

Derived from *Streptomyces roseosporus*, daptomycin is a 13-membered amino acid cyclic polypeptide with a decanoyl side-chain. It binds to the bacterial membrane and causes calcium-dependent potassium efflux and rapid depolarisation/cell death.

- Active against Gram-positive cocci, including staphylococci, streptococci and enterococci, including MRSA and VRE
- Reserved for difficult-to-treat skin/soft tissue infections, bacteraemia and endocarditis
- Requires the presence of free calcium to function
- Ineffective for pneumonias due to inactivation/calcium-dependent sequestration by surfactant

Pharmacokinetic Notes. Highly protein-bound. Low volume of distribution.

Cyclic Polypeptides (Colistin)

Derived from *Paenibacillus polymyxa*, these are pentacationic polypeptides with a fatty acid (hydrophobic) tail. The cationic polypeptide is attracted to the negatively charged lipopolysaccharide and displaces calcium/magnesium ions from the membrane, disrupting the membrane and causing leakage of cell contents and cell death in a detergent-like process.

- Active against most Gram-negative aerobic bacilli/coccobacilli, including *Acinetobacter baumanni*, *Enterobacteriaceae* species, including ESBL, and some carbapenemase-producing bacteria and *P. aeruginosa*
- Non-selective effect means compounds are potentially toxic, including causing nephrotoxicity, neurotoxicity and bronchoconstriction

Pharmacokinetic Notes. Not absorbed through the gastrointestinal tract. Administered as a pro-drug. Poor CNS penetration.

References and Further Reading

Cunha B, Torres D, Hage J, *et al.* Antibiotic pearls and pitfalls and antimicrobial drug summaries. In: CB Cunha, BA Cunha (eds). *Antibiotic Essentials*, 11th edn. Sudbury, MA: Jones & Bartlett; 2012. pp. 507–718.

Greenwood D, Finch R, Davey P, Wilcox M. General properties of antimicrobial agents. In: D Greenwood, R Finch, P Davey, M Wilcox (eds). *Antimicrobial Chemotherapy*, 5th edn. Oxford: Oxford University Press; 2008. pp. 13–67.

Kapoor G, Saigal S, Elongavan A. Action and resistance mechanisms of antibiotics: a guide for clinicians. *J Anaesthesiol Clin Pharmacol* 2017;**33**:300.

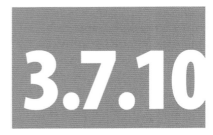

3.7.10

Antibiotic Prophylaxis, Resistance and Future Directions

James McKinlay and Alexander Fletcher

Key Learning Points

1. Antibiotic prophylaxis is used to prevent imminent/future infection.
2. Mostly importantly, it is used when a surgical implant is necessary.
3. A single dose can affect the gut flora and result in resistance.
4. Resistance to antibiotics is an ongoing problem.
5. New avenues are being trialled to reduce the problem of antibiotic resistance.

Keywords: resistance, prophylaxis, nano-antibiotics, phage, bacteria

Antibiotic Prophylaxis

Surgical antibiotic prophylaxis is now well established. It forms part of the World Health Organization's surgical safety checklist and is contained in the Scottish Intercollegiate Guidelines Network (SIGN) and National Institute for Health and Care Excellence (NICE) guidelines. The number needed to treat (NNT) to avoid infection varies by operative site (e.g. NNT = 4 for colorectal surgery, and 19 for Caesarean section). A recent meta-analysis found that surgical site infections are increased when prophylaxis is administered either >2 hours before or after incision. There was no overall difference if given within the 2-hour window. There may be procedure- or antibiotic-specific variation, however, and local guidelines should be followed. Commonly, they are given within an hour of skin incision, bearing in mind infusion duration (e.g. vancomycin). Prophylaxis should target the likely pathogenic bacteria which may proliferate following procedures. It should be given in the following situations:

- Surgery is clean but involves prosthesis implantation

- Clean-contaminated or contaminated surgery:
  - For example, high load of commensal bacteria introduced into the blood
- Surgery on dirty or infected wounds
- Consider for patients at high risk of infection, e.g. if immunocompromised

Prophylaxis may be repeated intraoperatively for prolonged procedures (e.g. longer than the antibiotic's half-life) or if massive haemorrhage occurs. Treatment of active sepsis should continue, but there is no evidence for ongoing 'prophylaxis' post-operatively for clean or clean-contaminated surgery. Even single-dose prophylaxis may lead to increased levels of resistant organisms.

Selective decontamination of the digestive tract (SDD) or selective oral decontamination (SOD) have been found to reduce infection rates and mortality in the ICU, with SDD appearing more effective than SOD. However, concerns primarily over Gram-negative bacterial resistance to, for example, aminoglycosides and colistin, have significantly limited uptake of these techniques.

Prophylaxis for dental procedures for infective endocarditis (IE) may be appropriate in specific patient groups, e.g. patients with previous IE, prosthetic heart valves or prosthetic repairs, cyanotic heart disease or prosthetically repaired congenital heart disease (for 6 months after or lifelong if residual shunt or regurgitant valve). Prophylaxis may include amoxicillin or clindamycin, but local guidance should be sought.

Antibiotic Resistance

Antibiotic resistance is increasing and is one of the world's greatest health threats, according to the World Health Organization. Resistance is an inherent and natural phenomenon in environmental bacteria; however, selection pressures in healthcare settings encourage resistance. Poor antibiotic management accelerates resistance, but effective antibiotic stewardship programmes (including strict hand hygiene) can help to reduce the spread of resistant organisms (see Chapter 4.2, Antibiotic Management and Monitoring).

Effectiveness of antibiotics in vivo relates to the intrinsic activity against the organism and the drug concentration at the infection locus (which is affected by the dose, route and site of infection). Multiple factors affect tissue penetration of drugs (see Chapter 4.2, Antibiotic Management and Monitoring). The same bacterium may be susceptible in one body site, but resistant in others if adequate concentrations cannot be achieved. Intrinsic resistance (or non-susceptibility) refers to the innate ability of a bacterium to resist an antibiotic's action (e.g. *Pseudomonas aeruginosa* has intrinsic resistance to flucloxacillin). Acquired resistance is less predictable and more worrying, but is usually agent-, not class-, specific. Some bacteria appear more prone to developing resistance than others. Relative resistance suggests organisms may be susceptible at higher, but achievable, antibiotic concentrations. Absolute resistance cannot be overcome with increasing doses. Resistance may be effective across multiple related agents via a single mechanism (cross-resistance) or against multiple unrelated agents (multiple resistance). It occurs in both Gram-positive and Gram-negative organisms.

Acquired resistance occurs through:

- Chromosomal mutations (single large-step or multi-step): occurrence of random base-pair alterations may confer resistance and then be selected when non-resistant organisms are killed by antibiotics
- Transmissible resistance: resistance genes are transferred to non-resistant bacterial cells. This occurs through transfer of plasmids or by bacteriophages (viruses which infect bacteria). Plasmids may confer resistance to several antibiotics

Resistance is effected through (examples of antibiotics affected given below each mechanism):

- Target modification (changing the antibiotic target site):
  ○ Aminoglycosides, fluoroquinolones, macrolides, penicillins, rifamycins, vancomycin
- Efflux (pumping antibiotics out of the bacterial cell):
  ○ Aminoglycosides, β-lactams, fluoroquinolones, macrolides, tetracyclines

- Immunity (antibiotics are bound by proteins, preventing binding to target sites):
  ○ Sulphonamides, tetracyclines, trimethoprim, vancomycin
- Enzyme-catalysed destruction (modifying the functional part of antibiotics):
  ○ Aminoglycosides, β-lactams, macrolides, rifamycins

Risk factors for drug-resistant organisms are noted in Table 3.7.10.1. In addition, overuse of broad-spectrum drugs, with unnecessarily long courses (including prophylaxis), repeated use of certain antibiotics and treating culture results, not the disease, may tend to select out resistant organisms. Infection with a resistant organism is associated with a worse prognosis, even if treated appropriately (possibly related to at-risk patient group characteristics). Table 3.7.10.1 lists some of the potentially resistant organisms seen in the ICU, along with antibiotic susceptibility information.

Future Directions

Point-of-care testing aims to reduce the time to diagnosis of pathological organisms. Various technologies are under assessment and may substantially reduce the need for prolonged broad-spectrum treatment.

There are a few new antibiotics on the horizon, including solithromycin (a macrolide), omadacycline and eravacycline (derived from tetracyclines), fifth-generation cephalosporins (in use in some countries), tedizolid (an oxazolidinone) and avibactam (a β-lactamase inhibitor), amongst others.

Nebulised antibiotics for ventilator-associated pneumonia (e.g. tobramycin, amikacin, colistin, aztreonam) may reduce systemic toxicity but carry practical challenges and must be non-pyrogenic, pH-adjusted, isotonic and preservative-free. Faecal transplantation for *C. difficile* infection and monoclonal antibodies for pseudomonal infection may prove useful.

Nano-antibiotic therapy, using nanoparticles of high surface area-to-volume ratios, may reduce resistance by electrostatically binding to the bacterial cell wall and catalysing the production of reactive oxygen species, inducing cell death without the need to enter the cell.

Lantibiotics, such as nisin, are bacteriocins which are lanthionine-containing peptides produced by Gram-positive bacteria with anti-microbial activity. They exhibit various forms of activity, including cell wall inhibition. They are potentially active against resistant Gram-postive bacteria, such as meticillin-resistant

Table 3.7.10.1 Resistance groups/bacteria of concern in intensive care

Acronym and name of group or organism	Examples of potentially resistant bacteria	Comments/resistance/sensitivity suggestions
Gram-positive bacteria		
GRE/VRE Glycopeptide/vancomycin-resistant enterococci	*Enterococcus faecium/faecalis*	Poorly pathogenic usually. Can be line/catheter-related or abdominal source. Consider ampicillin for *E. faecalis*. Otherwise consider tetracycline, cefipime, chloramphenicol, rifampicin or linezolid
MDR-Cdiff Multidrug-resistant *Clostridium difficile*	*C. difficile*	Anaerobic infection selected out following aerobic infection treatment, e.g. with clindamycin, cephalosporins, ciprofloxacin. May be resistant to clindamycin, fluoroquinolones, imipenem and rifampicin. Metronidazole- and vancomycin-resistant strains have been found but are still rare
PR-SP/MDR-SP Penicillin/multidrug-resistant *Streptococcus pneumoniae*	*S. pneumoniae*	Risk factors include prior antibiotics (e.g. macrolides) and smoking. Can be resistant to β-lactams (including carbapenems) (not via β-lactamases), macrolides, clindamycin, tetracyclines, Septrin® and fluoroquinolones. Consider above after testing or linezolid, tigecycline and daptomycin
MR-CNS Multi-resistant coagulase-negative staphylococci	*Staphylococcus epidermidis/haemolyticus/saprophyticus/lugdunensis*	Especially if indwelling prosthetic material. Forms biofilm. May be contaminant. *S. haemolyticus* may be resistant to glycopeptides. Consider vancomycin, linezolid, tigecycline, rifampicin, gentamicin, daptomycin ± combinations
MRSA/VRSA Meticillin/vancomycin-resistant *Staphylococcus aureus*	*S. aureus*	May secrete Panton–Valentine Leukocidin (PVL) toxin. May be sensitive to glycopeptides (not VRSA), clindamycin, rifampicin, fusidic acid, Septrin®, gentamicin + β-lactam. Consider linezolid, daptomycn, tigecycline, quinupristin or dalfopristin
Gram-negative bacteria		
AmpC Ambler class C β-lactamase	*Klebsiella pneumoniae, Escherichia coli, Proteus mirabilis, Enterobacter* spp.	Group C plasmid-mediated β-lactamase/cephalosporinase. Resistant to ceftriaxone, ceftazidime, clavulanic acid and aztreonam. Not inhibited by β-lactamases. Sensitive to fourth-generation cephalosporins/carbapenems. Consider temocillin
CPE Carbapenemase-resistant *Enterobacteriaceae*	*K. pneumoniae, E. coli*	Group A or B (metallo-β-lactamases or MBL) β-lactamases, e.g. *K. pneumoniae* carbapenemase (KPC), New-Delhi-Metallo-β-lactamase (NDM-1). Consider colistin, tigecycline, aminoglycoside ± combination therapy
ESBL Extended-spectrum β-lactamases	*K. pneumoniae, E. coli, Pseudomonas* spp., *Acinetobacter* spp.	Plasmid-mediated group A β-lactamases. There are many β-lactamase enzymes with differing activity (e.g. cefotaximase-Munich (CTX-M)). Affect Gram-negative organisms only (including coliforms/most *Enterobacteriaceae*, *Acinetobacter* and *Pseudomonas*). ESBLs resist third-generation cephalosporins. May be sensitive to β-lactamases. Sensitive to carbapenems. Consider temocillin
MDR-AB/XDR-AB Multi/extensively drug-resistant *Acinetobacter baumannii*	*A. baumannii*	Ambler class A–D β-lactamases can be present. Carbapenem-resistant. Previous carbapenem, third/fourth-generation cephalosporin or piperacillin/tazobactam exposure are risk factors. Clean environment. Consider colistin, tigecycline, sulbactam or ampicillin/sulbactam, glycopeptide ± combinations
Multi-resistant *Pseudomonas*	*Pseudomonas aeruginosa*	Has intrinsic resistance with AmpC β-lactamases and efflux pumps. Readily acquires resistance, even during treatment. May be β-lactam-, carbapenem-, fluoroquinolone- and aminoglycoside-resistant. Consider carbapenem with aminoglycoside or fluoroquinolone
Stenotrophomonas	*Stenotrophomonas maltophilia*	Related to *Pseudomonas*. Forms biofilm on foreign material. May be upper airway coloniser. Intrinsic β-lactam and aminoglycoside resistance. Consider Septrin®, levofloxacin or minocycline. Possibly tigecycline, colistin or ceftazidime
Mycobacterium		
MDR-TB/XDR-TB Multi/extensively drug-resistant tuberculosis	*Mycobacterium tuberculosis*	MDR resistant to isoniazid and rifampicin. XDR also resistant to fluoroquinolone and one of amikacin, kanamycin or capreomycin

Staphylococcus aureus and vancomycin-resistant *Enterococcus*, but are not in current use in humans.

Phage therapy, whilst not new, is seeing a resurgence of interest. It involves the use of lytic or lysogenic viruses (phages) to enter and destroy bacterial cells. It is attractive in that it does not rely on traditional anti-bacterial agents and can be highly specific, effective and safe and phages are modifiable. However, ongoing research is needed before standard clinical use is warranted.

References and Further Reading

Berríos-Torres SI, Umscheid CA, Bratzler DW, *et al.* Centers for Disease Control and Prevention guideline for the prevention of surgical site infection, 2017. *JAMA Surg* 2017;**152**:784.

de Jonge SW, Gans SL, Atema JJ, Solomkin JS, Dellinger PE, Boermeester MA. Timing of preoperative antibiotic prophylaxis in 54,552 patients and the risk of surgical site infection: a systematic review and meta-analysis. *Medicine (Baltimore)* 2017;**96**:e6903.

Greenwood D, Finch R, Davey P, Wilcox M. Resistance to antimicrobial agents. In: D Greenwood, R Finch, P Davey, M Wilcox (eds). *Antimicrobial Chemotherapy*, 5th edn. Oxford: Oxford University Press; 2008. pp. 119–69.

Vincent J-L, Bassetti M, François B, *et al.* Advances in antibiotic therapy in the critically ill. *Crit Care* 2016;**20**:133.

Wright GD. Q&A: Antibiotic resistance: where does it come from and what can we do about it? *BMC Biol* 2010;**8**:123.

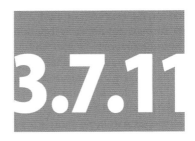

Anti-fungal Therapies

James McKinlay and Alexander Fletcher

Key Learning Points

1. Invasive fungal infections are associated with high mortality.
2. The majority of fungal infections are opportunistic in nature.
3. Resistance to anti-fungal agents is rare and difficult to detect.
4. *Candida* species are the most common cause of fungal infections.
5. Blood cultures have a low sensitivity for detecting fungaemias.

Keywords: anti-fungal, *Pneumocystis*, azoles, polyenes, echinocandins

Introduction

Unlike bacteria, fungi are eukaryotes, so anti-bacterials are mostly ineffective and anti-fungal agents may be toxic to the patient. Cellular differences exist, however (e.g. fungi use ergosterol, rather than cholesterol), which allow for anti-fungal selectivity.

Fungi may be classified as yeasts (e.g. *Candida albicans*, *Cryptococcus neoformans*), filamentous fungi (moulds) (e.g. *Aspergillus fumigatus*, *Mucorales*) or dimorphic fungi (either yeasts or filamentous fungi) (e.g. *Histoplasma capsulatum*, *Coccidioides immitis*, *Blastomyces dermatitidis*, *Paracoccidioides brasiliensis*, *Penicillium marneffei*). *Pneumocystis jirovecii* is a yeast-like fungus.

Candida is part of the normal flora of the skin, oropharynx, intestine and vagina, though each form is controlled by distinct immune mechanisms. *P. jirovecii* may be found normally in the upper respiratory tract. These, along with *Aspergillus* species (spp.) (in soil/airborne) and *Cryptococcus* spp. (from decaying wood/pigeon droppings), are opportunistic pathogens, causing illness when host defences are compromised. The dimorphic fungi are primary pathogenic fungi and generally originate from the soil.

Invasive fungal infection/systemic mycoses account for around 9–12 per cent of all bloodstream infections and are associated with prolonged ICU stay and high attributable mortality rates of around 10–49 per cent. *Candida* spp. account for the majority of invasive fungal infections and these are mostly *C. albicans* (around 56–60 per cent), though other species may carry higher crude mortality rates (e.g. *Candida glabrata*). The majority of candidaemias may be acquired whilst in the ICU, though only 5–30 per cent of colonised ICU patients develop candidaemia. Fungal infection should be suspected if pyrexia persists despite antibiotic treatment or when no other cause can be found, especially in the presence of risk factors (Table 3.7.11.1). Blood cultures have low sensitivity for fungi (*P. jirovecii* does not grow in culture) but, if grown, should not be assumed to be contaminants. *Candida* spp. grown in both urine and respiratory cultures together may indicate invasive infection. C-reactive protein (CRP) levels may be raised and can be as high as levels seen in bacterial infections. Fungal antigen levels, e.g. galactomannan (for *Aspergillus* and *Penicillium* spp.), mannan (for *Candida* spp.) and beta D-glucan (for *Candida*, *Aspergillus* and *Pneumocystis* spp.), and polymerase chain reaction tests may help guide the diagnosis.

The general principles of investigation/treatment are similar to those for antibiotic use; however, courses of treatment may be longer (e.g. for 2 weeks after clearance of candidaemia), so frequent blood culture sampling is recommended to monitor fungaemia. Fungaemia should also prompt ophthalmological examination within a week or a week after recovery from neutropenia. Evidence is limited for empirical systemic anti-fungal therapy, and there are many potential side effects and drug interactions (e.g. with statins, warfarin, calcium channel blockers, benzodiazepines, cyclosporine). However, treatment should not be delayed in

Table 3.7.11.1 Risk factors for invasive fungal infection

Pre-existing illness	Immunosuppression	Illness-related	Foreign material	Procedure-related	Other factors
Haematological malignancies	HIV with low CD4 count	Trauma/burns	Invasive lines	Ventilation/long ICU stay	Extremes of age
Diabetes	Neutropenia (especially >10 days)	Severe acute pancreatitis	Stem cell/organ transplant	Renal replacement therapy	Genetic predisposition
COPD	Prolonged corticosteroid use	Gastrointestinal surgery	Pathogen exposure, e.g. soil	Total parenteral nutrition	Recent antibiotic use

Abbreviations: HIV = human immunodeficiency virus; COPD = chronic obstructive pulmonary disease.

high-risk, critically unwell/shocked patients and should be based on the likely causative organism and body site involved. Consider stopping if no response and no evidence of invasive infection after 4–5 days. Expert advice is critical for effective management of invasive fungal infections. Invasive line removal should be considered, and underlying disease control is the key. Resistance is not commonly acquired during treatment; however, susceptibility testing is difficult.

Commonly used anti-fungal treatments, along with their mechanism of action and spectrum of activity, are listed in Table 3.7.11.2. In short summary, fluconazole should treat most common yeast and dimorphic fungal infections, except *C. glabrata/krusei*. Posaconazole also covers moulds. Amphotericin B will cover most important yeasts, moulds and dimorphic fungi. Echinocandins cover resistant *Candida* spp. and *Aspergillus* spp. Flucytosine may be added to amphotericin/azole treatment to extend cover with serious candidal and cryptococcal infections.

Note that *P. jirovecii* is not treated with standard anti-fungal drugs (partly as it does not synthesise ergosterol). Treatments may include co-trimoxazole, trimethoprim with dapsone or clindamycin, pentamidine,

Table 3.7.11.2 Description of the major classes of anti-fungal drugs used in intensive care

Group	Name example(s)	Mechanism of action	Spectrum of activity (with general examples)	Notes
Azoles (triazoles)	Fluconazole, voriconazole, itraconazole, posaconazole	Disrupt cell membrane by inhibiting CYP450-dependent lanosterol 14α-demethylase (needed for ergosterol synthesis). Some ergosterol damage	Varies by agent, e.g. fluconazole for *Candida albicans* and cryptococcal infections. All may be useful in mild *Blastomyces*, *Histoplasma*, *Coccidioides* and *Paracoccidioides* infections. Voriconazole/posaconazole for *Aspergillus fumigatus*. Posaconazole (broadest spectrum of azoles) for mucormycoses	Not first line if neutropenic/unstable. *Candida krusei* and most *Candida glabrata* are resistant to fluconazole (voriconazole may be effective). Generally fungistatic against *Candida* spp. Pharmacokinetics vary by the agent. Good CSF/urine penetration with fluconazole only. Major side effects include: hepatotoxicity and drug interactions (all); ↑ QTc/hallucinations with voriconazole; hypertension, hypokalaemia and oedema with itraconazole
Polyenes	Amphotericin B (standard, lipid-complexed and liposomal forms exist), nystatin (topical only)	Lead to pore formation in cell membrane by binding to ergosterol	Very broad cover, e.g. most *Candida* spp., *Cryptococcus*, most *Aspergillus* spp., *Mucorales*, *Histoplasma*, *Blastomyces*, *Coccidioides*, *Paracoccidioides*, *Penicillium*. Nystatin covers *Candida*, *Cryptococcus*, *Coccidioides* and *Histoplasma*	Amphotericin derived from *Streptomyces nodosus*. 'Amphoteric' = able to act as a base or an acid. Resistance to amphotericin B is rare. Major side effects include: renal toxicity (less in liposomal form), infusion reactions (test dose), anaemia and acidosis. For life-threatening cases. In practice, nystatin treats only topical/oro-gastrointestinal *Candida*

283

Table 3.7.11.2 (cont.)

Group	Name example(s)	Mechanism of action	Spectrum of activity (with general examples)	Notes
Echinocandins (cyclic hexapeptides)	Caspofungin, micafungin, anidulafungin	Cell wall interference by inhibiting β-1,3-glucan synthase	Similar between drugs. Severe candidal infections, including *C. glabrata* or if neutropenic. Aspergillosis (± voriconazole)	Fungicidal to *Candida* spp., fungistatic to *Aspergillus* spp. Poor oral bioavailability. Poor renal/CSF penetration. Major side effects (renal/hepatic impairment) uncommon. Expensive
Anti-metabolite	Flucytosine (5-FC)	Inhibits DNA/RNA synthesis, causing cell death	Invasive candidal infections or for cryptococcal meningitis. May have role in aspergillosis	Only used as adjunct to amphotericin B or azole. Serious cardiac/neurological/haematological/renal toxicity limits use

Abbreviations: CSF = cerebrospinal fluid; C. = *Candida*.

atovaquone and trimetrexate glucuronate with folinic acid.

Other factors such as pharmacokinetics and local resistance patterns must be taken into account when choosing appropriate treatment. Expert advice is the key.

References and Further Reading

Greenwood D, Finch R, Davey P, Wilcox M. General properties of antimicrobial agents. In: D Greenwood, R Finch, P Davey, M Wilcox (eds). *Antimicrobial Chemotherapy*, 5th edn. Oxford: Oxford University Press; 2008. pp. 67–77.

Lepak A, Andes D. Fungal sepsis: optimizing antifungal therapy in the critical care setting. *Crit Care Clin* 2011;**27**:123–47.

Moghnieh R, Kanafani ZA, Kanj SS. Antifungal use in intensive care units: another uncertainty that highlights the need for precision medicine. *J Thorac Dis* 2016;**8**:E1672–5.

Timsit J-F, Perner A, Bakker J, *et al.* Year in review in *Intensive Care Medicine* 2014: III. Severe infections, septic shock, healthcare-associated infections, highly resistant bacteria, invasive fungal infections, severe viral infections, Ebola virus disease and paediatrics. *Intensive Care Med* 2015;**41**:575–88.

Antiviral Therapies

3.7.12

James McKinlay and Alexander Fletcher

Key Learning Points

1. Viral infections are intracellular and more problematic in immunocompromised patients.
2. Apart from antiviral drugs, viral infections are also treated with immunomodulation.
3. Most serious viral infections in the intensive care unit involve the respiratory and/or neurological systems.
4. The mainstay of treatment of serious viral infections is supportive care.
5. Host toxicity from antivirals is likely due to the intracellular nature of infections.

Keywords: antiviral, intracellular, coronavirus, SARS, immune compromise

Introduction

Viruses, being obligate intracellular pathogens, exist as DNA within a protein shell and can only replicate within host cells. Most viral infections are managed by host defences but are much more problematic in immunocompromised states, as are often seen in intensive care patients.

The (known) prevalence of viral infections has risen with increasing availability of new tests to detect viruses. Outwith the context of tropical diseases, most serious acute viral infections in the intensive care unit involve the respiratory tract or central nervous system, but other systems may also be severely affected, e.g. the gastrointestinal and hepato-biliary systems. Immunocompromised patients may be taking antiviral prophylaxis, e.g. to reduce chances of cytomegalovirus (CMV) infection. Patients may present with undiagnosed HIV or viral hepatitis infection, but more usually patients with known disease on treatment regimens may present with concurrent illness. HIV

drugs are not discussed here. Specialist input is recommended when considering treatment of viral illnesses.

Regional Infection

Respiratory viruses which may cause pneumonia include: influenza A viruses (classified by haemagglutinin 1–18 and neuraminidase 1–11, e.g. H1N1, H5N1), influenza B virus, respiratory syncytial virus (RSV), CMV, herpes simplex virus (HSV), varicella-zoster virus (VZV), coronaviruses (severe acute respiratory syndrome (SARS) virus: SARS coronavirus 1 (SARS-CoV-1), SARS coronavirus 2 (SARS-CoV-2) – causing coronavirus disease 2019 (COVID-19), Middle East respiratory syndrome (MERS) virus) and adenovirus. Hospital-acquired viral pneumonias may be caused by, for example: rhinovirus, parainfluenza virus, human metapneumovirus, influenza and, more recently, SARS-CoV-2. Furthermore, latent viral reactivation (e.g. HSV/CMV) may occur in the context of bacterial ventilator-associated pneumonias and may or may not cause further parenchymal injury.

Nervous system infections may result in, for example, meningitis, encephalitis, seizures, reduced consciousness, Guillain–Barré syndrome and subsequent respiratory failure. The three most common viral causes include HSV, VZV and enteroviruses. Other viruses causing neuropathology include arboviruses, influenza viruses, West Nile virus, CMV, measles virus, mumps rubulavirus, rubella virus, rabies virus, acute HIV and likely also SARS-CoV-2.

Treatments

Supportive therapy is the mainstay of treatment for viral infections. Specific treatments can be aimed at any of the six stages in the replication cycle of viruses (often inhibiting viral DNA polymerase); however, host toxicity is likely due to the intracellular nature of viral infection. Furthermore, latent viruses have few active processes at which treatments can be targeted. However, there may be some antiviral treatments of

Table 3.7.12.1 Brief overview of major antiviral groups with examples

Mode of action	Compound	Spectrum of activity	Indication	Notes
Nucleoside analogue	Aciclovir	Narrow	HSV, VZV	Potent, specific and generally safe. Phosphorylated by virus
	Ganciclovir	Narrow	CMV	Less selective for viruses, causes bone marrow toxicity
	Cidofovir	Broad	CMV. Also HSV, VZV, EBV, HHV, adeno-/polyoma-/papilloma-/poxvirus	Once-weekly dosing. Nephrotoxicity limits use
	Entecavir	Narrow	Hepatitis B virus	Based on guanosine
	Ribavirin	Broad	Chronic hepatitis, RSV, Lassa fever	Inhaled or oral. Used in combination with interferon
	Lamivudine	Narrow	Chronic hepatitis	High levels of resistance
Uncoating of virus	Amantadine	Narrow	Influenza A virus	Tricyclic amine. Dopaminergic effects. High resistance levels
DNA polymerase inhibitor	Foscarnet	Broad	CMV, HSV, VZV, EBV, HHV	Pyrophosphate analogue. Alternative to aciclovir/ganciclovir. Nephrotoxic
Neuraminidase inhibitor	Oseltamivir/zanamivir	Narrow	Influenza A and B viruses	Neuraminidase aids new cellular infection. May reduce time to resolution by 1 day and reduce respiratory complications
Monoclonal antibodies	Palivizumab	Narrow	RSV	Better as preventative measure
Immuno-modulation	Interferon-α	Potentially broad	Chronic hepatitis	Activates several pathways, rendering cells resistant
Immuno-modulation	Intravenous immunoglobulin	Unclear	Unclear	May have role in some viral infections, but unclear
Vaccine (pre-/post-exposure)	rVSV-ZEBOV	Narrow	Zaire Ebola virus	Good efficacy pre-exposure. Unclear efficacy post-exposure

Note HSV 1 and 2, VZV, CMV, EBV and HHV 6–8 are all herpesviruses.
Abbreviations: HSV = herpes simplex virus; VZV = varicella-zoster virus; CMV = cytomegalovirus; EBV = Epstein–Barr virus; HHV = human herpesvirus; RSV = respiratory syncytial virus; rVSV-ZEBOV = recombinant vesicular stomatitis virus–Zaire Ebola virus.
Adapted from: Antimicrobial Chemotherapy 5th Edition, p. 98 with additions.

potential benefit. The major modes of action with some specific antiviral treatments are summarised in Table 3.7.12.1. The most common acute viral treatments include aciclovir given for 2–3 weeks for viral encephalitis, and oseltamivir given for 5 days for influenza (or inhaled zanamivir for 10 days if oseltamivir resistance or severe immunosuppression is present). Aciclovir has a low risk of side effects but can cause seizures and increase the nephrotoxicity of nephrotoxic drugs. Oseltamivir may cause nausea/vomiting and headaches, whilst zanamivir can cause bronchospasm in susceptible patients. Potential treatments for COVID-19 are not discussed as, at the time of writing, efficacy and safety have not yet been established.

References and Further Reading

Dandachi D, Rodriguez-Barradas MC. Viral pneumonia: etiologies and treatment. J Investig Med 2018;66: 957–65.

Dobson J, Whitley RJ, Pocock S, Monto AS. Oseltamivir treatment for influenza in adults: a meta-analysis of randomised controlled trials. Lancet 2015;385: 1729–37.

Greenwood D, Finch R, Davey P, Wilcox M (eds). Antimicrobial Chemotherapy, 5th edn. Oxford: Oxford University Press; 2008.

Kelesidis T, Mastoris I, Metsini A, Tsiodras S. How to approach and treat viral infections in ICU patients. BMC Infect Dis 2014;14:321.

3.7.13

Malaria and Tropical Diseases

Clare Morkane

Key Learning Points

1. Malaria is caused by a protozoan parasite of the *Plasmodium* genus, transmitted by mosquitoes.
2. There are five species of *Plasmodium* that regularly infect humans; *Plasmodium falciparum* is responsible for the vast majority of malarial deaths.
3. Severe malaria is a medical emergency, with mortality from untreated disease (particularly cerebral malaria) approaching 100 per cent. Early diagnosis and prompt, effective treatment are essential.
4. Parenteral artesunate is the treatment of choice for all severe malaria.
5. It is important to remember there are many causes of critical illness in the returning traveller, with a wide number of differentials, including, but not limited to: enteric fever (typhoid and paratyphoid), hepatitis, dengue or other arboviruses, avian influenza and viral haemorrhagic fever.

Keywords: malaria, *Plasmodium*, anopheles mosquito, artesunate, returning traveller

Introduction

Malaria remains one of the most common imported infections in the UK. Public Health England recorded 1683 cases in 2018, and 2–11 deaths are reported annually in the UK. Malaria is a serious and potentially life-threatening febrile illness, caused by obligate intra-erythrocytic protozoan parasites belonging to the *Plasmodium* genus. The primary vector for spread of infection is the female *Anopheles* mosquito in tropical and subtropical regions of the world.

Diagnosis

Four species of malarial parasite are classically considered to cause disease in humans (Table 3.7.13.1). A fifth – *Plasmodium knowlesi* – is now recognised as a zoonotic cause of malaria in parts of Malaysia. Approximately three-quarters of infections result from *Plasmodium falciparum*.

Malaria should be suspected in anyone with fever or a history of fever who has visited a malaria-endemic area. Falciparum malaria is most likely to occur within 3 months of return, whereas malaria caused by other species may be present >1 year following travel. It is important to remember that appropriate prophylaxis with full adherence does not exclude malaria. Symptoms are often non-specific and include fever/sweats/chills, headache, myalgia, diarrhoea and cough.

Table 3.7.13.1 Different species of plasmodia

Plasmodium species	Information	Incubation period
Plasmodium falciparum	Most common species identified Causes a more severe form of malaria and is responsible for the majority of malarial deaths worldwide	9–14 days
Plasmodium malariae	Less severe illness Causes fever at 3-day intervals May present with late recrudescence after many years	2–4 weeks
Plasmodium ovale	Relapsing malaria caused by a dormant parasite stage in the liver	12–18 days
Plasmodium vivax	Relapsing malaria caused by a dormant parasite stage in the liver	12–18 days
Plasmodium knowlesi	Parasite burden may expand rapidly, resulting in severe and sometimes fatal illness (short 24-hour asexual cycle) Very rarely imported at present	9–12 days

The gold standard investigation is examination of thick and thin blood smears by microscopy. However, because of the lack of out-of-hours access and expertise in some centres, rapid diagnostic tests (RDTs) based upon detection of parasite antigens are now commonly used, in addition to blood slides. Three negative diagnostic samples over a period of 24–48 hours are necessary to exclude malaria.

Pathophysiology

Manifestations of malarial illness result from infection of red blood cells by the asexual forms of the malaria parasite, the life cycle of which is as follows (shown in Figure 3.7.13.1):

1. *Plasmodium* parasites are introduced via the bite of an infected mosquito as sporozoites.
2. Sporozoites are taken up by hepatocytes where they mature over 7–10 days to form schizonts.
3. Schizonts rupture to release variable numbers of merozoites into the blood.
4. Merozoites rapidly invade erythrocytes, forming trophozoites.
5. Trophozoites mature into schizonts over a period of 24–72 hours, depending on the species.
6. Mature schizonts rupture, causing haemolysis and releasing further merozoites into the blood where they invade more erythrocytes.

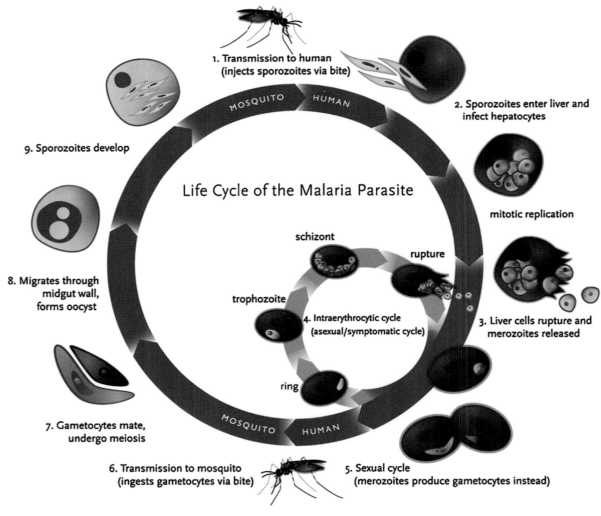

Figure 3.7.13.1 The life cycle of the malaria parasite.
Source: Reproduced with permission: Klein EY, *Int J Antimicrob Agents*. 2013 Apr; **41**(4): 311–317.

It is this periodic haemolysis that causes the majority of symptoms associated with malaria. Different species of malaria rupture red blood cells at different intervals, which leads to the diagnostic cycles of fever characteristic of malaria. *P. vivax*, for example, tends to produce cycles of fever every 2 days, whereas *P. malariae* produces fever every 3 days.

Severe Malaria

Criteria for severe falciparum malaria have been defined by the World Health Organization (WHO) and are defined in Table 3.7.13.2.

Table 3.7.13.2 Major features of severe falciparum malaria

Feature	Specifics
Impaired consciousness or seizures	GCS <11 in adults Blantyre coma score <3 in children >2 seizure episodes within 24 hours
Prostration	Generalised weakness such that the person is unable to sit, stand or walk without assistance
Pulmonary oedema	Radiologically confirmed or oxygen saturation <92% on room air with a respiratory rate >30 breaths/min, often with chest in-drawing and crackles
Severe malarial anaemia	Haemoglobin concentration ≤70 g/l or haematocrit ≤20% in adults (≤5 g/dl or haematocrit ≤15% in children <12 years old)
Acidosis	Base deficit >8 mEq/l or bicarbonate <15 mmol/l or lactate >5 mmol/l
Jaundice	Plasma or serum bilirubin >50 μmol/l (3 mg/dl), with a parasite count >100,000/μl
Renal impairment	Plasma or serum creatinine >265 μmol/l (3 mg/dl) or blood urea >20 mmol/l
Significant bleeding	Recurrent or prolonged bleeding from nose, gums or venepuncture sites Haematemesis Melaena
Shock	Systolic blood pressure <80 mmHg in adults or <70 mmHg in children, with evidence of impaired perfusion Secondary to complicating bacteraemia 'algid malaria'
Hypoglycaemia	Blood or plasma glucose <2.2 mmol/l
Hyperparasitaemia	*Plasmodium falciparum* parasitaemia >10%

Abbreviations: GCS = Glasgow Coma Score.
Source: Adapted from World Health Organization 2015 *Guidelines for the Treatment of Malaria*, third edition.

The initial parasite count is useful in estimating the potential future severity of disease; if >2 per cent of red blood cells are parasitised, there is an increased chance of developing severe disease, with 10 per cent parasitaemia representing severe disease.

Groups of patients at particular risk of developing severe malaria or deteriorating rapidly include pregnant women, the elderly and children. Other poor prognostic factors are: the presence of peripheral blood schizonts of *P. falciparum*, metabolic acidosis or elevated lactate, coma and renal impairment.

Management of Severe Malaria

Severe malaria is a medical emergency and patients with severe falciparum malaria must be admitted to the ICU/high dependency unit (HDU) for full monitoring. Urgent appropriate parenteral therapy with antimalarials has the greatest impact on survival in severe malaria; hence management should always be discussed with a specialist. Artesunate, intravenous (IV) or intramuscular (IM), is the treatment of choice for all adults and children (including infants and pregnant women) with severe malaria, and there is substantial evidence for its superiority over IV quinine. Artesunate is given for at least 24 hours and until patients can tolerate oral medication. Artesunate should be followed by a full dose of effective oral artemisinin-based combination therapy.

Careful attention to fluid balance is essential to avoid overfilling, as this may exacerbate the increased pulmonary capillary permeability that occurs in severe malaria. Intubation and mechanical ventilation may be indicated not only in those with respiratory failure, but also to facilitate airway protection and management of intracranial pressure (ICP) in cerebral malaria. A lumbar puncture should be performed in comatose patients to exclude bacterial meningitis. The cerebrospinal fluid (CSF) should be clear with white cells <10/μl and protein is often slightly raised. Blood glucose should be meticulously monitored, as malaria is associated with hypoglycaemia, complicated by quinine-induced hyperinsulinaemia.

Frequent parasite counts are not helpful in early management, as peripheral parasite counts will fluctuate, depending on the stage of parasite development, and a rise in count in the first 36 hours does not equate to treatment failure.

Exchange transfusion is no longer recommended in the management of severe malaria.

Key Critical Care Management Concepts

- Rapid administration of appropriate IV anti-malarials
- Meticulous attention to fluid balance
- Broad-spectrum antibiotics if evidence of shock
- Monitor closely for hypoglycaemia
- Low threshold for renal and respiratory support

Other Tropical Infections

When reviewing the critically ill returning traveller, it is important to consider other infections. The list of potential causes of fever in the returning traveller is long, but the following are of particular relevance: enteric fever (typhoid and paratyphoid), hepatitis, dengue or other arboviruses, avian influenza and viral haemorrhagic fever. Table 3.7.13.3 illustrates key features of other important tropical infection differentials.

Table 3.7.13.3 Other tropical disease differentials in the returning traveller

Name	Cause	Vector	Incubation period	Symptoms and classic features	Severe features	Management principles
Dengue fever	RNA flavivirus	*Aedes aegypti* mosquito	4–7 days	Fever, severe headache, arthralgia, myalgia, retro-orbital pain, rash, nausea and vomiting Low WBC count	Hypovolaemic shock secondary to vascular leakage Haemorrhage Multi-organ failure	Supportive No specific antivirals Prompt fluid resuscitation
Typhoid fever and parathyroid (enteric fever)	Typhoid: *Salmonella enterica* serovar typhi Paratyphoid: *Salmonella enterica* of the serotype paratyphi A, B or C	No non-human vectors Enteric spread	Typhoid: 8–14 days Paratyphoid: 1–10 days	Fever, malaise, diffuse abdominal pain and constipation Splenomegaly, leucopenia, anaemia, liver function abnormalities, proteinuria and coagulopathy are common Paratyphoid fever resembles typhoid fever	Delirium, coma Intestinal haemorrhage and DIC Bowel perforation Toxic myocarditis Multi-organ failure	Antibiotics: ceftriaxone, ciprofloxacin, azithromycin Nutrition (parenteral may be necessary) Fluid resuscitation Supportive care Prevention: vaccination
Viral haemorrhagic fever: Ebola virus	RNA virus of the *Filoviridae* family	No recognised reservoir. Transmitted via exposure to infected body fluids	2–21 days	Phase 1: fever, fatigue, myalgia Phase 2: diarrhoea, vomiting, abdominal pain Phase 3: bleeding, encephalopathy	Hypovolaemic shock Electrolyte disturbance Multi-organ failure Gastrointestinal haemorrhage, frequently fatal	Isolation IV fluid resuscitation Supportive care
Viral haemorrhagic fever: Crimean Congo haemorrhagic fever	Nairovirus of the *Bunyaviridae* family (RNA virus)	Tick bites or through contact with infected animal blood	5–13 days	Fever, myalgia, backache, headache, photophobia, nausea, vomiting, diarrhoea, abdominal pain early on, followed by sharp mood swings and confusion 2–4 days: depression and lassitude, detectable hepatomegaly	Large areas of severe bruising Severe nosebleeds and uncontrolled bleeding, beginning around the fourth day of illness and lasting for about 2 weeks In documented outbreaks, fatality rates in hospitalised patients have ranged from 9 to 50 per cent	Supportive care is the main approach The antiviral drug ribavirin has been used

Name	Cause	Vector	Incubation period	Symptoms and classic features	Severe features	Management principles
Yellow fever	Arbovirus of the *Flavivirus* genus	Mosquitoes: *Aedes* and *Haemagogus* species	3–6 days	Fever, muscle pain, backache, headache, loss of appetite, nausea/vomiting	Toxic phase in a small proportion of patients: within 24 hours of recovery from initial symptoms. Features: jaundice, dark urine, abdominal pain, vomiting. Bleeding can occur from the mouth, nose, eyes or stomach	Prevention: vaccination IV fluid resuscitation Supportive treatment for liver and kidney failure Antibiotics for associated bacterial infection
Amoebiasis	Protozoan *Entamoeba histolytica*	Humans are the only reservoir. Infection occurs by ingestion of mature cysts in food or water	2–4 weeks	Symptoms can range from mild diarrhoea to severe dysentery with blood and mucus	Amoebic colitis may lead to fulminant or necrotising colitis, toxic megacolon or amoeboma Amoebic liver abscess: may extend, rupture or disseminate and cause a brain abscess	Fluid and electrolyte replacement Metronidazole for acute invasive amoebic dysentery Tinidazole is also effective
African trypanosomiasis (sleeping sickness)	Two subspecies of the extracellular parasite *Trypanosoma brucei* (*gambiense* and *rhodesiense*)	Tsetse flies	3 weeks	Haemolymphatic stage: general malaise, fever, headache, pruritus, urticaria Meningoencephalitic stage: somnolence, insomnia, ataxia, behavioural changes, depression, stupor, coma	African trypanosomiasis leads to severe neuroinflammation and is fatal without treatment Meningoencephalitis with seizures	Airway support and close neurological observation Specific drug treatment depends on type of infection and disease stage There is no vaccine or effective prophylaxis

Abbreviations: RNA = ribonucleic acid; WBC = white blood cells; DIC = disseminated intravascular coagulation; IV = intravenous.

References and Further Reading

Karnad DR, Richards GA, Silva GS, *et al*. Tropical diseases in the ICU: a syndromic approach to diagnosis and treatment. *J Crit Care* 2018;**46**:119–26.

Lalloo DG, Shingadia D, Bell DJ, *et al*. UK malaria treatment guidelines 2016. *J Infect* 2016;**72**:635–49.

Marks M, Gupta-Wright A, Doherty J, *et al*. Managing malaria in the intensive care unit. *Br J Anaesth* 2014;**113**:910–21.

Public Health England. 2018. Malaria imported into the United Kingdom: 2018. Implications for those advising travellers. assets.publishing.service.gov.uk/government/uploads/system/uploads/attachment_data/file/812824/Malaria_imported_into_the_United_Kingdom_2018.pdf

Sinclair D, Donegan S, Isba R, Lalloo DG. Artesunate versus quinine for treating severe malaria. *Cochrane Database Syst Rev* 2012;**6**:CD005967.

World Health Organization. 2021. *WHO guidelines for malaria*. www.who.int/publications/i/item/guidelines-for-malaria

3.7.14

The COVID-19 Pandemic

Christopher Hellyar, Debashish Dutta and Carl Waldmann

Key Learning Points

1. Viral diseases continue to emerge and represent a serious issue to public health internationally.
2. A coronavirus is responsible for the coronavirus disease 2019 (COVID-19) pandemic. Other notable coronaviruses include severe acute respiratory syndrome coronavirus (SARS-CoV) and the Middle East respiratory syndrome coronavirus (MERS-CoV).
3. COVID-19 binds via the angiotensin-converting enzyme 2 receptor on type II alveolar cells and the intestinal epithelium in a similar manner to the SARS virus.
4. The World Health Organization's strategy of controlling a pandemic was challenged by COVID-19.
5. Many lessons have since been learnt regarding our ability in the NHS to react to a pandemic. These include the need for adequate personal protective equipment, rapid diagnostic testing of patients and staff and use of methods to communicate with relatives of patients who were seriously ill or dying in the intensive care unit.

Keywords: epidemic, pandemic, COVID-19, coronavirus, personal protective equipment

Introduction

Epidemic: 'the occurrence in a community or region of cases of an illness … clearly in excess of normal expectancy.'

Pandemic: 'an epidemic occurring worldwide, or over a very wide area, crossing international boundaries and usually affecting a large number of people.'

Viral diseases continue to emerge and represent a serious issue to public health internationally. In the last 20 years, three viruses have emerged, causing major respiratory disease epidemics: severe acute respiratory syndrome coronavirus (SARS-CoV) in 2003; H1N1 influenza in 2009; and Middle East respiratory syndrome coronavirus (MERS-CoV) in 2012.

In early December 2019, an epidemic of lower respiratory infections was identified in Wuhan, China and was initially classified as 'pneumonia of unknown aetiology' by the Chinese Center for Disease Control and Prevention. It was thought to be a zoonotic virus from a bat reservoir, and given its novel nature, nobody had prior immunity and thus everyone was at risk of potential harm.

The Virus

The virus was isolated on 30 December 2019, and genome sequencing identified the pathogen as a coronavirus (CoV) belonging to the beta subfamily (sarbecovirus). Other beta-CoV viruses include the severe acute respiratory syndrome coronavirus (SARS-CoV) and Middle East respiratory syndrome coronavirus (MERS-CoV). This novel virus was initially given the name '2019-nCoV'. However as it subsequently was seen to share 82 per cent of its genome with SARS, it was renamed SARS-CoV-2. In February 2020, the World Health Organization (WHO) announced that the novel coronavirus disease caused by SARS-CoV-2 would be called coronavirus disease 2019 (COVID-19).

Coronaviruses themselves are a large family of single-stranded RNA (+ssRNA) viruses, seven of which cause respiratory disease, ranging from the common cold to respiratory failure. It is estimated that coronaviruses are responsible for 5–10 per cent of acute respiratory infections globally. When compared to MERS-CoV (34 per cent) and SARS-CoV (10 per cent), SARS-CoV-2 is thought to have a lower case fatality rate (approximately 6.8 per cent). It is important to note, however, that we do not know how many people have been infected at this stage (i.e. unknown denominator) and early on in an epidemic, the sickest people seek care early and hence undergo testing and, as such, hospitalisation and case fatality rates are normally higher in the early period.

The standard method of diagnosis involves real-time reverse transcription polymerase chain reaction (rRT-PCR) from a nasopharyngeal swab; however, a greater yield is achieved from tracheal aspirates. Broncho-alveolar lavage is seldom used for diagnosis, as it carries the risk of aerosolisation and subsequent transmission.

Clinical Presentation and Pathophysiology

The classical clinical presentation is that of a respiratory infection with the severity of symptoms ranging from mild common cold-like illness to severe viral pneumonia leading to acute respiratory distress syndrome and multi-organ failure. Some people will also be asymptomatic when infected and demonstrate no signs.

COVID-19 binds via the angiotensin-converting enzyme 2 (ACE2) receptor on type II alveolar cells and the intestinal epithelium in a similar manner to the SARS virus. Viral replication occurs during the early phase of the illness with an innate immune response and direct viral cytopathic effects causing tissue damage. As the adaptive immune response occurs, viral titres reduce, but inflammation continues and the majority of tissue damage occurs.

Incubation is a median of 4 days (interquartile range 2–7) up to 14 days from exposure, and people are most infectious during the symptomatic period. It is thought, however, that the infectious period starts from 2 days before symptoms are present to 2 weeks after.

Eighty per cent of people recover from the disease without needing medical treatment, but for the remaining 20 per cent, a three-stage process has been widely documented.

- Stage 1: early infection is characterised by mild symptoms of fever (83–98 per cent), cough (59–82 per cent) and muscle aches (11–44 per cent). Ten per cent of patients present with gastrointestinal flu-like symptoms. Blood tests show lymphopenia, with increased prothrombin time and D-dimer and lactate dehydrogenase (LDH) levels. C-reactive protein (CRP) levels are elevated, but procalcitonin levels remain low unless there is a superadded bacterial infection.

- Stage 2: around day 8, the patient enters the second stage of disease (pulmonary phase). Shortness of breath (19–55 per cent) predominates and patients may develop pneumonia characterised on chest X-ray by bilateral, peripheral airspace opacities, predominantly in the lower zones. Some patients will experience 'silent hypoxaemia', with respiratory failure without dyspnoea.

- Stage 3: 17–29 per cent enter a third phase (hyperinflammation phase) with acute respiratory distress syndrome, and 5 per cent of all COVID-19 cases need admission to an intensive care unit for organ support. In this stage, patients may experience sepsis and multiple organ dysfunction, including cardiac and renal failure (70 per cent require advanced respiratory support, 23 per cent require renal support, and 28 per cent cardiovascular support). In some cases, it is also thought that an adaptive immune response may lead to a dysregulated immune–pathological 'cytokine storm', manifesting as a virally mediated haemophagocytic lymphohistiocytosis (HLH)-like syndrome, and there has also been documentation of widespread micro-emboli and micro-angiopathic changes and pulmonary emboli (PE) in 25 per cent of cases. Overall, the mortality rate in critical care ranges from 40 to 60 per cent.

COVID-19 and the Intensive Care Unit

Approximately 5 per cent of patients with COVID-19 require admission to intensive care. Without mitigating the rate of spread and incidence, this would lead to rapid saturation of critical care areas and trained staff. Previous experience from MERS, SARS, avian flu and flu A epidemics found that critical care beds were a precious resource. Initial reports from the experience in China suggested a case-fatality rate of 5.8 per cent in Hubei (the epicentre), compared to 0.7 per cent outside the province, suggesting that outcome was associated with health system capacity.

Concerns over a surge in critical care admissions led to planning at local, regional and national levels for how to best manage critical care resources such as hospital beds, ventilators, extracorporeal membrane oxygenation and renal replacement therapy. The majority of hospitals had to expand critical care services to deal with the increased demand. This involved reallocation of resources, restructuring of care services away from elective work and appropriate training of clinical staff.

The surge in admissions to critical care units and the associated morbidity and mortality brought intensive care medicine to the forefront of the global COVID-19 discussion. The role of the specialty had, until this time, been somewhat understated and elusive to the general public. With increasing publicity, it becomes more important to promote an understanding of the impact and consequences that admission to critical care and exposure to its therapies can have on patients and their families in the long term. This aspect of the patient journey is typically not well communicated to, or appreciated by, patients and relatives.

Recovery and rehabilitation for the thousands of patients being discharged from critical care after treatment for COVID-19 have also become an important consideration, with 30 per cent of patients likely to have complex rehabilitation needs. Aftercare therefore requires significant resources and effective coordination, even after hospital discharge. Models of integrated care have been suggested to deal with this pervasive issue.

The Search for a Vaccine

Within 4 months of the first case being identified, over 10,000 publications had been registered. In March 2020, the WHO issued the Coordinated Global Research Roadmap with nine research priorities. There were a total of 135 funded global projects on therapeutic interventions, including 41 on candidate vaccines. One of those trials is called the 'Recovery Trial' (Table 3.7.14.1) with five arms of treatments to compare. 'Repurposed' medications were tried, as they already have a proven safety profile.

Other treatments under trial include tocilizumab and convalescent plasma. Tocilizumab is a monoclonal antibody which has been used for treatment of rheumatoid arthritis. It binds to the interleukin-6 (IL-6) receptor and blocks it from functioning. IL-6 is a major pro-inflammatory cytokine implicated in the development of the cytokine storm. Convalescent plasma (immunoglobulins) from recovered previously infected patients has been used with SARS, MERS, Ebola and H1N1, with evidence of decreasing mortality and viral load. These trials are reflective of the desperation within the medical and scientific communities of the world to find a definitive treatment.

Vaccine development is normally a very long process to ensure vaccines are safe and effective as a prerequisite to licensing, before they can be distributed and used. Clinical trials are required for efficacy. Even with animal tests done in parallel with early human tests, this process is lengthy. Manufacturing a vaccine requires progression from a proof-of-principle to commercial development, with 95 per cent of vaccines failing at the first step. Thus, a large number of developers are required initially and need coordination through subsequent steps. Constraints on technologies, expertise, capacity and production mean that large pharmaceutical companies are required to see a product through its development. Global leadership and a coordinated and coherent response will be needed to ensure that any vaccine is distributed equitably. Vulnerable populations, such as those living in poverty or conflict areas, are especially at high risk of devastating impacts. Equitable access to the COVID-19 vaccine will be

Table 3.7.14.1 The Recovery Trial

Trial arm	Rationale
No additional treatment	There are currently no approved antiviral or host-directed treatments for COVID-19
Lopinavir–ritonavir	Lopinavir is a human immunodeficiency virus 1 (HIV-1) protease inhibitor, which is combined with ritonavir to increase lopinavir's plasma half-life. Lopinavir–ritonavir has shown activity against SARS-CoV and MERS-CoV
Low-dose corticosteroids	Favourable immune response modulation with low-dose corticosteroids might help treat severe acute respiratory syndrome coronavirus infections, including COVID-19, SARS and MERS
Hydroxychloroquine	Hydroxychloroquine, a derivative of chloroquine, has been used for many decades to treat malaria and rheumatological diseases. It has antiviral activity against SARS-CoV-2 in cell culture
Azithromycin	Azithromycin is a macrolide antibiotic with immunomodulatory properties that has shown benefit in inflammatory lung disease

Abbreviations: COVID-19 = coronavirus disease 2019; SARS-CoV = severe acute respiratory syndrome coronavirus; MERS-CoV = Middle East respiratory syndrome coronavirus.
Source: Recoverytrial.net

challenging where inequalities and unequal access to essential services have been compromised within some political systems. The WHO supports international vaccine coordination on COVID-19 through the International Coordinating Group (ICG) and several international partners to facilitate as procurement and distribution agencies. A global approach is the only feasible way of mobilising sufficient resources at a time of expected global recession.

Large-Scale Crisis Management of a Highly Contagious Disease

Epidemics are social problems as much as medical ones. The approach to management has to take into account the wider concerns of the community and society. The dynamics of epidemic diseases typically occur in four phases:

- **Phase 1:** introduction or emergence in a community
- **Phase 2:** localised transmission where sporadic infections with the pathogen occur
- **Phase 3:** amplification of the outbreak into an epidemic or pandemic
- **Phase 4:** reduced transmission when human-to-human transmission of the pathogen decreases

As the disease progresses through the phases, the required response also changes. This follows five stages involving the terminology defined below:

- **Stage 1:** anticipation of new and re-emerging diseases to facilitate faster detection and response
- **Stage 2:** early disease detection of emergence in animal and human populations
- **Stage 3:** containment of the disease at early stages of transmission
- **Stage 4:** control and mitigation of the epidemic during its amplification
- **Stage 5:** elimination of the risk of outbreaks or eradication of the infectious disease

Anticipation

The anticipation of risks focuses resources on the most likely threats – forecasting the most likely diseases to emerge, quick identification of the drivers that will worsen the impact or facilitate the spread and scenario planning.

Early Detection

With emerging diseases, rapid detection and investigation of the source enable proactive risk assessment. These are the key to reducing the risk of amplification and potential international spread. This involves training of healthcare workers and public health education, together with laboratory confirmation.

Containment

Early detection allows rapid implementation of containment measures in order to avoid a large-scale epidemic. Rapid containment should start as soon as the first case is detected, regardless of the aetiology, which is most likely to be unknown. It requires skilled professionals to safely implement the necessary countermeasures.

Control and Mitigation

Once the infectious disease threat reaches an epidemic or pandemic level, the goal of the response is to mitigate its impact and reduce its incidence, morbidity and mortality, as well as disruptions to economic, political and social systems.

Elimination or Eradication

Control of the disease alone may lead to its elimination where the disease is no longer considered as a major public health issue. Interventional measures are still required. Eradication of a disease involves permanent elimination of its incidence worldwide. There is no longer a need for intervention measures. Three criteria need to be met in order to eradicate a disease – there must be an effective and available intervention to interrupt its transmission; there must be efficient diagnostic tools to detect cases; and humans must be the only reservoir.

Countries, through their own public health organisations, identify the phase of infection and decide the appropriate staged response. Note that the response to a public health emergency needs to address medical, social, political and economic priorities peculiar to that area.

Given the wide-reaching effects of epidemics, the response must be coordinated on a national, regional and global level. The WHO provides an Emergency Response Framework (ERF) which requires the WHO to 'act with urgency and predictability' to best serve and be accountable to populations affected by emergencies. If WHO involvement occurs, then the organisation can activate the Incident Management System (IMS) which provides a standardised approach to emergency management, including operational oversight, assigning roles globally, standard operating procedures (SOPs) and technical support. In the case of COVID-19, the pandemic global response was somehow different. Different countries worldwide introduced different 'lockdown' measures to contain the spread of infection of COVID-19, resulting in inevitable social and economic consequences.

Conclusion

At the time of writing this chapter, the first phase of the UK COVID-19 pandemic is subsiding, but at the cost of an excess of 40,000 deaths. There are concerns about whether there will be a second phase. Guidance has been rapidly produced by the National Institute for Health and Care Excellence (NICE) (Quality Standard 159) to try and assist with decision-making about admission to the ICU during this pandemic.

Many lessons have since been learnt regarding our ability in the NHS to react to a pandemic. These include the need for adequate personal protective equipment, rapid diagnostic testing of patients and staff and use of methods to communicate with relatives of patients who were seriously ill or dying in the ICU. This has been aided by the provision of rapidly produced guidelines.

References and Further Reading

Lipsitch M, Donnelly CA, Fraser C, *et al*. Potential biases in estimating absolute and relative case-fatality risks during outbreaks. *PLoS Negl Trop Dis* 2015;**9**:e0003846.

National Institute for Health and Care Excellence. 2020. COVID-19 rapid guideline: critical care in adults. NICE guideline [NG159]. www.nice.org.uk/guidance/ng159

Siddiqu HK, Mehra MR. COVID-19 illness in native and immunosuppressed states: a clinical-therapeutic staging proposal. *J Heart Lung Transplant* 2020;**39**: 405–7.

The Faculty of Intensive Care Medicine. 2020. FICM Position Statement and Provisional Guidance: Recovery and Rehabilitation for Patients Following the Pandemic. www.ficm.ac.uk/sites/ficm/files/documents/2021-10/ficm_recovery_and_rehab_provisional_guidance.pdf

World Health Organization. 2018. Managing epidemics: key facts about major deadly diseases. apps.who.int/iris/handle/10665/272442

Wu Z, McGoogan JM. Characteristics of and important lessons from the coronavirus disease 2019 (COVID-19) outbreak in China: summary of a report of 72 314 cases from the Chinese Center for Disease Control and Prevention. *JAMA* 2020;**323**:1239–42.

Toxicology

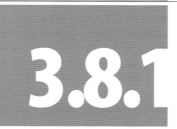

Timothy Snow

Key Learning Points

1. A systematic approach is needed for the assessment of a patient who has taken an overdose, and it should follow standard resuscitation algorithms.

2. Symptoms of drug overdose can produce a constellation of symptoms known as a 'toxidrome', knowledge of which aids identification and management when the specific drug is unknown.

3. Mixed overdose of multiple agents is common, and each agent may potentiate and prolong the effects of others.

4. Medications administered in the treatment of an overdose should be used judiciously. They too can potentiate some of the toxic effects.

5. Early engagement from both the psychiatric and the drug and alcohol liaison teams can aid step down from the intensive care unit.

Keywords: toxicology, drug overdose, poisoning, suicide

Introduction

Drug overdose and poisoning are a common presentation to the ICU, accounting for approximately 2000–3000 deaths per year. For an ICU physician, the resuscitation department will normally be the primary point of contact for these patients due to the adverse effect of the agents. A small subset of patients may require ICU input whilst as an inpatient, either due to the long-lasting or delayed effects of the drugs or from the iatrogenic effects of drugs given in the hospital environment.

This chapter addresses the initial management of an overdose and the ongoing management in the ICU.

It should be remembered, however, that when planning step-down of the patient to the ward, early involvement with psychiatry or the drugs and alcohol liaison services should be sought. These patients may also be under the Mental Health Act (in the UK) or may need to be placed under a Section if attempting to leave pre-psychiatric assessment (see Chapter 3.15.1, Capacity and Consent Issues in Intensive Care). Finally, it should be noted that in those patients we are unable to help, death by suicide (in the UK and many other countries) warrants a referral to the coroner for a post-mortem examination prior to issuing of a death certificate.

Initial Management of an Overdose

Initial management of a patient with a suspected overdose should always be the same – a structured ABCDE approach to sequentially identify any problems or concerns. Whilst the suspected causative agent may be known from the history, due to the risk of a mixed overdose involving multiple agents, an initial systematic broad approach will prevent task fixation on managing individual agents too early.

In patients where the causative agent or agents are unknown, an educated guess can be made on the basis of identifying a characteristic 'toxidrome' – a constellation of symptoms produced by certain groups of agents (Table 3.8.1.1).

Following a standard structured patient assessment, commonly encountered problems may include:

- Loss of a patent airway – commonly secondary to loss of normal protective airway reflexes from reduced consciousness or, far less commonly, through intentional bleach ingestion causing direct damage

- Hypoxia – may be due to a primary effect of the drug itself (e.g. cyanide) or as a consequence (e.g. aspiration pneumonitis). Hypercarbia may occur secondary to reduced/loss of normal respiratory drive (e.g. opiates) or due to patient exhaustion in severe metabolic disturbance (aspirin)

297

Table 3.8.1.1 Toxidromes

Toxidrome	Causative agents	Features
Anti-cholinergic	Anti-histamines, anti-psychotics, antidepressants, anti-Parkinson	Hypertension, tachycardia, dry skin, flushing, blurred vision, coma, delirium, hallucination, memory loss, mydriasis, myoclonus, psychosis, seizures, hyperthermia, urinary retention
Sympathomimetic	Salbutamol, amphetamines, cocaine, methamphetamines	Hypertension, tachycardia, anxiety, delusions, hyper-reflexia, mydriasis, seizures, sweating
Opioid	Heroin, morphine, fentanyl	Respiratory depression, coma, pinpoint pupils
Cholinergics	Organophosphates	Tachypnoea, bronchospasm, bronchorrhoea, bradycardia, confusion, miosis, seizures, fasciculations, diarrhoea, emesis, incontinence, hypothermia
Serotonin syndrome	Selective serotonin reuptake inhibitors, cocaine, amphetamines, monoamine oxidase inhibitors, tricyclic antidepressants, tramadol	Tachycardia, hypertension, ataxia, hyper-reflexia, confusion, hallucinations, agitation, seizures, rhabdomyolysis, coagulopathy

- Cardiac arrhythmias – bradycardias (e.g. beta-blockers), tachycardia (e.g. sympathomimetics) and QRS abnormalities (e.g. tricyclic antidepressants (TCAs)) may be seen. Hypotensive and hypertensive crises may also occur
- Altered consciousness – increased requiring sedation (e.g. sympathomimetics) or decreased requiring airway support (e.g. opiates)

Specific investigations which should always be considered include an ECG, full blood count/urea and electrolytes/creatinine/liver function tests/creatine kinase and glucose, arterial or venous blood gas and urine or serum drug assays. Calculation of the anion gap (raised with ethanol or salicylate) or osmolar gap (increased with alcohols) should also be undertaken.

General Treatment Strategies

General treatment strategies involve reducing further absorption of the drug, increasing elimination/excretion and supportive therapies.

1. **Reducing absorption:**
   a. Activated charcoal can be used within 1–2 hours of ingestion
   b. Gastric lavage may be indicated in severe overdose or in those who are unconscious and already intubated
   c. Decontamination: for chemical incidents, use barrier protection (with a mask if applicable) to prevent cross-contamination of medical staff, and then decontaminate the patient as per local protocols. Removal of clothing prior to skin cleansing tends to remove the majority

of the causative chemical, but remember to use tepid, rather than warm, water to minimise skin absorption

2. **Increasing elimination:**
   a. Antidote: use specific antidotes (Table 3.8.1.2)
   b. Urinary alkalinisation for salicylate poisoning
   c. Haemodialysis for severe poisoning with salicylates, ethylene, methanol, lithium, phenobarbital and chlorates

Table 3.8.1.2 Poison antidotes

Poison	Antidote(s)
Beta-blockers	Glucagon / Atropine
Carbon monoxide	Oxygen
Cyanide	Sodium nitrate or thiosulphate / Dicobalt edetate / Hydroxocobalamin
Digoxin	Digibind®
Ethylene glycol/methanol	Ethanol / Fomepizole
Iron	Desferrioxamine
Opioids	Naloxone
Organophosphates	Atropine / Pralidoxime
Paracetamol	Acetylcysteine / Methionine
Sulphonylureas	Glucose / Octreotide
Tricyclic antidepressants	Sodium bicarbonate / Intralipid®

3. **Supportive therapy:**
   a. Airway:
      i. Intubate if unconscious or risk of aspiration
   b. Breathing:
      i. Invasive ventilation for hypoxia or hypercarbia
   c. Circulation/cardiac:
      i. Head-down positioning and intravenous (IV) fluids should be the initial treatment for hypotension, with vasopressor use if refractory. Try to avoid inotropes as they may provoke arrhythmias
      ii. Arrhythmias: treat electrolyte or blood gas disturbances initially. Intralipid® infusions may be considered for some drugs (e.g. TCAs)
   d. Disability:
      i. For seizures of short duration, optimise electrolytes and blood gas abnormalities initially. Benzodiazepines can be used for longer-lasting or repeated seizures
   e. Exposure:
      i. Hypothermia from prolonged unconsciousness requires active warming, whilst hyperthermia caused by serotoninergics, amphetamines, monoamine oxidase inhibitors (MAOIs) or theophylline may need active cooling or dantrolene

Drugs: Over-the-Counter

Paracetamol

A common analgesic and anti-pyretic – if taken in overdose, it can cause severe liver damage. Presentation initially begins with nausea, vomiting and abdominal pain over the initial few hours, progressing to localised hepatic tenderness due to liver damage after 24 hours. Consequences of liver failure may become evident, with hypoglycaemia and coagulopathy initially, jaundice from 48 hours and hepatic encephalopathy from 3 days. Toxicity occurs due to direct cell damage by the paracetamol metabolite N-acetyl-p-benzoquinone imine (NAPQI) once hepatic stores of glutathione have been depleted.

Treatment with acetylcysteine (to replenish hepatic glutathione stores) is dependent on the timing of the overdose, and activated charcoal may be used within 1–2 hours of ingestion. Serum paracetamol levels should be sent at 4 hours post-ingestion or on arrival if presentation is delayed or staggered. If the patient has arrived within 8 hours, serum levels should be compared to the revised paracetamol overdose treatment nomogram (Figure 3.8.1.1), and treatment started if the level is at or above the toxicity line.

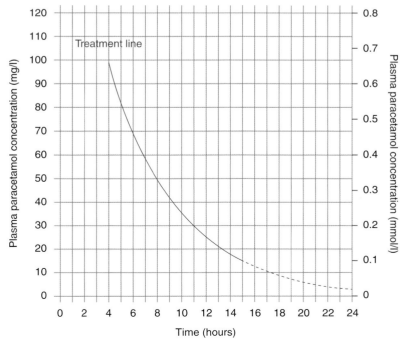

Figure 3.8.1.1 Revised paracetamol overdose treatment nomogram. The previous nomogram has been amended to a single treatment line (previously a high-risk line was also present), so all patients with a plasma paracetamol level above this are recommended to have treatment – regardless of risk factors for hepatoxicity.

Source: www.gov.uk/drug-safety-update/treating-paracetamol-overdose-with-intravenous-acetylcysteine-new-guidance

If presentation is delayed by >8 hours, then acetylcysteine should be started immediately and only stopped if serum paracetamol levels are below the nomogram. If >24 hours since ingestion, only stop treatment if serum paracetamol levels are <5 mg/l and there is no evidence of liver or renal impairment. Acetylcysteine is given as an infusion – initially 150 mg/kg body weight in 200 ml of 5% dextrose over 15 minutes, followed by 50 mg/kg in 500 ml over 4 hours, and finally 100 mg/kg in 1 l over 16 hours. An oral preparation is also available.

Despite severe liver failure, many cases of paracetamol overdose survive with supportive management. Liver function can be monitored biochemically, with a peak aspartate aminotransferase (AST)/alanine aminotransferase (ALT) seen at 3–4 days (often >10,000 IU/l), whilst bilirubin peaks at day 5. The international normalised ratio (INR) is the most sensitive marker, rising after 24 hours. Cases of severe liver failure should be discussed with local liver units, and transplantation may be considered according to the Kings College criteria: arterial pH <7.3, INR >6.7 (prothrombin time (PT) >100), creatinine >300 μmol/l and grade 3 or 4 encephalopathy.

Aspirin (Salicylic Acid)

The active ingredient in aspirin is salicylic acid, usually found at concentrations of 75–300 mg/tablet. Mild overdose (>150 mg/kg) presents with hyperventilation, vasodilation, dehydration, vomiting, tinnitus and deafness, progressing to confusion, convulsions and reduced Glasgow Coma Score (GCS) in severe cases (>500 mg/kg). Some preparations, including enteric-coated, may have a delayed or prolonged onset. Children are at risk of hyperpyrexia and hypoglycaemia, and rare presentations may include pulmonary and cerebral oedema or renal failure. Blood gases demonstrate respiratory alkalosis with metabolic acidosis (reversed in children) in moderate to severe poisoning, with hypokalaemia often present.

Initial treatment is aimed at reducing systemic absorption using activated charcoal. Further management is then based on plasma salicylate levels. Mild levels (<450 mg/l in adults, 350 mg/l in children) require observation only and increased oral fluids. In moderate poisoning (<700 mg/l), IV fluids are required – 1.26% bicarbonate is often utilised as this alkalinises urine-promoting excretion. (Aim for uri­nary pH >7.5, although this can be difficult to measure in uncatheterised or non-cooperative patients.)

Additionally, repeat salicylate levels should be sent to ensure there is no ongoing absorption. In severe poisoning (salicylate >700 mg/l, acidosis or central nervous system (CNS) features), mortality is significant. Intubation and ventilation may be required for coma or severe hyperventilation. Consider repeated activated charcoal via a nasogastric (NG) tube. Control the acidosis using a sodium bicarbonate infusion, and obtain central venous access to allow for haemofiltration – which can correct electrolyte imbalances, in addition to removing the salicylate. If any CNS features are present, this may be secondary to cerebral hypoglycaemia; hence, administer IV dextrose (even if serum levels are normal).

Drugs: Prescription
Opioids

Opioids are used commonly as analgesics (morphine and diamorphine (heroin)), cough suppressants (codeine) and anti-diarrhoeal agents (loperamide). Many, if not all, opiates may be abused as both prescription drugs and illicit preparations. Overdose classically presents with respiratory depression (sometimes progressing to cyanosis and apnoea), hypotension, reduced GCS (occasionally with convulsions) and characteristic pinpoint pupils.

Treatment primarily focuses on airway and ventilatory support (potentially requiring intubation) and use of naloxone as a reversal agent. Naloxone is usually given as IV boluses of 400–800 μg every 2–3 minutes (10 μg/kg in children) until the patient is breathing adequately, but not necessarily awake. The dose should be reduced in drug addicts to avoid precipitating opiate withdrawal syndrome, and can be dripped or sprayed intranasally (at the same dose) if IV access is difficult. It is important to remember that the half-life of naloxone is only 62 minutes, considerably less than that of many opiate preparations (especially methadone); thus, further doses may be required and patients should be observed for 6 hours following the last dose of naloxone. Additionally, it should also be remembered that some opiate-based analgesic formulations include paracetamol which may require separate management.

Antidepressants

Poisoning by TCAs presents with tachycardia, dry skin/mouth, dilated pupils, urinary retention, ataxia, limb jerking and drowsiness progressing to coma. Unconscious patients tend to have a divergent squint, increased muscular tone and reflexes, myoclonus and extensor plantar reflexes, although this can progress to muscle flaccidity and respiratory depression. Characteristic ECG changes include sinus tachycardia, progressing to PR and QRS prolongation, which can mimic slow ventricular tachycardia (VT). Convulsions, ventricular arrhythmias or bradycardias are pre-terminal events. Management involves activated charcoal, IV fluids for hypotension and intubation if unconscious. Arrhythmias may be controlled with sodium bicarbonate (50–100 ml boluses of 8.4%). If hypotension or arrhythmias are refractory, discussion with a toxicology expert is advised as anti-arrhythmics should be avoided. Glucagon or Intralipid® have been used successfully. Short, self-terminating convulsions should settle upon correcting hypoxia or acidaemia, but benzodiazepines can be used if they are persistent. Consciousness usually returns after approximately 12 hours. However, there remains a risk of delirium or hallucinations for the following 3 days, and these may require sedation.

Lithium overdose often occurs secondary to inadvertent drug interactions, and presents initially with nausea, vomiting and diarrhoea, followed by tremor, ataxia, confusion and clonus. Severe cases (serum lithium >1.5 mmol/l) may be complicated by convulsions, coma or renal failure, and can be delayed if prolonged-release preparations are used. Activated charcoal has no effect on lithium, but whole bowel irrigation may be considered if prolonged-release preparations are involved. Patients should be observed for >24 hours with supportive care, and benzodiazepines used for seizure control. In severe poisoning, haemodialysis may be used; however, prolonged use may be required due to redistribution of lithium sequestered in body tissues following initial plasma clearance.

Serotonin syndrome can be seen in patients recently started on selective serotonin reuptake inhibitors (SSRIs) or MAOIs or in those who take drugs which promote serotonin release, including cocaine, MDMA (3,4-methylenedioxymethamphetamine) and amphetamines. Symptoms may include autonomic changes (tachycardia, hypertension, flushing, hyperthermia), altered mental state (confusion, hallucinations, agitation, drowsiness or coma) and neuromuscular features (ataxia, rigidity, hyper-reflexia, teeth grinding and shivering). Severe cases may be complicated by convulsions, rhabdomyolysis, renal failure or coagulopathy. Treatment is supportive with glyceryl trinitrate (GTN), benzodiazepines and dantrolene, as indicated.

Benzodiazepines

When taken in overdose, benzodiazepines present with drowsiness, dizziness, ataxia and dysarthria. Activated charcoal is usually not necessary, and management is generally supportive. Benzodiazepines can, however, potentiate the effect of other depressant drugs taken at the same time, potentially necessitating airway protection and ventilation. Flumazenil is the specific antidote, but its short half-life of 1 hour and the risk of precipitating arrhythmias or convulsions in patients who have taken a combined overdose with TCAs mean that its use is reserved for severe cases only.

Sulphonylureas

These drugs are used for control of diabetes; thus, their main effect in overdose is hypoglycaemia. With long-acting preparations such as glibenclamide, the risk can last up to 72 hours. Glucose levels should be checked hourly, and 10% dextrose infusions used as a preventative measure. If higher concentrations of dextrose are needed, central access may be required. In severe cases, octreotide has been trialled to prevent pancreatic insulin release; however, discussion should be had with the toxicology service prior to considering this.

Beta-blockers

The primary concerns in overdose of beta-blockers are hypotension, bradycardia and cardiogenic shock; however, other risks include convulsions and bronchospasm. Rarely, propranolol can cause hypoglycaemia in children, and sotalol may induce polymorphic VT due to QTc prolongation. Management requires cardiac monitoring and activated charcoal. Atropine 1–2 mg IV may be trialled for bradycardia but tends to be ineffective. Glucagon 5–10 mg IV promotes rapid improvement; however, there is a risk of vomiting, and therefore aspiration. Repeated glucagon boluses (or an infusion) may be required, and adrenaline or dobutamine infusions are utilised as second-line therapies. Cardiac pacing may be attempted; however, it is often unsuccessful. Insulin may improve hypotension, and Intralipid® has been used successfully in cardiac arrest.

Calcium Channel Blockers

Initial symptoms of overdose are non-specific, with nausea, vomiting, dizziness and confusion, subsequently progressing to bradycardia, atrioventricular block, hypotension, metabolic acidosis and hyperkalaemia/glycaemia. Treatment is similar to that for beta-blockers, with potential addition of calcium gluconate (10 ml of 10%) (to improve atrioventricular dissociation) and/or high-dose glucose–insulin–potassium infusions (on which the toxicology service can advise if required).

Digoxin

Overdose can occur with both tablets and ingestion of glycosidic trees and plants such as yew or foxglove. Symptoms include nausea, vomiting, delirium, characteristic xanthopsia (yellowish visual discoloration) and arrhythmias ranging from bradycardia to VT. Hyperkalaemia can occur with metabolic acidosis, although this is secondary to poor tissue perfusion. Management includes activated charcoal – repeated doses of which may be warranted to reduce enterohepatic circulation – and control of acidosis and hyperkalaemia with bicarbonate and insulin–dextrose infusions. Atropine can be used initially for bradycardia; however, cardiac pacing may be required (often needing high voltages to achieve capture). VT may respond to lidocaine or beta-blockers. In severe cases, Digibind® (a specific antibody to digoxin) can be trialled, if available, following consultation with the toxicology service.

Theophylline

Poisoning with theophylline or aminophylline is often complicated by the predominance of prolonged-release preparations where signs and symptoms may thus be delayed by up to 24 hours following ingestion. These include hyperventilation, sinus tachycardia (deteriorating into supraventricular tachycardia, VT and ventricular fibrillation), headache, convulsions, coma, intractable vomiting, haematemesis, abdominal pain and hyperpyrexia. Blood gases are complex, with initial respiratory alkalosis, followed by metabolic acidosis, hypokalaemia and hypoglycaemia. Treatment is supportive, with activated charcoal, electrolyte replacement (although there is a risk of rebound hyperkalaemia) and benzodiazepines for seizures. Provided cardiac output is maintained, tachycardia may only require observation; however, if compromised, non-selective beta-blockers may be considered. Cautious use is warranted as they may precipitate bronchospasm, and for this reason, disopyramide is often used as the first-line anti-arrhythmic. Charcoal haemoperfusion can be considered in severe cases.

Iron

Serious poisoning tends to occur in children and requires levels of >60 mg/kg (normal preparations contain 35–110 mg/tablet). Symptoms of poisoning occur in two phases. In the early phase (<12 hours), most cases present with nausea, vomiting, abdominal pain and diarrhoea – with a greyish-black tinge to vomit or stool. In severe cases, patients also develop haematemesis, reduced GCS, convulsions, metabolic acidosis and shock in the early phase. Whilst the majority of cases will improve with supportive treatment after this first phase, some cases progress to a second phase 24–48 hours later. At this stage, metabolic acidosis, hypoglycaemia, liver failure, renal failure and bowel infarction may occur. Survivors are at future risk of gastric and post-pyloric strictures. Management of an overdose includes supportive measures and gastric lavage or whole bowel irrigation (but not activated charcoal if a large dose is ingested). In severe cases (usually characterised by coma or shock), liaise with the toxicology service and consider a desferrioxamine infusion (15 mg/(kg hr)), guided by the free iron:total iron-binding capacity ratio.

Clomethiazole

Overdose of this sedative can present with respiratory depression, hypotension, coma, hypothermia, hypersalivation and reduced muscle tone. It has a characteristic smell often noticed on the breath ('reminiscent of some sort of leafy garden plant'). Management is supportive, but intubation and ventilation may be required for airway and respiratory support.

Phenothiazines

In overdose, the anti-psychotics can cause arrhythmias, hypotension, reduced GCS, convulsions, dystonic reactions and hypothermia, although respiratory depression and coma are unlikely. Management includes activated charcoal, supportive therapy and correction of electrolytes and hypoxia prior to use of anti-arrhythmics. Procyclidine 5 mg IV can be used for dystonic reactions.

Barbiturates

Barbiturate poisoning presents with respiratory depression, hypotension, coma and hypothermia, with a risk of rhabdomyolysis secondary to prolonged unconsciousness. Initial management revolves around supportive treatment and repeated activated charcoal administration, and intubation for airway protection is not unusual. Charcoal haemoperfusion can be considered in the event of prolonged unconsciousness.

Angiotensin-converting enzyme inhibitors

Overdose may present with drowsiness, hypotension, hyperkalaemia and, rarely, renal failure. Normal dosing regimens are also associated with a risk of angio-oedema, initially affecting the face, and may cause airway obstruction. Occasionally misdiagnosed as allergy and anaphylaxis, angio-oedema often does not respond to steroids or adrenaline, instead requiring 2–4 units of fresh frozen plasma (which contains enzymes to break down the causative bradykinin accumulation).

Salbutamol

Beta-2 agonists, such as terbutaline, present with tachycardia, hypertension, palpitations, agitation, tremor, nausea and hypokalaemia. In severe cases, there may be arrhythmias, ischaemia, convulsions and hallucinations. Treatment is supportive, with electrolyte correction and activated charcoal, and in the event of severe tachy-arrhythmias with haemodynamic compromise, propranolol may be used.

Non-prescription
Amphetamines and Cathinones

Amphetamines, including MDMA/ecstasy, and cathinones (e.g. methedrone) are used as stimulants and can be ingested orally, sniffed or injected. Features of an overdose occur secondary to endogenous serotonin and catecholamine release, and may include tachycardia, hypertension, euphoria, agitation, mydriasis and headache. Severe features can also include arrhythmias, convulsions or coma, serotonin syndrome, hyperpyrexia and rhabdomyolysis (leading to renal failure), liver failure and cerebral haemorrhage. Biochemical abnormalities include hypoglycaemia, hyperkalaemia and hyponatraemia due to syndrome of inappropriate anti-diuretic hormone secretion (SIADH) or polydipsia. Treatment includes supportive care and activated charcoal, and in severe poisoning with hypertension, use of benzodiazepines with GTN. (Beta-blockers should be avoided due to the risk of unopposed alpha-adrenergic receptor stimulation.) Benzodiazepines may also be used to treat

agitation or prolonged convulsions, and if intubation is required, suxamethonium should be avoided due to concurrent hyperkalaemia. Bicarbonate infusions may be required for metabolic acidosis, and active cooling or dantrolene 1 mg/kg may be used for hyperpyrexia. Derangements of serum sodium are also common and should be actively monitored and treated accordingly.

Cocaine

When smoked, snorted or injected, cocaine causes the release of catecholamines and serotonin, and sodium channel blockade. This leads to tachycardia, hypertension, arrhythmias, euphoria, agitation, delirium, fits, mydriasis, sweating and vomiting. It can precipitate myocardial infarction, aortic dissection, cerebral haemorrhage, serotonin syndrome, rhabdomyolysis and renal failure. Treatment is with oxygen and benzodiazepines, and aspirin and GTN for chest pain. For hypertension, beta-blockers should be avoided, and instead GTN, calcium channel blockers or phentolamine should be used.

Gamma Hydroxybutyrate

Gamma hydroxybutyrate (GHB) is used in body building and as a psychedelic. Severe poisoning causes respiratory depression, bradycardia, hypotension, convulsions and coma. Treatment is supportive, with airway support, activated charcoal and benzodiazepines for convulsions, and in some case reports, naloxone has been shown to reverse some effects.

Lysergic Acid Diethylamide

Lysergic acid diethylamide (LSD) is a psychedelic agent which can cause hypertension, drowsiness or agitation. Severe overdose may cause respiratory arrest, coma or coagulopathy. Treatment is supportive.

Legal Highs

These new psychoactive substances are synthetic agents manufactured to produce similar effects to illegal drugs, whilst attempting to circumnavigate current drug legislation. Depending on the active agent, effects include stimulants, sedatives, hallucinogens and cannabinoid, or combinations thereof. Following a series of deaths amongst users, attempts have been made to ban the agents (such as the Psychoactive Substances Act 2016 in the UK). Management is predominantly supportive, though it should be tailored to the agent's predominant symptoms.

Plants/Fungi

Serious poisoning is relatively rare, with most symptoms being self-limiting and gastrointestinal in nature. The main exceptions are the glycosides (covered earlier in the 'Digoxin' section), and in the UK, the death cap mushroom (*Amanita phalloides*). This initially causes vomiting and diarrhoea; however, this may progress to liver and renal failure. Treatment is supportive.

Chemical

Alcohol

Overdose of alcohol (active ingredient ethanol) is common, particularly as part of mixed overdose where it can potentiate the depressant effect of other agents on the CNS. Severe cases may present with respiratory depression, hypotension, coma (with a risk of aspiration), hypothermia and metabolic acidosis (which may be secondary to lactate or ketones). Due to the high solubility of alcohol, measures to reduce absorption are ineffective; thus, management in severe cases primarily involves airway protection, blood sugar monitoring (with glucose as needed) and vitally exclusion of head injury as the primary cause for reduced GCS. Most hospitals have their own scare story about the drunken patient who was allowed to sleep off their intoxication, only to not wake up due to a missed intracranial haemorrhage.

Methanol and Ethylene Glycerol

Methanol and ethylene are encountered as constituents of methylated spirits or antifreeze. The toxic effects are caused by their active metabolite (including formaldehyde and glycolaldehyde, respectively); thus, severe symptoms tend to only present after 12 hours following ingestion.

Methanol initially presents with mild drowsiness. However, after 12 hours, symptoms progress to vomiting, abdominal pain, headache, dizziness, visual blurring and increasing drowsiness progressing to coma. Blood gas analysis shows severe metabolic acidosis and hyperglycaemia, and amylase levels may be raised. Treatment may include gastric lavage, but not activated charcoal. These patients should be discussed with the toxicology service early to guide commencement of fomepizole (an antidote) or ethanol. Both fomepizole and ethanol prevent the formation of the toxic metabolites by competitive inhibition of alcohol dehydrogenase. However, ethanol is often more readily available. Ethanol is given as 2 ml/kg of whiskey, vodka or gin orally (provided patients are awake), followed by a 12 g/hr ethanol IV infusion – increased in chronic alcoholics. Folic acid can also be used to further reduce metabolism. Sodium bicarbonate infusions should be used to control the metabolic acidosis, aiming for mild alkalosis (pH 7.5). In severe cases, haemodialysis can be used to enhance removal of methanol, although the ethanol infusion will need to be increased to counter its associated enhanced clearance. Ingestion of >30 ml is usually fatal, and in survivors, >10 ml causes permanent blindness.

Ethylene poisoning shares some similar features with methanol poisoning; however, severe features also include ataxia, dysarthria, convulsions and haematemesis. After 12 hours, pulmonary oedema, cardiac arrhythmias and failure can occur, and renal failure may be evident after 24 hours (secondary to acute tubular necrosis). Hypocalcaemia (which may be severe), with urinary calcium oxalate monohydrate crystals, is diagnostic. Treatment is as for methanol poisoning, with the addition of calcium gluconate to treat hypocalcaemia.

Petrol/Kerosene

The majority of symptoms during overdose are mild and self-limiting, unless pulmonary aspiration occurs. Hydrocarbon aspiration causes pneumonitis, with coughing, wheeze, breathlessness, cyanosis and fever. Chest X-ray signs may be present without symptoms. Severe cases can develop pulmonary oedema, drowsiness, convulsions or coma and renal failure. Treatment is with oxygen, bronchodilators and intubation and ventilation if necessary, and gastric lavage should be avoided due to increased risk of accidental aspiration.

Organophosphates

These anti-cholinesterases cause toxicity secondary to irreversible binding and inhibition of cholinesterases, which leads to accumulation of acetylcholine at nerve endings. They are highly soluble and easily absorbed through the skin, lung and gut mucosa, and are encountered as insecticides or nerve gas agents, e.g. sarin. Initial symptoms are predominantly from parasympathetic acetylcholine blockade (nausea, vomiting, headache, diarrhoea, miosis and hypersalivation), although sweating and muscle fasciculations may also be apparent. Severe poisoning progresses to pulmonary oedema, bronchospasm, cardiac arrhythmias, convulsions, coma and paralysis, as seen with nerve agents. The key feature in management is barrier precautions to prevent contamination of medical staff. Besides supportive care, atropine (2 mg IV) is administered at 5-minute intervals, aiming for a systolic blood pressure >80 mmHg, heart rate <80 bpm and a clear chest. Diazepam can be used to control seizures and agitation. In moderate to severe poisoning, irreversible binding can be prevented using pralidoxime, which 'reactivates' the cholinesterases by displacing the organophosphate.

Cyanide

Cyanide poisoning can occur from multiple sources. Whilst often considered the preserve of murder mystery novels, it can also be formed by certain drugs, such as sodium nitroprusside, and is found in nail polish remover and the kernels of some fruits. It is also formed during combustion of polyurethane foam which is found in household furnishings, thus should be borne in mind in burns patients presenting with severe metabolic acidosis. It is highly soluble and, like organophosphates, can be absorbed through the skin and mucosal surfaces. It causes toxicity by inhibiting the electron transport chain, thus preventing aerobic respiration, causing histotoxic hypoxia. Orally ingested cyanide reacts with gastric acid, producing hydrogen cyanide which can potentially poison any first-aiders who give mouth-to-mouth resuscitation. Presenting features occur due to hypoxia and include breathlessness, palpitations, dizziness, anxiety and headache, progressing to pulmonary oedema, arrhythmias, convulsions, coma, paralysis and metabolic acidosis. Bitter almonds are classically described on the breath of patients, although the ability to detect this is dependent on genetic polymorphisms. Management starts with avoiding health worker contamination, potentially with removal of clothing and decontamination. Activated charcoal may be of benefit, and in mild cases, only oxygen and monitoring may be required. In severe cases, specific antidotes are available, including dicobalt edetate, sodium thiosulphate/nitrate and hydroxocobalamin, although these should only be commenced following confirmation of diagnosis and in liaison with the toxicology service.

Household and Industrial Cleaners

These may be ingested deliberately (e.g. in a suicide attempt) or accidentally (e.g. by children when insecurely stored), and include bleach, chlorine, detergents and other cleaning products. Whether acidic or alkali, they cause caustic burns to the oropharynx, larynx, airway and oesophagus, and the degree of injury spread depends on whether the product is in the liquid or solid/powdered form. Powders and solids tend to adhere to the lips, oropharynx and larynx, producing a chemical burn injury which may present with stridor and airway compromise. Liquids can produce similar effects and damage to the oesophagus, airways and stomach, leading to ulceration, haematemesis and perforation or Boerhaave syndrome. A thorough airway assessment is thus indicated in all instances, with a low threshold for an expedited intubation – which should be anticipated (and thus prepared for) to be difficult. Discussion with the toxicology service often guides treatment and may involve dilution. (This is usually reserved only for powdered alkalis due to the high risk of vomiting and aspiration, and should never be used with acids as an exothermic reaction can occur, causing thermal burns.) Fine-bore NG tubes are sometimes suggested with large acid ingestion (as pyloric sphincter spasm can prolong agent contact time in the stomach), but due to the risk of damage and perforation to the oesophagus from insertion, some centres avoid such practice.

Paraquat

Whilst no longer available in many developed countries, this toxic weed-killer can be fatal with ingestions of as little as 10 ml. Paraquat initially produces complications, due to its corrosive nature, in the form of oral and airway burns (which peak in severity after 24 hours), abdominal pain and diarrhoea. Large overdoses are fatal within 24 hours, with pulmonary oedema, hypotension, convulsions and severe metabolic acidosis. Less severe overdoses do not produce symptoms of shock but are still fatal, with death due to hypoxia secondary to 'paraquat lung'. This is characterised by lung fibrosis and pulmonary oedema after approximately 5 days, leading to progressive respiratory failure and death within 1–6 weeks, depending on the amount ingested. In suspected overdoses, activated charcoal should be given, and gastric lavage considered. Gastric fluid or urine should be sent for microscopy where the presence of sodium dithionite is diagnostic, and plasma paraquat levels can be measured to aid prognostication. Importantly, oxygen should be avoided, as it enhances pulmonary toxicity. Therefore, in patients requiring oxygen or ventilatory support, as no treatment improves the outcome, palliative care may be the best course of action.

Carbon Monoxide

Carbon monoxide (CO), produced during incomplete combustion, is clear and colourless, and found in car exhaust fumes, fires and poorly maintained gas heaters. CO binds to haemoglobin and prevents it from carrying oxygen, and inhibits mitochondrial cytochrome oxidase. Early features are non-specific, but in severe poisoning (carboxyhaemoglobin (COHb) levels >15 per cent), hyperventilation, hypotension and convulsions, with increased muscle tone and reflexes, may be evident. Arrhythmias, cardiac ischaemia and pulmonary or cerebral oedema may also occur, and the skin may appear characteristically 'cherry red'. Management primarily involves removal of exposure, airway management and 100% oxygen – either through a tight-fitting face mask or via endotracheal intubation. In theory, hyperbaric oxygen chambers could be utilised. However, considering that the half-life of CO with 100% oxygen is approximately 1 hour, transfer is often not warranted in all but a select few patients.

References and Further Reading

Rasimas JJ, Sinclair CM. Assessment and management of toxidromes in the critical care unit. *Crit Care Clin* 2017;**33**:521–41.

Roberts TN, Thompson JP. Illegal substances in anaesthetic and intensive care practices. *Contin Educ Anaesth Crit Care Pain* 2013;**13**:42–6.

Wyatt J, Illingworth R, Graham CA, Hogg K, Robertson C, Clancy M. Toxicology. In: J Wyatt, R Illingworth, C Graham, K Hogg, C Robertson, M Clancy (eds). *Oxford Handbook of Emergency Medicine*, 4th edn. Oxford: Oxford University Press; 2012. pp. 179–217.

Zimmerman JL. Poisonings and overdoses in the intensive care unit: general and specific management issues. *Crit Care Med* 2003;**31**:2794–801.

Obstetric Emergencies

3.9.1

Shrijit Nair and Audrey Quinn

Key Learning Points

1. Critical illness in pregnancy is relatively uncommon; however, it carries a significant amount of morbidity and mortality when it does occur. The majority of patients will be admitted to the intensive care unit in the post-partum period.
2. Recent advances in the management of common direct obstetric causes of maternal critical illness have improved outcomes. Unfortunately, however, we have not seen similar advances in treating the indirect causes.
3. Managing this unique cohort of patients is challenging and requires an in-depth knowledge of both maternal physiological adaptations to pregnancy and how these may affect the course of the patient's illness.
4. In obstetric emergencies, the main priority must be to resuscitate the mother, which, in turn, will help resuscitate the fetus.

Keywords: pre-eclampsia, HELLP, massive obstetric haemorrhage, venous thromboembolism, obstetric sepsis, maternal collapse, amniotic fluid embolism, thrombotic thrombocytic purpura, acute fatty liver of pregnancy, AFLP, difficult obstetric airway

Introduction

Pregnancy is a normal physiological process where a complex maternal and fetal interface exists throughout pregnancy and childbirth – in most instances, without any significant complications. If, however, patients do become seriously ill, they pose a unique challenge, in part owing to the physiological changes during pregnancy (Table 3.9.1.1). A recent study on gestation-specific ranges for vital parameters for pregnant mothers (4Ps study) confirmed these but highlighted the absence of a clinically significant BP drop from 12 weeks of gestation. Evidence-based parameter ranges can therefore be used to identify sick mothers at an early stage, and the modified obstetric Early Warning Score (EWS) system is recommended by MBRRACE-UK (Mothers and Babies: Reducing Risk through Audits and Confidential Enquiries across the UK). A working party is currently undertaking a national obstetric EWS (Scotland obstetric EWS published in 2018).

In this chapter, we describe the more common obstetric emergencies that require critical care admission. The reader is directed to the Royal College of Obstetricians and Gynaecologists (RCOG) Green-top guidelines on thrombosis and embolism, obstetric haemorrhage, hypertensive disease, maternal collapse and bacterial sepsis. Cardiac disease is the most common indirect cause of death in pregnancy, and cardiac failure is discussed in Chapter 3.9.2, Pre-eclampsia and Eclampsia, and Chapter 3.9.3, Pre-existing Disease in Pregnancy.

Massive Obstetric Haemorrhage

Obstetric haemorrhage accounts for up to 50 per cent of maternal deaths in some developing countries, whilst in the UK, it is responsible for 10 per cent of all direct maternal deaths. Massive obstetric haemorrhage (MOH) is defined as blood loss of ≥2000 ml, whilst major haemorrhage is defined as blood loss of >1000 ml. A recent mortality report, however, underlined the significance of smaller volumes of blood loss – particularly in smaller women (<60 kg), and here close observation of blood losses and rapid replacement are vital. MOH occurs in approximately 0.6 per cent of maternities, antepartum haemorrhage (APH) in 3–5 per cent of pregnancies (e.g. placenta praevia, placental abruption, uterine rupture trauma) and post-partum haemorrhage (PPH) in up to 13 per cent of all maternities (e.g. uterine atony, retained products of

Table 3.9.1.1 Physiological changes in pregnancy

Physiological system	Increased	Decreased
Respiratory system	Tidal volume Minute volume Oxygen consumption (30%) Failed tracheal intubation and induction Hypoxia Pulmonary oedema Maternal 2,3-diphosphoglycerate	Lung volume Residual volume Functional residual capacity PAO_2–PaO_2 gradient
Cardiovascular system Impact of fetus delivery	Heart rate Stroke volume Cardiac output (30–50%) Plasma volume Uterine blood flow Aortocaval compression	Systemic vascular resistance Colloidal osmotic pressure
Renal system	Glomerular filtration rate Proteinuria (mild)	Plasma urea and creatinine
Haematological Immune system	Dilutional anaemia White cell count Coagulation: ↑ VII, VIII, IX, X, XII, fibrinogen, D-dimer	Coagulation: ↓ XI and protein S
Gastrointestinal system	Obesity Plasma glucose Metabolism	Lower oesophageal sphincter pressures

conception, clotting disorders, genital tract trauma, acute uterine inversion).

Management

- Treatment goals for transfusion include:
    - Haematocrit >0.3
    - Platelets >50 × 10^9/l
    - Fibrinogen >2 g/l
    - Ionised calcium >1 mmol/l
    - Temperature >36°C

- A multidisciplinary approach involves the obstetrician, anaesthetist and haematologist, with a low threshold for transferring the patient to the High Dependence Unit or the ICU for observations and invasive pressure monitoring.
- When the blood loss threshold is reached, the local MOH protocol should be activated, or even earlier if further extensive blood loss is anticipated. Syntocinon® bolus of 5 U, followed by an infusion of 125 ml/l (40 U in 500 ml), ergometrine (500 µg), tranexamic acid (1 g), carboprost prostaglandin 2 alpha (250 µg intramuscular every 15 minutes). First-line surgical manoeuvres include intrauterine balloon tamponade and uterine compression brace sutures.

- Other techniques include surgical uterine devascularisation and internal iliac artery ligation, or selective arterial occlusion or embolisation by interventional radiology. A peripartum hysterectomy may be necessary.
- Fibrinogen concentrate is increasingly used. Point-of-care-testing devices (e.g. ROTEM® for fibrinogen, HemoCue® for haemoglobin levels) are increasingly used, as well as TEG® for coagulation (Figure 3.9.1.1). Routine use of factor VIIa is not recommended.

Recent advances in MOH include:

- Cryoprecipitate or fibrinogen concentrate (the PITHAGORE6 study suggested that a low fibrinogen level (<3 g/l) at PPH diagnosis is an independent predictor of severe bleeding). Some centres recommend fibrinogen concentrate titrated to point-of-care testing.
- Tranexamic acid. The CRASH-2 trial showed all-cause mortality at 28 days was significantly reduced by tranexamic acid administration and there was no increase in thrombotic events in these patients.
- Cell salvage. Use of intraoperative cell salvage (IOCS) is well established in many types of surgery where it has been shown to reduce the

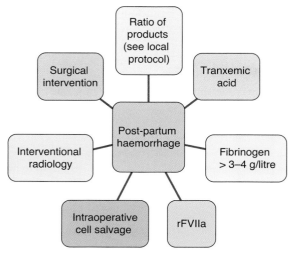

Figure 3.9.1.1 Summary of massive obstetric haemorrhage management.

need for allogeneic blood transfusions. The leucocyte depletion filter in the circuit seems to protect the mother against the risk of amniotic fluid embolus and red cell contamination. Large case series in the literature support its safe use in obstetric practice. The SALVO trial evaluated IOCS in obstetric practice and showed low complication rates and modest decrease in donor blood transfusions.

- Local haemorrhage guidelines recommend empiric plasma transfusion for PPH with haemostatic impairment.
- Fixed-ratio transfusion, as per trauma strategy, can result in unnecessary transfusion of fresh frozen plasma (FFP), associated with complications, and recent obstetric studies demonstrated FFP administration based on thromboelastometry results is feasible. Further research in this area is ongoing.

Venous Thromboembolism

Venous thromboembolism (VTE) in pregnancy is the leading direct cause of death in pregnancy. Careful assessment is important to look for congenital or acquired risk factors for VTE or thrombophilia such as age, obesity, multiple pregnancy, anti-phospholipid antibodies and past or family history, e.g. anti-thrombin, protein S or C deficiency. Low-molecular-weight heparin (LMWH) prophylaxis is frequently used, and so a safe window for regional techniques is carefully timed during labour and delivery. Warfarin causes

congenital abnormalities but rarely may still be seen in peripartum patients with mechanical heart valves.

Compression duplex ultrasound is used but is less specific in pregnancy; computed tomography pulmonary angiography (CTPA) or ventilation/perfusion (V/Q) scanning in some centres is used to diagnose pulmonary emboli (PEs). D-dimers are raised in normal pregnancy, which limits its usefulness.

Suspected VTE/PE should receive treatment with LMWH 1.5 mg/kg booking body weight until confirmation or otherwise. A heparin infusion may be indicated for antenatal PE, as it has a shorter half-life and can be reversed if major bleeding becomes a significant risk or if labour and delivery are likely. If maternal collapse occurs due to a PE, anticoagulation, thrombolysis or surgical embolectomy should be considered, depending on the severity. Intravenous unfractionated heparin is preferred and if a massive PE is diagnosed, lifesaving thrombolysis should be performed, irrespective of the higher bleeding risk from recent delivery or surgery. Bedside echocardiography is useful for rapid diagnosis. This test and/or CTPA should be done within 1 hour, with immediate referral to the senior medical team. An inferior vena cava (IVC) filter can be used in patients with iliac vein VTE and/or recurrent PE despite anticoagulation.

Obstetric Sepsis

Sepsis is a leading cause of morbidity and mortality worldwide, and genital tract infection by *Escherichia coli* is the most common cause. In high-income countries, overall all-cause sepsis mortality is 8 per cent; however, the morbidity-to-mortality ratio is 50:1.

Complex immunological changes occur in pregnancy and the roles of both the innate and adaptive systems are being increasingly understood. For example, the expansion of 'immunosuppressive' regulatory T cells in healthy pregnancy is implicated in a relative state of immunosuppression, with altered innate immune phenotype and gene expression. Risk factors for maternal sepsis include ethnic minority, operative vaginal or Caesarean delivery, febrile illness or pre-existing medical problem and recent antibiotics. Group A streptococcal (GAS) infection is an obstetric emergency. It is associated with progression to septic shock in <2 hours in 50 per cent of cases. Invasive infections such as endometritis, necrotising fasciitis and toxic shock syndrome require immediate treatment, confirmed by cultures from high vaginal and endometrial swabs.

309

Diagnosis of obstetric sepsis is confirmed by raised C-reactive protein (CRP) and white cell count (WCC), procalcitonin, lactate and positive blood cultures. The Society of Obstetric Medicine of Australia and New Zealand has proposed obstetrically modified Sequential Organ Failure Assessment (SOFA) and quick SOFA (qSOFA) scores to predict the need for higher levels of care. Treatment includes the 'Sepsis Six' pathway, inotropic support as required, close liaison with microbiology and source control. Rapid tests to identify pathogens, e.g. polymerase chain reaction (PCR) and matrix-assisted laser desorption/ionisation (MALDI), are being evaluated. Intravenous immunoglobulin is used in severe cases.

In the case of respiratory sepsis, pregnant women can be more vulnerable to influenza, as seen during the 2012 swine flu epidemic. Influenza vaccination is a priority, and Tamiflu® is often started early (Department of Health guideline). Transfer to a tertiary centre should be considered early if the patient deteriorates.

SARS-CoV-2 19

The impact of severe acute respiratory syndrome coronavirus 2 (SARS-CoV-2) on pregnancy (March to May 2020) was reported in an early UK Obstetric Surveillance System (UKOSS) study suggesting that women becoming severely ill tended to be in their third trimester, with risk factors including ethnicity, obesity and coexisting medical problems. Early results suggested women are no more likely to become ill than non-pregnant women. Continuation of pregnancy

throughout a severe respiratory illness and proning of the pregnant patient have been reported and discussed.

Neurological Disease

Epilepsy is the third most common cause of indirect maternal death in the UK. Generalised tonic–clonic seizures with associated periods of hypoxia carry the highest risk of sudden unexplained death in epilepsy (SUDEP). For women with pre-existing epilepsy, there is a risk of increased seizure frequency – thought to be due to faster plasma clearance of anti-epileptic agents, poor compliance, hyperemesis and poor sleep regulation. Epilepsy guidelines have been released by the RCOG, and women with epilepsy should be reviewed by a neurologist and an obstetric specialist prior to conception. The benefits of seizure control must be balanced against the teratogenic effects of anti-convulsants, and sodium valproate appears to invoke the highest risk of congenital malformations. In those who experience their first seizure in pregnancy, most cases are idiopathic. However, there are many secondary causes of new-onset seizures in pregnancy (Table 3.9.1.2).

A Caesarean section may be necessary for recurrent generalised seizures in late pregnancy, and an early epidural in labour will dampen the stress response and thus decrease the peripartum seizure risk. In the event of a seizure, patients should be treated with oxygen and diazepam (rectal or intravenous) or intravenous lorazepam. Status epilepticus may require propofol

Table 3.9.1.2 Causes of seizures in pregnancy

Cause	Potential distinguishing features
Eclampsia	High blood pressure, proteinuria
Thrombotic thrombocytopenic purpura	Symptoms that may include fever, low platelets, haemolytic anaemia and thrombosis causing renal and neurological impairment
Cerebrovascular accident	Ongoing neurological impairment and CT/MRI evidence of an infarct or haemorrhage
Cerebral venous or sinus thrombosis	Identified on CT venogram, often a history of severe headache
Hypoglycaemia	Neurological impairment should resolve once glucose is corrected (although this may depend on the period of hypoglycaemia)
Electrolyte imbalances	Typically hyponatraemia and hypocalcaemia
Posterior reversible leukoencephalopathy syndrome	Associated with visual symptoms. Can be associated with high blood pressure. Identified on MRI and symptoms usually resolve 1–2 weeks later
Reversible cerebral vasoconstriction syndrome	Typical history of thunderclap headache. Identified on CT/MR angiography. Presents post-partum and symptoms usually resolve in 3 weeks
Space-occupying lesion	Possible focal neurological deficit, depending on site of space-occupying lesion. Identified on CT/MRI

or thiopentone infusions, and a referral to preferably neuro-intensive care should be made.

Eclampsia is discussed in Chapter 3.9.2, Pre-eclampsia and Eclampsia.

Cerebrovascular Disease

There is an increasing incidence of thromboembolic stroke related to pregnancy, yet maternity mortality reports often describe delays in diagnosis and treatment of such events, as they are not expected in young pregnant patients. Cerebral venous thrombosis is a rare, but potentially devastating illness, which is more common in pregnancy. It must be excluded in any sick mother with a severe headache, with or without neurological signs and symptoms. Thrombolysis, thrombectomy, anticoagulation and neuro-radiological diagnosis and assessment must not be delayed.

Liver Disease in Pregnancy

The incidence of liver disease in pregnancy in the UK is 5 per 100,000 maternities. The differential diagnosis includes gallstones and cholecystitis, cholestasis of pregnancy, haemolytic uraemic syndrome (HUS), hepatitis and HELLP (haemolysis, elevated liver enzymes and low platelets) syndrome. The diagnosis of acute fatty liver of pregnancy (AFLP) utilises the Swansea criteria and the presence of six or more criteria in the absence of another explanation: vomiting, abdominal pain, polydipsia/polyuria, encephalopathy, elevated bilirubin, hypoglycaemia, elevated urate, leucocytosis, ascites or bright liver on scan, elevated transaminases and ammonia, renal impairment, coagulopathy; microvascular steatosis is seen on liver biopsy. AFLP and HELLP syndrome both can result in liver failure and carry a high incidence of fetal and maternal morbidity and mortality. Differentiating the two is difficult. However, AFLP is often seen in primiparous older women with a low body mass index (BMI), and is associated with prodromal vomiting, raised bilirubin, high white cells and low glucose levels (and lacks hypertension and thrombocytopenia seen in HELLP syndrome).

Diabetic Emergencies in Pregnancy

Diabetic ketoacidosis (DKA) carries high maternal and neonatal mortality. More commonly encountered in type 1 diabetes mellitus (DM), it is also seen in type 2 DM and gestational diabetes. Precipitating factors include hyperemesis gravidarum, infection, insulin non-compliance, drugs precipitating hyperglycaemia (steroids) and insulin pump failure. Clinical signs and symptoms are nausea, abdominal pain, polyuria, polydipsia, blurred vision, muscle weakness, lethargy, change in mental status, hyperventilation, tachycardia, tachypnoea, coma, shock and abnormal fetal heart trace. Physiological changes in pregnancy (e.g. respiratory alkalosis and low bicarbonate) can impair buffering capacity and increase lipolysis and insulin resistance, progesterone, cortisol and placental lactogen. Management includes insulin and intravenous fluid therapy, correction of electrolyte abnormalities (hyper- and hypokalaemia and hypophosphataemia), treatment of precipitating factors and careful maternal and fetal monitoring. Continuous fetal monitoring is required until the maternal condition stabilises, and level 2 care is often required. The aim is for blood ketone levels of <0.6 mmol/l, pH >7.3, bicarbonate >15 mmol/l and an anion gap of <12. This correction should be controlled with a decrease in blood ketone levels by 0.5 mmol/(l hr), an increase in venous bicarbonate levels by 3 mmol/(l hr) and a decrease in capillary glucose levels by 3 mmol/(l hr).

Maternal Collapse

Maternal collapse may be a life-threatening condition associated with various aetiologies (Figure 3.9.1.2), and cardiac arrests occur in approximately 1 in 36,000 pregnancies, with a case fatality rate of 42 per cent (Table 3.9.1.3). The most common causes of cardiac arrest in pregnancy requiring resuscitation are anaesthetic interventions (e.g. high spinal), venous thromboembolism and hypovolaemia. A recent MBRRACE report suggests that maternal morbidity has been increasing from year to year, with the most plausible reason being changing maternal demographics.

Particular consideration should be given to relief of aortocaval compression, and increasingly, left manual displacement of the uterus is the recommended technique for a visible bump above the umbilicus or gestation of >20 weeks. The same defibrillation levels are recommended as in non-pregnant patients. A peri-mortem Caesarean section (PMCS), or resuscitative hysterotomy, should be performed without delay within 4 minutes, and completed by 5 minutes if no return of spontaneous circulation (ROSC). Ultrasound may aid diagnosis but should not delay resuscitation. Figure 3.9.1.2 shows likely sources of collapse in pregnancy.

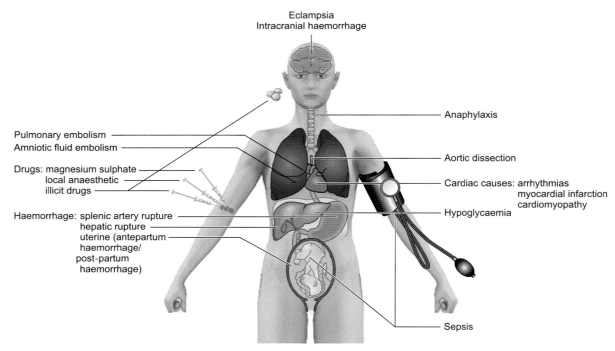

Figure 3.9.1.2 Causes of a maternal collapse.
Source: From *Maternal Collapse in Pregnancy and the Puerperium* (Green-top Guideline No. 56).

Table 3.9.1.3 Causes of 4 Hs and 4 Ts in pregnancy

Reversible causes	Causes in pregnancy
The 4 Hs	
Hypovolaemia	Bleeding (may be concealed) (obstetric or other) or relative hypovolaemia of dense spinal block, septic or neurogenic shock
Hypoxia	Pregnant patients can become hypoxic more quickly
Hypo-/hyperkalaemia and other electrolyte disturbances	No more likely
Hypothermia	No more likely
The 4 Ts	
Thromboembolism	Amniotic fluid embolus, pulmonary embolus, air embolus, myocardial infarct
Toxicity	Local anaesthetic, magnesium, other
Tension pneumothorax	Following trauma/suicide attempt
Tamponade	Following trauma/suicide attempt

Maternal collapse is often associated with poor maternal and fetal outcomes at any stage in pregnancy (and up to 6 weeks after delivery). However, timely resuscitation and PMCS can increase survival rates to 60 per cent. Management of maternal collapse involves a multidisciplinary team effort (involving input from obstetricians, anaesthetists, intensivists, neonatologists and midwives) and should follow the Resuscitation Council UK guidelines (Figure 3.9.1.3).

Thrombotic Thrombocytopenic Purpura

Thrombotic thrombocytopenic purpura (TTP) is a severe life-threatening haematological disorder affecting the microcirculation of multiple organ systems. It is caused by a deficiency (either acquired or inherited) in ADAMTS13, which is a specific von Willebrand factor (vWF) protease. The ensuing platelet plugs can cause kidney and heart failure in poorly treated cases, and acute

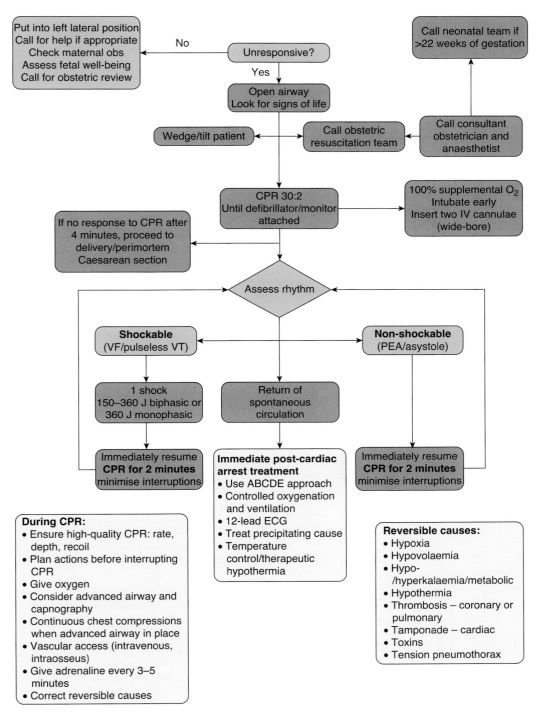

Figure 3.9.1.3 Resuscitation in pregnancy.
Source: Royal College of Obstetricians and Gynaecologists.

lung injury may be triggered by the associated inflammatory response. Treatment involves plasmapheresis, and the timing of labour and delivery, if occurring in the third trimester, requires careful multidisciplinary team planning, aiming for a platelet count of >50.

Amniotic Fluid Embolism

Amniotic fluid embolism (AFE) is a diagnosis of exclusion, with an incidence of 2 per 100,000 deliveries. It often presents as maternal collapse in labour/pregnancy or within 30 minutes of delivery, commonly preceded by acute hypotension, hypoxia and respiratory distress. Pulmonary hypertension may develop acutely, as may left ventricular failure and coagulopathy. Immediate delivery of the fetus will aid cardiovascular resuscitation but is obviously associated with an increase in bleeding complications. Management is supportive, with ABC and maintenance of oxygenation and cardiac output and correction of coagulopathy.

Trauma in Pregnancy

Maternal mortality and morbidity from penetrating trauma, accidental injury, domestic violence and suicide (often associated with mental health issues) has risen in recent years and was highlighted in the latest mortality report. Initial management for a pregnant woman is the same as for the non-pregnant patient, but the altered physiology and anatomy may affect responses to treatment. The main priority must be to resuscitate the mother, which, in turn, will resuscitate the fetus. Specialist equipment may be necessary (e.g. cardiotocography (CTG) for fetal monitoring), and immediate management may include a PMCS.

Anaesthetic and Airway Problems

Maternal, fetal, surgical and situational factors contribute to the increased incidence of failed intubation in around 1 in 400 obstetric general anaesthetics (GAs). Physiologically, the mucosa of the upper respiratory tract becomes more vascular and oedematous, leading to an increased risk of airway bleeding and swelling, exacerbated by fluids and oxytocin, and decreased functional residual capacity (FRC) and increased oxygen requirements in an often obese patient exacerbate desaturation during apnoea. The decline in incidence of obstetric GAs has resulted in reduced training opportunities, and concerns

regarding rapid delivery of the fetus often lead to time pressure, resulting in poor preparation, planning and communication and suboptimal performance of technical skills.

In light of this extremely difficult situation, the Obstetric Anaesthetists' Association and Difficult Airway Society have produced guidelines for the management of difficult and failed tracheal intubation in obstetrics.

References and Further Reading

Chu J, Johnston TA, Geoghegan J; Royal College of Obstetricians and Gynaecologists. 2019. Maternal collapse in pregnancy and the puerperium. Green-top guideline No. 56. obgyn.onlinelibrary.wiley.com/doi/10.1111/1471-0528.15995

Green LJ, Mackillop LH, Salvi D, et al. Gestation-specific vital sign reference ranges in pregnancy. *Obstet Gynecol* 2020;**135**:653–64.

Greer O, Shah NM, Johnson MR. Maternal sepsis update: current management and controversies. *The Obstetrician & Gynaecologist* 2020;**22**:45–55.

Knight M, Bunch K, Tuffnell D, et al.; MBRRACE-UK (eds). Saving lives, improving mothers' care. Lessons learned to inform maternity care from the UK and Ireland Confidential Enquiries into Maternal Deaths and Morbidity 2017–19. Oxford: National Perinatal Epidemiology Unit, University of Oxford; 2021. www.npeu.ox.ac.uk/assets/downloads/mbrrace-uk/reports/maternal-report-2021/MBRRACE-UK_Maternal_Report_2021_-_FINAL_-_WEB_VERSION.pdf

Knight M, Bunch K, Vousden N, et al.; UK Obstetric Surveillance System SARS-CoV-2 Infection in Pregnancy Collaborative Group. Characteristics and outcomes of pregnant women admitted to hospital with confirmed SARS-CoV-2 infection in UK: national population based cohort study. *BMJ* 2020;**369**:m2107.

Mushambi MC, Kinsella SM, Popat M, et al. Obstetric Anaesthetists' Asociation and Difficult Airway Society guidelines for the management of difficult and failed tracheal intubation in obstetrics. *Anaesthesia* 2015;**70**:1286–306.

Royal College of Obstetricians and Gynaecologists. 2011. Antepartum haemorrhage. Green-top guideline No. 63. www.rcog.org.uk/globalassets/documents/guidelines/gtg_63.pdf

Royal College of Obstetricians and Gynaecologists. 2012. Bacterial sepsis in pregnancy. Green-top guideline No. 64a. www.rcog.org.uk/globalassets/documents/guidelines/gtg_64a.pdf

Royal College of Obstetricians and Gynaecologists. 2012. Bacterial sepsis following pregnancy. Green-top guideline No. 64b. www.rcog.org.uk/globalassets/documents/guidelines/gtg_64b.pdf

Royal College of Obstetricians and Gynaecologists. 2015. Reducing the risk of venous thromboembolism during pregnancy and puerperium. Green-top guideline No. 37a. www.rcog.org.uk/globalassets/documents/guidelines/gtg-37a.pdf

Royal College of Obstetricians and Gynaecologists. 2016. Postpartum haemorrhage, prevention and management. Green-top guideline No. 52. www.rcog.org.uk/en/guidelines-research-services/guidelines/gtg52/

3.9.2

Pre-eclampsia and Eclampsia

Louise Swan and Audrey Quinn

Key Learning Points

1. Pre-eclampsia is a major cause of mortality in developing countries. It remains a cause of significant morbidity and is a common reason for critical care admissions in the obstetric population in the UK.
2. Careful adherence to national guidelines on the treatment and prevention of pre-eclampsia should be followed when a patient is admitted to critical care and this requires a multidisciplinary approach.
3. Acute pulmonary oedema occurs in 3 per cent of patients with severe pre-eclampsia, and early diagnosis is essential to differentiate between hypertensive disease of pregnancy and other causes.
4. Haemolysis, elevated liver enzymes and low platelets (HELLP) is associated with pre-eclampsia and carries high maternal and neonatal morbidity.
5. Eclampsia can complicate severe pre-eclampsia or occur in stable or undiagnosed pre-eclampsia. Prompt delivery of the fetus should occur as soon as the mother has been stabilised.

Keywords: pre-eclampsia, eclampsia, hypertension

Introduction

In 2016, mortality directly attributable to pre-eclampsia was at its lowest, as reported in the national maternal mortality report MBRRACE (Mothers and Babies: Reducing Risk through Audits and Confidential Enquiries across the UK). This improvement had been attributed to prompt diagnosis, close monitoring and standardised treatment pathways. However, the most recent report MBRRACE 2019 has reported increasing numbers. The multi-system disease still remains a common cause of maternal and neonatal mortality and is one of the common reasons a patient in the peripartum period is admitted into critical care.

Definitions

Pre-eclampsia

- Hypertension (systolic blood pressure ≥140 mmHg or diastolic blood pressure ≥90 mmHg) after 20 weeks' gestation in a previously normotensive patient, with proteinuria ≥0.3 g in 24-hour urine collection or a protein/creatinine ratio ≥0.30

Or

- New-onset hypertension with or without proteinuria and any of the following:
  - Platelet count <100,000/µl
  - Serum creatinine >97.2 µmol/l or doubling of creatinine concentration in the absence of other renal disease
  - Liver transaminases greater than twice the upper limit of normal concentrations
  - Pulmonary oedema
  - Cerebral or visual symptoms
  - Fetal growth restriction

Eclampsia

New-onset, generalised tonic–clonic seizures or coma in a woman with pre-eclampsia; 20 per cent will not have had a diagnosis of pre-eclampsia made and most occur post-partum within 12 hours of delivery.

Haemolysis, Elevated Liver Enzymes and Low Platelets (HELLP)

A severe form of pre-eclampsia, although hypertension and proteinuria may not coexist. Aspartate aminotransferase >70 IU/l or alanine aminotransferase >70 IU/l, platelet count <100 × 10⁻⁹/l and either hypertension, proteinuria or haemolysis (lactate dehydrogenase >600 IU/l, total bilirubin >20 mmol/l or schistocytes, burr cells or polychromasia on blood film). Mortality is 1–2 per cent, mostly due to intracranial haemorrhage.

Pathophysiology

Recent research into the pathophysiology and aetiology of pre-eclampsia is emerging with new theories. Pre-eclampsia occurs as a result of the response to stress of the syncytiotrophoblast. There are two sub-types: early- and late-onset pre-eclampsia. The former arises owing to defective placentation, whilst late-onset pre-eclampsia may reflect a maternal genetic predisposition to cardiovascular and metabolic disease, exacerbated by placental soluble factors.

The role of excess prolactin and use of predictive assays such as the ratio of serum Flt-1 to placental growth factor are being elucidated.

The cause of seizures in eclampsia is not known. It is hypothesised that it is a result of vasogenic and/or cytotoxic oedema from hypertension disrupting the cerebral autoregulatory system.

Prevention

Patients who have one high risk factor, or two or more moderate risk factors, are recommended to take aspirin 75 mg/day during their pregnancy. Major factors include hypertensive disease in previous pregnancy, chronic kidney disease, autoimmune disease, diabetes mellitus and chronic hypertension. Moderate risk factors include first pregnancy, ≥40 years, pregnancy interval of ≥10 years, family history of pre-eclampsia and multiple pregnancy.

Signs and Symptoms

Signs and symptoms of pre-eclampsia and eclampsia can be seen in Table 3.9.2.1.

Grading of Severity

The diagnosis of severe pre-eclampsia is met if the following are present:

- Severe hypertension (systolic blood pressure >160 mmHg or diastolic blood pressure >110 mmHg) not responding to treatment

Or

- Severe hypertension and any symptom described in Table 3.9.2.1 and/or an abnormal platelet count, raised transaminases or serum creatinine

Or

- Eclampsia

Differential Diagnosis

Prompt and early diagnosis of pre-eclampsia can still be missed if a woman does not exhibit the classical signs and symptoms. Most guidelines now remove the mandatory requirement for proteinuria, and eclampsia can occur without classical pre-eclampsia, so continued vigilance is required into the post-partum phase.

Other causes of hypertension, thrombocytopenia, liver abnormalities and renal abnormalities in pregnancy include acute fatty liver of pregnancy (AFLP), thrombotic thrombocytopenia purpura (TTP) and haemolytic uraemic syndrome (HUS).

In those with seizures, if there are atypical features present, other causes of seizures or headache need to be considered (e.g. post-dural puncture headache, cerebral venous thrombosis, subarachnoid haemorrhage, meningitis). These include those who do not meet the diagnostic criteria for pre-eclampsia and those with persistent neurological deficits, prolonged loss of consciousness or seizures not responding to magnesium sulphate.

General Treatment of Pre-eclampsia
Hypertension

Treat immediately with oral or intravenous labetalol, intravenous hydralazine or oral nifedipine, aiming for blood pressure of <150/100 mmHg. Fetal monitoring is required.

Table 3.9.2.1 Signs and symptoms of pre-eclampsia and eclampsia

Symptoms of pre-eclampsia	Signs of pre-eclampsia
Headache	Hypertension
Visual disturbance	Proteinuria
Vomiting	Papilloedema
Subcostal pain	Clonus (>2 beats)
Sudden swelling of face, hands or feet	Liver tenderness Thrombocytopenia (<100 × 10⁹/l) Abnormal liver enzymes (AST or ALT >70 IU/l) HELLP syndrome Pulmonary oedema
Symptoms of eclampsia	**Signs of eclampsia**
Prodrome of headache, visual disturbance and/or right upper quadrant or epigastric pain	Tonic–clonic seizure Coma

Abbreviations: AST = aspartate aminotransferase; ALT = alanine aminotransferase; HELLP = haemolysis, elevated liver enzymes and low platelets.

317

Anti-convulsants

Intravenous magnesium sulphate, as per the Collaborative Eclampsia Trial regimen, with a loading dose of 4 g over 5 minutes, followed by an infusion of 1 g/hr for 24 hours after delivery or the last seizure (whichever is later). Recurrent seizures require a further dose of 2–4 g given over 5 minutes.

Target blood magnesium levels are 2–4 mmol and the patient needs to be monitored for signs of toxicity, including loss of deep tendon reflexes and respiratory depression. If respiratory or cardiac arrest occurs due to magnesium toxicity, then alongside providing advanced life support management, give 10 ml of 10% calcium gluconate.

Magnesium sulphate is also used for fetal neuroprotection in preterm neonates and can be considered in those with severe pre-eclampsia.

Refractory seizures require a benzodiazepine (lorazepam) and neuroimaging to rule out other pathology.

Fluid and Electrolytes

In women with severe pre-eclampsia, maintenance fluids are 80 ml/hr of Ringer's lactate, unless there are other fluid losses (e.g. haemorrhage). Do not use volume expansion in women with severe pre-eclampsia, unless hydralazine is being used as the antenatal anti-hypertensive. Hyponatraemia can occur in severe cases.

Hypertensive Pulmonary Oedema

Acute pulmonary oedema is reported to occur in up to 3 per cent of cases with severe pre-eclampsia. Patients have raised left ventricular end-diastolic pressure, reduced lusitropy, decreased colloid osmotic pressure and increased endothelial permeability. Magnesium sulphate and tocolytic therapy such as terbutaline can also contribute.

Acute management involves an ABCDE assessment, supportive measures and early use of transthoracic echocardiography. The intensivist's skills in this area will be of immense help in aiding diagnosis, differentiating between this and pulmonary embolism in the pregnant woman with acute dyspnoea. Optimal non-invasive ventilatory support (continuous positive airway pressure, bi-level positive airway pressure or high-flow humidified nasal oxygen) is important and avoids the hypertensive response to laryngoscopy, reducing the risk of intracerebral haemorrhage. Management includes fluid restriction at 80 ml/hr, anti-hypertensives as discussed, a glyceryl trinitrate infusion (5 μg/min to a maximum of 100 μg/min), intravenous furosemide and morphine sulphate.

Mode and Timing of Delivery and Removal of the Placenta

This is ultimately curative for pre-eclampsia. Timing will depend on clinical circumstances, including speed of deterioration, presence of any coagulation abnormalities, cardiovascular stability and patient preference. A regional technique is usually preferred if clotting allows. Thromboelastography (TEG®) and rotational thromboelastometry (ROTEM®) with platelet mapping can be useful and a single-shot spinal is often preferred over insertion of an epidural catheter.

Role of Critical Care

Critical care input will vary from invasive blood pressure monitoring for those on intravenous anti-hypertensives to management of seizures and pulmonary oedema. NICE advises on level 2 care for patients for the following:

- Eclampsia
- HELLP syndrome
- Haemorrhage
- Hyperkalaemia
- Severe oliguria
- Coagulation support
- Intravenous anti-hypertensive treatment
- Initial stabilisation of severe hypertension
- Evidence of cardiac failure
- Abnormal neurology

Level 3 care is mandatory for those requiring intubation for pulmonary oedema.

Very few maternity units have designated level 2 care, and early referral to critical care and outreach is recommended. Recent changes in midwifery training incorporate a new set of Royal College of Midwives competencies for senior midwives called enhanced maternity care (EMC), which aim to bridge the gap between standard maternity care and designated critical care.

Fluids, Inotropic Support and Cardiac Output Monitoring in ICU

Fluid management in pregnancy usually follows guidance for crystalloids, colloids and major blood transfusion protocols in the non-pregnant population. Some situations, however, are unique in pregnancy. Women who suffer hyperemesis gravidarum may have extra electrolyte losses that can be severe enough to require admission and cause renal failure. Severe pre-eclampsia morbidity and mortality related to acute respiratory distress syndrome (ARDS) has been successfully reduced in recent decades by careful attention to fluid restriction (total 80 ml/hr). Physiological changes in pregnancy, labour and childbirth will also result in lower plasma sodium levels, and thus an increased risk of hyponatraemia. This was recently reported in an observational study of asymptomatic Swedish women where there was an 8 per cent incidence of plasma sodium level <130 mmol/l, and this can be compounded by water retention in the third trimester and exposure to the anti-diuretic hormone (ADH)-like effect of oxytocin. As a consequence, isotonic crystalloid solutions and low-concentration oxytocin solutions are routinely prescribed, and there should be plasma urea and electrolyte monitoring if diabetic regimes are used that prescribe dextrose solutions. Pregnant patients admitted with liver, renal and cardiac failure are all further predisposed to hypervolaemic hyponatraemia, and fluid restriction may be required. For symptomatic hyponatraemia from cerebral oedema (e.g. seizures or reduced consciousness), 150 ml of 3% saline can be given as an intravenous bolus over 30 minutes, with careful serial electrolyte sampling to avoid cerebral pontine myelinolysis associated with too rapid correction.

The optimal inotrope for use in pregnancy is unclear, as few comparative studies exist, but fetal well-being and umbilical artery blood flow are additional considerations. Phenylephrine and ephedrine are most commonly used in obstetric practice, but noradrenaline has compared favourably with phenylephrine in a recent obstetric study, albeit at relatively low doses. Of critical importance, however, is attention to avoiding aortocaval compression and care using cardio-active obstetric drugs such as oxytocin, carbocetin, prostin PGF2α, magnesium sulphate and ergometrine.

Extensive data and research on cardiovascular physiology are lacking in the critically ill obstetric population, owing to the small numbers of patients. This makes it difficult, but no less important, to measure responses to treatment regimens such as inotropes, fluids and drugs for heart failure. There have recently been excellent reports on the use of transthoracic echocardiography (TTE) and transoesophageal echocardiography (TOE) in pre-eclampsia. Suprasternal (USCOM) and oesophageal Doppler methods (CardioQ) have been reported for non-continuous cardiac output monitoring in the peripartum patient, but these have practical limitations – particularly in obese women at term. Other non-invasive continuous methods have been described such as bioimpedance techniques, and LiDCOplus monitoring has yielded useful information in women undergoing spinal anaesthesia and Caesarean section. Transpulmonary thermodilution (PiCCO) and pulmonary artery catheter thermodilution techniques have been described in case reports and may be indicated in ventilated patients with deteriorating cardiac function.

Prognosis

Despite a reduction in maternal mortality from pre-eclampsia and eclampsia, they still remain one of the most common causes of direct maternal death and are associated with significant maternal morbidity. Eclampsia is associated with intracerebral haemorrhage and cardiac arrest, and recurs in 2 per cent of subsequent pregnancies. It also increases the risk of other obstetric complications in future pregnancies, even if eclampsia does not develop. Counselling is advised for all future pregnancies, particularly if cardiomyopathy was present, as recurrence is common and can be severe and life-threatening.

References and Further Reading

Dennis AT, Solnordal CB. Acute pulmonary oedema in pregnant women. *Anaesthesia* 2012;**67**:646–59.

Knight M, Bunch K, Tuffnell D, *et al.*; MBRRACE-UK (eds). Saving lives, improving mothers' care. Lessons learned to inform maternity care from the UK and Ireland Confidential Enquiries into Maternal Deaths and Morbidity 2017–19. Oxford: National Perinatal Epidemiology Unit, University of Oxford; 2021. www.npeu.ox.ac.uk/assets/downloads/mbrrace-uk/reports/maternal-report-2021/MBRRACE-UK_Maternal_Report_2021_-_FINAL_-_WEB_VERSION.pdf

National Institute for Health and Care Excellence. 2019. Hypertension in pregnancy: diagnosis and management. NICE guideline [NG133]. www.nice.org.uk/guidance/ng133/chapter/Recommendations

Spasovski G, Vanholder R, Allolio B, *et al.*; Hyponatraemia Guideline Development Group. Clinical practice guideline on diagnosis and treatment of hyponatraemia. *Eur J Endocrinol* 2014;**170**:G1–47. Erratum in: *Eur J Endocrinol* 2014;**171**:X1.

The Regulation and Quality Improvement Authority. 2017. Guideline for the prevention, diagnosis and management of hyponatraemia in labour and the immediate postpartum period. www.rqia.org.uk/RQIA/files/df/dfd57ddd-ceb3-4c0d-9719-8e33e179d0ff.pdf

3.9.3 Pre-existing Disease in Pregnancy

Laura Vincent and Audrey Quinn

Key Learning Points

1. Direct obstetric deaths are those resulting from obstetric complications of the pregnancy state (pregnancy, labour and the puerperium) from interventions, omissions or incorrect treatment, or a chain of events resulting from any of the above.

2. Indirect obstetric deaths are those resulting from previous existing disease or disease that developed during pregnancy and which was not due to direct obstetric causes, but which was aggravated by physiological effects of pregnancy.

3. Indirect or pre-existing disease in pregnancy accounts for three-quarters of maternal deaths in the UK, and has remained stubbornly high in recent years.

4. Maternal morbidity is rising, owing to concurrent medical illness, increasing maternal age, socio-economic factors and obesity. Cardiac disease is the major cause, then death from thromboembolism, followed by neurological causes and all-cause sepsis.

5. Multidisciplinary teams care for the sick mother in different hospital sites. Recent national Royal College of Anaesthetists Maternal Critical Care Guidelines 2018 make general recommendations for optimal teamwork and collaboration on maternity and designated critical care units.

Keywords: pre-existing disease in pregnancy, indirect disease in pregnancy, maternal cardiac disease, maternal respiratory disease

Introduction

Demographics and health status of the obstetric population in the UK continue to change, with rising maternal age and prevalence of obesity and associated medical complications such as type 2 diabetes mellitus and cardiovascular disease. Whilst in the UK the rate of 'direct' maternal deaths (obstetric-related) has decreased over the past decade, the same cannot be said of 'indirect' or pre-existing disease, which accounts for approximately three-quarters of maternal mortality in the UK. Additionally, almost 50 per cent of direct deaths have associated pre-existing co-morbidity. A recent study on maternal risk modelling in critical care using a multivariable risk prediction model for death and prolonged intensive care highlights severe disease in the past medical history as a significant factor. Obstetric Intensive Care National Audit and Research Centre (ICNARC) data report an ICU admission rate of 2.3/1000 maternities. However, it is estimated that three times this number are managed on maternity units. This chapter should be read in conjunction with Chapter 3.9.1, Obstetric Emergencies and Chapter 3.9.2, Pre-eclampsia and Eclampsia, as there is much overlap.

Cardiac disease is the single largest cause of UK maternal deaths, followed by thromboembolism, neurological causes, other indirect causes and all-cause sepsis (Figure 3.9.3.1).

A recent focus on morbidity, as well mortality studies, revealed an even more complex interplay between the pathophysiology of pre-existing medical disorders, their treatments and the physiology of pregnant and recently pregnant women that mandates close coordination of both medical and obstetric issues and intensive care.

Cardiac Disease

Cardiac disease complicates 0.2–4 per cent of pregnancies in developed countries, and the incidence is rising due to increasing maternal age and risk factors such as diabetes, hypertension, pre-eclampsia, multiple pregnancies and more women with congenital heart disease (CHD) reaching childbearing age. The

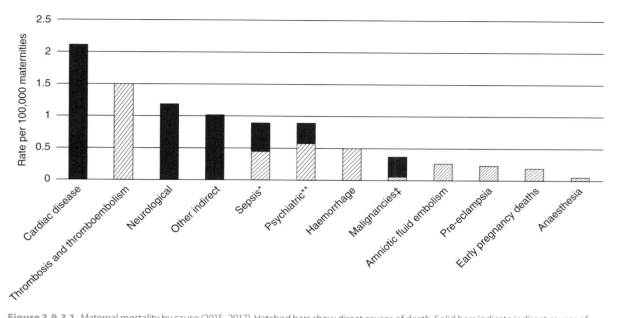

Figure 3.9.3.1 Maternal mortality by cause (2015–2017). Hatched bars show direct causes of death. Solid bars indicate indirect causes of death. *Rate for direct sepsis (genital tract sepsis and other pregnancy-related infections) is shown in hatched bars, and rate for indirect sepsis (influenza, pneumonia, others) in solid bar. **Rate for suicides (direct) is shown in hatched bar, and rate for indirect psychiatric causes (drugs/alcohol) in solid bar. ‡Rate for direct malignancies (choriocarcinoma) shown in hatched bar, and rate for indirect malignancies (breast/ovary/cervix) in solid bar.

Source: MBRRACE-UK.

main causes of cardiac mortality are often only first diagnosed in pregnancy, and include sudden adult death syndrome (SADS) (31 per cent), ischaemic heart disease (IHD) (21 per cent), myocardial disease/cardiomyopathy (14 per cent) and aortic dissection (12 per cent). These women often present with atypical symptoms and so are difficult to diagnose and easy to miss. Pregnant women with IHD have three times the mortality as compared to when they are not pregnant. Atherosclerosis is not universally a feature; instead coronary dissection, thrombosis or vasospasm are often implicated. With appropriate management, most pregnant women and their babies can be brought safely to term, but some high-risk cardiac conditions carry significant morbidity and mortality, and therefore should be managed in centres with specialist cardiac expertise. Cardiologists and a multidisciplinary team with obstetric expertise should regularly review these women, and investigations may include serial ECGs, transthoracic echocardiography, and cardiac CT or MRI for patients with aortopathies and complex CHD. Exercise stress tests are indicated in women with valve lesions, cardiopulmonary exercise testing (CPET) for complex CHD and continuous ECG monitoring

if there is a history of arrhythmia. Baseline and serial B-type natriuretic peptide (BNP) levels can screen for heart failure during pregnancy.

In women with pre-existing cardiac disease, the most common complications affecting women during pregnancy are arrhythmias, heart failure and thromboembolic events. In these cohorts of patients, early studies suggested functional status and cyanosis to be the most important determinants of outcome. However, several prospective risk stratification scores have since been validated, including the CARPREG score (Canadian Cardiac Disease in Pregnancy), the ZAHARA score and, most recently, the modified World Health Organization (WHO) risk classification (Table 3.9.3.1).

As seen, high-risk patients include those women with Fontan circulation, a systemic right ventricle, uncorrected cyanotic heart disease, pulmonary hypertension, failing prosthetic valves, fixed cardiac output conditions (e.g. severe mitral stenosis and aortic stenosis) and dilated cardiomyopathy with heart failure and aortopathies. In these instances, the timing, mode and site of delivery should be discussed in detail by the multidisciplinary team, and a robust system of

Table 3.9.3.1 Modified World Health Organization classification of maternal cardiovascular risk

CENTRAL ILLUSTRATION: High-Risk Heart Disease in Pregnancy

HIGH-RISK HEART DISEASE (HRHD) IN PREGNANCY

Pre-conception counseling and pregnancy risk stratification for all women with HRHD of childbearing age

In women considering pregnancy: Switch to safer cardiac medications and emphasize importance of close monitoring

In women avoiding pregnancy: Discuss safe and effective contraception choices or termination in early pregnancy

Valve disease	Complex congenital heart disease	Pulmonary hypertension	Aortopathy	Dilated cardiomyopathy
Pregnancy not advised in women with: • Severe mitral and aortic valve disease • Mechanical prosthetic valves if effective anticoagulation not possible	**Pregnancy not advised in women with:** • Significant ventricular dysfunction • Severe atrioventricular valve dysfunction • Failing Fontan circulation • O_2 saturation <85%	**Pregnancy not advised for:** • All women with established pulmonary arterial hypertension	**Pregnancy not advised in some women with:** • Marfan syndrome (MFS) • Bicuspid aortic valve (BAV) • Turner syndrome • Rapid growth of aortic diameter or family history of premature aortic dissection	**Pregnancy not advised in women with:** • Left ventricular ejection fraction <40% • History of peripartum cardiomyopathy
Pregnancy management: • Close follow-up • Drug therapy for heart failure or arrhythmias • Balloon valvuloplasty or surgical valve replacement in refractory cases	**Pregnancy management:** • Close follow-up	**Pregnancy management:** • Close follow-up • Early institution of pulmonary vasodilators	**Pregnancy management:** • Treat hypertension • Beta-blockers to reduce heart rate • Frequent echo assessment • Surgery during pregnancy or after C-section if large increase in aortic dimension	**Pregnancy management:** • Close follow-up • Beta-blockers • Diuretic agents for volume overload • Vasodilators for hemodynamic and symptomatic improvement
Delivery: • Vaginal delivery preferred • C-section in case of fetal or maternal instability • Early delivery for clinical and hemodynamic deterioration • Consider hemodynamic monitoring during labor and delivery	**Delivery:** • Vaginal delivery preferred • C-section in case of fetal or maternal instability • Consider hemodynamic monitoring during labor and delivery	**Delivery:** • Vaginal delivery preferred • C-section in case of fetal or maternal instability • Timing of delivery depends on clinical condition and right ventricular function • Early delivery advisable • Diuresis after delivery to prevent RV volume overload • Extended hospital stay after delivery	**Delivery:** • C-section in cases of significant aortic dilation MFS >40 mm BAV >45 mm Turner: ASI >20 mm/m²	**Delivery:** • Vaginal delivery preferred • C-section in case of fetal or maternal instability • Consider hemodynamic monitoring during labor and delivery • Early delivery for clinical and hemodynamic deterioration

Elkayam, U. *et al*. J Am Coll Cardiol. 2016;68(4):396–410.

communication and documentation throughout the pregnancy and peripartum phase is essential.

Peripartum cardiomyopathy (PPCM) is worthy of a mention, as patients present towards the end of pregnancy or, more classically, within the first few months post-partum; thus, the diagnosis should always be in the back of one's head when encountering a post-partum woman with left ventricular systolic dysfunction.

The aetiology is unclear, but predisposing factors include multiparity, family history, ethnicity, smoking, diabetes, hypertension, pre-eclampsia and increased (or very young) maternal age. Symptoms and signs are typical for heart failure, and PPCM is a diagnosis of exclusion. Women should be treated as per acute heart failure management under joint cardiac and obstetric care, and notably angiotensin-converting enzyme inhibitors are contraindicated during pregnancy due to fetotoxicity. Hydralazine and nitrates are an alternative in the first instance, but if the patient deteriorates, then inotropes, intra-aortic balloon pumps and ventricular assist device acutely, or even transplant in extreme circumstances, should be considered.

Respiratory Disease

Asthma

The Obstetric ICNARC data set reveals respiratory disease as the primary reason for admission to critical care in those patients who were currently pregnant (as opposed to recently pregnant). Asthma is the most common chronic condition in pregnancy, with a deterioration in 45 per cent, most likely in the second or third trimester. There is also association with pre-eclampsia, hypertension and complicated deliveries and adverse effects, including preterm labour, low birthweight, congenital malformation and neonatal death. Asthma exacerbations during pregnancy should be treated as in the non-pregnant population, including intravenous salbutamol, magnesium sulphate, theophylline and steroids. There should be a low threshold of admission to the ICU when exacerbations do not respond to maximal bronchodilator therapy. Close attention should be paid to left lateral positioning, oxygenation, hydration and nutrition. Difficulties and complications associated with intubation and ventilation should be anticipated, particularly dynamic hyperinflation due to gas trapping, which can, especially in the context of hypovolaemia, precipitate cardiac arrest. Restricted tidal volume and lung-protective ventilation, with a long expiratory time and a degree of permissive hypercapnia, may be necessary until bronchospasm improves, although the impact of acidaemia on the fetus should be borne in mind. Caesarean section should be considered, discussed and regularly reviewed by the multidisciplinary team if adequate ventilation cannot be achieved. The risk of asthma exacerbation is also increased by drugs used during labour and delivery. Histamine release in response to opiates or muscle relaxants (such as atracurium) may cause bronchospasm, as can uterotonic drugs used to treat post-partum haemorrhage such as ergometrine and prostaglandins. These should ideally be avoided in women with asthma.

Restrictive Lung Disease

Restrictive lung disease in pregnancy may result from a parenchymal interstitial process or from a chest wall or neuromuscular abnormality.

Interstitial lung disease is fortunately uncommon in pregnant women, as it mostly affects an older demographic group. Changes in lung volume and increased ventilatory requirement of pregnancy are poorly tolerated in women with a diffusion defect predisposing to hypoxaemia. This is exacerbated by the natural increase in cardiac output, and hence shorter alveolar capillary transit time, during pregnancy. Any associated pulmonary hypertension significantly increases the risk. Restrictive chest wall or neuromuscular disease may lead to respiratory failure in later pregnancy as the uterus size increases, but in the absence of interstitial pathology, hypoxaemia is less of a concern.

Whilst there are minimal data available, case series suggest restrictive lung disease is fairly well tolerated in pregnancy unless the vital capacity is <1 l. (In these cases, women should be advised to avoid pregnancy.) A multidisciplinary approach to care is vital and may include evaluation with pulmonary function tests, echocardiography and arterial blood gases. In patients with interstitial lung disease, oxygen saturations should be monitored regularly through later pregnancy and supplemental oxygen may be required. With neuromuscular or chest wall disease, nocturnal hypercapnia may be evident in advance of daytime compromise, and non-invasive ventilatory support may be needed in later pregnancy and during labour. In all of these groups, super-added pulmonary infections are more likely in the immune-compromised state of pregnancy.

SARS-CoV-2

The impact of severe acute respiratory syndrome coronavirus 2 (SARS-CoV-2) in pregnancy (March to May 2020) was reported in an early UK Obstetric Surveillance System (UKOSS) study, suggesting that women becoming severely ill tended to be in their third trimester, with risk factors including ethnicity, obesity and coexisting medical problems. The Royal College of Obstetricians and Gynaecologists (RCOG) have published guidelines on the impact of SARS-CoV-2 on medical disease in pregnancy.

Ventilatory Support in the Pregnant Patient

Endotracheal intubation in the pregnant patient is a high-risk procedure. The risk of failed intubation is eightfold higher in the pregnant population, with hypoxia and gastric aspiration exacerbated by obesity (Obstetric Anaesthetists' Association/Difficult Airway Society guidelines).

Non-invasive ventilation (NIV) via face mask may have a role in cases where short-term respiratory support is needed for rapidly reversible respiratory pathology. Any reduction in conscious level or the ability to protect the airway from aspiration should prohibit the use of NIV, and invasive ventilation via an endotracheal tube is indicated (although ongoing sedation will be required). Slightly higher airway pressures may be necessary to achieve desired tidal volumes towards term. Oxygenation must also be optimised for the benefit of the fetus too, as hyperoxia can exacerbate retinopathy of prematurity. Hyperventilation and respiratory alkalosis should be avoided due to uterine vasoconstriction and reduced placental blood flow. Similarly, permissive hypercapnia and lung-protective ventilation have not been assessed in pregnancy and could theoretically induce fetal acidosis and a rightward shift of the fetal oxygen–haemoglobin dissociation curve.

Unconventional Respiratory Support

Prone positioning has been employed successfully in pregnant patients with acute respiratory distress syndrome (ARDS). However, it is logistically challenging and requires continuous fetal monitoring and greater emphasis placed on minimising external abdominal pressure.

Extracorporeal membrane oxygenation (ECMO) is increasingly being used in dedicated centres for cases of refractory respiratory and cardiac failure in pregnant or post-partum women, and early referral to an ECMO centre is advised. Case reports and case series are emerging in support of the potential benefit to life of both the mother and child. However, bleeding due to systemic heparinisation is the main cause of mortality.

Obesity

More than 1 in every 1000 deliveries in the UK are to mothers with a body mass index (BMI) of >50. A careful history and examination are essential in these instances. There will be an increased incidence of diabetes, hypertension, obstructive sleep apnoea, hiatus hernia, gastric reflux and aspiration. Regular antacid therapy (H_2 blocker, proton pump inhibitor) should be prescribed. One should expect difficulty with the airway and rapid oxygen desaturation, bag/mask ventilation, endotracheal intubation and supraglottic airway insertion. There is an increased risk of aortocaval compression and cardiac complications, including cardiomyopathy of the morbidly obese. Thromboembolic prophylaxis is required, with a combination of appropriate-sized stockings and pneumatic compression devices. Peripheral and central venous access will be difficult, and invasive lines should be inserted early for repeated blood tests and accurate pressure readings.

Optimal delivery planning is advised, as there is a 50 per cent overall Caesarean section rate, even in non-complicated pregnancy of obese women. Early institution of a regional blockade for labour and delivery management may avoid emergency general anaesthesia, but a higher incidence of failed regional block and post-dural puncture headache rate can be expected. Finally, there may be practical nursing issues, including positioning, lifting and handling and dignity and respect considerations for the pregnant woman in an open-plan ICU environment.

Endocrine Disease

Diabetes

In the UK, approximately 5 per cent of women have either pre-existing diabetes or gestational diabetes. Of these, 87.5 per cent have gestational diabetes, and 7.5 per cent have type 1 and 5 per cent type 2 diabetes. The prevalence is increasing as a result of obesity and pregnancies in older women, in turn increasing stillbirth rates, congenital malformations, macrosomia, pre-eclampsia and preterm labour. Management requires careful monitoring of blood glucose and HbA1c, and regular input usually by a specialist obstetrician/physician and diabetic nurse and team. Diabetic retinopathy can worsen rapidly during pregnancy, as can renal function, thus requiring nephrologist input. For a diabetic woman admitted to the ICU, instructions on the insulin regime should be clearly documented in the case notes, and a protocol for labour, delivery and the post-partum period discussed with all the team in advance. Insulin requirements are usually immediately halved post-delivery.

Thyroid Disease

The most common form of thyroid disease in pregnancy is Graves' disease (80–85 per cent), and thyroid goitre occurs in iodine-deficient areas of the world. Women with active Graves' disease are at higher risk of a thyroid storm. Treatment is with anti-thyroid drugs (methimazole or propylthiouracil), surgery and beta-blockade for symptomatic palpitations. Radioiodine is contraindicated, as it crosses the placenta and can cause fetal hypothyroidism.

Renal Disease

The most common cause of renal failure in pregnancy is acute cortical necrosis following pre-eclampsia and haemorrhage, and this usually recovers to full function in the post-partum period. However, women who enter pregnancy with established chronic kidney disease (CKD) are less able to make the renal adaptations required for a healthy pregnancy, with blunted hormonal and circulatory responses and consequently an increased risk of acceleration in CKD progression and poor pregnancy outcomes. Seventy per cent of women with severe CKD pre-pregnancy will lose at least 25 per cent of their renal function during pregnancy; in 50 per cent of cases, this will persist to post-partum, and in 35 per cent will deteriorate to end-stage renal failure. Hypertension will advance this rate of decline, as well as predispose to pre-eclampsia; hence, good blood pressure control is essential. Aspirin should be prescribed in pre-eclampsia; erythropoietin is commonly required as pregnancy progresses, and thromboprophylaxis is advised – although this can be stopped for regional anaesthesia and delivery. Non-steroidal anti-inflammatory drugs (NSAIDs) are often prescribed in pregnancy and childbirth, but are absolutely contraindicated in CKD. Care is required in monitoring and avoiding magnesium toxicity.

The risk of fetal growth restriction, preterm labour, fetal and neonatal death and pre-eclampsia are all increased in women with pre-existing CKD, and the risk escalates with severity and coexisting factors such as hypertension and proteinuria or autoimmune diseases such as systemic lupus erythematosus. Indications for dialysis are no different in pregnancy, and include electrolyte imbalance, symptomatic uraemia and volume status that is not responding to medical therapy. For those women already receiving dialysis pre-pregnancy, their pregnancy needs careful monitoring in specialist units, with attention to dialysis adequacy, nutrition, anaemia management, hypertension control and thromboprophylaxis. Premature delivery is very common.

Renal Transplant

Renal allografts adapt similarly to native kidneys during pregnancy, with increasing volume, estimated glomerular filtration rate (eGFR) and creatinine clearance. Deterioration in allograft function during pregnancy requires the usual assessment for intrinsic renal disease, but also consideration of the development of pregnancy-related problems such as hypertension and pre-eclampsia, which occur in 30 per cent of cases (and are the main reasons for increased rates of preterm birth). Both mother and baby may experience complications during pregnancy relating to underlying diseases, suboptimal graft function and use of immunosuppressive therapy. Treated hypertension, proteinuria and elevated creatinine levels are strongly associated with graft loss or functional decline during pregnancy, though pregnancy itself has no impact on graft function in the absence of these factors. There are higher rates of Caesarean section (which can be technically difficult), preterm delivery and low birthweight, when compared to the general population. Careful consideration should be given to the choice and dose of immunosuppressive agent during pregnancy. The fetus is susceptible to drug toxicity, due to altered metabolism, teratogenicity and opportunistic infections. The risk:benefit ratio supports the use of tacrolimus, azathioprine and cyclosporine during pregnancy, and mycophenolate and cyclophosphamide should be avoided.

Haematological Disease

Pregnant patients may require ICU admission for severe inherited haemoglobinopathies such as homozygous sickle cell disease. In the event of deterioration, haematologists and multidisciplinary obstetric and anaesthetic teams need robust pathways of care for respiratory distress, acute chest syndrome, fever, headache and confusion. More rarely, inherited bleeding disorders can present in the peripartum period, requiring a clear plan of suitable care and availability of appropriate products.

Cancer in Pregnancy

As maternal age increases, there is a greater likelihood of women presenting with cancer during pregnancy and childbirth. In the last MBRRACE report 2019, the care of 30 women with breast cancer during the triennium was examined. Timing of surgery and chemotherapy requires careful planning with the multidisciplinary team and may require a higher level of nursing or midwifery care than available in maternity units. Close collaboration between teams, including critical care and outreach, for enhanced care is an important consideration, as well as considering the maternal needs during admission on designated critical care, e.g. encouraging breastfeeding, bonding and enabling the partner and baby to visit.

Maternal Critical Care Guidelines

The Maternal Critical Care Intercollegiate Group collated evidence-based guidelines published in 2018 by the Royal College of Anaesthetists on the management of the acutely unwell woman. These highlight the need for good communication and teamwork, as well as improvements in the organisation, teaching and training for all specialties.

References and Further Reading

Knight M, Bunch K, Tuffnell D, *et al.*; MBRRACE-UK (eds). Saving lives, improving mothers' care. Lessons learned to inform maternity care from the UK and Ireland Confidential Enquiries into Maternal Deaths and Morbidity 2017–19. Oxford: National Perinatal Epidemiology Unit, University of Oxford; 2021.

www.npeu.ox.ac.uk/assets/downloads/mbrrace-uk/reports/maternal-report-2021/MBRRACE-UK_Maternal_Report_2021_-_FINAL_-_WEB_VERSION.pdf

Royal College of Obstetricians and Gynaecologists. 2017. Management of inherited bleeding disorders in pregnancy. Green-top guideline No. 71. obgyn.onlinelibrary.wiley.com/doi/epdf/10.1111/1471-0528.14592

Royal College of Anaesthetists. 2018. Care of the critically ill woman in childbirth; enhanced maternal care. www.rcoa.ac.uk/sites/default/files/documents/2019-09/EMC-Guidelines2018.pdf

Simpson NB, Shankar-Hari M, Rowan KM, *et al.* Maternal risk modelling in critical care – development of a multivariable risk prediction model for death and prolonged intensive care. *Crit Care Med* 2020;**48**:663–72.

3.10.1 Disorders of Haemostasis in Intensive Care

Victoria Stables and Mari Thomas

Key Learning Points

1. Abnormal coagulation results are not uncommon in critically unwell patients.
2. In vitro tests do not always fully correlate with events in vivo, and so all results should be interpreted with reference to the clinical history, particularly any bleeding or thrombosis history.
3. The clinical severity of disseminated intravascular coagulation may not necessarily correlate with abnormalities seen in the laboratory tests, and an individualised plan should be made depending on the clinical scenario.
4. Patients with cirrhosis are at risk of thrombosis, as well as bleeding.
5. In a stable, non-bleeding patient with liver disease, there is no need for 'prophylactic' blood components unless procedures are required.

Keywords: haemostasis, disseminated intravascular coagulation, platelets

Haemostasis Simplified

Haemostasis involves a complex series of interactions between exposed collagen on the vascular endothelium, platelets and blood coagulation factors. It culminates in generation of thrombin, subsequent formation and stabilisation of a fibrin clot and prevention of excessive blood loss. Simultaneous antagonistic mechanisms exist to lyse the fibrin clots, thus preventing thrombosis. All elements and factors need to be present, both numerically and functionally, so the balance is not tipped adversely towards bleeding or thrombosis.

Common Laboratory Screening Tests

Screening coagulation tests that assess the gross integrity of haemostasis include those seen in Table 3.10.1.1.

These are 'in vitro' tests which do not always fully correlate with events in vivo. For example, a lupus anticoagulant or a deficiency of factor XII can cause a marked prolongation of the activated partial thromboplastin time (APTT), but with no associated increased bleeding risk. Conversely, the presence of a mild to moderate factor VIII, IX or XI deficiency may lead only to very mild prolongation of the APTT, but can be associated with a significant bleeding risk in surgery. In light of this, both normal and abnormal coagulation results need to be interpreted in the context of the clinical bleeding history, co-morbidities and examination.

Acquired Disorders of Haemostasis
Disseminated Intravascular Coagulation

Critically unwell patients may develop this disorder of haemostasis which leads to both depletion/consumption of coagulation factors/platelets and a predisposition to bleeding, and widespread fibrin deposition leading to microvascular thrombosis and a risk of

Table 3.10.1.1 Screening coagulation tests

Test	Explanation
Prothrombin time	A surrogate for the 'extrinsic' or 'initiation' phase of haemostasis
Activated partial thromboplastin time	A surrogate for the 'intrinsic' or 'amplification' phase of haemostasis
Fibrinogen	A glycoprotein that is converted to fibrin (main component of a blood clot)
International normalised ratio	A specific test for assessing the effect of warfarin. Not validated for use in any other setting

organ failure. The causes are widespread, including sepsis, malignancy, pancreatitis, trauma, burns, toxins and pregnancy-associated (e.g. placental abruption), and laboratory results may include those seen in Box 3.10.1.1.

A scoring system established by the International Society on Thrombosis and Haemostasis (ISTH) for disseminated intravascular coagulation (DIC) can aid diagnosis, taking into account the laboratory criteria (platelet count, prothrombin time (PT), fibrinogen and D-dimer). However, clinical severity may not necessarily correlate with abnormalities seen in the laboratory tests, and decisions with regard to product replacement are based on the clinical risk of bleeding and often necessitate discussion with haematology and the blood transfusion laboratory.

A pragmatic approach to treatment would be:
- To treat the underlying cause expeditiously
- At least twice-daily monitoring of activated partial thromboplastin time (APTT), PT, fibrinogen and platelet count
- Where there is spontaneous bleeding, or if procedures need to be undertaken, correct the PT and APTT with fresh frozen plasma (FFP) 10–15 ml/kg (pooled plasma from blood donors containing a mixture of coagulation factors)
- Correct fibrinogen if <1 g/l using cryoprecipitate (one adult dose is 2 × pools of 5 U per pool) or fibrinogen concentrate
- Keep platelets over 50×10^9/l in the event of bleeding
- Consider the use of the anti-fibrinolytic agent tranexamic acid at 1 g intravenously (IV) three times daily in the event of bleeding
- Complete a venous thromboembolism (VTE) risk assessment, and consider thromboprophylaxis if appropriate and after discussion with haematology

---

Box 3.10.1.1 Common Abnormalities in Laboratory Tests in Disseminated Intravascular Coagulation

- Prolonged prothrombin time and activated partial thromboplastin time
- Decreased fibrinogen (a late sign)
- Thrombocytopenia
- Fragmentation on blood film examination
- Raised D-dimers

- If thrombosis is the predominant feature of the clinical DIC (venous or arterial thrombosis, purpura fulminans, skin infarction, acral ischaemia), then consider anticoagulation with an agent with a short half-life. There may be difficulties in monitoring the therapeutic effect of unfractionated heparin if abnormalities of the laboratory tests exist at baseline and cases should be discussed with haematology.

Liver Disease

Most coagulation factors are produced in the liver, and as hepatocyte function is impaired and synthetic function diminishes, abnormalities in the coagulation tests are often seen. These include prolonged PT/APTT and hypofibrinogenaemia. Bone marrow function from alcohol toxicity, and hypersplenism from portal hypertension, can cause thrombocytopenia which can further increase the propensity of these patients to bleed. However, patients with cirrhosis are also at an increased risk of thrombosis due, in part, to lower levels of naturally occurring anticoagulants such as protein C and protein S.

In a bleeding patient, in addition to specific interventional haemostatic measures such as gastro-endoscopy and hepatology supportive care, consider correcting coagulopathy with:
- Platelets, aiming to keep $>50 \times 10^9$/l
- Cryoprecipitate or fibrinogen concentrate
- FFP 10–15 ml/kg or, in selected circumstances, prothrombin complex concentrate (PCC)
- Vitamin K 10 mg IV for at least 3 days or on alternate days if the patient has an ongoing admission
- Tranexamic acid can also be used up to 1 g IV or orally (PO) three times daily
- In ongoing bleeding, continued blood component support may be required

In a stable, non-bleeding patient, intermittent vitamin K can be given, but there is no need for 'prophylactic' blood components unless procedures are required.

Acquired Haemophilia and Acquired Platelet Function Defects

Rarer acquired problems leading to disordered haemostasis and a potentially severe bleeding phenotype include the development of antibodies to specific coagulation factors such as factor VIII (acquired haemophilia A) which can be idiopathic or associated with an underlying disorder such as malignancy or autoimmune disease. Although these bleeding disorders are beyond the scope of this chapter, it is useful to be aware of the abnormalities these disorders may cause to the widely used screening coagulation tests (outlined in Figure 3.10.1.1).

Acquired haemophilia A is often characterised by dramatic soft tissue bleeding, although haematuria, epistaxis, gastrointestinal bleeding and even intracranial haemorrhage may occur. Management involves

specialist haemophilia centre input and a combination of immunosuppression and factor replacement using an agent that bypasses the inhibitor and exogenously restores thrombin generation. Such agents include activated PCC (aPCC) or factor eight inhibitor bypassing agent (FEIBA). These products may not be stocked in all hospital blood banks and may require liaison with the local haemophilia centre.

The ability of platelets to function normally and contribute to haemostasis (despite having a normal or an increased numerical value) can be impaired in

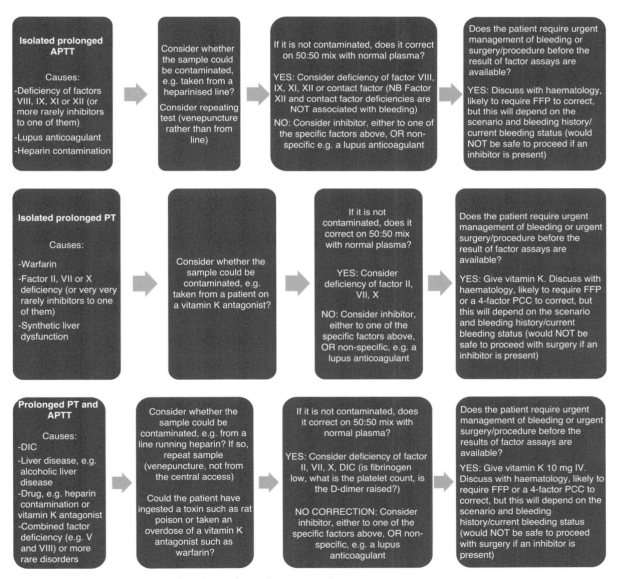

Figure 3.10.1.1 A pragmatic approach to abnormal coagulation test results in intensive care.

the presence of certain drugs (e.g. aspirin, clopidogrel) and over-the-counter medications (non-steroidal anti-inflammatory drugs (NSAIDs)), as well as in certain acquired medical conditions, e.g. essential thrombocythaemia (ET).

It is important to consider platelet function in the ICU setting either in the presence of bleeding or in anticipation of procedures, as prophylactic platelet transfusion may be indicated in the event of certain high-risk procedures (including lumbar puncture or neurosurgery) and such patients should be discussed with haematology.

Abnormal coagulation results are common in intensive care and critically ill patients who often require procedures with a bleeding risk. Figure 3.10.1.1 suggests a pragmatic approach to interpreting results.

References and Further Reading

Baker P, Platton S, Gibson C, *et al.*; British Society for Haematology, Haemostasis and Thrombosis Task Force. Guidelines on the laboratory aspects of assays used in haemostasis and thrombosis. *Br J Haematol* 2020;**191**:347–62.

Curry NS, Davenport R, Pavord S, *et al.* The use of viscoelastic haemostatic assays in the management of major bleeding: a British Society for Haematology Guideline. *Br J Haematol* 2018;**182**:789–806.

Levi M, Toh CH, Thachil J, Watson HG. Guidelines for the diagnosis and management of disseminated intravascular coagulation. British Committee for Standards in Haematology. *Br J Haematol* 2009;**145**:24–33.

Thachil J, Hill Q (eds). *Haematology in Critical Care: A Practical Handbook*. Chichester: John Wiley & Sons; 2014.

3.10.2

Thrombotic Disorders in Intensive Care

Victoria Stables and Mari Thomas

Key Learning Points

1. Heparin-induced thrombocytopenia (HIT) is very rare.
2. In suspected HIT, a low-risk pre-test probability score has a high negative predictive value, whilst some of the laboratory assays in use have a high rate of false positivity. The 4T score should therefore be calculated first.
3. Thrombotic thrombocytopenic purpura (TTP) is a haematological emergency, with high mortality if untreated. TTP and haemolytic uraemic syndrome (HUS) should be managed in an appropriate tertiary care centre with access to appropriate specialists and where 24-hour plasma exchange facilities are available.
4. Platelets should not be given, unless advised by a haematologist, in acute TTP and HUS, as it may precipitate worsening of the thrombotic complications.
5. Patients who receive eculizumab for HUS should have appropriate meningococcal vaccinations, and commence prophylactic antibiotics for the duration of therapy.

Keywords: heparin-induced thrombocytopenia, thrombotic microangiopathies, eculizumab

Heparin-Induced Thrombocytopenia

Heparin-induced thrombocytopenia (HIT) is a rare immune-mediated process occurring in a very small percentage of patients exposed to heparin. The thrombocytopenia may be asymptomatic or accompanied by clinical manifestations, which include:

- Venous thromboembolism
- Arterial thrombosis
- Skin lesions
- Acute systemic reaction
- Adrenal haemorrhage

The risk is highest in unfractionated heparin (UFH) exposure used, for example, in patients who have had cardio-thoracic bypass surgery. The heparin/platelet factor 4–antibody complex binds to platelets and leads to their activation and also leads to a pro-thrombotic state.

Many intensive care patients will experience both a low platelet count and a history of exposure to heparin within their admission, but only a very small proportion will have HIT.

The laboratory test used to diagnose HIT can be associated with high levels of false positivity, depending on the assay available. The '4Ts' pre-probability screening tool should be used to appropriately select those for whom the laboratory test will be suitable and takes into account:

- The degree of thrombocytopenia.
- The timing of the fall in platelet count in relation to the heparin exposure
- The presence of any type of thrombosis
- Any other possible causes of thrombocytopenia

This gives a score of high, intermediate or low. HIT can be excluded if the score is low, but if the score is intermediate or high, the laboratory tests available to a particular hospital should be requested and the patient switched to a non-cross-reacting alternative anticoagulant (i.e. NOT low-molecular-weight heparin (LMWH)), as per local policy (e.g. fondaparinux) pending test results. The tests should be sent and interpreted in liaison with haematologists, so a decision can be reached as to the likelihood of HIT, based on all the information available (the post-test probability of HIT). All sources of heparin must be stopped, including flushes, line locks, dialysis circuits, etc. Platelet transfusions should *not* be given.

Once the platelet count has returned to normal, the patient can be switched to an oral alternative, which should continue for 3 months if the patient has had HIT associated with thrombosis, and 4 weeks if there was no associated thrombosis. The patient should be counselled about the diagnosis and it should be documented in the medical records.

Thrombotic Microangiopathies

This group of disorders is characterised by microangiopathic haemolytic anaemia (MAHA), with red cell fragmentation, thrombocytopenia and microvascular thrombosis. They can be primary (thrombotic thrombocytopenic purpura (TTP) and haemolytic uraemic syndrome (HUS)), specific to pregnancy (haemolysis, elevated liver enzymes and low platelets (HELLP) or pre-eclampsia) or secondary to a number of conditions, including bone marrow transplant, drugs, malignancy, infections, malignant hypertension and catastrophic anti-phospholipid syndrome.

TTP and HUS are considered in more detail below.

Thrombotic Thrombocytopenic Purpura

TTP is a rare thrombotic microangiopathy caused by deficiency of ADAMTS13 (<10 per cent activity). ADAMTS13 is a von Willebrand factor (vWF)-cleaving protease and in the deficient state, there is an accumulation of ultra-large multimers of vWF which are highly platelet-adhesive, leading to the formation of platelet microthrombi in the microvasculature and critical organ dysfunction. It is usually caused by acquired antibodies to ADAMTS13 but may be secondary, e.g. underlying autoimmune disease, HIV or pancreatitis. Even more rarely, it can be congenital due to mutations within the gene encoding ADAMTS13, and diagnosis is then confirmed by ADAMTS13 antigen levels and genetic analysis.

TTP presents acutely with haemolysis (anaemia, red cell fragments on blood film examination, elevated lactate dehydrogenase, elevated bilirubin, elevated reticulocytes) and thrombocytopenia. Patients can also present with neurological, cardiac or abdominal symptoms or be asymptomatic. It is an acute haematological emergency, with an untreated mortality rate of over 90 per cent, and once identified, urgent tertiary referral to an appropriate haematology centre should be made so that lifesaving plasma exchange can be instituted, usually in the intensive care setting. Investigations to seek an underlying cause should be undertaken, including full autoimmune screen and virology, and disease severity assessed, including troponin measurement and a full neurological assessment.

Treatment comprises at least daily plasma exchange until platelet normalisation using solvent detergent fresh frozen plasma (FFP) and immunosuppression

with steroids and the monoclonal antibody rituximab. Platelets should *not* be given, as this exacerbates the thrombotic tendency, even to cover venous line insertions in the setting of often severe thrombocytopenia. Supportive care is with folic acid and blood transfusion, and aspirin and LMWH thromboprophylaxis are given once platelet count is >50 × 10⁹/l. Novel agents are emerging for clinical use, including the anti-vWF factor nanobody caplacizumab which prevents binding of the ultra-large VWF to platelets, and thus formation of new microthrombi. Recombinant ADAMTS13 is also in trial.

Haemolytic Uraemic Syndrome

In HUS, microangiopathic haemolytic anaemia and thrombocytopenia are accompanied by acute kidney failure. Typical cases are caused by Shiga-toxin producing *Escherichia coli* infection (STEC). Atypical HUS (aHUS) also presents with haemolytic anaemia, thrombocytopenia and acute kidney failure, but it is a disorder of complement overactivity as a result of specific genetic mutations or, more rarely, auto-antibodies. The differentiation from TTP is predominantly with laboratory investigation, but there may be clues with the clinical history and the degree of acute kidney failure. ADAMTS13 activity is normal or only mildly reduced in aHUS, unlike the severe ADAMTS13 deficiency which characterises TTP.

Management of aHUS is with terminal complement inhibition with eculizumab and renal replacement therapy, as well as supportive therapy with folic acid and blood transfusions. Prophylaxis with penicillin V, or a suitable alternative, is also important for the duration of eculizumab therapy, as well as vaccination against meningococcal disease.

References and Further Reading

Scully M, Hunt BJ, Benjamin S, *et al.*; British Committee for Standards in Haematology. Guidelines on the diagnosis and management of thrombotic thrombocytopenic purpura and other thrombotic microangiopathies. *Br J Haematol* 2012;**158**:323–35.

Thachil J, Hill Q (eds). *Haematology in Critical Care: A Practical Handbook*. Chichester: John Wiley & Sons; 2014.

Watson H, Davidson S, Keeling D; Haemostasis and Thrombosis Task Force of the British Committee for Standards in Haematology. Guidelines on the diagnosis and management of heparin-induced thrombocytopenia: second edition. *Br J Haematol* 2012;**159**:528–40.

3.10.3 Anticoagulation, Bridging and Emergency Reversal in Intensive Care

Victoria Stables and Mari Thomas

Key Learning Points

1. Urgent warfarin reversal is either with vitamin K or, in select emergency circumstances, with a 4-factor prothrombin complex concentrate.

2. Direct oral anticoagulants (DOACs) are being used increasingly, and their therapeutic effect is not excluded by normal coagulation screening tests.

3. There are specific reversal agents for dabigatran and factor Xa inhibitor anticoagulants.

4. If urgent heparin reversal is needed, in select cases, protamine sulphate can be considered after discussion with haematology, although low-molecular weight heparin will only be partially reversed.

5. Inferior vena cava filters are only recommended in select circumstances.

Keywords: warfarin, DOAC, IVC filter

Introduction

Anticoagulant medication is commonly used, either therapeutically or prophylactically. 'Bridging' is the term given to the temporary adjustment in anti-coagulation around an intervention to prevent bleeding, whilst being mindful of the risk of thrombosis. It takes into account the balance of risk pre-, peri- and post-operatively. In an emergency requiring intervention, there is no time for a 'bridging plan' and the effects of anticoagulation may need to be reversed rapidly. In the event of bleeding on anticoagulation, general measures of anticoagulant drug cessation, local haemostatic measures (e.g. applied pressure, surgical intervention to stop the bleeding source) and general pharmacological measures, such as anti-fibrinolytic agents (tranexamic acid intravenously, orally or topically), should be remembered, no matter which anticoagulant the patient has been taking.

Depending on the scenario and the ongoing thrombotic risk for which the patient was being anticoagulated, specific reversal agents or pro-thrombotic drugs may be indicated after discussion with haematology. The future underlying need for anticoagulation also needs to be considered, and appropriate bridging/restarting of therapy, according to local trust policy, at the earliest and safest time possible should be considered whenever anticoagulation is omitted.

Commonly used anticoagulants are considered in further detail below, with guidance on 'bridging' and reversal.

Warfarin

Warfarin is a vitamin K antagonist which leads to decreased activity of vitamin K-dependent coagulation factors. It needs to be ceased in advance of procedures (stopped usually 5–7 days pre-operation or pre-procedure), and higher-risk patients (i.e. those at significant risk of thrombosis if anticoagulation is stopped) need to be bridged pre-operatively once the international normalised ratio (INR) drops out of therapeutic range with full-dose or prophylactic-dose shorter-acting anticoagulation alternatives such as low-molecular-weight heparin (LMWH). Lower-risk patients (e.g. lower CHA_2DS_2VASc score in atrial fibrillation (AF)) do not require bridging pre-operatively, and risk stratification and planning will be according to local policy and a careful risk–benefit individualised assessment of bleeding risk versus thrombotic risk. Post-operative bridging/re-institution of warfarin depends on local policy and ongoing bleeding risk, but would usually comprise a prophylactic LMWH dose 6 hours post-procedure, increased gradually back to a treatment dose over 2–3 days, with re-institution of warfarin at days 3–5, with LMWH continuing until therapeutic range.

Should it be required, semi-urgent reversal can be achieved with small doses of oral/parenteral vitamin K, which takes up to 24 and 6 hours to work, respectively. This method of reversal is preferred where clinically feasible, to avoid unnecessary pro-thrombotic complications of prothrombin complex concentrate (PCC).

Certain situations, such as urgent surgery, intracerebral bleeding and acute life- or limb-threatening bleeding, necessitate more rapid reversal, which can be achieved with a 4-factor PCC. In such situations, discussion with haematology colleagues is indicated, so the most appropriate dose can be advised. Simultaneous vitamin K should be administered if ongoing reversal is likely to be needed, to avoid unnecessary repeated PCC dosing.

Direct Oral Anticoagulants

Direct oral anticoagulants (DOACs) (rivaroxaban, apixaban, edoxaban and dabigatran) are being used with increased frequency, and are licensed first line for non-valvular AF, venous thromboembolism (VTE) and thromboprophylaxis post-orthopaedic surgery. Unlike warfarin, their mode of action is more predictable in selected patients (documented assessment of bleeding risk, e.g. with HASBLED score, acceptable liver and renal function, no extremes of age or body weight, not pregnant, no drug interactions). Importantly, most do not have a uniform or predictable effect on normal screening coagulation tests, such that a normal activated partial thromboplastin time (APTT) or prothrombin time (PT) does not exclude a DOAC effect (and these should not be used to monitor or exclude an individual's risk of bleeding) and INR testing is not helpful. The only exception to this is with dabigatran only where a normal thrombin time (TT) excludes a significant anticoagulant effect.

DOACs should be ceased 24–72 hours prior to an intervention/procedure/surgery, according to local trust policy, and this depends on the DOAC in question, the nature of the procedure, the bleeding risk and the renal function (as measured by calculated Cockroft–Gault creatinine clearance). Post-operatively, thromboprophylaxis with LMWH is usually given once haemostasis is achieved until the DOACs are restarted 24–72 hours later, depending on the bleeding risk. (For minor procedures, DOACs can be restarted 6 hours post-procedure, assuming it is safe to therapeutically anticoagulate.)

Because of the relatively short half-life in the presence of normal renal function (rivaroxaban: 5–13 hours, depending on age; apixaban: 12 hours; dabigatran: 12–17 hours), reversal agents are rarely required. Specific antidotes do exist to reverse the effect of dabigatran (idarucizumab) and factor Xa anticoagulants (rivaroxaban, apixaban, edoxaban), but local availability varies and this requires discussion with haematology. In selected patients thought to have toxic effects of dabigatran, dialysis can be considered but would not be effective for the other DOACs as they are protein-bound. Very rarely, activated charcoal may be considered upfront in the event of bleeding and recent ingestion of a dose within 2 hours (or up to 6 hours if apixaban).

General management of bleeding on DOACs will be with basic haemostatic and resuscitative measures and consideration of PCC.

Heparins

Like DOACs, LMWH has a shorter half-life and a more predictable mode of action than warfarin. They are often used as anticoagulation in hospitalised patients, either at a full treatment dose or as a prophylactic dose for prevention against hospital-acquired venous thrombosis.

Accumulation or dose intensity can be assessed by undertaking an assay of plasma anti-Xa activity, and this may be useful at extremes of body weight, in renal impairment and in pregnancy. Testing should be done in conjunction with haematology, as interpretation of the results requires knowledge of how long post-dose the blood was taken (should be taken 4 hours post-dose and processed immediately by the laboratory) and the type of LMWH used.

For the purpose of surgery or higher-risk procedures, including lumbar puncture/spinal/epidural or arterial line insertion, it is advisable to wait at least 12 hours after a once-daily prophylactic dose, and 24 hours after a full treatment dose (including a split treatment dose), to allow time for LMWH to be cleared. This will be longer if renal function is abnormal and should be discussed with haematology. Protamine sulphate offers some reversal, depending on how soon after a dose it is administered, but must be discussed with haematology prior to its use to assess the perceived risk–benefit. In patients who are at high risk of bleeding requiring regular trips to theatre or procedures, split treatment dose of LMWH may help minimise bleeding and provide more flexibility. Unfractionated heparin may also rarely have a role in this instance, although monitoring is laborious and its use is limited.

Inferior Vena Cava Filters

There are very few occasions when temporary inferior vena cava (IVC) filters are recommended, and only after careful consideration and collaboration with haematology and radiology due to the risk of complications. Examples of scenarios where they may be considered include:

- Patients requiring urgent surgery in the first month post-acute proximal deep vein thrombosis (DVT)
- Patients with recent acute VTE where full anticoagulation is temporarily contraindicated due to a high bleeding risk

Anticoagulation should be resumed as soon as possible, and a date for IVC filter removal scheduled.

References and Further Reading

Keeling D, Tait RC, Watson H; British Committee of Standards for Haematology. Peri-operative management of anticoagulation and antiplatelet therapy. *Br J Haematol* 2016;**175**:602–13.

Kitchen S, Gray E, Mackie I, Baglin T, Makris M; BCSH Committee. Measurement of non-coumarin anticoagulants and their effects on tests of haemostasis: guidance from the British Committee for Standards in Haematology. *Br J Haematol* 2014;**166**:830–41.

Makris M, Van Veen JJ, Tait CR, Mumford AD, Laffan M; British Committee for Standards in Haematology. Guideline on the management of bleeding in patients on antithrombotic agents. *Br J Haematol* 2013;**160**: 35–46.

Thachil J, Hill Q (eds). *Haematology in Critical Care: A Practical Handbook*. Chichester: John Wiley & Sons; 2014.

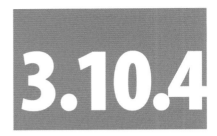

3.10.4

General Haematology for Intensive Care

Dunnya De-Silva, Emma Drasar and William Townsend

Key Learning Points

1. Anaemia in critical illness is often multifactorial. Careful assessment of history and trend of haemoglobin and full blood count parameters can help direct further investigations.

2. Restrictive red cell transfusion strategies are associated with lower mortality in the intensive care unit. The default transfusion threshold is 70 g/l unless there are specific conditions, e.g. cardiac disease.

3. Thrombocytopenia in critical illness is common and often reflects abnormal physiology; therefore, the mainstay of management is to treat the underlying cause.

4. Patients with sickle cell disease (SCD) have highly variable clinical presentations due to different sickle genotypes and clinical heterogeneity within each genotype. Therefore, the severity of previous sickle cell crises is the best indicator of severity of their condition. Management should be led by haematologists with experience in SCD.

5. Therapeutic plasma exchange removes harmful large molecules from the circulation. Protocols vary according to indication; therefore, management should be directed by the clinical team with expertise in the underlying condition.

Keywords: restrictive transfusion, sickle cell disease, plasma exchange, thrombocytopenia, anaemia

Anaemia

Anaemia in critical illness is common and often multifactorial (Table 3.10.4.1). Sixty per cent of patients admitted to the ICU are anaemic, and after 7 days, 80 per cent have a haemoglobin (Hb) level of <90 g/l. Early anaemia is usually iatrogenic, whilst impaired red cell production secondary to inflammation contributes to anaemia in prolonged illness.

Investigating Anaemia in the Intensive Care Unit

Mild anaemia in the context of critical illness does not require extensive investigation. The following investigations can be considered, depending on the clinical context, trend of Hb and other blood parameters:

Table 3.10.4.1 Causes of anaemia in the intensive care unit

Iatrogenic	• Blood tests – up to 70 ml/day venesected • Extracorporeal circuits • Haemodilution
Blood loss	• Traumatic • Occult gastrointestinal loss • Surgical/drain/line sites
Anaemia associated with inflammation (i.e. anaemia of chronic disease)	• Multiple mechanisms due to pro-inflammatory state – suppressed red cell production by cytokines, iron restriction (sufficient iron stores, but inability to be utilised), reduced responsiveness to erythropoietin
Impaired production	• Nutritional deficiency, e.g. haematinics • Renal impairment causing reduced erythropoietin production • Bone marrow infiltration/pathology – usually associated with pancytopenia
Haemolysis – immune	• Drugs, e.g. ceftriaxone, penicillin • Transfusion-associated, e.g. acute or delayed haemolytic reactions • Associated with haematological malignancies, e.g. chronic lymphocytic leukaemia
Haemolysis – non-immune	• Infections, e.g. malaria, *Mycoplasma* • Drugs, e.g. dapsone • Mechanical, e.g. mechanical heart valves, microangiopathic haemolytic anaemias • Systemic conditions, e.g. renal/liver failure • Rarely inherited red cell disorders, e.g. sickle cell disease, thalassaemia, glucose-6-phosphate dehydrogenase deficiency

- Repeat full blood count (FBC) – especially if unexpected acute drop in Hb
- History – review the FBC trend, drug and transfusion history (current and prior), travel, ethnic origin (inherited red cell disorders), jaundice and nutritional status
- Assessment of FBC:
  - Pancytopenia – consider impaired bone marrow function
  - Mean corpuscular volume (MCV) – can guide differential of isolated anaemia (Table 3.10.4.2)
- Blood film – evidence of haemolysis, bone marrow infiltration, inherited red cell pathology
- Iron profile – ferritin will be raised as an acute inflammatory marker; therefore, full iron profile needed to assess iron status
- Haematinics – B12, serum folate
- Thyroid function test
- Haemolysis screen: unconjugated bilirubin (raised in haemolysis), lactate dehydrogenase (LDH) (raised), haptoglobulins (suppressed), direct anti-globulin test (DAT) (positive in immune haemolysis; however, often falsely positive in acute illness/secondary to drugs)
- Reticulocyte count: appropriately raised in acute blood loss and haemolytic anaemia; inappropriately normal/reduced in impaired red cell production, e.g. haematinic deficiency
- Renal function
- Specific tests according to clinical history
  - Infective screens, e.g. malaria, parvovirus
  - Myeloma screen (protein electrophoresis, serum free light chains, urine Bence Jones

protein, urine protein:creatinine ratio), especially in acute illness presenting with anaemia, renal impairment, lytic bone disease and/or infection
  - Imaging for malignancy, especially if suggestion of bone marrow infiltration (common malignancies associated with bone metastases include prostate, breast, renal and thyroid); assess for lymphadenopathy and hepatosplenomegaly if suspected haematological malignancy, e.g. lymphoma
  - Flow cytometry of peripheral blood – at discretion of the haematologist if evidence of abnormal white cell population on FBC or film
  - Bone marrow biopsy – at discretion of the haematologist if suggestion of impaired bone marrow function or infiltration

Thresholds of Transfusions

The majority of red cell transfusions in the ICU are to correct anaemia. The Transfusion Requirements in Critical Care (TRICC) study showed that restrictive strategies of transfusion (threshold Hb 70 g/l) was associated with lower mortality (significant for patients aged <55 years and those less severely ill with APACHE II <20). As default, transfusion triggers should not exceed 70 g/l. Higher thresholds may be appropriate for specific conditions, e.g. early sepsis, neurological injury and acute coronary syndrome (Figure 3.10.4.1).

Key Considerations of Transfusion in Critical Care

- Does my patient need to be transfused?
  - Assess appropriate threshold for transfusions.
- How can I reduce the number of blood transfusions for my patient (i.e. prevention of anaemia)?
  - Consider iatrogenic blood loss and alternatives, e.g. reducing the number of blood tests or using paediatric bottles.
  - Address preventable causes of blood loss, e.g. stress ulcer prophylaxis, use of tranexamic acid to minimise bleeding, especially in major haemorrhage, correction of coagulopathy where appropriate.
  - Manage anticoagulation and anti-platelet therapy around elective procedures to minimise blood loss.

Table 3.10.4.2 Mean corpuscular volumes and their causes

Microcytic anaemia (MCV <80 fl)	Normocytic anaemia (MCV 80–100 fl)	Macrocytic anaemia (MCV >100 fl)
• Iron deficiency • Inherited red cell disorders, e.g. thalassaemia • Hyperthyroidism • Anaemia of chronic disease	• Anaemia of chronic disease • Haematinic deficiency • Blood loss • Dilutional	• Acute blood loss • Haemolysis • Megaloblastic anaemia (B12/folate) • Liver disease • Myelodysplasia (often chronic anaemia preceding acute illness) • Hypothyroidism

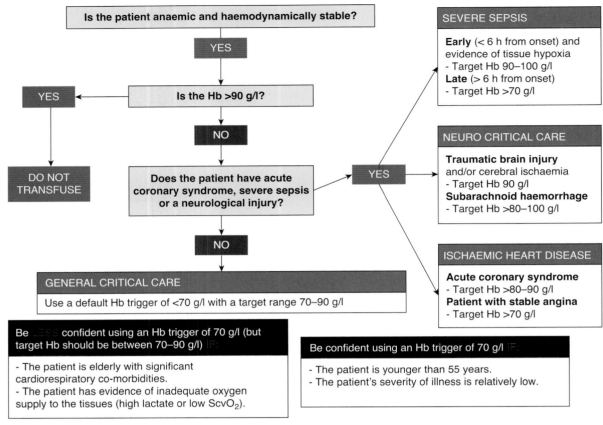

Figure 3.10.4.1 Suggested transfusion strategies for critically ill patients, according to British Society of Haematology guidelines. Source: *Guidelines on the management of anaemia and red cell transfusion in adult critically ill patients.* Retter *et al.* British Society of Haematology Guidelines.

- How much should I transfuse?
  - Transfusion-associated circulatory overload is a major cause of morbidity and mortality. Assess fluid status prior to each unit of blood transfused. One unit of blood (220–340 ml) increases Hb by approximately 10 g/l; however, this may be excessive in patients with low body weight when 4 ml/kg is sufficient.
- Are there any alternatives to transfusion?
  - Erythropoietin-stimulating agents (ESAs) – no evidence to support use and not licensed in critical care; associated with thrombosis.
  - Iron supplementation – indicated only in proven iron deficiency; due to inflammatory anaemia and inability to utilise iron; not

effective in correcting anaemia of chronic disease often seen in critical care.

Thrombocytopenia

Thrombocytopenia (platelets <150 × 10^9/l) is common and often multifactorial in the ICU. Up to 67 per cent of patients are thrombocytopenic on admission to the ICU, with 13–44 per cent of patients developing thrombocytopenia during their admission. Thrombocytopenia often reflects abnormal physiology; therefore, the mainstay of management is treating the underlying cause.

Clinical manifestations of spontaneous bleeding/bruising/petechiae are rare, unless platelet counts are <50 × 10^9/l (usually <20 × 10^9/l). However, these can occur at higher platelet counts due to coexisting coagulopathy or functional impairment of platelets, e.g. uraemia/drugs.

Table 3.10.4.3 Causes of thrombocytopenia in intensive care

Pseudothrombocytopenia	• Platelet clumping in EDTA impairs ability of automated FBC machines to quantify platelets. Consider if unexpected thrombocytopenia not consistent with previous results. Blood film confirms the presence of platelet clumps. Repeat FBC with citrated sample tube to avoid clumping
Haemodilution	• Intravenous fluids • Massive blood transfusion in major haemorrhage without transfusion of appropriate proportion of platelets
Platelet consumption	• Major trauma • Disseminated intravascular coagulation • Sepsis • Extracorporeal circuits
Platelet sequestration (pooling)	• Hepatosplenomegaly, e.g. portal hypertension, congestive cardiac failure
Impaired production	• Haematinic deficiency • Viruses, e.g. HIV, hepatitis B and C, CMV • Direct bone marrow toxicity by drugs, e.g. alcohol, chemotherapy • Bone marrow infiltration, e.g. acute leukaemia, non-haematological malignancy
Platelet destruction	• Drug-induced, e.g. penicillins, teicoplanin, proton pump inhibitors • Immune-mediated, e.g. autoimmune conditions (SLE), idiopathic thrombocytopenic purpura • Heparin-induced thrombocytopenic thrombosis • Thrombotic microangiopathic anaemias – TTP/HUS • Post-transfusion purpura – sudden thrombocytopenia after transfusion of any blood product due to anti-platelet antibodies (developed after pregnancy or previous transfusions)

Abbreviations: EDTA = ethylenediaminetetraacetic acid; FBC = full blood count; CMV = cytomegalovirus; SLE = systemic lupus erythematosus; TTP = thrombotic thrombocytopenic purpura; HUS = haemolytic uraemic syndrome.

Key Considerations When Investigating Thrombocytopenia in the Intensive Care Unit

- What was the patient's platelet count when they were well?
- Temporal course of thrombocytopenia, especially in relation to drug and transfusion history
- Clinical examination for petechiae, bruising and oozing from line sites, and for evidence of thrombosis, e.g. in thrombotic thrombocytopenic purpura (TTP) and heparin-induced thrombocytopenic thrombosis (HITT). Also consider hepatosplenomegaly and lymphadenopathy
- All patients should have blood film, haematinics, coagulation screen, fibrinogen and virology (Table 3.10.4.3) as a minimum
- Further specialist tests, e.g. for TTP, HITT and post-transfusion purpura (PTP), should be discussed with the haematologist. Sensitivity/ specificity of these assays are highly variable, and interpretation is often based on the clinical context

Management

- Treat the underlying cause.
- Avoid drugs associated with thrombocytopenia/ bone marrow suppression; for example, consider alternatives, especially antibiotics.
- Simple measures to minimise bleeding where possible, e.g. pressure dressings, tranexamic acid (topical/intravenous); avoid unnecessary procedures or use techniques which minimise bleeding risk, e.g. ultrasound-guided procedures.
- Where thrombocytopenia is transient, transfuse platelets to maintain adequate thresholds (Table 3.10.4.4).
- The duration of raised thresholds above the baseline for non-bleeding patients should be reviewed daily, depending on the clinical course and investigations. As a guide, the threshold should only be reduced if and when haemostasis is achieved.
- One pool of platelets usually increases the platelet count by 20–40×10^9/l. Therefore, recheck the platelet count after each pool before further transfusions, as often one pool is sufficient. For procedures, optimal dose and benefit of platelets

Table 3.10.4.4 Thresholds for platelet transfusions

Threshold	All patients	Procedures	Emergencies and trauma
No minimum platelet count		Bone marrow biopsy, PICC insertion, traction removal of tunnelled CVC line	
$>10 \times 10^9$/l	Non-bleeding patients		
$>20 \times 10^9$/l	Additional risk of bleeding, e.g. sepsis (platelet dysfunction)	Low-risk interventional procedures, e.g. ultrasound-guided CVC insertion	
$>30 \times 10^9$/l			Non-severe bleeding
$>40 \times 10^9$/l		Lumbar puncture	
$>50 \times 10^9$/l		Major surgery, percutaneous liver biopsy	Severe bleeding
$>80 \times 10^9$/l		Epidural catheter	
$>100 \times 10^9$/l		Neurosurgery	Multiple trauma, traumatic brain injury, spontaneous intracranial bleeding

Abbreviations: PICC = peripherally inserted central catheter; CVC = central venous catheter.

are achieved if transfused immediately prior to the procedure.

- Do not transfuse if suspected TTP/HUS/HITT, as this can exacerbate thrombotic complications.
- Exposure to frequent platelet transfusions can be associated with the development of anti-platelet alloantibodies, resulting in ineffective platelet transfusions in future. Therefore, carefully consider the necessity of each transfusion.

Sickle Cell Disease

Sickle cell disease (SCD) encompasses conditions resulting in clinical symptoms due to sickling of red blood cells secondary to polymerisation of haemoglobin S (HbS). HbS is caused by substitution of glutamic acid by valine in position 6 of the β-globin chain. HbS characteristically polymerises in deoxygenated states, with resultant sickle-shaped red cells causing vaso-occlusion and haemolytic anaemia. Inheritance of one HbS gene and one normal Hb gene (HbA) results in clinically silent sickle cell trait (HbAS). Inheritance of two HbS genes results in sickle cell anaemia (HbSS). HbS can be co-inherited with other variant haemoglobins, the clinical manifestation of which depends on the altered function of both variants; for example, inheritance of HbS and HbC genes (HbSC disease) results in a form of SCD which usually has fewer vaso-occlusive pain episodes, compared to HbSS, although a higher incidence of retinopathy. There is also clinical heterogeneity among patients with the same

genotype; for example, patients with HbSS range from presentations with infrequent painful episodes managed at home with oral analgesia to recurrent severe pain associated with significant morbidity. Therefore, a thorough clinical history of previous complications is essential in predicting the potential severity of acute episodes and assessing residual morbidity from previous events. Similar heterogeneity is found in the degree of haemolysis and presence of end-organ damage.

Key Principles for Management of Acute Sickle Cell Events

- Assess for trigger of acute presentation, e.g. cold weather, dehydration, infection, surgery, pregnancy
- Supportive measures – good hydration and analgesia. Patients often have a record of analgesic plans to manage acute episodes, as analgesic requirements are highly variable
- Low threshold for treating potential triggers, e.g. infections. Patients usually are functionally asplenic, and therefore prone to atypical infections
- Pro-thrombotic state – low threshold to assess and treat for venous thromboembolism
- Compare Hb level to the baseline for the patient – Hb of 70 g/l may not be abnormal for an individual and therefore may not require correction
- Management of these patients is complicated and must be led by a haematologist experienced in SCD

- Do not assume that complications are secondary to SCD – patients can get non-sickle-related issues also

Principles of Blood Transfusions in Sickle Cell Disease

- Transfusions can be used to simply correct anaemia to baseline (top-up transfusions) or as exchange transfusions. Transfusions may be part of management in the acute setting to treat a complication, or chronically to prevent or limit end-organ damage.
- Exchange transfusions reduce sickling by removing sickle red cells and replacing them with donor red cells. Exchange transfusions can be manual or automated. Automated exchanges result in more effective reduction of the proportion of sickle cells (HbS <15 per cent) and are not associated with iron overload. However, specialist equipment and training are required, often only available in tertiary centres. Manual exchange can be done in any hospital by any trained individual. This can reduce the proportion of sickle cells to a safe level (e.g. HbS <40 per cent) but is not iron-neutral and is associated with iron overload in the long term.
- Choice and frequency of exchange transfusion protocols should be directed by a haematologist experienced in managing SCD.
- Aim to minimise exposure to transfusions to reduce the risk of forming red cell alloantibodies that can limit the ability to transfuse in future (see 'Delayed Haemolytic Transfusion Reaction' section below).

Specific Complications

Acute Chest Syndrome

- Sickling affects the pulmonary vasculature, resulting in breathlessness and type 1 respiratory failure
- Haematological emergency with high mortality and morbidity
- Triggers: as above, but in particular infections, especially atypical chest infections (e.g. *Mycoplasma*). Consider travel history/flight history. Often preceded by a painful episode, particularly in adult patients
- Measure SpO_2 *on air* – the degree of hypoxia may not correlate with SpO_2; therefore, arterial blood gases (ABGs) required for assessment of PaO_2 if acute chest syndrome suspected, i.e. if SpO_2 ≤94 per cent on air or there is a fall in SpO_2 of ≥3 per cent from baseline
- Chest X-ray – bilateral consolidation/acute respiratory distress syndrome (ARDS)-type picture
- Good venous access – two green cannulae peripherally. Urgently, process cross-match samples (two if new to hospital) to allow provision of blood for red cell exchange
- Hydration, antibiotics, venous thromboembolism prophylaxis
- Red cell exchange – definitive management of chest crises. Automated, aiming to reduce the proportion of HbS to <15 per cent; or manual if automated unavailable
- Non-invasive ventilation can be beneficial in acute chest crises in avoiding intubation and invasive ventilation. Consider early, especially for patients with high-risk disease, e.g. poor pulmonary function reserve, multiple red cell antibodies limiting transfusions

Delayed Haemolytic Transfusion Reaction

- Multiple red cell antigens are present on blood cells, in addition to the ABO group
- Exposure to different red cell antigens by frequent blood transfusions can result in the patient developing antibodies against 'foreign' antigens (i.e. alloantibodies usually detected on group and screen)
- Further transfusion exposing the patient to foreign red cell antigen causes an immune response, ranging from an immediate/delayed haemolytic reaction to hyperhaemolysis
- Patients with SCD are more likely to develop red cell alloantibodies due to:
  - Different ethnicities to general blood donor population – therefore, more likely to have different red cell antigen profiles
  - Intact immune system capable of developing an immune response, compared to other regularly transfused patients (e.g. patients on chemotherapy)
  - Pro-inflammatory cytokine environment
- Hyperhaemolysis (or bystander haemolysis) is a clinical syndrome of acute intravascular haemolysis which destroys transfused cells,

as well as the patient's own red cells, causing severe anaemia with lower Hb, compared to pre-transfusion level

- Management:
  - Avoid unnecessary blood transfusions to avoid triggering hyperhaemolysis and developing further red cell antibodies
  - Immunosuppression: high-dose steroids (methylprednisolone) and intravenous immunoglobulin (IVIG)
  - If blood transfusion is required for severe systemic compromise due to anaemia, try to give blood matched to the patient's own red cell antigen profile. Due to rare blood groups and donor population, this requires early discussion with frozen blood banks (via the local hospital blood bank and haematology team; <8 hours to defrost and transport blood). In an emergency, however, give ABO-matched/O-neg blood, depending on clinical urgency
  - Novel therapies may be considered, e.g. eculizumab anti-C5 monoclonal antibody for inhibition of the complement pathway

Therapeutic Plasma Exchange

The aim of therapeutic plasma exchange (PEX) is to remove harmful large molecules, e.g. antibodies, from the circulation. Usually 1–1.5 plasma volumes are removed per procedure and replaced with 4.5–5% human albumin solution. PEX is usually an adjunct to definitive disease-directed therapy. The number and frequency of exchanges depend on the indications and should be guided by the clinical team managing the patient.

Complications of Plasma Exchange

- Transient hypocalcaemia secondary to binding of free plasma calcium to citrate anticoagulants – managed by adjusting the frequency and volume of PEX or by calcium supplements

- Hypovolaemia and vasovagal reactions uncommon, as PEX usually isovolaemic
- Transient depletion of coagulation factors and fibrinogen can cause mild prolongation of coagulation parameters, recovering within 24 hours. Rarely, this is associated with clinical bleeding. Some trusts recommend cryoprecipitate to replace fibrinogen if <0.5 g/l
- Risks associated with insertion of large-bore vascular access (femoral Vascath, central venous catheter line)
- Allergic reactions to plasma products

Therapeutic PEX with alternative replacement fluids and therapeutic apheresis, i.e. removal of other blood components, can be used for specific conditions, e.g. thrombotic thrombocytopenic purpura, SCD or leucostasis.

References and Further Reading

Estcourt LJ, Birchall J, Allard S, *et al.*; British Committee for Standards in Haematology. Guidelines for the use of platelet transfusions. *Br J Haematol* 2017;**176**:365–94.

Oteng-Ntim E, Pavord S, Howard R, *et al.*; British Society for Haematology Guideline. Management of sickle cell disease in pregnancy. A British Society for Haematology Guideline. *Br J Haematol* 2021;**194**: 980–95.

Retter A, Wyncoll D, Pearse R, *et al.*; British Committee for Standards in Haematology. Guidelines on the management of anaemia and red cell transfusion in adult critically ill patients. *Br J Haematol* 2013;**160**:445–64.

Schwartz J, Winters JL, Padmanabhan A, *et al.* Guidelines on the use of therapeutic apheresis in clinical practice-evidence-based approach from the Writing Committee of the American Society for Apheresis: the sixth special issue. *J Clin Apher* 2013;**28**:145–284.

Shander A, Javidroozi M, Lobel G. Patient blood management in the intensive care unit. *Transfus Med Rev* 2017;**31**:264–71.

3.10.5 Malignant Haematology in Intensive Care

Jenny O'Nions and William Townsend

Key Learning Points

1. Referral to the ICU should be made, considering the patient's previous performance score (PS), underlying disease, prognosis and treatment plan, as well as patient wishes. There are no absolute contraindications to ICU admission for haematology patients. A trial of intensive care is usually warranted in patients suitable for life-prolonging therapy.

2. The outcome of ICU admission is largely determined by the acute critical illness, not the underlying haematological malignancy.

3. Patients receiving treatment for haematological malignances are at high risk of infections and can have immune dysfunction in the absence of cytopenias (recovery of normal neutrophil levels after treatment does not guarantee normal functionality).

4. There are important differences between autologous haematopoietic stem cell transplants and allogeneic HSCT, which impact both complications and prognosis.

5. A tissue biopsy should usually be obtained in patients with suspected haematological malignancy prior to starting steroids. Histological diagnosis is critical in haematological malignancy.

Keywords: haematology, malignancy, autologous, allogeneic

Overview of Haematological Malignancy and ICU Admission

The aim of this section is to provide intensive care clinicians with an overview of the complications associated with haematological malignancies (HMs) and therapies. Patients with HM can develop critical illness relating to the underlying disease or due to anti-cancer therapies, including chemotherapy, immunotherapy (including chimeric antigen receptor (CAR) T-cell therapy), radiotherapy or haematopoietic stem cell transplant (HSCT). Most admissions to the ICU relate to treatment received for HMs. Outcomes are predominantly determined by the acute critical illness, as opposed to the underlying HM.

Historical data suggested that patients with HM have poor outcomes in the ICU (mortality rates reported of up to 90 per cent), previously leading some to advocate limitations to ICU admission and treatment. More recent data have shown improved outcomes, with significantly lower mortality (the ICNARC study of England, Wales and Northern Ireland reported a rate of 43.1 per cent in 2009). This is due to improvements in the ICU, infection prophylaxis and supportive care, reduction in therapy toxicity, use of novel (non-chemotherapeutic) agents and the introduction of reduced-intensity conditioning for allogeneic HSCT (alloHSCT). Many patients with HM have a long life expectancy if curative treatment is achieved, and accordingly the presence of an HM should not, in itself, be a barrier to ICU admission. The British Society for Haematology (BSH) guidance from 2015 recommended that referral for ICU admission should consider the patient's disease status, treatment plan and previous performance score (PS) (plus patient wishes), and a trial of ICU care should be considered in patients who are appropriate for life-extending treatment.

Complications of Haematological Malignancy and Treatment

Admission of patients with HM to the ICU may be required for a number of reasons. These include the following.

Infection

Patients with HM are at high risk of infection (the most common complication necessitating ICU admission) due to:

- Myelosuppression – secondary to bone marrow (BM) involvement or chemotherapy (or other therapy)
- Impairment of the adaptive immune system
- Breakdown of mucosal or skin barriers – translocation of bacteria into the bloodstream
- Indwelling central venous catheters
- Prolonged hospital stay
- Multiple, sometimes prolonged, courses of broad-spectrum antibiotics

Causative organisms are often not identified (blood cultures are negative in 70–75 per cent of cases of neutropenic sepsis).

Bleeding

Thrombocytopenia is a common complication. Prophylactic transfusions to target platelet counts of >10 are routine, or >20 if septic (higher if active bleeding).

Other

- Respiratory failure
- Fluid balance
- Electrolyte derangement

- Tumour lysis syndrome
- Complications following HSCT

Additionally, complications may arise from the haematological malignancy directly or secondary to the treatment (Table 3.10.5.1).

Introduction to Haematopoietic Stem Cell Transplantation

HSCT is the transfer of pluripotent haematopoietic stem cells (HSCs) to reconstitute haematopoiesis following intensive therapy (the 'conditioning regimen'). It is used to consolidate treatment in high-risk or relapsed HM, and less commonly to correct non-malignant disorders that may be otherwise life-threatening (e.g. immune deficiency, haemoglobinopathy, multiple sclerosis). HSCT can be categorised by donor type and intensity of conditioning. Conditioning regimens involve chemotherapy, radiotherapy and anti-lymphocyte agents, depending on HM type and patient co-morbidity. Transplant-related mortality (TRM) depends on the conditioning regimen, patient co-morbidities, previous treatment and the underlying HM.

Autologous Haematopoietic Stem Cell Transplantation versus Allogeneic Haematopoietic Stem Cell Transplantation

There are two broad categories – autologous HSCT (autoHSCT) and alloHSCT – with significant

Table 3.10.5.1 Complications arising from haematological malignancies and their treatment

Complications arising from haematological malignancy	Complications arising from treatment for haematological malignancy
Myelosuppression due to bone marrow infiltration – anaemia, thrombocytopenia, bleeding, neutropenia, reduced resistance to infection Disseminated intravascular coagulation Nervous system involvement 'B' symptoms – weight loss, fever, night sweats Hyperviscosity	Myelosuppression Mucositis – painful inflammation and ulceration of gastrointestinal tract mucosa; can occur from mouth to anus: • Poor oral intake, requirement for nasogastric/parenteral feeding • Nausea • Diarrhoea • Breakdown of protective mucosal barriers and translocation of gut commensals into the bloodstream Haemorrhagic cystitis (e.g. due to cyclophosphamide) Rashes/skin breakdown Allergic reactions Cytokine release syndrome (following immunotherapy, e.g. CAR T-cell therapy or bi-specific antibody therapy) Fevers in absence of infection (cytarabine) Organ impairment – renal/cardiac/pulmonary/liver Neurotoxicity – including intrathecal methotrexate-associated encephalopathy and CAR T-cell therapy-related neurotoxicity

Abbreviations: CAR = chimeric antigen receptor.

differences in the indications for each, and associated complications (Box 3.10.5.1; Table 3.10.5.2).

Autologous Haematopoietic Stem Cell Transplantation

AutoHSCT is most commonly used to consolidate treatment for myeloma and relapsed lymphomas. After HM-specific therapy is completed, the patient's HSCs are mobilised into the peripheral blood (PB) and

harvested by leukapheresis. AutoHSCT involves the use of very high-dose myeloablative chemotherapy followed by return of the patient's own HSCs to facilitate haematopoietic recovery.

The main complications of autoHSCT are those relating to chemotherapy used in conditioning and resulting myelosuppression, including risk of infections and severe mucositis. There is no risk of graft-versus-host disease (GVHD) or graft rejection, as the graft is autologous.

> **Box 3.10.5.1 Key Differences between AutoHSCT and AlloHSCT for ICU Staff**
>
> - Recipients of autoHSCT are most likely to require ICU support during the 3–4 weeks post-HSC re-infusion whilst awaiting count recovery. After count recovery, the risk of critical illness rapidly declines.
> - Recipients of alloHSCT may require ICU admission and support long after initial count recovery due to the added complications and ongoing immune dysfunction. The increased risk of alloHSCT is, however, offset by the increased potential for long-term cure.

Allogeneic Haematopoietic Stem Cell Transplantation

AlloHSCT offers potential cure for many HMs and utilises HSCs harvested from a human leucocyte antigen (HLA)-matched donor (by leukapheresis or BM harvest), usually a sibling (SIB) or unrelated donor (MUD). Umbilical cords and haploidentical (50 per cent matched) donors can also be used when no other suitable matched donor is available. Conditioning regimens can be myeloablative or 'reduced intensity' (RIC), which have lower toxicity, enabling older patients to undergo alloHSCT.

Table 3.10.5.2 Differences between autoHSCT and alloHSCT

	AutoHSCT	**AlloHSCT**
HSC source	Patient PB	Donor BM or PB
Donor available	Yes – but risk of failure to mobilise enough HSCs for reconstitution	Not always – time for search and matching required (limited in some ethnic groups)
Conditioning regiment	Usually chemotherapy, can involve radiotherapy	Chemotherapy, radiotherapy, anti-lymphocyte agents Myeloablative or RIC
Graft rejection	No	Yes (haplo > cord > MUD > SIB)
GVHD	No	Yes
GVT	No	Yes
Engraftment	Faster (8–12 days)	Slower (8–20 days, can be longer)
Immune reconstitution	Faster, patient's own IS	Slower, donor IS Immune deficiency persists after apparent haematological recovery
Immunosuppression	Not required	Yes
Complications	Related to previous chemotherapy/immunotherapy/myelosuppression, previous treatment, underlying disease	Related to chemotherapy, anti-lymphocyte agents and prolonged immune suppression
TRM	2–5%	10–20%
Increased risk of MDS	Yes	No
Risk of second malignancy	Yes	Yes

Abbreviations: PB = peripheral blood; BM = bone marrow; HSC = haematopoietic stem cell; RIC = reduced-intensity conditioning; MUD = matched unrelated donor; SIB = sibling; GVHD = graft-versus-host disease; GVT = graft-versus-tumour; IS = immune system; TRM = treatment-related mortality; MDS = myelodysplastic syndrome (a bone marrow failure disorder).

Therapeutic effect is from both intensive conditioning and graft-versus-tumour (GVT) effect. However, immunological complications of GVHD (where donor cells recognise the recipient's own cells as foreign) and graft rejection (recipient's cells target donor HSCs) can occur. Immune suppression (cyclosporine, tacrolimus or mycophenolate mofetil) is used to prevent these; hence, there is an increased risk of opportunistic infection and viral reactivation long after the initial transplant procedure (Table 3.10.5.3).

Graft-versus-Host Disease

GVHD can affect multiple organ systems, resulting in organ dysfunction and breakdown of the barriers to infection. GVHD increases with HLA mismatch and is an independent risk factor for ICU admission.

GVHD is graded in severity from 1 to 4 (with worse 100-day survival with increasing grade) and can be:

- Acute – occurring within the first 100 days of transplant; typically involves the skin, gut and liver
- Chronic – occurring after 100 days; can involve the gut, skin, liver, musculoskeletal system and eyes
  Features include:
- Mucositis
- Pneumonitis
- Colitis – diarrhoea, abdominal pain

- Hepatitis
- Jaundice
- Dermatitis – macular rash, blistering, desquamation
- Eyes – sicca
- Muscle, fascial and joint inflammation

GVHD is managed with immune suppression, which further increases the risk of infection. Treatment depends on the organ system affected and the severity of GVHD. Steroids are first line in acute flares (e.g. 1–2 mg/kg methylprednisolone).

Chimeric Antigen Receptor (CAR) T-Cell Therapy

CAR T-cell therapy is a new treatment modality for treating haematological malignancies. In CAR T-cell therapy, a patient's own lymphocytes are harvested by leukapheresis and their T cell receptors are genetically engineered to express a synthetic receptor for a target on malignant cells, e.g. CD19 on B lymphocytes. After receiving leucodepleting chemotherapy, the manufactured cells are re-infused. The cells hone to sites of disease where they recognise the tumour antigen, are activated and proliferate rapidly, exerting an antitumour effect.

This novel therapy is showing great promise in treating a range of HMs, including B cell acute

Table 3.10.5.3 Complications of alloHSCT

Early (3 months)	Late
Chemo-/radiotherapy:	**Chemo-/radiotherapy:**
• Nausea/vomiting	• Cardiac (or other organ) impairment
• Alopecia (reversible)	• Infertility
• Mucositis	• Endocrine insufficiency (hypothyroidism,
• Veno-occlusive disease	hypoadrenalism, hypogonadism)
• Dry skin	• Hyposplenism
• Fatigue	• Secondary malignancy
	• Cataracts
Infection	**Infection**
• Bacterial – Gram-negative/positive	• Bacterial – encapsulated
• Fungal – *Aspergillus, Candida*	• Fungal – *Aspergillus, Candida*
• Viral – reactivation (e.g. HSV, CMV, EBV, BK), acquired (rhino-/entero-/'flu/paraflu/norovirus)	• Viral – reactivation (e.g. HSV, CMV, EBV), acquired (rhino-/entero-/'flu/paraflu/norovirus)
• Atypical – PCP	• Atypical – PCP
• Protozoal – *Toxoplasma*	
Acute GVHD	**Chronic GVHD**
TMAs	**Transfusion-associated iron overload**

Admission to the ICU is more likely after myeloablative conditioning > reduced-intensity conditioning (RIC) > autologous haematopoietic stem cell transplant.

Abbreviations: PCP = pneumocystis pneumonia; HSV = herpes simplex virus; CMV = cytomegalovirus; EBV = Epstein–Barr virus; GVHD = graft-versus-host disease; TMA = treatment-related mortality.

lymphoblastic leukaemia (B-ALL), some B cell lymphomas and multiple myeloma.

CAR T-cell therapy and other treatments that engage T cells (e.g. bi-specific antibodies) have a unique and serious range of associated toxicities which can necessitate ICU admission (see 'Complications of CAR T-Cell Therapy' section below).

Management of Critical Illness in Malignant Haematology

Commonly encountered problems include:
- Neutropenic sepsis
- Tumour lysis syndrome
- Hyperleucocytosis and leucostasis
- Hyperviscosity
- Hypercalcaemia
- Spinal cord compression
- Superior vena cava obstruction (SVCO)
- Complications of T cell-engaging treatment – cytokine release syndrome and neurotoxicity

Neutropenic Sepsis

Neutropenic sepsis is the most common reason for ICU admission in haematology patients. Notably, it is important to remember:
- Neutrophil numbers can be normal, but with neutrophil function reduced (e.g. myelodysplastic syndrome)
- Patients on deffervescing agents (e.g. steroids) can be septic without pyrexia
- Some patients have an increased risk of renal impairment (e.g. myeloma, high-dose methotrexate, platinum-based chemotherapy); therefore, aminoglycosides should be used with caution – consider using alternative agents, e.g. ciprofloxacin, depending on local policy

All units should have specific local protocols for rapid diagnosis of infection (often involving early use of high-resolution CT) and early use of empirical broad-spectrum antibiotics (based on local sensitivities). Fungal infection risk is directly related to neutropenia duration; therefore, patients variably receive antiviral, anti-fungal and pneumocystis pneumonia (PCP) prophylaxis during their treatment. Early input from microbiology must be sought.

Diagnosis and treatment of neutropenic sepsis in patients receiving anti-cancer therapy can be seen Box 3.10.5.2.

Management

- Do not delay antibiotics pending full assessment or investigation; assessment and empirical antibiotics should be commenced within 1 hour of presentation
- Full clinical assessment (advanced life support (ALS) approach), including the chest, perineum, skin, CVC sites and fundi
- Investigations (may vary with local policy):
  - Full blood count (FBC), urea and electrolytes (U&Es), creatinine, liver function tests (LFTs), C-reactive protein (CRP)
  - Blood culture – peripheral and central lines
  - Swabs from any inflamed sites
  - Midstream urine (MSU) if symptomatic
  - Faeces if diarrhoea and/or if fungal infection suspected; check *Clostridium difficile* toxin, ova, cysts and parasites (OCP) and microscopy, culture and sensitivity (MC&S)

Box 3.10.5.2 NICE Diagnosis and Treatment of Neutropenic Sepsis in Patients Receiving Anti-cancer Therapy

Diagnosis
- Neutrophil count $<0.5 \times 10^9/l$
- Fever >38°C OR symptoms/signs consistent with clinically significant sepsis

Treatment
- Start empirical antibiotics (piperacillin/tazobactam, provided not penicillin-allergic) after septic screen sent; only use aminoglycoside if local microbiological or patient-specific indication) – *however, many protocols include empirical aminoglycoside use*
- No recommendation to empirically remove indwelling central venous catheter (CVC). However, there should be a low threshold for removing CVCs in patients who are not responding to antibiotics
- Do not switch empirical antibiotics unless clinical deterioration or microbiological indication
- Discontinue aminoglycoside after 24 hours if no evidence of Gram-negative infection
- Continue antibiotics until clinical response (use a validated scoring system to assess the risk of septic complications)
- Granulocyte colony-stimulating factor (G-CSF) is not always required but can shorten the duration of neutropenia in some circumstances

Source: NICE 2012 (guideline 151).

347

(consider viral polymerase chain reaction (PCR))

- ○ *Aspergillus* precipitins and PCR (beta *D*-glucan)
- ○ Serology, mouthwash, vesicle fluid for virology if indicated
- ○ Chest X-ray, sinus or dental X-rays if symptomatic

Translocation of Gram-negative organisms across disrupted mucosa is frequent.

Blood cultures are positive in 30 per cent, and 60 per cent of positive cultures are Gram-positive organisms.

Tumour Lysis Syndrome

Tumour lysis syndrome (TLS) results from breakdown of tumour cells, either spontaneously (in tumours with high cell division and turnover rates) or secondary to cytotoxic therapy, resulting in rising potassium, phosphate and urate levels and hypocalcaemia (Figure 3.10.5.1). This can result in potentially life-threatening biochemical disturbance and renal failure, seizures, coma, cardiac arrhythmias, multi-organ dysfunction and death if unrecognised or untreated.

Diagnosis may be based on clinical (Cairo and Bishop) or laboratory parameters (Table 3.10.5.4).

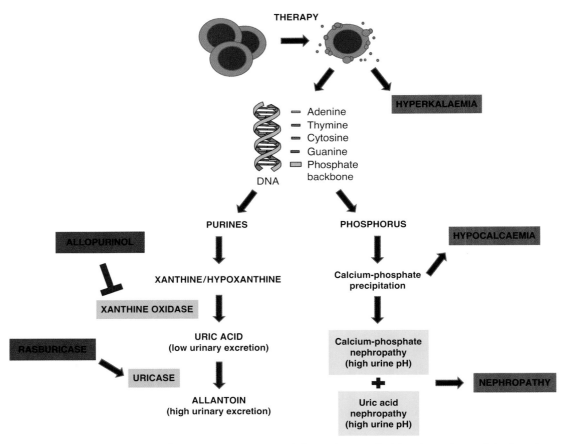

Figure 3.10.5.1 Pathophysiology of tumour lysis syndrome. Morbidity is a direct result of the release of intracellular electrolytes and DNA into the bloodstream and precipitation in the kidneys. Management involves hydration, electrolyte monitoring and management and uric acid inhibitors. Allopurinol inhibits xanthine oxidase, blocking synthesis of uric acid from hypoxanthine, reducing plasma (and therefore urine) uric acid levels and increasing plasma (and urine) levels of more soluble oxypurine precursors. Rasburicase is a recombinant urate oxidase (uricase), converting uric acid to allantoin, which is soluble and readily excreted by kidneys (drug elimination time 18 hours). Allopurinol blocks the synthesis of uric acid from xanthines, hence should not be used in conjunction with rasburicase.

- **Laboratory TLS:** ≥2 serum values of the following at presentation *or* a change by 25 per cent from −3 days to +7 days after cytotoxic therapy (most commonly 12–72 hours after commencement of treatment):
  - **Uric acid** – ≥ULN or 25 per cent increase from baseline (not included if rasburicase given in last 24 hours)
  - **Potassium** – ≥6.0 mmol/l or 25 per cent increase from baseline
  - **Phosphate** – ≥1.45 mmol/l or 25 per cent increase from baseline
  - **Corrected calcium** – ≤1.75 mmol/l or 25 per cent decrease from baseline
- **Clinical TLS:** laboratory TLS plus ≥1 of:
  - Creatinine >1.5 × upper limit of normal
  - Cardiac arrhythmia/sudden death
  - Seizure

Management involves risk stratification, hydration and hypouricaemic agents.

- Risk stratification – determines prophylactic management.
  - Low risk:
    - Monitoring, hydration (no potassium added to fluid, usually 3 l/(m² day) ± allopurinol (prevents uric acid formation in 24–72 hours)
  - Intermediate risk:
    - Monitoring, hydration and allopurinol
  - High risk:
    - Monitoring, hydration, rasburicase (reduces uric acid levels in 4 hours, variable dosing; 0.2 mg/kg for up to 7 days, check glucose-6-phosphate dehydrogenase (G6PD) – risk of haemolysis if deficient)
- Consider pre-phase of treatment or deferral of chemotherapy
- Monitor urine output, fluid balance and electrolytes (TLS bloods – renal profile, potassium, calcium, phosphate, urate every 6 hours initially, de-escalated as per clinical picture)
- Consider a loop diuretic if poor urine output
- There is no evidence for alkalinisation of the urine (can worsen nephropathy)
- Renal replacement therapy as required
- Management of seizure, cardiac arrhythmia

Table 3.10.5.4 Biochemical features of tumour lysis syndrome

Biochemical features	Clinical features
Hyperkalaemia	Lethargy, nausea, vomiting, diarrhoea, muscle weakness, paraesthesia, ECG changes (e.g. tall, tented T waves, widened QRS complex, ventricular arrhythmias).
Hyperphosphataemia and secondary hypocalcaemia	Anorexia, vomiting, confusion, carpopedal spasm, tetany, seizures, arrhythmias
Hyperuricaemia	Nausea, vomiting, anorexia and lethargy, renal injury (uric acid nephropathy – uric acid crystals deposit in renal tubules and collecting ducts)
Renal impairment	Reduced urinary excretion of potassium and phosphate, leading to fluid retention, pulmonary oedema and metabolic acidosis (predisposes to further renal urate deposition)

Hyperleucocytosis and Leucostasis

Hyperleucocytosis is the presence of increased numbers of circulating white blood cells (e.g. in leukaemias and myeloproliferative disorders). This is a laboratory abnormality and often does not require treatment.

Symptomatic hyperleucocytosis (leucostasis) is a pathological diagnosis (accumulation of white cells and fibrin in the lumen of blood vessels, forming plugs) and a medical emergency (1-week mortality 20–40 per cent). Commonly affected vascular beds are: central nervous system, eyes (central retinal artery occlusion), lungs, kidneys, heart, penis and spleen (infarction).

Leucostasis typically presents with respiratory or neurological distress, with features including:

- Dyspnoea and cough (pulmonary leucostasis)
- Confusion
- Decreased conscious level
- Isolated cranial nerve palsies (cerebral leucostasis)
- Visual symptoms
- Other symptoms, including pruritus, headache, hypertension and plethora

Management involves reduction of white cell concentration:

- **Conservative** – reduces mortality and need for leukapheresis:
  - Intravenous fluids

○ *Caution* with blood transfusion (can exacerbate hyperviscosity). If required (symptomatic anaemia, severe cardiovascular risk), peri-leukapheresis or exchange transfusion is preferable

- **Active:**
  ○ Leukapheresis/plasma exchange until white cell count $<50 \times 10^9/l$
  ○ Prompt administration of appropriate chemotherapy
  ○ Manage associated disseminated intravascular coagulation
  ○ Initiate the TLS protocol, including prophylaxis and monitoring

Treatment of asymptomatic patients is controversial and depends on age, co-morbidity and rate of white cell count increase.

Notably, there is an increased risk of intracerebral haemorrhage, with large reductions in white cell count and platelets usually maintained at $20–30 \times 10^9/l$.

Hyperviscosity

An increase in whole blood viscosity can occur as a result of:

- Red cells (e.g. polycythaemic rubra vera (PRV)):
  ○ Clinical features – lethargy, pruritus, headache, hypertension, plethora, arterial thrombosis (myocardial infarction, cerebrovascular accident), visual loss (central retinal artery occlusion)
  ○ Management – isovolaemic venesection (frequency varies), cytoreductive therapy (e.g. hydroxycarbamide)
- White cells (e.g. blasts):
  ○ Clinical features – hyperleucocytosis
  ○ Management – leukapheresis, cytoreductive therapy
- Plasma components, e.g. paraprotein (e.g. multiple myeloma or Waldenström's macroglobulinaemia):
  ○ Clinical features – headache, confusion, lethargy, seizure, memory loss, vertigo, visual disturbance (due to cerebral vessel 'sludging'), dizziness
  ○ Management – plasmapheresis, treatment of underlying disease

Spinal Cord Compression

In haematology patients, spinal cord compression most commonly occurs in multiple myeloma (at presentation, during treatment or at relapse) and some lymphomas.

Management includes:

- Dexamethasone
- Urgent magnetic resonance imaging (within 24 hours)
- Liaison with:
  ○ Neurosurgery (possible decompression, stabilisation, biopsy)
  ○ Clinical oncology for possible radiotherapy
- Steroid/chemotherapy may be sufficient treatment

Hypercalcaemia

Most commonly seen in multiple myeloma, and more rarely in some subtypes of lymphoma or acute lymphoblastic leukaemia (ALL).

Symptoms/signs include:

- Confusion, coma, obtundation
- Thirst, polyuria
- Constipation
- Muscle weakness
- Pancreatitis
- Acute renal failure

Treatment involves the following:

- Mild (2.6–2.9): oral/intravenous hydration
- Moderate/severe (>2.9): intravenous sodium chloride and bisphosphonates (zoledronic acid preferable to pamidronate)
- Steroids (e.g. dexamethasone 20–40 mg)
- Treat the underlying disorder
- Consider renal replacement therapy if calcium >4.5 mmol/l

Superior Vena Cava Obstruction

External compression of the superior vena cava (SVC) by a tumour mass, lymphadenopathy or an internal thrombus, resulting in dilation of contributory vessels, increased vascular pressure and tissue oedema. Presenting features include 'fullness' in the head, shortness of breath, cough, chest discomfort, dysphagia, dilated veins and cyanosis of the head, neck and upper body.

Treatment includes:

- Elevating the head of the bed
- Oxygen

- Steroids, e.g. dexamethasone 8 mg orally twice daily (note: discuss with the haematology consultant prior if no histological diagnosis)
- Imaging (computed tomography of the chest with contrast) to establish the level of SVCO
- Excluding a non-malignant cause, e.g. indwelling catheter
- Consider intravascular stenting (liaise with interventional radiology)
- Treat underlying malignancy

Complications of CAR T-cell Therapy
Cytokine Release Syndrome

After T cells engage and are activated, they proliferate rapidly, which can lead to a supra-physiological immune system reaction characterised by fever and increased production and release of a range of cytokines, e.g. tumour necrosis factor alpha (TNFα), interleukin (IL)-2, IL-6, IL-8, IL-10. This is termed cytokine release syndrome (CRS).

The clinical features of CRS are fever, hypotension and hypoxia. CRS can develop rapidly and may progress to a life-threatening scenario, in which ICU admission may be required for inotropic or ventilatory support.

The grading of CRS is according to the criteria shown in Table 3.10.5.5.

Neurotoxicity Associated with CAR T-cell Therapy
Immune Effector Cell-Associated Neurotoxicity Syndrome

A range of neurological toxicities have been described after CAR T-cell therapy termed immune effector cell-associated neurotoxicity syndrome (ICANS).

Manifestations include tremor, dysarthria, expressive dysphasia, seizures, raised intracranial pressure and reduced conscious level.

Management of CAR T-cell Toxicities

Prompt identification, grading and management of CRS and ICANS are required and ICU support may be required. Treatment should be initiated and guided by the specialist haematology team, and interventions may include the IL-6 receptor-blocking antibody tocilizumab, or corticosteroids.

Selection and Outcomes of Patients with Haematological Malignancy in the ICU

Approximately 7 per cent of hospitalised patients with HM have a critical illness and 13 per cent of patients undergoing HSCT require ICU admission. Patients with HM should be considered for an unrestricted trial of critical care.

Key British Society for Haematology Recommendations

- Patients with HM are at high risk of critical illness. Monitoring should include aggregate track-and-trigger systems (e.g. National Early Warning Score).
- Severe sepsis and respiratory failure are common reasons for ICU admission. In suspected sepsis, follow the Surviving Sepsis campaign recommendations and consider early removal of indwelling catheters.
- ICU referral should involve direct discussion between ICU and haematology consultants.

Table 3.10.5.5 Grading of cytokine release syndrome

CRS parameter	Grade 1	Grade 2	Grade 3	Grade 4
Temperature	≥38°C	≥38°C	≥38°C	≥38°C
WITH				
Hypotension	None	Not requiring vasopressors	Requiring vasopressors	Requiring multiple vasopressors
AND/OR				
Hypoxia	None	Requiring low flow by nasal cannula or blow-by	Requiring high flow oxygen	Requiring positive pressure (e.g. CPAP, BiPAP, intubation and mechanical ventilation)

Source: Lee *et al. Biol Blood Marrow Transplant.* 2019.

- Patients in the process of dying with irreversible illness or competent adults who decline treatment should not be referred.
- An unrestricted trial of critical care should be considered for all patients who are appropriate for life-extending treatment or with a good PS.
- Non-invasive ventilation should not normally be undertaken on the ward.
- Patients who have undergone alloHSCT should be managed in an ICU attached to a specialist haematology unit.
- Inter- and intra-hospital transfer should follow recommended procedures.

Factors Influencing Outcomes of Patients with HM Admitted to ICU

- **Organ failure** – single most important factor influencing survival; mortality increases directly with the number of organ systems affected (1 = 50 per cent; 3 = 84 per cent; 5 = 98 per cent)
- **Respiratory failure** – survival rates are 18–26 per cent in patients requiring invasive ventilation versus 60–80 per cent in those who do not. Duration of invasive ventilation and severity of hypoxaemia (prior to intubation and ventilation) are associated with worse outcomes
- **Age and disease status (stage/type)** – no evidence either affects outcomes. Age is important in long-term outcomes of treatment. Patients with refractory, relapsed or poor-risk disease have worse long-term outcomes following ICU admission
- **Neutropenia** – some evidence neutropenia is associated with worse outcomes. Granulocyte colony-stimulating factor (G-CSF) shortens neutropenia duration and is frequently used, but there is no evidence it improves ICU outcome

- **Type of HSCT** – in terms of survival, autoHSCT > alloHSCT and RIC > myeloablation
- **GVHD** – shown to be an independent predictor of mortality (with reduced survival in patients requiring invasive ventilation or renal replacement therapy who have GVHD)
- Standard ICU predictive scores (e.g. APACHE, SAPS) can be used but may underestimate mortality in this group

References and Further Reading

Foot C, Hickson L. Leadership skills in the ICU. In: A Webb, D Angus, S Finfer, L Gattinoni, M Singer (eds). *Oxford Textbook of Critical Care*, 2nd edn. Oxford: Oxford University Press; 2016. pp. 64–70.

Intensive Care Society. 2001. Guidelines for the transport of the critically ill adult. Standards and guidelines. www.baccn.org/static/uploads/resources/ICSStandardsTransport.pdf

Lee DW, Santomasso BD, Locke FL, *et al*. ASTCT consensus grading for cytokine release syndrome and neurologic toxicity associated with immune effector cells. *Biol Blood Marrow Transplant* 2019;**25**:625–38.

Matthey F, Parker A, Rule SA, *et al*. Facilities for the treatment of adults with haematological malignancies – 'levels of care': BCSH Haemato-Oncology Task Force 2009. *Hematology* 2010;**15**:63–9.

Thachil J, Hill Q (eds). *Haematology in Critical Care*. Oxford: Wiley-Blackwell; 2014.

Townsend WM, Holroyd A, Pearce R, *et al*. Improved intensive care unit survival for critically ill allogeneic haematopoietic stem cell transplant recipients following reduced intensity conditioning. *Br J Haematol* 2013;**161**:578–86.

Wise MP, Barnes RA, Baudouin SV, *et al*.; British Committee for Standards in Haematology. Guidelines on the management and admission to intensive care of critically ill adult patients with haematological malignancy in the UK. *Br J Haematol* 2015;**171**: 179–88.

3.10.6 Haemostasis, Coagulopathies and the Bleeding Patient

Ben Clevenger

Key Learning Points

1. Coagulation is a tightly regulated process controlled by interactions between the vessel, platelets, clotting factor enzymes, co-factors and inhibitors, aimed at stopping bleeding from damaged vessels.

2. Coagulation involves initiation, activation and propagation of platelet activity to generate a thrombin burst which polymerises fibrinogen to fibrin, plugging the vessel wall.

3. Coagulopathy is common in critically ill patients and is associated with increased illness severity and mortality.

4. The underlying cause of coagulopathy must be diagnosed and treated, whilst avoiding the unnecessary correction of laboratory test results, unless there is clinical bleeding or a surgical procedure required.

5. Disseminated intravascular coagulopathy is most commonly triggered by sepsis, leading to the consumption of clotting factors and platelets, which, in turn, causes bleeding and microthrombotic events. Treatment must be focused upon the underlying condition.

Keywords: coagulopathy, haemostasis, clotting, disseminated intravascular coagulopathy

Mechanisms of Coagulation and Haemostasis

Coagulation refers to the processes that result in blood clotting. This forms part of haemostasis, whereby bleeding from damaged vessels is stopped. Haemostatic systems initiate a rapid response to vessel injury, whilst attempting to maintain flow. Coagulation is a tightly regulated process resulting in the controlled formation of the enzyme thrombin (factor IIa) under the influence of clotting factor enzymes, co-factors and inhibitors. Thrombin initiates the formation of fibrin and stabilisation of a primary haemostatic plug.

Traditionally, coagulation was modelled simply by a classical cascade of activated serine proteases (coagulation factor enzymes), consisting of an intrinsic and extrinsic pathway, leading to the formation of a stable fibrin clot (Figure 3.10.6.1). This theory has been superseded by a cell-based model of coagulation occurring in three main stages: initiation, amplification and propagation (Figure 3.10.6.2), whereby platelet activation and adhesion are triggered, leading to the generation of thrombin and then fibrin deposition, plugging the disrupted vascular endothelium.

Primary haemostasis begins when the vessel wall is injured. Where a vessel wall is damaged, a pro-thrombotic state is initiated to stop bleeding, whilst smooth muscle cells coordinate local vasoconstriction. The increased shear stress increases the reactivity of platelets and von Willebrand factor (vWF). Where the vessel wall has been injured, sub-endothelial collagen is exposed. vWF binds to exposed collagen and it is unravelled to expose its main platelet-binding site, to which platelets bind and adhere to the collagen. The platelet is then activated, triggering the recruitment of more platelets. Activated platelets have an increased surface area and pseudopods to facilitate further binding. The activated platelets release alpha granules, dense bodies and lysosomes, which provide additional coagulation factors and energy to promote the formation of a platelet plug made up of the progressively recruited and bound platelets.

The coagulation pathway is triggered by exposed tissue factor (TF) in the vessel wall. TF is a protein expressed on fibroblasts and damaged or stimulated cells, including the endothelium. TF activates factor VII to stimulate the clotting cascade, leading to the generation of thrombin in a 'thrombin burst', which

353

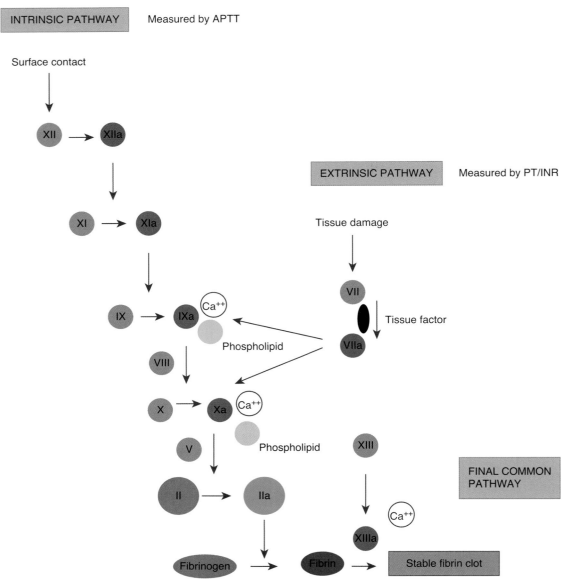

Figure 3.10.6.1 Coagulation cascade. APTT = activated partial thromboplastin time; Ca⁺⁺ = calcium; INR = international normalised ratio; PT = prothrombin time.

polymerises soluble fibrinogen to fibrin that stabilises the platelet plug.

The thrombin burst initiates a positive feedback loop, recruiting more platelets, generating more fibrin and converting more fibrinogen to fibrin. These processes are localised and protected from their inhibitors by localisation on the phospholipid surface provided by platelets. The developing thrombus is limited to the site of vessel injury by complex regulatory mechanisms

that involve anti-thrombin, activated protein C and plasmin.

The final step in haemostasis is removal of the thrombus on completion of wound healing. Fibrinolysis degrades the thrombus, mediated by plasmin. Tissue plasminogen activator (tPA) is secreted into the circulation from the endothelium and is present in a free form or bound to plasminogen activator inhibitor-1 (PAI-1). In the presence of a fibrin clot,

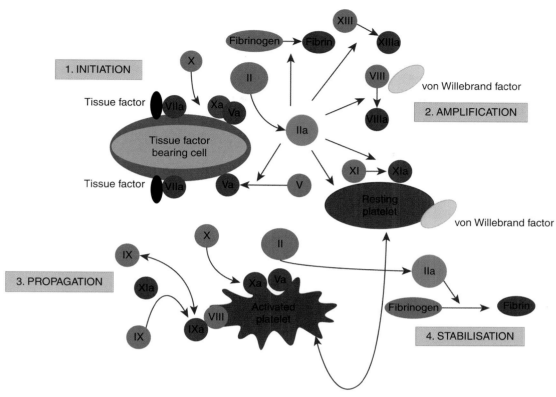

Figure 3.10.6.2 Cell-based model of coagulation.

tPA undergoes a conformational change, increasing its ability to convert plasminogen to plasmin. The main substrate of plasmin is fibrin, but it also hydrolyses fibrinogen and factors V and VIII, and activates the complement protein C3. Fibrinogen and fibrin are sequentially degraded to fibrin degradation products, which include D-dimers.

Coagulopathy

Coagulopathy means that the ability to form a clot and reduce bleeding is impaired. This is common in critically ill patients. Thrombocytopenia develops in up to 40 per cent of admissions, and an international normalised ratio (INR) of >1.5 is seen in almost two-thirds of patients. Coagulopathic patients are typically hospitalised for longer and are at an increased risk of acute kidney injury and multi-organ failure. Trauma patients have almost four times higher mortality if coagulopathic at presentation.

There are multiple pathophysiological causes of coagulopathy, as seen in Table 3.10.6.1.

The first principle of management of coagulopathies in critical care is to treat the underlying cause

Table 3.10.6.1 Pathophysiological causes of coagulopathy

Secondary to disruption of homeostasis
- Hypothermia (temperature <34°C)
- Severe acidosis (pH <7.25)
- Hypocalcaemia (ionised calcium <1 mmol/l)

Acquired platelet dysfunction
- Liver failure
- Renal failure
- Acquired dysfunction due to extracorporeal circuits and intra-aortic balloon pumps
- Iatrogenic due to anti-platelet agents

Thrombocytopenia
- Haemorrhage
- Dilutional secondary to massive transfusion
- Consumption in sepsis
- Direct myelosuppressant effect of medication
- Immune destruction
- Mechanical destruction secondary to extracorporeal circuits

Deranged coagulation pathways
- Disseminated intravascular coagulation
- Dilution and activation of coagulation factors
- Iatrogenic secondary to anticoagulants:
  - Vitamin K antagonists
  - Heparin and low-molecular weight heparin
  - Direct oral anticoagulants: direct thrombin inhibitors and direct factor Xa inhibitors
- Vitamin K deficiency
- Hyperfibrinolysis

without unnecessarily correcting laboratory abnormalities with blood products, unless there is a clinical bleeding problem or a surgical procedure is required, or both.

In the bleeding patient, a history must be taken to rule out bleeding disorders and the use of antithrombotic drugs. It must then be determined whether the bleeding is general or local, with reference to coagulation studies and platelet count, to diagnose the pathogenesis of bleeding in that patient.

Platelet function abnormalities or severe thrombocytopenia typically leads to bleeding immediately after trauma. Petechiae – small, discrete areas of capillary haemorrhage that develop due to increased venous pressure – are commonly seen with disorders of platelet function (Table 3.10.6.2). These are classically seen on dependent areas of the body. Patients with coagulation abnormalities often exhibit delayed bleeding such as ecchymoses – soft tissue haematomas that develop without a history of local trauma, due to the escape of blood into tissues.

Management of Coagulopathy

Vitamin K is required for the formation of coagulation factors II, VII, IX and X, as well as proteins C and S. An incidence of vitamin deficiency of up to 43 per cent has been shown in critical care populations. Dietary intake of vitamin K may be inadequate in intensive care, and therefore, supplementation may be required – either by supplementing nutrition or by intravenous administration.

Fresh frozen plasma (FFP) is indicated for treatment of patients with bleeding due to clotting factor deficiencies. When thawed, it contains normal levels of plasma proteins, including pro-coagulant factors and natural inhibitors of coagulation. A typical unit contains 250–300 ml and the recommended dose is 10–15 ml/kg. Much higher volumes may be required to produce therapeutic levels of coagulation factors, and volume overload can be a problem.

There is no evidence to support the use of prophylactic FFP to correct abnormal coagulation results prior to invasive procedures such as central line insertion.

Prothrombin complex concentrate (PCC) contains factors II, VII, IX and X. PCCs are recommended for rapid reversal of warfarin overdose with elevated INR and severe bleeding, instead of FFP, due to superior efficacy, ease of administration and lower risk of severe allergic reactions or fluid overload. Modern PCC formulations do not contain activated clotting factors and have a low risk of causing thrombotic complications. PCCs may also be used to treat bleeding due to coagulopathy associated with liver disease. The dose for reversal of warfarin is 25–50 IU/kg.

Management of Haemorrhage

Data from trauma and military cohorts have increasingly provided evidence which dictates the ratios of FFP:red blood cells to treat major bleeding. The PROPPR (Pragmatic, Randomized, Optimal Platelet and Plasma Ratios) trial of transfusion ratios in patients with severe trauma randomised patients to 1:1:1 versus 1:1:2 of plasma:platelets:red blood cells. No significant difference in mortality was noted at 24 hours or at 30 days. More patients in the 1:1:1 group achieved haemostasis, and despite increased use of plasma and platelets in these patients, there were no other predefined safety differences between the two groups.

Table 3.10.6.2 Platelet disorders in critical care

- Drugs:
  - Heparin (which may be associated with heparin-induced thrombocytopenia)
  - Glycoprotein IIb/IIIa inhibitors (e.g. abciximab, eptifibatide, tirofiban)
  - ADP receptor antagonists (e.g. clopidogrel)
  - Acute alcohol toxicity
- Sepsis – especially HIV infection, DIC
- Major blood loss and haemodilution
- Mechanical fragmentation – post-cardiac bypass, intra-aortic balloon pump, renal dialysis, ECMO
- Immune-mediated disorders – immune thrombocytopenic purpura, anti-phospholipid syndrome, HUS
- Hypersplenism
- Microangiopathic haemolytic anaemia – DIC, TTP, HUS
- Other – myelodysplastic syndrome, cancer, hereditary thrombocytopenia

Abbreviations: ADP = adenosine diphosphate; DIC = disseminated intravascular coagulation; ECMO = extracorporeal membrane oxygenation; HUS = haemolytic uraemic syndrome; TTP = thrombotic thrombocytopenic purpura.

Tranexamic acid (TXA) is increasingly used as an anti-fibrinolytic by competitively inhibiting plasminogen, thus inhibiting the breakdown of fibrin and fibrinogen by plasmin. TXA demonstrated a survival benefit in the CRASH-2 trial when administered early after traumatic injury. The National Institute for Health and Care Excellence (NICE) guidelines recommend TXA to be offered to adults undergoing surgery who are expected to have at least moderate blood loss of >500 ml.

Fibrinogen is critical in coagulation. It can become critically consumed or diluted, as well as degraded by fibrinolysis. Guidelines recommend supplementation of fibrinogen to 1.5–2.0 g/l in traumatic bleeding. Cryoprecipitate is the first-line product – as a concentrated source of fibrinogen, factor VII and vWF. Cryoprecipitate is appropriate when fibrinogen levels are <1.5 g/l and the patient is bleeding – the recommended adult dose being two bags of cryoprecipitate, which should increase the fibrinogen concentration by 0.5–1 g/l.

A goal-directed approach, based upon point-of-care and laboratory values, should be adopted to achieve haemostasis. Using an INR target of <1.5 and an activated partial thromboplastin time (APTT) ratio of <1.5 during major haemorrhage is advised. There is increasing interest in the use of factor concentrates in ratios dictated by rotational thromboelastometry (ROTEM®) or thromboelastography (TEG®).

Traumatic Coagulopathy

It is now understood that there is a specific pathophysiological state of acute traumatic coagulopathy (ATC) that develops after trauma. This is a multifactorial condition developing directly from the combination of bleeding-induced shock, tissue injury-related thrombin–thrombomodulin complex generation and activation of anticoagulant and fibrinolytic pathways. The additional influences of acidaemia, hypothermia, dilution, hypoperfusion and coagulation factor consumption contribute to the severity of the coagulopathy.

Thrombocytopenia

Thrombocytopenia is central to much of the coagulopathy seen in critical illness, due to decreased platelet production, increased destruction or sequestration in the spleen. The cause should be sought, in order to rule out those which require urgent action, including heparin-induced thrombocytopenia and thrombotic thrombocytopenic purpura (TTP) (Table 3.10.6.3). Low platelet count is independently correlated with illness severity, the presence of liver disease and sepsis. Patients with severe thrombocytopenia (platelet count <50 × 10⁹/l) are more likely to bleed in the ICU, receive any form of blood product and die following ICU discharge.

A platelet transfusion threshold of 10×10^9/l for stable patients is recommended. A higher threshold may be required for those with other haemostatic abnormalities or an increased platelet turnover. A typical transfusion trigger for actively bleeding patients is $30–50 \times 10^9$/l. Most recommendations suggest a platelet count of 100×10^9/l for those undergoing neurosurgery or those at risk of central nervous system bleeding. The British Society for Haematology guidelines suggest that the platelet count be maintained at $>50 \times 10^9$/l in patients who are bleeding. In patients with bleeding that is not considered life-threatening, the recommended transfusion threshold is 30×10^9/l.

The platelet count should be repeated 30 minutes after transfusion to ensure that the desired rise in platelets has occurred. This should be $30–50 \times 10^9$/l per pool. Failure to increment may be due to the presence of anti-platelet antibodies or ongoing consumption of platelets by either haemorrhage or thrombosis.

Table 3.10.6.3 Differential diagnosis of thrombocytopenia

Decreased platelet production
- Bone marrow failure
- Malignant infiltration
- Myelodysplasia
- Malnutrition (B12 and folate deficiency)
- Drugs
- Viral infection – HIV and hepatitis C

Increased platelet destruction
- Immune-mediated
- Immune thrombocytopenia
- Systemic lupus erythematosus
- Anti-phospholipid syndrome
- Heparin-induced thrombocytopenia
- HIV
- Non-immunological causes
- Microangiopathic haemolytic anaemia (TTP, HUS, DIC)

Increased sequestration in the spleen
- Portal hypertension with splenomegaly
- Liver cirrhosis
- Congestive cardiac failure

Abbreviations: TTP = thrombotic thrombocytopenic purpura; HUS = haemolytic uraemic syndrome; DIC = disseminated intravascular coagulation.

Disseminated Intravascular Coagulopathy

Disseminated intravascular coagulopathy (DIC) is defined as an acquired syndrome characterised by intravascular activation of coagulation, with loss of localisation arising from different causes. DIC leads to consumption of coagulation factors and platelets leading to bleeding, and microthrombotic events causing organ dysfunction.

In critical care, sepsis is the most common cause of DIC. An inflammatory response upregulates TF and impairs physiological anticoagulants and fibrinolysis. TF is critical in this process by activating coagulation, leading to widespread deposition of fibrin and causing microvascular thromboses which may contribute to multiple organ dysfunction.

Eventually, coagulation proteins are consumed, along with platelets. A rapidly decreasing or low platelet count is the most common haematological abnormality. Fibrin degradation products are produced, including D-dimers. Complex abnormalities of physiological anticoagulants occur as they are consumed whilst inhibiting activated coagulation factors.

The International Society on Thrombosis and Haemostasis (ISTH) scoring system can be used to assist the diagnosis of DIC, which can be difficult to accurately diagnose clinically. This is based upon platelet count, increase in fibrin markers, prothrombin time (PT) prolongation and fibrinogen level. Clinically, DIC leads to oozing at vascular access sites and wounds, and occasionally profuse haemorrhage. Treatment should focus upon supportive care and treating the underlying condition, with targeted replacement of coagulation proteins and platelets in those who are bleeding, aiming for platelet counts of $>50 \times 10^9/l$, PT and APTT <1.5 times the normal and fibrinogen levels of >1.5 g/l. Anti-fibrinolytic agents are generally contraindicated in DIC since the fibrinolytic system is required to recover from widespread fibrin production and deposition.

Heparin-Induced Thrombocytopenic Thrombosis

Heparin-induced thrombocytopenic thrombosis (HIT) is a transient drug-induced autoimmune prothrombotic disorder. Antibodies are formed to complexes of platelet factor 4 (PF4) and heparin, causing platelet activation. It is intensely pro-thrombotic and can be fatal.

Unfractionated heparin is more immunogenic than low-molecular weight heparin. The diagnosis of HIT is confirmed when the patient has the appropriate clinical picture and evidence of pathological heparin-dependent platelet-activating antibodies on assay testing. Thrombocytopenia is usually moderate – with a drop to $60 \times 10^9/l$ being usual. Timing is pathognomonic, usually 5–10 days after exposure to heparin. Clinical symptoms include venous thrombosis (deep vein or pulmonary thrombosis), as well as arterial thromboses, leading to limb ischaemia, cerebrovascular accidents and myocardial infarction, as well as necrotising skin lesions.

The '4Ts' score is utilised to predict the probability of HIT:

1. Timing of onset of thrombocytopenia
2. Presence or absence of thrombosis
3. Degree of thrombocytopenia
4. Other potential causes of thrombocytopenia

A maximum score of 2 per category is given, with a total score of: 3 or less = low; 4–5 = intermediate; and 6–8 = high. If the score is <3, then the risk of HIT is <1 per cent and antibody testing is not warranted. Patients with a score of 4 or more should have heparin discontinued and laboratory confirmation undertaken. The positive predictive value of a high score is poor – with only 50 per cent having HIT.

Another anticoagulant should be started, e.g. fondaparinux or argatroban. However, even after stopping heparin, a 30–50 per cent increased risk of thrombosis remains after 28 days. Once the antibody has waned – usually after 100 days – the patient can be successfully rechallenged with heparin. If the previous coexisting stimulus is not present and there is minimal or no PF4 release, the patient will not develop HIT.

Thrombotic Microangiopathies

Thrombotic microangiopathies lead to profound thrombocytopenia and microangiopathic haemolytic anaemia. Major causes are TTP, haemolytic uraemic syndrome and HELLP syndrome (pregnancy-related haemolysis, elevated liver enzymes and low platelets). TTP results in vWF-mediated platelet aggregation when subjected to high shear stress. Mortality is 95 per cent in untreated cases, reduced to 10–20 per cent with early plasmapheresis. Monoclonal antibody treatment with rituximab reduces the recurrence of autoimmune forms of the disorder. Death is usually due to platelet thrombi in the coronary arteries leading to myocardial infarction.

Liver Disease

Liver disease causes complex alterations to coagulation and haemostasis. The liver is responsible for the synthesis of thrombopoietin and most haemostatic proteins – both pro- and anticoagulant. Thus, patients with reduced synthetic function have abnormal coagulation tests (particularly INR and PT) and reduced platelet counts. However, there is a similar reduction of physiological anticoagulants, leading to rebalancing of haemostasis, with normal thrombin generation. Therefore, abnormal coagulation tests do not accurately represent the patient's bleeding risk. However, the reserve of the patient to be pushed into a prothrombotic or coagulopathic state is much reduced.

The failing liver does not metabolise tPA, increasing the fibrinolytic potential. Sialic acid is not removed from fibrinogen, resulting in dysfibrinogenaemia. In cholestatic liver disease, there is reduced absorption of lipid-soluble vitamins, reducing vitamin K-dependent coagulation factors. Portal hypertension leads to a reduction of circulating platelets due to splenic sequestration, whilst acute alcohol intake directly inhibits platelet aggregation.

Management of bleeding in the patient with liver disease should be based upon multiple tests, including platelet count, fibrinogen, APTT and PT and use of viscoelastic tests.

Upper Gastrointestinal Bleeding

A restrictive approach to blood products in patients with upper gastrointestinal bleeding should be adopted, including FFP, since the increase in plasma volume can raise portal pressures, increasing bleeding from varices. A survival benefit has been demonstrated in patients transfused to a restrictive haemoglobin threshold.

Renal Disease

Renal disease directly affects haemostasis. Uraemic bleeding symptoms classically are due to signs of impaired microvascular haemostasis, including ecchymoses, purpura, epistaxis and bleeding from puncture sites due to impaired platelet function. Uraemia causes dysfunction of vWF. Platelet dysfunction is a result of multiple changes: dysfunctional vWF, decreased production of thromboxane, increased levels of cyclic adenosine monophosphate (cAMP) and cyclic guanosine monophosphate (cGMP), uraemic toxins and altered platelet granules. Dialysis improves platelet function. Increasingly, citrate is a replacement anticoagulant for renal replacement therapy, with a reduction in bleeding, compared to heparinised circuits.

Patients with renal failure are typically anaemic. Anaemia leads to loss of laminar flow in arteries, so red cells no longer push platelets and plasma to the endothelium, leading to prolongation of the bleeding time. Therefore, correction of anaemia can improve haemostasis.

Fibrinolytic Bleeding

Hyperfibrinolysis can threaten the integrity of a haemostatic clot. Clinical suspicion should be high in cases where bleeding continues despite haemostatic replacement therapy, when platelet levels are relatively preserved, but fibrinogen levels are disproportionately low. TEG® can demonstrate fibrinolysis. Fibrinolytic bleeding should be considered in patients with liver disease and disseminated cancer. TXA is the most widely used anti-fibrinolytic in routine practice.

von Willebrand's Disease

Acquired von Willebrand's disease can be caused by several mechanisms, including autoantibodies, myeloproliferative and lymphoproliferative disorders and breakdown of high-molecular weight vWF due to high intravascular or extracorporeal circuit shear stresses. This can include intravascular shear stress from aortic valve disease and extracorporeal circuit use in extracorporeal membrane oxygenation (ECMO) and left ventricular assist devices (LVADs).

This can be treated with desmopressin, which stimulates the release of residual stores of vWF by endothelial cells, or vWF concentrates. Anti-fibrinolytics can be used to treat mucocutaneous bleeding. The cause of the shear stress must be removed as much as possible.

Bleeding Associated with Anti-thrombotic Drugs

Aspirin irreversibly inhibits platelet cyclo-oxygenase, whilst clopidogrel is a platelet adenosine diphosphate (ADP) $P2Y_{12}$ receptor antagonist – both require platelet transfusion to immediately reverse their effect.

Warfarin can be reversed using intravenous vitamin K (1–5 mg), with 25–50 IU/kg of PCC administered. FFP should only be used if PCCs are not available. Heparin can be treated with protamine.

Direct oral anticoagulant drugs include direct anti-Xa inhibitors (including rivaroxaban and apixaban) and the direct thrombin inhibitor dabigatran. Bleeding due to these agents can be challenging to treat due to limited availability of reversal agents. PCCs are generally regarded as the best method for reversing their action. The monoclonal antibody idarucizumab (Praxbind®) is now available for the reversal of dabigatran. It remains expensive and not universally available. However, the half-life of these drugs is short (dabigatran = 13 hours; rivaroxaban = 7–9 hours; apixaban = 9–14 hours), and thus the bleeding risk returns to normal within 24–48 hours, depending upon renal function.

Peripartum

Obstetric haemorrhage remains a common cause of maternal mortality in the UK, and the leading cause of maternal death worldwide. Haemostasis is altered during pregnancy, leading to a pro-coagulant state, which may reduce the risk of haemorrhage. However, the physiological anaemia of pregnancy and thrombocytopenia increase the risk of bleeding and blood transfusion requirements. Thrombocytopenia during pregnancy is multifactorial. Causes include gestational (75 per cent), pre-eclampsia, HELLP syndrome, acute fatty liver and DIC.

Blood losses of above 500 ml after vaginal delivery and 1000 ml after a Caesarean section represent peripartum haemorrhage. In the event of post-partum haemorrhage, the focus must include uterine atony as the major cause (75 per cent), the response to placental tissue, peripartum tissue damage and enhanced thrombin generation, hyperfibrinolysis and defibrination. Major obstetric haemorrhage protocols should be used, with efforts to increase uterine tone using uterotonics and surgical compression, with early administration of TXA, whilst maintaining normothermia, avoiding acidosis and replacing calcium. The WOMAN trial has demonstrated a significant reduction in mortality from post-partum haemorrhage with early administration of 1 g TXA.

Fibrinogen levels correlate with the severity of post-partum haemorrhage. A level of <2 g/l in early post-partum haemorrhage is associated with the development of severe bleeding and should be treated with PCCs, FFP and cryoprecipitate.

References and Further Reading

Estcourt LJ, Birchall J, Allard S, *et al.*; British Committee for Standards in Haematology. Guidelines for the use of platelet transfusions. *Br J Haematol* 2017;**176**:365–94.

Hoffman M, Monroe DM. A cell-based model of hemostasis. *Thromb Haemost* 2001;**85**:958–65.

Holcomb JB, Tilley BC, Baraniuk S, *et al.* Transfusion of plasma, platelets, and red blood cells in a 1:1:1 vs a 1:1:2 ratio and mortality in patients with severe trauma: the PROPPR randomized clinical trial. *JAMA* 2015;**313**:471–82.

Hunt B. Bleeding and coagulopathies in critical care. *N Engl J Med* 2014;**370**:847–59.

Retter A, Barrett NA. The management of abnormal haemostasis in the ICU. *Anaesthesia* 2015;**70**(Suppl 1):121–7, e40–1.

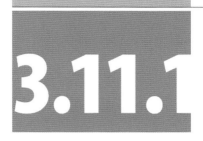

3.11.1

Acute Electrolyte Abnormalities – An Overview

Clare Morkane

Keywords: cation, anion, homeostasis, ECG changes

Introduction

The following chapter will address electrolyte abnormalities commonly encountered in the intensive care unit. Table 3.11.1.1 provides a general overview of the homeostatic mechanisms and the metabolism of the cations sodium, potassium, calcium and magnesium, as well as the anion phosphate. Table 3.11.1.2 provides a summary of the ECG changes that occur with various electrolyte abnormalities.

Table 3.11.1.1 Overview of major electrolytes

	Magnesium	Sodium	Potassium	Calcium	Phosphate
Normal serum level	0.7–1.0 mmol/l	135–145 mmol/l	3.5–5.0 mmol/l	2.2–2.6 mmol/l	0.85–1.4 mmol/l
Average daily requirement	0.1 mmol/(kg day)	1–2 mmol/(kg day)	0.8–1.2 mmol/(kg day)	0.1 mmol/(kg day)	20 mg/(kg day) of phosphorus
Absorption	Small intestine	Small intestine	Small intestine	Kidneys Small intestine Bone	Small intestine
Homeostasis	Found predominantly in bone, muscle and soft tissues The kidney predominantly regulates magnesium homeostasis	Sodium reabsorption is influenced by: • Renin–angiotensin–aldosterone system • ADH • Thirst	Na^+/K^+ ATPase controls potassium entry into cells and is regulated by: • Aldosterone • Insulin • Osmolality • β-adrenoceptor stimulation	Calcium is absorbed from the gut and reabsorbed from bones. Regulated by: • PTH • Vitamin D • Calcitonin	85% of phosphate is found in bone complexed with calcium Renal phosphate excretion is the principal mechanism for phosphate balance Hormonal control by: • PTH • Vitamin D
Excretion	1% of absorbed magnesium is excreted (renal and GI losses) Renal excretion is increased by: • Increased urinary flow • Aldosterone • Hypercalcaemia	>99% of sodium is reabsorbed by the kidney: • 70% in the PCT • 20% in the thick ascending loop of Henle • 5% in the DCT • 3% in the collecting duct	90% of absorbed potassium is renally excreted, influenced by: • Aldosterone and sodium reabsorption • β-adrenoceptor stimulation • Insulin • Bicarbonate • Urinary flow	GI tract Renal excretion (calcitonin inhibits tubular reabsorption of calcium which promotes renal loss) Deposition in bone	Renal excretion is influenced by: • PTH • Calcitonin • Vitamin D3 • Bicarbonate

361

Table 3.11.1.1 (Cont.)

	Magnesium	Sodium	Potassium	Calcium	Phosphate
Roles	Essential component of enzyme systems DNA, RNA and protein synthesis Regulation of calcium flux; natural calcium antagonist	Regulation of extracellular volume Preservation of osmolality, hence cellular integrity Maintenance of tubuloglomerular function by ensuring a hypertonic medullary interstitium	Regulation of acid–base balance Maintenance of resting membrane potential of excitable tissues Cardiac and skeletal muscle contraction Nerve conduction Tubuloglomerular function	Bone mineralisation Coagulation Co-factor for many enzymes (e.g. lipase) and proteins Essential in endocrine, exocrine and neuroendocrine function Important second messengers, signal transduction Muscle contraction	Energy production: ATP Phospholipid bilayer Red blood cell function (2,3-DPG) Phosphorylation Buffer Bone mineralisation

Abbreviations: ADH = anti-diuretic hormone; PTH = parathyroid hormone; GI = gastrointestinal; PCT = proximal convoluted tubule; DCT = distal convoluted tubule; ATP = adenosine triphosphate; 2,3-DPG = 2,3-diphosphoglycerate.

Table 3.11.1.2 ECG changes associated with electrolyte abnormalities

Electrolyte abnormality	ECG changes
Hyperkalaemia	K^+ >5.5 mmol/l: peaked T waves K^+ >6.5 mmol/l: • Wide, flat P wave • Prolonged PR interval, with eventual disappearance of P waves K^+ >7.0 mmol/l: • Wide QRS complexes • High-grade AV block • Conduction block (bundle branch blocks, fascicular blocks) • Brady-arrhythmias • Sine wave (a pre-terminal rhythm) • Cardiac arrest if left untreated
Hypokalaemia	Changes begin to appear when K^+ <2.7 mmol/l: • Tall, wide P waves • Prolonged PR interval • T wave flattening and inversion • ST depression • U waves • VT, polymorphic VT and VF
Hypermagnesaemia	• Prolonged PR interval, usually with normal P wave morphology • Wide QRS complexes • High-grade AV block • Conduction block (bundle branch blocks, fascicular blocks) • Brady-arrhythmias • Cardiac arrest
Hypomagnesaemia	• Prolonged QT interval • Signs of hypokalaemia: prolonged PR, T wave inversion, U waves • Supraventricular and ventricular ectopics and supraventricular tachy-arrhythmias • VT, polymorphic VT and VF (whether these changes are due to hypomagnesaemia or concurrent hypokalaemia is uncertain)
Hypercalcaemia	• Short QTc • Prolonged PR interval • Widened QRS • Wide T waves Ca^{2+} >3.75 mmol/l: • High-grade AV block and arrest
Hypocalcaemia	• Prolongation of QTc interval • AV block • Torsades de pointes may occur • Arrhythmias are uncommon

Abbreviations: K^+ = potassium; AV = atrioventricular; VT = ventricular tachycardia; VF = ventricular fibrillation.

3.11.2 Sodium

Clare Morkane

Key Learning Points

1. Disorders of sodium balance are frequently encountered in critically ill patients.
2. Measurement of serum and urinary electrolytes and osmolality and clinical assessment of volume status are essential components of the diagnostic approach to the patient with an abnormal serum sodium level.
3. Life-threatening neurological complications can arise from both an acute fall in sodium level (<120 mmol/l) and an overly rapid correction of hyponatraemia.
4. Treatment is based on severity of symptoms and underlying causes.

Keywords: sodium, hyponatraemia, hypernatraemia, SIADH, diabetes insipidus

Introduction

Sodium is the principal extracellular cation, and disorders of sodium balance are amongst the most common metabolic abnormalities seen in the ICU. The basic physiology underlying the abnormalities is often poorly understood, and mistakes in management are common, with the potential for serious consequences.

Hyponatraemia

Assessment

Hyponatraemia (serum sodium <135 mmol/l) is typically classified according to the tonicity of the extracellular fluid/plasma osmolality and the patient's volume status. Hyponatraemia in the context of a low serum osmolality (<285 mOsm/kg) should prompt clinical assessment of volume status and consideration of hypovolaemic, euvolaemic and hypervolaemic causes.

1. **Hypovolaemic hyponatraemia.** Total body water and total body sodium are both low; however, there is disproportionate loss of sodium, compared to water, e.g. increased anti-diuretic hormone (ADH) secretion in hypovolaemic states (vomiting, diarrhoea, etc.) and diuretic use.

   a. Urinary sodium differentiates renal versus extra-renal losses: urinary sodium <20 mEq/l suggests an extra-renal cause.

2. **Euvolaemic hyponatraemia.** This is the most common category of hyponatraemia seen in hospital inpatients. Causes include:

   a. Syndrome of inappropriate anti-diuretic hormome (SIADH), e.g. secondary to drugs, malignancy
   b. Adrenal insufficiency
   c. Hypothyroidism
   d. Psychogenic polydipsia

3. **Hypervolaemic hyponatraemia.** This is essentially dilutional hyponatraemia.

   a. There is a paradoxical increase in total body sodium, but a simultaneous and proportionally larger increase in total body water.
   b. Impairment in the ability of the kidney to excrete water maximally results in oedema.

Causes of hypervolaemic hyponatraemia with urinary sodium <20 mEq/l include:

1. Nephrotic syndrome
2. Congestive cardiac failure
3. Cirrhotic liver disease

Renal failure can cause hypervolaemic hyponatraemia with renal sodium loss, and hence a urinary sodium of >20 mEq/l.

Hyponatraemia occurring with a normal serum osmolality (285–295 mOsm/kg) is referred to as pseudohyponatraemia, and is usually secondary to elevated levels of lipids or proteins that essentially increase the non-water component of plasma.

Causes of hyponatraemia in the context of a high osmolality (>295 mOsm/kg) include hyperglycaemia and mannitol, which both cause water to move out of cells due to an osmotic gradient.

Syndrome of Inappropriate Anti-diuretic Hormone

SIADH is the most common cause of euvolaemic hyponatraemia and is associated with many different disorders (Table 3.11.2.1). Failure to suppress ADH production in lowered osmolality states is the main feature, resulting in disproportionate water retention, compared to sodium.

Treatment of SIADH should be guided by the following principles:

1. Fluid restriction, aiming for a slow rise in serum sodium of 1–1.5 mmol/(l day)

2. Consider hypertonic saline (1.8%) in symptomatic patients, administered via a central line

3. Demeclocycline 600–1200 mg/day to inhibit the renal response to ADH

4. ADH receptor antagonists are now available (e.g. conivaptan)

Table 3.11.2.1 Main causes of syndrome of inappropriate anti-diuretic hormone

Drugs	Psychotropics: • Anti-psychotics, e.g. haloperidol, chlorpromazine • Antidepressants, e.g. SSRIs, tricyclic antidepressants • Anti-epileptics, e.g. carbamazepine, valproate Opioids Chemotherapeutic agents (especially vincristine and cyclophosphamide) Recreational drugs: • MDMA
Malignancy	Lung (especially small cell lung cancer) Brain Gastrointestinal cancers (duodenum, pancreas) Lymphoma
CNS disorders	Haemorrhage Infarction Demyelination, e.g. Guillain–Barré syndrome
Infection	Pulmonary (pneumonia, TB, empyema) Cerebral (e.g. meningitis, abscesses)
Pain	Can mediate an increase in ADH secretion post-operatively

Abbreviations: SSRI = selective serotonin reuptake inhibitor; MDMA = 3,4-methylenedioxymethamphetamine; CNS = central nervous disorders; TB = tuberculosis; ADH = anti-diuretic hormone.

Management of Symptomatic Severely Hyponatraemic Patient

Neurological symptoms, such as seizures, result from the change in osmotic gradient that develops between the intracellular and extracellular fluid compartments, producing tissue oedema.

Specific management involves:

1. Administering hypertonic (3%) saline via a central line (and furosemide, if necessary, to promote free water excretion) until symptoms subside

   a. The aim is to address cerebral oedema, but not to normalise sodium level

2. Admission to the high dependency unit (HDU) and monitoring sodium level 1- to 2-hourly

3. An increase in serum sodium of 4–6 mmol/l, or exceeding the seizure threshold of 120 mmol/l, can reverse most severe manifestations of acute hyponatraemia

   a. Acute therapy can be slowed once this safe sodium level is attained

4. *The rate of sodium increase NOT exceeding 8–10 mmol/l in a 24-hour period*

Hypernatraemia

Defined as a plasma sodium concentration of >145 mmol/l, hypernatraemia indicates a decrease in total body water relative to sodium, and is associated with hyperosmolality (although total body sodium may be increased, decreased or normal).

Causes can be classified according to volume status, as illustrated in Table 3.11.2.2.

The clinical features depend on the severity and rapidity of hypernatraemia development, with

Table 3.11.2.2 Major causes of hypernatraemia

Volume status	Example
Hypovolaemic	Diuretic therapy Excessive sweating, burns Diarrhoea, vomiting, fistulae Lack of free water access DKA, HHS
Euvolaemic	Diabetes insipidus (central or nephrogenic)
Hypervolaemic	Hypertonic saline or bicarbonate administration Parenteral/enteral feeding Mineralocorticoid excess

Abbreviations: DKA = diabetic ketoacidosis; HHS = hyperosmolar hyperglycaemic state.

abnormal cognitive and neuromuscular function in many cases and the potential risk of haemorrhagic complications or death.

Management

Management of hypernatraemia focuses on restoration of normal plasma osmolality, alongside identification and correction of underlying causes of hypernatraemia.

1. Water replacement and sodium-containing hypotonic fluids are used to replace the free water deficit.
    a. Oral free water replacement guided by thirst is ideal, but intravenous (IV) replacement is often necessary.
2. Rate of correction depends on the rapidity of hypernatraemia development.
3. Frequent monitoring of plasma sodium levels is essential to ensure appropriate response and to adjust the rate of fluid replacement to prevent the risk of cerebral oedema.

Diabetes Insipidus

Cranial diabetes insipidus (DI) results from primary deficiency of ADH due to pituitary ischaemia/dysfunction. Nephrogenic DI is caused by an improper renal response to ADH, leading to a decrease in the ability of the kidney to concentrate urine by removing free water. Symptoms include extreme thirst and production of large volumes of very dilute urine.

DI is characterised by:

1. Urine output >4 ml/(kg hr)
2. Serum sodium >145 mmol/l
3. Serum osmolality >300 mOsm/kg
4. Urine osmolality <200 mOsm/kg

Treatment of DI involves fluid replacement with solutions containing minimal sodium. Desmopressin (DDAVP 0.1–0.4 μg IV) is the drug of choice for cranial DI.

Thiazide diuretics or indomethacin can be used to encourage salt and water uptake in the proximal tubule, hence improving nephrogenic DI.

References and Further Reading

Bradshaw K, Smith M. Disorders of sodium balance after brain injury. *Contin Educ Anaesth Crit Care Pain* 2008;**8**:129–33.

Cecconi M, Hochrieser H, Chew M, *et al.* Preoperative abnormalities in serum sodium concentrations are associated with higher in-hospital mortality in patients undergoing major surgery. *Br J Anaesth* 2016;**116**:63–9.

Ellison DH, Berl T. The syndrome of inappropriate antidiuresis. *N Engl J Med* 2007;**356**:2064–72.

Verbalis JG, Goldsmith SR, Greenberg A, *et al.* Diagnosis, evaluation and treatment of hyponatraemia: expert panel recommendations. *Am J Med* 2013;**126**:S1–42.

3.11.3

Potassium

Clare Morkane

Key Learning Points

1. Potassium is the principal intracellular cation and its concentration gradient greatly influences the resting potential of excitable membranes.
2. Potassium disorders are common in patients with low glomerular filtration rate and renal tubular disorders, and critically ill patients are at particular risk of alterations in serum potassium level.
3. Disorders of potassium balance predispose a patient to serious complications, in particular cardiac arrhythmias and muscle weakness.
4. Intravenous maintenance fluid alone should provide 1 mmol/(kg day) of potassium.
5. Concentrated potassium solutions given peripherally may cause pain, inflammation and venous thrombosis.

Keywords: hyperkalaemia, hypokalaemia, potassium, electrolytes, management

Introduction

As the principal intracellular cation, potassium plays a vital role in nerve conduction, skeletal and cardiac muscle contraction and glomerulotubular renal function. The characteristic ECG changes associated with both hyper- and hypokalaemia are listed in Chapter 3.11.1, Acute Electrolyte Abnormalities – An Overview.

Hyperkalaemia

Hyperkalaemia is defined as a serum potassium level of >5.5 mmol/l, and may be further subcategorised into mild (5.5–5.9 mmol/l), moderate (6.0–6.4 mmol/l) and severe (>6.5 mmol/l). The causes of hyperkalaemia are classified in Table 3.11.3.1.

Clinical features include gastrointestinal symptoms (nausea, vomiting), paraesthesia and weakness.

Complications are primarily cardiovascular; hypotension and fatal arrhythmias can occur. Arrhythmias are related to the *rate of rise* of serum potassium levels, rather than the absolute value.

Management

Treatment of acute hyperkalaemia is achieved by following Kidney Disease: Improving Global Outcomes (KDIGO) and the UK Kidney Association guidelines, and should ultimately be focused on treating the underlying cause. Figure 3.11.3.1 presents an algorithm for the management of acute hyperkalaemia taken from 2020 KDIGO executive conclusions.

1. **Protect the myocardium** (calcium increases cardiac conduction velocity and contractility in patients with ECG changes)

Table 3.11.3.1 Causes of hyperkalaemia

Impaired renal excretion	Addison's disease AKI, CKD Drugs: • Potassium-sparing diuretics • Aldosterone antagonists • ACE inhibitors, angiotensin 2 receptor blockers
Altered balance	Acidosis Insulin deficiency Tissue injury (rhabdomyolysis, tumour lysis syndrome, malignant hyperpyrexia) Drugs: • Suxamethonium • Digoxin
Increased intake	Potassium replacement therapy Blood transfusion
Pseudohyperkalaemia	Blood sample haemolysis

Abbreviations: AKI = acute kidney injury; CKD = chronic kidney disease; ACE = angiotensin-converting enzyme.

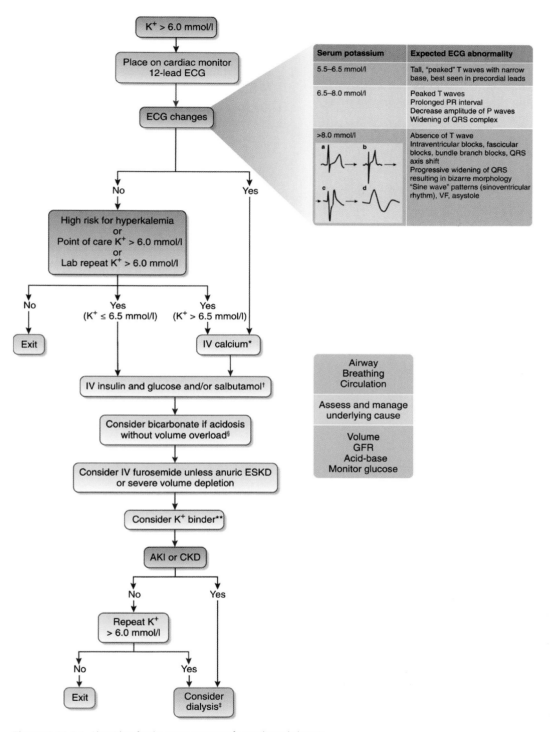

Figure 3.11.3.1 Algorithm for the management of acute hyperkalaemia

Source: *Kidney International* 2020 Jan; **97**(1): 42–61 DOI: (10.1016/j.kint.2019.09.018). Copyright © 2019 International Society of Nephrology. Reproduced with permission. (KDIGO executive conclusions 2020).

a. Give 1000–3000 mg calcium gluconate or 1000 mg calcium chloride intravenously (IV) over 5–10 minutes

   i. KDIGO guidelines recommend calcium gluconate as the first-line treatment, as calcium chloride has been associated with skin necrosis

2. **Shift potassium intracellularly** (short-term temporising measure whilst treating the underlying cause)

   a. Administration of insulin and glucose: 5 U of regular insulin appears as effective as the administration of 10 U

      i. Hypoglycaemia is a potential complication

   b. Administration of beta-agonists: 10 mg nebulised salbutamol results in significant reduction of potassium, with a peak at 120 minutes after use

3. **Consider potassium-binding agents and loop diuretics** – however, evidence of efficacy in the acute setting is lacking

4. **Potassium clearance**

   a. Consider renal replacement therapy (RRT) in cases of persistently elevated potassium levels of >6 mmol/l or ECG changes that are not responsive to medical management

5. **Monitoring**

   a. Regular serum potassium or blood gas measurements and continuous ECG monitoring

Hypokalaemia

Hypokalaemia is defined as a serum potassium level of <3.5 mmol/l. Acute and chronc causes of hypokalaemia are outlined in Table 3.11.3.2. Symptoms of more severe hypokalaemia include fatigue, muscle weakness, leg cramps, ileus, nausea and vomiting.

Diagnosis and Management

Observational studies suggest that the optimal range for potassium levels is 4–5 mmol/l. Acutely, treatment decisions generally depend on the severity of hypokalaemia and the presence of ECG abnormalities or symptoms.

1. **History and examination.** Elucidate medication-induced and gastrointestinal-related hypokalaemia. Suspect hyperaldosteronism in a patient with hypertension and normal glomerular filtration rate

2. **Stop all potassium-wasting drugs**

3. **Potassium supplementation**

   a. Oral potassium is suitable for mild and asymptomatic hypokalaemia

   b. IV potassium may be administered with maintenance IV fluids, concentrated via a central line, with continuous ECG monitoring, or added in parenteral nutrition. The maximum safe rate of replacement is 40 mmol/hr via a central route of administration, with continuous cardiac monitoring

      i. Caution with peripheral administration, as concentrated potassium solutions given via the peripheral route may cause pain, inflammation and venous thrombosis

   c. The maximum concentration of potassium for peripheral administration is generally accepted to be 40 mmol/l, with a rate of replacement not exceeding 10 mmol/hr

   d. If renal impairment is present, halve the initial replacement therapy

   e. Correct coexisting hypomagnesaemia

   f. Regular serum potassium or blood gas measurements are required

Table 3.11.3.2 Causes of hypokalaemia

Renal loss	Hyperaldosteronism • Primary: Conn's syndrome • Secondary Cushing's syndrome Renal tubular acidosis (types I and II) Diabetic ketoacidosis Hypomagnesaemia Bartter's and Gitelman's syndromes Drugs: • Diuretics, including acetazolamide • Carbapenems • Corticosteroids
Altered balance	Alkalosis Refeeding syndrome Hypothermia Familial hypokalaemic periodic paralysis Drugs: • Insulin • Catecholamines
Extra-renal depletion	Diarrhoea and vomiting Fistulae Use of laxatives Decreased intake (eating disorders, alcoholism)

References and Further Reading

Clase CM, Carrero JJ, Ellison DH, *et al.*; Conference Participants. Potassium homeostasis and management of dyskalemia in kidney diseases: conclusions from a Kidney Disease: Improving Global Outcomes (KDIGO) Controversies Conference. *Kidney Int* 2020;**97**:42–61.

Cook S-C, Thomas M, Nolan J, Parr M. Potassium. In: S-C Cook, M Thomas, J Nolan, M Parr (eds). *Key Topics in Critical Care*. London: JP Medical Publishers; 2014. pp. 273–5.

National Institute for Health and Care Excellence. 2013. Intravenous fluid therapy in adults in hospital. Clinical guideline [CG174]. www.nice.org.uk/guidance/cg174

Parikh M, Webb ST. Cations: potassium, calcium and magnesium. *Contin Educ Anaesth Crit Care Pain* 2012;**12**:195–8.

3.11.4

Calcium

Clare Morkane

Key Learning Points

1. Calcium is the most abundant mineral found in the human body and its numerous essential roles include exocrine, endocrine and neurocrine function, mediation of muscle contraction and coagulation.
2. Normal serum calcium concentrations are tightly regulated by the kidney, gastrointestinal tract and bone, under the influence of parathyroid hormone, vitamin D and calcitonin.
3. The effects of hypercalcaemia may be memorised as groans (constipation), bones (bone pain), stones (kidney stones) and moans (psychosis).
4. Treatment of hypercalcaemia is dependent on severity, with the mainstay involving hydration/intravenous administration of 0.9% saline to dilute plasma calcium, alongside treatment of the underlying cause.
5. One of the most frequent causes of hypocalcaemia in critical illness is hypoalbuminaemia.

Keywords: calcium, hypocalcaemia, hypercalcaemia, parathyroid hormone, vitamin D

Introduction

Calcium has numerous essential roles, including signal transduction, neurotransmitter release, muscle contraction, maintenance of potential difference across excitable membranes, protein synthesis and bone formation. More than 98 per cent of total body calcium is found in the bones. The plasma concentration is maintained between the narrow limits of 2.2–2.6 mmol/l as a result of tightly regulated ion transport by the kidney and gastrointestinal tract and bone, mediated

by parathyroid hormone (PTH), vitamin D and calcitonin. Calcium in plasma exists in three forms:

1. Free ions with a concentration of around 1.2 mmol/l, subject to tight hormonal control
2. Ions bound to plasma proteins, primarily albumin (40–50 per cent)
3. Diffusible complexes (<10 per cent)

The amount of total calcium in the plasma varies with the level of plasma albumin. However, it is the amount of ionised calcium that determines the biological effect. Profound effects on neurological, gastrointestinal and renal function can result in the context of abnormal calcium concentrations.

Hypercalcaemia

Defined as a serum calcium level of >2.6 mmol/l, the manifestations of hypercalcaemia are classically described by the phrase '*groans* (constipation), *bones* (bony pain), *moans* (psychosis) and *stones* (kidney stones)'. Cardiac arrhythmias can occur, and the characteristic ECG abnormalities associated with both hyper- and hypocalcaemia are listed in Chapter 3.11.1, Acute Electrolyte Abnormalities – An Overview. Coma or cardiac arrest may occur if plasma calcium concentration exceeds 3.75 mmol/l.

Table 3.11.4.1 presents a summary of symptoms and signs of hyper- and hypocalcaemia.

The main causes of hypercalcaemia are illustrated in Table 3.11.4.2.

Management

Treatment is dependent on the severity of hypocalcaemia and its underlying cause. Cancer-related hypercalcaemia can be treated with calcium-lowering agents such as glucocorticoids and mithramycin, and patients with raised PTH should be referred for urgent parathyroidectomy. Specific management of hypercalcaemia involves:

Table 3.11.4.1 Symptoms and signs of hyper- and hypocalcaemia

	Hypercalcaemia	Hypocalcaemia
Symptoms	Bony pain, fractures Renal colic Depression, hallucinations, confusion, coma Anorexia, nausea and vomiting, constipation, pancreatitis, peptic ulceration General malaise, weakness and hyporeflexia Nephrogenic diabetes insipidus	Numbness Muscle spasms Mental status changes
Signs	Dehydration Calcification in skin and cornea	Neuromuscular excitability: • Tetany • *Chvostek sign* (contracture of facial muscles produced by tapping the ipsilateral facial nerve) • *Trousseau sign* (carpopedal spasm with contraction of fingers elicited by inflating a blood pressure cuff) • Laryngospasm • Seizures

Table 3.11.4.2 Causes of hypercalcaemia

Endocrine	Primary hyperparathyroidism • Includes isolated adenoma and multiple endocrine neoplasia Tertiary hyperparathyroidism Familial benign hypocalciuric hypercalcaemia
Malignancy	Secondary deposits in bone Myeloma Ectopic parathyroid hormone and 1,25-dihydroxyvitamin D
Granulomatous diseases	Sarcoidosis Tuberculosis Leprosy Wegener's granulomatosis
Drugs	Thiazide diuretics Lithium Theophylline Vitamins D and A
Miscellaneous	Rhabdomyolysis Milk-alkali syndrome Renal failure (acute, chronic)

1. Stopping medications known to cause or worsen hypercalcaemia
   a. Calcium, vitamin D, thiazide diuretics
2. Intravenous (IV) hydration with 0.9% saline
   a. This forces diuresis – hence monitor potassium and magnesium
3. Bisphosphonate therapy
   a. Pamidronate 60–90 mg IV over 2–4 hours
4. Diuretics
   a. Furosemide can be used (promotes uptake of calcium from bones)
5. Additional therapies:
   a. Calcitonin, mobilisation, renal replacement therapy

Monitoring of haemodynamic and electrolyte status is necessary.

Hypocalcaemia

Hypocalcaemia is defined as a serum calcium level of <2.1 mmol/l. It is severe if calcium level is <1.9 mmol/l. Hypocalcaemia is frequently multifactorial in aetiology, with the more common causes including hypoalbuminaemia, hyperventilation and transfusion of citrated blood. Other causes are listed in Table 3.11.4.3.

Table 3.11.4.3 Causes of hypocalcaemia

Endocrine	Primary hypoparathyroidism Pseudohypoparathyroidism (resistance to parathyroid hormone) Vitamin D deficiency Congenital: di George syndrome
Malnutrition	Decreased dietary intake Intestinal malabsorption Vitamin D-dependent rickets Osteomalacia
Miscellaneous	Acute hyperphosphataemia Tumour lysis syndrome Rhabdomyolysis Acute renal failure Drugs: furosemide, bisphosphonates, phenytoin, aminoglycosides

Hypocalcaemia is treated with calcium supplementation (oral or parenteral, depending on severity).

References and Further Reading

Aguillera IM, Vaughan RS. Calcium and the anaesthetist. *Anaesthesia* 2000;**55**:779–90.

Bushinsky DA, Monk RD. Calcium. *Lancet* 1998;**352**:306–11.

Parikh M, Webb ST. Cations: potassium, calcium and magnesium. *Contin Educ Anaesth Crit Care Pain* 2012;**12**:195–8.

3.11.5

Magnesium

Clare Morkane

Key Learning Points

1. Magnesium is the second most important intracellular cation after potassium.
2. Magnesium antagonises the entry of calcium into cells, preventing excitation.
3. Treatment of hypomagnesaemia is important in critically ill patients for prevention of cardiac arrhythmias.
4. When treating hypomagnesaemia, coexisting hypokalaemia should also be corrected.
5. Magnesium has a role in the treatment of acute severe asthma, pre-eclampsia and eclampsia.

Keywords: magnesium, hypomagnesaemia, hypermagnesaemia, cation, electrolyte

Introduction

Magnesium is the second most important intracellular cation after potassium. It is an essential component of enzyme systems and is used in DNA, RNA and protein synthesis. Magnesium is crucial for the regulation of calcium flux by acting as a natural calcium antagonist.

Hypermagnesaemia

Hypermagnesaemia is rare, but almost invariably iatrogenic. Magnesium acts to antagonise the entry of calcium into cells, and therefore prevents excitation. The patient may complain of gastrointestinal symptoms (nausea, vomiting), with neurological signs, including weakness (that may progress to respiratory failure), and ultimately coma. The most rapidly detected sign is loss of deep tendon reflexes (seen at serum magnesium levels of >4–6 mmol/l). Cardiovascular complications of hypermagnesaemia include conduction abnormalities and cardiac arrest.

Management

A neurological examination and an ECG should be performed to assess clinical severity. Specific management involves:

- Calcium supplementation
  - Antagonises the effects of magnesium
  - 10 ml of 10% calcium chloride or 30 ml of 10% calcium gluconate intravenously (IV) over 5–10 minutes
- Magnesium excretion/clearance
  - Diuretics
  - Renal replacement therapy in severe cases
- Monitoring
  - Regular serum magnesium levels
  - Repeated examination of deep tendon reflexes to monitor clinical response to treatment
  - Continuous ECG monitoring

Hypomagnesaemia

Hypomagnesaemia, defined as a serum magnesium level of <0.7 mmol/l, is a common and frequently multifactorial electrolyte disorder which may be acute or chronic. Coexistence of other electrolyte abnormalities (e.g. hypocalcaemia, hypokalaemia, metabolic alkalosis) accounts for many of the clinical features.

Causes of hypomagnesaemia can be classified according to the underlying mechanism (Table 3.11.5.1).

Hypomagnesaemia mainly affects the nervous and cardiovascular systems. Neuromuscular hyperactivity may manifest as weakness, ataxia, tremor, stridor and dysphagia, and neurological disturbances can present as confusion progressing to generalised seizures and eventually coma. There may be hypertension, angina and rhythm disturbances.

Table 3.11.5.1 Causes of hypomagnesaemia

Renal loss	Hyperaldosteronism
	Diabetes
	Hypercalcaemia
	Alcoholism
Altered balance	Refeeding syndrome
	Phosphate depletion
Gastrointestinal loss	Diarrhoea and vomiting
	'Short bowel syndrome'
	Acute pancreatitis
	Laxative use
Drug-induced	Diuretics, aminoglycosides, angiotensin-converting enzyme inhibitors, cyclosporine
Reduced dietary intake	

Management

Oral magnesium replacement should be used wherever possible. However, in an emergency, IV administration is required as oral repletion takes significantly longer. Coexisting hypokalaemia should also be corrected.

- Emergency magnesium replacement
- 10–20 mmol (2.5–5 g) of magnesium sulphate by slow IV push over 10–15 minutes
  - Intravenous magnesium can be administered peripherally in 250 ml of normal saline or as a concentrated preparation via the central route
- Monitoring
- Regular serum magnesium and potassium levels
- Continuous ECG monitoring
- Magnesium infusion should be stopped if there is hypotension, bradycardia or loss of deep tendon reflexes or if serum magnesium level is >2.5 mmol/l

Therapeutic Use of Magnesium in Specific Emergency Scenarios

- Acute severe asthma
  - Magnesium is used in the treatment of acute severe asthma, in addition to other therapies. The British Thoracic Society recommends a single dose of magnesium sulphate (1.2–2 g IV infusion over 20 minutes) in patients with acute severe asthma (peak expiratory flow <50 per cent best or predicted) who have not had a good initial response to inhaled bronchodilators
- Pre-eclampsia and eclampsia
  - Magnesium has been advocated as prophylaxis and treatment of pre-eclampsia and eclamptic seizures. A standard regimen is a 4 g (16 mmol) loading dose, given IV over 5 minutes, followed by an infusion of 1 g/hr for 24 hours.

References and Further Reading

British Thoracic Society. 2021. BTS/SIGN British guideline on the management of asthma. www.brit-thoracic.org.uk/quality-improvement/guidelines/asthma/

Parikh M, Webb ST. Cations: potassium, calcium and magnesium. *Contin Educ Anaesth Crit Care Pain* 2012;**12**:195–8.

The Magpie Trial Collaborative Group. Do women with pre-eclampsia, and their babies, benefit from magnesium sulphate? The Magpie Trial: a randomised, placebo-controlled trial. *Lancet* 2002;**359**:1877–90.

Weisinger JR, Bellorín-Font E. Magnesium and phosphorus. *Lancet* 1998;**352**:391–6.

3.11.6

Phosphate

Clare Morkane

Key Learning Points

1. Phosphate and calcium are intimately related; both are under tight physiological control.
2. Phosphate plays a critical role in a number of processes, including energy metabolism, cellular signalling, bone mineralisation and membrane integrity.
3. Hypophosphataemia is a commonly encountered electrolyte abnormality in critically ill patients.
4. Disturbances in phosphate level are often multifactorial in aetiology.
5. Hypophosphataemia can result in respiratory failure and difficulty weaning from mechanical ventilation.

Keywords: phosphate, hypophosphataemia, hyperphosphataemia

Phosphate

In the presence of normal renal function and normal parathyroid hormone (PTH) activity, serum phosphate levels are under tight physiological control (normal adult range 0.85–1.4 mmol/l). Phosphorus plays an essential role in a number of diverse biological processes, including energy production (adenosine triphosphate), membrane function (phospholipid bilayer), red blood cell function (2,3-diphosphoglycerate) and bone mineralisation, and it also acts as an acid–base buffer.

Hyperphosphataemia

Hyperphosphataemia is defined as a serum phosphate level of >1.4 mmol/l. Hyperphosphataemia is predominantly asymptomatic, with morbidity more frequently a consequence of the underlying disease. The main causes can be classified as per Table 3.11.6.1.

Table 3.11.6.1 Main causes of hyperphosphataemia

Decreased renal clearance	Acute or chronic kidney disease Hypoparathyroidism Bisphosphonate use Vitamin D toxicity
Increased intake	Enteral/parenteral/enemas, intentional or accidental
Increased production/release	Rhabdomyolysis Tumour lysis syndrome Malignant hyperpyrexia Haemolysis Acidosis

Pseudohyperphosphataemia can occur due to interference with laboratory analysis, which is seen in conditions such as hyperlipidaemia and hyperbilirubinaemia.

Phosphate forms a complex with calcium and may therefore lead to hypocalcaemia (and consequential tetany) if the rate of rise is rapid. There may be nephrocalcinosis, renal calculi and ectopic calcification in tissues.

Management

Specific management is as follows:

- Binding agent (aluminium hydroxide)
  - Magnesium and calcium are also used
  - Caution regarding aluminium toxicity
- Phosphate depletion
  - Volume repletion and loop diuretics
  - Renal replacement therapy in severe cases
- *Monitor* serum phosphate and calcium

Hypophosphataemia

Hyphosphataemia (serum phosphate <0.85 mmol/l) is a very common electrolyte disorder in hospitalised patients, and causes of hypophosphataemia in critical illness, in particular, are multifactorial. It often coexists with other electrolyte abnormalities, which may

Table 3.11.6.2 Main causes of hypophosphataemia

Renal loss	Hyperaldosteronism
	Hyperparathyroidism
	Renal tubular acidosis
	Alcoholism
	Acetazolamide therapy
Altered balance	Refeeding syndrome
	Respiratory alkalosis
	Sepsis
	Effects of hormones:
	• Insulin
	• Glucagon
	• Cortisol
	• Adrenaline
Gastrointestinal loss	Antacid abuse
	Vitamin D deficiency
	Chronic diarrhoea

contribute to the clinical presentation. Mechanisms of phosphate deficiency include internal redistribution, increased renal excretion and reduced gastrointestinal absorption (Table 3.11.6.2).

Clinical features are usually only seen with severe hypophosphataemia (plasma phosphate <0.32 mmol/l) and include neuromuscular disturbance (proximal myopathy and weakness that may eventually progress to respiratory failure), symptoms of smooth muscle dysfunction (dysphagia, ileus) and acute cardiomyopathy. Failure to wean from mechanical ventilation is a feature, alongside impaired diaphragmatic contractility. Rhabdomyolysis may complicate severe cases, and phosphate release from necrotic skeletal muscle may mask the causative electrolyte disturbance.

Management

Management of severe symptomatic hypophosphataemia involves treatment of the underlying cause, alongside phosphate replacement.

- Phosphate supplementation
- Indicated if serum phosphate level is <0.5 mmol/l (depending on unit protocol), clinical evidence of hypophosphataemia or risk factors for phosphate depletion, e.g. alcoholism, malnutrition, refeeding
- The safest mode of replacement is oral, given in the form of Phosphate Sandoz® effervescent tablets. Each tablet contains phosphate 16.1 mmol, sodium 20.4 mmol and potassium 3.1 mmol. Up to six tablets daily can be given in divided doses
- Phosphate 10 mmol can be given intravenously over an hour and repeated as needed
- Phosphate Polyfusor® contains phosphate 50 mmol in 500 ml (alongside potassium 9.5 mmol and sodium 81 mmol) and should be infused via a dedicated port of a central line
- Correcting coexisting electrolyte disturbances
- Monitoring regular serum phosphate and calcium (risk of hypocalcaemia with intravenous phosphate replacement)

References and Further Reading

Gaasbeek A, Meinders AE. Hypophosphatemia: an update on its etiology and treatment. *Am J Med* 2005;**118**:1094–101.

Penido MG, Alon US. Phosphate homeostasis and its role in bone health. *Pediatr Nephrol* 2012;**27**:2039–48.

Wadsworth RL, Siddiqui S. Phosphate homeostasis in critical care. *BJA Educ* 2016;**16**:305–9.

Weisinger JR, Bellorín-Font E. Magnesium and phosphorus. *Lancet* 1998;**352**:391–6.

Diabetic Emergencies

3.12.1

Sridhar Nallapareddy and Jon Griffiths

Key Learning Points

1. Diabetic ketoacidosis (DKA) and hyperosmolar hyperglycaemic state (HHS) have a high mortality rate and require prompt identification and management.

2. Fluid resuscitation is often the most important therapeutic intervention in both groups, and patients with HHS often need no exogenous insulin at all.

3. The high mortality rate often results from electrolyte disturbances, particularly hypokalaemia in DKA. It should be very closely monitored, particularly in the early phase of treatment.

4. Thromboembolism is a life-threatening complication in both groups of patients, so always consider thromboprophylaxis early.

5. Look for common precipitating factors in all patients, but be aware that the white cell count and amylase, sodium and creatinine levels can all be abnormal in otherwise uncomplicated diabetic emergencies.

Keywords: diabetic ketoacidosis, hyperosmolar hyperglycaemic state, diabetic emergencies, treatment

Introduction

Three major forms of diabetic emergencies are especially relevant for intensive care physicians:
- Diabetic ketoacidosis (DKA)
- Hyperosmolar hyperglycaemic state (HHS)
- Hypoglycaemic coma

Diabetic Ketoacidosis

Definition and Introduction

DKA is an acute life-threatening complication of decompensated diabetes mellitus, which results from either absolute or relative insulin deficiency, together with excess stress hormones (mainly glucagon). It is most commonly seen in type 1 diabetes but is also possible in type 2 diabetes.

Pathogenesis

DKA occurs when the body is unable to metabolise glucose because of an absence of insulin. The subsequent switch to fatty acid metabolism via beta-oxidation leads to ketonaemia and acidaemia. Inability to metabolise glucose often (but not always) leads to hyperglycaemia and significant dehydration.

Diagnosis

Diagnosis requires:
- **D – Diabetes** – capillary blood glucose >11 mmol/l

(This may not be present in pregnancy, patients taking sodium–glucose co-transporter 2 (SGLT-2) inhibitors or those who have recently had insulin administered.)

- **K – Ketonaemia** – capillary ketones >3 mmol/l
- **A – Acidaemia** – venous pH <7.3 or bicarbonate <15

(A high anion gap acidosis is caused by accumulation of ketones – beta-hydroxybutyric and acetoacetic acids.)

Presentation

Patients can present in a number of ways. However, it often includes polyuria, polydipsia, weight loss, dehydration, hyperventilation (Kussmaul's respiration), a fruity 'pear drop' odour on their breath (ketones), abdominal pain, vomiting and confusion.

Investigations

- A finger prick is performed to measure capillary glucose. Hyperglycaemia should be confirmed with a serum glucose level. An electrolyte panel will reveal an elevated anion gap metabolic acidosis, and the blood pH can be determined by an arterial blood gas.
- Infection is a common precipitant of DKA; its presence is usually investigated with a full blood count (white cell count (WCC) can be elevated in DKA without infection), urinalysis and a chest radiograph.
- In older patients, an ECG should be done to look for myocardial ischaemia (as this can be painless).
- Increased amylase levels are common in the absence of pancreatitis.
- Blood urea nitrogen and creatinine may increase secondary to dehydration (pre-renal azotaemia).
- Serum electrolytes:
  - Potassium: may be high due to acidaemia causing extracellular shifts, but patients often have low total potassium levels due to increased urinary losses.
  - Pseudohyponatraemia due to osmotic movement of free water into blood resulting from hyperglycaemia. Total body sodium levels are usually normal.

Treatment

Treatment principles of DKA fall into three major categories:

1. Correction of fluid and electrolyte disturbances
2. Administration of insulin
3. Treatment of any precipitating cause

Fluids

In DKA, fluid and electrolyte deficits are invariably very high (approximately 100 ml/kg of water), and correcting these is the most important therapeutic intervention. The choice of fluids is somewhat controversial. However, there is a general consensus that crystalloids are preferred over colloids.

- If the patient is in shock, or systolic blood pressure is <90 mmHg, give a bolus of 0.9% sodium chloride (NaCl).
- Use 0.9% NaCl for resuscitation and rehydration, initially at 5–15 ml/(kg hr) (the rehydration

rate depends on clinical status, age and kidney function).
- Once the glucose level falls below 14 mmol/l, 10% glucose at 125 ml/hr should be run alongside other fluids to facilitate the use of a fixed-rate insulin infusion.
- Rehydrate steadily over 48 hours.
- Bicarbonate use is controversial and there is no documented benefit. It is not recommended unless the pH is <6.9.

Insulin

- A fixed-rate insulin infusion should be initiated at 0.1 U/(kg hr), and should continue until ketone levels are <0.6 mmol/l, pH is >7.3 and/or bicarbonate levels are >18 mmol/l.
- Variable-rate insulin infusions should not be used.
- If blood ketone levels are not falling by 0.5 mmol/ (l hr), then the fixed rate should be increased by 1 U/hr.
- If the patient is on long-acting insulin, this should be continued during DKA treatment.

Treatment of Cause

- Identify the trigger, and treat
- DKA is usually associated with triggers (do not forget to check the six 'I's')
  - Insulin deficiency: non-compliance, insufficient dose, new-onset diabetes
  - Iatrogenic: high-dose steroids, thiazide diuretics and atypical anti-psychotics
  - Infection
  - Inflammation: pancreatitis, cholecystitis
  - Ischaemia/infarction: myocardial infarction, stroke, gut ischaemia
  - Intoxication: alcohol, cocaine

Hypokalaemia/Hyperkalaemia

This deserves a special mention as it remains a significant cause of morbidity/mortality in patients with DKA.

Although potassium replacement is not normally required alongside the initial resuscitation fluid, 40 mmol potassium chloride (KCl) should be added to every subsequent 1-litre infusion as long as serum potassium levels are <5.5 mmol/l.

If the initial potassium level is <3.5 mmol/l, then insulin initiation should be temporarily delayed whilst additional potassium is given and the serum concentration increased.

Indications for Admission to Intensive Care Unit (Relative)

- Inability to protect the airway and altered sensorium (Glasgow Coma Score <8)
- Cardiovascular instability
- Presence of abdominal signs suggestive of acute gastric dilation
- Severe biochemical derangements: pH <7.0, bicarbonate <5 mmol/l, potassium <3.5 mmol/l on admission, anion gap >16, blood ketones >6 mmol/l
- Pregnancy
- Patient with co-morbidities

Complications of DKA

- Hypokalaemia
- Hypoglycaemia
- Cerebral oedema – if corrected too quickly

Hyperosmolar Hyperglycaemic State

Definition and Introduction

HHS is a state of extreme hyperglycaemia, characterised by severe dehydration, altered mental status and absence of severe ketoacidosis. It occurs more commonly in elderly type 2 diabetics.

Pathogenesis

In HHS, residual insulin secretion is usually enough to suppress ketogenesis and lipolysis, but not hyperglycaemia, thus leading to hyperosmolar dehydration.

Diagnosis

The diagnosis is less precise than with DKA, but the characteristic features of HHS are **hypovolaemia**, **hyperglycaemia** and **hyperosmolality** (usually >320 mOsm/kg), without significant ketonaemia (<3 mmol/l) or acidaemia (pH >7.3, bicarbonate >15 mmol/l). Blood glucose can often be >30 mmol/l, with fluid deficits in the region of 100–220 ml/kg.

Presentation

HHS presents somewhat differently to DKA. It tends to have a more insidious onset, and whilst DKA usually develops over 24 hours, HHS is often preceded by several days of polyuria, polydipsia, weight loss and increasing drowsiness.

Neurological features are more common in HHS (as a result of markedly higher osmolalities, when compared with DKA), with abdominal pain and hyperventilation less so. Additionally, the patient demographic is often >60 years.

Investigations

- Similar to DKA

Treatment

- The initial goal is expansion of the intravascular and extravascular volume deficits using crystalloids. This is often sufficient in itself to normalise the glucose level without use of insulin.
- Measure or calculate serum osmolalities hourly initially, and adjust the rate of fluid replacement to promote a gradual decline in osmolality over 24 hours.
- Hypotensive patients should receive isotonic intravenous fluids until stable haemodynamically; then this should be switched to hypotonic fluid. When the serum osmolality is >330, give 0.45% normal saline (1⁄2 NS) at a rate of 1–2 l/hr for 1–2 hours, then 1 l/hr for 3–4 hours, monitoring the response of blood pressure and urine output. Once these parameters have improved, 1⁄2 NS is given at a rate to replace half of the free water deficit over the first 12 hours, and the remainder in the next 24 hours. As soon as the patient is able to take water orally, this route should be used for ongoing replacements.
- If significant ketonaemia (>1 mmol/l) is present, then it is recommended to use a fixed-rate infusion, but half of that required for DKA, i.e. 0.05 U/(kg hr).
- Identify and treat the cause.
- All patients should receive prophylactic low molecular-weight heparin for the duration of their treatment due to an increased risk of thromboembolism (HHS > DKA).
- Indications to admit to the intensive care unit are similar to those in DKA.

Hypoglycaemic Coma

- Severe hypoglycaemia (blood glucose <1 mmol/l) is the most common cause of diabetic coma. It is usually a result of over-treatment with insulin.

- Clinically, it is characterised by varying degrees of neurological dysfunction (confusion to seizures and coma) and is responsive to the administration of glucose or glucagon.

References and Further Reading

Centers for Disease Control and Prevention. Diabetes data and statistics. www.cdc.gov/diabetes/data

Joint British Diabetes Societies Inpatient Care Group. 2013. The management of diabetic ketoacidosis (DKA) in adults, September 2013. www.diabetes.org.uk

Scott AR; Joint British Diabetes Societies (JBDS) for Inpatient Care; JBDS hyperosmolar hyperglycaemic guidelines group. Management of hyperosmolar hyperglycaemic state in adults with diabetes. *Diabet Med* 2015;**32**:714-24.

[No authors listed]. Use of glycated haemoglobin (HbA1c) in the diagnosis of diabetes mellitus: abbreviated Report of a WHO Consultation. Geneva: World Health Organization; 2011.

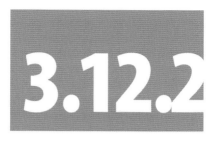

Syndrome of Inappropriate Anti-diuretic Hormone Secretion

Thomas Leith

Key Learning Points

1. The syndrome of inappropriate anti-diuretic hormone secretion is the most common cause of hyponatraemia in the hospital setting.
2. It is characterised by impaired water excretion in the setting of persistent or inappropriate release of anti-diuretic hormone.
3. There are a number of causes, the most common being respiratory disorders, malignancy, neurological disorders and drugs.
4. It should be suspected in patients with euvolaemic hyponatraemia who have a low plasma osmolality and a high urine osmolality.
5. Management involves treating the underlying condition and fluid restriction in the first instance.

Keywords: SIADH, hyponatraemia, hypertonic saline

Introduction

The syndrome of anti-diuretic hormone secretion (SIADH) is the most common cause of hyponatraemia in the hospital setting. It is characterised by impaired free water excretion in the setting of persistent or inappropriate release of anti-diuretic hormone (ADH). Water ingestion fails to suppress ADH, which is independent of haemodynamic or osmotic stimuli. Impaired water excretion leads to an increase in total body water, which results in hypotonic hyponatraemia. An increase in total body water transiently increases the extracellular fluid (ECF) volume and stimulates secondary natriuretic mechanisms. This promotes sodium and water loss, bringing the ECF

compartment back to its baseline volume and restoring euvolaemia.

Causes

The causes for SIADH are multiple and varied. These are outlined in Table 3.12.2.1.

Diagnosis

SIADH should be suspected in hyponatraemic patients with hypo-osmolality and a urine osmolality of above 100 mOsm/kg. Patients are typically euvolaemic and have a normal acid–base status and potassium balance and a urine sodium concentration of >30 mmol/l. The diagnostic criteria are summarised in Table 3.12.2.2.

The patient's volume status, although difficult to assess accurately, should be considered. If clinical features of volume depletion, such as poor skin turgor, dry mucous membranes and orthostasis, are present, it is reasonable to infuse up to 1 l of 0.9% saline, with close monitoring of serum sodium level. In hypovolaemic patients, the serum sodium level should increase with volume expansion. This is not recommended in euvolaemic patients where SIADH is strongly suspected, as it will likely further decrease the serum sodium level, as per the mechanism explained previously.

The results of urinary electrolytes and paired urine and serum osmolalities are often difficult to interpret, especially in the setting of diuretic use and intravenous (IV) fluid administration. An increased fractional excretion of uric acid (>12 per cent) has been shown to aid in the diagnosis of SIADH in patients receiving diuretics. However, this is not a widely available test.

Management

The underlying disease, if known, should be treated. This may include stopping any offending drugs, prescribing antibiotics for respiratory infections or correcting endocrine abnormalities.

Fluid restriction is generally accepted as first-line therapy for SIADH, unless the severity and acuity of

Table 3.12.2.1 Common causes of SIADH

Respiratory	Neurological	Malignant	Pharmacological	Intensive care-associated
Pneumonia	Intracranial haemorrhage	Small cell lung cancer	Selective serotonin reuptake inhibitors	Trauma
Tuberculosis	Malignancy	Head and neck cancer	Anti-psychotics	Pain
Cystic fibrosis	Traumatic brain injury	Prostate cancer	Cyclophosphamide	Anaesthesia
COPD	Guillain–Barré syndrome	Olfactory neuroblastoma	Vincristine	Positive pressure ventilation
Asthma	Stroke		NSAIDs	Nausea
	Delirium tremens			Hypoxia

Abbreviations: COPD = chronic obstructive pulmonary disease; NSAID = non-steroidal anti-inflammatory drug.

Table 3.12.2.2 Diagnostic criteria for SIADH

Major criteria
- Serum osmolality <275 mOsm/kg
- Urine osmolality >100 mOsm/kg in the context of normal renal function
- Clinical euvolaemia
- Urine sodium concentration >30 mmol/l, with normal dietary salt and water intake
- Absence of renal, thyroid, adrenal or pituitary dysfunction
- Absence of diuretic use

Minor criteria
- Fractional uric acid secretion >12%
- Correction of hyponatraemia with fluid restriction
- Failure to correct hyponatraemia with 0.9% saline infusion
- Serum uric acid <0.24 mmol/l (<4 mg/dl)
- Serum urea <3.6 mmol/l (<21.6 mg/dl)
- Fractional sodium excretion >0.5%
- Fractional urea excretion >55%

Source: Adapted from the European Clinical Practice guidelines 2014.

symptoms warrant hypertonic saline. Fluid intake should be limited to 500 ml less than the 24-hour urinary output, and should account for fluids used to co-administer medications, as well as parenteral and enteral nutrition.

Patients who present with profound symptomatic hyponatraemia (e.g. seizures or coma) should be treated urgently with 150 ml of hypertonic saline (3%) over 20 minutes (preferably via central venous access). The serum sodium level should be closely monitored during active correction, and whilst it is generally accepted that raising the serum sodium level by 4–6 mEq/l is enough to reduce intracranial pressure, thereby improving the neurological status, administration may be repeated, if necessary, until symptoms improve.

Further measures used treat SIADH include urea administration, oral sodium chloride and vaptans.

Urea promotes the excretion of electrolyte-free water, and has been recommended by the European Clinical Practice Guidelines as a second-line treatment at a dose of 0.25–0.50 g/(kg day). Notably, the unpleasant taste can be masked by sweeteners such as orange juice, or it may be given via an enteral tube with isotonic saline.

Oral sodium chloride may be used to increase the solute load, and this can be given with or without a low-dose loop diuretic (e.g. furosemide 20 mg twice a day), which acts to promote free water excretion by impairing the renal responsiveness to ADH.

The vaptans (e.g. tolvaptan, conivaptan) exert their action through antagonising the vasopressin type 2 (V_2) receptors in the distal nephron. They are referred to as aquaretics, because they cause free water excretion without the natriuresis and kaliuresis associated with diuretics. Their use in the intensive care setting is limited, however, due to their ability to cause rapid correction of the serum sodium level, and thus risk osmotic demyelination syndrome (ODS). They may also lead to hypovolaemia (and therefore must only be used once euvolaemia has been established) and hepatotoxicity.

Cerebral Salt Wasting

Cerebral salt wasting (CSW) may imitate SIADH, as both conditions cause hyponatraemia with raised urinary sodium excretion. Whilst also associated with neurological disease (especially subarachnoid haemorrhage), the pathophysiology of CSW is not fully understood. It is thought to result from increased secretion of atrial and B-type natriuretic peptide, which causes inappropriate sodium wasting and subsequent ECF depletion, leading to consequential release of ADH and free water retention.

SIADH can be extremely difficult to differentiate from CSW. However, the latter is more likely if there is evidence that volume depletion and increased urinary sodium excretion (i.e. salt wasting) preceded the development of hyponatraemia. As patients with CSW are usually volume-depleted, management involves volume resuscitation, with or without hypertonic saline, rather than fluid restriction.

References and Further Reading

Fenske W, Stork S, Koschker AC, *et al.* Value of fractional uric acid excretion in differential diagnosis of hyponatremic patients on diuretics. *J Clin Endocrinol Metab* 2008;**93**:2991–7.

Hannon M, Thompson CJ. The syndrome of inappropriate antidiuretic hormone: prevalence, causes and consequences. *Eur J Endocrinol* 2010;**162**:S5–12.

Spasovski G, Vanholder R, Allolio B, *et al.* Clinical practice guideline on diagnosis and treatment of hyponatraemia. *Eur J Endocrinol* 2014;**170**:G1.

Sterns RH, Hix JK, Silver SM. Management of hyponatremia in the ICU. *Chest* 2013;**144**:672–9.

Verbalis JG, Greenberg A, Burst V, *et al.* Diagnosing and treating the syndrome of inappropriate antidiuretic hormone secretion. *Am J Med* 2016;**129**:537.

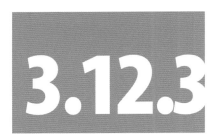

3.12.3

Diabetes Insipidus and Other Polyuric Syndromes

Thomas Leith

Key Learning Points

1. Polyuria is generally defined as urine output of >3 l/day in an adult of normal mass.
2. Water diuresis refers to the passage of large amounts of dilute urine, secondary to diabetes insipidus or primary polydipsia.
3. Solute diuresis is characterised by excess urinary solute, commonly due to hyperglycaemia or azotaemia or following the use of loop or osmotic diuretics.
4. Cranial diabetes insipidus is characterised by polyuria with a urine concentrating defect, due to a relative or absolute deficiency of arginine vasopressin (AVP).
5. Nephrogenic diabetes insipidus is characterised by polyuria due to renal resistance to the anti-diuretic effects of AVP.

Keywords: polyuria, diabetes insipidus, anti-diuretic hormone

Introduction

Polyuria is generally defined as urine output of >3 l/day in an adult of normal mass. Polyuria can rapidly lead to severe volume depletion and hyperosmolality in intensive care patients who are rarely in control of their fluid intake and/or may be unable to communicate thirst.

The causes of polyuria can be broadly defined as being due to water diuresis or solute diuresis.

Water Diuresis

Water diuresis refers to the passage of large amounts of dilute urine, with a urine osmolality of <300 mOsm/kg. The three main causes are:

• Primary (psychogenic) polydipsia
• Cranial diabetes insipidus (CDI)
• Nephrogenic diabetes insipidus (NDI)

Although excessive ingestion of water is pathological in primary polydipsia, water diuresis is an appropriate physiological response. These conditions are discussed below.

Solute Diuresis

A solute, or osmotic, diuresis, is caused by an excess of urinary solute which induces polyuria and hypotonic fluid loss. Normal solute excretion for an adult is 600–900 mOsm/day, and values above this represent solute diuresis. Glycosuria accounts for most of the causes seen in hospitalised patients. However, other common causes of solute diuresis encountered in intensive care are outlined in Table 3.12.3.1.

Physiological transient polyuria is often observed in the recovery phase of sepsis, when water and sodium (which has accumulated during the shocked state) are redistributed from the third space into the vascular compartment, and subsequently diuresed.

Management includes addressing the underlying condition and replenishing the extracellular fluid compartment. Solute diuresis is often associated with hypernatraemia, and rehydration should aim to gradually decrease the serum sodium level to avoid neurological injury.

Table 3.12.3.1 Causes of solute diuresis

Hyperglycaemia	Diabetic ketoacidosis, hyperosmolar hyperglycaemic state
Azotaemia (uraemia)	High protein enteral feed, catabolic states, acute tubular necrosis
Sodium	Loop diuretics, thiazide diuretics, hypertonic saline, sodium bicarbonate, high volume of normal saline, enteral feed
Renal	Fanconi syndrome, renal tubular acidosis, glomerulonephritis
Endocrine	Hyperaldosteronism, Addison's disease
Other	Paroxysmal tachycardia (increases atrial natriuretic peptide release)
Drugs	e.g. Mannitol, dextrose, magnesium sulphate

Assessment of Polyuria

- The history should be reviewed for evidence of recent neurosurgery, hypoxic–ischaemic encephalopathy or trauma. Pharmacological causes should be evaluated. Note should be made of the rapidity of onset of polyuria.
- Serum electrolytes, urine and serum osmolality, urinary electrolytes and specific gravity should be measured.
- If the urine osmolality is >300 mOsm/kg, solute diuresis is active and the presence of glycosuria, osmotic agents or diuretics should be sought.
- Polyuria with a urine osmolality of <300 mOsm/kg, in conjunction with a high serum osmolality of >300 mOsm/kg or in the presence of hypernatraemia, strongly suggests diabetes insipidus.

A therapeutic trial of 1 μg of desmopressin (DDAVP) can be administered intravenously to distinguish CDI from NDI. An increase in urine osmolality by 50 per cent or more confirms CDI. Failure of urine concentration suggests renal resistance to arginine vasopressin (AVP), and the causes of NDI should be considered. The water deprivation test, with measurement of plasma AVP levels, may be indicated in certain circumstances. Copeptin, the C-terminal glycoprotein cleaved from pro-AVP, is a stable marker that correlates well with AVP secretion. It is a promising new method of differentiating the causes of polyuric syndromes.

Diabetes Insipidus

Fluid and electrolyte homeostasis is maintained by the kidneys, which adjust urine volume and composition based on physiological requirements. AVP is secreted from the neurohypophysis in response to changes in serum osmolality and arterial blood volume. Activation of the vasopressin V2 receptors ($AVPR_2$) in the collecting duct, mediated by aquaporin (AQP), leads to water reabsorption and enables concentration of urine.

Cranial Diabetes Insipidus

This is characterised by polyuria and a urine concentration defect due to a relative or an absolute deficiency of AVP. The causes are outlined in Table 3.12.3.2. In intensive care, it is commonly encountered following damage to the hypothalamic–pituitary axis, often secondary to neurosurgery, trauma, intracranial haemorrhage or infection.

Table 3.12.3.2 Causes of cranial diabetes insipidus

Acquired	Congenital
• Trauma • Neurosurgery (especially trans-sphenoidal) • Ischaemic (hypoxic–ischaemic encephalopathy) • Vascular (cerebral haemorrhage, infarction, anterior communicating artery aneurysm or ligation, intrahypothalamic haemorrhage) • Neoplastic (craniopharyngioma, meningioma, germinoma, pituitary tumour or metastases) • Granulomatous (sarcoidosis, histiocytosis) • Infectious (meningitis, encephalitis) • Inflammatory/autoimmune • Drugs/toxins (ethanol, phenytoin, snake venom) • Other disorders (hydrocephalus, ventricular/suprasellar cyst, trauma, degenerative diseases) • Idiopathic	• Autosomal dominant: AVP-neurophysin gene mutations • Autosomal recessive: Wolfram syndrome (DIDMOAD)

Abbreviations: DIDMOAD = diabetes insipidus, diabetes mellitus, optic atrophy and deafness.

Management of CDI centres on replacing AVP and correcting the total body water deficit. DDAVP is a selective vasopressin type 2 (V_2) receptor agonist. It has a longer duration of action, compared to vasopressin, and is less likely to cause vasoconstriction. A standard dose is 1 μg, given intravenously or subcutaneously, 1–2 times a day.

Dehydration is uncommon in diabetes insipidus if a patient has an intact thirst mechanism and access to water. In intensive care, however, polyuria may be the only symptom of CDI and, if not recognised promptly, may lead to severe dehydration and hypernatraemia.

Nephrogenic Diabetes Insipidus

This is characterised by polyuria and a urine concentration defect due to renal resistance to the anti-diuretic effects of AVP. Although hereditary forms exist, acquired causes are far more frequent in intensive care, and are usually secondary to lithium use, biochemical abnormalities (especially hypercalcaemia) and post-obstructive uropathy (Table 3.12.3.3).

Management is directed at treating the underlying disorder, e.g. correcting biochemical abnormalities, relieving a urinary obstruction or amiloride therapy

Table 3.12.3.3 Causes of nephrogenic diabetes insipidus

Acquired	Congenital
• Lithium • Hypercalcaemia • Hypokalaemia • Post-obstructive uropathy • Multiple myeloma • Polycystic kidney disease • Infiltrative diseases (sarcoidosis, amyloidosis) • Sjögren's syndrome • Other drugs: demeclocycline, vaptans, aminoglycosides, amphotericin B, rifampicin, cisplatin	• X-linked recessive: *AVPR$_2$* gene mutations • Autosomal recessive: aquaporin 2 (AQP2) water channel gene mutations • Gitelman's syndrome, Bartter's syndrome

in lithium-associated NDI. Chronic NDI responds well to thiazide diuretics, and indomethacin and high-dose desmopressin are also used. Reducing the solute load by restricting protein and sodium intake may also improve polyuria. However, this is difficult to achieve in intensive care patients.

Gestational Diabetes Insipidus

Gestational diabetes insipidus (GDI) is characterised by excessive production of vasopressinase by the placenta, which degrades AVP. It is associated with an increased risk of complications in pregnancy, including pre-eclampsia and HELLP (haemolysis, elevated liver enzymes and low platelets). Desmopressin is resistant to vasopressinase and is therefore the treatment of choice.

Primary Polydipsia

Primary polydipsia is characterised by excessive water ingestion, usually due to psychiatric disease or, less commonly, hypothalamic lesions which affect the thirst centre. Infiltrative lesions, such as neurosarcoidosis, tuberculous meningitis and multiple sclerosis, have been implicated. Unlike DI, plasma osmolality is low or low-normal.

References and Further Reading

Bhasin B, Velez JC. Evaluation of polyuria: the roles of solute loading and water diuresis. *Am J Kidney Dis* 2016;**67**:507–11.

Bockenhauer D, Bichet DG. Pathophysiology, diagnosis and management of nephrogenic diabetes insipidus. *Nat Rev Nephrol* 2015;**11**:576.

Fenske W, Allolio B. Current state and future perspectives in the diagnosis of diabetes insipidus: a clinical review. *J Clin Endocrinol Metab* 2012;**97**:3426–37.

Robertson GL. Diabetes insipidus: differential diagnosis and management. *Best Pract Res Clin Endocrinol Metab* 2016;**30**:205–18.

Timper K, Fenske W, Kühn F, *et al.* Diagnostic accuracy of copeptin in the differential diagnosis of the polyuria-polydipsia syndrome: a prospective multicenter study. *J Clin Endocrinol Metab* 2015;**100**:2268.

3.12.4

Thyroid Emergencies

Sridhar Nallapareddy and Justin Ang

Key Learning Points

1. Severe hyperthyroidism or hypothyroidism should be identified and treated on clinical grounds, as laboratory tests are often delayed.
2. Always look for a trigger (e.g. infection, myocardial infarction).
3. When treating hypothyroidism, it is essential to consider if treatment of concomitant adrenal insufficiency is required.
4. Always give propylthiouracil at least 1 hour before iodides.
5. Avoid aspirin in hyperthyroid states.

Keywords: thyrotoxic storm, thyrotoxicosis, myxoedema coma, diagnosis, management

Introduction

Thyroid function tests are often abnormal in critical care patients. Thyroid emergencies are conversely extremely rare. However, if unrecognised and untreated, they are associated with high mortality rates.

Basic Physiology

Thyroid hormones are essential for normal functioning of most major organ systems. The thyroid hormones are tri-iodothyronine (T3) and thyroxine (T4), both of which consist of two tyrosine residues, conjugated with three and four iodine atoms, respectively.

Thyroid hormone synthesis occurs in the thyroid gland (Figure 3.12.4.1).

The process begins in the follicular cells where thyroglobulin is synthesised and iodide is taken up. Thyroglobulin is the precursor of thyroid hormones and serves to make tyrosine residues available to iodide. Thyroglobulin and iodide are exocytosed into

the colloid where iodide is oxidised to iodine and tyrosine residues are reduced to mono-iodothyronine (MIT) and di-iodothyronine (DIT). Iodinated tyrosine residues are then conjugated in a hydrolysis reaction to form T3 and T4. Synthesised thyroid hormone remains thyroglobulin-bound and is taken back into the follicular cell where proteolysis yields T3 and T4.

T4 is synthesised in the thyroid gland and has a half-life of 5–7 days. The majority of T3 is derived from de-iodination of circulating T4 in the peripheral tissues, and has a half-life of 10 hours. It is four times more potent than T4. If de-iodination of the inner ring occurs, metabolically inert reverse T3 (rT3) is formed. The proportion of rT3 formed increases in response to starvation, systemic illness and trauma (including surgery).

Circulating T3 and T4 are more than 99 per cent bound to proteins, predominantly thyroid-binding globulin (TBG), followed by albumin and pre-albumin. Only free T3 (fT3) and free T4 (fT4) are metabolically active. This provides both a reservoir and a buffer for thyroid hormones.

Thyroid hormones enter target cells by facilitated diffusion. T4 is de-iodinated to T3 by microsomal enzymes, and the rate of conversion varies in different cell types. fT3 binds to nuclear receptors, whereby gene expression is regulated to increase the basal metabolic rate and response to catecholamine.

Release and synthesis of thyroid hormone are dependent on thyroid-stimulating hormone (TSH) from the anterior pituitary, in turn stimulated by thyrotropin-releasing hormone (TRH) from the hypothalamus. Both are inhibited by T3 and T4.

Myxoedema Coma

Introduction

Myxoedema coma presents with exaggerated symptoms of hypothyroidism, including decreased consciousness and hypothermia. It is rarely encountered in recent times due to improved diagnosis of

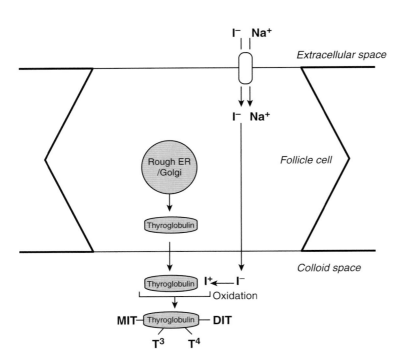

Figure 3.12.4.1 Initial steps in thyroid hormone synthesis.

hypothyroidism. However, mortality is still between 30 and 50 per cent, and is proportional to the degree of hypothermia. Myxoedema coma is more likely to affect older women, as this is the same group at risk of hypothyroidism.

Hyponatraemia is present in half of patients, due to vasopressin secretion and/or renal insufficiency, and may contribute to altered consciousness. Altered consciousness ranges from confusion to coma and seizures. Water retention also results in non-pitting oedema, affecting the face, tongue and limbs.

The number of beta-adrenergic receptors is reduced, whilst preservation of alpha-adrenergic receptors and circulating catecholamines results in beta/alpha-adrenergic imbalance, diastolic hypertension and reduced total blood volume. Hypotension may occur due to reduced myocardial contractility, bradycardia and decreased vascular tone, and concurrent adrenal insufficiency, if present, will contribute to dropping the blood pressure further. Pericardial effusion, if present, can result in cardiac tamponade.

Diagnosis

Initial diagnosis is a clinical one, with subsequent thyroid function tests revealing low T3 and T4 levels, and raised TSH levels in primary hypothyroidism, and low TSH levels in secondary and tertiary hypothyroidism. Plasma cortisol levels should also be checked.

Treatment

Treatment consists of supportive measures, steroids and thyroid hormone replacement. Hydrocortisone is nearly always recommended, as concurrent adrenal insufficiency is common. Combined T3 and T4 replacement has shown no benefit over T4 replacement alone. The intravenous route of administration is preferable to oral preparations, due to unpredictable absorption of the latter. A common regime used is a loading dose of 100–400 µg T4 intravenously (given to saturate TBG), followed by 50–100 µg daily.

Thyroid Storm

Introduction

Thyroid storms are rarely encountered, most likely due to improved diagnosis of hyperthyroidism and pre-operative optimisation of patients undergoing thyroid surgery. The mechanism by which a thyroid storm develops is often unclear, and total T3, T4 and TSH levels in patients with a thyroid storm are no different to those with hyperthyroidism and no storm.

Clinical manifestations of a thyroid storm are exaggerated signs and symptoms of hyperthyroidism.

Hyperpyrexia, which may be above 40°C, is a common finding, and the presence of a high fever in a hyperthyroid patient should raise suspicion of a thyroid storm. Tachycardia may present as either sinus tachycardia or atrial fibrillation and may result in high-output cardiac failure. Even in the presence of heart failure, thyroid storm patients are often hypovolaemic due to increased losses. Patients are more commonly hypertensive; however, this can rapidly progress to cardiovascular collapse. Central nervous system effects may range from tremor to agitated delirium and encephalopathy. Diarrhoea, nausea and vomiting are common and further contribute to fluid losses. A clinically acute abdomen should raise suspicion of perforation, and the presence of jaundice is a poor prognostic sign. Dyspnoea when present is due to increased metabolic requirements or impaired gas exchange secondary to pulmonary oedema. Rhabdomyolysis and global neuromuscular weakness have also been described.

Diagnosis

The diagnosis of a thyroid storm is based on clinical findings and is made using the Burch–Wartofsky Point Scale (BWPS) (Table 3.12.4.1).

- BWPS ≥45 is highly suggestive of a thyroid storm.
- BWPS 25–44 suggests an impending thyroid storm.
- BWPS <25 is unlikely to represent a thyroid storm.

Table 3.12.4.1 The Burch–Wartofsky Point Scale

Clinical finding	Value/degree of severity	Score
Temperature (°C) (°F)	37.2–37.7 (99–99.9)	+5
	37.8–38.2 (100–100.9)	+10
	38.2–38.8 (101–101.9)	+15
	38.9–39.2 (102–102.9)	+20
	39.3–39.9 (103–103.9)	+25
	>39.9 (>104)	+30
Heart rate (bpm)	90–109	+5
	110–119	+10
	120–129	+15
	130–139	+20
	>139	+25

Clinical finding	Value/degree of severity	Score
Central nervous system	Absent	0
	Mild (agitation)	+10
	Moderate (delirium, seizures)	+20
	Severe (coma)	+30
Gastrointestinal	Absent	0
	Moderate (diarrhoea, nausea, vomiting, abdominal pain)	+10
	Severe (unexplained jaundice)	+20
Heart failure	Absent	0
	Mild (pedal oedema)	+5
	Moderate (bibasilar crepitations)	+10
	Severe (pulmonary oedema)	+15
Presence of precipitating event		+10
Presence of atrial fibrillation		+10

Treatment

Treatment aims to:

- Mitigate the effects of thyroid hormone
- Prevent further synthesis of thyroid hormone
- Provide organ support
- Treat the precipitating cause

Beta-blockers effectively counteract the effects of thyroid hormones. Propranolol, a non-selective beta-blocker, is a common choice and inhibits the peripheral conversion of T4 to T3. Propranolol may be administered intravenously at 0.5–1.0 mg initially, followed by 1–2 mg at 15-minute intervals until an appropriate heart rate is achieved. Additional control of the heart rate may be achieved by administering digoxin, as long as hypokalaemia and hypomagnesaemia have been corrected to avoid digoxin toxicity.

Synthesis of thyroid hormone is blocked by thionamides. This class of medication includes propylthiouracil (PTU) and carbimazole. Both medications inhibit synthesis by blocking iodination of tyrosine residues. However, only PTU also inhibits peripheral conversion of T4 to T3. Neither medication is available as an intravenous preparation.

The release of thyroid hormones is inhibited by iodine-containing solutions such as Lugol's solution or sodium iodide. These must be given at least 60 minutes after thyroid hormone synthesis has been blocked, or the iodine may supplement thyroid hormone synthesis.

Corticosteroids are used as an adjunct to inhibit the peripheral conversion of T4 to T3 and, more importantly, to prevent adrenal insufficiency – in a hyperthyroid state, the metabolism of glucocorticoid is increased and the response to adrenocortico-stimulating hormone is attenuated.

Finally, in cases of resistant hyperthyroidism, clearance of thyroid hormone may be accelerated by using colestyramine (which binds to conjugated thyroid hormone and prevents its reabsorption) or plasmapheresis (which reduces the total concentrations of thyroid hormone).

References and Further Reading

Akamizu T, Satoh T, Isozaki O, *et al.*; Japan Thyroid Association. Diagnostic criteria, clinical features, and incidence of thyroid storm based on nationwide surveys. *Thyroid* 2012;**22**:661–79.

Burch HB, Wartofsky L. Life-threatening thyrotoxicosis. Thyrotoxic storm. *Endocrinol Metab Clin North Am* 1993;**22**:263–77.

Nayak B, Burman K. Thyrotoxicosis and thyroid storm. *Endocrinol Metab Clin North Am* 2006;**35**:663–86, vii.

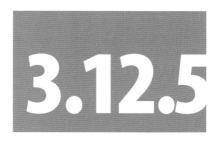

Adrenocortical Insufficiency in Critical Illness

Tom Parker

Keywords: sepsis, steroids, shock, critical illness-related corticosteroid insufficiency

The Role of Cortisol

Cortisol is a stress hormone which acts via intracellular receptors to alter gene expression. Its downstream effects include the liberation of metabolic substrate through the promotion of hepatic gluconeogenesis, lipolysis and muscle catabolism. Cortisol also exhibits anti-inflammatory and immunosuppressive effects (including decreased prostaglandin production and direct inhibitory effects on leucocytes), and a modest mineralocorticoid effect which promotes salt and water retention, and vasoconstriction (by sensitising the vasculature to vasoactive compounds such as angiotensin II, adrenaline and noradrenaline).

The Hypothalamic–Pituitary–Adrenal Axis

Endogenous cortisol secretion from the adrenal cortex occurs in response to adrenocorticotrophic hormone (ACTH) release from the anterior pituitary gland. This, in turn, is under the direct control of the hypothalamus, which stimulates ACTH release by secreting corticotrophin-releasing factor (CRF). At each step (Figure 3.12.5.1), a negative feedback relationship exists, such that cortisol inhibits the release of further ACTH, which, in turn, suppresses the release of CRF. This hypothalamic–pituitary–adrenal (HPA) axis functions to create the diurnal variation in plasma cortisol concentration observed in health.

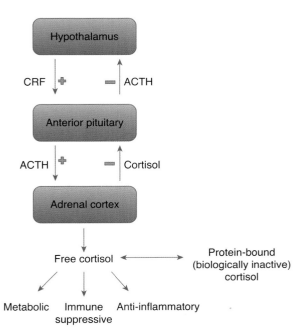

Figure 3.12.5.1 The hypothalamic–pituitary–adrenal axis.

A physiological response to the stress of acute illness is to increase the amount of free cortisol – generally in line with the severity of the insult. This occurs as a result of increased activation of the HPA axis and a loosening of the negative feedback control usually exhibited and through a reduction in circulating corticosteroid-binding globulin, which results in an increased biologically active free fraction of cortisol in circulation. This HPA axis response to metabolic stress may be perturbed during critical illness, resulting in relative glucocorticoid insufficiency.

Adrenocortical Insufficiency in Critical Illness

Critical illness-related corticosteroid insufficiency (CIRCI) is a form of relative adrenal insufficiency observed in critically unwell patients, usually characterised clinically by refractory vasoplegic shock, despite optimal filling and pressor support. The characteristic Addisonian biochemical picture of primary adrenal insufficiency, summarised as hyponatraemia, hyperkalaemia and acidosis, is typically not observed or, if present, is often better explained by other features of critical illness and its treatment, e.g. lactic acidosis and acute kidney injury.

CIRCI directly contributes to the pathophysiology of sepsis. Indeed it is in patients with sepsis that CIRCI is most described. Whilst not fully elucidated, a putative mechanism of CIRCI involves a dysregulated adrenocortical response to circulatory and metabolic stress, inadequate for the extreme conditions encountered during critical illness.

This may be compounded by other causes of adrenal suppression seen in the intensive care unit, including use of long-term steroids for the treatment of pre-existing conditions (inflammatory, rheumatological and transplant), administration of imidazole-derived drugs such as an induction agent, etomidate, pituitary infarction as a result of Sheehan's syndrome and pituitary apoplexy.

Interestingly, to date, there is no consensus definition, nor diagnostic criteria, for CIRCI. Furthermore, concerns regarding the reliability of the assay, not to mention the pulsatile nature of adrenal cortisol release, make plasma cortisol levels uninformative.

Poor Synacthen® responsiveness – a proposed definition of relative adrenal insufficiency – predicts mortality in critically unwell patients. However, subgroup analyses of CORTICUS (a trial aiming to answer the question 'Among critically ill patients with septic shock, does low-dose hydrocortisone therapy improve survival?') showed no survival benefit in Synacthen® non-responders versus Synacthen®-responsive controls. The same paper showed no survival benefit of intravenous hydrocortisone administration in the treatment of septic shock; however, it demonstrated earlier resolution of shock in those who survived and had received the steroid. These findings, alongside an increased adverse events rate in those who received hydrocortisone, were corroborated by the ADRENAL study in 2018.

Current Practice

The Surviving Sepsis Guidelines make a pragmatic 2b recommendation (i.e. based on weak evidence of moderate quality) to administer hydrocortisone to patients who remain hypotensive despite filling and vasopressors. Additionally, they do not advise Synacthen® testing in the context of sepsis.

References and Further Reading

Annane D, Sebille V, Charpentier C, *et al.* Effect of treatment with low doses of hydrocortisone and fludrocortisone on mortality in patients with septic shock. *JAMA* 2002;**288**:862–71.

Messotten D, Vanhorebeek I, Van den Berghe G. The altered adrenal axis and treatment with glucocorticoids during critical illness. *Nat Clin Pract Endocrinol Metab* 2008;**4**:496–505.

Rhodes A, Evans LE, Alhazzani W, *et al.* Surviving Sepsis Campaign: international guidelines for management of sepsis and septic shock 2016. *Crit Care Med* 2017;**45**:486–552.

Sprung CL, Annane D, Keh D, *et al.* Hydrocortisone therapy for patients with septic shock. *N Engl J Med* 2008;**358**:111–24.

Venkatash B, Finfer S, Cohen J, *et al.* Adjunctive glucocorticoid therapy in patients with septic shock. *N Engl J Med* 2018;**378**:797–808.

Traumatic Brain Injury

3.13.1

Wilson Fandino

Key Learning Points

1. Critical care management of traumatic brain injuries aims to avoid the development of secondary insults, which may impact on survival outcomes.

2. Intracranial hypertension is associated with increased mortality in patients with traumatic brain injury.

3. Interventions proposed to control intracranial hypertension should be made after balancing the associated risks and benefits.

4. Avoidance of corticosteroids in traumatic brain injuries is the only Grade I recommendation included in the Brain Trauma Foundation Guidelines.

5. Further research is needed to make clear recommendations regarding the role of decompressive craniectomy on functional outcomes.

Keywords: craniocerebral trauma, intracranial hypertension, decompressive craniectomy

Introduction

Traumatic brain injury (TBI) is a major cause of death and hospital admissions worldwide. In the European Union, it has been estimated that nearly 57,000 TBI-related deaths occurred in 2012, whilst long-term disabilities amongst survivors are related to decreased life expectancy and a significant economic burden. Although the management of TBI has changed relatively little over the last few years, most of the interventions are not supported by strong evidence, but rather by clinical experience and expert opinions.

Pathophysiology

Immediately following the primary insult, a cascade of pathophysiological events (including axonal demyelination, release of glutamate and other excitatory neurotransmitters, increase of calcium influx, generalised cell depolarisation and augmentation of anaerobic metabolism) leads to the development of secondary injury. These pathophysiological changes, along with disruption of the blood–brain barrier and an increase of vascular permeability, as well as water accumulation, elicit the development of cytotoxic and vasogenic oedema. In addition, impaired autoregulation worsens intracranial elastance, and all these changes eventually increase the intracranial pressure (ICP).

Catecholamines are released following acute TBI, and can elicit neurogenic pulmonary oedema, myocardial ischaemia and neurogenic stunned myocardium syndrome. Pro-inflammatory cytokines, neuroendocrine and autonomic derangements, electrolyte abnormalities and hypothalamic–pituitary–adrenal axis dysfunction can also lead to systemic complications.

Clinical Examination

The Glasgow Coma Score (GCS) has long been used to classify TBI as mild (GCS 13–15), moderate (GCS 9–12) and severe (GCS <9). It is, however, not always possible to undertake a full GCS assessment, as facial and ocular injuries may prevent eye opening evaluation, and in sedated, comatose or intubated patients, verbal response assessment is not possible. In addition to this, a sedation hold is not always feasible, particularly in patients with severe TBI. Motor response is thus the most important component of the GCS, and it is related to survival outcomes. The pupil diameter and reactivity to light are also important to diagnose both uncal herniation (which is related to survival) and lesions causing compression to the third cranial nerve. Neurological assessments during sedation holds give valuable information regarding progress of the injury, the presence of brainstem impairment and the development of neurological motor deficits.

Imaging

Intracranial lesions observed on the first CT scan are classified into skull fractures, parenchymal contusions and vascular lesions, with the latter including traumatic subarachnoid haemorrhage and extradural and subdural haematomas. It is crucial to evaluate the midline shift, basal cistern effacement and the volume of the intracranial lesion. In 1991, Marshall *et al.* developed and validated a classification based on these findings, and it remains one of the most common systems used to predict mortality in these patients. A second CT scan is indicated in comatose patients with acute clinical worsening or consistently raised ICP despite appropriate management, in order to rule out the need for surgical intervention.

Thrombosis/dissection of intracranial vessels and perfusion impairments can be evaluated with CT angiography and perfusion CT, respectively. On the other hand, cerebral oedema and lesions caused by diffuse axonal injury are typically evaluated with MRI.

Neuromonitoring Techniques

Several modalities have been proposed to monitor patients with TBI. They involve invasive (e.g. ICP, cerebral microdialysis, brain tissue oxygen measurement, intra-parenchymal thermal diffusion flowmetry, electrocorticography, jugular bulb oximetry) and non-invasive (e.g. electroencephalography, transcranial Doppler, near-infrared spectroscopy) techniques, and evaluate focal and global brain physiology, respectively. These techniques are discussed in detail in the 'Neuromonitoring Techniques' section.

Intracranial Hypertension

Normal ICP values range from 5 to 15 mmHg. Raised ICP is associated with increased mortality in patients with TBI. Young patients with parenchymal contusions or subdural haematomas, or both, are at highest risk of developing intracranial hypertension. In contrast, elderly patients are at low risk, presumably due to age-related atrophy. Increased ICP in this population may therefore indicate worse injuries, compared with younger patients.

ICP can be monitored via an external ventricular drain (EVD) or an intra-parenchymal catheter. The

EVD also allows cerebrospinal fluid (CSF) collection, at the cost of an increased risk of complications, including infection, since this is a more invasive intervention. The ICP waveforms and trends also provide valuable information about intracranial compliance and impending uncal herniation.

Interventions intended to control the ICP should take into account the potential harm associated with each, and therefore should be considered in a rigorous sequence. Use of consistent protocols appears to improve outcomes. For instance:

- Stage 1: head elevation, ventilation, sedation, analgesia, paralysis
- Stage 2: hyperosmolar therapy, loop diuretics, inotropes, temperature control, EVD insertion
- Stage 3: barbiturates, decompressive craniectomy

Decompressive Craniectomy

In 2011, Cooper *et al.* reported the results of a trial evaluating the functional outcomes of early (during the first 72 hours) bilateral and extended decompressive craniectomy, as compared with standard care, in patients with diffuse TBI (excluding intracranial haematomas) refractory to first-tier treatment (DECRA study). Although stay in the ICU was shorter and ICP was lower in the surgical arm, patients undergoing surgery had a greater risk of unfavourable outcomes at 6 months. Mortality at that point was, however, similar between groups. Five years later, a trial of decompressive craniectomy for traumatic refractory intracranial hypertension (RESCUEicp) was published. Patients who underwent this procedure (either unilateral or bilateral) as a last-tier treatment had lower mortality at 6 months, when compared with those receiving treatment with barbiturates, at the expense of higher vegetative state. Thus, the role of decompressive craniectomy in the improvement of functional outcomes and mortality in these patients remains debatable.

Critical Care Management

Table 3.13.1.1 provides critical aspects for the initial assessment of the patient with TBI. Table 3.13.1.2 summarises updated recommendations for the management of severe TBI included in the Brain Trauma Foundation Guidelines. Pulmonary complications, including pneumonia and acute lung injury (ALI), are common following TBI. Therefore, low tidal volume ventilation, with normocapnia and moderate levels of positive-end expiratory pressure (PEEP) of

Table 3.13.1.1 Initial assessment of the patient with traumatic brain injury, based on the 'ABCDE' approach

Airway	• Administer supplemental oxygen
	• Ensure airway protection and prevent airway occlusion
	• Maintain spinal stabilisation
	• Consider endotracheal intubation if:
	  ○ GCS ≤8
	  ○ Severe extracranial injuries
	  ○ Agitation
	  ○ Intoxication
	• Consider rapid sequence intubation (RSI)
	• Monitor $ETCO_2$ and SaO_2

Breathing	• Obtain $PaCO_2$ and adjust $ETCO_2$, considering the ventilatory dead space • Consider transient hyperventilation ($PaCO_2$ 3.5–4.5 kPa) if clinical signs of impending herniation are observed • Individualise use of PEEP
Circulation	• Insert large-bore cannulae • Consider intraosseous needle insertion if difficult intravenous access • Aim for systolic blood pressure ≥100 mmHg • Administer anticoagulant reversals if appropriate • Avoid hypotonic fluids

Disability	• When possible, evaluate GCS before administering hypnotics
	• Examine pupils: size, reactivity and symmetry
	• Document focal neurology deficits
	• Evaluate CT scan images:
	  ○ Extra-axial lesions
	  ○ Midline shift
	  ○ Grey and white matter differentiation
	  ○ Basal cisterns/ventricles effacement
	  ○ Volume of intracranial haematoma
	• Provide sedation/analgesia (e.g. propofol, alfentanyl)
	• Obtain early neurosurgical consultation
	• Consider seizure prophylaxis in high-risk patients (Table 3.13.1.2)

Exposure	• Avoid hypothermia • Administer empirical antibiotics if contaminated wound, CSF leaking or multiple injuries • Rule out concomitant lesions • Check blood glucose levels

Abbreviations: GCS = Glasgow Coma Score; $ETCO_2$ = end-tidal carbon dioxide; PEEP = positive end-expiratory pressure; CSF = cerebrospinal fluid.
Source: Adapted from: Garvin, R. and Mangat, H.S. Emergency Neurological Life Support: Severe Traumatic Brain Injury. *Neurocritical Care*, 2017;**27**(1):159–69.

Table 3.13.1.2 Recommendations included in the Brain Trauma Foundation Guidelines for the management of severe traumatic brain injury in the critical care unit

Topic	Intervention	Background	Recommendations	Comments
ICP control	Hyperosmolar therapy	Mannitol (0.25–1 g/kg) and 5% hypertonic saline (2 ml/kg) have long been used for relieving intracranial hypertension	ICP-guided administration, unless impending transtentorial herniation or progressive neurological deterioration Careful intravascular volume replacement	Cardiovascular stability and sodium blood concentration may dictate the selection of appropriate agent Superiority of these agents, compared to each other, is uncertain Effects on mortality are unknown
	Hypothermia	Hypothermia has been proved to be protective in animal models	Insufficient evidence to recommend its use in humans, either prophylactically or therapeutically	Risks include coagulopathy, immunosuppression, dysrhythmia and death

Topic	Intervention	Background	Recommendations	Comments
	Hyperventilation	$PaCO_2$ is the most important factor of CBF	$PaCO_2$ should be maintained within normal range (4.5–6 kPa) Transient hyperventilation is only indicated in cases of impending herniation	In order to prevent cerebral ischaemia, transient hyperventilation should be avoided during the first 24 hours of admission and ideally used along with cerebral oxygen delivery monitoring
	Barbiturates	Barbiturates optimise CBF (via $CMRO_2$ effect), resulting in decreased CBV and ICP improvement	High-dose barbiturates are recommended to treat refractory intracranial hypertension Prophylactic barbituric coma is not effective and may cause metabolic disturbances	Reduction of CPP by means of hypotension and decreased cardiac output may preclude its potential benefits. Therefore, cardiovascular stability is essential
	CSF drainage	An EVD is usually placed in patients with TBI and GCS <6, in order to drain CSF or monitor ICP, or both	Continuous, rather than intermittent, drainage is more effective to lower ICP Anti-microbial-impregnated catheters can be used to reduce the risk of infections	Midbrain level should be the reference to zero the system Whether EVD insertion reduces mortality in these patients is unknown
Prophylaxis	Prevention of DVT	Hypercoagulability, prolonged immobilisation and focal motor deficits render TBI patients at high risk of developing DVT	Heparin (unfractioned or low-molecular-weight) can be used along with mechanical compression stockings	Due to the risk of intracranial haemorrhage, the decision of using pharmacological prophylaxis should be made on a case-by-case basis
	Prevention of post-traumatic seizures	Post-traumatic seizures are common in elderly people	Phenytoin can be used to diminish the risk of early (i.e. occurring during the first week), but not late, post-traumatic seizures in high-risk patients[a] for no more than 2 weeks	Plasmatic phenytoin levels should be closely monitored Levetiracetam has not been proved to be more effective than phenytoin to prevent early seizures
Monitoring	ICP	Raised ICP has detrimental effects on the survival outcomes following TBI	The need for monitoring ICP in all patients following TBI is not supported by current evidence Maintain ICP of <22 mmHg (<18 mmHg in women and patients aged >55 years)	ICP monitoring may not always be available in developing countries Clinical judgement and image findings should not be replaced by ICP readings
	CPP	CPP is defined as the difference between MAP and TCP	Maintaining SBP of >100–110 mmHg and CPP between 60 and 70 mmHg has been demonstrated to decrease mortality	Patients with intact brain autoregulation or pre-existing hypertension may have the benefit of higher thresholds, but that may also increase the risk of ARDS and cardiovascular complications
Metabolism	Nutrition	Stress and metabolic expenditure following TBI render patients with higher requirements for calories	Transpyloric jejunal feeding started during the first week following injury decreases mortality and diminishes the risk of VAP	Tight glycaemic control is not recommended, as it does not improve mortality and increases the risk of hypoglycaemic episodes
Cerebral oedema	Corticosteroids	Corticosteroids are useful for treatment of vasogenic oedema	There is no evidence to recommend the use of corticosteroids in the context of TBI High-dose methylprednisolone increases mortality in these patients	Avoidance of corticosteroids in TBI is the only Grade I recommendation included in the Traumatic Brain Foundation Guidelines

[a] High-risk patients: GCS <10, immediate seizures, penetrating injury, intracranial haematoma, cortical contusion or age >65 years.

Abbreviations: ICP = intracranial pressure; CBF = cerebral blood flow; CBV = cerebral blood volume; CPP = cerebral perfusion pressure; EVD = external ventricular drain; CSF = cerebrospinal fluid; GCS = Glasgow Coma Score; DVT = deep vein thrombosis; MAP = mean arterial blood pressure; SBP = systolic blood pressure; VAP = ventilator-associated pneumonia.

<15 cmH$_2$O, are recommended. Analgesia and sedation are usually provided with short half-life opioids (remifentanil or alfentanil) and propofol infusions. Midazolam infusion also can be added to minimise propofol doses. Sodium disturbances are common, and distinction should be made between syndrome of inappropriate anti-diuretic hormone secretion (SIADH), cerebral salt wasting syndrome (CSW) and central diabetes insipidus.

References and Further Reading

Carney N, Totten AM, O'Reilly C, *et al.* 2016. Guidelines for the management of severe traumatic brain injury, 4th edn. braintrauma.org/uploads/13/06/ Guidelines_for_Management_of_Severe_ TBI_4th_Edition.pdf

Cooper DJ, Rosenfeld JV, Murray L, *et al.* Decompressive craniectomy in diffuse traumatic brain injury. *N Engl J Med* 2011;**364**:1493–502.

Hawthorne C, Piper I. Monitoring of intracranial pressure in patients with traumatic brain injury. *Front Neurol* 2014;**5**:121.

Hutchinson PJ, Kolias AG, Timofeev IS, *et al.* Trial of decompressive craniectomy for traumatic intracranial hypertension. *N Engl J Med* 2016;**375**:1119–30.

Stocchetti N, Carbonara M, Citerio G, *et al.* Severe traumatic brain injury: targeted management in the intensive care unit. *Lancet Neurol* 2017;**16**:452–64.

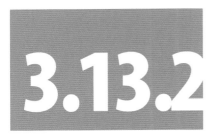

Maxillofacial and Upper Airway Injuries

Rajamani Sethuraman

Key Learning Points

1. Maxillofacial injuries are always associated with difficult airway management.
2. Delay in early airway management can be fatal.
3. Early tracheostomy in difficult and extensive injuries can be lifesaving.
4. Surgical management is sometimes delayed until there is resolution of oedema from the injuries.
5. Beware of associated base of skull fractures.

Keywords: LeFort fractures, facial–maxillary trauma, base of skull injuries

Maxillofacial Injuries

Severe blunt or penetrating trauma resulting in maxillofacial injuries is often associated with injuries of the upper airway, head, cervical spine and thorax. Bones commonly involved include the maxilla, orbital bones, zygoma, nasal bones, mandible, teeth and alveolar ridge, and also the temporomandibular joint. Maxillofacial trauma is commonly seen in younger age groups between 15 and 40 years, with a male predominance. Seventy-five per cent of all cases of blunt injuries are from road traffic accidents (RTAs), whilst other causes include falls, assault, sports and industrial injuries. RTA-related injuries have, however, decreased as a result of legislation on drink driving and the use of seat belts and airbags.

Mandible Fractures

These commonly occur at the mandibular ramus and body, usually at the level of the first and second molar teeth. Two-thirds of fractures, however, can be at multiple sites and may lead to airway obstruction due to lack of support of the tongue and facial oedema. An 'Andy Gump fracture', for example, describes a bilateral mandibular angle fracture which leads to obstruction of the upper airway due to the tongue falling back into the oropharynx.

The temporomandibular joint may be disrupted due to condylar and zygomatic arch fractures. Such fractures are essential to diagnose, especially if they require intubation, as these result in restricted mouth opening which is not relieved by muscle relaxants.

Bifacial Fractures

These are often best described using LeFort's classification (Figure 3.13.2.1) where LeFort I describes a low-level fracture, LeFort II a pyramidal or sub-zygomatic fracture and LeFort III a high transverse or supra-zygomatic fracture.

A LeFort III fracture is of particular concern, as it results in an unstable craniofacial disjunction – often associated with significant soft tissue injuries with bleeding and oedema. Airway management can be extremely difficult and surgery is often delayed until the facial oedema subsides.

Life-threatening bleeding can occur in up to 10 per cent of patients with mid-facial fractures and, in itself, can obstruct the airway and cause pulmonary aspiration. It often occurs as a result of disruption of internal carotid artery branches (e.g. lacrimal, zygomatic and anterior and posterior ethmoidal arteries); however, bleeding from the intraosseous branches may be most problematic as these are difficult to control, since it is hard to identify the source due to soft tissue oedema.

Orbital Injuries

Zygomatic and orbital injuries are common with LeFort's fractures. The severity of injury varies considerably, in a spectrum ranging from mild ecchymosis and subconjunctival haemorrhage through to permanent loss of vision due to globe rupture and optic nerve

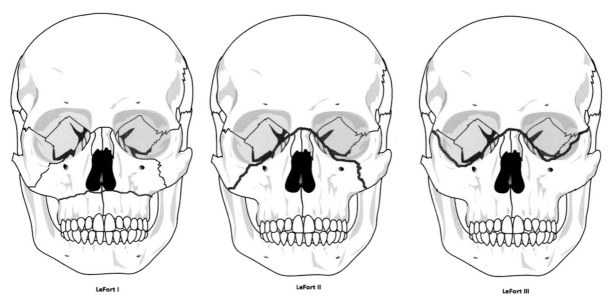

Figure 3.13.2.1 LeFort's classification of mid-facial fractures.
Source: Maxillofacial and upper airway injuries Chapter 66. Butterworth Heinemann. *Oh's Intensive Care Manual* 5th edition 2003.

injury. Orbital blowout fractures occur due to a direct globe injury or secondary to a force being transmitted through the eyeball to the surrounding bones. They present as enophthalmos, epistaxis (fractured nasal bones), ophthalmoplegia, diplopia and infraorbital sensory disturbances.

Other Associated Injuries

As maxillofacial injuries are often associated with trauma, they are frequently associated with other injuries, some of which may be more anatomically distinct. Having an awareness of these, however, is important, as they should be actively assessed for and ruled out.

- A cerebrospinal fluid (CSF) leak occurs in 10–30 per cent of base of skull fractures. CSF rhinorrhoea can present at the time of injury, or up to a week later, and may be due to anterior cranial fossa fractures, middle ear injury with CSF exiting through the Eustachian tube and sphenoid sinus fractures.
- Soft tissue injuries include those to the cheek, lacrimal ducts, ear, parotid, facial nerve, tongue, palate and pharynx. Early airway management is advised, as the resultant oedema may be considerable, often to the extent it can obstruct the airway over 24–48 hours.

- Intracranial head injuries occur in up to 15 per cent of patients with maxillofacial injuries and should be ruled out with CT.
- Cervical spine fractures occur in 11 per cent of patients, most often those who were involved in RTAs and falls. C1/2 and C5–7 are most at risk, especially with mandibular injuries.
- Thoracic, abdominal and/or musculoskeletal injuries occur in up to 40 per cent of patients.
- A carotid–cavernous fistula may occur and present as pulsating exophthalmos and an orbital bruit.
- Carotid artery dissections may present with neurological disturbances, but not necessarily with an associated head injury.

Management

Immediate management of maxillofacial injuries and their associated pathologies revolves around following the advanced trauma life support (ATLS) protocol to identify and treat any immediate life-threatening injuries using an ABCDE approach. It is also important on the patient's arrival in the emergency department to ask for a history from on-scene witnesses, the police and ambulance crew members, as these can give clues to possible injuries sustained. Signs of maxillofacial injuries may include those seen in Box 3.13.2.1.

Box 3.13.2.1 Signs of Maxillofacial Injuries

- Facial asymmetry
- Enophthalmos
- Dental malocclusion
- Nasal septum defects
- Diminished jaw opening
- Signs of base of skull fractures, including Battle sign
- Raccoon eyes
- Cerebrospinal fluid leaks
- Loss of visual acuity
- Facial nerve palsy
- Bruit over carotids

Airway Management

This is often extremely difficult and expert help should be sought early. Due to the unstable nature of max-illofacial injuries, especially LeFort III, securing a definitive airway is crucial so as to relieve airway obstruction – most often caused by the tongue fall-ing back into the oropharynx. Bag–mask ventilation may be tricky, and even hazardous in a craniofacial disjunction, and early definitive interventions are required. Nasopharyngeal airways and nasotracheal intubations (and nasogastric tubes) are usually con-traindicated due to the risk of basal skull fractures, and thus options are either tracheal intubation with rapid sequence induction or awake tracheal intubation, or immediate tracheostomy. Immediate tracheostomy is performed in about 22 per cent of maxillofacial injury patients; thus, it is essential to have surgical exper-tise present. Table 3.13.2.1 highlights airway prob-lems encountered in maxillofacial trauma and their management.

Laryngotracheal Injuries

Laryngotracheal injuries (LTi) may be caused by numerous different mechanisms – examples of which are demonstrated in Table 3.13.2.2, alongside possible signs and symptoms.

Investigations of LTi may include anteroposterior (AP) and lateral X-rays of the neck (looking at the C-spine and soft tissue), CT with reconstruction or MRI. Additionally, direct examination by an ear, nose and throat (ENT) or maxillofacial surgeon using a flex-ible fibrescope (under local or general anaesthesia) can provide valuable information about laryngeal cartilage and vocal cord injuries.

In terms of management, use of dexamethasone can be beneficial to decrease oedema. Mask ventila-tion can lead to subcutaneous emphysema; thus, aim to maintain spontaneous ventilation as much as pos-sible. When obtaining a definitive airway, cricothy-roidotomy is not advised due to possible anatomical disruption, and as such, awake surgical tracheostomy is often utilised.

Table 3.13.2.1 Airway problems encountered in maxillofacial trauma and their management

Airway problem	Management
Haemorrhage and debris: Impaired laryngoscopy, aspiration risk from swallowing, clot inhalation and airway obstruction, teeth and bone fragments	Suction, volume replacement, head down, definitive haemorrhage control, Magill forceps
Soft tissue oedema and haematoma: Increases over 48 hours, results in mask fitting poorly	Monitor airway closely, head up 30°, maintain spontaneous ventilation during airway manipulation, laryngeal mask ventilation
Bilateral mandibular body/angle fractures: Posterior displacement of tongue	Anterior traction of the tongue or jaw using towel clip or suture to elevate the tongue
Temporomandibular joint impairment: Mandibular condyle and zygomatic arch involved, mouth opening limited	Nasotracheal intubation or surgical airway
Mid-facial fracture: Mask seal poor, soft palate collapses against the pharynx	Anterior traction on mobile segment
Basal skull fracture: Nasotracheal intubation contraindicated, pneumocephalus from mask ventilation	Avoid nasal intubation
Cervical spine injury: At risk of neurological injury, with associated risks	Orotracheal intubation with in-line stabilisation of the C-spine, fibreoptic intubation, surgical airway

Source: *Oh's Intensive Care Manual* 5th edition, chapter 66.

Table 3.13.2.2 Examples of laryngotracheal injuries, signs and symptoms

Examples of laryngotracheal injury	Signs and symptoms
• Extension of neck (e.g. from trauma or clothes line) • Strangulation • Direct injury to larynx and trachea (e.g. from a stab wound or gunshot fragments)	• Respiratory distress • Hoarse voice • Dysphonia • Stridor • Dysphagia • Cough • Surgical emphysema • Ecchymosis • Haemoptysis • Additionally, be mindful of the possibility of major vascular injuries in the neck and thoracic injuries

Source: *Oh's Intensive Care Manual* 5th edition, chapter 66.

References and Further Reading

Ardekian L, Samet N, Shoshani Y. Life threatening bleeding following maxillofacial trauma. *J Craniomaxillofac Surg* 1993;**21**:336–40.

Bajwa JSB, Kaur J, Singh A, *et al.* Clinical and critical care concerns of craniofacial trauma: a retrospective study in a tertiary care institute. *Natl J Maxillofac Surg* 2012;**3**:133–8.

Le Fort R. Experimental study of fractures of the upper jaw. *Rev Chir Paris* 1901;**23**:208–27 [reprint: *Plast Rconstr Surg* 1972;**50**:497–506].

Marentette LJ, Valentino J. Traumatic anterior cranial fossa cerebrospinal fluid fistulae and craniofacial considerations. *Otolaryn Clin North Am* 1991;**24**: 151–63.

3.13.3 Traumatic Chest Injuries

Harish Venkatesh and Sanjeev Ramachandran

Key Learning Points

1. Thoracic trauma accounts for a large proportion of trauma-related mortality, with many patients not even surviving to reach hospital.
2. Multi-system injuries are common, and as such, a systematic advanced trauma life support assessment must be carried out to ensure nothing is missed.
3. The location, velocity and type of trauma inflicted (e.g. blunt versus penetrating) are important factors for predicting the extent and severity of an injury.
4. Bedside investigations through focused echocardiography, invasive monitoring and appropriately timed computed tomography scans are essential in aiding clinicians' diagnosis of life-threatening injuries.
5. Effective management involves the presence of a multidisciplinary team, including anaesthetists, intensivists, general surgeons and thoracic surgeons.

Keywords: thoracic, cardiothoracic, chest, trauma, imaging

Introduction

It is estimated that thoracic trauma accounts for approximately 25 per cent of all trauma-related deaths. Of those encountered in the emergency department, only a small proportion go on to receive early operative input; instead the mainstay of management involves delivery of effective medical resuscitation and timely completion of necessary technical procedures, with the end-goal being ventilatory and cardiovascular stability.

Cardiothoracic trauma can be broadly categorised as either blunt or penetrating trauma, with other injuries resulting as a consequence of these initial insults. Hypoxia, hypercarbia and acidaemia are common acute sequelae. However, the most common cause of mortality is exsanguination and coagulopathy. It is not uncommon to have multi-system injuries, and as such, a thorough advanced trauma life support (ATLS) assessment is recommended to guide initial resuscitation. Findings in the primary and secondary surveys generally guide acute management, and this may include endotracheal intubation, mechanical ventilation, thoracostomy tube insertion and fluid resuscitation. Further management may include anaesthetic input for intraoperative stabilisation and/or subsequent intensive care input for post-operative care or advanced medical management if operative management is not indicated.

Timely imaging plays an essential role in the diagnosis and treatment of thoracic injuries. Focused echocardiography and lung ultrasound can be used to identify pericardial effusions, myocardial injury, pneumothoraces and pleural effusions. CT scans are useful for visualising the thoracic cavity, mediastinum and visceral organs to see if there has been any damage sustained (e.g. contusions, lacerations), in addition to identifying the origin of any pneumomediastinum (i.e. aerodigestive versus alveolar tract).

Assessment and Management of Life-Threatening Thoracic Injuries

The primary survey aims to identify immediate issues related to the airway, breathing and circulation. Any problems encountered should be dealt with as soon as they are identified. The secondary survey serves to find and treat other potentially life-threatening injuries.

Airway

Upper airway obstruction due to primary laryngeal injury, or secondary to obstruction from other structures, can be subtle. Key clinical features to elicit include any change in breathing pattern (e.g. stridor), acute vocal changes (e.g. hoarseness) and subcutaneous emphysema.

A tracheobronchial injury is rare, and these patients usually do not make it to hospital alive. In patients who have imminent airway obstruction, endotracheal intubation or a surgical airway is indicated (tracheostomy recommended over cricothyroidotomy). Less severe injuries may be assessed using imaging prior to anaesthetic intervention, whilst urgent surgical input is sought. If time permits and the patient is stable enough, an awake fibreoptic intubation might be useful, especially as it allows visualisation of any damage to the airway. During this time, 100% oxygen should be administered to the patient, and a plan for a large-bore intercostal drain should be made. Adequate ventilation through a single-lumen endotracheal tube may not be possible with severe trauma. Therefore, an experienced anaesthetist may consider the use of a dual-lumen tube to stabilise the bronchi. If the latter is utilised, then immediate operative input is normally required.

Chest Wall

Rib fractures commonly occur secondary to blunt trauma. Clinical examination of the chest should look for local tenderness and crepitations at the site of injury, with palpable or visual deformity of the chest wall signifying the presence of rib fractures. The site of rib fractures is also important, as fractures of the first to third ribs may indicate possible underlying injury to the great vessels and bronchi, whilst additional diminished pulses/blood pressure in one arm may indicate the presence of a mediastinal haematoma. Lower rib fractures, in turn, are associated with abdominal organ damage, e.g. liver, kidney or spleen lacerations. Pain associated with rib fractures can splint the thorax and prevent effective ventilation, oxygenation and coughing. This is particularly important in the elderly in whom the rate of pneumonia and mortality is twice as high as in younger patients and, therefore, effective analgesia is essential.

Flail chests occur when a portion of the chest wall does not have bony continuity. It usually occurs secondary to multiple rib fractures where two or more adjacent ribs are damaged in two or more places. In such instances, underlying pulmonary contusions are often present, and during ventilation, paradoxical movement of the affected area occurs. Injury to the lung, impaired ventilation and restricted chest wall movement due to pain all contribute to hypoxia. Effective management of a flail chest begins with good analgesia (e.g. intercostal blocks, thoracic epidurals, patient-controlled analgesia) allowing adequate ventilation, administration of humidified oxygen and careful fluid resuscitation (avoiding volume overload). A short period of intubation and lung-protective ventilation in the ICU may be required in more severe cases.

Lungs

Exposure of the whole neck and chest is mandatory to enable thorough examination of the respiratory system. Hypoxia and tachypnoea are early and important signs of respiratory distress, whereas cyanosis is a late sign. Situations where immediate resuscitation is necessary include:

1. Pneumothoraces (including tension and open wound)
2. Massive haemothorax
3. Pulmonary contusion

Pneumothoraces occur when a one-way valve air leak occurs into the pleural space from the lung or through the chest wall. Tension pneumothoraces occur when increased intra-pleural pressure causes lung collapse, mediastinal shift, decreased venous return and subsequent collapse of the contralateral lung. A common cause of this is positive pressure mechanical ventilation in patients with a visceral pleural injury, but it can also be caused primarily by blunt or penetrating trauma. If suspected on clinical examination, immediate treatment should be initiated – do not wait for radiological confirmation. This involves large-bore needle decompression into the second intercostal space in the mid-clavicular line. Subsequent definitive management involves insertion of a chest drain tube into the fifth intercostal space, just anterior to the mid-axillary line.

Open pneumothoraces, also known as sucking chest wounds, occur when there are large open defects in the chest wall. As air tends to follow along the path of least resistance, if the wound diameter is approximately two-thirds or larger than the trachea, air preferentially passes through the defect on inspiration. Initial management of open pneumothoraces involves application of a square, sterile occlusive dressing over the defect, which is taped over three edges to make a flutter-type valve effect. In this way, air does not track into the pleural space on inspiration and, on expiration, residual air is expelled out through the defect/valve. A chest tube should be inserted at the earliest opportunity at a site away from the open defect.

Massive haemothoraces occur due to accumulation of blood and fluid in the pleural space. This hinders ventilation and significantly worsens hypovolaemia and hypoxia. Immediate chest tube insertion is required in order to offset this and re-expand the lung, with steps taken to replace the lost blood volume either through autotransfusion or with type-specific blood administration. Indications for an emergency thoracotomy include an initial drainage of ≥1500 ml of blood or continued blood drainage of ≥200 ml/hr for 2–4 hours whilst being guided by the patient's clinical status. Whilst both penetrating and blunt injuries can lead to a massive haemothorax, penetrating chest wounds (in particular, those medial to the nipple line and posterior wounds medial to the scapula) should alert clinicians to the possible need for a thoracotomy due to the proximity of the injury to key mediastinal structures, including the great vessels.

Pulmonary contusions are perhaps the most commonly encountered traumatic chest injury, with the potential for causing death. They are more common in younger patients, as their compliant lungs withstand more energy transfer without sustaining rib fractures. The earliest sign of a contusion is hypoxaemia, and whilst supplemental oxygen may be sufficient for some patients, others may require non-invasive ventilation or intubation and mechanical ventilation. Lung-protective ventilation with small tidal volumes and positive end-expiratory pressure (PEEP) is recommended to prevent volutrauma, along with cautious fluid resuscitation to prevent fluid overload. Management is largely supportive.

Heart

Blunt cardiac injury can lead to myocardial contusion, chamber rupture, vessel dissection/thrombosis and valvular disruption. Rupture usually presents with cardiac tamponade, and this may be identified in the primary survey, either clinically (Beck's triad of hypotension, distended neck veins and muffled heart sounds) or through focused echocardiography. If sternal fractures are identified, then cardiac tamponade must be proactively ruled out. Tamponade would be managed through pericardiocentesis and should cardiac arrest occur, emergency thoracotomy must be considered. Decisions relating to this and other cardiac pathologies should involve discussion with the vascular and cardiothoracic specialists.

Major Vessels

Any patient who has sustained a decelerating blunt chest injury is at risk of damage to the thoracic aorta, and these patients have very high mortality (approximately 75 per cent) without surgery. Two-thirds of such patients die secondary to delayed rupture within 2 weeks. The most common site of injury involves the aortic isthmus at the level of the ligamentum arteriosum. Large shear forces here cause partial or complete tears in the intima and media of the aorta, and blood can subsequently escape into the mediastinum. Total transection of the aorta is usually fatal unless repair is done in a matter of minutes. However, those with partial tears may survive due the presence of a contained haematoma. As clinical diagnosis of a traumatic aortic disruption is difficult, chest radiographs can be used as adjuncts (Box 3.13.3.1).

Helical contrast-enhanced CT scans are the gold standard initial investigation and have a high sensitivity for picking up aortic injuries.

Management of major vessel injuries is mainly surgical, involving either a primary repair or a resection of the torn segment and replacement with an interposition graft. Endovascular repair is also an acceptable option in the more stable patient.

Oesophagus

Oesophageal trauma is more commonly due to penetrating injuries. However, blunt injuries to the upper abdomen may cause an expulsion of gastric contents and tearing of the lower oesophagus. Gastric contents can irritate the mediastinum, causing mediastinitis, and this is associated with high mortality. Conscious patients may complain of severe chest or abdominal

---

Box 3.13.3.1 Features of Major Vascular Injury on Chest X-ray

- Widened mediastinum
- Obliteration of the aortic knob
- Tracheal deviation
- Depression of left main bronchus and elevation of right main bronchus
- Obscuration of the aortopulmonary window
- Oesophageal deviation
- Presence of pleural or apical cap
- Left haemothorax
- First/second rib or scapular fractures

pain, and pneumomediastinum may be evident on chest radiographs. If patients have chest tubes *in situ*, they may drain gastric contents.

Pre-operatively, the patient should be stabilised in the ICU with chest drainage, intravenous fluid replacement and invasive monitoring, and early repair of these injuries (usually involving direct repair of the structure via a thoracotomy) leads to a better prognosis.

Diaphragm

Diaphragmatic ruptures can occur in up to 5 per cent of patients sustaining a blunt injury to the trunk, and such injuries are usually picked up late due to difficulty in clinically diagnosing them. Chest and abdominal pain, diminished breath sounds and respiratory distress may be evident, but such symptoms are not obviously specific. Gastric organs tear through the diaphragm and herniate into the chest cavity, and ruptures occur more frequently on the left side as the presence of the liver may dampen the injury on the right side. An elevated right hemidiaphragm may be the only feature seen on radiographs with right-sided ruptures.

If a laceration is suspected, a nasogastric tube may be passed, then imaged with a chest radiograph. If the tube is in the chest cavity, then a definitive diagnosis can be made by instilling contrast media and re-imaging with a radiograph or CT scan. Definitive management is usually surgical via direct repair.

References and Further Reading

Albert JM, Smith CE. Advanced anesthetic considerations for thoracic trauma. *ASA Monitor* 2015;**79**:24–8.

Allman KG, Wilson IH. Traumatic chest injuries. In: K Allman, I Wilson, A O'Donnell (eds). *Oxford Handbook of Anaesthesia*, 4th edn. Oxford: Oxford University Press; 2016. pp. 856–8.

American College of Surgeons. *ATLS® Advanced Trauma Life Support®. Student course manual*, 9th edn. Chicago, IL: American College of Surgeons; 2012. pp. 94–111.

Parry NG, Moffat B, Vogt K. Blunt thoracic trauma: recent advances and outstanding questions. *Curr Opin Crit Care* 2015;**21**:544–8.

Schellenberg M, Inaba K. Critical decisions in the management of thoracic trauma. *Emerg Med Clin North Am* 2018;**36**:135–47.

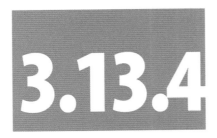

Traumatic Spinal Cord Injuries

Manpreet Bahra and Sachin Mehta

Key Learning Points

1. Traumatic spinal cord injury (TSCI) is a devastating event which can lead to transient or permanent nerve damage, with a peak incidence in young adult males.
2. The American Spinal Injury Association (ASIA) impairment scale is a helpful tool for diagnosing and classifying the severity of cord injury.
3. Initial management should follow established advanced trauma and life support (ATLS) guidance using a systematic approach.
4. Early priorities include prevention of secondary spinal injury and timely identification of an unstable fracture.
5. TSCI can cause organ dysfunction, depending on the level of injury, and may require support to optimise physiological parameters.

Keywords: trauma, spinal cord injury

Classification

Traumatic spinal cord injury (TSCI) is trauma-induced damage to the spinal cord which results in transient or permanent motor, sensory or autonomic disturbances. Injury can occur at any level, though approximately 50 per cent involve the cervical cord. The American Spinal Injury Association (ASIA) impairment scale is a recognised tool for diagnosing and classifying the severity of cord syndromes. The assessment consists of a motor, sensory and anorectal examination. The last is vital to establish completeness of the injury and ascertain the presence of spinal shock. Injury grade and neurological level can be deduced from the findings of these examinations.

Epidemiology

In the UK, the main causes of TSCI are falls, road traffic accidents and sports injuries. Globally, the peak incidence of TSCI occurs amongst young adults (males: 20–29 years; females: 15–19 years), with a minimum male-to-female predominance of 2:1. However, increasing incidence after the age of 65 is an emerging phenomenon.

Pathophysiology

Mechanisms of TSCI can be divided into primary and secondary injury. Primary injury refers to cell death occurring as an immediate effect of pathological forces induced by the initial trauma. Secondary injury, which can start within minutes, refers to a complex cascade of biochemical effects propagated by the original insult. Ischaemia, hypoxia, inflammation and oedema are all implicated and continue to evolve over several hours, causing further tissue damage. Patients who initially present with incomplete cord injury may show clinical evidence of neurological deterioration secondary to these cellular processes. Neurogenic shock (hypotension often with bradycardia) can occur from disruption of autonomic pathways in lesions above T6 and may further exacerbate secondary injury. Efforts to limit secondary injury are crucial, to improve the prognosis for patients with TSCI, and ultimately their quality of life.

Diagnosis

Clinical presentation of TSCI differs from patient to patient, depending on the mechanism of trauma and extent of injury. Pain and immobility may be unreliable features, especially if there are coexisting brain or systemic injuries. A targeted history and examination are therefore vital to establish completeness and determine the neurological level of TSCI. The approach to this is defined by the advanced trauma and life support (ATLS) guideline. A multidisciplinary 'Trauma Team' conducts a primary survey, simultaneously identifying and managing life-threatening injuries based on an ABC approach. Once resuscitation efforts are in progress and the patient is stabilised, a secondary survey evaluating the patient from head to toe can commence. Further imaging is dictated on the basis of this assessment. This may range from plain X-rays to full-body CT scanning and MRI.

Management of Suspected Traumatic Spinal Cord Injuries

All trauma patients with sufficient mechanism of injury should be managed as having a spinal injury until proven otherwise. Patients may arrive at the emergency department with spinal protection measures in place – in a neutral position on a firm surface, ideally with a rigid cervical collar to maintain C-spine alignment, side head supports and strapping. The adequacy of these measures should be reviewed, or initiated if not already in place. Patients with lesions to C5 and above are at risk of respiratory failure and may arrive intubated or in urgent need of intubation. This should be done using manual in-line stabilisation or fibre-optic intubation if time, availability of equipment and expertise allow. Initial priorities in suspected TSCI are to minimise any further damage to the spinal cord and confirm the diagnosis in a timely manner. In the context of a patient with impaired conscious level, negative imaging should be interpreted cautiously and clinical correlation sought when conscious level improves.

Physiological parameters should be optimised in order to maintain an adequate spinal cord perfusion pressure and limit secondary injury. This involves achieving an acceptable mean arterial pressure (MAP), avoiding hypoxia and aiming for $PaCO_2$ levels between 4 and 4.5 kPa to ensure adequate delivery of oxygen. Hypotension attributed to neurogenic shock requires initial fluid resuscitation, followed by titration of vasopressors to achieve an appropriate MAP. Temperature and blood glucose should be maintained at normal levels, as derangement of these parameters can worsen neurological injury.

Management of Confirmed Traumatic Spinal Cord Injuries

Spinal protection precautions (as above) should continue, depending on the site and stability of TSCI, with continuation of log-rolling manoeuvres during nursing care. These strategies are appropriate only in the short term. Surgical fixation is necessary where confirmed unstable injuries exist. Neurosurgical teams should be involved early, as prompt transfer to a specialist neurosurgical centre may improve outcomes. Use of methylprednisolone remains a contentious issue, with limited evidence, and should be guided by a senior neurosurgeon.

In addition to optimisation of physiological parameters previously mentioned, general principles of intensive care should be instigated. These include venous thromboembolism prophylaxis (anticoagulants must be appropriately risk-assessed regarding bleeding and potential surgical/procedural interventions), stress ulcer prophylaxis, ventilator-associated pneumonia prevention, nutritional support, aperients and titrated levels of sedation and analgesia.

Long-Term Management

TSCI is often devastating for the patient and their family, with long-term physical and psychosocial sequelae. Autonomic hyper-reflexia is a life-threatening condition which can occur 4–6 weeks following TSCI. It is characterised by massive sympathetic outflow initiated by reflex stimulation from a variety of triggers (commonly bladder and rectal distension). Management involves identifying and avoiding triggers, as well as using alpha-blockers to control hypertension.

Long-term ventilated patients are especially prone to depression and anxiety, and liaison psychiatry should be involved early. This group are also particularly at risk of nosocomial infections. Therefore, necessary precautions must be taken to avoid these. Ongoing care should continue in a regional spinal rehabilitation centre. Prognosis is determined by the level and completeness of neurological injury. Patients with higher and complete injuries suffer the poorest prognosis.

References and Further Reading

ATLS Subcommittee; American College of Surgeons' Committee on Trauma; International ATLS working group. Advanced trauma life support (ATLS®): the ninth edition. *J Trauma Acute Care Surg* 2013;**74**: 1363–6.

Bonner S, Smith C. Initial management of acute spinal cord injury. *Contin Educ Anaesth Crit Care Pain* 2013;**13**:224–31.

Denton M, McKinlay J. Cervical cord injury and critical care. *Contin Educ Anaesth Crit Care Pain* 2009;**9**:82–6.

World Health Organization. International perspectives on spinal cord injury. Geneva: World Health Organization; 2013.

3.13.5 Traumatic Abdominal and Pelvic Injuries

Karina Goodwin

Key Learning Points

1. Abdominal and pelvic trauma may be concealed.
2. Exsanguination into the abdominal or pelvic cavity should be managed in the resuscitation phase.
3. Obvious abdominal distension is an indication for laparotomy.
4. Post-operative ileus should be anticipated and managed appropriately.
5. Abdominal compartment syndrome is a serious complication of abdominal/pelvic trauma.

Keywords: abdominal, pelvic, FAST scan, compartment syndrome, laparotomy

Introduction

Abdominal and pelvic trauma may result in visceral, vascular or bony injuries. A direct blow, deceleration, shearing, crush or penetrating injury can lead to blunt or penetrating trauma. Combined blunt and penetrating injuries must be considered.

Damage to organs or large blood vessels can be life-threatening and concealed. Obvious injuries can distract from concealed trauma. Advanced trauma life support (ATLS) primary and secondary surveys are designed for rapid, systematic assessment in trauma to identify and rule out life-threatening injuries.

Trauma can occur from rupture of a hollow viscus, bleeding from a solid organ or fracture of the bony pelvis. The abdomen and pelvis are large cavities with major blood vessels and vital organs that can be damaged in trauma. Due to their size, and as a result of the sympathetic response to trauma, blood loss and pain, significant haemorrhage and damage may be present before a physiological response is seen, abdominal dimensions are altered or signs of peritoneal irritation occur. Injuries to retroperitoneal visceral structures, in particular, are hard to recognise due to their location. They are difficult to physically examine and may not present with signs or symptoms of peritonitis.

The method of assessing possible abdominal and pelvic trauma is determined by the mechanism of injury, injury forces, the location of injury and the patient's haemodynamic status.

Of patients with stab wounds that penetrate the anterior peritoneum, 55–60 per cent have hypotension, peritonitis or evisceration of the omentum or small bowel. This requires an emergency laparotomy. Hypotension should be assumed to be caused by hypovolaemia until proven otherwise. Suspicion of abdominal and/or pelvic trauma should be raised where there is hypovolaemia and no obvious external haemorrhage.

The Initial Examination

Examination of the abdomen involves:

- Inspection – bruising, lacerations and distension
- Auscultation – bowel sounds (free intra-peritoneal fluid can produce ileus)
- Percussion – peritonitis
- Palpation – tenderness (superficial or deep), guarding, high-riding prostate gland (significant pelvic injury)

A pelvic radiograph should be performed in the resuscitation room for all patients with blunt trauma. Springing the iliac crests may detect a severely disrupted pelvis. It should be done once only due to the risk of worsening trauma. The effect of gravity on an unstable hemi-pelvis causes outward rotation and migration cephalad due to muscular forces. An unstable pelvis can be closed manually by pushing on the iliac crests at the level of the anterior iliac spine. An external fixator device should be applied to close the pelvis and reduce haemorrhage.

Urethral, perineal and rectal examinations complete the physical assessment of abdominal and pelvic trauma. This may occur during the log roll where flanks should also be inspected. Blood at the urethral meatus, swelling, bruising and laceration of the perineum, vagina, rectum or buttocks raise suspicion of pelvic fracture.

During examination, remember to cover the patient with warmed blankets to help prevent hypothermia. Hypothermia may contribute to coagulopathy of major trauma and is associated with high mortality.

Investigations

Marked abdominal distension indicates the need for a laparotomy as part of the resuscitation phase. An indeterminate abdominal examination requires investigation by CT or ultrasound.

A focussed assessment with sonography in trauma (FAST) scan can be performed by a trained emergency physician, to rapidly assess the four Ps: pericardial, perihepatic, perisplenic and pelvic regions. This is good for detecting blood in the abdominal and pelvic cavities. A second scan may be performed after 30 minutes to detect progressive haemoperitoneum. Notably, a negative FAST scan cannot exclude significant intra-abdominal injury.

A CT scan generally provides information related to specific organ injury. However, some diaphragmatic, pancreatic and gastrointestinal pathologies can be missed. Free fluid in the abdominal cavity in the absence of hepatic or splenic injury is suggestive of injury to the gastrointestinal tract or mesentery, and an indication for operative intervention.

Specific contrast studies, including urethrography, cystography, intravenous pyelography or gastrointestinal contrast studies, can support a diagnosis of specific injuries. They should not delay management of haemodynamically unstable patients.

Initial Management

Exsanguinating pelvic haemorrhage should be managed in the resuscitative phase with involvement of an orthopaedic surgeon and an interventional radiologist if required. Definitive management of ongoing haemorrhage related to pelvic fractures may require angiographic embolisation. Resuscitative endovascular balloon occlusion of the aorta (REBOA) is a method used to control haemorrhage and improve afterload. It is used in some regions, either pre-hospital and/or in the emergency department, as a lifesaving intervention in the event of catastrophic pelvic haemorrhage.

For abdominal injuries, an emergency laparotomy may be required. A rapid sequence induction of anaesthesia with manual in-line stabilisation will be required, as gastric stasis will prolong gastrointestinal transit time, such that even if no food is eaten within the 6 hours preceding the traumatic event, regurgitation and aspiration may still occur at induction. Maintenance of cardiovascular stability is essential, and the degree of pre-induction haemodynamic compromise will determine the anaesthetic technique, including induction agents and doses. Invasive monitoring, including invasive blood pressure and cardiac output monitoring, may be useful to guide fluid and inotrope requirements intraoperatively. However, insertion of arterial and central lines prior to induction of anaesthesia may be more difficult in someone who is hypovolaemic and peripherally shut down.

Ongoing Management in Critical Care

The extent of injuries and physiological response of the patient will determine whether the patient is transferred to a local or regional ICU, and as either a level 2 or a level 3 patient. Once there, a number of considerations arise, including:

1. In haemodynamically unstable patients, invasive blood pressure and cardiac output monitoring should be used to enable goal-directed fluid therapy and monitor cardiovascular response. Thermodilution, dye dilution, ultrasound Doppler with Swan–Ganz catheter and LiDCO and PiCCO methods are available in different units

2. Ileus may develop post-surgery involving the abdomen and pelvis. Some degree of postoperative ileus is a normal physiological response to surgery and resolves without complications. Prolonged ileus leads to discomfort and extended hospitalisation. More serious complications of surgery must be ruled out prior to management of the ileus, which generally involves:

   a. Large-bore nasogastric (Ryles) tube (free drainage and regular aspiration)
   b. Prokinetics – erythromycin and metoclopramide may improve gut motility and aid absorption
   c. Laxatives
   d. Chewing gum – not generally used in the critical care setting

3. Adequate analgesia is essential to minimise diaphragmatic splinting, to support physiotherapy and facilitate mobilisation. These are important factors in prevention of respiratory tract infections and rehabilitation. Major abdominal or pelvic surgery may involve intraoperative placement of an epidural, which provides excellent post-operative pain relief. However, hypovolaemia and/or coagulopathy may restrict their use. If one has been placed, it is important to monitor blood pressure closely and check the level of motor and sensory block regularly in the ICU. Alternative analgesia may utilise intravenous opiates (either nurse-administered or using patient-controlled analgesia). These obviously have a number of side effects, including contributing to post-operative ileus and nausea. However, non-opiate analgesia is unlikely to be sufficient in the post-operative setting

4. Nutritional requirements in the trauma patient should be assessed early on by a dietitian, and enteral or parenteral nutrition commenced as soon as tolerated. Gastric ulcer prophylaxis should also be commenced on admission to the ward

5. Monitoring for primary abdominal compartment syndrome (ACS). This is associated with injury in the abdominopelvic region and may be a complication of trauma or surgery in the post-trauma setting. It is defined as an intra-abdominal pressure (IAP) >20 mmHg with new organ failure. In an awake patient, signs include increasing pain and abdominal distension, and in a ventilated patient, it may be recognised by rising peak pressures, reduced ventilatory compliance and abdominal distension. IAPs may be measured using intravesicular pressure (through the indwelling urinary catheter), and intra-abdominal hypertension (IAP >12 mmHg) may be the first sign of impending ACS. In brief, medical management options that can be instigated in the ICU include:

a. Improved abdominal wall compliance (sedation, analgesia, neuromuscular blockade, bed <30°)
b. Evacuation of intraluminal contents (nasogastric and rectal decompression, prokinetics)
c. Correction of positive fluid balance (diuretics, avoiding excessive fluid resuscitation, haemodialysis/ultrafiltration)
d. Evacuation of abdominal fluid collections (paracentesis, percutaneous drainage)
e. Organ support (optimising ventilation and alveolar recruitment)

Despite this, surgical interventions, such as laparotomy, are often required; however, this is often done as a last resort, as it is associated with increased morbidity, mortality and prolonged recovery.

References and Further Reading

American College of Surgeons. *ATLS® Advanced Trauma Life Support®. Student course manual*, 9th edn. Chicago, IL: American College of Surgeons; 2012.

Kalff JC, Wehner S, Litkouhi B. 2021. Postoperative ileus. www.uptodate.com/contents/postoperative-ileus

Kirkpatrick AW, Roberts DJ, De Waele J, *et al.* Intra-abdominal hypertension and the abdominal compartment syndrome: updated consensus definitions and clinical practice guidelines from the World Society of the Abdominal Compartment Syndrome. *Intensive Care Med* **39**:1190–206.

Smith T, Pinnock C, Lin T, Jones R (eds). *Fundamentals of Anaesthesia*, 3rd edn. Cambridge: Cambridge University Press; 2009.

3.13.6

Mediastinitis

Arun Krishnamurthy

Key Learning Points

1. Mediastinitis is an infection of the whole or part of the mediastinum.
2. The mediastinum lies between the right and left pleura. It extends from the posterior aspect of the sternum to the anterior surfaces of the vertebral bodies, and contains all the thoracic viscera, except the lungs.
3. Mediastinitis is usually a result of instrumentation, trauma or surgery.
4. Broad-spectrum antibiotics should be commenced as soon as possible, with both Gram-positive and Gram-negative cover included.
5. Mediastinitis is associated with a significant increase in mortality (11–35 per cent) and a prolonged hospital stay.

Keywords: mediastinitis, cardiac surgery, antibiotics

Introduction

Mediastinitis is a life-threatening condition which carries extremely high mortality if recognised late or if treated inadequately. It usually results from an infective process, leading to inflammation of any of the mediastinal structures. It can be acute or chronic, and lead to signs of sepsis, bleeding and compression.

Anatomy

The mediastinum lies between the right and left pleura. It extends from the posterior aspect of the sternum to the anterior surfaces of the vertebral bodies, and contains all the thoracic viscera, except the lungs. Inferiorly, it is bounded by the diaphragm and extends to the thoracic inlet superiorly. It may be divided into an upper portion (above the upper level of the pericardium), which is named the **superior mediastinum**, and a lower portion (below the upper level of the pericardium), which is subdivided into three parts as follows.

The **anterior mediastinum** extends from the posterior surface of the sternum to the anterior surface of the pericardium. It normally contains the thymus gland, adipose tissue and lymph nodes.

The **middle mediastinum** includes the bronchi, the heart and pericardium, the hila of both lungs, the lymph nodes, the phrenic nerves, the great vessels and the trachea.

The **posterior mediastinum** includes the descending aorta, the oesophagus, the azygos vein, the thoracic duct and the vagus and sympathetic nerves.

Aetiology

These can be divided into acute and chronic (Box 3.13.6.1).

Chronic fibrosing mediastinitis is the deposition of thick fibrous tissue that encases any of the various mediastinal structures outside of the mediastinal lymph nodes.

Some groups of patients are more at risk of mediastinitis, e.g. those who have diabetes or are immunocompromised.

Box 3.13.6.1 Causes of Acute Mediastinitis

- Cardiothoracic surgery:
  - Post-sternotomy
  - Sternal wound dehiscence
- Oesophageal perforation
- Tracheobronchial perforation
- Blunt trauma to the chest or abdomen
- Direct spread of infection from the lungs
- Descending infection from the head and neck:
  - Tonsillitis
  - Pharyngitis
  - Sinusitis
  - Dental abscess

Epidemiology

In the UK, mediastinitis is relatively rare, and following cardiac surgery, the incidence is <1 per cent. In developing countries, it is still a common complication of head and neck infection. However, with the advent of antibiotics, descending necrotising mediastinitis has become rarer.

Microbiology

Mediastinitis commonly occurs following cardiac surgery. In the majority of these cases (50–60 per cent), the causative organisms are Gram-positive cocci – mainly *Staphylococcus aureus* and *Staphylococcus epidermidis*. Isolates in the remainder of cases tend to show mixed Gram-positive and Gram-negative growth.

Presentation

There may be a history of recent instrumentation to the airway, e.g. endoscopy, bronchoscopy, intubation, or recent thoracic surgery. Most patients normally experience symptoms (Box 3.13.6.2) for a couple of days prior to presentation. However, occasionally, with a fulminant course, symptoms may have only lasted a few hours.

Differential Diagnosis

Box 3.13.6.3 shows the differential diagnosis for mediastinitis.

Investigations

The following investigations should be considered:
- **Full blood count:** elevated white cell count
- **Blood cultures**
- **Swabs for microbiology:** look for a source of sepsis in the oropharynx, and take swabs as appropriate

---

Box 3.13.6.2 Common Symptoms in Patients with Mediastinitis

- Fever and rigors
- Shortness of breath
- Cough
- Sore throat
- Pleural and retrosternal chest pain radiating to the neck or back
- Swelling in the neck

Box 3.13.6.3 Differential Diagnosis

- Myocardial infarction
- Pulmonary embolism
- Aortic aneurysm dissection
- Pneumonia/empyema/lung abscess
- Cellulitis/necrotising fasciitis of the neck
- Mediastinal tumour
- Mallory–Weiss tear
- Myocarditis

- **Chest X-ray:** look for pneumomediastinum and air–fluid levels. You may see areas of consolidation or pleural effusions. Mediastinal widening has also been described, but it is not a reliable sign
- **X-ray of the neck:** may show widening of the pre-cervical, retropharyngeal and paratracheal soft tissues
- **Computed tomography/magnetic resonance imaging of the thorax:** can better delineate mediastinal abnormalities and may find evidence of the source of descending infection

Management

Patients with mediastinitis can be critically ill. Initial management should therefore focus on resuscitation.

Airway

- Ensure adequate oxygenation with supplementary oxygen.
- Intubation for airway protection or worsening hypoxia may need to be considered.
- Intubation may be difficult, so take the necessary precautions and prepare for a difficult intubation.

Breathing

- Ensure adequate ventilation

Circulation

- Intravenous fluid resuscitation

Specific Management

Broad-spectrum antibiotics should be commenced as soon as possible, with both Gram-positive and Gram-negative cover included. Due to the polymicrobial nature of the infection, seek microbiological advice. Your antibiotic regime may be modified when culture results become available, and usually involves a prolonged course.

Surgical referral is required, with input from ear, nose and throat (ENT) surgery in cases of descending infection. Surgery usually consists of a thoracotomy or access via a cervical approach. Drainage of pus and necrotic material and tissue debridement are carried out. A source of infection should actively be looked for, and this may involve drainage of an oropharyngeal or cervical infective focus, or closure of a tracheobronchial or oesophageal rupture. All material drained or debrided should be sent for culture and sensitivities.

Currently, there is no general consensus as to the best strategy to aid wound healing. Strategies therefore include open wound treatment, vacuum and irrigation drainage, vacuum-assisted closure (VAC) therapy and reconstructive plastic surgery with vascularised soft tissue flaps.

Complications

- Sepsis/septic shock
- Bleeding from major vessels or the heart
- Pneumothorax/pneumomediastinum
- Pleural effusions
- Empyema

Prognosis

Mediastinitis is associated with a significant increase in mortality (11–35 per cent) and a prolonged hospital stay.

References and Further Reading

Athanassiadi KA. Infections of the mediastinum. *Thorac Surg Clin* 2009;**19**:37–45.

El Oakley RM, Wright JE. Postoperative mediastinitis: classification and management. *Ann Thoracic Surg* 1996;**61**:1030–6.

Ennker IC, Ennker JC. Management of sterno-mediastinitis. *HSR Proc Intensive Care Cardiovasc Anesth* 2012;**4**: 233–41.

Drowning

Tom Parker

3.14.1

Key Learning Points

1. Drowning is a leading global killer of children and young adults.

2. Outcomes from drowning are uncertain, principally determined by the time of cerebral anoxia, and not the extent of pulmonary aspiration and soiling.

3. Trauma should be considered as a potential cause or consequence of drowning; hence, protective C-spine measures should be considered.

4. Rescue breaths should be administered to both adult and paediatric drowned patients with or without spontaneous circulation.

5. Hypothermia is commonplace in drowned patients and should be managed with active rewarming to 34°C.

Keywords: drowning, aspiration, hypoxia, hypothermia, cardiac arrest

Definition

Drowning refers to the respiratory impairment experienced as a result of submersion or immersion in liquid. Outcomes from drowning include death or survival with or without morbidity.

Epidemiology

The 2014 World Health Organization (WHO) 'Global report on drowning: preventing a leading killer' estimates 372,000 people die as a result of drowning each year, mostly children predominantly in the global south. Drowning is therefore a major global health concern to be considered, alongside malaria and malnutrition, as a cause of preventable deaths.

In the UK, the National Water Safety Forum reports 321 deaths by accidental drowning in 2015. The incidence of non-fatal drowning is unknown.

Pathophysiology

Drowning occurs when an individual's airway is submerged in liquid. An initial period of voluntary breath-holding occurs, during which time the victim becomes increasingly hypoxaemic, hypercapnic and acidaemic. A depressed level of consciousness ensues, enabling water ingress into the naso-oropharynx.

The presence of liquid in the upper airway, combined with often exaggerated primitive airway-protective reflexes associated with impaired consciousness, may result in laryngospasm. Respiratory effort, driven by the potent combined stimulus of hypoxaemia and hypercapnia, continues at this point, with 'see-saw' chest movement against an obstructed upper airway.

Profound hypoxaemia eventually terminates laryngospasm, allowing pulmonary macro-aspiration of the drowning medium and continued failure of gas exchange. Cerebral hypoxia, resulting in coma and apnoea, supervenes, with the final common mode of death being cardiac dysrhythmia – bradycardia, pulseless electrical activity and asystole.

The term 'dry drowning' has been used to explain post-mortem findings suggesting the absence of pulmonary aspiration in up to 15 per cent of those who had apparently drowned. However, these findings have now been called into question and the term should be avoided.

Management

Management of the drowned patient begins at the scene and, in accordance with the advanced trauma life support (ATLS) principles, adopts a systematic ABC approach. Cardiopulmonary resuscitation (CPR) should not be attempted in the water. Rescue breaths may be administered by those trained to do so, in the presence of spontaneous circulation. The patient should be retrieved from the water horizontally in order to maintain cardiac preload, thus avoiding potential circulatory collapse with the release of water pressure.

C-spine injury is uncommon (approximately 0.5 per cent). Nevertheless, spinal precautions should be instituted if there is reason to suspect C-spine injury as either a cause or a consequence of drowning. A history of diving, waterslide use, intoxication or other apparent trauma can all be associated with C-spine injury. In cardiac arrest scenarios, basic life support, with five rescue breaths followed by 30:2 chest compressions, should begin immediately with advanced life support when available. Wet clothing should be removed as this can worsen hypothermia, and the patient should be wrapped in dry blankets. The Heimlich manoeuvre should not be attempted.

In-hospital management begins in the resuscitation room and should continue in a critical care setting. Resuscitative measures to support the airway, breathing and circulation should continue, in addition to the following special considerations.

Hypothermia and Neuro-protection

Hypothermia is a common finding, which has implications for management of the drowned patient. During CPR, clinicians should be prepared for a prolonged resuscitation attempt; the old adage 'you're not dead until you are warm and dead' applies here.

Following return of spontaneous circulation (ROSC) in the patient who remains comatose, active rewarming to 34°C and avoidance of pyrexia for 12–24 hours are recommended by the 2002 World Congress on Drowning as part of a neuro-protective strategy for the prevention of secondary brain injury.

Other 'neuro-protective measures', including aiding venous drainage of the head through 30° head-up patient positioning, tight control of respiratory gas tensions, maintenance of an adequate perfusion pressure, avoidance of metabolic or electrolyte derangements and early treatment of seizures should also be instituted.

Ventilation and Pulmonary Infection

Drowning may lead to a variety of pulmonary complications, including negative-pressure pulmonary oedema from inspiratory effort against an obstructed upper airway and bronchospasm resulting from aspiration of an airway irritant. Large-volume aspiration also causes surfactant dysfunction and washout, resulting in alveolar collapse, atelectasis, worsening ventilation/perfusion (V/Q) inequality and reduced lung compliance.

Osmotic gradients occur across the alveolar membrane, with aspiration of both fresh and salt water. These changes damage membrane integrity, resulting in cellular dysfunction, fluid shifts and pulmonary oedema. The clinical picture is often one of acute respiratory distress syndrome (ARDS), and should be managed accordingly with lung-protective strategies detailed elsewhere in this book.

There is no real difference in the severity of lung injury between those who drown on land and those who drown at sea, though the bacterial, fungal and protozoal burden of fresh water is greater and the intensive care specialist should be mindful of the potential for atypical causes of pulmonary infection in these patients. Positive cultures should be actively sought and treated if in keeping with the clinical picture.

Renal and Electrolytes

Electrolyte disturbances resulting from bulk aspiration of water are rare and often overstated. Exceptions include aspiration of uncommonly electrolyte-rich solutions. Life-threatening electrolyte disturbances have been reported in patients who drowned in the Dead Sea, for example.

Hyperlactataemia and acidosis are common and due to tissue hypoxia. Acute kidney injury can occur, and its aetiology is probably multifactorial; hypoxia–ischaemia, hypovolaemia secondary to fluid shifts and redistributive shock, in addition to reperfusion injury and damage from reactive oxygen species are all likely to contribute, as does myoglobinaemia from damaged muscle in rhabdomyolysis, seen more in the context of trauma.

Close attention to fluid balance and monitoring and correction of electrolytes are therefore paramount. Volume status can be difficult to assess clinically – if in doubt, some form of cardiac output monitoring may help to guide fluid therapy.

Cardiovascular

Drowned patients can exhibit cardiovascular instability due to myocardial stunning as a result of tissue hypoxia and post-cardiac arrest syndrome. In addition, cardiac dysrhythmias are common, particularly in association with hypothermia and as a result of high levels of circulating catecholamines. Management is largely supportive with inopressor support and rhythm control.

Outcomes

Outcomes from drowning are principally determined by the duration of cerebral anoxia. An immersion time of >10 minutes, cardiac arrest on presentation, delayed initiation of CPR or prolonged CPR attempt and the presence of asystole are all predictors of poor outcomes.

References and Further Reading

Layon AJ, Modell JH. Drowning update 2009. *Anesthesiology* 2009;**110**:1390–40.

World Health Organization. *WHO Global Report on Drowning: preventing a leading killer*. Geneva: World Health Organization; 2014.

Burns

3.14.2

Behrad Baharlo

Key Learning Points

1. Burn injury manifests as a local and systemic inflammatory response.
2. Under- and over-resuscitation and 'fluid creep' worsen the prognosis and must be avoided.
3. Expeditious surgery improves outcomes and mitigates septic complications.
4. Septic complications are highly likely and can be difficult to diagnose.
5. Patients with severe burns are hypermetabolic, with a significant nutritional deficit.

Keywords: burn, fluid, sepsis, inhalation, nutrition

Introduction

In 2016–2017, 12,395 hospital admissions in England were due to burn injuries (63 per cent males; 37 per cent females), of which 9067 were emergencies. About one-third required regional burns service input, and 1–2 per cent of emergencies resulted in admission to critical care.

Pathophysiology

Following a burn injury, an immediate local response, followed by a systemic pro-inflammatory reaction, develops. In 1947, Jackson described the local response as three discrete zones around the focus of the burn-injured area. Identifying these zones is important in assessing the extent of injury.

The **zone of coagulation** is at the focus of the burnt area where maximal damage has occurred. The **zone of stasis** immediately surrounds the zone of coagulation and is tissue suffering from hypoperfusion that is potentially salvageable with resuscitation. The zones of stasis and coagulation are included in calculating the percentage of total body surface area (TBSA) burnt. The **zone of hyperaemia** surrounds the zones of coagulation and stasis, and is characterised by increased tissue perfusion. These areas are likely to recover from injury, so do not contribute to any calculation of the percentage of TBSA burnt.

The systemic response is characterised by microvascular injury secondary to the developing milieu of pro-inflammatory mediators, e.g. histamine, bradykinin, prostaglandin, leukotrienes. This results in an increase in capillary permeability, protein loss and fluid leak. Clinically, it manifests as hypovolaemic and distributive shock, though an evolving hypothesis is of a direct effect on the heart, causing cardiogenic shock.

Complications of Burns

- Burn oedema
- Abdominal compartment syndrome
- Limb compartment syndrome
- Acute respiratory distress syndrome (ARDS)
- Electrolyte deficiencies
- Acute kidney injury
- Hypothermia
- Poisoning (carbon monoxide (CO) or cyanide)
- Sepsis
- Deep vein thrombosis
- Stress ulceration
- Chronic pain, depression, post-traumatic stress disorder

Death is more likely in larger burns, extremes of age and the frail, and with concurrent inhalation injury. Where burn injury and critical illness are so severe and rehabilitation is not possible, withdrawal decisions should be the subject of multidisciplinary input and governed by legal frameworks.

Ongoing and Critical Care Management

In those needing ongoing mechanical ventilation, lung-protective ventilation strategies, as described by the ARDS network, should be employed. Whilst ARDS is likely to develop, inadequate ventilation and/or rising airway pressures may also be caused by abdominal compartment syndrome or circumferential burns to the abdomen or thorax (necessitating escharotomy), and these therefore must be excluded.

Select patients may require a tracheostomy tube in due course, and most burns surgeons are well versed with this technique. In keeping with non-burn populations, there is no consensus as to the optimal timing of performing this procedure.

The Parkland formula (2–4 ml/(kg % TBSA)) offers a guide to burn shock resuscitation in the first 24 hours, and resuscitation endpoints should be reviewed regularly to avoid under- and over-resuscitation. Conversely, fluids may be required, in addition to that described by Parkland, e.g. in inhalation injury, electrical burns, delayed resuscitation, concurrent rhabdomyolysis.

After the initial 24 hours, fluid requirements should be titrated to clinical signs (heart rate, mean arterial pressure, central venous oxygen saturation >60 per cent), though daily evaporative losses can be estimated using the formula [3750 ml × BSA (m²) × (% TBSA burnt/100)] to aid calculating overall requirements. A urine output of 0.5 ml/(kg hr) in adults, and 1 ml/(kg hr) in paediatrics, is commonly targeted as a surrogate of adequate organ perfusion.

Fluid Creep

A potential pitfall of ongoing fluid management is the iatrogenic phenomenon of 'fluid creep'. Described by Pruitt as 'fluid resuscitation in excess of that predicted by the Parkland formula and which is associated with compartment syndrome', it has been shown that the risk of compartment syndrome increases with larger volumes of fluid employed (>250–300 ml/kg per 24 hours). Factors implicated in 'fluid creep' are the use of semi-invasive cardiac output measures, over-sedation and analgesia ('opioid creep'), over-estimate of burn size and overzealous or inattentive resuscitation.

Notably, persistent hypotension in an adequately resuscitated burn patient should alert the clinician to possible unrecognised bleeding, poisoning, associated inhalational injury, sepsis, myocardial infarction or heart failure.

Inhalation Injury

Inhalation injury is the aspiration of superheated gases, liquids or noxious products (typically smoke or chemical fumes). It poses unique challenges in respect of airway and lung injury.

Injury can affect the upper airway (above the larynx) and lower airway (below the larynx), or be due to sequelae of noxious substances.

Smoke inhalation injury is characterised by fibrin deposits in the alveolar spaces (which inhibits surfactant), and carbonaceous deposits are commonly seen on bronchoscopy.

Management of inhalation injury includes pulmonary toileting, nitric oxide, nebulised heparin (potentiates anti-thrombin III-mediated inactivation of thrombin and is a free radical scavenger), nebulised 20% N-acetylcysteine, bronchodilators and oral mucolytics.

Surgery

Burnt tissue is a bacterial and fungal culture medium acting as a source of inflammatory mediators. The aim of surgery is to excise non-viable tissue and provide wound coverage, thus reducing septic and metabolic sequelae. Typically, deep partial-thickness and full-thickness burns require early surgical management, aiming for complete excision within 72 hours. Staged strategies (approximately 20 per cent TBSA excised per visit to theatre) are employed to mitigate the challenges posed by blood loss (estimated at 50–100 ml per percentage area excised) and hypothermia in larger burns. Blood transfusions are often required, and though the TRICC trial did not include burns populations, the American Burn Association (ABA)-sponsored TRIBE trial recently reported no difference in rates of organ dysfunction or mortality between 'restrictive' or 'liberal' strategies in burns.

The application of biological dressings serves to reduce fluid, protein and electrolyte loss, and reduce infection and pain in the interim prior to proceeding to grafting when appropriate. Circumferential burns result in 'eschars' (scars) that act analogous to a tourniquet where, in the presence of oedema and swelling, ischaemia of the tissue ensues. Escharotomies (incision through burnt skin) are needed urgently. Fasciotomies may be needed for similar reasons in limb compartments.

Nutrition

The patient with burns of >20 per cent TBSA is hypermetabolic and catabolic, leading to a net loss of protein and lean body mass which is proportional to the burn size. This state can persist for many months (peaks from days 5 to 21 post-injury). Nutritional support, in conjunction with attenuation of this hypermetabolic response, is needed.

Strategies include enteral nutrition (preferred), total parenteral nutrition, beta-blockade with propranolol (to attenuate the sympathetic response) and the anabolic steroids oxandrolone and nandrolone. There is significant loss of trace elements, and replacement of zinc, copper and selenium is associated with better wound healing and fewer infections. Nursing in a warm environment (ambient temperature of 30°C) and optimal analgesia and sedation reduce lean body mass loss.

High protein nutrition (1.5–2 g/(kg day) in adults and 3 g/(kg day) in children) is necessary, and input from dietetics should be sought for tailored regimens. Whilst indirect calorimetry is the gold standard to determine energy requirements, use of recognised formulae, such as the Toronto formula, can be employed.

Enteric nutrition has well-rehearsed benefits (e.g. improved splanchnic perfusion, prevention of bacterial translocation) and is preferred to total parenteral nutrition (TPN). Duodenal feeding facilitates continued nutrition during surgery where breaks in enteral nutrition delivered conventionally (pre-pyloric) due to multiple visits to the operating theatre have been implicated as a cause of failure to meet calorific requirements.

TPN is indicated if >60 per cent of calculated calorific requirements are not met for four consecutive days.

Sepsis in Burns

Infection is highly likely in the burn patient, though diagnosis poses unique challenges because the usual signs of sepsis are common in the severely burnt patient (tachycardia, tachypnoea and a rise in baseline temperature). The most common sites of infection are wound site and pulmonary.

In 2007, the ABA published diagnostic criteria in adults to aid the diagnosis of sepsis in burns. Three of these criteria should trigger concern of an infection (Table 3.14.2.1).

Table 3.14.2.1 The American Burn Association criteria for sepsis in burns

Sepsis trigger is three or more of the following
Temperature >39°C or <36°C
Tachycardia >110 bpm
Tachypnoea >25 bpm (spontaneously ventilating) or minute ventilation >12 l/min (if ventilated)
Thrombocytopenia <100,000/µl (not applied until 3 days after initial resuscitation)
Hyperglycaemia in the absence of diabetes mellitus of >11.1 mmol/l or >7 U/hr of intravenous insulin or >25% increase in insulin dose over 24 hours
Feed intolerance for >24 hours (abdominal distension, high gastric residual volumes of more than twice the feeding rate or diarrhoea of >2500 ml/day)

C-reactive protein (CRP), white cell count (WCC) and erythrocyte sedimentation rate (ESR) remain valuable markers of infection. More recently, procalcitonin has been demonstrated as a marker of sepsis in burns (less so in the paediatric population).

Broad-spectrum anti-microbials are best avoided in favour of narrow-spectrum targeted therapy. Guidance from a microbiologist is invaluable in establishing local pathogen and resistance patterns and the significance of positive wound swabs (colonisation versus active source of infection). Specimens should only be sent when indicated, and the value of baseline cultures on admission is debatable. A septic screen is advocated with any change or introduction of anti-microbial therapy.

Due to high rates of colonisation, cultures from arterial and central venous catheters should not be taken. Furthermore, because of the high prevalence of transient bacteraemia of unlikely significance, cultures should be avoided around the time of dressing changes and wound surgery. Though not universal, the practice of regular rotation of lines (every 7 days) is common, though in the severely burnt patient, this can be difficult to achieve.

There is no role for prophylactic antibiotics. The key to prevention of sepsis is early surgical excision and subsequent skin grafting. Furthermore, patients should be nursed in isolation, with meticulous attention to contact prevention and hand hygiene (high risk of spread of multidrug-resistant organisms).

Acute Kidney Injury

Acute kidney injury is common, and its severity correlates with the severity of burn injury. The need for renal replacement therapy is associated with increased mortality (>80 per cent). Other aetiologies include sepsis, intra-abdominal hypertension, rhabdomyolysis and use of nephrotoxic drugs. A small ABA-sponsored study (RESCUE) recently suggested that compared to standard care, high-rate (70 ml/(kg hr)) continuous renal replacement therapy in burn patients with septic shock and acute kidney injury may reverse shock severity more expeditiously.

Analgesics and Anxiolysis

A multi-modal analgesic approach is advocated to include opioids, N-methyl-D-aspartate (NMDA) receptor antagonists (ketamine) and gamma amino-butyric acid (GABA) analogues (pregabalin). The need for analgesia reduces as the burn heals; however, abrupt cessation of analgesia, especially opioids, should be avoided to prevent withdrawal. In combating 'opioid creep' (increasing opioid requirements), opioid rotation is employed.

Carbon Monoxide

CO poisoning should be considered in cases of entrapment, burns sustained in an enclosed space or those presenting with a reduced conscious level. Carboxyhaemoglobin (COHb) avidly binds haemoglobin and displaces oxygen, and signs of poisoning relate to levels of COHb – escalating from headaches and dyspnoea (CO levels 10–20 per cent) to syncope, coma and convulsions (CO levels >40 per cent). Note that oxygen saturations measured by pulse oximetry will be normal because of similar absorption spectra of COHb and oxyhaemoglobin. Pregnant women are particularly vulnerable, as CO binds more readily to fetal haemoglobin than to adult haemoglobin.

Treatment is with 100% oxygen to reduce the half-life of COHb. Hyperbaric oxygen is rarely used or accessible.

Electrical Burns

Electrical burns occur due to current passing through the body, resulting in prolonged muscle contraction and dissipation of heat energy. Concurrent fractures are common. The severity of burns injury is related to the voltage exposed to, resistance of the patient (e.g. presence of moisture reduces resistance), the route taken through the body by the current and the duration of the contact.

There is a significant risk of cardiac conduction abnormalities and rhabdomyolysis associated with electrical burns, and careful monitoring of the electrocardiogram, muscle compartments, creatine kinase, myoglobin and potassium levels is necessary.

Cyanide

Cyanide poisoning is a further sequela of fires (cyanide inhibits cytochrome C oxidase, thus disrupting the mitochondrial electron transport chain and aerobic respiration). It is a diagnostic challenge due to the paucity of readily available diagnostic tests. It presents with varying neurological signs and should be suspected in any victim of entrapment and/or smoke inhalation (especially in the context of lactataemia and absence of an attributable head injury). Baud et al. showed that lactate concentration increases proportionally with the amount of cyanide, and this can often be the only indicator in a critically ill patient. Treatment is with high-flow oxygen and the antidote hydroxocobalamin (70 mg/kg IV) which chelates cyanide to cyanocobalamin. Administration of hydroxocobalamin turns urine, and sometimes skin, purple.

Acknowledgements

The author would like to thank Dr Tomasz Torlinski, Consultant in Intensive Care Medicine, Queen Elizabeth Hospital, Birmingham for his review of, and suggestions to, this chapter.

References and Further Reading

Clarey A, Trainor D. Critical care management of severe burns and inhalational injury. *Anaesth Intensive Care Med* 2017;**18**:395–400.

Guttormsen A, Berger M, Sjoberg F, Heisterkamp H. 2012. Burns injury. European Society of Intensive Care Medicine (ESICM) PACT module.

Midlands Burn Care Network. www.mcctn.org.uk/burns .html

Snell J, Loh N-H, Mahambrey T, Shokrollahi K. Clinical review: the critical care management of the burn patient. *Crit Care* 2013;**17**:241.

3.14.3 Thermal Disorders

Behrad Baharlo

Key Learning Points

1. Disturbance of the body's thermoregulatory processes can have profound systemic sequelae, including multi-organ failure.
2. Numerous underlying disease states can cause hyperthermia or hypothermia.
3. Heatstroke is a medical emergency requiring immediate cooling measures.
4. A number of syndromes due to drugs manifest with hyperthermia.
5. Neuroleptic malignant syndrome differs from serotonin syndrome in its onset.

Keywords: hypothermia, hyperthermia, heatstroke, neuroleptic, serotonin

Introduction

Body temperature is controlled by the hypothalamus via dynamic thermoregulatory processes. Normal core temperature is between 35.5°C and 37.5°C, and exhibits diurnal variations.

Hypothermia

A common definition is that of a core temperature of <35°C. It is further classified as mild (32–35°C), moderate (28–32°C) and severe (<28°C).

Risk factors for hypothermia include: extremes of age (elderly and neonates), immobility, drugs (e.g. alcohol, barbiturates, antidepressants), malnutrition, endocrine causes (e.g. hypothyroidism, adrenal insufficiency, hypothalamic lesions), sepsis, trauma, spinal cord injury, burns and water immersion.

The body's response to hypothermia includes behavioural changes, peripheral vasoconstriction, reduced sweating and shivering.

Consequences of hypothermia include reduced respiratory rate, bradycardia and arrhythmias, reduced reflexes, confusion, coma, hyperglycaemia, coagulopathy, disseminated intravascular coagulation (DIC), pancreatitis, reduced drug clearance, electrolyte disturbances and renal failure.

ECG manifestations include prolonged PR and QT intervals, characteristic J waves (seen with temperatures of <32°C), widening of QRS and risk of ventricular fibrillation (VF).

Techniques used to aid rewarming include heated and humidified oxygen, warm intravenous (IV) fluids, active warming blankets or mattresses, body cavity lavage and extracorporeal blood warming (e.g. renal replacement or cardiopulmonary bypass).

Hyperthermia

Hyperthermia is defined as a core temperature of >38°C. Fever (>38.3°C) describes hyperthermia when the thermoregulatory set point is increased due to an underlying condition, e.g. infection. Hyperpyrexia is a temperature of >40°C.

The most common cause of hyperthermia in the ICU is sepsis, being a natural (and possibly beneficial) response. Notwithstanding infection, hyperthermia occurs in severe burns, thyrotoxicosis, phaeochromocytoma, hypothalamic disturbance, heatstroke or secondary to drugs. There exist a number of syndromes due to drugs that manifest as hyperthermia. These include neuroleptic malignant syndrome, serotonin syndrome, anti-cholinergic syndrome, sympathomimetic syndrome and malignant hyperthermia.

The body's response to hyperthermia includes behavioural changes, peripheral vasodilation, sweating and reduced piloerection.

Consequences of hyperthermia include tachycardia, high cardiac output, low systemic vascular resistance (SVR), increased oxygen demand and carbon dioxide (CO_2) production, and a right shift of the oxygen dissociation curve. Uncontrolled, it can lead to multi-organ failure, cerebral oedema, seizures, coma, rhabdomyolysis and DIC.

Treatments include paracetamol (a cyclo-oxygenase 3 (COX-3) inhibitor), non-steroidal anti-inflammatory drugs (NSAIDs) or pharmacotherapy specific to the underlying cause, e.g. antibiotics, dantrolene, bromocriptine, cyproheptadine, neuromuscular blockers, analgesics or sedatives. Cooling measures include surface cooling with ice pack and cooling blankets, cooled IV fluids, body cavity lavage with cold fluids, renal replacement therapy (RRT) and cardiopulmonary bypass.

Heatstroke

This is a medical emergency characterised by hyperthermia (due to failure of the thermoregulatory system) and a change in mental state. It can progress to multi-organ failure and carries a mortality rate of up to 50 per cent. Heatstroke is the severest on a spectrum of heat-related disorders which includes heat syncope, heat cramp, heat exhaustion and heatstroke.

Risk factors include obesity, concurrent febrile illness, lack of sleep, food or water, recent alcohol ingestion, lack of fitness, male sex, lack of acclimatisation and use of exacerbating drugs (e.g. anti-cholinergics, anti-histamines, TCAs).

It manifests as one of two cardiovascular entities – either hyperdynamic or hypodynamic. The common presentation is that of a hyperdynamic circulation – high cardiac output with hypotension. The rarer hypodynamic presentation of low cardiac output and paradoxical vasoconstriction carries a poorer prognosis. Consistent with both cardiovascular presentations are hypovolaemia, arrhythmias and a prolonged QT interval (which is the most common ECG abnormality). Neurologically, the patient presents with lethargy, delirium, seizures or coma. Intracranial haemorrhage has been reported. Lactataemia occurs, which often worsens with fluid resuscitation due to skeletal muscles being reperfused when hypovolaemia is corrected. Acute kidney injury is common, which can be due to direct thermal injury, hypovolaemia or rhabdomyolysis. Liver dysfunction on a spectrum from transaminitis through to acute failure has been described, whilst DIC is common in severe heatstroke.

Management is supportive with use of an ABCDE approach. Active cooling should be initiated immediately, the modality of which is dependent on availability. The aim should be to cool rapidly (within 30 minutes of presentation) to <38.9°C, which has been shown to improve survival. A combination of approaches may be necessary to achieve this goal (e.g. surface cooling, cold IV fluids, bladder lavage ± RRT). Dantrolene is not effective.

Poor prognostic markers include inability to cool to <38.9°C within 30 minutes of presentation, hypodynamic circulation on presentation and raised lactate dehydrogenase, creatine kinase (CK), aspartate aminotransferase (AST) or alanine aminotransferase (ALT) on admission. In survivors, concentrations of these enzymes fall at 24 hours.

Malignant Hyperthermia

This autosomal dominant condition results in a defect on the ryanodine receptor, causing an increase in intracellular calcium concentrations when the patient is exposed to triggering agents, typically volatile anaesthetics and suxamethonium. The resultant sustained skeletal muscle contractions manifest clinically as masseter spasm (an early sign), muscle rigidity, a high end-tidal carbon dioxide ($ETCO_2$), tachycardia, hypoxia (due to increased demand) and pyrexia (often a late sign). Hyperkalaemia, metabolic acidosis and rhabdomyolysis (myoglobinaemia) ensue which, if untreated, can progress to multi-organ failure. Though prompt treatment with dantrolene has improved prognosis, malignant hyperthermia is an anaesthetic emergency with significant mortality (up to 20 per cent despite treatment with dantrolene). The Association of Anaesthetists of Great Britain and Ireland (AAGBI) published treatment guidelines for cases of suspected malignant hyperthermia, which include removal of the offending agent, active cooling and administration of dantrolene (2.5 mg/kg IV bolus, then repeat 1 mg/kg bolus up to a maximum of 10 mg/kg). Ongoing management is supportive, and suspected cases should be referred to the malignant hyperthermia unit in Leeds for testing.

Neuroleptic Malignant Syndrome

This is an idiosyncratic drug reaction to anti-psychotic medications which inhibit central dopaminergic receptors (e.g. haloperidol, droperidol, promethazine), or after withdrawal of a dopamine receptor agonist.

It presents with bradykinesia or akinesia, agitation, coma or seizures, autonomic disturbance (hypertension) and pyrexia. In contrast to serotonin syndrome, symptoms occur over days or weeks.

Management is supportive, ensuring withdrawal of the offending agent. Dantrolene and the dopamine

423

agonist bromocriptine are specific therapies used in management.

Serotonin Syndrome

This is due to serotonin toxicity in those taking serotonergic medications (e.g. selective serotonin reuptake inhibitors, TCAs). In contrast to neuroleptic malignant syndrome, onset is within 24 hours, presenting as a triad of neurological signs (hyper-reflexia, clonus and tremor, leading to agitation, seizures or coma) autonomic disturbance and pyrexia. (Refer to Hunter serotonin syndrome criteria.)

Management is supportive, though the anti-histamine and anti-serotonergic drug cyproheptadine is used in severe cases.

Anti-cholinergic Syndrome

This occurs due to inhibition of central and peripheral muscarinic receptors. It presents with tachycardia, mydriasis, dry and flushed skin, dry mouth, myoclonus, urinary retention, agitation, delirium, seizures and pyrexia. Offending agents are anti-histamines, anti-Parkinsonian medications, atropine, TCAs and sleep aids (e.g. doxylamine). Management is supportive, with physostigmine being used in severe cases.

Sympathomimetic Syndrome

Sympathomimetic syndrome is typically present due to ingestion of recreational drugs (e.g. ecstasy, MDMA, (3,4-methylenedioxymethamphetamine), cocaine, amphetamines, PMA (paramethoxyamphetamine), mephedrone).

Presentations are variable but include pyrexia, sweating, dehydration, arrhythmias, tachycardia, hypertension, hyper-reflexia, confusion or seizures which can progress to multi-organ failure. As well as the generic sequelae of sympathomimetic toxicity, specific manifestations of the underlying drug may be present, e.g. hyponatraemia associated with ecstasy poisoning.

2,4 Dinitrophenol (illegal in the UK, but purchased from overseas suppliers over the internet) has grown in popularity as a weight loss adjunct in recent years and has been related to a number of deaths. A phenol-based product, it causes uncoupling of oxidative phosphorylation. Toxicity presents with sympathomimetics such as signs of severe hyperthermia, tachycardia and diaphoresis.

Acknowledgements

The author would like to thank Dr Tomasz Torlinski, Consultant in Intensive Care Medicine, Queen Elizabeth Hospital, Birmingham for his review of, and suggestions to, this chapter.

References and Further Reading

Association of Anaesthetists. 2020. Malignant hyperthermia 2020. anaesthetists.org/Portals/0/PDFs/Guidelines%20 PDFs/Guideline%20Malignant%20hyperthermia%20 2020.pdf?ver=2021-01-13-144236-793

Dunkley E, Isbister G, Sibbritt D, Dawson A, Whyte I. The Hunter serotonin toxicity criteria: simple and accurate diagnostic decision rules for serotonin toxicity. *QJM* 2003;**96**:635–42.

Grogan H, Hopkins P. Heat stroke: implications for critical care and anaesthesia. *Br J Anaesth* 2002;**88**:700–7.

Musselman M, Saeley S. Diagnosis and treatment of drug-induced hyperthermia. *Am J Health Syst Pharm* 2013;**70**:34–42.

Walter E, Carraretto M. Drug-induced hyperthermia in critical care. *J Intensive Care Soc* 2015;**16**:306–11.

3.14.4

Envenomation

Timothy Snow

Key Learning Points

1. Whilst venomous creatures are endemic to specific regions, travel and exotic pets may cause envenomated patients to appear where not expected.
2. Anaphylaxis is the leading cause of death from envenomation.
3. Whilst creature identification can aid management, attempted capture by untrained individuals can create more problems, and thus should not be encouraged.
4. Management is primarily good basic first aid, anaphylaxis treatment and organ support.
5. Anti-venoms are available but can themselves be the cause of anaphylaxis.

Keywords: anaphylaxis, venoms, anti-venoms, snake bites

Introduction

Despite the multitude of phobias regarding creatures which swarm, swim, scuttle or slide, humans are at risk of coming into contact with them, knowingly or unknowingly. Whilst many are envenomous creatures, the majority are relatively harmless to humans, causing minimal or localised reactions only. Of the few that cause systemic effects, those intensivists working in endemic areas should have an awareness of presentations and management. However, even for those of us working in non-endemic areas, with the rise in global travel and the desire for exotic pets, envenomation may occur when we least expect it. It should also be remembered that death can occur from envenomation-induced anaphylaxis, even from those creatures that cause minimal local irritation.

Difficulties that arise in the management of envenomation include extraction of affected individuals from the potential remote or marine environments where the envenomation occurred and preventing other individuals from attempting to catch the offending animal (and being bitten or stung themselves). Specific treatments are listed below, but in most cases, it broadly involves removal of the patient from the environment, analgesia and supportive care. In some cases, however, use of a specific anti-venom is indicated.

Anaphylaxis

Anaphylaxis due to envenomation should be managed no differently to other causes of anaphylaxis – follow the standard Resuscitation Council UK algorithm, with prompt adrenaline administration being the key treatment. It should be remembered, however, that anti-venoms themselves may also cause anaphylaxis, and thus should only be administered where adrenaline is also available. Lastly, whilst some histamine-releasing venoms (e.g. scromboid) may be mistaken for anaphylaxis, unless the diagnosis is certain, it is prudent to treat as presumed anaphylaxis until proven otherwise.

Aquatic Creatures

Poisonous Fish

Ciguatera fish poisoning occurs as a consequence of ingestion of toxins produced by *Gambierdiscus toxicus*, a flagellate organism. The toxins accumulate in the animals at the top of the food chain (e.g. large carnivorous warm-water fish, including snapper and mackerel), and after ingestion, inactivation of sodium channels ensues. Initial presentation of gastrointestinal symptoms is usually self-limiting but may quickly progress to respiratory paralysis or cardiac arrhythmia, with death occurring in approximately 0.1 per cent of cases. In severe cases, ventilatory support or anti-arrhythmics may be required. However, drugs with their mechanism of action involving sodium channels (e.g. lidocaine or amiodarone) should be avoided. Intravenous (IV) mannitol 0.5–1 g/kg may be of benefit in severe cases.

Tetrodotoxin, produced by scaleless porcupine, sun and classically poorly prepared puffer fish in Japan, is a powerful neurotoxin. Symptoms present within 10–45 minutes of ingestion, with death by respiratory paralysis 2–6 hours later. Ventilatory support is the mainstay of treatment, as no antidote is available.

Scromboid toxicity presents with a histamine-like syndrome and can be mistaken for anaphylaxis. Bacterial contamination of tuna, mackerel and canned fish leads to decomposition and release of histamine. Symptoms occur early – initially buccal tingling, followed by flushing, sweating, urticaria and abdominal symptoms. Severe cases may be complicated by hypotension or bronchospasm. Treatment is similar to that for anaphylaxis, with anti-histamines, bronchodilators and adrenaline.

Paralytic shellfish poisoning occurs when bivalve molluscs, such as cockles and mussels, are exposed to toxic dinoflagellate algal blooms, characterised by a 'red tide'. Paralysis begins within 30 minutes of ingestion, with death by respiratory paralysis within 12 hours in approximately 8 per cent of cases. Management is with respiratory support, including intubation and ventilation.

Fish Stings

Venomous fish have a series of spines on their gills, fins or tail, and tend to cause stings when stood on. Most cause localised pain and swelling. However, in some cases, a neuro-toxidrome of vomiting, diarrhoea, sweating, dysrhythmia, hypotension and muscle spasm can occur. Larger stingrays, with their barbed tails, may cause fatal trauma from haemorrhage or pneumothorax. Management is pain relief, with immersion in hot (<45°C) water or local anaesthetic, and supportive care. An anti-venom exists for the most dangerous – the stone fish. Sea urchin spines, also venomous when stood on, rarely produce a systemic effect.

Jellyfish

Common stinging jellyfish have tentacles studded with millions of nematocysts – capsules which fire venomous hairs into the skin upon contact. Features include severe localised pain and erythematous wheals, which, in turn, lead to skin necrosis. Systemic reactions include severe muscle pain, sweating, tachycardia, arrhythmias, hypertension and pulmonary oedema. Anaphylaxis may occur, and urticarial reactions can recur for months following the initial sting. Management is aimed at preventing further nematocyst discharge with weak acids, such as vinegar (the old surfers' tale of peeing on the sting therefore only works if the person's urine is acidic – usually somewhat difficult to prove!), pain relief and supportive care. An anti-venom exists for the Indo-Pacific Box jellyfish which boasts the title of the 'most venomous marine animal'.

Reptiles
Snakes

Excluding a select few countries such as Ireland (thanks to St Patrick), most parts of the world have resident venomous snakes. Whilst there are hundreds of different types, knowledge of those local to your area is usually sufficient. Envenomation occurs in only 50 per cent of venomous snakebites and usually takes hours to occur. Snake venom tends to produce a specific characteristic envenomation syndrome, although pit viper and viper venom can cause all types. These syndromes are listed in Table 3.14.3.1.

Table 3.14.3.1 Syndromes related to snake bites

'Syndrome'	Type of snake	Signs and symptoms
Skin	Asps and cobras	Localised swelling, bruising, blistering and lymph node enlargement, progressing to tissue necrosis
Coagulopathy	Boomslang, vine and elapids	Spontaneous bleeding from mucosal surfaces, skin and the genitourinary tract occurs due to clotting factor consumption. Diagnosed using the 20-minute whole-blood clotting test
Cardiovascular instability	Elapids and asps	Hypotension and arrhythmias
Paralysis	Elapids	Follows a descending pattern with ptosis, ophthalmoplegia, bulbar palsy and respiratory paralysis, followed by generalised flaccid paralysis

'Syndrome'	Type of snake	Signs and symptoms
Rhabdomyolysis	Sea snakes, elapids and kraits	Myalgia and myoglobinuria, which may progress to acute kidney injury
Acute kidney injury	Sea snakes and elapids	May occur as a direct consequence of the venom or secondary to another syndrome

Initially, first aid should be used to manage bites (immobilisation, simple analgesics and direct pressure in case of elapid bite). Specific anti-venom is indicated in the case of rapidly spreading or severe envenomation syndrome. Prophylactic adrenaline should be given subcutaneously (0.25 mg), whilst monitoring for development of anaphylaxis (which should be managed as standard). Supportive management, including IV fluids, haemofiltration and ventilatory support, should be provided if required. Coagulopathy usually settles within 6 hours of anti-venom administration (secondary to new clotting factor synthesis by the liver).

Insects

Scorpions

Found in dry desert or dusty terrains, scorpion stings are both extremely painful and contain autonomic neurotransmitters which cause significant systemic effects. As a general rule, scorpions with small pincers, but large tails are the most toxic. Acetylcholine causes vomiting, abdominal pain, sweating and hypersalivation, with bradycardias, bulbar palsy, weakness or respiratory paralysis in severe cases. Catecholamines cause hypertension, tachycardia, pulmonary oedema, heart failure and arrhythmias. The toxin produced by the *Tityus trinitatis* scorpion is famously a rare cause of pancreatitis, as many medical students may remember! Management requires local anaesthetics for pain, anti-venoms if available and supportive treatments, including intubation and ventilation (respiratory failure is the primary cause of death), vasodilators and IV fluids.

Spiders

The most dangerous spiders include the black or brown widows, brown recluse, Australian funnel web and South American wandering, armed or banana spiders. The majority of symptoms occur due to neurotoxin envenomation causing abdominal pain, muscle spasm or weakness, sweating, salivation, arrhythmias and hypo- or hypertension. Other syndromes include necrosis and a systemic effect with fever, rash, haemoglobinuria, coagulopathy and acute kidney injury. Management is primarily supportive, although some specific anti-venoms exist.

Other Insects

Wasps, hornets, bees and ants may all cause local reactions from stings and bites, and anaphylaxis may occur in sensitised individuals. Other invertebrates, including ticks and mosquitoes, whilst causing local reactions, may induce a systemic infection from parasitic organisms such as typhoid and malaria, respectively.

Leeches

Leech bites are painless, thus allowing the leech to ingest blood undetected before dropping off. Land leeches, found on rainforest floors, attach to exposed ankles or legs, whilst aquatic leeches can attach anywhere, including the anus, oropharynx, vagina and urethra. The main risk following a leech bite is blood loss. The bite contains hirudin, an anticoagulant; thus, upon detachment, the fragile clot may break down, leading to significant haemorrhage. Pharyngeal leeches may cause stridor, haemoptysis or airway obstruction. Finally, cases exist of peritonitis from leeches entering via the anus and causing sigmoid perforation. Treatment is removal of the leech with salt, heat or turpentine, with bleeding controlled using pressure dressings or silver nitrate. Endoscopic removal with dilute adrenaline or concentrated saline spray may be required for penetrating aquatic leeches.

References and Further Reading

Ahmed AM, Ahmed M, Nadeem A, *et al.* Emergency treatment of a snake bite: pearls from literature. *J Emerg Trauma Shock* 2008;**1**:97–105.

Bane V, Lehane M, Dikshit M, *et al.* Tetrodotoxin: chemistry, toxicity, source, distribution and detection. *Toxins (Basel)* 2014;**6**:693–755.

Cegolon L, Heymann WC, Lange JH, *et al.* Jellyfish stings and their management: a review. *Mar Drugs* 2013;**11**:523–50.

Eddleston M, Warrell D. Poisoning and envenoming. In: R Davidson, A Brent, A Seale (eds). *Oxford Handbook of Tropical Medicine*, 4th edn. Oxford: Oxford University Press; 2014. pp. 882–91.

Montgomery L, Seys J, Mees J. To pee or not to pee: a review on envenomation and treatment in European jellyfish species. *Mar Drugs* 2016;**14**:127.

3.14.5

Ballistic Injuries

Tim Hartley

Keywords: ballistic injury, intensive care, gunshot wound, blast radius, barotrauma

Introduction

Whilst encounters with patients who have sustained ballistic injuries and trauma are relatively rare in the UK, intensivists are often involved in their care, either in the assessment and resuscitation stage in the emergency department or subsequently on/after admission to the ICU. Knowledge of the different types of ballistic trauma and initial and ongoing management of such patients are therefore important.

Categories of Blast Injuries

The categories of blast injuries can be seen in Figure 3.14.5.1.

Primary Blast Injury

These are caused by blast wave 'overpressure' on tissues and organs. Associated injuries include those seen in Table 3.14.5.1.

Secondary Blast Injury

These are caused by high-energy fragments, from bomb casings, debris or projectiles. These tend to cause penetrating and soft tissue injuries but can also cause fractures. There may also be a risk of viral transmission from fellow victims or suicide bombers.

Tertiary Blast Injury

These are caused by the body being thrown by the blast wind. Injuries include fractures, head injuries and traumatic amputations.

Quaternary Blast Injury

These are injuries caused by everything else. Examples include: burns, trauma from falling debris, acute coronary syndromes, acute asthma attacks and inhalation of toxic fumes.

Table 3.14.5.1 Primary blast injuries

Type of trauma	Examples of injuries
Pulmonary barotrauma	Pulmonary contusion, pneumothorax, haemothorax, air embolism, fat embolism, acute respiratory distress syndrome
Abdominal barotrauma	Bowel perforation, haemorrhage, solid organ laceration, bowel necrosis
Acoustic barotrauma	Tympanic membrane rupture, ossicle fracture, haemotympanum
Traumatic amputation	Of any limb or digit

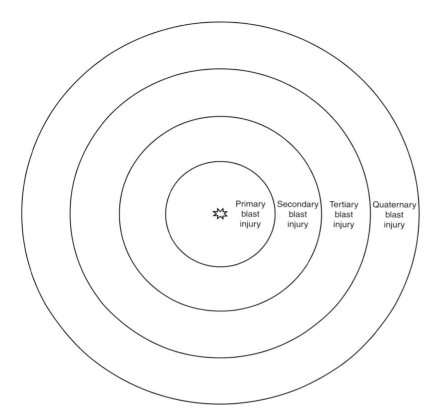

Figure 3.14.5.1 Categories of blast injuries.

Gunshot Wounds

Gunshot wounds are increasingly encountered in the Western world; thus, knowledge of their pathophysiology is important. There are two major mechanisms of injury that occur via a gunshot wound: crushing tissue destruction by the path of the projectile, and stretching and shock by the formation of a temporary cavity. A temporary cavity is formed by a preceding shock wave, which forces tissue away from the course of the projectile. It is important to note that this shock wave can also cause damage to the area surrounding the temporary cavity and tissue necrosis, haemorrhage or fractures can occur.

Gunshot wounds usually become infected quickly due to the negative pressure exerted by the temporary cavity pulling in environmental debris and skin organisms. It is essential to consider prophylactic antibiotic usage in all cases.

The path of a bullet is very unpredictable and, as such, must be extensively investigated radiologically to see the full path and extent of the damage. Also keep in mind secondary missiles such as bone fragments, bullet fragments and teeth.

Treatment Steps for Management of a Patient with Ballistic Injuries

Treatment of patients with ballistic injuries can be simplified into three main steps (Figure 3.14.5.2).

Step 1: Resuscitation and Primary Surgery

The first steps of treatment are done in the pre-hospital setting, the emergency department and the operating theatre. The main aims are to fluid-resuscitate, control haemorrhage, control contamination and minimise abnormal physiology.

Step 2: Restoration of Normal Physiology in the Intensive Care Unit

There are three main physiological areas that need to be addressed by the ICU team in the ballistic trauma patient: acidosis, hypothermia and coagulopathy.

Acidosis

Adequate oxygen delivery is imperative in trying to establish restoration of normal physiology. Haemoglobin levels, oxygen carriage and cardiac output all need to be normalised for adequate oxygenation and reversal of acidosis.

Hypothermia

Hypothermia inhibits enzymes in the clotting cascade. Correcting hypothermia reduces coagulopathy and contributes to improved survival in patients with exsanguinating penetrating abdominal injuries.

Coagulopathy

There are a number of factors that may be responsible for coagulopathy in the ballistic trauma patient, including massive transfusion, dilution, hypothermia and disseminated intravascular coagulation. It is therefore essential to correct any abnormality early and support all areas of the clotting cascade to achieve haemostasis.

Step 3: Return to Theatre

If appropriate, the patient may need to be taken back to theatre for removal of packs, closure of wounds, washouts or less urgent surgery.

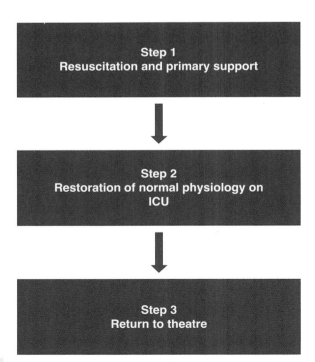

Figure 3.14.5.2 The three treatment steps for the patient with ballistic injuries.

Intensive Care Management of the Patient with Ballistic Injuries

On Admission to the Intensive Care Unit

- **Thorough repeat examination:** including log rolling of the patient and temporary removal of any supportive equipment, such as a hard collar, for visualisation. Investigate for wounds that may have been missed or upon signs of worsening injury and patient deterioration
- **Full history of the injury:** type of injury, type of weaponry, time of injury, other victims and any secondary injury occurred
- **Full history of all resuscitation:** care provided in the pre-hospital setting, resuscitation area and theatre; the amount of blood products, antibiotics, fluids, inotropes, tetanus, analgesics and sedatives given
- **Full review of all investigations already performed:** all radiological investigations and echocardiography must be reviewed. It is important for the ICU team to understand all projectile trajectories to ensure all injuries have been identified. All blood investigations must also be reviewed, paying close attention to haemoglobin levels, coagulation parameters, pH, lactate levels, base deficit and bicarbonate levels. Ensure adequate cross-matching of the patient's blood has been done
- **Full medical history from the patient or relatives:** past medical history, past surgical history, drug history and allergies. If the patient is incapacitated, then try to obtain this from the patient's friends or relatives
- **Reassessment of all invasive lines and support equipment:** definitive securing of the endotracheal tube, if present, and its placement checked with X-ray; central line and arterial line placement checked and properly secured, and peripheral intravenous lines changed. Chest drains checked for security; placement and drainage monitored. Urinary catheter placed, if not already done. Any further drains to be assessed and monitored
- **Insertion of invasive cardiac monitoring equipment:** useful if there is anticipated large-volume resuscitation and to determine the need for inotropes
- **Discussion with different specialties:** there should be a multidisciplinary approach to

the patient's treatment, including surgery, haematology and radiology teams

- **Repetitive examination is a necessity:** further injuries, such as compartment syndrome, may develop. Regular examination of the patient is therefore a necessity
- **Family update:** relatives should be updated and allowed to visit the patient if appropriate

Ongoing Care in the Intensive Care Unit

Ongoing ICU care is a multidisciplinary approach. Repeat examinations and assessments should be performed by all specialties, and their directed investigations are necessary for the well-being of the patient. Some considerations for the ICU team are mentioned below:

- **Analgesia and sedation:** adequate analgesia and sedation for the patient must be considered, and sedation holidays are important to further assess the patient's neurological state
- **Inotropic support:** it is important to maintain sufficient mean arterial pressure. Invasive and non-invasive methods can direct the clinician to decide which inotropes are appropriate for ongoing support
- **Repetitive blood work:** haemoglobin levels, coagulation parameters, infective markers, renal and liver function, pH, gas exchange and lactate levels should all be repeated at regular intervals
- **Chest X-ray:** ongoing chest radiographs are useful in the early detection of acute respiratory distress syndrome (ARDS), pneumonia, pneumothorax and effusions
- **Cardiac monitoring:** regular electrocardiography and directed echocardiography help pick up arrhythmias and cardiac ischaemia
- **Ventilatory modes:** frequent measurements of gas exchange, compliance and regular X-rays help decide the pressure and mode of ventilation in the sedated patient. Muscle relaxants may also be necessary to achieve adequate ventilation
- **Anticoagulation:** deep vein thrombosis prophylaxis should be considered in all patients; however, thought needs to be assigned to ongoing surgical treatment, occult haemorrhage and spinal cord or solid organ injury. Compression stockings and devices should be used where appropriate

- **Nutritional support:** malnutrition has been shown to increase susceptibility to poor wound healing and poor immunological response. Enteral or parenteral nutrition should therefore be started as soon as is appropriate
- **Stress gastritis prophylaxis:** this should be considered in all patients
- **Glucose control:** maintenance of euglycaemia, whilst avoiding hypoglycaemic episodes, has been shown to reduce mortality in the intensive care patient
- **Antibiotics:** prophylactic antibiotics may be necessary, especially in gunshot wounds. This should be directed by ongoing cultures and microbiology advice
- **Hypothermia:** normothermia is essential for cessation of non-surgical bleeding by helping the enzymes involved in the coagulation cascade. Use of internal temperature probes is advised. Passive and active warming methods can be used – blankets, warming blankets, fluid warmers, humidified ventilator circuits and body cavity lavage if appropriate
- **Intra-abdominal pressure monitoring:** patients with intra-abdominal injuries, or who have received massive volume resuscitation, should have intra-abdominal pressures measured frequently to pick up abdominal compartment syndrome early. This can be done easily via the intravesicular route

References and Further Reading

Brett S. Blast injury and gunshot wounds: pathophysiology and principles of management. In: AD Bersten, N Soni (eds). *Oh's Intensive Care Manual*, 6th edn. Elsevier; 2009. pp. 867–76.

Frangos SG, Freitas M, Frankel H. Intensive care of the trauma patient with ballistic injuries. In: PF Mahoney, JM Ryan, CW Schwab (eds). *Ballistic Trauma*. London: Springer; 2005. pp. 445–64.

Goorah S, Hindocha S. Management of ballistic soft tissue injuries: a review. *IOSR Journal of Dental and Medical Sciences* 2013;**8**:28–35.

Hull JB, Bowyer GW, Cooper GJ, *et al.* Pattern of injury in those dying from traumatic amputation caused by bomb blast. *Br J Surg* 1994;**81**:1132–5.

Rabinovici R, Frankel H, Kaplan L. Trauma evaluation and resuscitation. *Cure Probl Surg* 2003;**40**:599–681.

3.15.1 Capacity and Consent Issues in Intensive Care

Ruth Taylor and Peter Byrne

Key Learning Points

1. The four components of capacity concern a patient's ability to understand, retain, weigh and communicate a decision.
2. It is the responsibility of the lead clinician to ensure that capacity has been assessed and to make the final decision regarding capacity, even where a professional opinion has been sought.
3. The Mental Capacity Act (MCA) 2005 allows treatment of patients for MEDICAL conditions only, under the 'best interests' principle.
4. All patients admitted to the intensive care unit should be considered at risk of deprivation of liberty, and a Deprivation of Liberty Safeguards (DoLS) assessment should be considered.
5. The Mental Health Act (MHA; 1983) allows treatment of patients for PSYCHIATRIC conditions only.

Keywords: capacity, restraint, MCA, best interests, liberty

Introduction

Informed consent describes a process of communication between a clinician and a patient that results in the patient agreeing or refusing to undergo a specific intervention.

To give informed consent, a patient must have mental capacity to make this decision.

If there are concerns around a patient's capacity to consent, then a capacity assessment must be carried out. In emergency medical situations, urgent decisions and immediate action must be taken in the patient's best interests.

The use of patient restraints is commonly deployed under relevant legislation to facilitate safe intensive care. This section provides an overview of current legislation.

'Lacks Capacity'

A person lacks capacity if:

- They have an impairment or a disturbance that affects the way their mind or brain works *and*
- The impairment means that they are unable to make a specific decision at the time it needs to be made

Capacity is decision-specific – at a particular time, a person may have capacity to make some decisions, but not others.

Loss of capacity may be partial or temporary and may change over time. Other patients, e.g. those with irreversible brain injury, may always lack capacity to make some types of decisions.

A person is unable to make a decision if they cannot:

1. **Understand** information about the decision to be made
2. **Retain** that information in their mind
3. **Weigh** that information as part of the decision-making process or
4. **Communicate** (their decision)

The Assessment Process

The starting assumption should always be that the person *has capacity* to make the decision.

They must be provided with all relevant information they need to make a decision in a way that is appropriate to the individual, as well as be made aware of all the different options.

The test of capacity is two-stage:

- **First:** proof is required to show that the person has an impairment of the mind or brain, or a disturbance that affects the way their mind or brain works

- ○ Examples include: dementia, learning difficulties, effects of brain damage, medical conditions causing confusion, drowsiness or loss of consciousness, delirium, concussion, alcohol or drug intoxication and some conditions associated with mental illness
- **Second:** does the impairment or disturbance mean that the person is unable to make a specific decision when they need to?

Who Should Assess Capacity?

If a doctor proposes a treatment, they must assess the person's capacity to consent. It is the responsibility of every clinician to ensure that capacity has been assessed.

For more complex decisions, a professional opinion by a psychiatrist, for example, might be necessary.

The final decision must be made by the person intending to carry out the treatment, *not* the advising professional.

Following a Capacity Assessment

1. If the person passes the test of capacity and has made the right decision, then the decision is respected.
2. If the person passes the test of capacity but has NOT made the right decision, explain that the best possible decision has not been made, express concerns, make clear the decision is contrary to medical advice, encourage further consideration of the decision and offer further information and support. The decision made by the patient must be respected, and reasonable alternatives offered.
3. If the test of capacity is not passed, the person may be treated under the Mental Capacity Act (MCA) 2005.

The Mental Capacity Act 2005 (England and Wales)

The MCA provides the legal framework for acting and making decisions on behalf of individuals who lack mental capacity to make particular decisions for themselves.

The MCA has five statutory principles:

1. A person is assumed to have capacity unless it is established that they lack capacity.

2. Lack of capacity is established only if all practical steps to help the person make a decision have failed, e.g. interpreters or visual aids for people who cannot read.
3. Lack of capacity cannot be assumed on the basis of an unwise decision.
4. An act or decision must be made in the person's best interests.
5. The least restrictive option must have been considered.

The MCA provides a checklist to cover when acting in a person's best interests:

- Encourage participation of the person lacking capacity.
- Try to identify all relevant circumstances.
- Consider the person's views, beliefs, values and other personal factors.
- Avoid discrimination based on age, appearance, condition or behaviour.
- Assess whether the person might regain capacity.
- If decisions concern life-sustaining treatment, they must not be motivated by a desire to bring about death.
- Consult others (e.g. relatives, friends) and whether there is an appropriate lasting power of attorney, any deputy of the court of protection or an Independent Mental Capacity Advocate (IMCA).
- Has the person made a relevant advance directive?
- Avoid restricting the person's rights.

These must be considered in order to decide what would be in the person's best interests *before* an action is taken.

The MCA provides those acting on behalf of patients who lack capacity with protection from liability. There are important limitations to this such as use of inappropriate restraint and when a person is deprived of their liberty.

Restraint

The action of restraint will be protected from liability *only* if:

1. The person taking the action believes it is necessary to prevent harm and
2. The amount or type of restraint is considered a proportionate response to the likelihood and seriousness of harm

Deprivation of Liberty

The MCA does not protect from liability an act that results in someone being deprived of their liberty, as defined by Article 5(1) of the European Convention on Human Rights.

The Mental Health Act (MHA) 2007 made amendments to the MCA 2005 to include Deprivation of Liberty Safeguards (DoLS).

Deprivation of Liberty Safeguards

DoLS came into force in 2009 (England and Wales) to provide protection for the human rights of vulnerable people who lack capacity to decide about their care and treatment.

A DoLS authorisation allows lawful deprivation of a person's liberty when they lack capacity.

Most patients in the ICU would be considered to be deprived of their liberty, except when:

- They have capacity to decide to be admitted to the ICU
- They consent to the restrictions applied to them
- They consented to ICU admission prior to losing capacity

  Note that those under the MHA 1983 are already subject to deprivation of liberty under that Act.

  Why deprive a patient of their liberty?

- To protect from harm
- Proportional response, compared to potential harm faced by the person
- No less restrictive alternative

Actions which constitute deprivation of liberty include:

- Restraint
- Medication/treatment against one's will
- Taking decisions on a person's behalf

Provision of life-sustaining treatment is allowed by the MCA, and not considered a deprivation of liberty.

Deprivation of Liberty Safeguards Authorisation

An application is made to the local authority to grant DoLS authorisation.

There are two types:

- Standard: granted within 21 days of application (lasts a maximum of 12 months, with regular review)
- Urgent: completed by hospital staff, takes immediate effect and lasts 7 days. There must be a simultaneous application for standard DoLS

Within intensive care, it is likely that all DoLS authorisations will initially be made as urgent authorisations.

Six Criteria for DoLS Authorisation

1. Age assessment: over 18 years?
2. Mental health assessment
3. Mental capacity assessment
4. Eligibility assessment: is (or should) the person be subject to treatment under the MHA 1983?
5. 'No refusals' assessment: has the person refused treatment or made a relevant advance decision?
6. Best interests assessment

The local authority may refuse a DoLS application if:

- There is a less restrictive option
- A DoLS is not felt to be in the patient's best interests
- The patient requires detention under the MHA 1983 (see 'The Mental Health Act 1983' section)

Summary of Recommendations for the Lead Clinician

- DoLS should not delay emergency treatment.
- Every patient in the ICU should be considered at risk of deprivation of liberty.
- DoLS should be regularly reviewed.
- Avoid DoLS and use least (less?) restrictive options when possible.
- Apply for urgent DoLS *and* standard DoLS as soon as possible.
- If DoLS does not authorise treatment, this is under the MCA principle of best interests.
- If DoLS refused, you cannot deprive a person of their liberty.
- Deaths of patients under DoLS must be reported to the coroner.

The Mental Health Act 1983

The MHA is designed to ensure the safety, protection and treatment of people with mental illness, and the MHA can be used only to treat psychiatric illness.

Detention of a patient under the MHA will be considered if:

1. They are suffering from a mental disorder of a nature or degree that warrants hospital admission for assessment and/or treatment
2. They ought to be detained in the best interests of their own health and safety or that of others

435

Treatment of physical illness in patients who lack capacity must be under the MCA.

The two exceptions, tested in the court, are:

1. Feeding and supplementation may be administered to a patient with anorexia nervosa under the MCA
2. It is also lawful to treat the effects of a disorder, e.g. overdose, in an emergency

Delirium can be treated under the MHA.

Patients may be admitted to the ICU under a Section of the MHA, or during admission, they may warrant a MHA assessment, and the psychiatric liaison team should be involved at the earliest opportunity.

Section 5(2): The Doctor's Holding Power

If there are immediate concerns about a patient and their safety, they can be placed on a Section 5(2), which takes immediate effect.

Any doctor is able to place a patient on a Section 5(2), according to the MHA 1983. However, individual trusts may have a policy in which a particular doctor is assigned for this.

Section 5(2) permits detention of a patient in hospital for 72 hours whilst a MHA assessment is arranged. It does not allow patients to be treated against their will.

Section 2: Admission to Hospital for Assessment

This allows detention in hospital for up to 28 days for assessment and/or treatment. The patient can appeal within 7 days, and a MHA tribunal will be arranged within 14 days of the commencement of the section.

Section 3: Admission to Hospital for Treatment

This allows detention in hospital for up to 6 months. For the first 3 months, the patient can be treated by the responsible clinician. Beyond this, another opinion must be sought from a second opinion approved doctor (SOAD).

A patient may be discharged early from a section by the responsible clinician or hospital managers, or following a tribunal or an appeal by the nearest relative.

References and Further Reading

Crews M, Garry D, Phillips C, *et al*. Deprivation of liberty in intensive care. *J Intensive Care Soc* 2014;**15**:320–4. www.mentalcapacitylawandpolicy.org.uk/wp-content/uploads/2014/04/1504320.pdf

Department of Constitutional Affairs. *Mental Capacity Act 2005: Code of Practice*. London: The Stationery Office; 2007. www.gov.uk/government/uploads/system/uploads/attachment_data/file/497253/Mental-capacity-act-code-of-practice.pdf

e-learning for healthcare. 2017. e-Learning deprivation of liberty safeguards. Health Education England in partnership with the Royal College of Psychiatrists. www.e-lfh.org.uk/programmes/deprivation-of-liberty-safeguards/

legislation.gov.uk. 1983. Mental Health Act 1983. www.legislation.gov.uk/ukpga/1983/20/contents

Macovei M. The right to liberty and security of the person. A guide to the implementation of Article 5 of the European Convention on Human Rights. Strasbourg: Council of Europe; 2002. web.archive.org/web/20110707041600/http://www.echr.coe.int/NR/rdonlyres/D7297F8F-88DB-42B0-A831-FB4D1223164A/0/DG2ENHRHAND052004.pdf

White DB. 2017. Ethics in the intensive care unit: informed consent. www.uptodate.com/contents/ethics-in-the-intensive-care-unit-informed-consent

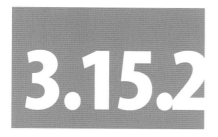

3.15.2

Managing Aggression in Intensive Care

Ruth Taylor and Peter Byrne

Key Learning Points

1. All busy hospitals receive violent patients. Staff should be trained in appropriate reduction and response practices. Make the environment as safe as possible, and plan for a 'worst case scenario'.
2. For patients who understand their behaviours, set limits to expressions of anger. Aggression must not compromise others' care.
3. Identify specific groups at risk of 'unpredictable aggression'.
4. Reducing aggression requires: (1) coordinated, multi-level action; (2) treatment of pain, review of medication and safe prescription of sedatives; (3) consistent nursing staff, extra staffing and a multidisciplinary team approach; (4) family involvement; and (5) psychiatric liaison.
5. After violent events, document and report events accurately, and debrief all staff involved.

Keywords: aggression, precipitants, risk, debrief

Introduction

All healthcare staff should receive training on how to respond to angry and aggressive patients. This includes:

- Management strategies for aggression:
  ○ Keep yourself safe: know your exit route from the bedside for each intervention; remove sharp objects and potential missiles
  ○ Keep other patients and staff safe
- Have clear escalation strategies, e.g. inform security about the individual, consider a visible security presence. If security cannot help, consult hospital managers and consider seeking police assistance. Consider the appropriate level of observation
- For many patients, a male primary nurse may be necessary
- Know your patient – past violence predicts future violence. Find the old notes, and seek out psychiatric summaries. Identify any pattern or triggers (e.g. attacks only female staff, hates noise, increased late night activity). Create a plan to anticipate aggression
- Some patients have little control over anger outbursts. Understanding *why* they are refusing treatments and acting out against staff will set the tone for how staff respond. In general, there is a spectrum of escalating aggression where the person is unable to control this (cognitive impairment, learning difficulties, psychosis)

Patients Who Understand Their Behaviours

Communication problems are often at the root of aggressive behaviour, including obvious issues such as language barriers.

Avoid jargon – frustration can be reduced by using simple lay terminology for technology and procedures.

Most people can articulate *why* they become angry, once they step back from the moment. Acknowledge anger without agreeing with the patient (e.g. 'I can see why this upsets you', rather than 'yes, that surgeon *is* incompetent').

Remain consistent that expressing anger (shouting, swearing, throwing things, assaults) is never acceptable on a hospital ward.

437

Possible Precipitants of Aggression (When There Is No Clear Precipitant)

- **Physical symptoms:** for example, pain, constipation, urinary symptoms/uncomfortable catheter, immobility, too hot or too cold
- **Pharmacology:** for example, stimulant drugs, paradoxical effect of benzodiazepines, low glucose may contribute to agitation
- **Alcohol, smoking, drug use:** sudden/unplanned withdrawal can cause significant agitation. Consider substitutes, e.g. nicotine inhalator or electronic cigarette
- **The focus of anger:** is the anger related to a particular team, individual or event? Take any complaint seriously. Consider whether informal routes (e.g. explanation/apology/conversation with the relevant individual) may be appropriate and sufficient. Inform the patient of formal complaints procedures if appropriate
- **Aggression following adverse events (emergency admission, surgery):** consider whether the anger is proportionate to events. Consider the possibility of an untreated anxiety disorder. Consult relatives
- **Bipolar disorder patients:** patients who relapse can go 'high' with extreme irritability, perhaps precipitated by a traumatic event. Many medications contribute to relapse and propagation of manic symptoms: anti-retrovirals, steroids and other anti-immune medication, even antidepressants. Refer to the psychiatric team at the earliest possible time
- **Psychosis:** violence is not a symptom of psychosis, but its symptoms (paranoid ideas, disinhibition, activation by voices) sometimes make aggression more likely in stressful settings. Low doses of patients' usual anti-psychotics are useful here. Cognitive impairment is likely in angry patients who are disorientated and fluctuate (worse at night), and who cannot remember the cause of their distress or are disinhibited (frontal lobe involvement). Follow protocols for delirium – whether it is acute or acute-on-chronic (pre-existing dementia), basic management principles apply

Specific Groups at Risk of Unpredictable Aggression

Disproportionate anger might indicate abnormal personality traits (e.g. impulsivity, dissocial personality) and/or a pre-existing episode of depression. With some exceptions below, behaviours are modifiable and depression is always treatable.

Take time with the patient's family to learn about what usually happens when the patient is ill or restricted. List the person's usual relaxation routines, e.g. reading, music, television, computing – and try to incorporate these into the ICU.

These are especially useful as distraction techniques in patients who are retraumatised by the ICU (see 'Post-Traumatic Stress Disorder and ICU' section in Chapter 3.15.5).

Head Injury

New-onset cognitive impairment is a major challenge – it is unpredictable, even for close family. Agitation is associated with increased cerebral metabolic rate of oxygen consumption and should be managed with medication.

Intellectual (Formerly Learning) Disability

A spectrum from mild to severe – many will carry a 'patient passport', with likes and dislikes and pointers to persuading them towards interventions they may not understand. Some are also on the autistic spectrum and have problems with communication, new situations and changes to routine. Their frustrations will generally be directed at themselves, not others. Family and regular support workers will guide ICU staff. Familiar ICU staff and fixed routines (no moving) are helpful too.

Aggression Reduction

Consider the level of observation required for any patient deemed at risk of being aggressive.

To help identify triggers to aggression, and to help create personal interventions to reduce the behaviour, consider an ABC approach:

- **A**ntecedents – event or activity immediately preceding the behaviour
- **B**ehaviour – observation of the behaviour
- **C**onsequences – events that follow

Recognition of indicators that a person may *become* aggressive is important. These include:

- Changes in tone of voice and volume of speech
- Changes in posture and body language
- Psychomotor agitation, e.g. pacing or restlessness
- Inappropriate eye contact
- Verbal threats

Specific triggers may be routine (meals, changes of staff, bathing) or particular events (venesection, physiotherapy). Restrictions placed on a patient can cause anger and frustration.

Poor sleep will lower aggression thresholds. Ideal sleep happens at night (turning down machine alarms, earplugs, minimising nursing interventions). Avoid medications, such as benzodiazepines and Z drugs, that will lower thresholds further, impair cognition and give poor quality sleep.

When managing aggression, consider using 'rewards', e.g. quiet time, visitors, music/television time. Where practical, short periods off ICU (visitors' room even) can break the monotony.

For psychiatric liaison team referral, contact the team if aggression is thought to relate to a past psychiatric problem or if the person has become so aggressive that their behaviour requires pharmacological intervention. Psychiatric liaison can obtain the past psychiatric history, including treatments, build up relationships with families, create behavioural (ABC) charts and advise on pharmacology. Linking to existing services will help support admission in vulnerable patients with cognitive impairment, intellectual disability or psychiatric disorders.

Pharmacology

Pharmacology for aggression should be a last resort – after identification of underlying medical and/or psychiatric disorders and verbal de-escalation attempts.

Drugs are used to treat specific symptoms (insomnia, anxiety), not simply to sedate.

The ideal medication is short-acting, with parenteral administration, low side effects (especially cardiovascular) and minimal drug interactions.

Avoid benzodiazepines, unless there are alcohol/drug withdrawals or the patient is already addicted to them.

In emergencies, lorazepam 1–2 mg given intravenously may be necessary, but try to avoid this as a regular preparation – patients build up tolerance quickly.

These drugs/classes are especially useful in the ICU – all four can be used in extreme cases:

- Promethazine (anti-histamine) for night sedation, 25–50 mg oral/intramuscular
- Anti-psychotics (especially if delirium and/or paranoia) – olanzapine 2.5 mg, titrating upwards to a maximum of 15 mg as once-daily dose. Oral and dissolvable buccal preparations are available
- Use olanzapine *or* haloperidol, not both. Haloperidol is in the moderate group for prolongation of the QTc interval. The advantage is oral or IV preparations – older people will settle on low doses of haloperidol (0.5 mg given once at night), and most adults start on 1–2 mg at night. The IV preparation has twice the potency of the oral dose, and going beyond a total oral dose of 10 mg (5 mg IV equivalent) will not confer advantages, but only its potential toxicity: extra-pyramidal symptoms, cardiovascular effects
- Bespoke anti-psychotics for special populations: quetiapine for dementia of Lewy bodies (severe reactions seen with other anti-psychotics), amisulpride for people in liver failure

As with all anti-psychotics, give most of the dose at night and use sparingly by day.

Clonidine is an alpha-adrenergic blocker that is profoundly sedating and useful in haemodynamically stable patients who can tolerate its hypotensive and tachycardic effects. It can be given 4–6 times a day, starting at 25 µg and titrating upwards.

Valproate has a small evidence base for reducing aggression. It is never given to fertile women due to its teratogenicity. It is sedating, and the long-acting preparation at night-time at 500 mg, titrating upwards to a maximum of 2 g (send plasma levels), is useful as part of the other interventions listed above.

After the Event

Always make a clear note about violence – what, when and the response. New staff coming on shift, visiting colleagues and staff in the destination ward all need to know the details.

References and Further Reading

Hallman MR, Joffe AM. ICU management of traumatic brain injury. *Curr Anaesthesiol Rep* 2013;**3**:89–97.

Helmy A, Vizcaychipi M, Gupta AK. Traumatic brain injury: intensive care management. *Br J Anaesth* 2007;**99**:32–42.

National Institute for Health and Care Excellence. 2010. Delirium: prevention, diagnosis and management. Clinical guideline [CG103]. www.nice.org.uk/ guidance/cg103/chapter/1-guidance#treating-delirium

National Institute for Health and Care Excellence. 2015. Violence and aggression: short-term management in mental health, health and community settings. NICE guideline [NG10]. www.nice.org.uk/guidance/ ng10/chapter/recommendations#terms-used-in-this-guideline

National Institute for Health and Care Excellence. 2015. Challenging behaviour and learning disabilities: prevention and interventions for people with learning disabilities whose behaviour challenges. NICE guideline [NG11]. www.nice.org.uk/guidance/ng11/chapter/ 1-Recommendations#general-principles-of-care–2

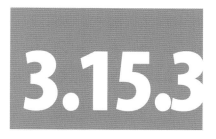

Overdose, Serotonin Syndrome and Neuroleptic Malignant Syndrome

Ruth Taylor and Peter Byrne

Key Learning Points

1. Features of overdose depend on the type of antidepressant or anti-psychotic agent taken.
2. All patients suspected of overdose must be monitored for QRS/QT prolongation.
3. In some overdoses (monoamine oxidase inhibitors, hypoglycaemic agents, long-acting insulin, anticoagulants), onset of symptoms may be delayed; an asymptomatic patient may still require admission and treatment in the intensive care unit.
4. Serotonin syndrome is a medical emergency defined as an adverse reaction to serotonergic agents.
5. Neuroleptic malignant syndrome is a medical emergency caused by an idiosyncratic reaction to neuroleptic medication.

Keywords: salicylate, anti-cholinergic, serotonergic agent, neuroleptics

Introduction

Psychiatric medications can be dangerous in overdose (OD), resulting in admission to the ICU. This section will provide an overview of the management and treatment of OD of antidepressants and anti-psychotics, including life-threatening conditions of serotonin syndrome (SS) and neuroleptic malignant syndrome (NMS).

Antidepressants

The features of OD depend on the type of antidepressant.

Signs and Symptoms

- **Selective serotonin reuptake inhibitors (SSRIs):** generally well tolerated, often no symptoms of OD, occasionally gastrointestinal (GI) symptoms. Seizures can occur but are rare. Prolongation of the QT interval can occur and is most likely with citalopram/escitalopram
- **Serotonin–noradrenaline reuptake inhibitors (SNRIs):** central nervous system (CNS) depression, seizures, tachycardia. Venlafaxine is associated with QRS prolongation and ventricular arrhythmias
- **Tricyclic antidepressants (TCAs):** symptoms generally occur within 6 hours. CNS depression, hypotension, seizures and anti-cholinergic toxicity. QRS prolongation is caused by sodium channel blockade, and QT prolongation is caused by potassium channel blockade
- **Monoamine oxidase inhibitors (MAOIs):** asymptomatic for many hours post-ingestion; may require admission to the ICU, although asymptomatic. After 24 hours, symptoms include tachycardia, hypertension, stroke, cardiovascular collapse with hypotension and bradycardia and CNS depression and seizures

Diagnosis

All patients suspected of OD should have:

- A 12-lead ECG
- Bloods, including full blood count (FBC), urea and electrolytes (U&Es), liver function tests (LFTs), glucose, C-reactive protein (CRP) and creatine kinase (CK)
- Paracetamol and salicylate levels
- Urinary drug screen (benzodiazepines will contribute to CNS depression)

History is key to diagnosis; however, supportive care should not be delayed whilst trying to obtain a history. The patient's family may be able to list available drugs or substance misuse; signs may point towards what agent has been taken – for example, anti-cholinergic symptoms with QT prolongation may suggest TCA OD.

Differential Diagnosis

This depends on exact signs and symptoms; seizures of any cause can present with similar features to OD. There are no confirmatory tests, and a urine drug screen cannot confirm or exclude an OD.

Management

The first step in any overdose is to secure the airway – endotracheal intubation may be required. Respiratory distress must be treated, followed by hypotension. Any patient with altered mental status should have capillary glucose checked. Subsequent management depends on the offending agent, examination findings and results of investigations.

General Points

- Supportive care is paramount.
- Monitor the 12-lead ECG for QRS and QT changes.
- Hyperthermia due to increased neuromuscular excitability should be treated with benzodiazepines ± neuromuscular blockade.
- **SSRIs:** patients usually discharged from the emergency department following an observation period (as per TOXBASE®). Treat isolated seizures with benzodiazepines.
- **SNRIs:** monitor as per TOXBASE®, specifically the ECG for QRS/QT changes.
- **TCAs:** treat hypotension with crystalloid fluid resuscitation ± vasopressors. Treat seizures with sodium bicarbonate and benzodiazepines. Treat QT prolongation with sodium bicarbonate bolus ± bicarbonate infusions, aiming for pH 7.5–7.55. If no response, hypertonic saline can be used. Lipid infusions are reserved for patients with profound haemodynamic instability.
- **MAOIs:** only treat hypertension if severe; treat with short-acting agents. Treat hypotension with fluids and infusion of vasopressor (indirect-acting vasopressors are unlikely to benefit, as hypotension is caused by depletion of pre-synaptic catecholamines).

Serotonin Syndrome

SS is an adverse reaction to serotonergic agents (5HT agonists), and is a manifestation of excessive stimulation of the CNS and peripheral serotonin receptors.

SS can range from mild symptoms to life-threatening illness.

Causes

SS can occur with therapeutic drug use, due to drug interactions, or drug OD. All antidepressants are implicated in SS; there is an increased risk with combination therapy and particularly MAOIs. Lithium can contribute to SS, and other drugs known to cause SS include analgesics (tramadol, pethidine, fentanyl, dextromethorphan), anti-emetics (ondansetron, metoclopramide) and recreational agents (cocaine, MDMA (3,4-methylenedioxymethamphetamine), amphetamine, LSD (lysergic acid diethylamide)).

Signs and Symptoms

A triad of autonomic instability, neuromuscular changes and fluctuating mental state. Not all features are required for a diagnosis.

- **Autonomic instability:** hypertension, tachycardia, mydriasis, excessive sweating, increased bowel sounds
- **Neuromuscular change:** tremor, clonus, ocular clonus, hypertonia, hyper-reflexia
- **Mental state changes:** anxiety, agitation, confusion, coma

Symptoms occur within 6 hours. Tremor, akathisia and diarrhoea are early features, and acute delirium is a feature in severe cases.

Diagnosis

Diagnosis is clinical – all suspected patients should have:

- Bloods – FBC, U&Es, LFTs, CK, toxicology screen
- Blood cultures
- Chest X-ray (CXR)
- CT head – if trauma, seizures or focal neurology
- Lumbar puncture

Differential Diagnoses

Include NMS, catatonia, dystonia, malignant hyperthermia, anti-cholinergic poisoning, recreational drug toxicity, encephalitis and rhabdomyolysis.

Management

The first step is to stop the offending agent. In large OD, activated charcoal may be used to prevent absorption. Supportive treatment to manage haemodynamic instability is the mainstay of treatment. Benzodiazepines can be given for agitation, and cyproheptadine can be used as an adjunct (do not give if anti-cholinergic toxicity is also present). Chlorpromazine can assist in reducing SS. Sedation, neuromuscular paralysis and ventilatory support may be required. Severe hyperthermia should be managed with paralysis, ventilation and ice baths.

Complications include:
- Hyperthermia-induced metabolic acidosis
- Seizures
- Aspiration pneumonia
- Respiratory failure

Prognosis

Most deaths occur within the first 24 hours. However, if diagnosed and treated promptly, then the outcome is good.

Anti-psychotics

Anti-psychotics can be divided into typical and atypical agents.

The typical agents (e.g. haloperidol, chlorpromazine, prochlorperazine) generally have a high affinity for the D_2 receptor.

Atypical agents (e.g. olanzapine, risperidone, clozapine, aripiprazole, quetiapine) have less affinity for dopamine receptors, and higher affinity for serotonin receptors. The symptoms of OD are generally an exaggeration of the adverse effects observed at therapeutic doses.

Signs and Symptoms

Presentations vary between agents; each drug has different binding affinities to the different receptors, which predict the effects observed in OD.
- H_1 antagonism: leads to CNS depression
- Anti-cholinergic effects: urinary retention, altered mental state, tachycardia, hyperpyrexia, dry mucous membranes (with the exception of clozapine, which presents with sialorrhoea)
- Hypotension
- QT prolongation
- Seizures (all anti-psychotics lower the seizure threshold)
- Extra-pyramidal side effects occur, including akathisia and acute dystonia. Rarely, pharyngeal or laryngeal muscle spasm can cause respiratory distress

Diagnosis

There are no confirmatory tests – all patients with suspected OD should be investigated, as described in 'Antidepressants' section.

Management

As outlined above in 'Antidepressants' section, the first step is to secure an airway and provide supportive treatment. Subsequent management depends on the offending agent and the status of the patient. Patients with a QT interval of >500 ms should be given 2–4 g of magnesium sulphate. Seizures should be treated with benzodiazepines, and refractory seizures with phenobarbital.

Neuroleptic Malignant Syndrome

NMS is rare, but potentially life-threatening. It is caused by an idiosyncratic reaction to neuroleptic drugs associated with central D_2 receptor blockade. It presents as a diagnostic challenge, given its shared features with SS and malignant hyperthermia.

Causes

NMS is caused by the use of neuroleptic drugs, most commonly (but not always) at initiation or following dose increase. Risk factors for the development of NMS include:
- Genetic susceptibility
- Metabolic susceptibility
- High-dose anti-psychotic depot preparations
- Agitation
- High ambient temperature
- Dehydration
- History of NMS
- Other agents implicated include:
  - Promethazine
  - Metoclopramide
  - Lithium

Signs and Symptoms

Onset is usually gradual over 1–3 days, and symptoms can persist for 5–10 days after discontinuation of the offending drug (up to 21 days if depot medication).

Patients may complain of dyspnoea, dysphagia, gait problems and tremor.

Signs include pyrexia, muscular rigidity (always present), altered mental state (agitation and confusion), autonomic instability, pallor, tachycardia, fluctuating blood pressure, excessive sweating, tremor and incontinence.

443

Diagnosis

Diagnosis of NMS is clinical. Diagnostic features include:

- Neuroleptics within 1–4 weeks
- Hyperthermia
- Muscle rigidity
- Five of the following:
  - Raised CK
  - Altered mental state
  - Tachycardia
  - Fluctuating blood pressure
  - Tremor
  - Incontinence
  - Diaphoresis or sialorrhoea
  - Metabolic acidosis
  - Leucocytosis, mostly neutrophil peaks that mirror the rise in CK

If NMS is suspected, the following investigations should be undertaken:

- Bloods
- CK – raised
- FBC – leucocytosis
- U&Es – acute kidney injury (AKI)
- Serum calcium – hypocalcaemia
- LFTs – raised transaminases and lactate dehydrogenase
- Clotting
- Urine myoglobin
- Blood cultures
- CXR
- CT head
- ± lumbar puncture

Management

As with SS, the first step is to stop the offending drug. Supportive treatment is the mainstay of treatment, as described in sections above.

Additionally, points of consideration include:

- Physical restraint should be avoided/minimised as it can worsen hyperthermia
- Cooling devices to treat hyperthermia
- If evidence of rhabdomyolysis and AKI, alkalinisation of urine and dialysis may be required
- In severe cases, dopaminergic drugs (bromocriptine, amantadine) and muscle relaxants (dantrolene) may be used, although there is limited evidence regarding their efficacy
- Electroconvulsive therapy (ECT) may be considered if medication fails

  Complications include:

- Cardiac arrest
- Rhabdomyolysis
- AKI (due to rhabdomyolysis and dehydration)
- Seizures
- Disseminated intravascular coagulopathy
- Deterioration in mental state following withdrawal of anti-psychotics
- Hepatic failure
- Pulmonary embolism

Prognosis

Prognosis is good when there is early detection and treatment. Mortality is around 10 per cent. However, AKI increases mortality up to 50 per cent. Death is usually caused by cardiovascular or respiratory collapse and arrhythmias.

References and Further Reading

Ambulkar RP, Patil VP, Moiyadi AV. Neuroleptic malignant syndrome: a diagnostic challenge. *J Anaesthesiol Clin Pharmacol* 2012;**28**:517–19.

Boyer EW, Shannon M. The serotonin syndrome. *N Engl J Med* 2005;**352**:1112–20.

Kateon H. Differentiating serotonin syndrome and neuroleptic malignant syndrome. *Mental Health Clinician* 2013;**3**:129–33.

National Organization for Rare Disorders. 2004. Neuroleptic malignant syndrome. rarediseases.org/rare-diseases/neuroleptic-malignant-syndrome/

Sternbach H. The serotonin syndrome. *Am J Psychiatry* 1991;**148**:705–13.

3.15.4

Suicidal Patients in Intensive Care

Ruth Taylor and Peter Byrne

Key Learning Points

1. Emergency medical treatment should not be delayed and is provided in the patient's best interests.
2. Informed consent must be sought for further medical interventions. Capacity assessments are carried out where necessary.
3. A risk assessment should be carried out at the earliest opportunity, whether the patient is conscious or not.
4. Intensive care staff work closely with the psychiatry team to provide combined medical and psychiatric care.
5. Ongoing training for intensive care staff caring for psychiatric patients improves confidence and reduces risk.

Keywords: self-harm, suicidal, risk, psychology

Introduction

Whether post-overdose or suicide attempt, or new suicidal ideas, the suicidal patient in the ICU presents challenges in management for ICU staff. Capacity and consent issues require careful consideration, and treatment must be provided under the correct legal framework.

Following a suicide attempt, factors associated with an increased risk of ICU admission include:

- Drug overdose
- Older age
- History of suicide attempts
- Life-threatening injuries

Management of Patients Admitted to the ICU Following a Suicide Attempt

The patient's physical health comes first, and emergency treatment should not be delayed.

The psychiatry liaison team should be involved at the earliest opportunity. They should be involved whether or not the patient is conscious, to both advise on risk management and contact the community psychiatry team for further information on the patient.

Medical Management

Emergency Treatment

Emergency treatment should be provided, and the patient stabilised. This can be done without consent under the principle of (the patient's) best interests.

Further Medical Care

Where a patient is unconscious, they can be treated under the Mental Capacity Act (MCA) 2005, following the principle of best interests. Informed consent should be sought from the patient at the earliest opportunity. Document capacity (present or not) for each important decision.

A conscious patient who refuses treatment complicates capacity assessment, especially in the context of ongoing suicidality. A psychiatrist should assess whether there is a mental disorder and whether this affects the patient's decision to refuse treatment. The Mental Health Act (MHA) 1983 provides a legal basis to treat mental disorders and their effects, including overdose (e.g. antidotes and supportive treatments to preserve life).

Psychiatric Management

Contact the psychiatry liaison team for a psychiatric assessment to ascertain:

- Evidence of mental disorders
- Ongoing suicidal intent
- Immediate and medium-term risks
  Following assessment, the patient may:
- Agree to stay in hospital and accept treatment on an informal basis

- Refuse admission and treatment, and have capacity to do so
- Be found to be suffering from a mental illness, and lack capacity to make decisions about *psychiatric* care. Under these circumstances, they can be detained under an appropriate Section of the MHA 1983

In the context of fluctuating mental states (voices, delusions, varying mood or anxiety), capacity to make decisions can change and should be regularly reviewed.

ICU staff may need to contact the on-call doctor to assess a patient for a MHA Section 5(2) if there are immediate concerns for the patient. This authorises detention of a patient in hospital for up to 72 hours, to allow a MHA assessment by two senior doctors and an approved mental health professional (AMHP). All three must agree to achieve legal detention under MHA 'Section'. The patient can be sectioned to either or both a general hospital and the person's local psychiatric unit.

Risk Assessment and Management

Immediate and further risks to the patient and to others must be assessed and kept under review.

Following a suicide attempt, general risk management suggestions include:

- Not leaving the patient alone. A 1:1 registered mental health nurse (RMN) may be required
- Making clear the level of observation – if concerned, specify 'eye-level observation 24/7'
- Removing potential means of making further self-harm attempts
- Balancing the level of observation of the patient against privacy and dignity
- Encouraging the patient to engage with staff – recording what the patient says
- Speaking to relatives and friends. Even if the patient refuses requests to disclose information, we can still receive and record important information about them
- Considering admission to a psychiatric unit by persuasion or using MHA 1983

Short-Term Management

The patient needs ongoing support and regular review from the psychiatry liaison team.

If the patient is known to a community mental health team, advice can be sought from the local consultant regarding management.

Where mental disorder is evident, it should be treated with appropriate medication and psychological therapies, in accordance with the National Institute for Health and Care Excellence (NICE) guidelines.

- Emotional support – 1:1 nursing can also provide emotional support. Family members should be involved where possible
- Pharmacology requires special consideration if the patient has previously taken an overdose. Advice should be sought from the psychiatry team
- Brief psychological therapy. ICU is not always an appropriate setting, but it is still important to consider and facilitate such therapies, if possible

Long-Term Management

The full mental health multidisciplinary team should be involved to ensure a biopsychosocial approach to management of the patient. The patient should be made aware of how they can access help if there is another crisis, including 24-hour crisis support.

On discharge from the ICU, the full psychiatric management plan and risk assessment can be clearly handed over to nursing staff on the receiving ward. Staff should know to contact the psychiatry liaison team if they have any concerns.

Staff Attitudes

Clinical staff attitudes towards patients who self-harm, and their knowledge about self-harm and psychiatric patients, have been shown to influence clinical practice, as well as patients' experience and outcomes.

Studies show that general hospital staff can hold negative views of patients who self-harm, which mirrors the patients' experience of care. Negative attitudes are more common amongst doctors than nursing staff. Appropriate staff training has a positive impact on both staff and patients.

Support for ICU Staff

Physical health nurses receive little training in looking after psychiatric patients and patients following a suicide attempt. ICU staff should be supported to manage personal reactions, attitudes and beliefs towards patients and to develop a collaborative and therapeutic relationship with the patient.

Senior nurses in the psychiatry liaison team may provide teaching for physical health nurses to help them manage patients on their ward.

Support for Family Members

Admission to the ICU is distressing for family and friends, particularly following a suicide attempt. Families can be angry, perplexed, hurt and/or anxious about what happens next.

Whilst arrangements vary amongst hospitals, support and information are available from:

- ICU-attached psychologist
- The psychiatric liaison team
- ICU relative support team
- The charity ICUsteps (www.icusteps.org)

References and Further Reading

Bongar B, Berman AL, Maris RW, Silverman MM, Packman W, Harris EA. *Risk Management with Suicidal Patients.* New York, NY: The Guildford Press; 1998.

Davidhizar R, Vance A. The management of the suicidal patient in a critical care unit. *J Nurs Manage* 1993;**1**: 95–102.

Saunders KEA, Hawton K, Fortune S, Farrell S. Attitudes and knowledge of clinical staff regarding people who self-harm: a systematic review. *J Affect Disord* 2012;**139**:205–16.

Walker X, Lee J, Koval L, *et al*. Predicting ICU admissions from attempted suicide presentations at an Emergency Department in Central Queensland. *Australas Med J* 2013;**6**:536–41.

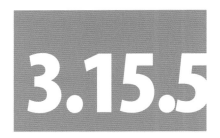

3.15.5 Anxiety, Psychological Trauma and the Difficult Patient in Intensive Care

Ruth Taylor and Peter Byrne

Key Learning Points

1. No one chooses to become an intensive care patient – adjusting well draws both on coping skills and on experienced, empathic staff to help vulnerable people.

2. Anxiety is the norm, not the exception, in a busy, noisy ICU. Even high-standard ICU care can bring back memories of previous bad experiences, especially psychological traumas such as childhood abuse.

3. Early identification of anxiety disorders (including trauma-generated) and multi-level interventions will reduce anxiety amongst patients, their carers and staff.

4. Experienced ICU staff deal with a range of personality traits and diverse reactions to illness. Staff supporting one another is the most effective intervention.

5. Up to 25 per cent of discharged ICU patients have post-traumatic stress disorder (PTSD) symptoms – there are subgroups more likely to get PTSD and minimising ICU benzodiazepine use has been shown to diminish it.

Keywords: PTSD, relaxation, insomnia, splitting, personality

Anxiety

High stress level and anxiety are generated by unexpected, unwanted admission to the ICU. Anxiety is increased by machine sounds, instrumentation (needles, suction) and ICU activity that professionals perceive as routine. Anxiety, defined as being 'prolonged and/or out of proportion with the perceived threat', is best understood as comprising two components:

- **Cognitive:** fearful (of real or perceived threat), poor concentration, difficulty relaxing, sensitive to noise, racing thoughts (in people with obsessionality as a trait, ruminations and obsessions) and irritability

- **Physical:** dry mouth, abdominal discomfort ('butterflies'), difficulty breathing (at extreme, during a panic attack, hyperventilation with tetany/contracture of the hands), chest restriction, palpations (tachycardia), dizziness, tremor, urinary frequency and insomnia

Management of Anxiety

When questioning patients about anxiety, engage patients first with open questions (inviting any response, e.g. 'do you want to ask me anything? Are you OK? Are you worried about something?'), and then move to closed questions seeking a specific answer. Ask in detail about previous hospital experiences and, if rapport builds, previous stressful life events that may mirror current anxiety: 'does this remind you of something that happened to you before?'. Talking usually helps, but document if reassurance lasts for seconds, rather than minutes/hours.

If anxiety is long-standing, the patient may have 'paired' physical sensations they are experiencing now with past anxiety episodes. Some of these may have been generated by current medication: dry mouth (anti-cholinergics), tachycardia (bronchodilators), abdominal discomfort (lipid-lowering drugs), urinary frequency (diuretics), etc. Explain that these things happen for appropriate reasons, and try to 'unpair' them from the person's ongoing anxiety. Explain that stress is best understood as an emotional state that happens when our perception of what we must overcome (illness) is overwhelmed by our perception of our ability (reserve) to overcome it. Human nature overestimates the threat and underestimates our reserves. Challenging these thoughts is a great start. Be proactive.

- Identify each individual's stress reduction activities (hobbies, activities, which of their visitors), and help them schedule these.
- Relaxation exercises are useful – slow breathing, mindfulness techniques.
- Cut down ICU noise, give earplugs by night and minimise night-time interruptions; consider giving morning medications later, if possible.
- Mind your language – it is better to talk of agreed solutions or respond to 'setbacks' that are part of ICU experience, rather than 'complications' or 'doctors running out of options'. Tell patients what usually happens (anonymise a patient's experience), to avoid their default response of uncertainty and worry.

Insomnia

Anxious people have difficulty getting to sleep (too much to think/worry about) and have broken sleep during the night. Depressed patients experience early morning wakening, characteristically with their mood worse at the start of each day (diurnal mood variation). For anxious patients, a vicious cycle begins of poor sleep by night and excessive worrying and activation by day. Their inner turmoil is noticeable, but we often overlook anxiety's distressing adrenaline-driven physical effects (see above).

Treating Insomnia

- Cut down noise.
- Dim lights at night.
- Visible clocks orientate patients by day but lead to 'clock watching' insomnia at night.
- Ration caffeine – tea or coffee after 6 p.m. will keep people awake.
- Consider nicotine replacement therapy doses (and timings) in smokers.
- Review medications that may affect sleep – antidepressants, such as some selective serotonin reuptake inhibitors (SSRIs) and venlafaxine, should not be given at night.
- Try to keep your patient awake and active by day – rigorous physiotherapy mobilises and promotes sleep.

In terms of medications, avoid benzodiazepines and Z drugs (zopiclone, zolpidem), which provide poor-quality sleep and risk tolerance and addiction. Promethazine or quetiapine (licensed in anxiety) has been found to be useful.

Patients who remain anxious despite these interventions may be clinically depressed (most common cause of new anxiety in people aged over 40, and treatable) or have a history of psychological trauma and post-traumatic stress disorder (PTSD).

Post-Traumatic Stress Disorder and ICU

Around one in four patients experience PTSD post-ICU admission. Evidence shows a link between ICU admission and PTSD, irrespective of the events leading to ICU admission.

ICU patients are at risk of PTSD as they suffer life-threatening illness, undergo stressful procedures and interventions and receive a cocktail of psychoactive medications. It is likely that ICU-related PTSD results from a complex interaction of the following factors:

- Long-term sedation
- Sleep disturbance
- Delirium
- Memory of the ICU experience, including delusional memories
- Changes in regulation of the adrenal axis (due to administration of corticosteroids and catecholamines)

Increased benzodiazepine use and increased psychological distress seem to be the biggest risk factors for developing PTSD. However, other risk factors include female gender, previous psychiatric history and longer duration of stay in the ICU.

Interventions

Studies suggest that psychological support for patients in the ICU can reduce the prevalence of PTSD. However, the National Institute for Health and Care Excellence (NICE) advises not to use cognitive behavioural therapy (CBT) within 1 month of symptoms. Psychological care should be proactive. Simple changes in nursing practice are likely to improve psychological outcomes, and relieve fear and worry through caring behaviour. ICU diaries, which record the patient's stay, including pictures shown to the patient 1 month post-discharge, can help them make sense of their stay. This has been shown to have a positive effect; however, evidence is limited. Strategies to reduce sleep disturbance and restore physiological sleep patterns, reduce delirium and optimise analgesia and sedation should be routine. Most importantly, limit use of benzodiazepines and sedation where possible.

Difficult Patients in ICU

ICU admission imposes restrictions on an individual, with uncertainty about when or if their stay will end. Anxious patients may have dependence traits, reaching out excessively for reassurance. Avoidant patients are likely to be silent and unlikely to interact until in crisis. Others (schizotypal, paranoid) have different inner worlds, with faulty reality testing focused on the least important detail of information/interventions. Most, however, know their responses are not helping, and staff should acknowledge this without them losing face. Medication rarely helps.

Dissocial (Antisocial) Personality Disorder

Characteristics include a disregard for the rights of others and lack of empathy or guilt for actions. They are unlikely to feel remorse and will blame others for past negative consequences of their actions. In the ICU, they have a need to feel 'special'.

Responses and rules must be clear and consistent across the team.

- Patients need to be made aware of the impact of their behaviours on other patients and staff.
- Set limits, and document excessive demands; repeat what has been agreed, and avoid splitting (staff turned against each other by manipulation).
- Be clear about rules/procedures that prioritise tasks, and that sometimes others need assistance before they do.
- Under-stimulate both their sense of entitlement and expressions of rage.

Abuse and aggression need clear responses (sanctions, hospital security, police), and if ignored, serious violence may result.

Most will behave as they do when incarcerated – as 'model prisoners' who know how to get the most out of the system. The exception to this is those who have borderline traits and behaviours.

Borderline (Emotionally Unstable) Personality Disorder

Characterised by unstable relationships (absent social boundaries, love–hate interactions), affect (mood swings, but not bipolar mood disorder) and impulsivity (bad decisions, self-harm). Collateral history from close relatives or partner will identify abnormal past behaviours and likely flashpoints. General practice or local psychiatric service may provide a summary of what to expect. Liaison psychiatry are not usually contacted in the early stages.

Consider the following:

- A person with borderline traits can bring out the worst in staff and evoke anger, even punitive behaviours from caring staff, with the patient concluding: 'I told you that X (staff member, previously idealised) does not like me'
- Think about risk of self-harm or violence to others – past behaviours (suicide attempts, charges for violence) predict future behaviours
- If 1:1 nursing is indicated, brief the nurse about the diagnosis and known dysfunctional behaviours
- A symptomatic approach is useful (low mood, anxiety, insomnia as targets for intervention), but medication is unlikely to help as it becomes a symbol of how much patients think staff 'like or dislike' them
- The point of transfer or discharge may provoke dysfunctional behaviours intended to prolong admission. The liaison team should acknowledge the underlying (personality) problems will not be fixed, acknowledge the patient's perception of 'bad treatment' (minimising their bad behaviours, but perceiving the medical case as punishment) and signpost to therapy after discharge

A system of informal debriefs for staff following transfer of difficult patients should maintain morale and prevent staff burnout.

References and Further Reading

Bienvenu OJ, Neufeld KJ. Post-traumatic stress disorder in medical settings: focus on the critically ill. *Curr Psychiatry Rep* 2010;**13**:3–9.

Groves JE. Difficult patients. In: TA Stern, GL Fricchione, NH Cassem (eds). *Massachusetts General Hospital Handbook of General Hospital Psychiatry*, 5th edn. Philadelphia, PA: Elsevier; 2004. pp. 78–81.

Hatch R, McKechnie S, Griffiths J. Psychological intervention to prevent ICU-related PTSD: who, when and for how long? *Crit Care* 2011;**15**:141.

Mealer M, Jones J, Moss M. A qualitative study of resilience and post-traumatic stress disorder in United States ICU nurses. *Intensive Care Med* 2012;**38**:1445–51.

Myhren H, Ekeberg O, Toien K, Karlsson S, Stokland O. Posttraumatic stress, anxiety and depression symptoms in patients during the first year post intensive care unit discharge. *Crit Care* 2010;**14**:R14.

Wade D, Hardy R, Howell D, Mythen M. Identifying clinical and psychological risk factors for PTSD after ICU: a systematic review. *Minerva Anestesiol* 2013;**79**:944–63.

Wake S, Kitchiner D. Post-traumatic stress disorder after intensive care: a patient's journey. *BMJ* 2013;**346**:3232.

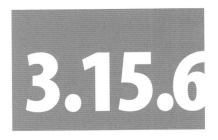

3.15.6

Substance Misuse and Withdrawal in Intensive Care

Ruth Taylor and Peter Byrne

Key Learning Points

1. All patients should be considered at risk of withdrawal syndromes.
2. Prompt recognition and treatment are key to its management.
3. Treatment for withdrawal syndromes is generally supportive, alongside the use of benzodiazepines.
4. Alcohol withdrawal syndrome is a medical emergency, with 20 per cent mortality if untreated.
5. The specialist drugs team should be contacted for advice prior to the prescription of methadone.

Keywords: withdrawal syndrome, delirium tremens, opiates, methadone

Introduction

Withdrawal syndromes in patients in the ICU are a cause of significant morbidity and some are fatal if missed. They are difficult to diagnose and manage. All ICU patients should be considered at risk, withdrawal syndromes promptly recognised and individualised treatment given. Withdrawal from multiple agents occurs and can be complicated by therapeutic interventions. Withdrawal from novel psychoactive substances should also be considered.

Alcohol Withdrawal Syndrome

Alcohol is the most common, clinically significant addiction, and excess/dependence is frequently denied. Management can be complicated by iatrogenic and medical co-morbidities. Unexplained changes in

mental state (fearful affect), body temperature and haemodynamic instability should lead to a suspicion of alcohol withdrawal syndrome (AWS).

If possible, the clinician should elicit an alcohol history, including:

- Recent drinking pattern – amount, frequency, time of last drink
- History of withdrawal symptoms, e.g. needing a drink to get going each day, the 'eye opener'
- History of need for detoxification
- History of withdrawal seizures
- Concurrent drug use

It is important to distinguish between delirium tremens (DTs) (which can lead to death) and alcoholic hallucinosis (when the sensorium is intact/no disorientation and the patient experiences visual, auditory or tactile hallucinations). Withdrawal syndrome can occur 6–48 hours after alcohol use. DTs can occur from 48 to 96 hours after alcohol use.

Factors associated with an increased risk of DTs include:

- Chronic alcohol use
- Previous history of DTs
- Older age
- Co-morbid physical illness
- Increasing time since last drink

Mortality is associated with older age, lung disease, higher temperatures and hepatic failure, owing to worsening dehydration, decreased cerebral blood flow and hypokalaemia, hypomagnesaemia and hypophosphataemia.

Treatment

Treatment is largely supportive, combined with a course of reducing-dose benzodiazepines. Supportive treatment should include:

- Hydration
- Correction of electrolyte imbalance

- Thiamine, folate and multi-vitamin supplementation – **always give intravenous thiamine before glucose**

Thiamine should be given early to prevent Wernicke's and Korsakoff's syndromes. Benzodiazepines are prescribed to manage withdrawal symptoms and prevent seizures.

It is common practice to prescribe a standard reducing regimen of chlordiazepoxide. However, evidence suggests that symptom-triggered administration is preferred, as generally requiring less medication and shorter treatment. Symptom-triggered administration requires careful monitoring of the patient with a validated measure, e.g. the Clinical Institute Withdrawal Assessment for Alcohol (CIWA). This measures symptoms such as agitation, anxiety, nausea, sweating and orientation, with a maximum score of 67. Sometimes, in critically ill patients or those with gastrointestinal malabsorption, parenteral benzodiazepines are necessary – a change to oral should be attempted when possible.

Chlordiazepoxide should be avoided in hepatic failure, and lorazepam should be prescribed instead.

Multiple agents have been trialled as an adjunct therapy to treat symptoms of AWS, including beta-blockers, alpha-agonists, neuroleptics, carbamazepine and ethyl alcohol infusions. These have shown little benefit and risk masking early signs of withdrawal.

All patients should be referred to the hospital drugs and alcohol team for review, with a view to formulating a long-term management plan.

Opiates

Heroin/Opiate Overdose

Admission to hospital is rare and usually associated with complications of heroin use, rather than with the overdose itself. Direct effects of heroin on the central nervous system (CNS) (critically respiratory arrest) are reversible with naloxone. No response to naloxone should prompt further exploration of the cause. Re-sedation may occur if large doses of heroin have been used due to differing half-lives of opiates and naloxone.

Admission to the ICU is indicated in the following circumstances:

- Patient requiring respiratory support
- Life-threatening arrhythmia
- Shock

- Recurrent seizures
- Continuous naloxone infusion required
- Non-cardiogenic pulmonary oedema

Recurrent seizures require further investigation of the cause. Seizures caused by heroin/narcotic overdose should respond to benzodiazepines. Prolonged seizures and coma can lead to rhabdomyolysis, which should be treated with fluid resuscitation, alkalinisation of the urine and forced diuresis. Following treatment of the overdose, the patient should be referred to the drugs and alcohol team for assessment and discussion around support with abstinence and maintenance treatment.

Heroin/Opiate Withdrawal

Any patient admitted to the ICU could be at risk of withdrawal syndromes from drugs.

Withdrawal symptoms from heroin begin 8–24 hours after last use and continue for up to 10 days. Withdrawal symptoms from methadone begin 12–48 hours after last use and can continue for up to 20 days.

Suspect opiate withdrawal if:

- Known drug user or needle marks/infection on the limbs or femoral vein
- Nausea and vomiting
- Diarrhoea
- Insomnia
- Thermodysregulation
- Sweating
- Rhinorrhoea
- Myalgia

Opiate withdrawal is not life-threatening, unlike alcohol withdrawal. It usually requires treatment for symptomatic relief such as metoclopramide for nausea and non-steroidals for pain relief. More severe withdrawal symptoms can be treated with clonidine, with close monitoring of the heart rate and blood pressure.

Following initial treatment, the patient should be referred to the drugs and alcohol team.

According to the National Institute for Health and Care Excellence (NICE) guidelines, methadone is first line for maintenance treatment in opiate substitution. Methadone substitution can be started in the hospital. However, advice must be sought from the drugs and alcohol team regarding dosing regime and follow-up. (Give small amounts, and divide into twice-daily dosing to reduce 'walkouts' in patients who want a large loading dose before leaving hospital.) For a patient

453

already taking methadone, the dose should be confirmed by their issuing pharmacy before methadone is prescribed and administered. Out of hours, the drugs and alcohol team/psychiatry liaison team should be contacted for advice.

Other Substances

Mushrooms

Mushrooms containing atropine and muscarinic alkaloids can cause poisoning. Severe poisoning can occur with two specific types:

- *Gyromitra esculenta* – causes nausea and vomiting, abdominal pain, liver failure, seizures, coma and death in up to 40 per cent of cases. Management is supportive, plus intravenous pyridoxine hydrochloride
- *Amanita phalloides* – causes gastrointestinal irritability, hepatic and renal failure leading to encephalopathy and death in up to 50 per cent of cases. Management includes gastric lavage, penicillin G and plasmapheresis

Street Drugs and Novel Psychoactive Agents

All street drugs (including cocaine, amphetamines, gamma hydroxybutyrate (GHB) and phencyclidine) can lead to ICU admission in extreme cases. Early recognition and treatment are paramount. There are no specific antidotes to these drugs and treatment is largely supportive, with benzodiazepines given for sedation. Importantly, GHB taken with alcohol has an increased sedative effect, and a number of deaths have been associated with cardio-respiratory arrest.

Novel Agents in ICU to Treat Withdrawals

Benzodiazepines are the mainstay of treatment for AWS. However, there have been a number of case reports when large doses of benzodiazepines have failed to prevent or shorten the duration of DTs. Benzodiazepines bind at the gamma aminobutyric acid (GABA) benzodiazepine receptor in the CNS. These receptors can become saturated, and as such, patients may tolerate a high dose but gain no benefit

from further administration. After high-dose therapy, benzodiazepines are also sequestered into fat stores, leading to residual sedation and longer ICU stays. Though liver-friendly, lorazepam can also cause renal problems. Propofol has been successfully used in patients refractory to large doses of benzodiazepines. Propofol binds to GABA receptors and inhibits N-methyl-D-aspartate (NMDA) glutamate receptors, which are known to play a central role in both alcohol and substance dependence and withdrawal states. Propofol has also been successfully used for sedation for rapid opioid detoxification, with the benefits of reduced haemodynamic impairment and a reduction in dose of medication used. Patients are generally responsive after 20 minutes of stopping a propofol infusion. In a number of case reports, propofol has proved safe and effective, and it is preferable to both haloperidol (which can lower the seizure threshold) and clonidine (which has less effect on hallucinations and may provoke hypotension and/or tachycardia).

References and Further Reading

Garimella PS, Joffe A, Velho V. Street drug abuse leading to critical illness. *Intensive Care Med* 2004;**30**:1526–36.

Habal R. 2016. Heroin toxicity treatment and management. emedicine.medscape.com/article/166464-treatment

National Institute for Health and Care Excellence. 2019. Alcohol withdrawal management for acute admissions to hospital. www.nice.org.uk/sharedlearning/alcohol-withdrawal-management-for-acute-admissions-to-hospital

Royal College of Physicians. 2012. Alcohol dependence and withdrawal in the acute hospital. www.rcplondon.ac.uk/guidelines-policy/alcohol-dependence-and-withdrawal-acute-hospital

Subramaniam K, Gowda RM, Jani K, Zewedie W, Ute R. Case report: propofol combined with lorazepam for severe poly substance misuse and withdrawal states in intensive care unit: a case series and review. *Emerg Med J* 2003;**21**:632–4.

Tetrault JM, O'Connor PG. Substance abuse and withdrawal in the critical care setting. *Crit Care Clin* 2008;**24**:767–88, viii.

World Health Organization. 2009. Clinical guidelines for withdrawal management and treatment of drug dependence in closed settings. www.ncbi.nlm.nih.gov/books/NBK310654/

3.15.7

Staff Burnout in Intensive Care

Ruth Taylor and Peter Byrne

Key Learning Points

1. Up to 45 per cent of critical care physicians report severe burnout.
2. Up to 33 per cent of critical care nurses report severe burnout. The majority report at least one isolated symptom of burnout.
3. Both personal and environmental factors are implicated as causal factors for burnout.
4. Both individual- and organisational-level interventions are helpful, although organisational-level interventions have longer-lasting effects.
5. It is our responsibility to look after our own health and to support colleagues in doing so.

Keywords: exhaustion, satisfaction, depersonalisation, effectiveness, self-care

Introduction

Staff burnout is a persistent and significant issue, threatening the individual, patients and the organisation.

Burnout comprises a prolonged response to interpersonal and emotional job stressors, leading to exhaustion, feelings of cynicism and detachment from the job, a sense of ineffectiveness and a lack of accomplishment. It is recognised in the International Statistical Classification of Diseases and Related Health Problems (ICD) as a 'state of vital exhaustion' within the category of 'problems related to life-management difficulty'.

Ford (*Nursing Times*, 2016) found that critical care staff have amongst the highest burnout rates. The Critical Care Societies Collaborative in the United States published a report which found that up to one in three critical care nurses suffer severe burnout. The majority of staff reported at least one of 'exhaustion, depersonalisation and reduced personal accomplishment'. The report quotes that 45 per cent of critical care doctors, and up to 71 per cent of paediatric critical care specialists, report severe burnout.

Consequences for the Unit

- Absenteeism
- Stated intention to leave the post
- Negative impact on patient care – medical errors and increased morbidity and mortality
- Reduced productivity and effectiveness
- Reduced job satisfaction and commitment
- Reduced patient satisfaction
- Consequences for the individual, including: post-traumatic stress disorder (PTSD), harmful use of alcohol and substances, chronic pain, diabetes and cardiovascular disease and resignation or loss of job

Risk Factors

- Stressful environment of the ICU
- Inherently emotional quality of ICU interventions
- Personal characteristics – age, gender, job status
- Empathic traits
- Personality traits – 'vulnerable personality' (as rated by neuroticism (vulnerability), extroversion (intensity) and control and compulsiveness) is positively correlated with burnout
- Dysfunctional coping mechanisms, e.g. alcohol, drugs, gambling
- Organisational factors – flexibility of working patterns, days off in between shifts, staff turnover, organisational insensitivity and bullying
- Interpersonal difficulties –conflicts with patients, relations with senior nurse and clinicians
- End-of-life factors, e.g. caring for the dying patient and decisions to forgo life-sustaining treatments, addressing the emotions of family members
- Lack of social support networks outside employment

Interventions

The Critical Care Societies Collaborative suggests that interventions should be based on enhancing the ICU environment and supporting individuals to cope with the environment. Staff should be provided with pastoral care in the form of supervision by senior staff where discussion about burnout should be made welcome. Organisational interventions, such as changes to workload and work practices, have been shown to produce longer-lasting effects (although these are less common).

Mitigating factors and interventions can include:

- An ICU team in which each member feels respected and listened to
- Recognition that potential burnout is a shared responsibility and individual burnout negatively impacts the function of the whole ICU
- A 'no blame' or 'shared blame' culture (balanced with the demands of individual responsibility)
- A safe space for emotional expression, and the valuation of self-awareness and emotional literacy as an asset for both medical care and career progression
- Individuals may benefit from structured pastoral care, small group workshops, cognitive behavioural therapy (CBT) training and stress management, meditation and mindfulness practices
- Practical support for staff where possible, not least flexibility with shifts and time off, may significantly help a work–life balance

Duty of Self-Care

Healthcare professionals are notoriously poor at looking after their own health. The General Medical Council (GMC)'s 'Good Medical Practice' guide for all registered doctors states our responsibility to ensure that:

- Doctors' own health does not negatively impact upon their work
- Doctors recognise the signs of our own burnout
- Doctors obtain guidance and support from colleagues when needed
- Doctors support others – there is an ethical and moral obligation to act, should we suspect that colleagues are struggling at work

Sources of Help

All literature agrees that there is a need for further research into initial burnout, diagnosis and effective interventions for staff burnout as a means to protect the mental and physical health of healthcare professionals. Sources of help include:

- NHS trusts' occupational health department
- Psychiatry liaison teams – these can offer advice about local services, and may provide staff training sessions on stress management and other coping skills as a preventative measure

References and Further Reading

Bagnall AM, Jones R, Akter H, Woodall J. 2016. Interventions to prevent burnout in high risk individuals: evidence review. www.gov.uk/government/uploads/system/uploads/attachment_data/file/506777/25022016_Burnout_Rapid_Review_2015709.pdf

Ford S. 2016. Critical care nurses at higher risk of burnout. *The Nursing Times.* www.nursingtimes.net/news/workforce/critical-care-nurses-at-higher-risk-of-burnout/7006269.article

General Medical Council. 2013. Good Medical Practice: risks posed by your health. www.gmc-uk.org/guidance/good_medical_practice/your_health.asp

Myhren H, Ekeberg O, Stokland O. Job satisfaction and burnout among intensive care unit nurses and physicians. *Crit Care Res Pract* 2013;**2013**:786176.

Poncet MC, Toullic P, Papazian L, *et al.* Burnout syndrome in critical care nursing staff. *Am J Respir Crit Care Med* 2006;**175**:698–704.

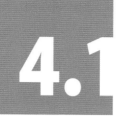
Principles of Safe Prescription of Drugs and Therapeutics (Including Pharmacokinetics, Pharmacodynamics and Drug Monitoring)

4.1

Caroline Moss

Key Learning Points

1. Understanding how the patient will handle a drug (pharmacokinetics) and how the drug will affect the patient (pharmacodynamics) is crucial to prescribing any drug safely.

2. It is important to consider both how the drugs may interact with other drugs being co-administered and how their effect/handling may be affected by the patient's critical illness and associated organ dysfunction.

3. The loading dose, repeat doses and/or dosing interval may need to be adjusted, and in some cases monitoring of drug levels may be possible/necessary.

4. Critical illness is a rapidly changing dynamic state. Daily medication chart review, considering if drugs are still indicated and/or if their dosing needs reviewing, depending on the changing clinical condition of the patient, is essential.

5. Prescribing in critical illness can be a complex area; however, there are comprehensive resources available to guide practice. Seeking support and advice from your pharmacist when in doubt is a very useful and sensible approach.

Keywords: pharmacokinetics, pharmacodynamics, absorption, distribution, metabolism, excretion, clearance

Introduction

Provision of intensive care involves administration of a wide range of therapeutic medications which can both facilitate necessary organ support (e.g. sedation, inotropes, vasopressors) and provide specific treatment for the underlying diagnosis (e.g. anti-microbials). An understanding of some basic principles is fundamental in ensuring that all drugs are used safely and effectively. Critically unwell patients may be affected by drugs differently and may handle them differently, so some special considerations are important to bear in mind. This chapter will provide only a brief overview of some key concepts, with further reading recommended to explore the topics in more detail.

There are two broad areas to consider, and we will discuss each briefly in turn:

1. Pharmacokinetics (PKs) – 'how the body handles the drug'
2. Pharmacodynamics (PDs) – 'how the drug affects the body'

Pharmacokinetics

PKs can be broken down into four main processes.

Absorption

To render their effect, drugs must be taken up from the site of administration and reach their site of action. Within intensive care, the intravenous (IV) route will most often be used, resulting in direct reliable systemic delivery. The oral route may sometimes be used, when bioavailability (percentage of the drug reaching the systemic circulation, compared to the IV dose) will need to be considered. Factors to consider affecting oral bioavailability include first-pass metabolism in the liver, and gastrointestinal failure resulting in reduced/delayed absorption.

Distribution

The extent of drug distribution following administration and absorption is dependent on the properties of the drug (molecular size, lipid solubility, protein binding, ionisation) and regional blood flow to organs.

High-blood flow organs (brain, kidney, heart) → moderate blood flow (muscle) → lowest blood flow (fat)

When considering the dose of drug to give, the volume of distribution (V_D) is important, which is how much the drug distributes within and between the various body compartments.

V_D = theoretical volume into which a drug distributes following administration (often expressed in litres per kilogram)

The relationship between the immediate drug concentration following IV administration and the V_D can be seen in Figure 4.1.1.

Small, lipid-soluble, poorly protein-bound drugs distribute more widely than large, polar, lipid-insoluble drugs, and so have a larger V_D, which has implications for the loading dose of the drug needed to be given.

Loading dose = V_D × [plasma] required

Changes in lean body mass, total body water and plasma pH (with its effects on protein binding) can all alter the active plasma concentration of the drug and impact drug dosing in the critically unwell patient.

Metabolism

Drug metabolism mainly (though not exclusively) occurs in the liver, usually reducing the activity of the drug, aiming to produce more water-soluble molecules for biliary or renal excretion.

Phase 1 metabolism involves oxidation, reduction and hydrolysis, commonly via the cytochrome P450 system of enzymes.

Phase 2 metabolism (synthetic) includes glucuronidation, sulfation, acetylation and methylation.

In patients with hepatic failure, phase 1 metabolism is often affected before phase 2 processes, so prescribing may need modifying in patients with liver impairment.

Excretion

Elimination refers to removal of a drug from the plasma (including distribution and metabolism), whereas excretion is removal of a drug from the body. Clearance of a drug includes elimination and excretion, and is defined as:

Clearance = volume of plasma from which a drug is removed per unit time (ml/min)

Factors which impact clearance of a drug (such as increased V_D, reduced hepatic metabolism, renal impairment and reduced renal excretion) are important to consider when deciding on dose and interval between doses. Dosing in renal failure, and in patients requiring renal replacement therapy where clearance of medications is altered, is a complex area, but specific guidance exists to guide practice.

Pharmacodynamics

Drugs can exert their actions in a variety of ways:
- Physiochemical, e.g. antacids
- Structural interaction with target proteins:

  ○ Receptors (most commonly G-protein-coupled receptors)
  ○ Ion channels (such as voltage-gated sodium (Na$^+$) channels)
  ○ Enzymes (such as acetylcholinesterase)

Drugs that act on enzymes are most commonly enzyme inhibitors, with the result of increasing the concentration of the substrate and reducing the concentration of the product.

Most commonly used drugs act via receptor interactions in three main classes:

1. Altering permeability of the cell membrane to ions (inotropic receptor interactions, e.g. muscle relaxants acting on nicotinic acetylcholine receptors)
2. Effect on intracellular second-messenger systems (metabotropic G-protein-coupled receptor

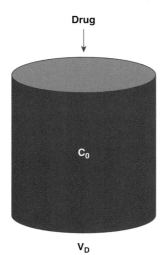

Drug

Figure 4.1.1 Diagram depicting the relationship between the immediate drug concentration following intravenous administration (C_0) and the volume of distribution (V_D). C_0 = immediate [drug] following IV administration, which is an extrapolated value at $t = 0$ from early first plasma concentrations.

C_0

V_D

interactions, e.g. catecholamines acting on α- and β-adrenoreceptors)

3. Regulation of gene transcription (via cytoplasmic intracellular receptors, e.g. steroid action)

Drug–receptor interactions are described by the ability of the drug (ligand) to bind the receptor (affinity), and by the magnitude of the effect caused once the ligand is bound to the receptor (intrinsic activity (IA) or efficacy). Drugs can be:

- Full agonists: high affinity, IA = 1
- Partial agonists: high affinity, IA <1
- Antagonists: high affinity, IA = 0

These properties can be graphically represented by dose–response and log dose–response curves (where the scale is adjusted as $\log_{10}$ dose to render the middle portion of the curve linear, and thus make interpretation easier). Figures 4.1.2, 4.1.3 and 4.1.4 demonstrate dose–response curves.

Drug Interactions

Polypharmacy is common within intensive care, with potentially significant interactions between drugs administered. Some anticipation and understanding of these interactions are important, as they can be advantageous or, more concerningly, harmful. These interactions can be:

1. **Physiochemical:**
   a. For example, sugammadex reversal of paralysis by rocuronium

2. **Pharmacokinetic:** administration of a drug which alters how the body deals with another, altering:
   a. **Absorption:** for example, adrenaline administered with local anaesthetics causes vasoconstriction and reduced systemic absorption

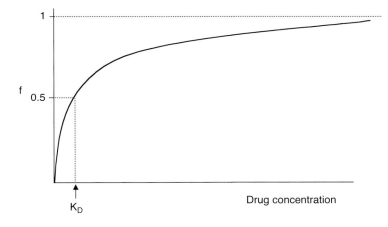

Figure 4.1.2 Normal agonist dose–response curve. A normal agonist dose–response curve is hyperbolic.

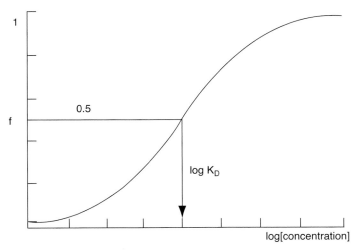

Figure 4.1.3 Log dose–response curve. This curve is plotted using a log scale for the dose and produces the classic sigmoid shape.

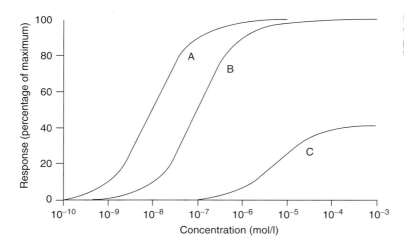

Figure 4.1.4 Log dose–response curves for three drugs. A and B are full agonists; B is less potent than A. C is a partial agonist that is unable to elicit a maximal response.

b. **Distribution:** for example, aspirin competes for protein binding sites, increasing the free fraction and activity of warfarin

c. **Metabolism:** drugs which induce hepatic enzyme systems (e.g. phenytoin, barbiturates) accelerate the breakdown of drugs metabolised by these enzymes. The converse is true for enzyme inhibitors (e.g. omeprazole)

d. **Excretion:** drug elimination can be enhanced by co-administration of drugs; for example, bicarbonate administration alkalinises the urine, increasing elimination of salicylates

3. **Pharmacodynamic:** occurs when the action of one drug on the body is altered by administration of another in the following ways:

a. **Summation:** each drug has independent activity, but effects are additive (1 + 1 = 2)

b. **Synergism:** combined action of two drugs administered together is greater than would be expected by a purely additive effect (1 + 1 = >2) (e.g. administration of propofol and remifentanil for sedation in the ICU)

c. **Antagonism:** action of one drug blocks or inhibits the action of another (e.g. morphine is reversed by administration of naloxone, a competitive antagonist)

Therapeutic Drug Monitoring

Drugs are administered in order to cause a therapeutic effect. Therapeutic drug monitoring (TDM) is important for two main reasons:

- To reduce toxicity from the drug
- To ensure that plasma concentrations are therapeutic

Some drugs have a narrow therapeutic index where toxic effects occur at concentrations close to therapeutic levels. Examples of commonly used drugs in the ICU include antibiotics (aminoglycosides), digoxin, phenytoin and theophylline. TDM is particularly important with regard to anti-microbials to improve clinical outcome from infection and reduce resistance.

Summary

We have a huge armamentarium of drugs available in intensive care to support and treat critically unwell patients. To use them safely and effectively, an understanding of some basic pharmacological principles, and how these can be impacted in disease states, is fundamental. The principles briefly touched on here can be built on and explored further in the recommended reading below.

References and Further Reading

Ashley C, Dunleavy A. *The Renal Drug Handbook: The Ultimate Prescribing Guide for Renal Practitioners*, 4th edn. London: Radcliffe Publishing; 2014.

Bangash MN, Kong ML, Pearse RM. Use of inotropes and vasopressor agents in critically ill patients. *Br J Pharmacol* 2012;**165**:2015–33

Peck TE, Hill S, Williams M. *Pharmacology for Anaesthesia and Intensive Care*, 3rd edn. Cambridge: Cambridge University Press; 2008.

Rowe K, Fletcher S. Sedation in the intensive care unit. *Contin Educ Anaesth Crit Care Pain* 2008;**8**:50–5.

Varley AJ, Sule J, Absalom AR. Principles of antibiotic therapy. *Contin Educ Anaesth Crit Care Pain* 2009;**9**:184–8.

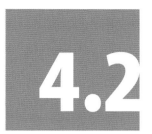

Antibiotic Management and Monitoring

4.2

James McKinlay and Alexander Fletcher

Key Learning Points

1. Poor anti-microbial stewardship and selection pressure encourage antibiotic resistance.
2. Pharmacokinetics may be altered significantly and unpredictably by critical illness.
3. Optimal dosing of antibiotics is difficult. Many patients are likely under-dosed.
4. Different antibiotics require different approaches to achieving optimal antibiotic exposure.
5. Therapeutic drug monitoring is standard for aminoglycosides and glycopeptides, but may be helpful for β-lactams, linezolid and some 'azole' anti-fungal agents.

Keywords: stewardship, anti-microbial, pharmacokinetics, pharmacodynamics, dose

Introduction

Antibiotics should be given at the right dose and for the right duration. Suboptimal antibiotic exposure may contribute to therapy failure and resistance. Some antibiotics are routinely administered based on weight and/or the renal function of the patient. However, in adults, most are given at relatively standard doses. This is unlikely to be the best approach in critically unwell patients whose physiology may be changing rapidly, and giving a more individualised dose, tailored to each patient's physiology and drug pharmacokinetics, for the duration of therapy would be ideal. Drugs with narrow therapeutic windows and significant risk of toxicity are routinely monitored using plasma levels and are discussed below, along with future considerations for monitoring of other commonly used anti-microbials. Drug monitoring should be part of an anti-microbial stewardship programme, which also includes auditing local anti-microbial use, delivering policies and guidelines for anti-microbial regimens, education and monitoring resistance patterns in the local patient population.

Pharmacological Principles of Monitoring

Effective and appropriate antibiotic use requires an antibiotic with efficacy against the pathogen, to be delivered to the target site at an effective concentration for an adequate period of time. This is determined by the concentration in blood, which, in turn, is affected by absorption, distribution, metabolism and elimination of the drug.

The pharmacological principles underlying the absorption, distribution, metabolism and elimination of drugs are covered comprehensively in other texts. To summarise very briefly:

- The intravenous (IV) route avoids first-pass metabolism and ensures bioavailability. Drugs with high oral bioavailability include: ciprofloxacin, clindamycin, chloramphenicol, fluconazole, linezolid, metronidazole and rifampicin
- High levels of protein binding reduce the free portion of drug available to diffuse to the tissues and have its effect, but may also assist with delivery to inflamed areas with proteinaceous fluid leak. Most bacteria are located in the extracellular space and antibiotics may reach these areas, unless 'protected' by non-fenestrated capillaries, e.g. the central nervous system or prostate
- Lipophilic drugs tend to be more widely distributed and can pass into tissue more easily. They are generally eliminated via the hepato-biliary route (except fluoroquinolones and trimethoprim), as opposed to hydrophilic drugs which are nearly all cleared by the kidneys. Furthermore, the volume of distribution (V_D)

461

for lipophilic drugs appears to be quite well maintained in critical illness, unlike the V_D for hydrophilic drugs which is likely to increase. Some infective organisms (e.g. *Chlamydia pneumoniae*, *Legionella pneumophila*, *Listeria monocytogenes*, *Mycobacterium tuberculosis*) may be intracellular and require specific antibiotics for treatment (e.g. fluoroquinolones, macrolides, lincosamides, meropenem, rifampicin)

Clearance of a drug depends on metabolism (usually by the liver) and elimination (usually renal, with some intestinal elimination). Elimination half-life of a drug is related to the V_D and inversely to the clearance. A steady-state plasma level may be achieved after five 'bolus' doses with a dosing interval of one half-life, or after five half-lives for continuous infusions. Loading doses (calculated by the desired plasma concentration multiplied by the V_D, and approximated from twice the maintenance dose with a dosing interval of one half-life) are used to achieve steady-state levels rapidly in drugs with a long half-life or large V_D, within safe limits of maximal bolus doses. Loading doses are not reduced in renal failure but may be increased in sepsis for hydrophilic drugs, and for lipophilic drugs in sepsis with severe hepatic dysfunction. Table 4.2.1 illustrates how a knowledge of drug properties and pharmacokinetic variables, as well as an understanding of patients' physiology, is important in achieving effective anti-microbial treatment.

Pharmacological Characteristics of Antibiotics

Some antibiotics exhibit so-called time-dependent killing characteristics; others exhibit concentration-dependent properties, and some exhibit both (Table 4.2.2). Their likely effect is estimated with reference to a factor (e.g. time, concentration or total drug exposure), compared to the minimum inhibitory concentration (MIC) (as opposed to minimum bactericidal concentration (MBC)). MICs are derived in vitro and can vary widely for the same drug, depending on the bacterial genera/species targeted. In general, pathogens with higher MICs require higher concentrations of an antibiotic to achieve inhibition. Increasing MICs of a pathogen equate to decreased sensitivity to that antibiotic.

Time Dependence

This implies that effective action (inhibition of bacteria) occurs with prolonged time above the MIC for that antibiotic. β-Lactams generally require around 50–60 per cent of dosing time, with free drug concentration above the MIC for adequate bactericidal effect, though this varies with antibiotic group. There is evidence, however, that maintaining a concentration above the MIC for 100 per cent of the dosing period, especially for pathogens needing higher MICs,

Table 4.2.1 Various drug/physiological states and likely effects on pharmacokinetic parameters

Drug property/ physiological state	Volume of distribution	Clearance	Elimination half-life ($T_{1/2}$)	Protein binding	Plasma drug concentration	Tissue/cellular penetration
Lipophilic	Generally high Little change in critical illness	Mostly hepato-biliary	Tends to be longer	Generally ↑	Generally ↓	Generally ↑
Hydrophilic	Generally low ↑ in critical illness	Mostly renal	Tends to be shorter	Generally ↓	Generally ↑	Generally ↓
Highly protein-bound	V_D ↓ (apparent)	Cl ↓	↑		Generally ↓ (measure free drug)	Generally ↓
Capillary leak/altered protein binding/RRT	V_D ↑	RRT may ↑ Cl of some drugs	May ↑[a]	Variable	Generally ↓	Generally ↑
High cardiac output		Cl ↑	May ↓[a]		↓	Depends on local perfusion
Organ dysfunction/↓ perfusion		Cl ↓	May ↑[a]	May ↓ if synthetic function ↓	↑	↓

[a] Dependent on multiple inter-related factors. More likely to be the case in the absence of other physiological derangements (e.g. isolated high cardiac output state without capillary leak).

Abbreviations: V_D = volume of distribution; Cl = clearance; $T_{1/2}$ = elimination half-life; ↑ = high or increased; ↓ = low or decreased; RRT = renal replacement therapy.

Table 4.2.2 Killing characteristics and lipophilicity of various antibiotics/antibiotic classes

Time-dependent (T > MIC)	Concentration-dependent (C_{max}:MIC)	Concentration-dependent with time dependence (AUC_{0-24}:MIC)
β-Lactams	Aminoglycosides	**Azithromycin**
Carbapenems	Daptomycin	**Fluoroquinolones**
Clarithromycin	**Metronidazole**	Glycopeptides
Clindamycin	Polymyxins	**Tetracyclines**
Erythromycin	**Quinupristin/**	**Tigecycline**
Linezolid	**dalfopristin**	
	Telithromycin	

Antibiotics in bold are lipophilic (colistin, a polymyxin, may be both hydro- and lipophilic).

Abbreviations: MIC = minimum inhibitory concentration; T > MIC = time with plasma concentration above MIC; C_{max} = maximum plasma concentration; AUC_{0-24} = area under concentration/time curve in a 24-hour period.

results in maximal bactericidal effect. For this reason, frequent dosing or infusions may be preferable. Furthermore, concentrations maintained at 4–5 times the MIC for 90–100 per cent of dosing time may also be more effective.

Concentration Dependence

These drugs achieve rapid inhibitory effect with higher concentrations, up to a maximal point. For example, aminoglycosides work best with maximal concentrations (C_{max}) 8–10 times the MIC. For this reason, generally 'large' doses are used, but given less frequently.

Concentration and Time Dependence

For drugs with both properties, the total amount of drug exposure is important, and the total area under the drug concentration/time curve (AUC) in 24 hours divided by the MIC is the relevant pharmacokinetic/dynamic parameter. For example, an AUC:MIC ratio of 400 may be needed for meticillin-resistant *Staphylococcus aureus* (MRSA) infection treated with vancomycin.

AUC may be estimated from the formula:

$$AUC = dose/clearance = (dose \times elimination\ half\text{-}life)/(ln2 \times V_D)$$

However, in critically unwell patients, the V_D and clearance (and hence half-life) are unpredictable and may vary with, for example, renal and liver dysfunction, capillary leak and/or volume overload.

Post-antibiotic Effects

Persistence of inhibition of bacterial growth after the concentration of an antibiotic has fallen below the MIC can be a feature of all antibiotics. However, the magnitude/duration vary, depending on the specific antibiotic/bacteria combination (Figure 4.2.1). Prolonged post-antibiotic effects (PAEs) (e.g. several hours) tend to occur more commonly with inhibitors of nucleic acid/protein synthesis such as aminoglycosides. However, carbapenems also exhibit prolonged PAEs.

Therapeutic Drug Monitoring for Specific Drugs

Some drugs display significant inter-individual variation in pharmacokinetics, whilst others may have a narrow therapeutic window with significant side effects/toxicity. Along with antibiotics exhibiting concentration-dependent inhibition, these types of drugs may be suitable for therapeutic drug monitoring (TDM). The antibiotics routinely monitored currently are: gentamicin, amikacin, vancomycin and sometimes teicoplanin. Some anti-fungal agents may potentially be monitored. Close liaison with intensive care pharmacists and microbiologists is recommended for patients requiring TDM, especially if patients are receiving renal replacement therapies where drug dosing/interval changes are more complex to manage. More specific examples of monitoring practice can be seen in Table 4.2.3.

Gentamicin/Amikacin

The main side effects are dose-related, including irreversible nephrotoxicity. However, this may be more

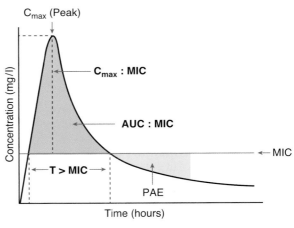

Figure 4.2.1 Representation of pharmacokinetic/pharmacodynamic parameters for antibiotic dose optimisation.

Table 4.2.3 Examples of monitoring regimes for specific drugs

Drug	Loading dose	Usual dose	'Usual' interval	Level timing	Target	Action if level high
Gentamicin (nomogram)		5 mg/kg	24-hourly	6–14 hours after first dose	Use nomogram	Extend interval
Gentamicin (trough levels)		2–5 mg/kg	24-hourly	Trough 18–24 hours after first dose	<1 mg/ml	Extend interval or reduce dose. Re-check levels
Gentamicin (multiple daily dosing)		1 mg/kg bd	12-hourly	Trough 1 hour before third dose. Peak 1 hour post-third dose. Do not await level for next dose	Trough <1 mg/ml Peak 3–5 mg/ml	Withhold subsequent dose 10% dose reduction
Amikacin	25 mg/kg once-off if severe infection	15 mg/kg	24-hourly	Trough 1 hour before second dose	<5 mg/l	Extend interval
Vancomycin (trough)	25–30 mg/kg if severe infection	Weight-based, e.g. 750 mg–1.5 g	12- to 24-hourly (CrCl-based)	Trough 1 hour before third or fourth dose. Await level before next dose	10–15 mg/l 15–20 mg/l if severe infection	Extend dosing interval. Repeat per dose if CrCl changing
Teicoplanin (standard) (line sepsis) (bone/IE)	(12-hourly) 6 mg/kg × 3 10 mg/kg × 5 12 mg/kg × 5	(Then) 6 mg/kg 10 mg/kg 12 mg/kg	24–72 hours (CrCl-based)	If, for example, >7 days/ severe infection/renal impairment Trough 1 hour pre-dose Do not await levels	>20 mg/l and <60 mg/l	

'Usual interval' refers to initial interval with standard dosing in young (e.g. <65 years) patients with normal renal function. Renal function/ CrCl should be assessed using the Cockcroft–Gault formula. Follow local protocols and liaise with microbiology/pharmacy for specific advice. This should not be used in place of formularies/prescribing guidelines.

Abbreviations: CrCl = creatinine clearance; IE = infective endocarditis.

frequently encountered when used in conjunction with other drugs (e.g. high-dose flucloxacillin) or when used in older patients. Ototoxicity appears to occur more frequently in patients receiving longer courses of gentamicin and in those with increasing age. Courses should generally be short (e.g. 3–5 days or less) and extended interval dosing (24- to 48-hourly) is recommended, unless used in severe burns, endocarditis, meningitis, ascites/liver failure or cystic fibrosis. To predict the dosing interval, the calculated creatinine clearance (CrCl) should be used (using, for example, the Cockroft–Gault formula), using ideal bodyweight for obese patients. Local protocols should be followed for monitoring. Doses are usually given over at least half an hour (gentamicin) or an hour (amikacin).

Vancomycin/Teicoplanin

Vancomycin monitoring has been shown to increase the rate of clinical efficacy and to reduce the rate of nephrotoxicity. Under-dosing also contributes to resistance. There is limited evidence for a direct causal link between vancomycin and nephrotoxicity. However, risk factors for its development include: pre-existing

renal impairment, use of other nephrotoxic agents (e.g. aminoglycosides) and elderly and dehydrated patients. Renal impairment is usually reversible on discontinuation of treatment. Ototoxicity may occur but again is rarely associated with vancomycin when used alone. Risks for ototoxicity include other ototoxic medications (e.g. aminoglycosides), pre-existing hearing loss and excessive doses – hearing should ideally be monitored in these cases. Hearing loss may be transient or permanent, and antibiotic treatment should be stopped if signs occur. Neutropenia can occur with prolonged usage (e.g. >7 days), and full blood counts should be monitored.

Vancomycin is commonly given by intermittent infusion. Continuous infusions are utilised in some centres, though despite theoretical advantages there is limited evidence of an outcome benefit. Various nomograms based on age, CrCl and/or weight may be used to suggest initial dosing and interval timings. Trough levels are the most reliable and practical method for monitoring efficacy as they serve as a surrogate for AUC calculations, and dangerous peak levels are unlikely with normal trough levels. Various nomograms are available to make dosing and interval adjustments, and local protocols (based on trough levels) should be followed.

Teicoplanin may be preferable to vancomycin if CrCl is poor (e.g. <30 ml/min). Loading doses (× 3–5) are normally used and separated by 12 hours, followed by 24- to 72-hourly dosing, depending on CrCl. Again, local protocols should be followed.

Other Potential Drug Classes for Monitoring

β-Lactam antibiotics may be given by continuous or extended infusion. This may increase the proportion of time spent with concentrations above the MIC, and evidence has demonstrated higher steady-state concentrations and reduced treatment failures, though an outcome benefit is not clear. There is concern that using continuous infusions could lead to increased time with antibiotic concentrations in the so-called mutant selection window (MSW) – a range between the MIC and the mutant prevention concentration (MPC) (the concentration above which emergence of resistance strains is inhibited). Achieving concentrations above the MPC may be difficult and associated with potential toxicity; hence, TDM would be important. The MSW concept may not be relevant for all pathogen–antibiotic combinations.

Linezolid may be amenable to TDM to optimise dosing, rather than to minimise toxicity. A continuous infusion in association with TDM may be able to aid this and minimise inadequate dosing (which is thought to occur in approximately 60 per cent of patients). However robust clinical evidence of improved outcomes is required for this approach to become standard practice.

Anti-fungal monitoring is not routinely used, as agents demonstrate a high degree of inter-patient variability in the dose–exposure relationship. Current evidence only suggests potential TDM use for the mould-active 'azole' group (namely, voriconazole, itraconazole and possibly posaconazole) and for flucytosine (due to toxicity). In critically unwell patients with extensive/multi-site disease, monitoring of these agents may be suitable and should be discussed with local pharmacy/microbiology teams.

Special Circumstances
Continuous Renal Replacement Therapy

Renal replacement therapy in the intensive care unit is not standardised and, therefore, guidelines are challenging. Pharmacokinetics may vary, depending on many factors, including: whether filtration or dialysis, or a combination, is used; the type of membrane used; the dose/ultrafiltrate rate; duration; and patient factors. Discussion with an intensive care unit pharmacist and reference to specialist texts is thus advised.

Extracorporeal Membrane Oxygenation

Extracorporeal membrane oxygenation may affect pharmacokinetics, specifically the V_D and clearance. There are, however, very limited data regarding this, with most studies available involving paediatric populations. Specialist pharmacist/microbiologist advice is therefore recommended, but in general, most agents probably do not require dose adjustment, bar notably meropenem, fluconazole and caspofungin which probably require higher-dosing regimens.

Antibiotic Stewardship

Antibiotic stewardship is defined as 'an organisational or healthcare-system-wide approach to promoting and monitoring judicious use of antimicrobials to preserve their future effectiveness'. Stewardship is embedded within the Health and Social Care Act 2008, and is monitored by the Care Quality Commission. The 'Start Smart – Then Focus' campaign and toolkit offer guidance for an effective stewardship programme and are published by the Department of Health/Public Health England. Stewardship consists of multiple components, including: performing prospective audit with feedback; antibiotic restriction; antibiotic de-escalation; education; guideline use; optimal antibiotic dosing and duration; microbiologist, pharmacist and clinician input; and computer-aided clinical support. The overall aim is to ensure the right drug is given at the right time at the right dose and for the right duration, with a view to eradicating infection and minimising collateral damage (e.g. nosocomial infection, drug toxicity, resistant organisms, increased costs). This process is discussed in more detail in Chapter 3.7.8, Principles of Antibiotic Use In Intensive Care. TDM forms an integral part of stewardship, with its role in helping to establish the correct dose and timing.

Other notable aspects of stewardship include the following:

1. Limiting prescribing to a set formulary restricted by clinical area/specialty/seniority of the prescriber can be effective at limiting widespread use of certain antibiotics. It may, however, lead to delayed administration and compensatory increases in non-restricted antibiotics may occur. Alternatively,

465

locally developed guidelines based on local resistance/sensitivity patterns for empirical antibiotic choice, administration, monitoring and de-escalation or 'rescue' suggestions can improve appropriate antibiotic use.

2. Consideration/use of newer pathogen identification technologies may lead to more rapid identification of pathogens. Examples include automated mass spectrometry, real-time polymerase chain reaction (PCR) and matrix-assisted laser desorption/ionisation time-of-flight (MALDI-TOF) techniques.

Acknowledgements

The authors would like to thank James Clayton, Consultant Microbiologist, for all his help with this chapter.

References and Further Reading

Abdul-Aziz M, Lipman J, Mouton J, Hope W, Roberts J. Applying pharmacokinetic/pharmacodynamic principles in critically ill patients: optimizing efficacy and reducing resistance development. *Semin Respir Crit Care Med* 2015;**36**:136–53.

Cotta MO, Roberts JA, Lipman J. Antibiotic dose optimization in critically ill patients. *Med Intensiva* 2015;**39**:563–72.

Johnson I, Banks V. Antibiotic stewardship in critical care. *BJA Education* 2017;**17**:111–16.

National Institute for Health and Care Excellence. 2015. Antimicrobial stewardship: systems and processes for effective antimicrobial medicine use. www.nice.org.uk/guidance/ng15/chapter/1-Recommendations

Vincent J-L, Bassetti M, François B, *et al.* Advances in antibiotic therapy in the critically ill. *Crit Care* 2016;**20**:133.

Administration of Blood and Blood Products in Intensive Care

4.3

Ben Clevenger

Key Learning Points

1. Right blood, right patient, right time and right place is the key message for safe blood administration.
2. Accidental transfusion of ABO-incompatible blood is classified as a 'never event'.
3. Most errors could be prevented by a final bedside check when performed correctly.
4. Patient blood management has three pillars of focus to reduce unnecessary transfusions: recognition and treatment of anaemia, minimisation of bleeding and blood loss and optimisation of anaemia and transfusion thresholds.
5. Unnecessary delays in transfusion can lead to death and major morbidity.

Keywords: blood transfusion, transfusion reaction, anaemia, patient blood management, haemorrhage

Introduction

Blood transfusion is now very safe when best practice is followed (Table 4.3.1).

Donors are screened for infectious disease, including hepatitis B, HIV, hepatitis C, human T cell lymphotropic virus and syphilis – and in some circumstances, cytomegalovirus, malarial antibodies, West Nile virus antibodies and *Trypanosoma cruzi* antibodies. Precautions to reduce transmission of prion-associated diseases are taken by deferring blood donation from some people at high risk, including those who have received a blood transfusion since 1980. All blood donations are filtered to remove white blood cells (pre-storage leucodepletion) and processed into blood components (Table 4.3.2).

Table 4.3.1 Principles of safe and effective blood transfusion

Ten principles of transfusion

1. Transfusion should only be used when the benefits outweigh the risks and there are no appropriate alternatives.
2. Results of laboratory tests should not be the sole deciding factor for transfusion.
3. Transfusion decisions should be based on clinical assessment, underpinned by evidence-based clinical guidelines.
4. Not all anaemic patients need transfusion (there is no universal 'transfusion trigger') – this should be based upon an individual patient basis.
5. Discuss the risks, benefits and alternatives to transfusion with the patient and gain their consent.
6. The reason for transfusion should be documented in the patient's records.
7. Timely provision of blood component support in major haemorrhage can improve outcome – good communication and teamwork are essential.
8. Failure to check patient identity can be fatal. Confirm identity at every stage of the transfusion process. If there is any discrepancy, do not transfuse.
9. The patient must be monitored during transfusion.
10. Education and training support safe transfusion practice.

Source: Adapted From: *Handbook of Transfusion Medicine*: 5th Edition, 2013.

Table 4.3.2 Blood components

Red cells in additive solution
- Saline, adenine, glucose and mannitol additive solution (SAG-M)
- Irradiated – for patients at risk of transfusion-associated graft-versus-host disease
- Washed red cells – for patients with recurrent or severe allergic or febrile reactions

Platelets

Plasma; fresh frozen plasma (FFP)
- One-donor exposure per pack
- Solvent detergent (SD)-treated FFP (Octaplas) – pooled (up to 1520 donors). SD treatment inactivates bacteria and most encapsulated viruses, including hepatitis B and C and HIV. Sourced from countries at low risk of variant Creutzfeldt–Jakob disease (vCJD)
- Methylene blue-treated FFP (MB-FFP) – single-donor pathogen-reduced component

Cryoprecipitate
- Thawed FFP producing cryoglobulin rich in fibrinogen, factor VIII and von Willebrand factor

Table 4.3.2 (cont.)

Human albumin solution
- Cross-matching not required
- Isotonic (4.5% and 5%) and concentrated (20%)

Clotting factor concentrates
- Single-factor concentrates for most inherited coagulation deficiencies available (except factors V and II (prothrombin))
- Fibrinogen concentrate (factor I)
- Prothrombin complex concentrate (PCC) – factors II, VII, IX and X

Immunoglobulin solutions, granulocytes and plasma derivatives

Blood Groups and Cross-Matching

Blood group antigens are molecules present on the surface of red blood cells (RBCs). ABO antibodies naturally occur after the first 3 months of life. Anti-A or anti-B antibodies in the recipient's plasma bind to transfused cells, activating the complement pathway, which leads to destruction of transfused red cells (intravascular haemolysis) and release of inflammatory cytokines that can cause shock, renal failure and disseminated intravascular coagulation (DIC).

ABO-incompatible red cell transfusions are often fatal and their prevention is the most important step in clinical transfusion practice. There are >300 human blood groups, but only a minority cause clinically significant transfusion reactions. The two most important in clinical practice are the ABO and rhesus (Rh) systems.

Alloantibodies produced by exposure to blood of a different group by transfusion or pregnancy can cause transfusion reactions, haemolytic disease of the fetus and newborn (HDFN) or problems in selecting blood for regularly transfused patients. To prevent sensitisation and the risk of HDFN, RhD-negative or J-Kell (K)-negative girls and women of childbearing potential should not be transfused with RhD- or K-positive red cells, except in an emergency.

Traditional cross-match involves a serological test of the patient's plasma and a sample of red cells from the units of blood to be transfused, looking for evidence of an incompatibility reaction. However, modern electronic 'computer cross-matching' relies on establishing the patient's ABO and RhD groups. With a negative antibody screen, the possibility of incompatible blood being issued is negligible. All compatible units can then be identified from the blood bank database.

Safe Transfusion

Preventable incidents due to patients receiving the 'wrong blood' are nearly always caused by human error and can result in fatal reactions. The crucial final opportunity to prevent mistransfusion is the identity check between patient and blood component. Positive patient identification, excellent communication and good documentation at all stages are required, which can be enhanced by electronic systems such as barcoding.

Where possible, patients should give consent for transfusion, based upon appropriate information and discussion. The National Institute for Health and Care Excellence (NICE) guidance suggests patients be consented for transfusion, including the risks and alternatives. Signed consent is not a legal requirement and the need for consent should not delay the administration of urgent blood transfusion.

Monitoring the patient is essential, including pre-transfusion observations of pulse, BP and temperature 15 minutes after the start of the transfusion, a post-transfusion observation and then observation over the next 24 hours.

Blood should be transfused through a 170- to 200-μm integral mesh filter. A dose of 4 ml/kg should raise the haemoglobin (Hb) concentration by approximately 10 g/l. One adult therapeutic dose of platelets (pool of 4 units) typically raises the platelet count by $20–40 \times 10^9/l$. Platelets can be administered through special administration sets; however, it is safe to use a standard blood administration set. If red cells have previously been used in that set, it should not then be used for platelets.

Adverse Effects of Transfusion

Blood transfusion is very safe overall. In 2018, for over 2.3 million units of blood components (over 1.69 million units of RBCs) issued within the UK, there were 4037 reports submitted to the Serious Hazards of Transfusion (SHOT) database – equating to 16.3 reports per 10,000 components issued in England. SHOT reporting of adverse events and near misses is voluntary. These reports included 20 deaths where transfusion was implicated. Delays in transfusion and pulmonary complications are the most common cause of death and major morbidity. Around 1 in 13,000 blood component units is transfused to the wrong patient, and up to 1 in 1300 pre-transfusion blood samples are taken from the wrong patient. The risk of death from transfusion is approximately 1 in 200,000 in the UK.

Severe acute transfusion reactions are the most common cause of major morbidity (Table 4.3.3). These include immunological reactions (allergy, anaphylaxis,

Table 4.3.3 Non-infectious acute transfusion reactions

Acute transfusion reactions	Signs and symptoms	Further information	Management
Febrile non-haemolytic transfusion reactions	Usually clinically mild Fever, sometimes shivering, muscle pain, nausea	Can occur up to 2 hours post-transfusion	Slow or stop transfusion; give anti-pyretic Monitor closely for signs of more severe transfusion reaction If pyrexia >2°C above baseline or >39°C, stop transfusion
Allergic transfusion reactions	Range from mild urticaria to life-threatening angio-oedema or anaphylaxis	May occur with all blood components, but most commonly with plasma-rich components, including fresh frozen plasma and platelets	Resuscitate as appropriate. All staff carrying out transfusions must be trained in management of anaphylaxis and emergency drugs must be available, particularly intramuscular adrenaline
Acute haemolytic transfusion reactions	For example, ABO incompatibility (1 in 180,000 RBC units transfused) 5–10% of episodes contribute to death of a patient Shock, acute renal failure and disseminated intravascular coagulation ensue	ABO-incompatible red cells react with patient's anti-A or -B antibodies Destruction of transfused RBCs, release of inflammatory cytokines	Call for urgent medical help Resuscitation ABC Discontinue transfusion, maintain venous patency with crystalloid Monitor vital signs Inform transfusion department Return unit and giving set to transfusion laboratory
Bacterial contamination of blood unit	Range from mild pyrexial reactions to rapidly lethal septic shock Rigors, fever, hypotension and shock ensue, with decreased level of consciousness	Acute severe reaction soon after starting transfusion	As above, take blood cultures and immediately treat with intravenous broad-spectrum antibiotic against Gram-positive and -negative bacteria
Transfusion-associated circulatory overload (TACO)	Acute or worsening pulmonary oedema within 6 hours of transfusion Acute respiratory distress, tachycardia, raised BP and positive fluid balance Traditionally under-reported	Small patients such as the elderly or patients most at risk due to inappropriately high volume and rapid blood transfusions Single-unit transfusion practice should be instituted	Supportive treatment Stop transfusion Oxygen and diuretic therapy
Transfusion-related acute lung injury (TRALI)	Usually presents within 2 hours of transfusion with breathlessness and pulmonary oedema (up to 6 hours) 1 in 150,000 units transfused (most commonly plasma-rich components, usually from female donors sensitised during pregnancy)	Classically due to antibodies in donor blood reacting with patient's neutrophils, monocytes or pulmonary endothelium. Inflammatory cells sequestered in lungs, causing plasma leak into alveolar space	Supportive treatment with high-concentration oxygen therapy and ventilatory support as required. Steroids are ineffective and diuretics may increase mortality. Recovery is usual within 1–3 days Retrospective confirmation with demonstration of antibodies in donor plasma that react with patient's white blood cells

Delayed transfusion reactions

Delayed haemolytic transfusion reactions	Occur >24 hours after transfusion in a patient previously 'alloimmunised' to a red cell antigen by a blood transfusion or pregnancy. Falling Hb or failure to increment, jaundice, fever, haemoglobinuria or acute renal failure	Secondary immune response to transfusion of antigen-positive red cells, leading to haemolysis of transfused cells. Apparent up to 14 days post-transfusion	Confirm by laboratory investigation, blood film, repeat blood group and antibody screen Supportive treatment Patient should be given an antibody card

Table 4.3.3 (cont.)

Acute transfusion reactions	Signs and symptoms	Further information	Management
Transfusion-associated graft-versus-host disease (TA-GvHD)	Rare and usually fatal. At-risk patients usually have impaired cell-mediated immunity, including intrauterine transfusions to the fetus, inherited immunodeficiency disorders, and iatrogenic immunosuppression such as stem cell transplantation or purine analogue chemotherapy Only one case since 2000 in the UK due to routine leucodepletion	Viable lymphocytes in blood donation engraft in patient and mount an immune response against recipient's cells of a different human leucocyte antigen type Symptoms 7–14 days post-transfusion – fever, skin rash, diarrhoea, abnormal liver function tests, worsening bone marrow aplasia	Seek specialist transfusion medicine advice
Post-transfusion purpura	Very low platelet count and bleeding 5–12 days post-transfusion	Re-stimulation of platelet-specific alloantibodies in patient that also damage their own platelets Rare since routine leucodepletion	Seek specialist transfusion medicine advice

Table 4.3.4 Infectious hazards of transfusion

Viral infections	Estimated risk per million blood donations[a]	Comments
Hepatitis B	0.79	Readily transmitted by blood or bodily fluids. Perinatal transmission common in endemic areas Initial acute hepatitis; sometimes chronic carrier-state cirrhosis and hepatocellular carcinoma risk
Hepatitis C	0.035	Often symptomless initial infection; however, 80% develop chronic carrier state, leading to cirrhosis, liver failure and liver cancer
HIV	0.14	Very rare due to modern donor selection and screening Two incidents since SHOT reporting both from HIV antibody-negative window period donations prior to screening for HIV RNA
Hepatitis E	Since May 2017, all red cells and platelet components are routinely screened for hepatitis E virus	Small, non-enveloped RNA virus. Increasing incidence in the UK since 2011
Bacteria	Most contamination from donor at the time of collection, which can proliferate during storage	*Staphylococcus aureus*, *Escherichia coli*, *Klebsiella* and *Pseudomonas* spp. More common with platelets due to storage at 20–24°C
Variant Creutzfeldt–Jakob disease (vCJD)	Fatal neurological disease due to a prion protein 174 recorded cases in the UK	No practical screening for blood donors Risk reduction measures by importation of some products and exclusion of at-risk donors (including those who have received a blood transfusion since 1980)

[a] All have dropped dramatically due to the introduction of donor screening, making transmission very rare in the UK.

haemolytic reactions and lung injury), circulatory overload and rare bacterial contamination. Transfusion-transmitted infection is very rare; however, awareness for new threats is necessitated (Table 4.3.4). Variant Creutzfeldt–Jakob disease (CJD) transmission by blood had a major impact upon transfusion in the UK, though this risk appears to be receding.

If a serious transfusion reaction is suspected, the transfusion should be stopped, and the patient assessed and resuscitated as appropriate. The patient's details on their ID band should be checked and matched with the component label. There is a legal requirement to report serious adverse events and reactions to the Medicine and Healthcare products Regulatory Agency (MHRA).

Patient Blood Management

The aim of patient blood management (PBM) is to prevent unnecessary and inappropriate blood transfusions, with the aim of improving transfusion safety and patient outcomes. PBM has three pillars of focus:

- Recognition and treatment of anaemia
- Minimisation of bleeding and blood loss
- Optimisation of anaemia and transfusion thresholds

Preoperative anaemia is now a recognised independent, yet modifiable risk factor for both increased morbidity and mortality after surgery. Iron deficiency is the most commonly detected cause in the preoperative period, and there is increasing understanding of the role of inflammation in the production of a state of functional iron deficiency, as well as absolute iron deficiency, which is increasingly treated using high-dose intravenous (IV) iron preparations.

Intraoperatively, blood loss should be minimised using multi-modal interventions, including anti-fibrinolytic drugs, intraoperative cell salvage, minimally invasive surgical techniques and point-of-care monitoring of bleeding and coagulation. The efficiency of cell salvage is improved with use of anti-fibrinolytic drugs, and tranexamic acid with cell salvage is recommended by NICE.

The TRICC trial in 1999 strongly influenced the practice of blood transfusion, demonstrating that there was a trend towards lower mortality in patients randomised to a restrictive policy, along with lower rates of new organ failure and acute respiratory distress syndrome. These findings have been replicated in many patient populations subsequently. Post-operatively, restrictive transfusion thresholds have been shown to be non-inferior to liberal thresholds, whilst reducing the volume and costs of transfused blood in patients. However, in those patients with ischaemic heart disease, a higher transfusion threshold has been demonstrated to be beneficial.

In the haemodynamically stable, non-bleeding patient, transfusion should only be considered if the Hb concentration is 80 g/l or lower. A single red cell unit should be transfused, and the patient reassessed before further transfusions take place. This should happen after each unit of blood.

Treatment of anaemia post-operatively and in critical care is an area of current research focus. The IRONMAN study of IV iron versus placebo in critical-illness anaemic patients admitted to critical care (excluding those with severe sepsis) randomised patients to either IV ferric carboxymaltose or placebo. No significant difference in the number of RBCs transfused was demonstrated, although IV iron showed a significantly higher Hb concentration on hospital discharge (107 g/l versus 100 g/l; $p = 0.02$).

Post-operative red cell salvage and re-infusion from drains can be utilised in relevant surgeries, and there is increasing focus on the use of post-operative iron infusions to improve post-operative Hb mass.

Effective Transfusion in Surgery and Critical Care

More than half of all patients admitted to critical care are anaemic, of whom 30 per cent have an initial Hb concentration of <90 g/l. This can be exacerbated by haemorrhage, haemodilution and frequent blood sampling. Reduced red cell production due to inflammation becomes an important factor and after 7 days, 80 per cent of patients have a Hb concentration of <90 g/l. Most critical care transfusions are to treat low Hb concentrations, rather than active bleeding. Strategies such as minimising blood sampling and use of paediatric sampling tubes have been shown to reduce transfusion rates.

Major Haemorrhage

This can be defined as loss of >1 blood volume within 24 hours, loss of >50 per cent of total blood volume in <3 hours or bleeding in excess of 150 ml/min, and practically by bleeding that leads to hypotension or tachycardia. Early recognition and intervention are essential.

Successful transfusion support in major haemorrhage depends on the rapid provision of compatible blood, a protocol-driven multidisciplinary team approach and excellent communication between the clinical team and the transfusion laboratory. The benefit of routinely transfusing fresh frozen plasma (FFP) in a fixed ratio to red cells in traumatic haemorrhage and early administration of tranexamic acid has been shown to reduce mortality.

Management of Patients Who Do not Accept Transfusion

The values and beliefs of all patients must be respected. Jehovah's Witnesses decline the transfusion of blood and blood products, yet individuals will have different preferences as to what products or autologous procedures they are willing to accept. It is important to clearly establish the preference of each patient, and when possible, refer to an advance decision document that must be respected. Emergency transfusion of critically ill patients with temporary incapacity must be given, unless there is clear evidence of prior refusal such as a valid advance decision document. No one can give consent on behalf of a patient with mental capacity.

References and Further Reading

Hébert PC, Wells G, Blachman MA, *et al*. A multicenter, randomized, controlled clinical trial of transfusion requirements in critical care. *N Engl J Med* 1999;**340**:409–17.

Klein AA, Arnold P, Bingham RM, *et al*. AAGBI guidelines: the use of blood components and their alternatives. *Anaesthesia* 2016;**71**:829–42.

National Institute for Health and Care Excellence. 2015. Blood transfusion. NICE guideline [NG24]. www.nice .org.uk/guidance/ng24

Norfolk D (ed). *Handbook of Transfusion Medicine*, 5th edn. Norwich: The Stationery Office; 2013.

Serious Hazards of Transfusion (SHOT). SHOT publications – articles. www.shotuk.org/shot-publicati ons-2/750-2/

4.4 Monitoring Coagulation, Including Thromboelastography

Ben Clevenger

Key Learning Points

1. Coagulopathy is common in the ICU and abnormal results should be interpreted in the context of the patient's clinical condition.
2. Conventional coagulation tests monitor the intrinsic and extrinsic pathways of coagulation and are the mainstay of haemostatic monitoring.
3. Full blood count and conventional coagulation tests have a turnaround time that renders them unhelpful in acute bleeding scenarios.
4. Point-of-care viscoelastic tests, such as thromboelastography (TEG®) and rotational thromboelastometry (ROTEM®), can provide a rapid overview of coagulation from clot formation to lysis, demonstrating both hypo- and pro-coagulant states.
5. Algorithms based upon viscoelastic tests in bleeding patients have demonstrated a reduction in blood transfusion requirements.

Keywords: coagulopathy, coagulation, clotting, laboratory tests, point of care, thromboelastography, TEG®, ROTEM®

Introduction

The usual screening tests to investigate abnormal haemostasis are full blood count and laboratory-based conventional coagulation tests (CCTs). CCTs include the activated partial thromboplastin time (APTT), prothrombin time (PT) and international normalised ratio (PT-INR). These tests were developed based upon the classical intrinsic and extrinsic pathways of coagulation. PT or APTT results do not reflect clot stability and activity of the fibrinolytic system, nor do they adequately reflect pro-thrombotic states.

The ideal coagulation test would be easily performed and interpreted, with results rapidly available, which are reliable and robust. These would ideally give evidence towards both the risk of bleeding and the risk of thrombosis in the critically ill patient.

Point-of-care tests (POCTs) give rapid results at the bedside upon which to base coagulation management. Viscoelastic tests (VETs) of coagulation, such as thromboelastography (TEG®) and rotational thromboelastometry (ROTEM®), analyse whole blood to give a complete assessment of haemostasis from clot formation to fibrinolysis.

When abnormal coagulation tests arise in an otherwise stable patient, consideration must be made of a sampling error or testing problem, e.g. blood taken from an inadequately flushed heparinised arterial line or blood clotting within a sample tube leading to spurious results. If a repeat result is similar, then further investigation of coagulation and liaison with a haematologist should take place as required.

Conventional Coagulation Tests

Conventional coagulation tests remain the mainstay of haemostatic monitoring in intensive care (Table 4.4.1). However, there remain several deficiencies to these tests. The PT measures the extrinsic pathway of coagulation and is relatively insensitive, remaining normal until single factor levels are <50 per cent of normal values (remaining more sensitive to multiple factor deficiencies).

APTT is used commonly in the ICU to monitor those patients receiving unfractionated heparin. This can remain normal in mild deficiencies of the intrinsic and common pathways of coagulation, including factor deficiency, mild von Willebrand disease, platelet dysfunction and factor XIII deficiency. A normal platelet count does not exclude platelet dysfunction – including in those taking anti-platelet therapy.

If the APTT and/or PT are prolonged, a mixing test is performed. The patient's plasma is mixed with normal plasma in a 1:1 ratio to distinguish between a clotting factor deficiency and an inhibitor. If the result

Table 4.4.1 Conventional tests of coagulation

Test	Method	Measurement	Normal range	Prolonged by
PT/PT-INR	The time for fibrin strand formation when platelet-poor plasma is added to calcium and thromboplastin (tissue factor and phospholipid) The INR is the ratio of the test PT sample compared to a normal PT (patient PT/control PT), used because of the variability between laboratory reagents and instruments	• Extrinsic pathway • Prothrombin (factor II) • Factors I, V, VII and X	PT: 13–15 seconds INR: 0.9–1.2	• Factor I, II, V, VII and X deficiency • Vitamin K deficiency or inhibition (e.g. warfarin) • Fibrinogen deficiency • High-concentration heparin • Direct thrombin inhibitors (e.g. lepirudin) • Dilutional coagulopathy
APTT	APTT reagent contains phospholipid, but no tissue factor. Platelet-poor plasma is added to the reagent and a contact activator (e.g. silica or ellagic acid) before calcium is added to initiate clotting. APTT is the time taken for a fibrin clot to form once calcium is added	• Intrinsic and common coagulation pathways • Fibrinogen • Factors II, V, VIII, IX, XI and XII • Does not test factors VII and XIII	27–35 seconds	• Factor VIII, IX, XI and XII deficiency • Lupus anticoagulant • Acquired clotting factor inhibitors • Vitamin K deficiency • Liver disease • Direct thrombin inhibitors • DIC • Dilutional coagulopathy • Unfractionated heparin
Thrombin time (TT)	Measures the conversion of fibrinogen to fibrin after the addition of thrombin (which cleaves fibrinogen) to platelet-poor plasma, comparing the rate of clot formation to that of normal pooled plasma	Functional fibrinogen levels (qualitative or quantitative deficiency)	13–15 seconds	• Dysfibrinogenaemia • DIC • Liver disease • Malignancy • Unfractionated heparin • Elevated fibrin degradation products (e.g. DIC) • Paraproteinaemia • Hypoalbuminaemia
Fibrinogen	Fibrinogen can be measured by several assays, including the commonly used Clauss assay, based upon the time for fibrin clot formation, allowing the fibrinogen concentration to be calculated against a calibration curve of reference plasma with known concentrations of fibrinogen	Fibrinogen concentration	1.5–5.0 g/l	
Factor assays	Specific factor assays can be requested in the light of an abnormal screening test	Individual factors selected, including prothrombin (factor II) and factors VII and X	Dependent upon selected test	

Abbreviations: PT = prothrombin time; PT-INR = international normalised ratio; INR = international normalised ratio; APTT = activated partial thromboplastin time; TT = thrombin time; DIC = disseminated intravascular coagulation.

remains abnormal, the plasma contains an 'inhibitor' – such as heparin, anti-phospholipid antibodies or coagulation factor-specific inhibitors. If the mixture corrects the values, then the patient has a factor deficiency – which can then be investigated by factor assay.

Point-of-Care Tests

POCTs can be performed at, or near, the patient's bedside, providing real-time information to inform goal-directed treatments and monitor the effects of therapeutic interventions.

Activated Clotting Time

The activated clotting time (ACT) is used to monitor the effect of unfractionated heparin in patients undergoing cardiac (particularly those on cardiopulmonary bypass) or vascular surgery, and those receiving haemofiltration or extracorporeal membrane oxygenation (ECMO) where heparin is administered. Fresh whole blood is added to an activator of coagulation, via the intrinsic pathway. The normal reference range is between 70 and 180 seconds. In cardiopulmonary bypass, heparin is usually given to maintain an ACT of >400 seconds, to prevent clotting within the bypass circuit.

Viscoelastic Tests – Thromboelastography (TEG®) and Rotational Thromboelastometry (ROTEM®)

These tests allow a global assessment of coagulation, utilising whole blood. It has been shown that use of POCT-based coagulation and transfusion management algorithms intraoperatively reduces transfusion requirements. TEG® and ROTEM® assess haemostatic function from clot formation and strengthening, then retraction and fibrinolysis. Whole blood is added to a cuvette, into which a pin is suspended, connected to a detector. The cup is rotated around the pin (TEG®), or the pin rotated within the cup (ROTEM®). As the blood clots, fibrin strands form between the cup and pin, altering the rotation, forming characteristic traces as this is transmitted to the detector (Figure 4.4.1), which can be read to provide additional information on the real-time clotting process (Table 4.4.2). Native tests use whole blood alone, or activators (e.g. kaolin or tissue factor) can be added to accelerate the coagulation process. Heparinase can be added to reverse the action of heparin to assess haemostasis in heparinised patients.

Functional fibrinogen concentration can be measured using a platelet inhibitor (abciximab for TEG® or cytochalasin D in the FIBTEM test using ROTEM®).

The uptake of viscoelastic POCT devices has historically been hindered by the need for training in pipetting blood, mixing reagents and loading cuvettes. However, these have been eliminated by the modern generations of these devices such as the TEG6s® and ROTEM Sigma®. These no longer require the pipetting of blood and can perform a range of assays using a single blood sample. The TEG6s® uses novel resonance-frequency viscoelasticity measurements and microfluidic cartridges. A standard cartridge will provide four results: a citrated kaolin (CK)-activated TEG trace; a citrated kaolin heparinase (CKH) trace to remove any effect of heparin; a citrated rapid TEG (CRT) trace which rapidly assesses clot strength, including a 10-minute indicated maximum amplitude (MA) value (called A10) and a final MA value; and a citrated functional fibrinogen (CFF) trace for the isolated contribution of fibrinogen to clot strength.

The ROTEM Sigma® retains a cup and pin that have been incorporated into a fully automated system. These newer devices reduce the training and time required to perform VETs, increasing their accessibility to clinicians, and may also improve the validity of results by reducing sample preparation errors.

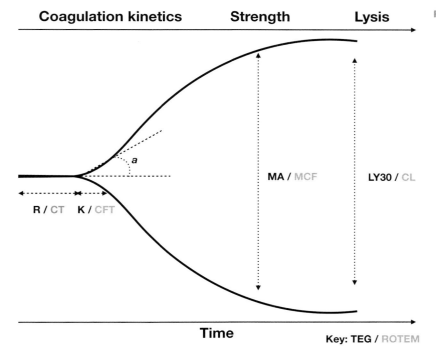

Figure 4.4.1 Traces of TEG®/ROTEM®.

Table 4.4.2 Parameters of TEG®/ROTEM®

	TEG®	ROTEM®	Description
Clotting time	R (minutes)	CT	Relates to concentration of soluble clotting factors in the plasma, the period of initial fibrin formation (time to reach 2-mm amplitude on the tracing)
Clot kinetics	K (minutes)	CFT	Measure the kinetics of clot formation Measures the speed to reach a specific level of clot strength (period for amplitude to increase from 2 to 20 mm)
	Alpha angle (angle in degrees)	α	Measures the rate of clot formation and reflects the rate of fibrin build-up and cross-linking (angle between a tangent to the tracing at 2-mm amplitude and the horizontal midline)
Clot strength	MA (mm)	MCF	Represents the ultimate strength of the clot (platelets and fibrin), the maximum dynamic properties of fibrin and platelet bonding via glycoprotein IIb/IIIa receptors (greatest vertical width of tracing)
Clot stability	LY30	CLI	Relates to clot stability and lysis Measures the rate of amplitude reduction from MA at 30 minutes (in per cent)

Abbreviations: R = reaction time; CT = clotting time; K = K-value; CFT = clot formation time; MA = maximum amplitude; MCF = maximum clot firmness; LY30 = lysis at 30 minutes as a ratio of MA; CLI = clot lysis index.

Platelet Tests

The platelet count is part of the routine full blood count, with a normal range of 150–400 × 10^9/l. However, patients with a normal quantitative platelet count can suffer from functional disorders due to disease or anti-platelet drugs. Additionally, there is marked individual variability in response to anti-platelet drugs. Platelet function can be assessed by a variety of tests, including light transmission aggregometry (LTA), flow cytometry and impedance aggregometry.

Standard VETs cannot be used to assess the effect of anti-platelet drugs. However, platelet mapping assays can be undertaken using TEG®, measuring the MA reduction occurring with anti-platelet therapy and reporting the percentage inhibition and percentage aggregation. The inhibiting effects of the different types of anti-platelet agents, including thromboxane A2 inhibitors (e.g. aspirin) and adenosine diphosphate (ADP) inhibitors (e.g. clopidogrel), are measured using arachidonic acid or ADP agonists to create an adjusted MA which is compared to the patient's baseline. A result of <30 per cent platelet inhibition is associated with an increased risk of in-stent thrombosis, but it can be assumed that there is no increased risk of bleeding at this level of inhibition.

Thrombin Generation Tests

Thrombin generation is the key event in coagulation and the formation of a thrombus. Such tests are an established research tool, with increasing interest in their clinical application. Thrombin generation tests can give information regarding the lag time (to start thrombin generation), time to peak, peak height and endogenous thrombin potential in samples, helping to quantify an individual's risk of bleeding or thrombosis beyond the start of coagulation, as measured by CCTs, and beyond when a fibrin clot is generated, as measured by VETs.

References and Further Reading

Haas T, Fries D, Tanaka KA, *et al.* Usefulness of standard plasma coagulation tests in the management of perioperative coagulopathic bleeding: is there any evidence? *Br J Anaesth* 2015;**114**:217–24.

Kozek-Langenecker SA, Ahmed AB, Afshari A, *et al.* Management of severe perioperative bleeding. *Eur J Anaesthesiol* 2017;**34**:332–95.

Lancé MD. A general review of major global coagulation assays: thromboelastography, thrombin generation test and clot waveform analysis. *Thromb J* 2015;**13**:2607.

Levi M, Hunt BJ. A critical appraisal of point-of-care coagulation testing in critically ill patients. *J Thromb Haemost* 2015;**13**:1960–7.

Mallett SV, Armstrong M. Point-of-care monitoring of haemostasis. *Anaesthesia* 2014;**70**(Suppl 4):73–7, e25–6.

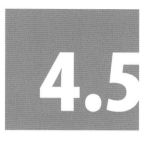

Fluids, Inotropes and Vasopressors, Vasodilators and Anti-hypertensives

Ed McIlroy

Key Learning Points

1. Try to avoid high chloride-containing solutions as they worsen peri-operative outcomes and, in particular, can cause acute kidney injury.
2. There is currently no evidence to support the use of albumin over crystalloids.
3. Multiple studies have found no evidence of superiority of early goal-directed therapy with dobutamine.
4. Bicarbonate will denature inotropes if infused together.
5. Beta-blocker initiation should be used cautiously in the critical care population but may have benefit in the sickest patients.

Keywords: fluid therapy, inotropes, vasopressors, inodilators, anti-hypertensives, vasodilators, beta-blockers

Fluids

Intravenous fluids are prescribed to replace water, electrolytes and blood components, resuscitate and improve tissue/organ perfusion. They are used in the majority of hospital admissions.

Fluid Physiology

Water is freely distributed across all body compartments, and thus has very little effect on intravascular volume. Sodium-containing solutions are distributed across extracellular spaces, resulting in moderate effects on intravascular space, whilst solutions containing large molecules (e.g. gelatins/starches/proteins) remain in the intravascular space to a greater degree. Starling's forces provide a simple model of how fluids move between vessels and the extravascular space. However, it is thought that the colloid osmotic pressure of the endothelial glycocalyx and its disruption in disease states also contribute significantly to fluid distribution.

The ICU Patient and Fluid Treatment

An ICU admission is often associated with liberal fluid prescription. Positive fluid balance has been related to poor outcomes in some pathologies (e.g. acute respiratory distress syndrome (ARDS) and sepsis), secondary to tissue/organ oedema (Box 4.5.1).

Despite best intentions to titrate fluid therapy carefully, insensible losses/third space collections and deranged fluid dynamics often make this difficult. Causes of fluid derangements in ICU patients include:

- Oncotic pressure gradient loss (low albumin)
- Loss of musculoskeletal pump (venous and lymphatic return impaired by prolonged immobility)
- Leaky capillaries due to inflammation (water movement from intravascular to interstitial compartment)
- Inflamed serosal surfaces which are leaky, allowing potential space fluid collection

In light of this, there are some advocates for 'de-resuscitation' (i.e. fluid restriction) by days 3–7 of critical illness.

Box 4.5.1 Effects of Tissue/Organ Oedema

- Impaired oxygen and metabolite diffusion
- Distortion of tissue architecture
- Impeded capillary blood flow and lymphatic drainage
- Disturbed cell–cell interactions
- Raised intra-abdominal pressure
- Reduced perfusion of swollen/encapsulated organs
- Oedema of anastomotic sites
- Damage to endothelial glycocalyx

Cystalloids

These are used as 'maintenance' and 'resuscitation' fluids, and for electrolyte replacement. They are cheap, freely available, easily stored and not allergenic.

- Sodium chloride (NaCl) 0.9%
- Hartmann's/Ringer's lactate
- Dextrose solutions
- Dextrose/saline solutions (0.9% or 0.45% NaCl with 5% dextrose)
- Hypertonic saline
- Bicarbonate and phosphate solutions

The electrolyte concentrations and pH of crystalloids can be seen in Table 4.5.1.

The routine use of 'normal' saline has been superseded by 'balanced' solutions (e.g. Hartmann's), predominantly due to their lower chloride content reducing the incidence of hyperchloraemic acidosis (with lower incidence of post-operative infection and blood transfusion) and renal injury or the need for renal replacement therapy. It is also thought the higher acidity and chloride content of 0.9% NaCl damages the endothelial glycocalyx.

Balanced solutions contain buffers (either lactate or acetate), which are metabolised by the liver or kidney to bicarbonate. The dextrose/saline solutions should be used in paediatrics (possibly with the exception of during acute resuscitation).

Things to Consider

- Crystalloids potentially spend limited time in the intravascular space, resulting in volume overload/tissue oedema (due to increased extravascular space diffusion).
- Glucose solutions, in particular, are the equivalent of giving free water (once glucose is metabolised), and thus do little to increase intravascular volume and have added potential to dilute electrolytes.
- Dextrose 20% and 50% can cause phlebitis, necessitating large vein delivery.

Sodium Bicarbonate

Useful in

- Hyperkalaemia
- Sodium channel blocker overdose (e.g. tricyclic antidepressant overdose)
- Urinary alkalinisation (salicylate poisoning)
- Bicarbonate replacement

Adverse effects of sodium bicarbonate include those seen in Box 4.5.2.

Table 4.5.1 Electrolyte concentrations and pH of various crystalloids

Fluid	Na^+ (mmol/l)	K^+ (mmol/l)	Cl^- (mmol/l)	HCO_3^- (mmol/l)	Ca^{2+} (mmol/l)	Mg^{2+} (mmol/l)	Oncotic pressure (mmH$_2$O)	Typical plasma half-life	pH
5% dextrose	–	–	–	–	–	–	0	–	4.0
0.9% NaCl	154	0	154	0	0		0	–	5.0
Ringer's lactate (Hartmann's)	131	5	111	29[a]	2	1	0	–	6.5
4% NaHCO$_3$	1000	0	0	1000	0	0	–	–	8.0
Haemaccel (succinylated gelatin)	145	5.1	145	0	6.25		370	5 hours	7.4
Gelofusine® (polygeline gelatin)	154	0.4	125	0	0.4	0.4	465	4 hours	7.4
Hetastarch	154	0	154	0	0		310	17 days	5.5
Human albumin solution 4.5%	150	0	120	0	0		275	–	7.4
Human albumin solution 20%	50–120	<10	<40	0	0	0			6.4–7.4

[a] Lactate or acetate added to solutions is rapidly metabolised by the liver to form bicarbonate ions. Bicarbonate cannot be added directly as it is unstable and would precipitate.

Abbreviations: Na^+ = sodium ions; K^+ = potassium ions; Cl^- = chloride ions; HCO_3^- = bicarbonate ions; Ca^{2+} = calcium ions; Mg^{2+} = magnesium ions.

Box 4.5.2 Adverse Effects of Sodium Bicarbonate

- Hypernatraemia (1 mmol of Na^+ for every 1 mmol of HCO_3^-)
- Hyperosmolality
- Hypokalaemia
- Hypocalcaemia
- Volume overload
- Rebound or 'overshoot' alkalosis
- Impaired oxygen unloading due to left shift of the oxyhaemoglobin dissociation curve
- Hypercapnia (worsens intracellular acidosis)
- Tissue necrosis (if extravasation occurs)
- Denatures catecholamines if delivered with same infusion line

Box 4.5.3 Complications of Hypertonic Saline

- Hyperosmolality
- Overshoot hypernatraemia
- Congestive heart failure and pulmonary oedema
- Hypokalaemia
- Normal anion gap metabolic acidosis
- Coagulopathy
- Phlebitis
- Renal failure due to vasoconstriction
- Decreased level of consciousness
- Rebound intracranial hypertension
- Seizures
- Central pontine myelinolysis
- Subdural and intra-parenchymal haemorrhage

Things to Consider

- Metabolic acidosis leads to adverse cardiovascular effects, so endeavour to correct the underlying cause of acidosis and give supportive care, rather than treat the numbers with sodium bicarbonate.
- Due to the Henderson–Hasselbalch equation, increased amounts of carbon dioxide will be produced; thus, ensure adequate ventilation to ensure elimination.

Hypertonic Saline

(Preparations: 2%, 3%, 5%, 7% and 23%)

Useful in

- Acute intracranial hypertension (osmotic diuretic)
- Correction of hyponatraemia (may be used when fluid restriction/conservative measures have failed, or acutely if the patient is symptomatic (seizures, coma, confusion)). In the latter instance, recent European guidelines recommend raising the sodium level by 5 mmol/l by using 150 ml of 3% NaCl over 20 minutes. The risk–benefit is thought to tip in favour of avoiding cerebral oedema versus osmotic demyelination

Complications of hypertonic saline include those seen in Box 4.5.3.

Colloids

This broad term covers a number of fluids, including gelatins, starches, albumin and blood products (packed red blood cells, platelets, fresh frozen plasma, cryoprecipitate and blood product concentrates).

Gelatins

- Constituents: large-molecular-weight proteins (bovine, heat-treated and then cooled), suspended in saline solutions
- Uses: plasma replacement; increasing plasma colloid oncotic pressure
- Benefits: 95 per cent excreted unchanged in urine; it is thought to maintain glycocalyx integrity
- Problems and considerations: anaphylactoid/anaphylaxis reactions; triggers coagulopathy

Hydroxyethyl Starches

Mentioned here for completion, but these have since been withdrawn from the market due to safety concerns, including acute kidney injury, coagulopathy, anaphylaxis and accumulation in the reticuloendothelial system causing pruritus. Contained a derivative of amylopectin (a branched starch).

Albumin

- Uses: fluid resuscitation, intravascular protein replacement, extravascular buffer; possible free radical scavenger (oxygen and nitrite peroxidases)
- Preparations: 4% and 20% solutions
- Problems and considerations: risk of allergic reactions. As a resuscitation fluid, albumin has no evidence to support its use over crystalloids such as normal saline (SAFE study data). Albumin passes through the septic leaking microvasculature into the extravascular space, and thus may exacerbate tissue oedema. It should be avoided in traumatic brain injury as it is associated with increased mortality. This may be secondary to increasing intracranial pressure via an oncotic effect

479

Inotropes, Vasopressors and Inodilators

When fluids fail to optimise cardiac output, pharmacological interventions may be required (dependent on pathology). Initiating these potent pharmacological agents requires careful titration according to clinical assessment and cardiac output monitoring. These drugs work on various receptors (e.g. α- and β-adrenoreceptors) (Table 4.5.2) and have varying effects on the cardiovascular system (Box 4.5.4). The receptors/mechanisms of action, metabolism, doses, uses, effects, side effects and cautions of inotropes, vasopressors and inodilators, as well as their respective reference studies, can be seen in Table 4.5.3.

Vasodilators

In general, vasodilators reduce systemic vascular resistance and may therefore be used to counteract vasoconstriction and dilate stenosed vessels (Table 4.5.4).

Miscellaneous Vasodilators

These drugs are often used as vasodilators. Some of their mechanisms are not well described, and others do not function by increasing nitric oxide, blocking calcium channels or activating potassium channels (Table 4.5.5).

Anti-hypertensives
Alpha (α) Antagonists

These are used to treat hypertension (acute and chronic) and Raynaud's disease, as well as relax bladder and prostate smooth muscle in prostatic hypertrophy. They function by manipulating central autonomic control as well as peripheral arterioles and smooth muscle. They can be selective for $α_1$ and $α_2$, and also be non-selective. There is sometimes a 'first-dose' effect where there is a profound decrease in blood pressure with the first dose that can induce orthostatic hypotension (Table 4.5.6).

Beta (β) Antagonists

These are commonly used for the treatment of blood pressure, tachycardia, secondary cardiac protection, anxiety, glaucoma and migraine prophylaxis. They are competitive antagonists (Table 4.5.7), and prolonged administration may result in upregulation of β-adrenoreceptors. Different agents have varying degrees of receptor selectivity, with desirable $β_1$ effects and generally undesirable $β_2$ effects (Box 4.5.5).

Table 4.5.2 Physiological response to receptor activation

Receptor	Effect
α1	• Vasoconstriction • Inotropy
α2	• Vasoconstriction • Sedation • Inhibition of lipolysis
β1	• Inotropy • Chronotropy • Dromotropy (increased speed of atrioventricular conduction)
β2	• Inotropy • Bronchodilation • Vasodilation
Dopamine (DA)	• Natriuresis • Splanchnic vasodilation

> **Box 4.5.4 General Effects of Inotropes, Vasopressors and Inodilators**
>
> - Inotropes: increase myocardial contractility, e.g. adrenaline, dobutamine, dopamine, ephedrine
> - Vasopressors: cause vasoconstriction, thus increasing systemic (SVR) and pulmonary vascular resistance (PVR), e.g. noradrenaline, vasopressin, metaraminol, methylene blue
> - Inodilators: cause inotropy and peripheral vasodilation (i.e. reduced SVR/PVR), e.g. milrinone, levosimendan
>
> NB. Some of these agents overlap in their effects, generally in a dose-dependent manner.

Table 4.5.3 Inotropes, vasopressors and inodilators

Drug	Receptors/ mechanism of action	Metabolism	Dose	Uses	Effects	Side effects	Cautions	Literature
Adrenaline (= *epinephrine*)	β > α (at low dose); α > β (at high dose) *G receptor-increased* Ca^{2+} *and* ↑ *cAMP*	Onset: minutes COMT/MAO $T_{1/2}$: 2 minutes	Stat: 0.1–1 mg/ml in ALS/anaphylaxis Infusion: 0.01–0.5 µg/ (kg min)	ALS Low CO Cardiac surgery	Increased CO Increased myocardial O_2 consumption Coronary and cerebral artery dilation Bronchodilation Increased SVR	Increased metabolic rate Lactic acidosis Increased glucose Low K^+ and PO_4	Central line required Degraded in alkaline environment (i.e. do not run with $NaHCO_3$) Avoid in HOCM	PARAMEDIC 2, Perkins *et al., N Engl J Med* (2018) – adrenaline versus placebo for out-of-hospital cardiac arrest: increased 30-day survival in adrenaline group, with possible worse neurological outcome CATS, Annane *et al., Lancet* (2007) – adrenaline versus noradrenaline ± dobutamine first-line agent in septic shock: NO DIFFERENCE (possible trend towards harm in adrenaline group) CENSER, Permpikul *et al., Am J Resp Crit Care Med* (2019) – low-dose noradrenaline versus standard therapy in early shock: may improve shock control by 6 hours
Noradrenaline (= *norepinephrine*)	α > β *G receptor-increased* Ca^{2+} *and* ↑ *cAMP*	Onset: minutes COMT/MAO $T_{1/2}$: 2 minutes	Infusion: 0.05–0.5 µg/ (kg min)	Septic shock Vasodilation	Increased SVR Improved coronary perfusion Increased myocardial O_2 consumption Increased venous return	Reflex bradycardia HTN Peripheral ischaemia May increase PVR Decreased hepatic/ splanchnic/ uterine blood flow	Central line required Degraded in alkaline environment (i.e. do not run with $NaHCO_3$) Avoid in HOCM Caution in patients on MAOIs = exaggerated/prolonged effects	
Dopamine	DA > β > α *D1 and D2 – G receptor-increased* Ca^{2+} *and* ↑ *cAMP*	Onset: minutes COMT/MAO $T_{1/2}$: 3 minutes	Infusion: 1–5 µg/(kg min) = DA 5–10 µg/(kg min) = β >10 µg/(kg min) = α	Cardiac surgery First-line paediatric inotrope	At low rates: β1: Increased HR Increased contractility Increased CO Increased coronary flow At higher rates (>10 µg/(kg min)): α1: Increased SVR Increased venous return D1: Vasodilated mesenteric vessels ? Increased UO due to increased CO and inhibition of proximal tubule Na^+ re-absorption	Increased PVR Attenuated carotid body response to hypoxia Nausea and vomiting Arrhythmias Immune dysregulation	Caution in patients on MAOIs = exaggerated/prolonged effects	Ventura *et al., Crit Care Med* (2015) – dopamine versus epinephrine as first-line in paediatric septic shock: possible increased mortality in dopamine group, increased time to resuscitation, greater need for RRT and hospital-acquired infections also noted. Single centre, low patient number Bellomo *et al., Lancet* (2000) – low-dose dopamine in early renal dysfunction: no place for dopamine to prevent renal dysfunction in SIRS De Backer *et al., N Engl J Med* (2010) – dopamine versus noradrenaline in shock: increased tachydysrhythmias in dopamine group

Table 4.5.3 (cont.)

Drug	Receptors/ mechanism of action	Metabolism	Dose	Uses	Effects	Side effects	Cautions	Literature
Dobutamine	β1 and β2 Gs-adenylyl cyclase – ↑cAMP	Onset: minutes Liver methylation and conjugation Urinary and biliary excretion $T_{1/2}$: 2 minutes	Infusion: 0.5–20 μg/ (kg min)	Low CO Cardiac surgery	Increased contractility Increased HR Increased myocardial O_2 requirement	Mild β2-mediated decrease in SVR Arrhythmias	Avoid in patients prone to AF/flutter (increased AV conduction) Avoid in cardiac outflow obstruction (AS/tamponade/ HOCM/Takotsubo)	ARISE, N Engl J Med (2014) and PROMISE, N Engl J Med (2015): no benefit (or harm) in EGDT (including dobutamine) and SCVO₂ sampling. Also not cost-effective See above for CATS (2007)
Milrinone	Phosphodiesterase III inhibitor ↑cAMP = net Ca^{2+} influx	Minimal metabolism $T_{1/2}$: 2–3 hours (prolonged in RF)	Loading dose: 50 μg/kg Infusion: 0.375–0.75 μg/ (kg min)	Low CO Cardiac surgery Chronic β receptor down-regulation/ beta-blocked patients (CCF) Pulm HTN/RV failure	Decreased SVR Increased contractility Decreased PVR	Hypotension may require vasopressor Thrombocytopenia Liver impairment	Accumulation in RF	Yamada et al., J Cardiothorac Vasc Anesth (2000): more successful wean from cardiopulmonary bypass OPTIME-CHF, J Am Coll Cardiol (2003): milrinone may be deleterious in IHD, neutral to beneficial in non-IHD cardiomyopathy
Vasopressin	V1: vasoconstriction V2: renal/ endothelium V3: pituitary oxytocin receptors	Peptidases Increased effect: TCAs, opiates, NSAIDs, barbiturates, catecholamines Decreased effect: ethanol, phenytoin, corticosteroids, haloperidol	Infusion: 0.01–0.1 units/min (doses above 0.08 units/min associated with increased cardiac ischaemia and no additional benefit in CO)	Septic shock Cardiac surgery Catecholamine resistance Vasopressor refractory shock	Increased SVR Constriction preserved in acidosis	Increased PVR Splanchnic/ mesenteric ischaemia Uterine contraction Increased intestinal motility Increased ACTH release Anti-diuresis = H_2O/ hyponatraemia	Reflex bradycardia > noradrenaline Doses >0.04 units/ min may decrease CI Relative contraindications: hyponatraemia, coronary artery disease, SAH/ cerebral vasospasm, late pregnancy (due to uterine contractions)	Liu et al, Intensive Care Med (2018) – terlipressin (> V1-selective agent) versus noradrenaline as first line in septic shock: no mortality benefit as first line, possibly more serious SE (digital ischaemia) in terlipressin group VASST, Russell et al, N Engl J Med (2008): no mortality benefit in adding vasopressin if MAP maintained with conventional vasopressors VANISH, Gordon et al, JAMA (2016): early vasopressin maintains MAP and reduces requirement for noradrenaline and RRT. Does not reduce RRT-free days or mortality rate

Drug	Receptors/mechanism of action	Metabolism	Dose	Uses	Effects	Side effects	Cautions	Literature
Levosimendan	Modulates troponin C to maintain contraction Activates vascular K⁺ channels (to cause vasodilation)	Slow onset (loading dose can be given) Liver and renal metabolism $T_{1/2}$: 1 hour Active metabolites for 1 week	Loading dose: 6–24 µg/kg (over 10 minutes) Infusion (24 hours): 0.05–0.2 µg/(kg min)	Heart failure Sepsis Post-resuscitation Peri-operative optimisation of cardiomyopathy Beta-blocker overdose Catecholamine resistance	Increased SV Increased HR Increased coronary flow Decreased SVR Decreased pulmonary arterial pressure Anti-inflammatory/anti-apoptotic	Headache Low BP Tachycardia N&V	Do not use in liver/renal failure Caution in LVOTO	CHEETAH, Landoni et al., N Engl J Med (2017): low-dose levosimendan does not improve survival in patients with LV dysfunction undergoing cardiac surgery LEVO-CTS, Mehta et al., N Engl J Med (2017): no benefit of prophylactic use in patients undergoing cardiac bypass surgery LeoPARDS, Gordon et al., N Engl J Med (2017): in adults with sepsis, a 24-hour infusion of levosimendan (in addition to standard treatment) not associated with less severe organ dysfunction, possibly higher incidence of haemodynamic instability
Methylene blue	Inhibits guanylyl cyclase (NO)-mediated vasodilation, reducing catecholamine requirements MAO inhibition Reduces methaemoglobin (Hbᵐᵉᵗ) (Fe³⁺) to Hb (Fe²⁺)	Converted to leucomethylene blue by Hbᵐᵉᵗ reductase Excreted in urine	1% preparation In vasoplegia: 1.5–2 mg/kg over 30–60 minutes In methaemoglobinaemia: 1–2 mg/kg IV over 5 minutes (repeat 30–60 minutes if Hbᵐᵉᵗ not falling) Can be repeated 6–8 hours in prolonged Hbᵐᵉᵗ	Methaemoglobinaemia Vasoplegic shock (post-bypass) Hepatopulmonary syndrome Septic shock	Decreases NO release and may increase sensitivity to catecholamines Vasoplegia	Increased PVR Skin discoloration Increased ALT/AST Dizziness, headache, confusion, chest pain, N&V	Contraindicated in G6PD deficiency, renal impairment, Hbᵐᵉᵗ reductase deficiency, nitrate-induced methaemoglobinaemia due to cyanide poisoning Can cause hypersensitivity/anaphylaxis Difficulty monitoring SpO₂ Extravasation = tissue necrosis Paradoxical methaemoglobinaemia due to iron oxidation at high dose (>7 mg/kg)	El Adawi et al., J Anaesthesiol (2016) – methylene blue versus vasopressin in sepsis-induced vasoplegia: suggests methylene blue may reduce noradrenaline/adrenaline requirement. Single-centre study with methodological flaws

Abbreviations: Ca^{2+} = calcium; cAMP = cyclic adenosine monophosphate; COMT = catechol-O-methyltransferase; MAO = monoamine oxidase; $T_{1/2}$ = half-life; ALS = advanced life support; CO = cardiac output; O_2 = oxygen; SVR = systemic vascular resistance; K^+ = potassium; PO_4 = phosphate; $NaHCO_3$ = sodium bicarbonate; HOCM = hypertrophic obstructive cardiomyopathy; HTN = hypertension; PVR = pulmonary vascular resistance; MAOI = monoamine oxidase inhibitor; DA = dopamine; HR = heart rate; UO = urine output; Na^+ = sodium; RRT = renal replacement therapy; SIRS = systemic inflammatory response syndrome; AF = atrial fibrillation; AV = atrioventricular; AS = aortic stenosis; EGDT = early goal-directed therapy; SCVO₂ = central venous oxygen saturation; RF = renal failure; CCF = congestive cardiac failure; RV = right ventricular; IHD = ischaemic heart disease; TCA = tricyclic antidepressant; NSAID = non-steroidal anti-inflammatory drug; ACTH = adrenocorticotrophic hormone; H_2O = water; CI = cardiac index; SAH = subarachnoid haemorrhage; SE = side effects; MAP = mean arterial pressure; SV = stroke volume; N&V = nausea and vomiting; LVOTO = left ventricular outflow tract obstruction; LV = left ventricular; NO = nitric oxide; Fe^{3+} = ferric ion; Hb = haemoglobin; Fe^{2+} = ferrous ion; IV = intravenous; Hbᵐᵉᵗ = methaemoglobin; ALT = alanine aminotransferase; AST = aspartate aminotransferase; G6PD = glucose-6-phosphate dehydrogenase; SpO_2 = oxygen saturation.

Table 4.5.4 Vasodilators

	Drug	Uses	Mechanism of action	Preparation/dose	Effects	Things to consider
Nitrates/NO donors	Sodium nitroprusside	Vascular surgery Rapid BP titration (e.g. hypertensive crisis, aortic dissection)	Metabolised → NO → activates guanylyl cyclase = increased cGMP → decreased intracellular Ca^{2+} = arteriolar and venous dilation	IV drug only 0.5–6 µg/(kg min)	↓ SVR ↑ Venous capacitance ↓ Preload ↓ Ventricular wall tension ↓ Myocardial O_2 consumption No direct effect on contractility	Tachyphylaxis Inhibits hypoxic vasoconstriction (shunt) Vasodilation ↑ intracranial blood volume → ICP (cerebral autoregulation maintained) Cyanide formed due to metabolism→ causes cytotoxic hypoxia in toxicity Degrades in light (needs special preparation and opaque lines)
	GTN	Cardiac/vascular surgery Myocardial ischaemia/angina HTN Oesophageal spasm	Venodilator > arteriodilation Increases NO (see sodium nitroprusside above)	IV Sublingual (300–600 µg) Tablets (immediate- and modified-release, buccal) Transdermal patches (can explode with DCCV)	Vasodilation of capacitance vessels ↓ Preload ↓ Ventricular end-diastolic pressure and wall tension ↓ Myocardial O_2 demand ↑ Subendocardial blood flow	Tachyphylaxis >48 hours (loss of sulfhydryl groups in vascular endothelium) → may require daily drug-free period Increased ICP (causing headache) Relaxation of GI sphincters Can cause methaemoglobinaemia
	ISMN	Angina/IHD prophylaxis	(See Sodium nitroprusside above) 100% oral bioavailability ISMN $T_{1/2}$ 4.5 hours → angina prophylaxis	Oral 30–120 mg once daily/twice daily		Prepared with mannitol and lactulose to reduce risk of explosion Caution with phosphodiesterase V inhibitors → profound vasodilation
Calcium channel antagonists	Verapamil	SVT (not AF or WPW) HTN	Blocks Ca^{2+} L-type channels on vascular smooth/ myocardial muscle/cardiac nodal tissue (SA and AV nodes) → ↓ intracellular Ca^{2+} via cAMP-dependent protein kinase	20–240 mg tablets (some modified-release) IV (2.5 mg/ml)	↓ Conduction from SA to AV node Vasodilates peripheral vascular smooth muscle Mild coronary vasodilator	Heart block Heart failure VF in WPW syndrome After chronic use → potentiates effect of muscle relaxants
	Nifedipine	Angina HTN Raynaud's	Tablets 5–10 mg Sublingual and oral		↓ Peripheral and coronary artery tone ↓ SVR ↑ Coronary blood flow ↑ HR Can cause reflex ↑ HR and contractility	

Drug	Uses	Mechanism of action	Preparation/dose	Effects	Things to consider
Nimodipine	Vasospasm prophylaxis in SAH	IV and tablet (60 mg/4- to 6-hourly)		More lipid-soluble analogue of nifedipine → can penetrate blood–brain barrier	
Diltiazem	Angina HTN	60–200 mg tablets, some as slow release	↑ AV conduction ↓ Contractility (< verapamil) ↓ SVR ↑ Coronary blood flow (vasodilation)		
Potassium channel activators	Angina CCF HTN	Arterial and venodilation → activates ATP-sensitive K⁺ channels In the open state, K⁺ passes down the concentration gradient → hyperpolarises cell → closes Ca²⁺ channels = less Ca²⁺ available for contraction Relaxes venous capacitance smooth muscle via nitrate moiety	Nicorandil: Tablets (10–30 mg/ twice daily)	↓ Pre- and afterload ↓ LVEDP ↑ Coronary blood flow Good suppression of torsades in prolonged QTc states Contractility and AV conduction not affected	

Abbreviations: NO = nitric oxide; cGMP = cyclic guanosine monophosphate; IV = intravenous; SVR = systemic vascular resistance; O_2 = oxygen; ICP = intracranial pressure; GTN = glyceryl trinitrate; HTN = hypertension; DCCV = direct current cardioversion; GI = gastrointestinal; ISMN = isosorbide mononitrate; IHD = ischaemic heart disease; $T_{1/2}$ = half-life; SVT = supraventricular tachycardia; AF = atrial fibrillation; WPW = Wolff–Parkinson–White; Ca^{2+} = calcium; SA = sinoatrial; AV = atrioventricular; cAMP = cyclic adenosine monophosphate; VF = ventricular fibrillation; HR = heart rate; SAH = subarachnoid haemorrhage; CCF = congestive cardiac failure; ATP = adenosine triphosphate; K^+ = potassium; LVEDP = left ventricular end-diastolic pressure.

Table 4.5.5 Miscellaneous drugs

Drug	Uses	Mechanism of action	Preparation/dose	Effects	Things to consider
Hydralazine	HTN Pre-eclampsia CCF	Uncertain ? Activation of guanylyl cyclase → increase in cGMP= ↓ intracellular Ca^{2+} = vasodilation	Tablets (25–50 mg) Powder for IV (20 mg; do not reconstitute with 5% dextrose = breakdown) IV dose: 5- to 10-mg boluses (can be run as infusion)	↓ Arterial tone (SVR), capacitance vessels less affected Increased ICP Seems to be safe in pregnancy	Fluid retention, oedema Reduction in urine output Nausea and vomiting common Drug-induced SLE (slow acetylators) Peripheral neuropathy and blood dyscrasias have been described
Minoxidil	Severe HTN Alopecia areata		Tablets (2.5–10 mg) 5 mg initial dose, increasing to max 100 mg/day (over days) 2% IV solution 5% topical lotion	↓ Arterial tone (SVR)	Avoid in acute porphyrias Contraindicated in phaeochromocytoma Fluid retention, oedema
Diazoxide	IV for hypertensive crisis associated with renal disease (1–3 mg/kg) Intractable hyperglycaemia and malignant islet cell tumours	Vasodilator chemically related to thiazide diuretics Alters levels of cAMP → Ca^{2+} influx in arterioles = vasodilation Biochemical effects due to inhibition of insulin secretion and increased catecholamines	Tablets 50 mg IV 15 mg/ml	Arterial dilation, no obvious effect on capacitance vessels Reflex ↑ in HR and CO ↑ glucose, catecholamines, renin and aldosterone (= fluid retention)	Nausea and vomiting Extra-pyramidal effects (including oculogyric crisis) Thombocytopenia Hyperuricaemia
Sildenafil	Pulmonary HTN RV failure Erectile dysfunction	Potent cGMP type 5 inhibitor. Vascular smooth muscle in respiratory arteries and corpus cavernosum relaxed as cGMP levels ↑	20 mg three times daily for pulmonary HTN	Pulmonary arterial vasodilator	Marked hypotension with nitrates
Bosentan	Pulmonary HTN Scleroderma (digital ulceration)	Dual endothelin receptor antagonist	62.5 mg twice daily for 4 weeks, increasing to 125 mg twice daily	Decreases PVR and SVR	Teratogenicity Liver injury

Abbreviations: HTN = hypertension; CCF = congestive cardiac failure; cGMP = cyclic guanosine monophosphate; Ca^{2+} = calcium; IV = intravenous; SVR = systemic vascular resistance; ICP = intracranial pressure; SLE = systemic lupus erythematosus; cAMP = cyclic adenosine monophosphate; HR = heart rate; CO = cardiac output; RV = right ventricular; PVR = peripheral vascular resistance.

Table 4.5.6 Alpha (α) antagonists

Drug	Uses	Mechanism of action	Preparation/dose	Effects	Things to consider
Phentolamine	Hypertensive crises Excessive sympathomimetics: MAOI interactions Phaeochromocytomas (especially during tumour handling)	Competitive, non-selective α-blocker $α_1 > α_2$ (3:1)	10 mg mesylate reconstituted to IV preparation Dose 1–5 mg, titrated to effect	$α_1$ blockade: vasodilation, hypotension $α_2$ blockade: tachycardia, ↑ CO, nasal congestion	Sulphites in preparation exacerbate asthma Increases gut motility Hypoglycaemia due to ↑ insulin secretion
Phenoxybenzamine	Pre-operative phaeochromocytoma management → allows expansion of intravascular compartment Occasionally used as adjunct to severe shock	Long-acting, non-selective α-blocker with high affinity for $α_1$ adrenoreceptor Also ↓ neuronal and extra-neuronal uptake of catecholamines	Tablets 10 mg 10 mg/once daily increased daily until control gained (usually 1–2 mg/(kg day)) IV 50 mg/ml Via CVC 1 mg/(kg day) slow infusion	Hypotension Reflex tachycardia	Sedation Miosis
Prazocin	Hypertension Raynaud's Benign prostatic hypertrophy	Highly selective $α_1$ adrenoreceptor antagonist	0.5–2 mg tablets (dose can be increased to 20 mg/day)	Causes vasodilation of arteries and veins, with no reflex tachycardia Diastolic pressures fall the most	Severe postural hypotension/syncope may follow first dose Relaxes the bladder but may cause impotence and priapism

Abbreviations: MAOI = monoamine oxidase inhibitor; CO = cardiac output; IV = intravenous; CVC = central venous catheter.

Table 4.5.7 Beta (β) antagonists

Drug	Lipid solubility	$T_{1/2}$ (hours)	Dose	Cardioselectivity	Tips/uses	Evidence
Acebutolol	++	6	400 mg/bd Up to 1.2 g/day	Cardioselective – β1		Martin et al., J Trauma (2005) – beta-blockers given to patients with high troponin: showed 50% reduction in mortality Christensen et al., Crit Care (2011) – cohort study: critically ill patients on beta-blockers prior to admission had improved 30-day mortality
Atenolol	+	7	50–100 mg/day (PO) 2.5 mg IV (slow bolus)	Cardioselective – β1		
Esmolol	+++	0.15	50–200 μg/(kg min) (infusion) 10-mg boluses (IV)	Highly cardioselective – β1 No intrinsic sympathomimetic activity	Rapid onset/offset Treatment of peri-operative HTN/tachycardia SVT Tissue necrosis if extravasation	Morelli et al., JAMA (2013) – RCT: HR control with esmolol on haemodynamic and clinical outcomes in septic shock: esmolol group mortality = 49.4% versus 80.5% in control
Metoprolol	+++	3–7	50–200 mg/day (PO) Up to 5 mg (IV)	Relatively cardioselective – β1 > β2 No intrinsic sympathomimetic activity	Early use in MI reduces infarct size Adjunct to thyrotoxicosis Migraine prophylaxis High lipid solubility= crosses BBB and enters breast milk	
Propranolol	+++	4	160–330 mg/day (PO) 0.5–10 mg IV	Non-cardioselective	Racemic mixture S-isomer most of effects R-isomer prevents peripheral conversion of T4 → T3 (thyrotoxicosis) Essential tremor Displaced from protein by strong binding with heparin	Ko et al., J Trauma Acute Care Surg (2016) – non-randomized study, propranolol given in first 24 hours of TBI: 18% had mortality benefit (other studies have been equivocal of benefit)
Sotalol	+	15	80–160 mg/bd (PO) 50–100 mg over 20 minutes (IV)	Non-cardioselective	Class III anti-arrhythmic SVT (and prophylaxis) Can precipitate torsades (high doses → prolonged QTc)	
Labetalol	+++	5	100–800 mg/bd (PO) 5–20 mg (IV) to max 200 mg	α and β α:β ratio: IV – 1:7 PO – 1:3	Angina Pregnancy: HTN, pre-eclampsia	

Abbreviations: $T_{1/2}$ = half-life; bd = twice daily; RCT = randomised controlled trial; HR = heart rate; TBI = traumatic brain injury; PO = oral; IV = intravenous; HTN = hypertension; SVT = supraventricular tachycardia; MI = myocardial infarction; BBB = blood–brain barrier; T4 = thyroxine; T3 = tri-iodothyronine.

Box 4.5.5 Physiological Effects of β Antagonists

- Cardiac:
  - Negative chronotropy and inotropy
  - Slowing of sinoatrial node automaticity and atrioventricular conduction time
  - Bradycardia increases diastolic coronary filling time
  - Increases oxygen supply
  - Decreases oxygen consumption
  - Decreased cardiac output
  - Inhibition of renin–angiotensin system
  - Desensitised baroreceptors
  - Pre-synaptic β2 receptor inhibition reduces noradrenaline release
- Respiratory:
  - Bronchoconstriction; caution in asthma
- Metabolic:
  - Non-selective β-blockade obtunds normal blood sugar response to exercise = hypoglycaemia
  - Increase in resting sugar levels in diabetics, and may mask symptoms of hypoglycaemia
- Central nervous system (increases with increasing lipid solubility):
  - Depression
  - Hallucinations
  - Nightmares
  - Fatigue
- Ocular:
  - Reduced intra-ocular pressure (decreased aqueous humour production)
- Gut:
  - Dry mouth
  - Gastrointestinal disturbance

Drugs that Affect the Renin–Angiotensin–Aldosterone System

The renin–angiotensin–aldosterone system (RAAS) mediates its effects via a cascade of enzyme reactions triggered by the release of renin from the juxtaglomerular apparatus in response to:

- Direct sympathetic (β_1) fibre stimulation
- Decreased renal perfusion
- Decreased presentation of Na^+ to the macula densa

Drugs that inhibit various steps (enzymes/receptors) in this cascade are central to the management of hypertension and heart failure (Table 4.5.8).

Miscellaneous Anti-hypertensives

Miscellaneous anti-hypertensives include those seen in Tables 4.5.8 and 4.5.9.

Table 4.5.8 Drugs that affect the renin–angiotensin–aldosterone system

Drug	Mechanism of action	Dose	Uses	Effects	Cautions/side effects
Ramipril	ACE inhibitor (pro-drug)	1.25 mg/day Up-titrated to 10 mg/day (PO)	HTN CCF Secondary prevention of MI	↓ SVR No effect on HR Baroreceptor reflex unaffected Transient hypotension on initiation of symptoms Renal hypoperfusion in renal artery stenosis/renal failure ↓ Aldosterone release = ↑ renin release, leading to hyperkalaemia Raised urea/Cr Unexplained hypoglycaemia in type 1/2 diabetes	Do not use in conjunction with NSAIDs = renal impairment CI in pregnancy Angio-oedema (0.2%) Agranulocytosis Thrombocytopenia Cough (decreased bradykinin breakdown) Loss of taste Fever Aphthous ulcers
Enalapril	ACE inhibitor (pro-drug)	2.5 mg/day Up-titrated to max 40 mg/day	HTN CCF Secondary prevention of MI		
Losartan	Angiotensin II receptor antagonist	25–50 mg/day	HTN CCF (use when ACE inhibitor cough intolerable)		
Spironolactone	Aldosterone receptor antagonist (competitive)	50–100 mg once daily (PO)	HF Ascites Nephrotic syndrome Conn's syndrome	↓ Na$^+$ re-absorption in distal tubule K$^+$ excretion significantly reduced	Gynaecomastia Irregular menstruation Hyperkalaemia CI in Addison's

Abbreviations: ACE = angiotensin-converting enzyme; PO = oral; HTN = hypertension; CCF = congestive cardiac failure; MI = myocardial infarction; SVR = systemic vascular resistance; HR = heart rate; Cr = creatinine; NSAID = non-steroidal anti-inflammatory drug; CI = contraindicated; PO = oral; HF = heart failure; Na$^+$ = sodium; K$^+$ = potassium.

Table 4.5.9 Miscellaneous anti-hypertensives

Drug	Uses	Mechanism of action	Dose	Effects	Cautions/things to remember
Guanethidine	Anti-hypertensive Sympathetically mediated pain	Adrenergic antagonist Displaces NA from binding sites and prevents further neuronal release	10 mg/day Up-titrated to 50 mg/day 20 mg IV for chronic pain	Hypotension Postural hypotension Fluid retention Diarrhoea Failure to ejaculate	TCAs/cocaine prevent guanethidine uptake (via uptake 1 mechanism) Upregulation of adrenoreceptors with chronic use → ↑ sensitivity to direct-acting sympathomimetic amines

Table 4.5.9 (cont.)

Drug	Uses	Mechanism of action	Dose	Effects	Cautions/things to remember
Methyldopa	Hypertension (especially in pregnancy)	Centrally acting anti-hypertensive Crosses BBB Decarboxylated → α methyl-NA, a potent α_2 agonist → ↓ centrally mediated sympathetic tone	250 mg/tds Increasing to 3 g/day	↓ SVR Postural hypotension CO not changed Rebound HTN on cessation	Sedation Dizziness Depression Nightmares Decreased MAC with volatile anaesthesia Positive direct Coombs' test (10–20%) Leucopenia, thrombocytopenia (rare) Liver function may deteriorate after long-term use Gynaecomastia Constipation May interfere with urinary catecholamine assays
Clonidine	Hypertension Pain adjunct Opiate-sparing Sedation	α_2 agonist ↓ Central sympathetic outflow Augments endogenous opiate release Modulates ascending NA stimulation of central α_2 receptors K+ channels also activated	25–300 µg/day (PO) 15–150 µg boluses/ infusions Transdermal patch available	May have transitory ↑ in BP after administration (α_1 agonism), followed by hypotension Bradycardia Obtunds stress response to surgery	PR prolongation Slowing of AV conduction Sedation Reduction in MAC with volatile anaesthesia Anxiolysis at low dose, anxiogenic at high dose ADH inhibition can lead to diuresis Therapeutic doses do not cause platelet aggregation (via α_2 platelet receptor)

Abbreviations: NA = noradrenaline; IV = intravenous; TCA = tricyclic antidepressant; BBB = blood–brain barrier; tds = three times daily; SVR = systemic vascular resistance; CO = cardiac output; HTN = hypertension; MAC = minimum alveolar concentration; PO = oral; AV = atrioventricular; ADH = anti-diuretic hormone.

References and Further Reading

Belletti A, Castro ML, Silvetti S, *et al*. The effect of inotropes and vasopressors on mortality: a meta-analysis of randomized clinical trials. *Br J Anaesth* 2015;**115**:656–75.

Coppola S, Froio S, Chiumello D. β-blockers in critically ill patients: from physiology to clinical evidence. *Crit Care* 2015;**19**:119.

Finfer S, Myburgh J, Bellomo R. Intravenous fluid therapy in critically ill adults. *Nat Rev Nephrol* 2018;**14**:541–57.

Jackson R, Bellamy M. Antihypertensive drugs. *BJA Education* 2015;**15**:280–5.

Martin G, Bassett P. Crystalloids vs. colloids for fluid resuscitation in the intensive care unit: a systematic review and meta-analysis. *J Crit Care* 2019;**50**:144–54.

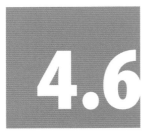

4.6

Principles of Mechanical Circulatory Support in the Acute Setting

Susanna Price and Stephane Ledot

Key Learning Points

1. Mechanical circulatory support is not a treatment per se.
2. Treating the underlying cause for cardiogenic shock is vital.
3. Early discussion and referral provide the best chance for a successful outcome.
4. Matching the patient and the device demands significant expertise.
5. High-quality evidence for benefit is lacking.

Keywords: mechanical circulatory support, cardiogenic shock, VA ECMO, percutaneous left or right ventricular assist device, intra-aortic balloon pump

Introduction

Despite advances in interventional therapies for cardiogenic shock (CS), mortality remains high (40–80 per cent, depending on the aetiology). Providing the underlying cause for CS is treated (most commonly myocardial ischaemia/infarction), patients recover, with a good quality of life. The intra-aortic balloon pump (IABP) has previously been extensively used to provide mechanical circulatory support (MCS) in CS. However, evidence of its lack of efficacy, together with increasing use of extracorporeal membrane oxygenation (ECMO) following the H1N1 pandemic, has led to a resurgence of interest in alternative MCS in adult patients. This chapter outlines the current evidence and recommendations for MCS in the critically ill.

Aims and Indications for Mechanical Circulatory Support

The aims of MCS are resuscitation (maintaining end-organ perfusion and minimising harm from high-dose vasoactive agents), stabilisation (allowing revascularisation or other cardiac intervention) and offloading the heart. Therefore, in the acute setting, MCS must be safe, relatively simple and rapid to institute, providing good haemodynamic support whilst protecting the myocardium. Current recommendations are that in CS (INTERMACS (Interagency Registry for Mechanically Assisted Circulatory Support) I), short-term MCS (days/weeks) may be used to support patients with left/biventricular failure until cardiac function has recovered. In addition, MCS can be used to support the patient as a 'bridge-to-decision' in acute/rapidly deteriorating CS.

Types of Mechanical Circulatory Support

The various devices recommended for use in the acute setting vary according to access route/size, mechanism of action, which side of the heart is failing, whether oxygenation can be provided and the level of support required. They share a number of potential major complications (Table 4.6.1), and all require anticoagulation, although the level required varies according to the device and the individual clinical scenario.

Intra-aortic Balloon Pump

The IABP is a 30–50 cm^3 balloon placed in the descending aorta, timed to inflate in diastole and deflate in systole, thereby increasing coronary perfusion and reducing left ventricular (LV) afterload. Despite its use for >40 years, data demonstrating lack of mortality benefit means it is no longer recommended for routine use in CS complicating myocardial infarction (MI). The IABP may still be used in CS for patients with mechanical complications of MI or in severe mitral regurgitation and/or in combination with other MCS.

Percutaneous Left Ventricular Assist Devices

A number of percutaneous **left ventricular assist devices** (pLVADs) are available to provide MCS to the left heart. The Impella® is a microaxial rotatory device,

Table 4.6.1 Types of mechanical circulatory support

Type of support	Level of support (maximum)	Ventricle (left/right)	Oxygenation? (yes/no)	Main complications
IABP	0.5–1 l/min	L	N	A, B, T, H
Impella®	2.5, 4, 5 l/min	L	N	A, B, C, T, H
Impella® RP	4 l/min	R	N	B, V, C, T, H
Tandem Heart®	3–4.5 l/min	L	N	A, B, V, C, T, H
Protek Duo®	4 l/min	R	Y/N	B, V, C, T
ECMO	8 l/min	L and R	Y	A, B, V, T, H

Abbreviations: IABP = intra-aortic balloon pump; L = left; N = no; A = arterial trauma; B = bleeding; T = thrombocytopenia; H = haemolysis; R = right; C = cardiac perforation; V = venous trauma; Y = yes; ECMO = extracorporeal membrane oxygenation.

positioned retrogradely across the aortic valve, taking blood from the left ventricle (LV) and returning it to the ascending aorta. Depending upon the size of the device and the degree of support provided, implantation is either percutaneous (Impella® 2.5 and CP) or surgical (Impella® 5). By contrast, the Tandem Heart® (TH) is a percutaneously inserted device that works by draining oxygenated blood from the left atrium (via trans-septal puncture) and returning it to the level of the aortic bifurcation via a low-speed centrifugal pump. Both the Impella® and the TH require preserved right ventricular (RV) function to work, as no right-sided support is provided (Table 4.6.1). Although theoretically attractive, delivering superior haemodynamic support, complications (primarily vascular access-related) are high, and there is no mortality benefit compared with the IABP. They are currently not recommended in CS, although they may still be used to support the circulation in high-risk angioplasty.

Percutaneous Right Ventricular Assist Devices

RV dysfunction causing CS has a high mortality, with few evidence-based therapies to guide support. Two percutaneous right ventricular assist devices (pRVADs) are currently available: the Impella® RP (working on the same principle as the left-sided Impella®, but inserted via the femoral vein and inferior vena cava (IVC)), which drains blood from the right atrium (RA) and returns it to the pulmonary artery, and the Protek Duo® (inserted via the internal jugular vein), which drains blood from the RA, returning it to the pulmonary artery, and has the option to add an oxygenator to the circuit, thereby providing additional respiratory support if required (Table 4.6.1). These

relatively new devices have little evidence to support their use. However, their relative ease of insertion and application and effective right-sided support, as well as the lack of alternative mechanisms to manage catastrophic RV failure, mean it is likely that evidence will emerge to guide their use in future.

Veno-arterial Extracorporeal Membrane Oxygenation

Percutaneous veno-arterial ECMO (VA-ECMO) provides rapid high-level cardiac/cardio-respiratory support to both sides of the heart, although it is not full cardiopulmonary bypass (Table 4.6.1). Using femoral venous access, deoxygenated blood is drained from the IVC and pumped through an oxygenator to be returned to the descending aorta. In addition to its use in CS, VA-ECMO has been used as an adjunctive therapy in refractory cardiac arrest and may be considered as an option in advanced life support in selected patients (extracorporeal life support (ECLS)). Current recommendations are that VA-ECMO may be used to support patients with left/biventricular failure until cardiac and other organ function have recovered, or where cardiac function does not recover, as a bridge-to-decision (longer-term device or transplantation). The Survival After VA-ECMO (SAVE) score may be used to help predict survival (www.save-score.com/). Contraindications include severe aortic regurgitation, acute aortic dissection, severe and irreversible survival-limiting non-cardiac organ failure and irreversible cardiac failure where transplantation or long-term ventricular assist devices (VADs) are not possible (absolute), and severe coagulopathy, contraindication to anticoagulation and limited vascular access (relative).

493

Despite its increasing use, there is no high-quality evidence from randomised controlled trials that VA-ECMO improves patient outcomes, with data coming from only small retrospective cohort studies, case series and registries. Published survival after VA-ECMO varies from 20 to 68 per cent, varying according to a number of factors, including age, underlying aetiology of CS, requirement for cardiopulmonary resuscitation (CPR), preceding co-morbidities and physiological status of the patient at the time of institution of support. The major studies and registry data from the Extracorporeal Life Support Organisation (ELSO) are summarised in Table 4.6.2.

Implementation and Monitoring of Mechanical Circulatory Support

A patient with CS not responding to standard supportive therapies (INTERMACS I or SCAI (Society for Cardiovascular Angiography and Interventions) C/D/E), after/simultaneous with treating the underlying cause, should *urgently* be considered/referred for MCS, before multi-organ failure supervenes.

Choice of device will be determined by:

- Requirement for right and/or left heart support
- Requirement for oxygenation
- Presence of absolute/relative contraindications to each type of device
- Predictions as to the ability of the heart to support the device
- Potential impact of the heart on the device

Table 4.6.2 Outcomes from ECMO from ELSO registry data/ published series

Underlying pathology	Survival (%)
Acute myocarditis	59[a]
ACS/AMI	50[a]
e-CPR	29[a]
Septic shock	71
Post-cardiotomy	16–43.6[a]
Post-cardiac transplantation	Primary graft dysfunction: 46–100; late graft failure: 79[a]
Pulmonary embolism	57 (hospital), 47 (90-day)

Outcomes from VA-ECMO from ELSO registry data[a] or published series.
Abbreviations: ACS = acute coronary syndrome; AMI = acute myocardial infarction; e-CPR = extracorporeal cardiopulmonary resuscitation.

- Access routes
- Experience of the team
- Availability of equipment/devices

Once MCS is commenced, echocardiography is used to confirm the aims of support have been achieved, primarily in terms of adequacy of cardiac output, reduction in filling pressures and offloading of the left heart. If not already addressed, the underlying cause for CS should be treated. Where the desired aims of support are not achieved, support should be upgraded to a higher level, or additional devices used in combination (i.e. IABP/Impella® with VA-ECMO to increase LV offloading).

The patient should be assessed and monitored at least daily, specifically to exclude complications, ensure the aims of support are still met and assess whether it is possible to wean from MCS. Where the heart does not recover, a strategy for withdrawal of therapy to longer-term support (e.g. left or right VAD, biventricular VAD or total artificial heart) or transplantation should be made.

Summary and Conclusion

The use of MCS in CS is increasing. However, evidence to support its benefit is lacking. Key to successful patient outcomes are appropriate patient selection, early treatment of the underlying reversible pathology and rapid institution of appropriately matched support before the patient develops multi-organ failure.

References and Further Reading

Brechot N, Luyt CE, Scmodt M, *et al.* Venoarterial extracorporeal membrane oxygenation support for refractory cardiovascular dysfunction during severe bacterial septic shock. *Crit Care Med* 2013;**41**:1616–26.

Corsi F, Lebreton G, Brechot N, *et al.* Life-threatening massive pulmonary embolism rescued by venoarterial extracorporeal membrane oxygenation. *Crit Care* 2017;**21**:76.

Ponikowski P, Voors AA, Anker SD, *et al.* 2016 ESC Guidelines for the diagnosis and treatment of acute and chronic heart failure. *Eur Heart J* 2016;**37**:2129–200.

Stub D, Bernard S, Pellegrino V, *et al.* Refractory cardiac arrest treated with mechanical CPR, hypothermia, ECMO and early reperfusion (the CHEER trial). *Resuscitation* 2015;**86**:88–94.

Van Herck JL, Claeys MJ, De Paep R, *et al.* Management of cardiogenic shock complicating acute myocardial infarction. *Eur Heart J Acute Cardiovasc Care* 2015;**4**:278–97.

4.7 Mechanical Ventilation: Initiation, Maintenance and Weaning

Ranil Soysa and Kate Tatham

Key Learning Points

1. Indications for initiating mechanical ventilation are multifactorial and patient-specific.
2. Various modes of ventilation are available and can be modified, depending on individual patient requirements.
3. A systems-based approach to patient care during mechanical ventilation may reduce the risk of associated complications.
4. Application of therapies such as proning may improve outcome.
5. Weaning from mechanical ventilation should be a team-based decision, and use of a structured protocol is recommended.

Keywords: mechanical ventilation, weaning, proning, SIMV, APRV

Initiating Mechanical Ventilation

Mechanical ventilation assists with, or replaces, spontaneous breathing in the management of life-threatening respiratory failure.

Ventilatory support may be indicated in patients with airway impairment and/or respiratory dysfunction or failure. Support should also be considered in patients with neurological impairment, which may result in reduced level of consciousness, respiratory and pharyngeal muscle weakness and risk of aspiration.

Commencement and the appropriate mode of ventilator support can be determined using a combination history, examination, investigations and resultant diagnoses. Clinical indices used (often in combination) to determine when to use ventilatory support, and which forms to use, vary, but broadly the respiratory parameters include those listed in Box 4.7.1.

> **Box 4.7.1** Indices of Respiratory Function Indicating Requirement for Ventilatory Support
>
> - Symptoms/signs:
>   - Airway compromise, e.g. stridor, trauma, failure to clear secretions
>   - Ventilatory compromise, e.g. reduced Glasgow Coma Score (GCS), apnoea, flail chest, (respiratory muscle) fatigue
> - Parameters:
>   - Respiratory rate >30 breaths/min
>   - Minute ventilation <3 or >10 l/min
>   - Vital capacity <10–15 ml/kg
>   - Oxygen saturations <90 per cent, with supplementary oxygen
>   - PaO_2 <8 kPa (60 mmHg) with supplementary oxygen
>   - $PaCO_2$ >6.5 kPa (50 mmHg), with pH <7.25

Maintenance of Ventilation
Types of Ventilation

Ventilation can be largely split between invasive and non-invasive ventilation (NIV). Invasive ventilation requires insertion of a definitive airway (e.g. an infraglottic tracheal tube – either endotracheal or tracheostomy), whereas NIV utilises the application of a mask that fits over either the nose or the nose and mouth, or a hood/helmet interface.

NIV utilises two means of delivering positive airway pressure – continuous positive airway pressure (CPAP) and bi-level positive airway pressure (BiPAP). CPAP delivers a constant pressure throughout the respiratory cycle; no additional inspiratory support is delivered above this level. It is proposed that CPAP can reduce shunt, via recruitment of alveoli, whilst delivering a set concentration of inspired oxygen, thus improving delivery. With BiPAP, positive airway pressure is pre-assigned for both the inspiratory and expiratory phases ('IPAP' and 'EPAP', respectively) of a patient's spontaneous respiratory cycle. The difference between these two settings is known as the 'pressure support' and correlates to end-tidal volumes. A rate of delivery can be set (in breaths per minute), and the concentration of oxygen adjusted, thus aiding oxygenation, in addition to carbon dioxide clearance. It has been demonstrated as especially beneficial in exacerbations of chronic obstructive pulmonary disease (COPD) and cardiogenic pulmonary oedema.

Invasive ventilation is delivered via a tracheal tube (e.g. nasal, oral or tracheostomy), which, in adults, are predominantly cuffed, thus providing protection of the airway.

Modes of Ventilation

Ventilators vary, offering a multitude of proprietary modes and settings. However, broadly speaking, most can be set to deliver either a constant volume ('volume-controlled') or a constant pressure ('pressure-controlled'), or a combination of both, in a mandatory and/or supportive fashion.

Volume-controlled ventilation delivers a set tidal volume to the patient at a pre-determined rate. However, this volume is achieved, regardless of the pressure required to do so.

Pressure-controlled ventilation delivers a set inspiratory pressure over the inspiratory phase only, and a set respiratory rate governs the timings of the remaining phases. The subsequent tidal volume achieved with each breath is thus dependent on both the resistance and the compliance of the respiratory system. Additional safety features, i.e. pressure and volume limiters, are built into most makes of ventilators, however.

Pressure support relies on patient-triggered breathing. The ventilator supplies a set positive end-expiratory pressure (PEEP) continuously, and as the patient initiates a breath, a supplementary pressure is administered on top of this. This pressure, combined with the PEEP, is the total amount of support given to the patient during inspiration. This mode is entirely dependent on the patient initiating each breath, so if patients are not reliably doing so, assist modes of ventilation, whereby the ventilator will deliver a minimum set number of breaths per minute, can be utilised. Often ventilators can perform a combination of assist and support modes, ideal for lightly sedated patients or those weaning from ventilatory support.

Synchronous intermittent mandatory ventilation (SIMV) provides a combination of mandatory breaths (e.g. set at 12/minute) if no patient inspiratory effort

is detected, whilst also allowing patient-triggered supported breaths. If the latter occur, the ventilator delivers a mandatory breath in response to their effort, and thus the patient will still achieve the minimum selected (i.e. 12/minute). The patient will also receive supported breaths above this rate.

Ventilatory parameters (partial pressure of end-tidal CO_2 ($PETCO_2$), partial pressure of arterial oxygen (PaO_2)) can be targeted directly with the use of more advanced modes such as INTELLiVENT®-ASV®. This has the ability to automatically alter the ventilatory settings, breath-to-breath, based on the patient's parameters.

Airway pressure release ventilation (APRV) is a mode of ventilation that was originally described as continuous CPAP phase, with an intermittent release phase. APRV applies CPAP, known as 'P-high', for a period of time known as 'T-high'.

This phase recruits alveoli, promoting oxygenation and carbon dioxide removal, during a time-cycled release phase following T-high. This short phase is set to a user-defined pressure 'P-low' for a specified period of time 'T-low'. APRV can therefore be used to augment oxygenation, and reduce ventilation/perfusion (V/Q) mismatch and dead space, thus being potentially of benefit in patients with acute lung injury and acute respiratory distress syndrome (ARDS). Some studies have shown a reduced need for vasopressors and improved end-organ perfusion whilst requiring lesser amounts of sedation. Others suggest that with early application of APRV in the appropriate patient subgroups, there may be more ventilator-free days, reduced length of stay in the ICU and fewer tracheostomies.

It is thought to be most effective in spontaneously breathing patients. It is generally not used for patients with high sedation requirements and patients with obstructive lung disorders who tend to benefit from prolonged expiratory times, as opposed to the short 'T-low' utilised in APRV.

Ventilation Considerations

Adopting a simple systems-based ('ABC') approach highlights some of the factors that should be considered when ventilating a patient.

Airway

Patient tolerance of a tracheal tube is key to preventing patients from, for example, biting on and thus obstructing them, or stimulation of excessive coughing. Additionally, for effective ventilation to occur, synchronising patient respiratory efforts with the ventilator is desirable. This can be achieved with titrated use of sedatives (e.g. propofol, midazolam, opiates), with or without the addition of neuromuscular blockade. The latter is avoided where possible, owing to an association with ICU-acquired weakness.

The airway should be secured well enough to withstand accidental removal (e.g. with movement when transferring or rolling of the patient). Care must be taken, however, to ensure tracheal tube-anchoring devices, or ties, do not induce pressure injuries.

Patency of the tube must be maintained – not only to allow gas exchange, but also to permit pulmonary hygiene and suctioning, and sampling of the bronchial tree.

Breathing

1. There are several features of mechanical ventilation that may be utilised to allow clinicians to reach their desired ventilatory targets (e.g. PaO_2, $PaCO_2$, pH).

   a. The fraction of inspired oxygen (FiO_2) is set to achieve a specified target peripheral oxygen saturation and PaO_2. Efforts should be made to administer the lowest possible FiO_2 to avoid the harmful effects of hyperoxia.

   b. PEEP is used to increase functional residual capacity, preventing small airway closure, reducing shunt and improving oxygenation. It can be a useful adjunct to limit excessive FiO_2. Typical values for PEEP start at 5 cmH_2O and it is titrated up, as tolerated, to achieve target oxygenation. Rarely, PEEP will reach 20 cmH_2O.

   c. The inspiratory/expiratory ratio (I:E) refers, as the name suggests, to the time spent in the inspiratory and expiratory phases of ventilation. In normal spontaneous breathing, the expiratory time is about twice the inspiratory time. In mechanical ventilation, the I:E ratio can be adjusted to assist gas exchange in certain conditions. For example:

      i. Asthmatic patients may benefit from smaller I:E ratios, i.e. increasing expiration time (e.g. 1:4) to avoid air-trapping and auto-PEEP

      ii. Larger I:E ratios (1:1) can be used to increase gas distribution in patients requiring high peak airway pressures

      iii. Inverse I:E ratios may be employed in patients with reduced lung compliance such as those in ARDS. This can assist by reducing dead space ventilation, thereby reducing shunt and improving V/Q mismatch. Notably, however, it can leave the patient at risk of barotrauma and worsen pulmonary oedema, so it should only be used in patients where conventional methods have failed

2. Lung-protective ventilatory strategies are advocated to prevent, for example, aspiration of gastric contents, ventilator-associated pneumonia, ventilator-induced lung injury (VILI) and ARDS.

Suggested strategies include:

- Maintenance of tidal volumes at 6 ml/kg (ideal body weight), plateau pressures of 30 cmH_2O and use of PEEP and recruitment manoeuvres to aid oxygenation

- Avoidance of hypoxaemia may take preference over aiming for normocapnia, via 'permissive hypercapnia', in the absence of severe acidosis, e.g. in severe ARDS, asthmatics and patients with COPD

- Patients should be assessed for aspiration risk. Swallow assessment and facilitating gastric emptying and/or drainage should be considered to reduce the risk of such an eventuality

- It is recommended that patients are nursed in a semi-recumbent position, to prevent ventilator-acquired pneumonia (VAP)

- In addition, changing the ventilator circuits regularly, use of humidifiers, utilisation of endotracheal tubes with closed-circuit suction ports and maintaining appropriate endotracheal cuff pressures may also avoid colonisation of the respiratory tree and minimise the risk of developing VAP

Circulation

Critically ill patients requiring mechanical ventilation frequently also have cardiovascular compromise. Furthermore, the medications required to facilitate intubation and ventilation may be negatively inotropic and reduce systemic vascular resistance, thus significantly impacting on cardiac output, and hence end-organ perfusion/oxygenation. Careful consideration should therefore be taken prior to initiation of ventilation, as to how best to optimise and maintain the

497

cardiac output whilst ventilated. Judicious use of intravenous fluid therapy and appropriate selection and (e.g. pre-emptive) administration of inotropes and/or vasopressors may be warranted.

Moreover, both invasive ventilation and NIV impact the physiological dynamics of the cardio-respiratory system. High levels of CPAP or PEEP can increase intrathoracic pressure, which may reduce venous return. This negative effect on the preload can reduce stroke volume and mean arterial pressures, and consequently cardiac output.

Special Considerations

Proning has been shown to convey a survival benefit in patients with severe ARDS. In the prone position, it is hypothesised that improved ventilation is governed by favourable changes in pleural pressure and lung atelectasis. In ventilated patients with ARDS, exposing the ventral areas of the lung to higher pleural pressures reduces atelectasis throughout the larger-volume dorsal lung tissue, with less diaphragmatic splinting, caused by displacement of abdominal contents. As lung parenchymal blood flow is relatively uniform in ARDS, proning can be effective against V/Q mismatch, hence improving oxygenation in these patients.

High-frequency oscillatory ventilation (HFOV) has been used as a rescue strategy for adult patients with ARDS. HFOV delivers breaths at a high frequency with low tidal volumes, generating high mean airway pressures, with passive expiratory phases. Through this method, the potential disadvantages of mechanical ventilation such as overdistension, volutrauma, atelectauma and barotrauma could, in theory, be avoided. This makes HFOV a potential strategy in managing patients with ARDS or ventilator-associated lung injury. After setting the mean airway pressure, tidal volumes are altered based on driving power (P), and a frequency generally set between 3 and 10 Hz. Carbon dioxide clearance is directly proportional to the tidal volume and frequency. Oxygenation, as with other modes of ventilation, is governed by the FiO_2, mean airway pressure and lung volumes. However, two large trials indicated a signal to harm when comparing HFOV to conventional ventilation, and it has thus fallen out of favour as a rescue technique in ARDS.

Barotrauma, volutrauma and biotrauma are examples of inadvertent harm to the lungs as a result of ventilation, or 'VILI'. Volutrauma and barotrauma are terms used to describe lung injury caused by alveolar overdistension and high transpulmonary pressure, respectively. It is important to consider that high airway pressures alone do not cause VILI. The injury is caused by high transpulmonary pressure, which is the difference in pressure between forces acting within the lung and those outside. So factors such as chest wall stiffness, pleural pressures, (dyssynchronous or high-volume) spontaneous breathing and intra-abdominal pressures need to be considered in avoidance of volu- and barotrauma. The resultant effect of this strain upon the lung can cause injury at a cellular level also. Exposure to these forces can cause cellular detachment from the basement membrane, epithelial and endothelial junction breaks and alveolar and interstitial oedema. Biotrauma refers to systemic mediator release from injured ventilated lungs, resulting in distal organ dysfunction.

Gas trapping is abnormal retention of air in the alveoli at the end of expiration. This results in development of intrinsic continuous positive alveolar pressure – a condition known as 'auto-PEEP'.

Auto-PEEP can be caused by obstructive diseases such as COPD or asthma, or it can be as a result of insufficient time for ventilated lungs to return to functional residual capacity after the expiratory phase. Factors contributing to auto-PEEP are reduced expiratory time due to increased respiratory rate, increased tidal volume and increased inspiratory time. Auto-PEEP subjects patients to increased work of breathing, barotrauma and haemodynamic instability.

Weaning from Ventilation

Weaning refers to the process by which patients are liberated from mechanical ventilation. The decision as to whether to attempt to wean a patient from a ventilator should be explored on a daily basis, as limiting time spent on the ventilator reduces associated complications such barotrauma, volutrauma, air-trapping, haemodynamic instability, VAP and inadvertent tracheal tube displacement.

An 'ABCDE' system-wise approach to guide weaning can be used.

- Airway and breathing: weaning can be considered when the reasons for intubation and ventilation have been adequately addressed, though complete resolution may not be entirely necessary. Ideally,

FiO_2, PEEP and pressure support will be minimal, gas exchange/pH will have normalised, and the patient will have adequate cough and swallowing function.

- Cardiovascular system: ideally, the patient should be stable haemodynamically, and not requiring high levels of vasoactive drugs nor showing signs of cardiac failure.

- Disability: neurologically, the patient must be appropriate and cooperative when sedation is held, with optimised overall strength and the ability to generate appropriate tidal volumes. Systematically, this can be explored with sedation holds or with a gradual reduction in sedation levels as their physiology improves. The effects of any neuromuscular blockade should have been allowed to wear off completely and pain should be well controlled.

- Exposure: ensure the patient is not systemically unwell, e.g. fever/signs of sepsis, nor has any biochemical abnormalities.

Once patients have been weaned to appropriate levels of sedation, a spontaneous breathing trial can be attempted, typically using a pressure support mode. Spontaneous breathing trials may need to be carried out over gradually increasing lengths of time, so as to allow the patient to build up their respiratory musculature (e.g. if they have been ventilated for a prolonged period of time).

Once extubated, or following discontinuation of ventilatory support, the patient should be monitored closely, as the risks and sequelae of re-intubation are not insignificant in this population. The use of a bridging therapy, such as NIV or high-flow nasal oxygen, may be employed for those recently extubated, to aid the transition.

Recommendations for weaning patients from mechanical ventilation are listed in Box 4.7.2.

Box 4.7.2 American Thoracic Society Recommendations for Liberation of Patients who Have Been Mechanically Ventilated for >24 Hours (2017)

- Use of ventilator liberation protocols
- Daily spontaneous breathing trials, with pressure augmentation
- Protocolised early mobilisation/rehabilitation
- Protocolised sedation liberation
- Cuff leak test and pre-extubation steroid administration, where indicated
- Extubation to non-invasive ventilation (or high-flow nasal oxygen)

Source: Adapted from Fan E, Del Sorbo L, Goligher EC *et al.* An Official American Thoracic Society/European Society of Intensive Care Medicine/Society of Critical Care Medicine Clinical Practice Guideline: mechanical ventilation in adult patients with acute respiratory distress syndrome. *Am J Respir Crit Care Med* 2017;**195**:1253–63.

References and Further Reading

Fan E, Del Sorbo L, Goligher EC, *et al.* An Official American Thoracic Society/European Society of Intensive Care Medicine/Society of Critical Care Medicine Clinical Practice Guideline: mechanical ventilation in adult patients with acute respiratory distress syndrome. *Am J Respir Crit Care Med* 2017;**195**:1253–63.

Girard TD, Alhazzani W, Kress JP, *et al.* An Official American Thoracic Society/American College of Chest Physicians Clinical Practice Guideline: liberation from mechanical ventilation in critically ill adults rehabilitation protocols, ventilator liberation protocols, and cuff leak tests. *Am J Respir Crit Care Med* 2017;**195**:120–33.

Goligher EC, Douflé G, Fan E. Update in mechanical ventilation, sedation and outcomes 2014. *Am J Respir Crit Care Med* 2015;**191**:1367–73.

Guerin CJ, Reignier J, Richard J-C, *et al.* Prone positioning in severe acute respiratory distress syndrome. *N Engl J Med* 2013;**368**:2159–68.

Slutsky AS, Ranieri VM. Ventilator-induced lung injury *N Engl J Med* 2013;**369**:2126–36.

4.8 Renal Replacement Therapy in Critical Care

Nuttha Lumlertgul, Marlies Ostermann and
Gursharan Paul Singh Bawa

Key Learning Points

1. Conventional indications for renal replacement therapy (RRT) are refractory hyperkalaemia, refractory metabolic acidosis, pulmonary oedema, uraemia and sustained oliguria or anuria with fluid overload.
2. Two major principles of RRT are diffusion and convection.
3. Intermittent haemodialysis (IHD), prolonged intermittent renal replacement therapy (PIRRT) and continuous renal replacement therapy (CRRT) are commonly used in intensive care units. These modalities differ in regard to the duration of therapy and blood flow rate, hence the rapidity of solute and fluid removal. They are used to supplement one another according to each patient's status and clinical settings.
4. When prescribing CRRT, the modality, vascular access, blood flow rate, dose, anticoagulation, target fluid balance and fluid composition should be considered.
5. RRT-related complications, such as vascular access complications, hypotension and electrolyte imbalances, should be frequently monitored, prevented and appropriately managed.

Keywords: renal replacement therapy, acute kidney injury, haemofiltration, ultrafiltration haemodialysis

Introduction

Renal replacement therapy (RRT) is a common practice in ICUs to manage critically ill patients with acute kidney injury (AKI). Whilst conventional indications for RRT initiation have long been recognised, when to initiate RRT in patients without conventional indications remains debatable. Various modalities of RRT are available in the ICU. Factors to consider when prescribing RRT include vascular access, dose, target fluid removal and anticoagulation. In addition, initiation of RRT may impact other therapies, including drug dosing, nutrition and physiotherapy. This chapter aims to summarise practical points of RRT in critical care, with focus on continuous renal replacement therapy (CRRT).

Indications

RRT is classically indicated in patients with solute and/or electrolyte disturbances, fluid overload and complications from uraemic toxin accumulation, e.g. pericarditis or encephalopathy. The term 'renal replacement' might be misleading, as this therapy merely facilitates removal of excess fluid and solutes and does not replace other native kidney functions, including vitamin D regulation, erythropoietin production or gluconeogenesis. For non-traditional indications, RRT is used to remove dialysable toxic substances, correct acidosis and regulate electrolyte disturbances. It often forms an integral component of multi-organ support therapy (MOST) in multiple organ failure (MOF) (Table 4.8.1).

Table 4.8.1 Conventional and non-conventional indications for renal replacement therapy

Conventional indications	Non-conventional indications
Severe hyperkalaemia (plasma $K^+ \geq 6.0$ mmol/l and/or ECG changes) refractory to medications	Drug intoxication, e.g. salicylates, methanol, barbiturates, lithium
Severe metabolic acidaemia (pH <7.15) refractory to medications	Severe electrolyte disturbances, e.g. hyponatraemia or hypernatraemia
Refractory fluid overload, including pulmonary oedema	Prevention of fluid overload in patients with limited respiratory reserve (i.e. ARDS)
Uraemic complications, e.g. pericarditis, encephalopathy	

Abbreviations: ARDS = acute respiratory distress syndrome.

Principles and Techniques of RRT

All treatment modalities are based on the principle of allowing water and solute clearance through a semi-permeable membrane (haemofilter) and removal of waste products. The process of solute (e.g. urea, creatinine) removal from the blood is via two mechanisms – diffusion and convection – or both.

- **Diffusion:** technique whereby a solute moves down a concentration gradient across a semi-permeable membrane. It provides efficient clearance of low-molecular-weight molecules (<500–1500 Da), e.g. creatinine, urea, potassium. Diffusive clearance decreases with increased solute molecular weight.
- **Convection:** technique whereby a hydrostatic pressure gradient is set across a semi-permeable membrane and water is pushed across this membrane containing dissolved solutes. The solute clearance is determined by the pore size of the haemofilter.

Blood is pulled from the venous circulation via a peristaltic 'blood pump' through one port of a double-lumen cannula. The blood flow rate of the blood pump ranges from 150 to 300 ml/min and the blood passes through the filter. The blood pump generates a perfusion pressure that drives the ultrafiltrate across the semi-permeable membrane, thus removing volume and solutes. Then the blood is subsequently returned to the patient via the other port of the catheter. For dialysis, a dialysate solution passes in an opposite direction of blood flow to create a concentration gradient. In convection, replacement fluid is administered pre- or post-filter to create pressure and drive solutes and water across the membrane. The effluent contains fluid and waste products. The rate of ultrafiltration can be adjusted by setting the 'ultrafiltration pump' at a specified rate of fluid removal. The total amount of dialysate fluid, ultrafiltrate and fluid removal is called the 'effluent volume', which determines the dosing of RRT.

Nomenclatures for Continuous RRT

Continuous Venovenous Haemofiltration (CVVH)

The principal method is ultrafiltration via a haemofilter with larger pores. The ultrafiltration rate is created by a hydrostatic gradient. Solutes are transported across the membrane as a result of 'solvent drag' along with water. The ultrafiltrate is discarded and replaced by replacement fluid pre- or post-filter (Figure 4.8.1a).

Continuous Venovenous Haemodialysis (CVVHD)

The principal method is diffusion of molecules across a semi-permeable membrane along a concentration gradient. A dialysate fluid is pumped countercurrent to the blood through a filter. Depending on the concentration gradient, solutes are drawn from the blood across the membrane into the dialysate and removed from the body. The diffusive principle is more effective at removing small-size solutes. There is no need for replacement fluid (Figure 4.8.1b).

Continuous Venovenous Haemodiafiltration (CVVHDF)

The principal method is a combination of diffusion and convection. The replacement fluid can be administered pre- or post-filter (Figure 4.8.1c).

Slow Continuous Ultrafiltration (SCUF)

The principal method is ultrafiltration to remove excess fluid from the body. The filter pores are generally smaller than in CVVH. The main indication for SCUF is fluid overload (Figure 4.8.1d).

Modalities of RRT

There are a number of options available for providing RRT in the acute setting, mainly categorised into continuous RRT or intermittent RRT (Table 4.8.2).

Intermittent RRT systems are in the form of intermittent haemodialysis (IHD) or prolonged intermittent RRT (PIRRT) or slow low-efficiency dialysis (SLED). Continuous forms can be extracorporeal (CRRT) or intra-corporeal (peritoneal dialysis) (Table 4.8.3).

All types of RRT have advantages and disadvantages (Table 4.8.4). IHD provides rapid solute clearance and fluid removal during a short period (3–5 hours). In contrast, CRRT gradually removes solute and fluid over a prolonged period (optimally 24 hours). PIRRT is a hybrid of CRRT and IHD where fluid and solutes are removed over a 6- to 12-hour period. PIRRT can be performed using IHD or CRRT equipment, but with blood flow, dialysate flow rate and replacement fluid rates in between. PIRRT combines advantages of CRRT and IHD and facilitates improved haemodynamic stability, with gradual solute and volume removal as in CRRT. Peritoneal dialysis in AKI has

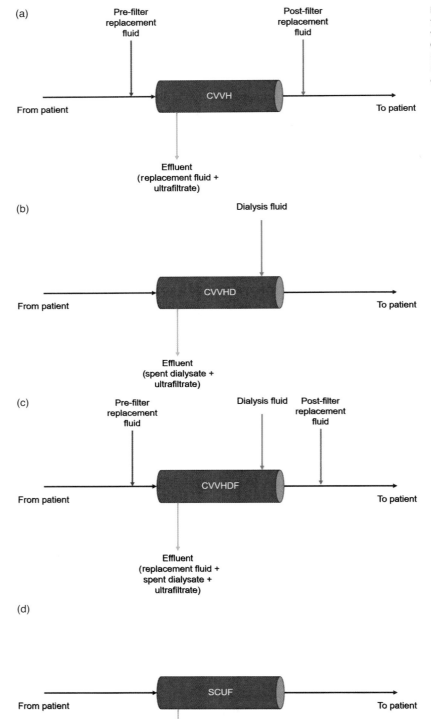

Figure 4.8.1 Principles of different types of continuous RRT. (a) Continuous venovenous haemofiltration (CVVH). (b) Continuous venovenous haemodialysis (CVVHD). (c) Continuous venovenous haemodiafiltration (CVVHDF). (d) Slow continuous ultrafiltration (SCUF).

Table 4.8.2 Benefits of intermittent and continuous RRT

Continuous RRT	Intermittent RRT
Continuous removal of toxins and electrolytes	Rapid clearance of toxins and electrolytes
Slower removal of excess fluid (i.e. better haemodynamic tolerability)	More time for diagnostic and therapeutic procedures
Fewer fluid and metabolic fluctuations	More time for physiotherapy/ rehabilitation
	Reduced exposure to anticoagulation
	Lower financial costs

Abbreviations: RRT = renal replacement therapy.

shown comparable outcomes to CRRT and IHD in resource-limited settings, but is beyond the scope of this review.

Current evidence has not shown differences in mortality between each modality of treatment, although CRRT is observed to increase long-term renal recovery. CRRT allows slow and continuous removal of fluids and toxins. Therefore, it is recommended in patients with haemodynamic instability or increased intracranial pressure, e.g. brain oedema, liver failure. Intermittent modalities are suitable in haemodynamically stable patients who require rapid fluid and electrolyte removal, e.g. dialysable intoxication or hyperkalaemia. In addition, IHD or PIRRT allows patients to mobilise and rehabilitate in between sessions.

In certain clinical situations, the use of one modality may be preferred; factors influencing this decision therefore include the primary goal of therapy (removal of solute or fluid, or both) and practical

Table 4.8.3 Characteristics of different renal replacement therapy modalities used for acute kidney injury in intensive care units

Parameter	Modality			
	IHD	Hybrid RRT SLED/ EDD/PIRRT	CRRT	PD
Duration (hours)	4–6	6–16	24	24
Frequency	Daily/alternate days	Daily/alternate days	Daily	Daily
Solute transport	Diffusion	Diffusion or convection, or both	Diffusion or convection, or both	Diffusion
Blood flow (ml/min)	200–350	100–300	100–250	NA
Dialysate flow (ml/min)	300–800	200–300	0–50	25–40
Urea clearance (ml/min)	150–180	90–40	20–45	15–35
Access	Central venous dialysis catheter	Central venous dialysis catheter	Central venous dialysis catheter	Peritoneal dialysis catheter
Need for anticoagulation	Usually, but not absolutely necessary	Usually, but not absolutely necessary	Yes	No
Fluctuations of osmotically active metabolites	++	+	Fewer; can occur in case of treatment interruptions	No
Fluctuations of intravascular fluid volume	++	+	Fewer; can occur in case of treatment interruptions	No
Effect on ICP in patients with acute brain injury	Increased	Potential increase	Usually no change	No change
Effect on serum concentrations of renally cleared drugs	Major fluctuations	Some fluctuations	Fewer fluctuations	Fewer fluctuations
Infection risk	Line infection/ bacteraemia	Line infection/ bacteraemia	Line infection/ bacteraemia	Exit site infection; tunnel infection; peritonitis
Loss of nutrients into dialysate/ filtrate	Yes	Yes	Yes	Yes

Abbreviations: ICP = intracerebral pressure; RRT = renal replacement therapy; SLED = slow low-efficiency dialysis; EDD = extended daily dialysis; PIRRT = prolonged intermittent renal replacement therapy.

Table 4.8.4 Advantages and disadvantages of different modalities of renal replacement therapy

	Modality			
	IHD	**SLED**	**SCUF**	**CRRT**
Advantages	• Allows more rapid removal of low-molecular-weight substances and toxins • Reduced anticoagulation exposure • Lower cost than CRRT • More time for rehabilitation and mobilisation	• More haemodynamic stability than with IHD • Decreased anticoagulation requirements • Time when not receiving treatment may be used for diagnostic or therapeutic procedures or rehabilitation	• Gentler fluid removal and control of fluid balance in volume overload • Decreased anticoagulation requirements	• Haemodynamic stability as a result of gentler fluid removal • Continuous removal of toxins and better metabolic homeostasis • Gentler fluid removal and better control of fluid balance
Disadvantages	• Hypotension with rapid fluid removal • Dialysis disequilibrium syndrome with risk of cerebral oedema • Usually not provided by ICU team • More complex drug dosing • Possibly higher risk of long-term dialysis dependency • Loss of micronutrients	• May not be tolerated by extremely unwell unstable patients	• No clearance of solutes or toxins • Can only be used in patients with fluid overload	• Slower clearance of toxins • Need for anticoagulation • Risk of hypothermia • Higher costs compared to IHD • Immobilisation • Loss of micronutrients

Abbreviations: IHD = intermittent haemodialysis; SLED = slow low-efficiency dialysis; SCUF = slow continuous ultrafiltration; CRRT = continuous renal replacement therapy.

issues (e.g. convective therapies give better clearance of molecules with a large molecular weight). However, there are not enough data to recommend one modality over another. The selection of one therapy over another often depends on local expertise, availability of staff and equipment and conditions of each individual patient. Multiple modalities can be used in one patient, based on the circumstances and condition of the individual.

Timing of RRT Initiation

The optimal timing of initiation of RRT in patients without life-threatening indications remains unclear. Theoretically, early initiation of RRT has the advantage of achieving control of fluid overload, toxin accumulation and electrolyte disturbances earlier. However, early initiation may expose patients to unnecessary RRT-related complications such as vascular access complications or haemodynamic instability. By contrast, a 'late' or 'delayed' strategy of starting RRT only in case of absolute indications avoids utilising resources in those patients whose kidney function might recover spontaneously.

To date, there is no consensus on the definition of 'early' or 'late' initiation. Some studies used serum biochemistry levels or AKI staging and others used timing

from diagnosis of AKI or timing from ICU admission to start RRT. The issue of timing of initiation remains one of the most controversial topics in RRT.

Three large randomised controlled trials have been recently published (Table 4.8.5).

The Artificial Kidney Initiation in Kidney Injury (AKIKI) trial included over 600 patients with severe AKI, predominantly medical patients. No significant difference in mortality was observed at 60 days between the early (AKI stage 3) or late groups (RRT by conventional indications). Further analysis showed just under 50 per cent in the delayed group never needed RRT and the mortality rate in patients who received no RRT was the lowest at 37 per cent.

The Early versus Late Initiation of Renal Replacement Therapy in Critically Ill Patients with Acute Kidney Injury (ELAIN) trial was a single-centre randomised controlled trial in Germany which included 231 patients. The study consisted of primarily post-operative patients, of whom 47 per cent were post-cardiac surgery. The 90-day mortality rate was 25 per cent lower in the early group (AKI stage 2), compared to the late group (AKI stage 3).

The Initiation of Dialysis Early Versus Delayed in the Intensive Care Unit (IDEAL-ICU) randomised

Table 4.8.5 Comparison between large randomised controlled trials in different timing of the initiation of renal replacement therapy

Studies	ELAIN	AKIKI	IDEAL-ICU
Number of patients enrolled	231	620	488
Population (%)	Surgery, 94.8 (post-operative)	Sepsis, 79.5	Septic shock, 100
Criteria for early RRT	KDIGO stage 2	KDIGO stage 3	RIFLE (failure stage)
Criteria for standard RRT	KDIGO stage 3	By indications	1. Emergency condition 2. 48 hours after AKI diagnosis
SOFA score at initiation of RRT	15.8	10.9	12.3
Received RRT in the late group (%)	91	51	62
Time to RRT (hours)	6 versus 25	2 versus 57	7 versus 51
Mode of RRT (%)	CRRT, 100	IHD, 50; CRRT, 30	IHD, 34; CRRT, 46; both, 20
Primary endpoint (%)	90-day mortality 39 versus 55 ($p = 0.03$)	60-day mortality 49 versus 50 (NS)	90-day mortality 58 versus 54 (NS)
Secondary endpoints	Early strategy • Shorter RRT duration, mechanical ventilation and hospital length of stay • More renal recovery	Early strategy • Delayed diuresis • Higher risk of catheter-related bloodstream infections	Early strategy • Shorter RRT-free days

Abbreviations: RRT = renal replacement therapy; KDIGO = Kidney Disease: Improving Global Outcomes; RIFLE = Risk, Injury, Failure, Loss, End-stage kidney disease; AKI = acute kidney injury; SOFA = Sequential Organ Failure Assessment; CRRT = continuous renal replacement therapy; IHD = intermittent haemodialysis; NS = not significant.

488 sepsis patients. There were no differences in mortality between the early (failure stage defined by the Risk, Injury, Failure, Loss, End-stage kidney disease (RIFLE) criteria) and late groups. Of note, 21 per cent of all patients in the late group never met the conventional criteria for RRT and spontaneously recovered.

Major limitations of these trials included the different modalities for RRT used, inclusion criteria and definitions of early versus late initiation. The largest multi-centre randomised controlled trial (STARRT-AKI) consisting of over 3000 patients (ClinicalTrials.gov identifier: NCT02568722) has recently been completed and may shed light on this area of interest.

For now, there are no absolute urea or creatinine cut-off values for RRT initiation. Clinicians should consider the severity of AKI, the severity of illness and the trajectories, the patient's metabolic and fluid demands, the kidney's capacity to cope with complications of AKI and the risks of RRT. The presence of other co-morbidities and the prognosis of overall illness, with respect to the patients' and families' wishes, need to be considered too. Finally, the availability of staff and machines should be taken into account for modality selection.

Vascular Access

The patient will need a temporary large-bore central venous catheter (11–14 Fr) to allow for sustained blood flows >100 ml/min. These are called 'non-tunnelled' vascular catheters, or known as 'Vascath'. They can be either a double-lumen catheter where the red port is 'arterial' (blood leaving the body to the circuit) and the blue port is 'venous' (blood returning to the patient), or a triple-lumen catheter with an additional narrow port for fluid and drug administration or sampling of blood. When not in use, both ports need an anticoagulant solution, such as citrate or heparin, to avoid intraluminal thrombus formation. Central venous approaches used are the internal jugular, subclavian and femoral veins. The lengths should be appropriate for each site: 12–15 cm for the right internal jugular vein; 15–20 cm for the left internal jugular vein; and at least 19–24 cm for the femoral veins (Table 4.8.6).

The right internal jugular vein is recommended as first-line access. Femoral access is acceptable as the risks of colonisation, bacteraemia and thrombosis are similar to internal jugular venous access, with the exception of patients with a body mass index (BMI) >28.4 kg/m^2 where femoral vein cannulation is associated with more

505

Table 4.8.6 Preferential insertion site of RRT catheters and corresponding catheter length

Insertion site	Catheter length (cm)
Right internal jugular vein	15
Femoral vein	24–25
Left internal jugular vein	20
Subclavian vein	Right: 15–20 Left: 20

complications. Cannulation of the left internal jugular vein is associated with a higher risk of complications and catheter malfunction. Lastly, the subclavian veins are not recommended for temporary RRT access due to increased risk of subsequent stenosis.

Insertion of a vascular catheter should be performed under ultrasound guidance. Ideally, the catheter tip for internal jugular catheters should be at the junction of the superior vena cava and right atrium, or in the atrium. If patients eventually require transition to long-term dialysis, tunnelled catheters should be placed.

Dose of RRT

CRRT dose is based on the effluent flow rate, which is derived from the dialysate flow rate, replacement flow rate plus fluid removal rate. Two large multi-centre randomised controlled studies (the VA/NIH Acute Renal Failure Trial Network (ATN) study and the Randomised Evaluation of Normal versus Augmented Level (RENAL) study) have shown that the mortality rates between the standard delivered dose of CVVHDF (20–25 ml/(kg hr) of effluent) or IHD/PIRRT three sessions per week and higher dose (35–40 ml/(kg hr)) and IHD/PIRRT six sessions per week were similar. Higher-intensity RRT does not reduce mortality or improve renal recovery or non-renal organ failure. It is also associated with more hypotensive episodes requiring a vasopressor, more hypophosphataemia, a higher nursing workload and increased loss of vitamins and trace elements.

The Kidney Disease: Improving Global Outcomes (KDIGO) guideline has recommended a minimum of delivered effluent flow rate of 20–25 ml/(kg hr). RRT downtime, defined as a period of treatment interruption due to interventions, radiology or circuit change, should be accounted for in dosing calculations. For practicality, a higher dose of 25–30 ml/(kg hr) should be prescribed to account for the RRT downtime. IHD should be prescribed to deliver a Kt/V_{urea} of at least 1.2–1.4 on a thrice-weekly schedule, with more frequent treatments provided when the target dose is not achieved. More frequent IHD treatments may also be required to remove excess fluid and optimise volume management. In IHD and CRRT, higher treatment doses may be required in hypercatabolic individuals or to control severe hyperkalaemia or acidaemia.

Fluid Balance and Management

Fluid balance is an important component of RRT management, as fluid overload is a well-established risk factor for increased mortality in AKI and RRT patients. There is no clear guideline for volume management, but the fluid balance goal should be set daily based on the patient's volume status. The rate of fluid removal should be adjusted accordingly. There are variable methods to adjust for fluid balance, by either maintaining a fixed replacement rate and varying the net ultrafiltration rate or by maintaining a fixed ultrafiltration rate and varying the replacement rate. The overarching goal is to achieve euvolaemia whilst maintaining haemodynamic stability.

Anticoagulation

There are different types of anticoagulation available to keep the circuit patent (Table 4.8.7).

Regional citrate anticoagulation (RCA) is recommended as the first line anticoagulant for CRRT. Sodium citrate is added to the arterial port where it chelates calcium (and magnesium) and inhibits the coagulation cascade. Approximately half of the calcium citrate complexes are removed across the membrane and any complexes entering the body are metabolised to bicarbonate in a 1:3 ratio in the liver and skeletal muscle. Systemic calcium infusion is added to the venous port to replace lost calcium. Compared with systemic heparin, citrate is associated with longer filter lifetime and fewer bleeding complications.

Unfractionated heparin (UFH) is effective, inexpensive and easily accessible. It can be administered systemically or via the circuit. Typical complications include dosing variabilities, induced thrombocytopenia, heparin resistance and increased bleeding.

Low-molecular-weight heparins (LMWH), thrombin antagonists and platelet-inhibiting agents have been used, with little robust data to support their use universally. LMWH has a lower risk of bleeding and heparin-induced thrombocytopenia (HIT) than UFH. However, it requires serial factor Xa monitoring and has a higher bleeding risk, compared with RCA. Non-heparin

Table 4.8.7 Characteristics of commonly used anticoagulants

Characteristics	Unfractionated heparin	Low-molecular-weight heparin	Epoprostenol	Citrate
Mode of action	Inactivation of thrombin and other proteases involved in the clotting cascade	Inactivation of thrombin and other proteases involved in the clotting cascade	Inhibition of platelet function	Chelation of calcium
Extent of anticoagulation	Systemic	Systemic	Systemic	Regional
Most common side effects	Bleeding HIT	Bleeding HIT	Vasodilation	Citrate accumulation Metabolic alkalosis Hypo-/hypercalcaemia
Absolute/relative contraindications	Bleeding HIT	Bleeding HIT	Severe haemodynamic instability due to vasodilation	Severe liver failure Severe intracellular hypoxia

Abbreviations: HIT = heparin-induced thrombocytopenia.

anticoagulants, including argatroban, lepirudin and danaparoid, are viable options in patients with HIT. Epoprostanol (prostacyclin) is a weak anticoagulant with anti-platelet effects but is associated with a higher risk of hypotension, increased intracranial pressure and short haemofilter survival. It may be used to spare heparin doses in centres where UFH is utilised.

Anticoagulation may be omitted in patients with contraindications to citrate and heparin, e.g. severe thrombocytopenia, coagulation disorders. However, this is associated with a shorter circuit lifetime. Haemofilter life can be prolonged by using high blood flow rates (200–300 ml/min) and pre-filter replacement fluid and minimising the fluid removal rate.

CRRT Prescription and Monitoring

Every patient should have an RRT prescription in order to standardise care and also for audit purposes to improve care in the future.

The prescription should include the following components.

- **Modality:** CVVH or CVVHD or CVVHDF can be chosen. SCUF should be prescribed in patients with only pulmonary oedema.
- **Anticoagulation:** citrate anticoagulation is the first-line agent, followed by heparin and/or no anticoagulation if contraindicated.
- **Vascular catheter:** optimal catheter function should be ensured to minimise interruptions in blood flow and circuit.
- **CRRT dose:** the prescribed dose should be at least 25–30 ml/(kg hr).

- **CRRT blood flow rate:** this should be maintained at 150–250 ml/min. A high blood flow rate of >300 ml/min can damage the circuit and the pump, and increase the risk of thrombus formation. A low blood flow rate of <150 ml/min without anticoagulation can cause blood stasis and increase the risk of clots.
- **CRRT solutions:** these are used for replacement fluid and dialysate. They can be either lactate- or bicarbonate-based, with varying concentrations of potassium.
- **Patient fluid removal rate:** this should be adjusted, depending on the clinical condition, and can be adjusted hourly for a net positive or negative balance.

'Filtration fraction' is another important term which describes the ratio of ultrafiltration rate to plasma water flow rate. It is usually kept below 20 per cent. Filtration fractions >20 per cent are associated with circuit thrombus formation. The filtration fraction can be adjusted by increasing the blood flow rate, decreasing the ultrafiltration rate or increasing the pre-filter to post-filter ratio.

During CRRT, there must be close monitoring of the technical equipment, the patient's cardiovascular status and regular blood gas and electrolyte analysis, including magnesium and phosphate, of which the frequency will depend on the clinical status.

Complications of CRRT

The associated complications of CRRT can be related to the extracorporeal treatment or to the disease process.

507

Complications Associated with Vascular Access

- Haemorrhage
- Infection
- Venous thrombosis
- Venous stenosis
- Traumatic arteriovenous fistula
- Pneumothorax
- Haemothorax
- Air embolism
- Visceral injury

Haemofilter Clotting

Despite anticoagulation, microthrombi may form in the haemofilter over time, reducing its efficiency, and thus the clearance of solutes reduces. The filter life can depend on the type of anticoagulation used and, in turn, the type of membrane used.

Haemodynamics

Haemodynamic instability may occur during RRT due to the underlying disease process, the rate of fluid removal and underlying myocardial dysfunction. There is minimal change when minimising blood flow, compared with standard blood flow rate.

Bioincompatibility and Haemofilter Reactions

As blood comes into contact with the haemofilter membrane, microthrombi may form due to activation of leucocytes, complement and the coagulation cascade. This bioincompatibility can depend on the type of dialysis filter used. Cellulose or natural filters (e.g. cuprophane) are associated most with bioincompatibility. Synthetic filters (e.g. polysulfone, polyacrylonitrile) are generally more biocompatible. Rarely, patients may have allergic reactions to haemofilters, ranging from rash, wheezing and hypotension to anaphylaxis.

Air Embolism and Micro-bubbles

Air embolism can happen anywhere in the circuit when the connection is loose or broken, but micro-bubbles can be formed within the circuit and these may give rise to obstruction of capillary blood flow, leading to tissue ischaemia, hypotension and cardiac arrest. Air embolism in the brain can lead to brain anoxia, seizure and coma.

Bleeding and Anaemia

The risk of bleeding from insertion of the vascular catheter site, inadvertent disconnections of equipment, frequent dialysis filter changes and systemic anticoagulation can lead to a decrease in haemoglobin levels.

Electrolyte Imbalance

CRRT can lead to hypokalaemia, hypophosphataemia and hypomagnesaemia. If citrate is used as the anticoagulant, a high citrate buffer may lead to hypernatraemia, hypocalcaemia and metabolic alkalosis. Wide-gap metabolic acidosis can be found in patients with liver failure who may have a reduced ability to metabolise citrate or in patients with lactataemia. Ionised calcium, electrolytes and pH should be monitored frequently. Citrate accumulation should be suspected if the ratio of systemic total calcium to ionised calcium is >2.5.

Drug Removal

Drug removal during RRT depends on numerous factors, including the modality used, the type of dialysis filter, the membrane's surface area and ultrafiltrate and dialysis flow rates. The amount of drug removed on a daily basis can also vary during the course of the treatment, in line with changes in total body fluid and changes in the protein component of the blood. Low-molecular-weight non-protein-bound drugs can be cleared by CRRT, dependent on the effluent flow rate. High-molecular-weight drugs that are highly protein-bound or have large volumes of distribution are rarely cleared by CRRT; therefore, dosing adjustment is not required.

Hydrophilic antibiotics (e.g. aminoglycosides, β-lactams, glycopeptides) tend to be removed more than lipophilic antibiotics (e.g. fluoroquinolones, oxazolidinones). It is important to be aware of this anomaly, as clinically there is a risk of under-treatment of infection or over-treatment, leading to side effects of the antibiotics.

Nutritional Losses

During RRT, nutrients and water-soluble vitamins are removed and lost into the effluent. Total daily calories of approximately 35 kcal/(kg day) should be targeted, with a target protein intake of 1.7 (up to 2.5) g/(kg day).

Hypothermia

Thermal losses during CRRT cause vasoconstriction and may mask fever. Significant hypothermia may occur, necessitating external warming.

Weaning from RRT

There are no universally accepted criteria for RRT discontinuation. RRT is usually continued until kidney function returns or the goals of care change. Renal recovery is suspected if urine output increases. Discontinuation of RRT should be considered if the patient's spontaneous urine output is >400 ml without diuretics, and 2000 ml with diuretics. In the ATN trial, patients with urine output of >750 ml/day underwent measurement of 6-hour timed urine creatinine clearance (CrCl). RRT was discontinued when CrCl was >20 ml/min, continued when CrCl was <12 ml/min, and left to the clinicians' discretion if CrCl was between 12 and 20 ml/min. After RRT is discontinued, patients should be monitored for signs of relapse such as worsening of overall clinical status, rising urea and creatinine, a new onset of oliguria and worsening hyperkalaemia and/or acidosis. If there are no signs of recovery after 2–3 weeks, a tunnelled semi-permanent catheter placement may be considered.

Patients with a history of AKI have higher risks of recurrent AKI, chronic kidney disease (CKD), end-stage renal disease (ESRD) and long-term mortality. Therefore, nephrologists should be consulted before patient discharge from critical care to arrange appropriate post-AKI follow-up. For patients requiring multiple types of organ support, decisions about continuing or withdrawing RRT should be considered as part of multiple organ support.

Conclusion

RRT has become an integral part in the treatment of severe AKI in critically ill patients and its use has increased over the last few decades. There is no clear evidence as to the best modality to use, when the optimum time is to initiate treatment prior to life-threatening indications and when to discontinue RRT. Prescription should be personalised in each patient regarding solute control, fluid removal and timing of initiation. Finally, RRT should be considered as part of overall life-sustaining treatments, with goals of care in mind.

References and Further Reading

Barbar SD, Clere-Jehl R, Bourredjem A, *et al*. Timing of renal replacement therapy in patients with acute kidney injury and sepsis. *N Engl J Med* 2018;**379**:1431.

Bellomo R, Ronco C, Mehta RL, *et al*. Acute kidney injury in the intensive care unit: from injury to recovery: reports from the 5th Paris International Conference. *Ann Intensive Care* 2017;**7**:49.

Gaudry S, Hajage D, Schortgen F, *et al*. Initiation strategies for renal replacement therapy in intensive care units. *N Engl J Med* 2016;**375**:122–33.

RENAL Replacement Therapy Study Investigators; Bellomo R, Cass A, Cole L, *et al*. Intensity of continuous renal-replacement therapy in critically ill patients. *N Engl J Med* 2009;**361**:1627–38.

VA/NIH Acute Renal Failure Trial Network. Intensity of renal support in critically ill patients with acute kidney injury. *N Engl J Med* 2008;**359**:7–20.

Zarbock A, Kellum JA, Schmidt C, *et al*. Effect of early vs delayed initiation of renal replacement therapy on mortality in critically ill patients with acute kidney injury: the ELAIN Randomized Clinical Trial. *JAMA* 2016;**315**:2190–9.

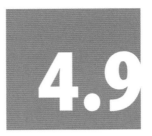

4.9 Nutritional Assessment and Support in Intensive Care (Enteral and Parenteral Nutrition)

Liesl Wandrag

Key Learning Points

1. Intubated patients should usually receive nutritional support within 24–48 hours of admission.
2. Enteral nutrition is the preferred route of feeding, where feasible.
3. The National Patient Safety Agency (NPSA) advises that nasogastric tubes (NGTs) should be checked after initial placement and daily before use with either chest X-ray or pH paper (pH <5.5) to ensure correct stomach placement.
4. Feeding protocols are strongly encouraged to ensure that nutritional support is initiated, increased and monitored appropriately.
5. Parenteral nutrition should start early when enteral nutrition is not feasible in high-risk or poorly nourished patients.

Keywords: enteral nutrition, parenteral nutrition, feeding protocols

Introduction

Robust evidence for nutritional practices in the ICU is often limited due to heterogeneity of study populations, methodological challenges in the ICU research setting, difficulty in estimating nutritional requirements in the critically ill and variation in nutritional interventions studied in terms of dose, timing and duration, and by limited consensus as to agreed core outcome sets for nutritional studies. These limitations to study design have led to opposing study findings, and also to variation observed in international ICU nutrition guidelines.

Critically ill patients are catabolic, often hypermetabolic and hyperinflammatory, and as such, nutritional support would aim to support patients through this period. Current thinking is that nutritional support should be tailored according to the phase of critical illness: acute, chronic and recovery phase. However, the exact dose of nutrition to give in each phase and the mechanism to determine transition between each of these phases have yet to be defined.

In critically ill patients, the benefits of enteral nutrition support include:

- Improved wound healing
- Decreased catabolic response to injury
- Improved gastrointestinal structure and function
- Improved clinical outcomes, including a reduction in complication rates and length of stay

Feeding protocols should be used in which enteral nutrition can be commenced based on patient weight, to ensure early feed delivery is achieved. Interruptions to feeding should be minimised to ensure optimal feed delivery, and many ICUs use guidelines for stopping and restarting enteral nutrition pre-and post-procedures/surgery to minimise delays in feeding.

Nutritional Assessment in the ICU

Assessing the nutritional status of a critically ill patient is challenging, as traditional screening tools and assessment methods are not validated in the ICU setting. Nutritional assessment, usually conducted by a specialist critical care dietitian, includes assessment of weight, height, body mass index (BMI), biochemistry, clinical history and nutritional intake history. The concept of 'nutrition risk' has been developed as a method to determine the patients who may benefit the most from aggressive nutritional support. This scoring system (NUTRIC score) includes variables for age, severity of illness, co-morbidities and hospital length of stay prior to ICU admission, and has been recommended for use by the American Society for Parenteral and Enteral Nutrition (ASPEN) and the Society of Critical Care Medicine (SCCM).

More traditional anthropometric measures, such as weight, mid-arm circumference, skinfold thickness and bio-electrical impedance analysis, are inaccurate due to the enormous daily fluid shifts seen in these patients. Additional methods to assess lean body mass, such as muscle volume measurement via ultrasound or computed tomography, are available, but these are largely restricted to research settings at present.

How to Provide Nutritional Support

Nutritional support in critical care is usually provided as enteral or parenteral nutrition. However, oral nutritional support, in addition to oral diet (nutritional supplements or food fortification), may also be appropriate in some cases. Critical care dietitians would be the main contact and provider of nutritional support; they may work embedded within the critical care multidisciplinary team (MDT) or occasionally work in conjunction with nutritional support teams consisting of gastroenterologists, nutritional support nurses and pharmacists. A critical care dietitian (or nutrition team) will play a vital role in minimising complications that may arise from either enteral or parenteral nutrition.

Enteral Nutrition

All intubated patients should usually receive enteral feeding within 24–48 hours of admission once haemodynamically stable (local guidelines may differ on the exact timings).

Enteral Access Routes

National Patient Safety Agency (NPSA)-compliant nasogastric tubes (NGTs) must be used (Ryles tubes are not usually used for enteral feeding, hydration or medication):

- Nasogastric feeding tubes (most commonly used enteral feeding tube)
- Oro-gastric feeding tubes for patients with a base of skull fracture or facial trauma where an NGT cannot be passed
- Post-pyloric (duodenal or jejunal) feeding for poor gastric feed tolerance or upper gastrointestinal obstruction
- Gastrostomy for longer-term enteral feeding (although these are not commonly placed in most institutions)

Management of NGTs

Only trained healthcare professionals should insert feeding tubes. The NPSA advises that NGTs should be checked after initial placement and daily before use with either chest X-ray or pH paper (pH <5.5) to ensure correct stomach placement. The NEX (nose, earlobe, xiphisternum) measurement is usually taken and documented for all new NGT insertions. This measurement is a guide as to where the final position of the NGT should be. The final position should not be shorter than the NEX measurement but may be longer, if required, after review of the chest X-ray.

Administration

The head of the bed should be elevated to 30–45°, except when clinical position prevents it. Continuous delivery of enteral nutrition or volume-based delivery could be provided. Drug administration via enteral feeding tubes may also determine timing of feeding or feed breaks.

Complications Associated with Enteral Nutrition

- Misplaced enteral feeding tubes, in particular NGTs, and aspiration pneumonia
- NGT insertion trauma
- Refeeding syndrome if feed is titrated up too fast in at-risk patients
- Gastric intolerance

Parenteral Nutrition

Parenteral nutrition (PN or total PN (TPN)) is considered when patients:

- Do not have a functioning gastrointestinal tract
- Cannot tolerate full volumes of enteral nutrition due to poor absorption or prolonged ileus
- Have high-output or entero-cutaneous fistulae
- Present with short bowel syndrome
- Have severe oral mucositis
- Have prolonged intestinal failure, i.e. radiation enteritis or necrotic bowel
- Need 'top-up' nutritional support where enteral feeding is not deemed adequate.

The potential risk outweighs any perceived benefit if PN is provided for <5 days (National Institute for Health and Care Excellence, 2006).

Parenteral Access Routes

Central access routes include:

- A dedicated lumen in a multi-lumen central line
- Subclavian or internal jugular vein access for shorter-term PN

- A dedicated peripherally inserted central catheter (PICC line) for medium-term access
- Tunnelled lines for long-term access (e.g. Hickman or Portacath)

Management

Trained healthcare professionals who are competent in catheter placement should place catheters. Adequately trained professionals should monitor access sites and the administration of PN.

Administration

Continuous administration is the preferred method when PN is initiated and when patients are critically ill. Unless contraindicated, some trophic enteral feed (10–30 ml/hr) should be administered to maintain gastrointestinal integrity (to reduce villous atrophy). PN should **not** be disconnected if patients leave the ward for investigations, as this increases the likelihood of line infections. PN should be weaned gradually to avoid rebound hypoglycaemia. Patients should have approximately 50 per cent of their requirements met by enteral nutrition before PN is discontinued. It is prudent to monitor blood glucose levels whilst PN is weaned and once it is discontinued.

Parental Nutrition Preparations

PN is usually provided as an all-in-one preparation consisting of amino acids, lipids, glucose, electrolytes and micronutrients. Hospitals either buy in pre-mixed compounded PN or compound PN themselves in an aseptic unit in the pharmacy. Here lipid, glucose, amino acids, electrolytes, vitamins and minerals are mixed together under aseptic conditions. If required, lipid-free or electrolyte-free preparations can be compounded or bought in. In most ICUs, the critical care dietitian and aseptics pharmacist would take responsibility for PN monitoring and ordering, although this may vary per institution.

Complications Associated with Parenteral Nutrition

- Catheter-/insertion-related complications (discussed elsewhere in the textbook)
- Nutritional/metabolic:
  - Hyperglycaemia
  - Hypoglycaemia
  - Refeeding syndrome
  - Liver dysfunction
  - Lipaemia
  - Electrolyte imbalance

Energy Targets

Indirect calorimetry is deemed the gold standard method to determine energy expenditure in the critically ill. However, it is mostly used in a research setting in the UK. Various predictive equations are used, each with its own inherent limitations. Commonly used equations include:

- 20–25 kcal/kg (American College of Chest Physicians)
- 25–30 kcal/kg (European Society for Clinical Nutrition and Metabolism)
- Penn State equation, 2009 (age, gender, weight, maximum body temperature and minute ventilation required. Mifflin St Jeor equation is used first to determine the basal metabolic rate)

For patients with BMI >30 kg/m^2, ESPEN recommends:

- 25 kcal/kg adjusted body weight

Non-feed energy sources should be considered – propofol 1% and 2% (approximately 1.1 kcal/ml) and regional citrate anticoagulation used in haemofiltration could both contribute to additional caloric load, particularly if significant volumes are used for an extended duration.

Protein Targets

Critically ill patients are unlikely to be in positive nitrogen balance, with weight loss and muscle wasting commonly observed in survivors of critical illness. Protein recommendations are currently based on observational data only.

Protein recommendations include:

- 1.2 g/(kg day) in the general ICU population
- 1.5–2.5 g/(kg day) for patients on CRRT and obese patients (SCCM, ASPEN, ESPEN)

Carbohydrate Requirements and Glucose Control

Excessive carbohydrate intake may cause hyperglycaemia, hypertriglyceridaemia, fatty liver and hypercapnia. To avoid excess carbon dioxide production from surplus carbohydrate, the glucose oxidation rate can be calculated (4–7 mg/(kg bodyweight min day)). Blood glucose levels should be maintained between 6 and 10 mmol/l in patients receiving enteral nutrition and/or PN.

Micronutrients

There are insufficient data to make recommendations for routine supplementation of vitamins and minerals in the critically ill. Burns patients or those on continuous renal replacement therapy (or patients with high alcohol consumption or at risk of refeeding syndrome) should be supplemented in accordance with local and national guidelines.

Refeeding Syndrome

Severe fluid and electrolyte shifts with metabolic complications may occur in malnourished patients undergoing refeeding. This could occur via enteral, parenteral or oral nutrition and via intravenous glucose provision.

- **At-risk patients:**
  - Those with poor nutritional intake for >5 days, especially if already malnourished (BMI <20 kg/m² or unintentional weight loss of >5 per cent in the last 3–6 months)
- **High-risk patients – patients have <u>one or more</u> of the following:**
  - BMI <16 kg/m²
  - Unintentional weight loss of >15 per cent within 3–6 months
  - Little or no nutrition for >10 days
  - Low levels of potassium, phosphate or magnesium prior to feeding
- **High-risk patients – patients have <u>two or more</u> of the following:**
  - BMI <18.5 kg/m²
  - Unintentional weight loss >10 per cent within the last 3–6 months
  - Little or no nutritional intake for >5 days
  - A history of alcohol abuse or drugs, including insulin, chemotherapy, antacids and diuretics

Management of Refeeding

- Supplement vitamins prior to starting feed, for 10 days: Pabrinex® I + II, one pair once daily, or oral thiamine 200–300 mg daily, vitamin B co strong one or two tablets three times a day (or full-dose daily intravenous vitamin B preparation) and a balanced multi-vitamin/trace element supplement once daily.
- Introduce nutritional support very slowly at 10 kcal/kg; aim to meet energy requirements over 4–7 days.
- Monitor and supplement potassium, phosphate and magnesium, as required (National Institute for Health and Care Excellence guideline, 2006).

Protocols

The use of evidence-based protocols is encouraged to ensure that nutritional support is initiated, increased and monitored appropriately.

Protocols should:

- Promote early feeding
- Indicate gradual increases in enteral nutrition; this may include a volume-based feeding approach
- Suggest gastric residual volume handling instructions. There is no evidence to recommend a specific value – some units have abandoned the practice of measuring these altogether
- Encourage the use of prokinetic agents if gastric feed is not tolerated
- Advocate the use of post-pyloric feeding tubes for feeding intolerance

Volume-Based Feeding

Volume-based feeding protocols focus on delivering daily volumes of feed, rather than on a target rate of feed per hour. Nursing staff calculate the remaining daily feed volume to be delivered and then adjust the rate of feeding to accommodate for time lost to investigations, procedures and theatre.

Summary

- Optimum macro- and micronutrient requirements for ICU patients are still not known; it remains unclear whether meeting requirements of these nutrients would lead to improved ICU outcomes.
- Both over- and underfeeding should be avoided.
- Early nutritional support should be considered (24–48 hours after ICU admission).
- Feeding protocols may allow for a more optimum nutrient delivery.
- In the absence of indirect calorimetry or a specialist critical care dietitian, approximately 25 kcal/(kg day) would be appropriate for most general ICU patients. Once patients are in the recovery phase, 30 kcal/kg can be used.
- A total of 1.2–1.5 g/(kg day) protein should be provided.

References and Further Reading

Elke G, van Zanten ARH, Lemieux M, *et al.* Enteral versus parenteral nutrition in critically ill patients: an updated systematic review and meta-analysis of randomized controlled trials. *Crit Care* 2016;**20**:117.

Heyland DK, Dhaliwal R, Drover JW, Gramlich DA, Dodek P; Canadian Critical Care Clinical Practice Guidelines Committee. Canadian practice guidelines for nutrition support in mechanically ventilated, critically ill adult patients. *JPEN J Parenter Enteral Nutr* 2003;**27**:355–73. [Guidelines updated: 2009]

McClave SA, Taylor BE, Martindale RG, *et al.* Guidelines for the provision and assessment of nutrition support therapy in the adult critically ill patient: Society of Critical Care Medicine (SCCM) and American Society for Parenteral and Enteral Nutrition (A.S.P.E.N.). *JPEN J Parenter Enteral Nutr* 2016;**40**:159–211.

Preiser JC, van Zanten AR, Berger MM, *et al.* Metabolic and nutritional support of critically ill patients: consensus and controversies. *Crit Care* 2015;**19**:35.

Singer P, Reintam Blaser A, Berger MM, *et al.* ESPEN guideline on clinical nutrition in the intensive care unit. *Clin Nutr* 2019;**38**:48–79.

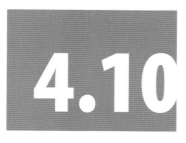

4.10 Neuromonitoring and Cerebral Protection

Wilson Fandino

Key Learning Points

1. The physiological changes governing the Monro–Kellie doctrine become quickly exhausted when the intracranial volume reaches a critical value, thus expediting intracranial hypertension.

2. The main factors influencing the balance between cerebral oxygen delivery and consumption are cerebral blood flow (CBF), arterial oxygen saturation (SaO_2), haemoglobin concentration and cerebral metabolic rate of oxygen ($CMRO_2$).

3. In the critical care unit, the most common advanced neuromonitoring technique involves measurement of intracranial pressure (ICP) and estimation of cerebral perfusion pressure (CPP). However, brain tissue oxygen tension ($PtiO_2$), jugular venous oxygen saturation ($SjvO_2$), cerebral microdialysis, transcranial Doppler ultrasound and continuous electroencephalography are also helpful to detect early complications.

4. Jugular venous oxygen saturation ($SjvO_2$) values <55 per cent may indicate elevated $CMRO_2$, low CBF, systemic oxygen desaturation or cerebral ischaemia. Conversely, readings >75 per cent may represent high CBF, metabolic suppression or massive cerebral infarction.

5. Cerebral microdialysis is an evolving technique that can help to diagnose cerebral ischaemia, traumatic axonal injury and inflammatory insults at early stages. However, more research is needed to validate its clinical use.

Keywords: neurophysiology, neurophysiological monitoring, intracranial hypertension

Introduction

The cerebral vault is a rigid structure containing the brain parenchyma, cerebrospinal fluid (CSF) and blood. According to the Monro–Kellie doctrine, under normal circumstances, the three components self-regulate to maintain a constant intracranial volume. However, when the uncompressible volume reaches a critical value, the intracranial compliance (Δ volume/pressure) suddenly decreases and the intracranial pressure (ICP) dramatically rises with further small increases in intracranial volume.

In patients with intact autoregulation, despite the subsequent drop in cerebral perfusion pressure (CPP) (which is defined as the difference between mean arterial blood pressure (MAP) and ICP), the cerebral blood flow (CBF) will initially be maintained by means of vasodilation of cerebral arterioles, resulting from decreased cerebral vascular resistance (CVR):

$$CBF = \frac{CPP}{CVR} = \frac{(MAP - ICP)}{CVR}$$

Nonetheless, this mechanism quickly becomes overcome, and CBF eventually decreases. Cerebral arterioles are also vasodilated in response to a drop in the MAP. In patients with impaired autoregulation, or if the MAP is out of the vasoregulation range (usually between 50 and 150 mmHg), the CBF will be entirely dependent on the CPP. Thus, a drop in CPP will result in cerebral hypoperfusion.

The balance between oxygen delivery and consumption (the latter expressed as the cerebral metabolic rate of oxygen, or $CMRO_2$) can be evaluated using several parameters, including parenchymal tissue oxygen tension ($PtiO_2$) and jugular venous oxygen saturation ($SvjO_2$), which reflect local and global changes, respectively. Oxygen delivery is defined as the product of CBF and arterial oxygen content (CaO_2). The CaO_2 is, in turn, mainly dependent on haemoglobin (Hb) concentration and arterial oxygen saturation (SaO_2). The main factors influencing these variables are summarised in Fig. 4.10.1.

515

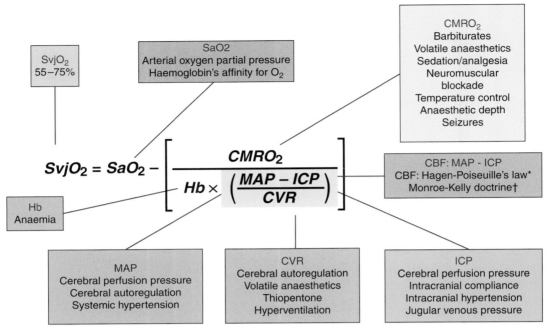

Figure 4.10.1 Estimation of jugular venous oxygen saturation ($SjvO_2$) and the main factors influencing the variables. The equation has been adapted from the Fick's principle for oxygen consumption. * The cerebral blood flow (CBF) follows the Hagen–Poiseuille's law, which states that the laminar flow is directly related to the fourth power of the ratio and the pressure difference registered in the cerebral vessels. † According to the Monro–Kellie doctrine, any effect of an increase in CBF will be compensated to maintain a constant intracranial volume. SaO_2 = arterial oxygen saturation; $CMRO_2$ = cerebral metabolic rate of oxygen; Hb = haemoglobin; MAP = mean arterial blood pressure; ICP = intracranial pressure; CVR = cerebrovascular resistance.

Intracranial Pressure

Whilst normal ICP ranges from 5 to 15 mmHg, intracranial hypertension is usually diagnosed with values >20–22 mmHg. ICP can be monitored through the placement of an external ventricular drain (EVD) or an intra-parenchymal bolt. Although the former is considered the gold standard for global ICP monitoring in some institutions, it is mainly used for draining CSF. Placement of an EVD entails a significant risk of complications, including infection (5–20 per cent) and haemorrhage (2 per cent). Alternatively, intra-parenchymal monitors are useful to monitor regional ICP, with a minimal risk of bleeding or infection. Some of them also allow access to monitor other variables, including $PtiO_2$, cerebral microdialysis and brain temperature.

Brain Tissue Oxygen Tension

The normal values of $PtiO_2$ range from 20 to 35 mmHg, with ischaemia thresholds between 10 and 15 mmHg. Oxygen tension is measured (either with luminescent or polarographic methods) through a catheter placed

in radiographic normal brain of the ipsilateral affected hemisphere (usually in the frontal lobe) or in the non-dominant hemisphere (in cases of diffuse brain injury).

Several surrogate biomarkers, including CPP and ICP, have failed to demonstrate utility to predict brain hypoxia, probably because improvement of oxygenation mainly depends on the status of cerebral autoregulation. Low brain $PtiO_2$, by contrast, has been clearly associated with poor outcomes. Nevertheless, normal low levels can be found when the metabolic demands of the brain are diminished in response to metabolic autoregulation (e.g. hypothermia, anaesthesia), and high levels may indicate hyperaemia.

Jugular Bulb Oximetry

$SjvO_2$ can be estimated with retrograde insertion of a small fibreoptic catheter in the dominant jugular vein. It should be placed at the level of the jugular bulb, to avoid mixture with the external jugular blood. Figure 4.10.1 provides the variables influencing the estimation of $SjvO_2$, along with the main factors determining its measurement. Values <55 per cent may indicate elevated $CMRO_2$, low CBF, systemic oxygen desaturation or cerebral ischaemia. By contrast, values >75 per cent may represent high CBF, metabolic suppression or massive cerebral infarction. $SjvO_2$ is also inversely related to the cerebral oxygen extraction ratio ($CERO_2$).

Cerebral Microdialysis

Dialysis is defined as the process of removing particles across a semi-permeable membrane, applying the principles of diffusion of solutes and ultrafiltration of fluids. Similar to the conventional dialysis used to remove toxins from the blood, cerebral microdialysis generates a chemical gradient in the cerebral parenchyma, to evaluate the brain extracellular fluid. A microdialysis catheter consists of two concentric tubes and a semi-permeable membrane with 20 or 100 kDa molecular weight cut-offs. Whilst the outer tube contains a perfusion fluid (artificial CSF), the inner tube carries the microdialysate collected in the tip of the catheter to be analysed. The catheter should be placed in the most at-risk tissue (ipsilateral to the lesion) or in the non-dominant hemisphere (in diffuse injuries).

Cerebral ischaemia, which is accompanied by low levels of glucose and parenchymal tissue oxygen tension ($PbtO_2$), can elicit the anaerobic glycolysis pathway, thus resulting in a high lactate/pyruvate ratio (LPR >25–40 mmol/l). Other microdialysis measurements include glucose (>2 mmol/l), glutamate (<15 mmol/l) and tau protein (which has been correlated with traumatic axonal injury). The significance and clinical applications of these findings still remain debatable. Neuroinflammatory substances, such as cytokines and chemokines, can also be recovered from 100-kDa cut-off catheters.

Transcranial Doppler Ultrasound

The CBF can be estimated by measuring the mean flow velocity (MFV) of the vessels (usually at the junction of the middle and anterior cerebral arteries) with transcranial Doppler ultrasound (TCD), assuming that the calibre of the vessels remains unchanged. However, the diameter of the blood vessels is heavily influenced by the state of cerebral autoregulation. The main indications for TCD in the neurocritical care unit are detection of vasospasm in patients with subarachnoid haemorrhage and estimation of cerebral autoregulation, and in some countries it has been used as a confirmation test for brain death. The sensitivity and specificity of TCD are highly variable, depending on the artery evaluated, the status of the intracranial vasculature, the angle of insonation, the indication for the test and the experience of the clinician.

Continuous Electroencephalography

Electroencephalography (EEG) is useful in the setting of neurocritical care for detecting non-convulsive seizures, inducing burst suppression and confirming brain death. The bispectral index (BIS) can also be used to monitor burst suppression and sedation depth, but this has not been validated for neurosurgical or intensive care use.

Table 4.10.1 summarises the main indications, advantages, disadvantages and critical values for the most common neuromonitoring modalities used in clinical practice. The majority of these recommendations, however, are based on expert opinions and therefore have low to moderate quality of evidence.

Table 4.10.1 Indications for neuromonitoring techniques, including advantages, disadvantages and critical values of each modality

Modality	Critical values	Indications	Advantages	Disadvantages
ICP[a]	>20–22 mmHg	Patients at risk of elevated ICP, based on clinical or radiologic findings	Accurate and reliable readings, with both EVD and parenchymal ICP monitors	ICP cannot be used as a surrogate marker for functional outcome or an indicator of quality of care
$PbtO_2$[b]	<20 mmHg	Patients deemed at risk of regional cerebral ischaemia and/or hypoxia Therapy guidance in patients with TBI and GCS score <9 Detection of delayed cerebral ischaemia Following SAH in patients with MCA or ICA aneurysms	Strong predictor of mortality and functional outcome, when values consistently abnormal	Data influenced by probe location, CBF, PaO_2, $PaCO_2$, temperature and oxygen consumption/delivery

Table 4.10.1 (cont.)

Modality	Critical values	Indications	Advantages	Disadvantages
SjvO$_2$[b]	<50–55%	Patients deemed at risk of global cerebral ischaemia and/or hypoxia	Strong predictor of mortality and functional outcome, when values consistently abnormal	Requires frequent re-calibrations Complications include catheter misplacement, colonisation and infection Not reliable to detect regional ischaemia SjvO$_2$ does not improve outcomes following TBI
Cerebral microdialysis[b]	Glucose <2 mmol/l Glutamate >15 mmol/l Lactate/pyruvate >25–40 mmol/l	Patients at risk of cerebral ischaemia, hypoxia, energy failure or glucose deprivation May be used to estimate clinical prognosis in patients with TBI and/or SAH May be used to guide systemic glycaemic control	Consistently low brain glucose and/or elevated lactate/pyruvate ratio are strong predictors of mortality and poor functional outcome	Only useful for regional metabolic derangements 2–3 mm around probe Not useful if probe is placed in infarcted tissue or haematoma
Transcranial Doppler ultrasound	Cerebral blood flow velocity >80–100 cm/s (MCA)	May be helpful to detect vasospasm in patients with SAH Can be used to estimate cerebral autoregulation and carbon dioxide reactivity	Non-invasive technique Real-time assessment of cerebral haemodynamics	Measures CBF velocity (cm/s), but cannot be used to estimate CBF (cm³/s) Significant learning curve; reliability of measures is dependent on clinician's experience and skills
Continuous EEG	NA	Patients with persistent altered consciousness not explained by acute brain injury Patients with refractory status epilepticus Comatose patients following cardiac arrest undergoing therapeutic hypothermia within 24 hours, to rule out non-convulsive status	Early detection of convulsive and non-convulsive seizures	Time and resource-consuming EEG has not been proved to be useful to diagnose cerebral ischaemia in patients with acute ischaemic stroke

[a] Consider starting treatment on an individual basis. Monitor cerebral perfusion pressure along with ICP.

[b] Should be used as part of multi-modal monitoring or in combination with ICP.

Abbreviations: ICP = intracranial pressure; EVD = external ventricular drainage catheter; PbtO$_2$ = parenchymal tissue oxygen tension; TBI = traumatic brain injury; GCS = Glasgow Coma Scale; SAH = subarachnoid haemorrhage; MCA = middle cerebral artery; ICA = internal carotid artery; CBF = cerebral blood flow; PaO$_2$ = partial pressure of arterial oxygen; PaCO$_2$ = partial pressure of arterial carbon dioxide; SjvO$_2$ = jugular venous oxygen saturation; EEG = electroencephalography; NA = non-applicable.

Modified from: Le Roux, P., Menon, D.K., Citerio, G., Vespa, P., Bader, M.K., Brophy, G. *et al.* The international multidisciplinary consensus conference on multimodality monitoring in neurocritical care: a list of recommendations and additional conclusions. *Neurocritical Care*, 2014;**21**(2): 282–296.

References and Further Reading

De Georgia MA. Brain tissue oxygen monitoring in neurocritical care. *J Intensive Care Med* 2015;**30**:473–83.

Frontera JA. Multimodality monitoring in critically ill neurologic patients. In: DL Reich, RA Kahn, AJ Mittnacht, AB Lebowitz, ME Stone, JB Eisenkraft (eds). *Monitoring in Anesthesia and Perioperative Care.* New York, NY: Cambridge University Press; 2011. pp. 237–48.

Makarenko S, Griesdale DE, Gooderham P, Sekhon MS. Multimodal neuromonitoring for traumatic brain injury: a shift towards individualized therapy. *J Clin Neurosci* 2016;**26**:8–13.

Stocchetti N, Roux P, Vespa P, *et al.* Clinical review: neuromonitoring – an update. *Crit Care* 2013;**17**:201.

Tisdall MM. Cerebral microdialysis: research technique or clinical tool. *Br J Anaesth* 2006;**97**:18–25.

Practical Procedures

5.1.1

Oxygen Administration in Intensive Care

Jo Hackney

Key Learning Points

1. The choice of method of oxygen administration is dependent largely on the desired fraction of inspired oxygen (FiO_2).
2. To ensure delivery of a high FiO_2 and avoid entrainment of room air, the delivery flow rate of oxygen must exceed the patient's peak inspiratory flow rate.
3. Oxygen administration devices can be fixed or variable performance.
4. Variable performance devices can be adapted to allow for delivery of increased flows and/or higher FiO_2.
5. Consideration of patient preference and comfort is an important deciding factor when selecting an oxygen administration device.

Keywords: oxygen administration, variable performance, fixed performance

Introduction

The primary reason for oxygen administration in critical care is for correction of hypoxaemia. However, oxygen therapy is also utilised to increase pulmonary oxygen reserves, absorb pneumothoraces and increase the fraction of dissolved oxygen, e.g. in carbon monoxide poisoning.

The choice of oxygen administration device is largely dependent on the desired fraction of inspired oxygen (FiO_2), which is intrinsically linked with the peak inspiratory flow rate of the patient. An average 70-kg patient breathing normally will exceed the inspired FiO_2 of fresh gas once their peak inspiratory flow rate exceeds the fresh gas flow rate (FGF). At this point, the patient will entrain room air, thus diluting the FiO_2.

It must also be considered that during the respiratory cycle, an active inspiratory breath does not have a consistent flow rate, accelerating towards the peak flow rate in the middle of the inhalation. Other factors influencing the delivered FiO_2 include the presence of a respiratory pause, the mask volume and fit and resistance to ventilation. When unintentional room air entrainment occurs, the FiO_2 the patient is breathing is unknown.

Classification of Devices

There are several ways to classify the methods of administration of oxygen. The focus here shall be on the performance of the device – fixed or variable.

Fixed-Performance Devices

FiO_2 is constant, despite changes in the patient's respiratory rate and inspiratory flow rate. Fixed-performance devices include:

- Venturi mask
- Anaesthetic breathing circuit

Venturi Mask

Venturi masks use the Bernoulli principle and Venturi effect to deliver a set FiO_2 value at a given oxygen flow rate. The face mask feeds have a narrow orifice, with holes incorporated in their design, to allow jet mixing of room air at a set fraction into the oxygen stream. A pressure drop caused by an increase in velocity at the narrowing of the orifice leads to room air entrainment. Different connectors (indicated by their colour) produce specific set FiO_2 values secondary to both the oxygen flow rate and the size of the aperture open to room air – which sets the entrainment ratio (Table 5.1.1.1).

The reliability of this system depends on the patient's peak inspiratory flow rate not exceeding the total gas flow rate. If this occurs, the patient will entrain further room air through other apertures in or around the face mask, and consequently the FiO_2 will fall.

Anaesthetic Breathing Circuit

Anaesthetic breathing circuits can provide a fixed FiO_2 at low flow rates via a face mask, as long as the mask is tight-fitting. The flow rates must be adequate to ensure

Table 5.1.1.1 Different flow rates and FiO$_2$ associated with Venturi masks

Venturi mask (colour)	Flow rate (l/min)	FiO$_2$ delivery (%)
Blue	2	24
White	4	28
Yellow	6	35
Red	8	40
Green	12	60

there is no re-breathing, and this is dependent on both the classification of the circuit (Mapleson) and the minute volume of the patient.

Variable Performance Devices

These include:

- Nasal cannulae
- High-flow nasal oxygen therapy
- 'Classic' face masks:
  - Simple Hudson mask
  - Non-rebreathe face mask (reservoir)

Nasal Cannulae

These deliver 100% oxygen at low flow rates (usually 1–4 l/min) into the nasopharyngeal space. The oxygen is subsequently diluted on inspiration by entrained room air, delivering an FiO$_2$ of approximately 24–35%, depending on the flow and the patient's respiratory pattern. Obvious advantages to this method of administration include patient comfort and tolerance, and the ability of the patient to eat and drink. Drying of the nasal mucous membranes and a limit on the flow rate of oxygen delivered are some disadvantages of standard nasal cannulae. However, these can be overcome with high-flow nasal oxygen therapy.

High-Flow Nasal Oxygen Therapy

High-flow nasal oxygen therapy provides high concentrations of humidified oxygen to patients. Its use has been implemented in a variety of hospital settings, including the emergency department, the ICU and perioperatively in the theatre environment. More recently, it has been used not only to pre-oxygenate patients during rapid sequence inductions, but also to maintain oxygenation and ventilation in anaesthetised patients undergoing operations such as bronchoscopy and glottic surgery.

The improved comfort attributed to the humidification increases patient compliance, and as such, it

is often preferred over more invasive and distressing forms of ventilation.

The equipment features nasal prongs, a heating and humidifying system, an oxygen flow meter, a gas analyser and an air–oxygen gas blender. Flows of 40–60 l/min can be delivered, with a positive end-expiratory pressure (PEEP) of around 5 cmH$_2$O and humidity of 95–100% at temperatures of 33–43°C. An FiO$_2$ of close to 1.0 can be achieved.

'Classic' Face Masks

Face masks are available in a variety of designs, ranging from simple face masks (e.g. Hudson mask) to non-rebreathe face masks with a reservoir. Hudson masks deliver oxygen at a variety of flow rates (classically 1–15 l) and allow entrainment of room air when the peak inspiratory flow rate exceeds the FGF. The Hudson mask's variable oxygen delivery is therefore dependent on the patient's tidal volume and respiratory rate and the flow of oxygen.

Non-rebreathe face masks use a reservoir bag, which fills with oxygen when the patient's inspiratory flow rate is lower than the oxygen delivery rate. Thus, when the the peak inspiratory flow rate exceeds the FGF, the patient will preferentially inhale 100% oxygen from the bag instead of entraining room air.

Both the classic face mask and non-rebreathe face mask demonstrate a significant deterioration in performance with increased minute ventilation.

Other methods of oxygen administration include continuous positive airway pressure (CPAP) and bi-level positive airway pressure (BiPAP), variations of mechanical ventilation and hyperbaric therapy.

References and Further Reading

Ashraf-Kashani N, Kumar R. High flow nasal oxygen therapy. *BJA Education* 2017;**17**:63–7.

Ely J, Clapham M. Delivering oxygen to patients. *Br J Anaesth CEPD Rev* 2003;**3**:43–5.

O'Driscoll BR, Howard LS, Earis J, *et al.* British Thoracic Society guidelines for oxygen use in adults in healthcare and emergency settings. *Thorax* 2017;**72**(Suppl 1):ii1–90.

Wagstaff TAJ, Soni N. Performance of six types of oxygen delivery devices at varying respiratory rates. *Anaesthesia* 2007;**62**:492–503.

Yentis S, Hirsch NP, Smith GB. Oxygen therapy. In: S Yentis, NP Hirsch, GB Smith (eds). *Anaesthesia and Intensive Care A–Z: An Encyclopedia of Principles and Practice*, 4th edn. London: Churchill Livingstone; 2009. p. 438.

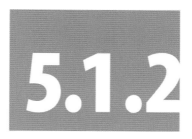

Emergency Front of Neck Airway Management

Jo Hackney

Key Learning Points

- Emergency cannula cricothyroidotomies are associated with high failure rates.
- Airway management in an emergency or a remote location is associated with a higher risk of complications.
- Anatomy of the neck is key to success in oxygenating via emergency front of neck access.
- There is now a single recommended technique for performing emergency cricothyroidotomy agreed by both surgeons and anaesthetists.

Keywords: NAP4, airway emergency, cricothyroidotomy, Difficult Airway Society

Introduction: The 4th National Audit Project

The 2011 report from the Royal College of Anaesthetists 4th National Audit Project (NAP4) entitled '*Major Complications of Airway Management*' identified several important clinical themes which contributed to adverse events and/or poor outcomes. Amongst these were:

- Failure to plan for failure
- Difficult intubations managed by repeated intubation attempts
- High failure rates of emergency cannula cricothyroidotomy (60 per cent)
- At least one in four major airway events reported was from intensive care or the emergency department

Emergency airway management is associated with higher complication and failure rates than planned elective intubation. This is not specific to the frequency of encountering a difficult airway but takes into account the simultaneous management of a critically ill patient. Limited time to assess and plan for potential airway complications, reduced respiratory reserve and functional residual capacity, increased risk of aspiration, cardiovascular instability and occasionally an unfamiliar environment with poor support are all factors which can lead to worse outcomes in the emergency setting.

In the event of a 'Can't Intubate Can't Oxygenate' scenario in an emergency setting, front of neck access may be required. Cricothyroidotomy is an emergency airway management technique that, as a whole, is poorly conducted by anaesthetists. High failure rates are encountered, and common complications include:

- Hypoxia
- Subcutaneous or mediastinal emphysema
- Haemorrhage
- Damage to surrounding anatomical structures
- Air embolus
- Pneumothorax
- Barotrauma

Anatomy

To appropriately discuss the approaches to front of neck access, an understanding of the anatomy is essential. A cricothyroidotomy involves a puncture of the cricothyroid membrane. This passes between the thyroid cartilage (which lies above) and the cricoid cartilage (which lies below). The thyroid cartilage is the protruding cartilage commonly referred to as the 'Adam's apple'. More prominent in males than females, it can be a useful anatomical landmark. Above the thyroid cartilage, the next palpable hard mass is the hyoid bone, which is joined to the thyroid cartilage by the thyrohyoid membrane. The cricothyroid cartilage is felt below the thyroid cartilage, with the membrane being palpated as a slight dip felt between the two more solid structures. This is best identified in most patients with them lying in the supine position, with their head and neck extended and shoulders bolstered. The cricothyroid membrane is avascular and approximately 10–20 mm. Important vessels relating to the cricothyroid membrane are the venous tributaries arising laterally from the inferior thyroid and anterior jugular veins, and the overlying superior thyroid artery. The vocal cords are roughly 1 cm above the cricothyroid membrane.

Approaches

There are two main recognised approaches to performing a cricothyroidotomy: needle and surgical (scalpel). Whilst these two techniques will not be discussed in detail in this chapter, as the focus will be on the approach now recommended by the Difficult Airway Society (DAS), Table 5.1.2.1 provides a comparison of the two methods.

Difficult Airway Society's Recommended Technique

In 2015, DAS updated their guidelines for management of an unanticipated difficult airway in adults. One of the notable changes to the algorithm was the adaptation to 'Plan D' which relates to the 'Can't Intubate Can't Oxygenate' scenario for emergency front of neck access.

DAS suggests a didactically taught method of effectively securing front of neck access in an emergency, with the aim of increasing the success rate of

Table 5.1.2.1 Needle and surgical cricothyroidotomy

Needle cricothyroidotomy	Surgical cricothyroidotomy
Simple technique	Generally more complex technique
Quick to perform	May take longer to perform
Less chance of haemorrhage	Increased haemorrhage risk
Equipment for procedure in pre-made pack	Equipment for procedure may take longer to set up
More equipment required to provide oxygenation	Can be used with simple endotracheal tube and anaesthetic circuit
Used for oxygenation only	Can be used for oxygenation and ventilation
Barotrauma more common, particularly in upper airway obstruction	Barotrauma less likely

cricothyroidotomy through both repetitive practising and reducing confusion by limiting the number of suggested approaches. Figure 5.1.2.1 shows the procedure.

References and Further Reading

Cook T, Woodall N, Frerk C. NAP4: Major complications of airway management in the United Kingdom. Report and findings March 2011. 4th National Audit Project of The Royal College of Anaesthetists and The Difficult Airway Society. London: The Royal College of Anaesthetists; 2011.

Scalpel cricothyroidotomy

Equipment: 1. Scalpel (number 10 blade)
2. Bougie
3. Tube (cuffed 6.0mm ID)

Laryngeal handshake to identify cricothyroid membrane

Palpable cricothyroid membrane

Transverse stab incision through cricothyroid membrane
Turn blade through 90° (sharp edge caudally)
Slide coude tip of bougie along blade into trachea
Railroad lubricated 6.0mm cuffed tracheal tube into trachea
Ventilate, inflate cuff and confirm position with capnography
Secure tube

Impalpable cricothyroid membrane

Make an 8–10cm vertical skin incision, caudad to cephalad
Use blunt dissection with fingers of both hands to separate tissues
Identify and stabilise the larynx
Proceed with technique for palpable cricothyroid membrane as above

Figure 5.1.2.1 Scalpel cricothyroidotomy. Source: Reproduced with permission of the Difficult Airway Society.

Difficult Airway Society. 2015. DAS guidelines for management of unanticipated difficult intubation in adults 2015. das.uk.com

Goon SSH, Stephens RCM, Smith H. Practical procedures. The emergency airway. www.ucl.ac.uk/anaesthesia/sites/anaesthesia/files/Airway.pdf

Gudzenko V, Bittner EA, Schmidt UH. Emergency airway management. *Respir Care* 2010;**55**:1026–35.

Pracy JP, Brennan L, Cook TM, *et al.* Surgical intervention during a Can't intubate Can't Oxygenate (CICO) event: emergency front-of-neck airway. *Br J Anaesth* 2016;**117**:426–8.

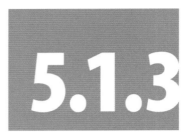

Difficult Intubation Guidelines and Failed Airway Management

Jo Hackney and Benjamin Post

Key Learning Points

1. Poor airway assessment and planning and failure to follow guidelines were highlighted as major issues in the Royal College of Anaesthetists 4th National Audit Project (NAP4). A lack of equipment was identified as an issue particularly prevalent in the intensive care environment.

2. Factors which enable prediction of a difficult airway should be assessed for early to allow appropriate forward planning.

3. It is important to have a well-organised, appropriately stocked and signposted difficult airway trolley, with regular teaching and updates to ensure all staff groups are familiar with the equipment.

4. Thorough knowledge of the Difficult Airway Society's guidelines on how to manage an unpredicted difficult airway in adults is essential. As of 2018, these include one specific to the intensive care unit – 'Guidelines for the management of tracheal intubation in critically ill adults'.

5. One must be able to appreciate the differences in emergency management of a tracheostomy (with a patent upper airway) and a laryngectomy (without a patent upper airway).

Keywords: difficult airway, difficult airway trolley, guidelines, tracheostomy, airway emergency

Introduction: NAP4

The 4th National Audit Project (NAP4), conducted by the Royal College of Anaesthetists and Difficult Airway Society (DAS), looked at the major complications of airway management and identified recurrent clinical themes. With particular reference to difficult intubations and failed airway management, they found:

- Poor airway assessment and poor planning contributed to poor airway outcomes
- Failure to plan for, and use, the guidelines available in the event of a difficult airway
- Difficult intubation was managed by repeated attempts, leading to further problems
- Lack of suitable equipment being immediately available was a problem prevalent in the ICU
- A theme of poor judgement arose

How to Predict an Anatomically Difficult Airway

NAP4 highlighted the importance of early identification of potentially difficult airways, advanced planning for failure, knowing the guidelines for a failed intubation and ensuring, prior to beginning anaesthesia, that the necessary equipment is available. In elective surgery where time is not of the essence, the elective patients are generally optimised and not critically unwell; more help is available in the event of encountered difficulty, and the option of waking the patient in the event of failure exists – the process may therefore be relatively straightforward. In intensive care, however, this is generally not the case. Early identification of potentially problematic patients is thus essential. This includes identifying anatomical patient factors that help predict a difficult airway:

- Mallampati classification
- Decreased thyromental distance/sternomental distance
- Buck teeth and poor dentition
- High body mass index (BMI)
- Poor mouth opening (inter-incisor gap <4 cm)
- Decreased range of movement of the head and neck
- Poor jaw protrusion (class 2/3) or upper lip bite test
- Previous surgery/radiotherapy
- High-arched palate

Equipment

The 2012 Association of Anaesthetists of Great Britain and Ireland (AAGBI)'s safety guidelines on checking anaesthetic equipment state that 'equipment for the management of the anticipated or unexpected difficult airway must be available and checked regularly in accordance with departmental policies.' A difficult airway trolley (DAT) should be adequately stocked, well organised and readily available from a suitable location (Figure 5.1.3.1).

ICUs should have a designated person, or persons, responsible for checking the DAT on a daily basis. (That said, if a piece of equipment is used, the user should ensure they have informed the appropriate person or restocked it themselves.) Many trusts choose to adopt the DAS algorithm to order the drawers of the trolley, which both allows for ease of use and acts as an aide memoire. There is a wide variety of equipment available on the market, and DAS recommendation is that whatever the piece of kit or brand chosen, there is: (1) consistency in its use; and (2) thorough, continuous training of both the user

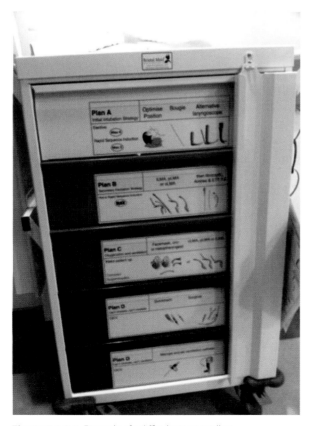

Figure 5.1.3.1 Example of a difficult airway trolley.
Source: Reproduced with permission of the Difficult Airway Society.

and assistants – intensive care nurses, operating department practitioners, emergency department staff, etc. An audit published in the *Journal of the Intensive Care Society* in 2010 suggested that the ability to deal with difficult airways in critical care across the UK was inadequate. One of the subsequent recommendations from NAP4 was that the DAT should be standardised nationally.

Difficult Airway Society Guidelines and Airway Management in Critically Ill Adults

Airway management in the critically ill patient poses a unique challenge, as concurrent illness and physiological precarity dramatically increase task complexity when compared to elective airway manipulation. Airway assessment is difficult in the uncooperative and obtunded patient, and airway anatomy may be dynamic (e.g. head and neck surgery or trauma, airway oedema from fluid resuscitation, prolonged ventilation). Airway aside, due attention must also be paid to the patient's risk of cardiovascular compromise, respiratory failure, fasting status and altered pharmacokinetics. Human and environmental factors play a role in task complexity, and contributed to the deficiencies in airway management identified in the critical care environment by the NAP4 study. Overall, this cohort of patients have a higher risk of failed 'first-pass success', hypoxaemia, cardiovascular complications and cardiac arrest. As such, whilst a DAS guideline exists for the '*Management of unanticipated difficult airway in adults (2015)*' (Figure 5.1.3.2), a new guideline and algorithm have been introduced for critically ill adults – '*Guidelines for the management of tracheal intubation in critically ill adults (2018)*' (Figure 5.1.3.3).

The DAS recommends a four-stage (Plan A–D) approach to airway management in the critically ill patient, mirroring the standard guidelines for difficult intubation, but with several key modifications. Preparation should include the use of a team brief, intubation checklist, consideration of cardiovascular stability and early enlistment of senior personnel. A modified airway assessment tool – the MACOCHA score – is recommended in this cohort. 'Awakening' patients, in view of failure of intubation, may not be feasible and should be discussed before induction of anaesthesia. Pre-oxygenation may include advanced techniques such as high-flow nasal oxygen or non-invasive ventilation. The concept of 'per-oxygenation' is also introduced, which includes maintaining oxygen

527

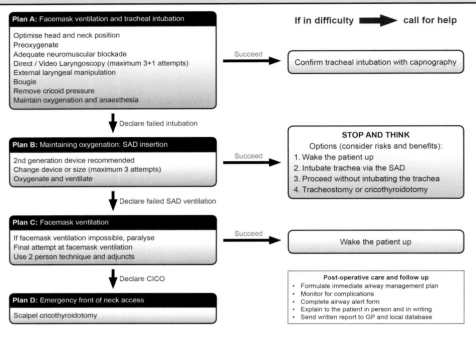

Figure 5.1.3.2 Management of unanticipated difficult tracheal intubation in adults.
Source: *Management of unanticipated difficult intubation in adults.* Reproduced with permission from the Difficult Airway Society.

delivery (e.g. nasal oxygen at 15 l/min) after induction of anaesthesia/neuromuscular blockade and throughout airway manipulation. Choice of induction agent and neuromuscular blockade needs to be patient- and situation-specific, and non-traditional rapid sequence induction drugs, such as ketamine and rocuronium, may be considered. For laryngoscopy, early use of a videolaryngoscope is encouraged, and a single failed attempt at intubation should prompt retrieval of the 'front of neck access' set. Failed intubation should lead to the use of second-generation supraglottic airways and/or face mask ventilation. In the event of a 'Can't Intubate Can't Oxygenate' (CICO) scenario, a 'scalpel–bougie–tube' cricothyroidotomy technique is recommended.

Tracheostomy difficulties

Intensive care patients may also require emergency airway management in the presence of a tracheostomy, presenting a unique set of challenges. The National Tracheostomy Safety Project is a group of intensive care doctors who aim to improve the management of patients with tracheostomies. They have since incorporated the expertise of multidisciplinary groups (e.g. Intensive Care Society, Royal College of Anaesthetists, ENT UK, British Association of Oral and Maxillofacial Surgeons, etc.) to create guidelines for the management of both tracheostomy and laryngectomy airway emergencies. For the majority of tracheostomies in the ICU (e.g. to facilitate a respiratory wean), the upper airway is theoretically patent, in contrast to the laryngectomy patient where tracheal access through the upper airway is not possible. Two separate algorithms have been produced for management of an airway emergency in these patients, with accompanying nationally recognisable colour-coded signs to differentiate between patients with a laryngectomy and those without.

The algorithms seen in Figures 5.1.3.4 and 5.1.3.5 are designed to help the responder manage common tracheostomy issues, prompt them to call for help and equipment and proceed with more invasive actions if no improvement is seen.

Tracheal intubation of critically ill adults

Difficult Airway Society | intensive care society | The Faculty of Intensive Care Medicine | RCoA Royal College of Anaesthetists

Pre-oxygenate and Checklist

Position: head up if possible
Assess airway and identify cricothyroid membrane
Waveform capnograph
Pre-oxygenate: facemask / CPAP / NIV / nasal O_2
Optimise cardiovascular system
Share plan for failure

Note the time

Plan A: Tracheal Intubation

Laryngoscopy
Maximum 3 attempts

Maintain oxygenation
- **Continuous nasal oxygenation**
- **Facemask ventilation between attempts**

Neuromuscular block
Video or direct laryngoscopy +/- bougie or stylet
External laryngeal manipulation
Remove cricoid

Succeed → Confirm with capnography

First failure →
Call HELP
- Video laryngoscopy
- Get Front Of Neck Airway (FONA) set

Fail | Declare "failed intubation"

EXPERT: one extra attempt if appropriate
Video / direct laryngoscopy
Facemask or supraglottic airway
Front Of Neck Airway

Plan B/C: Rescue Oxygenation

2nd generation supraglottic airway ⇄ Facemask
- 2 person
- adjuncts

Maximum 3 attempts each
Change device / size / operator
Open Front Of Neck Airway set

Succeed →
Stop, think, communicate
Options
- Wake patient if planned
- Wait for expert
- Intubate via supraglottic airway x1
- Front Of Neck Airway

Fail | Declare "can't intubate, can't oxygenate"

Plan D: Front Of Neck Airway: FONA

Use FONA set
Scalpel cricothyroidotomy

Extend neck
Neuromuscular blockade
Continue rescue oxygenation

Trained expert only

Other FONA techniques

Non-scalpel cricothyroidotomy
Percutaneous tracheostomy
Surgical tracheostomy

This flowchart forms part of the DAS, ICS, FICM, RCoA Guideline for tracheal intubation in critically ill adults and should be used in conjunction with the text.

Can't Intubate, Can't Oxygenate (CICO) in critically ill adults

  intensive care society   The Faculty of **Intensive Care Medicine**   RCoA

CALL FOR HELP

Declare "Can't Intubate, Can't Oxygenate"

Plan D: Front Of Neck Airway: FONA

Extend neck

Ensure neuromuscular blockade

Continue rescue oxygenation

Exclude oxygen failure and blocked circuit

Scalpel cricothyroidotomy

Equipment: 1. Scalpel (wide blade e.g. number 10 or 20)
2. Bougie (≤ 14 French gauge)
3. Tube (cuffed 5.0-6.0mm ID)

Laryngeal handshake to identify cricothyroid membrane

Palpable cricothyroid membrane

Transverse stab incision through cricothyroid membrane

Turn blade through 90° (sharp edge towards the feet)

Slide Coudé tip of bougie along blade into trachea

Railroad lubricated cuffed tube into trachea

Inflate cuff, ventilate and confirm position with capnography

Secure tube

Impalpable cricothyroid membrane

Make a large midline vertical incision

Blunt dissection with fingers to separate tissues

Identify and stabilise the larynx

Proceed with technique for palpable cricothyroid membrane as above

---

Trained expert only

Other FONA techniques

Non-scalpel cricothyroidotomy
Percutaneous tracheostomy
Surgical tracheostomy

Post-FONA care and follow up
- Tracheal suction
- Recruitment manoeuvre (if haemodynamically stable)
- Chest X-ray
- Monitor for complications
- Surgical review of FONA site
- Agree airway plan with senior clinicians
- Document and complete airway alert

This flowchart forms part of the DAS, ICS, FICM, RCoA Guideline for tracheal intubation in critically ill adults and should be used in conjunction with the text.

Figure 5.1.3.3 Algorithm for tracheal intubation of critically ill adults.
Source: *Algorithm for tracheal intubation of critically ill adults.* Reproduced with permission from the Difficult Airway Society.

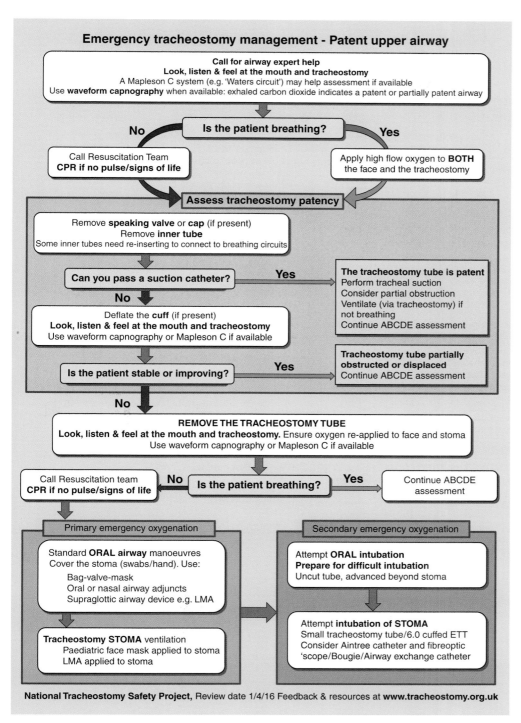

Emergency tracheostomy management - Patent upper airway

Call for airway expert help
Look, listen & feel at the mouth and tracheostomy
A Mapleson C system (e.g. 'Waters circuit') may help assessment if available
Use **waveform capnography** when available: exhaled carbon dioxide indicates a patent or partially patent airway

Is the patient breathing?

No → **Call Resuscitation Team**
CPR if no pulse/signs of life

Yes → Apply high flow oxygen to **BOTH** the face and the tracheostomy

Assess tracheostomy patency

Remove **speaking valve** or **cap** (if present)
Remove **inner tube**
Some inner tubes need re-inserting to connect to breathing circuits

Can you pass a suction catheter?

Yes → **The tracheostomy tube is patent**
Perform tracheal suction
Consider partial obstruction
Ventilate (via tracheostomy) if not breathing
Continue ABCDE assessment

No → Deflate the **cuff** (if present)
Look, listen & feel at the mouth and tracheostomy
Use waveform capnography or Mapleson C if available

Is the patient stable or improving?

Yes → **Tracheostomy tube partially obstructed or displaced**
Continue ABCDE assessment

No →

REMOVE THE TRACHEOSTOMY TUBE
Look, listen & feel at the mouth and tracheostomy. Ensure oxygen re-applied to face and stoma
Use waveform capnography or Mapleson C if available

Is the patient breathing?

No → Call Resuscitation team
CPR if no pulse/signs of life

Yes → Continue ABCDE assessment

Primary emergency oxygenation

Standard **ORAL airway** manoeuvres
Cover the stoma (swabs/hand). Use:
Bag-valve-mask
Oral or nasal airway adjuncts
Supraglottic airway device e.g. LMA

Tracheostomy STOMA ventilation
Paediatric face mask applied to stoma
LMA applied to stoma

Secondary emergency oxygenation

Attempt **ORAL intubation**
Prepare for difficult intubation
Uncut tube, advanced beyond stoma

Attempt **intubation of STOMA**
Small tracheostomy tube/6.0 cuffed ETT
Consider Aintree catheter and fibreoptic
'scope/Bougie/Airway exchange catheter

National Tracheostomy Safety Project, Review date 1/4/16 Feedback & resources at **www.tracheostomy.org.uk**

Figure 5.1.3.4 Emergency tracheostomy management – patent upper airway.

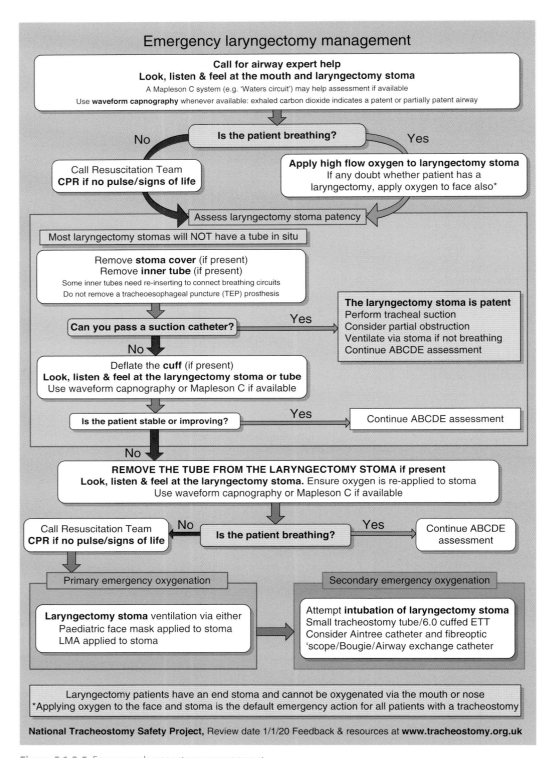

Figure 5.1.3.5 Emergency laryngectomy management.

Source: Reproduced from McGrath BA, Bates L, Atkinson D, Moore JA. Multidisciplinary guidelines for the management of tracheostomy and laryngectomy airway emergencies. *Anaesthesia*. 2012 Jun 26. doi: 10.1111/j.1365-2044.2012.07217, with permission from the Association of Anaesthetists of Great Britain & Ireland/Blackwell Publishing Ltd.

In summary, airway management in the critically ill patient should always be considered high risk and assistance from airway experts should be sought early. Regular training, careful patient assessment and thorough preparation are essential.

References and Further Reading

Cook T, Woodall N, Frerk C. NAP4: Major complications of airway management in the United Kingdom. Report and findings March 2011. 4th National Audit Project of The Royal College of Anaesthetists and The Difficult Airway Society. London: The Royal College of Anaesthetists; 2011.

Crawley SM, Dalton AJ. Predicting the difficult airway. *Contin Educ Anaesth Crit Care Pain* 2015;**15**:253–7.

Frerk C, Mitchell VS, McNarry AF, *et al.*; Difficult Airway Society intubation guidelines working group. Difficult Airway Society 2015 guidelines for management of unanticipated difficult intubation in adults. *Br J Anaesth* 2015;**115**:827–48.

Higgs A, McGrath BA, Goddard C, *et al.* Guidelines for the management of tracheal intubation in critically ill adults. *Br J Anaesth* 2018;**120**:323–52.

McGrath BA, Bates L, Atkinson D, *et al.* Multidisciplinary guidelines for the management of tracheostomy and laryngectomy airway emergencies. *Anaesthesia* 2012;**67**:1025–41.

Seo S-H, Lee J-G, Yu S-B, *et al.* Predictors of difficult intubation defined by the intubation difficulty scale (IDS): predictive value of 7 airway assessment factors. *Korean J Anesthesiol* 2012;**63**:491–7.

5.1.4

Principles of Performing Fibreoptic Bronchoscopy and Broncho-alveolar Lavage in the Intubated Patient

Nicola Rowe and Ramprasad Matsa

Key Learning Points

1. Fibreoptic bronchoscopy (FOB) is generally a safe procedure that is performed at the bedside in the ICU, thus avoiding potentially dangerous transfers out of the ICU.
2. FOB is utilised for both diagnostic and therapeutic purposes.
3. FOB-guided broncho-alveolar lavage (BAL) and protected brush specimen (PSB) are extremely valuable procedures and have a high diagnostic yield in identification of the causative organism in pneumonia.
4. FOB is increasingly used in managing difficult airway and in inserting percutaneous tracheostomy devices.
5. In intubated patients, FOB increases airway resistance during the procedure. This causes an increase in the peak inspiratory pressure (PIP) and peak end-expiratory pressure (PEEP), which may result in barotrauma.

Keywords: fibreoptic bronchoscopy, broncho-alveolar lavage, respiratory

Introduction

Flexible fibreoptic bronchoscopy (FOB) is an invasive procedure widely used in intensive care. The procedure examines the tracheobronchial tree and helps to diagnose and treat pulmonary pathology. The bronchoscope has mechanisms to flex or extend its distal end, making it easier to intubate narrow bronchi and navigate difficult angulations, which serve to minimise any damage caused. It contains an enclosed fibreoptic system and a light source that transmits views from the distal end to the eyepiece (Figure 5.1.4.1). A camera system is attached to the eyepiece which displays images on a screen.

Indications for Bronchoscopy in the ICU

Indications for bronchoscopy (Table 5.1.4.1) can be broadly divided into diagnostic and therapeutic.

Certain important indications are described below.

Pneumonia

FOB is helpful in identifying the causative organisms in pneumonia. It has a high diagnostic yield in diagnosing *Pneumocystis jirovecii*, mycobacteria and fungal pneumonia. FOB-guided broncho-alveolar lavage (BAL) and protected specimen brush (PSB) are extremely valuable in this regard.

Broncho-alveolar Lavage and Protected Specimen Brush

After isolating the specific airway lumen with FOB, at least 120 ml (the European Task Force recommends 240 ml) of isotonic saline is instilled in several aliquots through the working channel of the bronchoscope, followed by suction to retrieve the aspirate. The amount of fluid aspirated (usually about 50–70 per cent of the instilled fluid) is proportional to the yield of the results. The collected BAL fluid should be processed within 30 minutes for microbiological analysis. PBS involves the use of a double-lumen catheter brush system with a distal occluding plug to prevent contamination from airway secretions during passage of the catheter through the flexible bronchoscope channel.

Whilst analysing the sample, it is important to differentiate a contaminated specimen from that of a true infection. Differential cell count and quantitative cultures are of paramount importance in this regard. The samples should be rejected if >1 per cent of total cellularity is squamous or bronchial epithelial cells. The diagnostic thresholds for BAL and PBS samples are 10^4 colony-forming units (CFU)/ml and 10^3 CFU/ml, respectively. The sensitivity of BAL ranges from 60 to 90 per cent for bacterial infections; 70–80 per cent for mycobacterial, fungal and most viral infections; and 90–95 per cent for *P. jirovecii*. False positive results

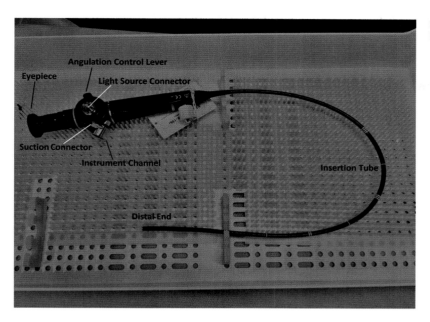

Figure 5.1.4.1 Flexible fibreoptic bronchoscope.

Table 5.1.4.1 Indications for fibreoptic bronchoscopy

Diagnostic	Therapeutic
1. Pneumonia	1. Airway management
2. Airway trauma (intubation injury, blunt thoracic injury, post-operative)	2. Foreign bodies
	3. Haemoptysis/haemorrhage
	4. Atelectasis, lobar collapse and excessive secretions
3. Acute inhalational injury or burns	5. Strictures and stenosis
4. Tracheo-oesophageal fistula	
5. Diffuse or focal lung disease	

Source: Tai DYH. Bronchoscopy in the intensive care unit (ICU). *Ann Acad Med Singapore.* 1998;**27**:552–559.

can be minimised by using an aseptic technique and avoiding tracheal and main bronchial aspiration. As lidocaine can inhibit bacterial growth, its use should be restricted. It should be noted that the diagnostic yield will be affected if the patient is under antibiotic cover.

Mini-BAL sampling is a blinded technique (non-bronchoscopic) that uses a telescopic plugging catheter. The aspirate collected after instilling about 20–150 ml of normal saline is analysed. Mini-BAL is essentially performed for the diagnosis of ventilator-associated pneumonia (VAP). A count of $\geq 10^3$–10^4 CFU/ml is considered as the cut-off to differentiate infection from colonisation. The sensitivity and specificity values are 63–100 per cent and 66–96 per cent, respectively. The mini-BAL sampling methodology is not standardised and should be restricted to units where FOB is not readily available.

Haemoptysis

FOB is helpful in identification of the source and to treat mild to moderate haemoptysis through instillation of cold saline, diluted adrenaline and fibrin precursors. FOB is used to tamponade the bleeding bronchial segment using a Fogarty balloon-tipped catheter. In massive haemoptysis, rigid bronchoscopy is preferred due to better visualisation and aspiration of clots. In cases of unilateral massive bleeding, selective endobronchial intubation using FOB of the non-bleeding lung can be a lifesaving measure.

Thoracic Trauma

FOB helps to visualise tracheal lacerations, bronchial transection or lacerations at any point of the bronchial tree, pulmonary haemorrhage and contusions of mucous membranes.

Airway Inhalation Injury

FOB is useful in the assessment of both upper and lower airways in inhalational injuries to assess the extent of damage. FOB is indicated in patients with carbonaceous sputum, facial or nasal cilia burns, suspected acute obstruction of the airway and inhalation of toxic vapours or fumes. Endoscopic visualisation of the lower airway shows scaly and necrotic areas, with carbon particles and focal areas of ulceration, alternating with areas of normal mucosa (mosaic or leopard skin appearance).

Atelectasis

The advantage of bronchial aspiration in lung collapse using FOB versus aggressive chest physiotherapy is unclear. However, specific groups of patients who derive maximum benefits include patients with spinal cord and brain injury and those with neuromuscular disorders. The best results of FOB are found in lobar atelectasis caused by a central mucus plug rather than by sub-segmental atelectasis.

Percutaneous Tracheostomy

FOB-guided percutaneous tracheostomy is safe and frequently performed. FOB guidance helps direct visualisation, thereby preventing paratracheal insertion of the tracheal tube and damage to the posterior wall of the trachea, and aids endotracheal tube (ETT) positioning during the procedure.

Management of Difficult Airways

FOB-guided endotracheal intubation is performed in patients with suspected difficult airway and is usually done as an elective procedure. The oral route is preferred to the nasal route due to potential damage to the nasal mucosa. FOB is also helpful in assessment of glottis damage associated with prolonged intubation.

Contraindications

Apart from patient refusal and in uncooperative patients, contraindications are generally relative and should be weighed against risk and benefit (Table 5.1.4.2).

Procedure
Procedural Aspects – Key Technical Issues

Procedural aspects and key technical issues can be seen in Box 5.1.4.1.

Table 5.1.4.2 Contraindications for fibreoptic bronchoscopy

Absolute contraindications	Relative contraindications
Patient refusal	Severe hypoxaemia
Uncooperative patient	Active bronchospasm
Endotracheal tube with small internal diameter	Significant haemodynamic instability
	Uncontrolled arrhythmia
	Coagulopathy
	Raised intracranial pressure

Box 5.1.4.1 Carrying out the Procedure

1. Gain consent (if possible). If the patient is unable to give consent, perform in the patient's best interests. Risk versus benefit must be considered prior to carrying out the procedure.
2. Equipment check, including bronchoscope, monitoring equipment and emergency airway trolley. Ensure availability of appropriate staff, including airway-competent person.
3. Check for contraindications prior to starting the procedure.
4. Pre-oxygenate using fraction of inspired oxygen (FiO$_2$) 100% prior to the procedure and continue this during the procedure.
5. Ensure the patient is appropriately sedated.
6. The ventilator should be set to the mandatory mode.
7. A special adaptor is used in mechanically ventilated patients (Figure 5.1.4.2) that helps to perform bronchoscopy without disconnecting the ventilator.
8. The trachea is identified by the presence of tracheal rings. Tracheal rings are C-shaped, with the posterior gap being closed by the trachealis muscle. The fibreoptic bronchoscope is therefore further advanced, assessing the anatomical landmarks.
9. Clean the bronchoscope after use, using an appropriate cleaning solution.
10. Check the patient's vital parameters and monitor post-procedure.

Pathophysiological Effects that Occur during FOB

1. FOB increases the peak inspiratory pressure (PIP) and the positive end-expiratory pressure (PEEP).
2. Suctioning and/or instillation of saline during BAL washes out the surfactant and leads to alveolar collapse, affecting the compliance of the lungs.
3. Both hypoxaemia and hypercapnia can develop during the procedure. These changes affect the vascular tone, which, when associated with raised intrathoracic pressure, can alter the haemodynamics.
4. FOB can increase the intracranial pressure.

Bronchoscope Adaptor

In ventilated patients, a special adaptor is used (Figure 5.1.4.2) to facilitate the introduction of the

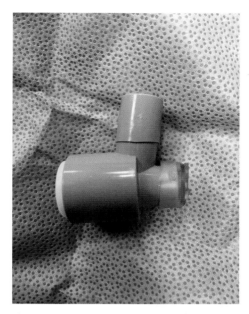

Figure 5.1.4.2 Special adaptor for the fibreoptic bronchoscope.

bronchoscope into the airway without disconnection of mechanical ventilation.

The adaptor valve provided allows continued ventilation and maintenance of PEEP during the technique. To maintain adequate minute volume and minimise barotrauma, it is recommended to use an ETT with a probe diameter of at least 2 mm larger than the bronchoscope diameter.

Complications

Complications of fibreoptic bronchoscopy may be seen in Table 5.1.4.3.

Generally, FOB is a safe procedure, with an associated mortality rate of 0.01 per cent and major complication rates of 0.08–2 per cent.

Table 5.1.4.3 Complications of fibreoptic bronchoscopy

Anaesthesia-related	Procedure-related	Post-procedure
Cardiovascular instability	Infection	Bleeding
Arrhythmias	Arrhythmias	Pneumothorax
Bronchospasm and laryngospasm	Hypoxaemia	Post-bronchoscopy fever
Seizures	Hypercapnia	
	Bleeding	
	Pneumothorax	
	Bronchospasm	
	Raised intracranial pressure	

Conclusion

FOB is an extremely useful procedure in critical care, and is used for both diagnosing and treating tracheobronchial pathologies. It is a safe procedure. Understanding the pathophysiological effects that occur during the procedure is important to minimise complications.

References and Further Reading

Bonella F, Ohshimo S, Bauer P, Guzman J, Costabel U. Bronchoalveolar lavage. *Eur Respir Mon* 2010;**48**:59–72.

Bonnet M, Monteiro MB. Fiberoptic bronchoscopy in intensive care—particular aspects. *Rev Port Med Int* 2003;**12**:17–19.

Liebler JM, Markin CJ. Fiberoptic bronchoscopy for diagnosis and treatment. *Crit Care Clin* 2000;**16**:83–100.

Marini J, Pierson D, Hudson L. Acute lobar atelectasis: a prospective comparison of fiberoptic bronchoscopy and respiratory therapy. *Am Rev Respir Dis* 1979;**119**:971–8.

Raoof S, Mehrishi S, Prakash UB. Role of bronchoscopy in modern medical intensive care unit. *Clin Chest Med* 2001;**22**:241–61.

Tai DYH. Bronchoscopy in the intensive care unit (ICU). *Ann Acad Med Singapore* 1998;**27**:552–9.

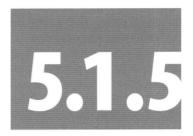

5.1.5 Percutaneous Tracheostomies and Management of Tracheostomy Emergencies

Ramprasad Matsa

Key Learning Points

1. Percutaneous dilatational tracheostomy (PDT) is generally a safe procedure when performed appropriately, and may be conducted in the intensive care unit setting, thereby avoiding a needless transfer to the theatre facility.
2. The single dilator technique is the most commonly used method to perform percutaneous tracheostomy in the UK.
3. The use of fibreoptic bronchoscopy and ultrasound guidance has increased the procedural safety and decreased failure rates.
4. Education and training in tracheostomy emergency management are mandatory and should remain as part of the governance policy.
5. Adequate humidification and regular suctioning are important components of the post-tracheostomy management, and both have been shown to reduce the subsequent complication rates.

Keywords: percutaneous tracheostomy, single dilator technique, national tracheostomy project

Introduction

A tracheostomy is an artificial opening made in the anterior wall of the trachea. The methods used to achieve this include surgical tracheostomy (ST) and percutaneous dilatational tracheostomy (PDT). ST involves placement of a tracheostomy tube under direct vision (open-operative) and is usually performed in the operating theatre. PDT is often performed in the ICU and utilises the Seldinger's technique followed by dilatation of the trachea.

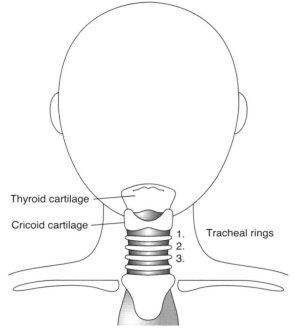

Figure 5.1.5.1 Tracheal anatomy.

Pre-procedural Considerations

Anatomy

The trachea is made of cartilaginous rings and extends from the larynx (C5 vertebra) to the tracheal bifurcation. The first ring is broader and connected to the cricoid cartilage. A tracheostomy is normally performed between the second and third tracheal rings (Figure 5.1.5.1), although some prefer between the third and fourth rings.

Important anterior relations to the trachea include the thyroid gland and isthmus, the thyroid ima artery and branches of the anterior thyroid vein.

Anatomical landmarks can be altered due to scars, burns, obesity, radiotherapy, thyroid goitre and in conditions associated with difficult neck extension (ankylosing spondylitis, unstable cervical spine, etc.). In such patients, careful assessment should be made with regard to suitability for PDT, and perhaps ST is a more suitable and safer option.

Percutaneous Tracheostomy versus Surgical Tracheostomy

PDT is preferred to ST in the ICU, as it has a good safety profile when performed correctly and eliminates the myriad of problems associated with transferring an unstable patient to the theatre. PDT has less cosmetic disfigurement, compared to ST, and is less prone to wound infection. That said, careful patient selection is vital for procedural success and safety, and if in doubt, consult a ear, nose and throat surgeon for their opinion.

Indications and Contraindications

PDT is an elective and planned procedure. Patients should therefore be carefully chosen based on indications and contraindications (Table 5.1.5.1).

The main indication for tracheostomy is to secure a definitive airway in upper respiratory tract obstruction (actual or potential). Other indications include:

- Facilitating weaning in prolonged ventilation
- Minimising sedation requirements in anticipated difficult wean
- Facilitating tracheobronchial toileting in patients with a high risk of aspiration (e.g. neuromuscular disorders, head injuries, stroke, etc.)

Timing of Tracheostomy

The benefits of early versus late tracheostomy (>10 days) are widely debated and there has not been

Table 5.1.5.1 Contraindications of percutaneous dilatational tracheostomy

Absolute	Relative
Patient or family refusal	Significantly high ventilatory requirements (FiO$_2$ >0.6; PEEP >10)
Operator inexperience	
Emergency situations	Difficult anatomy (short neck, obesity, limited neck extension)
Infants and small children	Tracheomalacia
	Suspected or known difficult airway
	High-riding innominate artery
	Previous tracheostomy
	Midline neck mass
	Coagulopathy
	Infection at the insertion site
	Unstable C-spine injury

Abbreviations: FiO$_2$ = fraction of inspired oxygen; PEEP = positive end-expiratory pressure.

a clear consensus in this regard. The TracMan study compared early (4 days) versus late (>10 days) tracheostomy and demonstrated a moderate reduction in sedation requirements for tracheostomy performed early, but did not demonstrate any difference in either length of stay or ventilator-associated pneumonia (VAP) rates. Recently published guidelines do not provide any strong recommendation on timings but do advise early tracheostomy for patients with acute cervical spinal cord injury.

Selection of Tube Size

Tube selection is based on the outer diameter. The preferred sizes for adult men and women are 11 mm and 10 mm as outer diameter, respectively. The ideal length of a tracheostomy tube is such that the tube tip lies a few centimetres above the carina. Short tubes carry a higher risk of accidental decannulation and partial airway obstruction due to poor positioning. Long tubes may, however, impinge on the carina, leading to discomfort and coughing. Patients with long necks and those who are obese may thus require tracheostomy tubes with a longer stem.

Procedure

There are several techniques used to perform PDT. These include Ciaglia serial dilatational technique, Seldinger single dilator technique (SDT), guidewire forceps (Griggs) technique and translaryngeal (Fantoni's) technique. The commonly used method in the UK is the SDT. The SDT consists of a single-bevelled, curved hydrophilic dilator. The advantages of the SDT are that there is less loss of tidal volume and it also reduces damage to the posterior tracheal wall due to the curved shape of the dilator (Figure 5.1.5.2).

Patient Positioning and Assessment

Appropriate positioning of the patient is important (Figure 5.1.5.3).

Neck extension using pillows between the shoulder blades helps to identify the landmarks for the procedure. Ultrasound use should be encouraged to assess the neck anatomy (e.g. enlarged thyroid gland), localise the tracheal rings and aid identification of aberrant vessels.

Procedural steps

The Seldinger single dilator technique for performing PDT may be seen in Box 5.1.5.1.

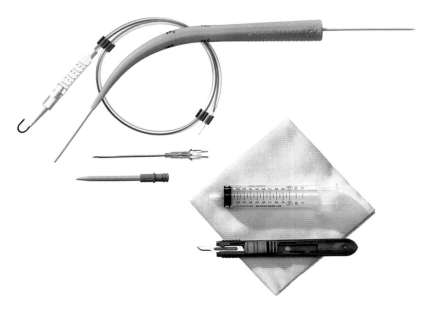

Figure 5.1.5.2 Single dilator percutaneous tracheostomy kit. Source: Picture Courtesy: ©TRACOE medical GmbH.TRACOE experc Dilation Set.

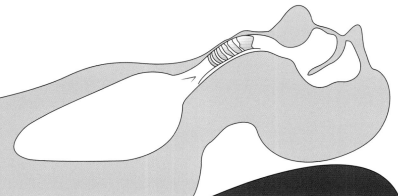

Figure 5.1.5.3 Positioning the patient.

Box 5.1.5.1 Procedural Steps for Performing Percutaneous Dilatational Tracheostomy (Seldinger Single Dilator Technique)

1. Preliminary checks: consent, assessment of the patient and neck anatomy, equipment and monitoring checks.
2. Ensure 100% FiO_2 and the ventilator is set on the mandatory mode.
3. Ensure that the patient is adequately sedated and paralysed.
4. Deflate the endotracheal tube cuff, and under direct visualisation through the laryngoscope, withdraw the endotracheal tube until the cuff is visualised just below the vocal cords; re-inflate the cuff then.
5. Re-check the anatomy of the neck and site of insertion.
6. Sterilise the area of operation using 2% chlorhexidine.
7. Infiltrate the skin with local anaesthetic containing a vasoconstrictor (2% lidocaine with 1 in 200,000 adrenaline).
8. Blunt dissection following a 2.5-cm transverse incision at the chosen site using mosquito forceps until the tracheal rings are seen.
9. Introduce the bronchoscope through the endotracheal tube until the tracheal lumen is visualised.
10. Insert the 14 G sheathed introducer needle through the midline of the trachea.

Box 5.1.5.1 (cont.)

11. Confirm placement of the needle in the trachea by confirming air can be aspirated into a saline-filled syringe and by direct visualisation using the bronchoscope.
12. Withdraw the needle and introduce the Seldinger guidewire through the plastic sheath.
13. Dilate the insertion site with the help of a small tracheal dilator.
14. A single graduated dilator is lubricated with saline and then loaded over the guiding catheter. Bronchoscopic guidance ensures that the dilator is in the trachea.
15. After adequate dilation, remove the dilator, leaving the guidewire *in situ*.
16. The whole tracheostomy assembly is then loaded over the guiding catheter, and advanced as a unit into the trachea in a sweeping action.

Table 5.1.5.2 Complications related to percutaneous dilatational tracheostomy

Immediate complications	Delayed complications	Late complications
Haemorrhage	Tube blockage with secretions or blood	Granulomata of trachea
Misplacement of tracheostomy tube – within tissues around trachea	Partial or complete tube displacement	Tracheal dilatation, stenosis, persistent sinus or collapse
Pneumothorax	Infection of stoma site	(tracheomalacia)
Tube occlusion	Ulceration and/or necrosis of trachea	Scar formation
Surgical emphysema	Mucosal ulceration by tube migration	Blocked tubes
Loss of upper airway	Tracheo-oesophageal fistula formation	Haemorrhage
	Haemorrhage	

Post-procedure

Complications

Complications related to PDT may be seen in Table 5.1.5.2.

Tracheostomy Emergencies

Major emergencies that can occur following tracheostomy insertion include:

- Obstructed tubes
- Partial or complete dislodgement of tracheostomy tubes
- Haemorrhage

Key Concepts in Managing Tracheostomy Emergencies

Careful assessment of the patient and escalation should be done if they develop any of the red flag signs (Box 5.1.5.2).

The 'tracheostomy emergency algorithm' (Figure 5.1.5.4) should be followed when needed.

Tracheostomy emergency equipment (Box 5.1.5.3) should be easily accessible.

In the case of tracheostomy emergency, assessment should involve clinical examination, observation of the capnography trace and assessment of the tracheostomy

Box 5.1.5.2 Tracheostomy – 'Red Flag' Signs

- Apnoea or respiratory distress
- Vocalisation when cuff inflated (cuff up) and associated grunting, snoring and stridor
- Unable to maintain oxygen saturations
- Cyanosis
- Restlessness, confusion, agitation and anxiety
- Blood or bloodstained secretions via tracheostomy
- Cuff requires recurrent inflation

Box 5.1.5.3 Recommended Bedside and Emergency Airway Equipment for Tracheostomised Patients

- Mapleson C circuit
- Suction catheters
- Spare tracheostomy tubes
- Clean pot for spare inner cannula
- Sterile water for cleaning suction tube
- Scissors
- Tracheal dilators
- Difficult intubation trolley
- Fibreoptic bronchoscope

lumen patency. Use of a 'Water's circuit' can also be helpful to rule out ventilator-associated problems and to get a feel of the ventilation. All devices connected

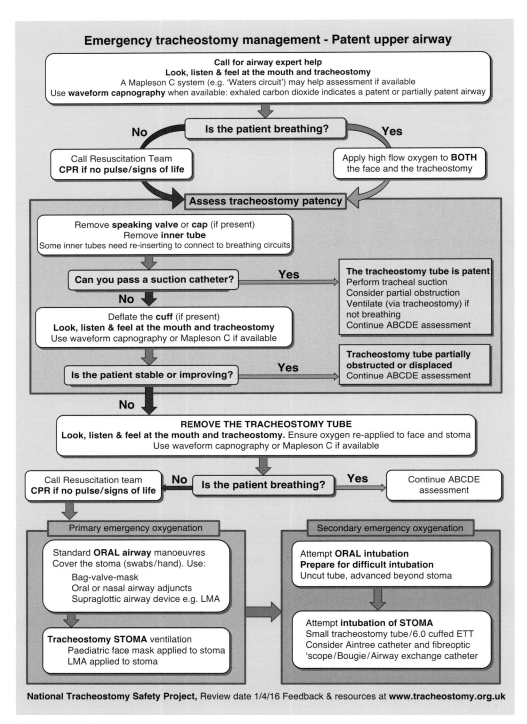

Figure 5.1.5.4 Tracheostomy emergency algorithm.

Source: McGrath *et al.*, National Tracheostomy Safety Project. www.tracheostomy.org.uk.

to the tracheostomy tube (e.g. speaking valves or a Swedish nose) should be looked for and removed, and a suction catheter may be passed down the tracheostomy tube. Gum-elastic bougies or other stiffer introducers should be avoided owing to the risk of creating a false passage (especially in partially displaced tubes).

In the event of a blocked tracheostomy, removing the inner tube may help to resolve the obstruction. In partial obstruction, vigorous attempts at ventilation via a displaced tracheostomy tube can lead to significant surgical emphysema and can complicate airway management further. Deflating the cuff may allow airflow past a partially displaced tracheostomy tube to the upper airways.

If a suction catheter cannot be passed and deflating the cuff fails to improve the clinical condition, the tracheostomy tube should be removed. Primary emergency oxygenation may be achieved via the oro-nasal route and/or the tracheostomy stoma, until a definitive airway is achieved. If this fails, secondary emergency oxygenation manoeuvres are required, including advanced airway management. In the event of postprocedural haemorrhage, leaving the cuff inflated may cause a tamponade effect, thereby reducing bleeding.

Post-tracheostomy Care

Understanding the physiological changes that occur following tracheostomy (Box 5.1.5.4) helps to guide post-tracheostomy care.

Provision of humidification (heat and moisture exchanger (HME) filter) and regular suctioning are important to avoid blockage of tracheotomy tubes. The

---

Box 5.1.5.4 Physiological Changes with Tracheostomy

- Reduction in anatomical dead space of up to 50 per cent
- Loss of natural warming and humidification, and filtering of air that usually takes place in the upper airway is lost
- The patient's ability to speak is removed
- The ability to swallow is adversely affected
- Sense of taste and smell can be lost

---

inner tube should be regularly checked and cleaned. Tube cuff pressure should be maintained in the range of 20–25 mmHg. Cuff pressures of >25 mmHg are associated with mucosal ischaemia, whilst low cuff pressures of <15 mmHg are associated with leak and micro-aspiration.

Decannulation

If the patient has not required mechanical ventilation for at least 24 hours, has a good cough (enough to protect the airway from aspiration) and has been able to maintain adequate oxygenation, decannulation should be considered. If the tracheostomy has been *in situ* for more than a few days, then speech and language therapy (SALT) input is important to help assess for swallowing difficulties prior to decannulation.

Acknowledgements

The author would like to thank Dr E. Shackel for providing the graphic images on illustrations of the tracheal anatomy (Figure 5.1.5.1) and positioning of the patient during the tracheostomy procedure (Figure 5.1.5.3).

References and Further Reading

Madsen KR, Guldager H, Rewers M, Weber SO, Kobke-Jacobsen K, Jensen R; Danish Society of Intensive Care Medicine; Danish Society of Anesthesiology and Intensive Care Medicine. Guidelines for percutaneous dilatational tracheostomy (PDT) from the Danish Society of Intensive Care Medicine (DSIT) and the Danish Society of Anesthesiology and Intensive Care Medicine (DASAIM). *Dan Med Bull* 2011;**58**:C4358.

McGrath BA, Bates L, Atkinson D, *et al.* Tracheostomy management guidelines. *Anaesthesia* 2012;**67**:1025–41.

Mehta C, Mehta Y. Percutaneous tracheostomy. *Ann Card Anaesth* 2017;**20**:S19–25.

Raimondi N, Vidal MR, Calleja J, *et al.* Evidence based guidelines for the use of tracheostomy in critically ill patients. *J Crit Care* 2017;**38**:304–18.

Young D, Harrison DA, Cuthbertson BH, Rowan K; TracMan Collaborators. Effect of early vs. late tracheostomy placement on survival in patients receiving mechanical ventilation: the TracMan randomized trial. *JAMA* 2013;**309**:2121–9.

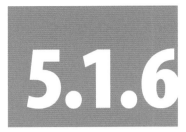

Chest Drain Insertion

5.1.6

Jonathan Barnes

Key Learning Points

1. Clear British Thoracic Society guidelines exist for optimal management of a pneumothorax.
2. Different techniques exist for chest drain insertion, each with its own advantages and disadvantages.
3. Chest drains must be secured adequately, otherwise they will fall out.
4. Be careful to avoid re-expansion pulmonary oedema.
5. Always send samples if a fluid is drained.

Keywords: chest drain, pneumothorax, pleural effusion, Seldinger technique

Introduction

Chest drains are poly-vinyl-chloride tubes inserted into the intra-pleural space to drain air (pneumothorax) or fluid (pleural effusion, haemothorax, etc.). Drains may be narrow (8–14 Fr), medium (16–24 Fr) or large (>24 Fr) bore, and may be inserted via a thoracostomy created by blunt dissection (open/surgical drain) or via a Seldinger 'over the wire' approach.

Drains have a distal port and fenestrations to aid drainage and prevent blockage, and are attached to an underwater seal to prevent air from being drawn back into the intra-pleural space (Figure 5.1.6.1).

Indications

- Pneumothorax
- Symptomatic unilateral pleural effusion
- Decompensated/refractory bilateral pleural effusion
- Haemothorax
- Chylothorax
- Bronchopleural fistula
- Empyema
- For pleurodesis (obliteration of the intra-pleural space via instillation of an irritant agent)

Contraindications (Relative)

- Infection over the area of insertion
- Coagulopathy (platelets $<50 \times 10^9/l$, international normalised ratio (INR) >1.5)
- Pulmonary bullae or adhesions
- Loculated effusion

Technique for Insertion
Equipment Required

- Sterile drapes, gown, gloves, mask
- Chlorhexidine 2%
- Local anaesthetic for skin (lidocaine 1% or 2%, 5–10 ml), syringe and 25 G and 19 G needles
- Seldinger chest drain kit:
  - Needle, syringe, wire, dilators, scalpel
- Open chest drain kit:
  - Scalpel, blunt dilators (e.g. straight artery forceps), forceps
- Chest drain tube
- Suture kit (silk or similar)
- Dressings
- Underwater seal:
  - Tubing, bottle(s), water, three-way tap (if compatible)

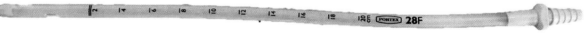

Figure 5.1.6.1 Chest drain tube.

- Syringes for samples:
  - If for fluid aspiration (e.g. effusion)
- Ultrasound, jelly and probe cover (if used, see below)

Point of Insertion

Chest drains should be inserted into the 'triangle of safety' (Figure 5.1.6.2), as this minimises complications. For fluid drainage, experienced operators using ultrasound may deviate from this; however, this is not standard practice. The triangle of safety is the area bordered by the mid-axillary line posteriorly, the pectoral groove anteriorly and the fifth intercostal space (approximately nipple level) inferiorly.

When inserting a chest drain through the intercostal space, insertion should be along the superior aspect of the rib in question, rather than on the inferior aspect where the neurovascular bundle is situated.

Technique for Insertion – Seldinger

1. Consent and position the patient. A 30° head-up positon, with the arm abducted and elbow flexed (as if relaxing in the sunshine) is most commonly used.
2. Identify and palpate the 'triangle of safety' to identify the insertion point. Ideally, this should be confirmed using ultrasound.
3. Clean and drape the skin.
4. Instil local anaesthetic.
   a. Use your 25 G needle to instil a few millilitres of local anaesthetic subcutaneously.
   b. Then, with your 19 G needle, advance the needle and syringe perpendicular to the skin, applying negative pressure as you advance. When the pleura is breached, air (pneumothorax) or fluid (effusion, etc.) will be aspirated, thus confirming localisation.

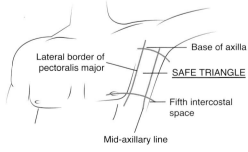

Figure 5.1.6.2 The 'triangle of safety'.

c. Slowly withdraw your needle, instilling plenty of anaesthetic into the intercostal muscles. This will reduce the pain of dilation, which can be exquisitely painful, and helps spread the muscle fibres, aiding drain insertion.

5. Now insert the Seldinger needle and syringe along the line of the 19 G needle, again applying negative pressure until the pleura is breached.
   a. Ideally, this should be done with one hand, whilst using the other hand to hold the ultrasound probe, keeping the needle in view and ensuring it enters the correct space.
6. Advance the needle a few more millimetres, and remove the syringe.
7. Insert the guidewire through the needle.
   a. For a pneumothorax, the drain should point cephalad, so have the needle bevel facing upward and insert the guidewire with its natural coil taking it upward.
   b. For an effusion/haemothorax, etc., the drain should point caudad; therefore, do the reverse (bevel down, wire coiling downward).
8. With the wire inserted, remove the needle and use the scalpel to make a small incision in the skin (approximately 5 mm) above it.
9. Insert the dilator.
   a. Keeping the wire straight and ensuring the dilator is aimed along the line of insertion, gently, but firmly, advance the dilator over the wire and through the skin and muscle.
   b. It is worth warning an awake patient before doing this, as it can be extremely uncomfortable.
   c. Gentle rotation of the dilator may aid insertion.
   d. If you have multiple dilators, use them. Start with the smallest and build up sequentially.
   e. Do not be too forceful, and keep your original line of insertion, or else you will kink the wire.
10. Once dilated, gently remove the dilator and insert the drain over the wire, angling it in the desired direction.
11. Remove the wire and, if present, the stylet from the drain.
12. Attach the three-way tap to the drain, then attach the tubing.

13. Suture the drain securely in place.

    a. An anchor suture should be placed to the skin, followed by a run of sutures up the drain, wrapping around and tying off every few turns.

14. Apply an occlusive dressing.

Technique for Insertion – Open (Classically Surgical)

1. As before, consent and position the patient. Clean and drape, and apply local anaesthetic.

2. Make an incision, approximately 2–3 cm (depending on drain size) in the skin at the point of insertion.

    a. Notably, whilst commonly done, making an excessively large hole increases the risk of subsequent complications.

3. Place your closed blunt dilators into your incision, orientating them so that they will open along the anterior–posterior line (rather than superior–inferior).

4. Gently advance the dilators, opening them up as you move forward. Close them and repeat.

5. Gently dilate through the muscle until you breach the pleura (you may feel a small 'pop').

6. Remove your dilators; insert your index finger through the hole created, and perform a 'sweep' (with your finger slight flexed, run it around the inside of the hole).

7. Remove your finger and insert your drain.

    a. Clamp your forceps onto the drain tip to guide it through your hole.

    b. Do not use the trocar in the drain (if there is one) due to the risk of complications.

    c. As with the Seldinger drain, aim cephalad for a pneumothorax, and caudad for a collection of fluid.

8. Suture in place, and dress as above.

Seldinger Technique versus Open Technique

Advantages of the Seldinger approach include:
- Better seal
- Improved patient comfort and recovery time
- Facilitating use of ultrasound for improved safety
- Reduced infection and subcutaneous emphysema

Advantages of the open approach include:
- Drains are often larger and less prone to blockage
- Finger sweep allows clearance of the pleura, preventing trauma
- Potentially less risk of local structure puncture (no sharp needles/wires/dilators)

Role of Ultrasound

Ultrasound has been shown to be more accurate than chest radiography for detecting pleural fluid, and use of ultrasound for pleural aspiration and drain insertion is associated with reduced complication and failure rates. The British Thoracic Society (BTS) recommends using real-time ultrasound guidance for all pleural procedures.

Drainage Bottles

The chest drain is connected to an underwater seal which creates a valve, allowing air/fluid to leave the pleural space, but preventing its return. The tubing connecting the drain to the bottle should be long enough to allow the bottle to sit at least 80–100 cm below the patient, and the volume of tubing should be at least 50% of the patient's vital capacity to prevent water from the bottle from being drawn back into the chest.

The standard drainage bottle set up is a one-bottle system, although a three-bottle system may also be employed (Figure 5.1.6.3). The one-bottle system involves connecting the drain to a tube that sits 2–4 cm underwater, with the bottle also having an opening to the atmosphere on top. An underwater seal is thus created, and the hole on top equalises pressure or can be used to apply suction (<20 cmH$_2$O) to aid lung re-inflation.

The three-bottle system involves connecting the tubing to a bottle with no underwater seal, but which is connected to a second bottle that creates the underwater seal in the same way as a one-bottle system. A third bottle contains a suction port (if needed) and a further underwater seal.

Re-expansion Pulmonary Oedema

Overly rapid re-expansion of a collapsed lung may lead to pulmonary oedema. Although rare, this can be a serious and avoidable complication. BTS guidelines recommend pausing drainage after 1.5 l have been drained, although many practitioners will temporarily halt drainage after anything from 500 ml to 1 l.

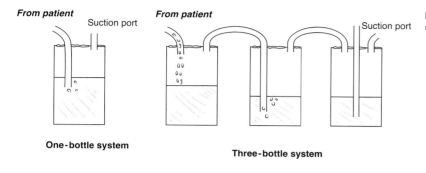

From patient   Suction port   From patient   Suction port

One-bottle system

Three-bottle system

Figure 5.1.6.3 One- and three-bottle underwater seal drainage systems.

Pneumothorax Management

Pneumothorax

A pneumothorax is a collection of air in the intra-pleural space. It may be primary (spontaneous) or secondary (on a background of respiratory disease). Signs and symptoms include dyspnoea, tachypnoea and hypoxia, with reduced breath sounds and hyper-resonance on examination of the affected side. Diagnosis is via chest radiography, although ultrasound scanning may be more sensitive. Computed tomography is the gold standard imaging modality.

Management of a pneumothorax varies, depending on the clinical situation, but may include supportive care, chest aspiration and/or chest drain insertion. Below is a simple approach to managing spontaneous pneumothorax, based on BTS guidelines (Figure 5.1.6.4).

Tension Pneumothorax

A tension pneumothorax is a pneumothorax that leads to significant respiratory and/or cardiovascular compromise. It is normally associated with a rapidly expanding pneumothorax that has occurred in association with the formation of a one-way pleural valve, thereby allowing the pneumothorax to increase in size with inspiration (air is sucked in), but not decompress with expiration. It is often seen in association with trauma or assisted ventilation.

In addition to the signs and symptoms associated with a 'simple' pneumothorax, patients may be

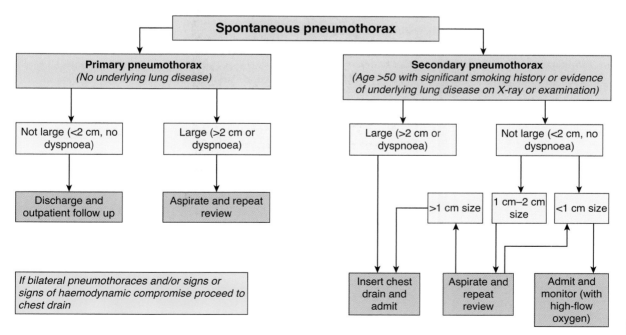

Figure 5.1.6.4 British Thoracic Society guidelines for pneumothorax management.

547

cardiovascularly compromised. The classical signs of neck vein engorgement and tracheal deviation away from the affected side are rarely seen.

Management of a tension pneumothorax should include ABCDE assessment, including oxygen therapy and chest drain insertion. In an unstable patient, immediate decompression of the chest, by insertion of a large-bore cannula through the second intercostal space in the mid-axillary line, should be performed. To aid placement, the cannula may be inserted with a syringe of saline attached to it, so that if negative pressure is applied, bubbles will be seen upon entry into the air collection.

Analysis of Fluid

For drains inserted for fluid collection, it is important to diagnose the aetiology of the fluid. In the first instance, one should assess whether it is an exudate (infection, thromboembolism, malignancy, connective tissue disease, pancreatitis, haemothorax, etc.) or a transudate (cardiac, renal or liver failure, hypothyroidism, Meig's syndrome, etc.). This is most commonly done using Light's criteria. This states that a fluid is likely to be an exudate if:

- Pleural:serum protein >0.5
- Pleural:serum lactate dehydrogenase (LDH) >0.6
- Pleural LDH > two-thirds the upper limit of normal serum LDH

  Indicators of specific pathology include:
- Frank pus: suggests empyema
- Bloodstained pleural:serum haematocrit >0.5: haemothorax

- Bloodstained pleural:serum haematocrit <0.5: often embolism or malignancy
- Pro-B-type natriuretic peptide (BNP) levels: raised in cardiac failure
- Triglyceride level >110 mg/dl: chylothorax (although approximately 10 per cent of chylothoraces may have normal levels)
- Amylase level: raised in pancreatitis

  To further investigate the cause of an effusion, samples should also be sent for microscopy, culture and sensitivity (MC&S), cytology, glucose and pH.

Complications

- Acute:
  - Pain
  - Damage to local structures
  - Pneumothorax
  - Infection
  - Subcutaneous emphysema
- Chronic:
  - Bronchopleural fistula
  - Scarring

References and Further Reading

Aston D, Rivers A, Dharmadasa A. *Equipment in Anaesthesia and Critical Care*. Banbury: Scion; 2014.

Havelock T, Teoh R, Laws D, Gleeson F. Pleural procedures and thoracic ultrasound: British Thoracic Society pleural disease guideline 2010. *Thorax* 2010;**65**:61–76.

MacDuff A, Arnold A, Harvey J. Management of spontaneous pneumothorax: British Thoracic Society pleural disease guideline 2010. *Thorax* 2010;**65**:18–31.

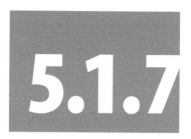

Lung Ultrasound

Arthur W. E. Lieveld and Andrew P. Walden

Key Learning Points

1. Bedside lung ultrasound has similar diagnostic properties to computed tomography in the diagnosis of acute respiratory failure.
2. A scan can be performed in under 5 minutes, reducing time to diagnosis and treatment.
3. It can be useful in monitoring lung aeration and guiding weaning of mechanical ventilation.
4. It can help in assessing and draining pleural effusions.
5. It can differentiate between pneumonia, acute respiratory distress syndrome and cardiac pulmonary oedema.

Keywords: lung ultrasound, ARDS, BLUE protocol, A-line, B-line

Introduction

For many years, it was felt that ultrasound was of no value in imaging the lung due to low acoustic impedance of air. However, imaging of the pleura and the patterns of common artefacts found on lung ultrasound – A-lines and B-lines – can be correlated with particular lung diseases (Figures 5.1.7.1 to 5.1.7.6). Lung ultrasound diagnostic accuracy is better than that of physical examination and conventional radiography (chest X-ray (CXR)), and comparable to that of chest CT in diagnosing acute respiratory pathologies, ranging from (ventilator-associated) pneumonia to acute respiratory distress syndrome (ARDS). Furthermore, it has a steep learning curve for physicians and other (para)medical personnel. The focus of this chapter is on the role of ultrasound in imaging the lung.

Figure 5.1.7.1 Normal lung.

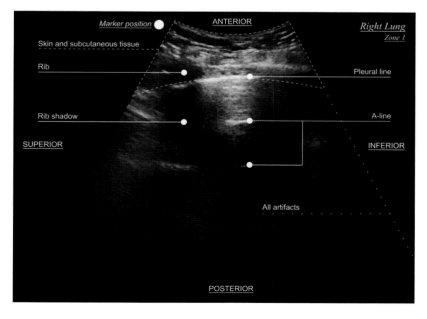

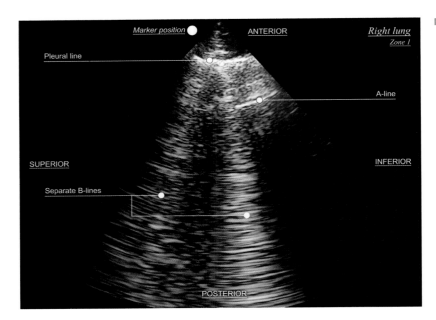

Figure 5.1.7.2 Discrete B-lines.

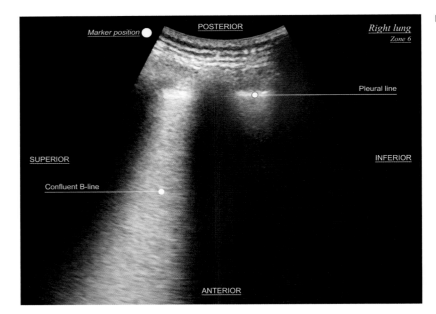

Figure 5.1.7.3 Confluent B-lines.

Diagnosis of Acute Respiratory Failure

In patients presenting with acute respiratory failure, lung ultrasound has a high diagnostic accuracy. Bedside lung ultrasound is a rapid, reproducible, dichotomous decision-making tool to come to a clear and reliable diagnosis. The most commonly used protocol is the Bedside Lung Ultrasound in Emergency (BLUE). It uses an algorithmic approach that employs three scan points per hemi-thorax that can differentiate between causes of acute respiratory failure in under 5 minutes (Figure 5.1.7.7).

The upper and lower BLUE points are identified and scanned, looking for evidence of pleural sliding. This is the lateral sideways movement of the pleura that is easily visualised. Once pleural sliding has been confirmed and a pneumothorax excluded, the presence of A-lines

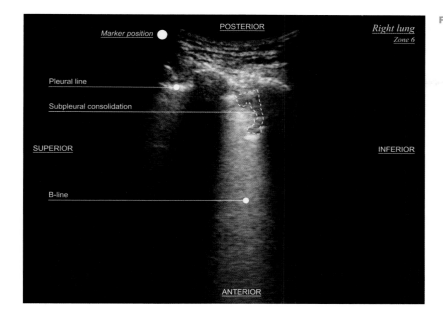

Figure 5.1.7.4 Subpleural consolidation.

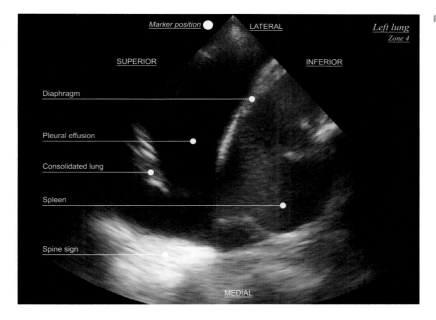

Figure 5.1.7.5 Uncomplicated effusion.

and B-lines is determined. In the presence of bilateral A-lines, a venous compression test of the lower limb veins is performed to rule out venous thromboembolic disease and if this is negative, a scan of the posterolateral alveolar and/or pleural syndrome (PLAPS) point is made. The PLAPS point is either normal or abnormal, maintaining the dichotomous nature of the decision tree. In the original study, the diagnostic accuracy was found to be over 90 per cent for common causes of acute respiratory failure such as pneumonia, pulmonary embolism, chronic obstructive pulmonary disease and pneumothorax, even without considering the history, clinical examination or laboratory results. Other studies have shown it is reproducible in clinical practice and that it reduces time to diagnosis and appropriate treatment.

551

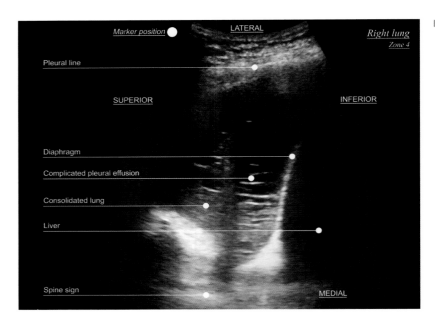

Figure 5.1.7.6 Complicated effusion.

Ultrasound in the Role of Weaning from Mechanical Ventilation

Weaning and discontinuation of mechanical ventilation are pivotal moments in the management of a critically ill patient. Failure to wean is failure of a spontaneous breathing trial or re-intubation 48 hours following discontinuation of mechanical ventilation. Up to 30 per cent of patients fit these criteria, with an associated increase in mortality and morbidity. In longer-stay patients, the causes are multi-faceted, including respiratory, cardiac and neuromuscular factors. A structured approach is essential and ultrasound can be very helpful.

Diaphragmatic Function

There are two proposed diaphragm sonographic predictors of weaning outcome – the diaphragmatic excursion (DE) and the diaphragm thickening fraction (DTF). However, a recent meta-analysis does not support the use of DE in prediction of weaning outcome, and has shown that DTF is, by itself, a modest predictor of weaning outcome.

Lung Aeration

Conversely, by semi-quantifying lung aeration with the global lung aeration score, ultrasound can predict weaning outcome. It uses 12-zone scanning of the lung, apportioning a score of 0 to 3 for each zone and adding the scores for a maximum of 36 (Table 5.1.7.1). Zones 1, 2 and 6 are analogous to, respectively, the upper and lower BLUE points and PLAPS of the BLUE protocol (Figure 5.1.7.7). A dynamic re-aeration score based on the same four patterns can be computed before and after treatments, aimed at improving lung aeration. Both scores can be used to determine the likely success of liberation from mechanical ventilation or veno-venous extracorporeal membrane oxygenation (VV-ECMO). It can also guide fluid resuscitation and re-aeration after ARDS or ventilator-associated pneumonia (VAP).

Pleural Effusions

In case series, about 50 per cent of patients on mechanical ventilation will develop pleural effusions within the first 48 hours of their intensive care stay. Using ultrasound, both quantitative and qualitative considerations can be made about the need to drain the effusions.

Qualitatively, septation or loculation of pleural fluid should, at the very least, trigger a diagnostic pleural tap to look for evidence of infection or empyema. Flattening or inversion of the hemidiaphragm means it will be on an adverse portion of the length/tension curve and affect its function. Stimulation of stretch receptors in this situation is also likely to drive respiratory rate.

Quantitatively, the intra-pleural distance (IPD) at the base of the lung can be correlated with effusion volume. With the patient supine, an IPD of 45 mm on the

Table 5.1.7.1 Lung aeration score

Number of points	Aeration	Description	Appearance
0	Normal	A-line pattern with <3 B-lines per zone	(Figure 5.1.7.1)
1	Moderate loss	Multiple regularly spaced B-lines or confluent B-lines in <50% of the zone	(Figure 5.1.7.2)
2	Severe loss	Confluent B-lines in >50% of the zone	(Figure 5.1.7.3)
3	Total loss	Lung consolidation or pleural effusion in >50% of the zone	Subpleural consolidation with shred sign (Figure 5.1.7.3) Uncomplicated pleural effusion with consolidated lung (Figure 5.1.7.4) Complicated pleural effusion with consolidated lung (Figure 5.1.7.5)

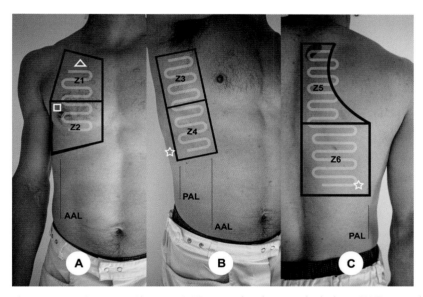

Figure 5.1.7.7 Scan zones. The upper BLUE point is the white triangle; the lower BLUE point is the white square and the PLAPS point is the white star.

left or 50 mm on the right reliably predicts a volume of >800 ml. With a patient supine at 15° elevation, IPD measured in the posterior axillary line in millimetres approximates to fluid volume by a factor of 20. It is unclear at what volume the fluid should be drained, but it has been shown to be safe and lead to improvements in gas exchange.

Distinguishing Atelectasis from Pneumonia

The characteristic features of consolidation due to obstruction, VAP or resorption atelectasis can be very similar as lung aeration is lost. It is especially important to be able to differentiate VAP from the rest.

VAP develops in about 25 per cent of mechanically ventilated patients – who are not on selective digestive tract decontamination – with a 50 per cent mortality rate. It increases the length of hospital stay by more than a week, adds costs and the mortality rate of about 50 per cent increases when adequate treatment is delayed.

Interestingly, similar to the CXR, we find (hemi)-lobar infiltrates in all of the above-mentioned diagnoses. These are therefore totally non-specific for VAP. Conversely, the small subpleural hypoechoic or tissue-like consolidations, or 'shred-sign', are very specific for VAP (Figure 5.1.7.4). Specificity increases if more regions are affected. Interestingly, these tend to occur anteriorly and upper laterally.

The most specific feature of VAP, however, is the dynamic bronchogram. Dynamic air bronchograms represent air in distal bronchi(oles) and are displayed as hyper-echoic linear or arborescent and mobile arte-facts (>1 mm) within consolidations. They prove there is a patent airway and therefore exclude atelectasis. With re-aeration of atelectasis, these will, however, reappear. Dynamic fluid bronchograms are hypo-echoic linear or arborescent anechoic images, which represent fluid-filled bronchi(oles) and are indicative of post-obstructive pneumonia. Static air broncho-grams can be seen in both resorption atelectasis and pneumonia, and therefore cannot be differentiated.

Further evidence demonstrates that in consolida-tion with concomitant effusion, a complex effusion and consolidation-to-pleural effusion ratio >1 was more likely to be due to an infiltrative process, whilst a rhomboid-shape consolidation increased the chance of compression atelectasis. Combining ultrasound with procalcitonin (PCT) has been suggested to increase specificity. However, current guidelines do not recom-mend the use of PCT in the diagnosis and treatment of VAP.

Ultrasound to Distinguish ARDS from Cardiac Pulmonary Oedema

Bedside lung ultrasound assessment has proven to be more accurate than physical examination, N-terminal pro-BNP (NT-pro-BNP) and CXR in assessing patients with suspected acute cardiogenic pulmonary oedema (CPO). Although ARDS, pneumonia and CPO can produce a B-line pattern, differentiation of the B-pattern can help further distinguish among several entities with often similar clinical pictures. A unilateral B-pattern suggests pneumonia. If homogeneous, bilat-eral and diffuse (i.e. at least two regions per hemi-thorax are affected), accompanied by a thin pleura and (bi)-lateral effusion, it orients to CPO (Figure 5.1.7.2). By contrast, the B-pattern in ARDS and viral pneumonia (e.g. coronavirus disease 2019 (COVID-19)) is more heterogeneous, patchy and asymmetrical. ARDS is fur-ther characterised by a thickened, irregular pleura and small subpleural consolidations in gravity-dependent areas (Figures 5.1.7.3 and 5.1.7.4). The C-profile, with its anterior consolidations, also points towards ARDS. Bedside ultrasound has, in fact, been incorporated in the Kigali modification of the Berlin definition of ARDS. Of note, this ARDS pattern is also seen in COVID-19 pneumonia, which gives an ARDS-like clinical picture in severe disease. In a different popula-tion, parenchymal lung disease (i.e. fibrosis, silicosis, sarcoidosis) exhibited a homogeneous B-pattern, but an irregular and thickened pleura.

Further Reading and References

Lichtenstein DA. BLUE-Protocol and FALLS-Protocol. *Chest* 2015;**147**:1659–70.

Llamas-Álvarez AM, Tenza-Lozano EM, Latour-Pérez J. Diaphragm and lung ultrasound to predict weaning outcome: systematic review and meta-analysis. *Chest* 2017;**152**:1140–50.

Mojoli F, Bouhemad B, Mongodi S, Lichtenstein D. Lung ultrasound for critically ill patients. *Am J Respir Crit Care Med* 2019;**199**:701–14.

Staub LJ, Biscaro RRM, Maurici R. Accuracy and applications of lung ultrasound to diagnose ventilator-associated pneumonia: a systematic review. *J Intensive Care Med* 2018;**33**:447–55.

Staub LJ, Mazzali Biscaro RR, Kaszubowski E, Maurici R. Lung ultrasound for the emergency diagnosis of pneumonia, acute heart failure, and exacerbations of chronic obstructive pulmonary disease/asthma in adults: a systematic review and meta-analysis. *J Emerg Med* 2019;**56**:53–69.

Lung Function Testing

5.1.8

Lola Loewenthal

Key Learning Points

1. Lung function testing is important in the diagnosis, severity assessment and monitoring of lung diseases.
2. Spirometry measures forced vital capacity (FVC), forced expiratory volume in 1 second (FEV$_1$) and FEV$_1$/FVC ratio. Its uses include: screening for airflow limitation, assessing disease progression and diagnostic purposes (in combination with further lung function testing).
3. Lung volume measurements provide additional information to help differentiate restrictive, obstructive and mixed lung diseases.
4. Transfer factor for carbon monoxide (TLCO) (diffusion capacity of carbon monoxide (DLCO)) measures the ability of the lungs to transfer inhaled gas from the alveoli to red blood cells in the pulmonary capillaries. It can be used alongside the carbon monoxide transfer coefficient (KCO) for diagnostic purposes and to monitor disease progression.
5. Lung function testing is subject to a number of limitations and, as such, should be interpreted with flow–volume loops and clinical context.

Keywords: spirometry, flow loop, gas transfer, restrictive lung disease, obstructive lung disease

Introduction

Lung function testing is used in the diagnostic pathway for patients with respiratory symptoms (i.e. cough, dyspnoea and wheeze), an algorithm for which can be seen in Figure 5.1.8.1. Lung function testing can evaluate disease severity, monitor progression or screen those at risk such as in pre-operative assessment or occupational exposures.

Lung function testing mainly comprises spirometry, lung volumes and gas transfer. All readings should be interpreted with examination of flow–volume loops and predicted values. Abnormally low results are generally taken to be below the lower limit of normal (LLN) or 80% predicted. Predicted values are produced from reference ranges/equations (based on the subject's age, height, gender and sometimes ethnicity). The LLN is defined as below the fifth percentile in a normal healthy population, providing the data have a normal distribution.

Spirometry

Spirometry provides a simple, readily available test of respiratory function and is often used as a screening tool in symptomatic patients. It is one of the most reproducible and objective measures of airflow limitation but should be used in clinical context with lung volumes. Volume is recorded against flow (Figure 5.1.8.2) and time. Patients are normally asked to omit their bronchodilators prior to testing to provide baseline results.

There are three main measurements, each recorded in their units and percentage predicted:

1. **Forced vital capacity (FVC):** total forced volume (in litres) during maximal expiration after maximal inspiration
   a. A low FVC may indicate restrictive lung disease. It can also provide a prognostic marker in restrictive lung diseases such as interstitial lung disease (ILD)
2. **Forced expiratory volume in 1 second (FEV$_1$):** expired volume (in litres) during the first second of maximal expiration
   a. Useful as a prognostic marker in airways diseases such as chronic obstructive pulmonary disease (COPD)

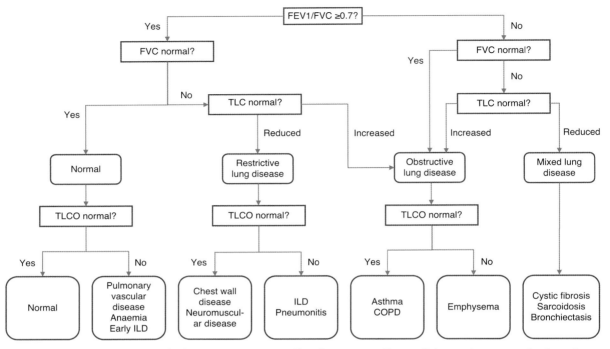

Figure 5.1.8.1 Simplified algorithm for diagnostic interpretation of lung function tests. Abnormally low results are generally taken to be below the lower limits of normal, or 80% predicted.

Source: Adapted from Figure 5.1.8.2 in Pellegrino R, Viegi G, Brusasco V, *et al*. Interpretive strategies for lung function tests. *Eur Respir J* 2005;**26**(5):948–68.

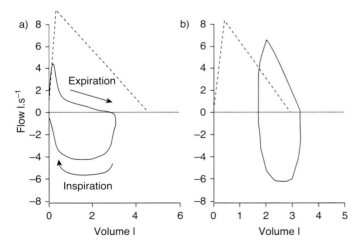

Figure 5.1.8.2 Spirometry flow–volume curves. (a) Obstructive lung disease. (b) Restrictive lung disease. Normal predicted expiratory curves are denoted by the dotted line.

Source: Fig 1a and c from Pellegrino R, Viegi G, Brusasco V, *et al*. Interpretive strategies for lung function tests. *Eur Respir J* 2005;**26**(5):948–68.

3. **FEV_1/FVC ratio:** percentage of total exhaled volume in 1 second of a forced expiratory manoeuvre

   a. Useful in differentiating between obstructive and restrictive lung disease

   b. A ratio of <0.7 is suggestive of obstructive lung disease

   c. The FEV_1/FVC ratio decreases with age, resulting in over-diagnosis of obstructive lung disease in the elderly. The LLN should therefore also be considered in older age groups

Characteristic flow–volume curves may be seen with restrictive and obstructive disease (Figure 5.1.8.2).

Spirometry can also provide further information on upper airway obstructions and reversibility.

Inspiratory and Expiratory Flow–Volume Loops in Upper Airway Obstruction

Inspiratory and expiratory flow–volume loops can be performed with forced inspiration immediately after full expiration (standard spirometry only provides the expiratory portion). Significant upper airway obstruction can produce characteristic flow–volume shapes (Figure 5.1.8.3).

These vary according to the obstruction's location (above or below the thoracic inlet) and whether it changes the airway calibre on ventilation (fixed or variable); they are described below:

- Fixed obstructions (Figure 5.1.8.3a), such as post-intubation strictures, fixed tracheal tumours and goitres, will limit both inspiratory and expiratory air flow. Both flow loops will therefore have a flattened/truncated appearance.
- Variable intrathoracic obstructions (Figure 5.1.8.3b), such as tracheomalacia and some tracheal tumours, have a flattening of the expiratory curve. The inspiratory curve is preserved as intra-tracheal pressure exceeds pleural pressure on inspiratory flow. However, expiratory flow is reduced as increased pleural pressure causes the obstructing lesion to reduce the lumen's calibre.

- Variable extra-thoracic obstructions (Figure 5.1.8.3c), such as vocal cord dysfunction, strictures of the glottis and mobile tumours above the thoracic inlet, have a flattening of the inspiratory curve. This is due to reduced intraluminal pressure relative to the atmospheric pressure on forced inspiration.

These patterns require obstructions to reduce the tracheal calibre by over 50 per cent and can be affected by poor technique. Clinical correlation with imaging and/or direct visualisation should therefore always be performed.

Bronchodilator Response and Reversibility

Reversibility should be performed in the diagnosis and stratification of patients with asthma and COPD. Patients are asked to withhold bronchodilators prior to testing. Spirometry is then performed prior to, and 15 minutes after, administration of a short-acting beta agonist (salbutamol) via an inhaler or a nebuliser.

A positive bronchodilator response is defined as:

- An absolute percentage improvement in FEV_1 of >12%

$$[(\text{Post-bronchodilator } FEV_1 - \text{pre-bronchodilator } FEV_1)/\text{pre-bronchodilator } FEV_1] \times 100 = {>}12\%$$

- And/or an FEV_1 increase of >200 ml.

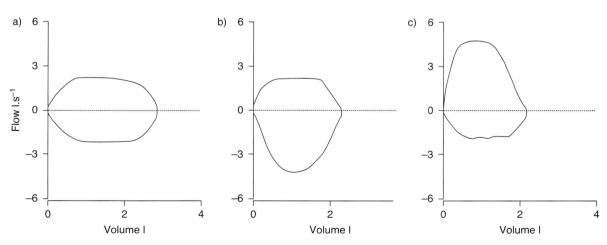

Figure 5.1.8.3 Flow–volume loops in upper airways obstruction. (a) Fixed obstructions. (b) Variable intrathoracic obstructions. (c) Variable extra-thoracic obstructions.
Source: Figure 5.1.8.3 in Pellegrino R, Viegi G, Brusasco V, *et al*. Interpretive strategies for lung function tests. *Eur Respir J* 2005;**26**(5):948–68.] but with 3b and 3c switched.

Both asthma and COPD may show a bronchodilator response, but an FEV_1 increase of >400 ml is highly suggestive of asthma.

Patients with normal or near-normal spirometry may not demonstrate a bronchodilator response and a provocation challenge to induce airway hyper-responsiveness might be considered.

Lung Volumes

Measurement of lung volumes alongside spirometry provides further diagnostic information (Figure 5.1.8.1). Lung volumes are needed to diagnose restrictive lung disease and hyperinflation. Lung volume measurements are normally performed in lung function laboratories and are not available as bedside tests.

The key measurements (all recorded in litres) are detailed below:

1. Vital capacity (VC):
   a. Total forced volume during maximal expiration after maximal inspiration
   b. Can be recorded as FVC or slow vital capacity (SVC)
   c. The difference between FVC and SVC is normally small; however, airway collapse causing gas trapping in severe obstructive lung disease can significantly lower the FVC

2. Total lung capacity (TLC):
   a. Volume of gas in lungs after maximal inspiration
   b. May be increased with hyperinflation such as in COPD
   c. Always decreased in restrictive lung disease

3. Residual volume (RV):
   a. Volume of gas remaining in the lungs after maximal expiration
   b. May be increased in obstructive lung disease
   c. RV/TLC is increased with hyperinflation
   d. May be decreased in restrictive lung disease

4. Functional residual capacity (FRC):
   a. Volume of gas remaining in the lungs at the end of normal expiration

Disease Patterns

Ventilatory lung diseases can be differentiated into obstructive, restrictive and mixed patterns. These are outlined below.

Obstructive Lung Disease

Obstructive lung diseases result in increased airway resistance, with a reduction in FEV_1 and FEV_1/FVC ratio. Flow–volume curves may show 'kinking' or 'scalloping' of the expiratory flow loop due to a reduction in airflow velocity (Figure 5.1.8.2a). Obstructive lung disease can occur with COPD, asthma, laryngeal disease, tracheal compression or central bronchial tumours.

COPD is characterised by a post-bronchodilator FEV_1/FVC ratio of <0.7. The severity of airflow limitation can be defined by FEV_1 and forms part of the Global Initiative for Chronic Obstructive Lung Disease (GOLD) classification for COPD.

Lung volume measurements are important in the diagnosis of obstructive lung disease. Air-trapping and/or hyperinflation in obstructive lung disease may result in an increased RV and reduced FVC normalising of the FEV_1/FVC ratio. Air-trapping is implied when the FRC or RV is >120% predicted. Hyperinflation is implied when the TLC is >120% predicted. Measurement of volumes therefore helps differentiate between obstructive lung disease with preserved FEV_1/FVC and mixed obstructive and restrictive disease.

Restrictive Lung Disease

Restrictive lung disease is defined as a reduced TLC less than the LLN or 80% predicted. Spirometry shows a reduced FVC with a preserved FEV_1/FVC ratio and a normal-shaped flow–volume curve. The FVC can be used to monitor disease progression. Restrictive lung disease has multiple aetiologies, examples of which are outlined below:

- Diseases of the lung: ILD/acute pneumonitis
- Disease of the chest wall: pleural diseases, kyphoscoliosis and other chest wall deformities
- Neuromuscular disease: myasthenia gravis, motor neurone disease

Gas transfer measurement can play an important role in differentiating between the causes of restrictive lung disease.

Mixed Obstructive and Restrictive Lung Disease

Reductions in TLC and FEV_1/FVC ratio are suggestive of mixed obstructive and restrictive lung disease. Common causes include cystic fibrosis, sarcoidosis and bronchiectasis.

A summary of how to interpret lung function tests is given in Figure 5.1.8.1.

Gas Transfer

Measurement of gas transfer across the alveolar–capillary membrane can be used to identify altered oxygen uptake capacity. It can be used to help identify causes of dyspnoea, as well as to monitor disease progression in ILD, and for complications such as pulmonary hypertension.

Carbon monoxide (CO) is normally used for diffusion measurements due to its high affinity binding to haemoglobin (>200 times that of oxygen). Gas transfer measurements can be reduced in smokers (as the subject has already inhaled CO), so subjects should not smoke for 24 hours prior to measurement. Measurements are also reduced in pregnancy. Three main measurements are recorded:

1. Transfer factor for carbon monoxide (TLCO), also known as diffusion capacity of carbon monoxide (DLCO):
   a. TLCO (DLCO) measures the ability of the lungs to transfer inhaled gas from the alveoli to red blood cells in pulmonary capillaries
   b. Recorded in mmol/(min kPa) and percentage predicted
   c. Affected by anaemia, carboxyhaemoglobin levels, altitude and lung volume, so adjustments for these factors may be required

2. Alveolar volume (VA):
   a. Volume of contributing alveolar units providing a gas exchange surface area
   b. Recorded in litres
   c. Measured during the single breath method and using a tracer gas (normally helium)

3. Carbon monoxide transfer coefficient (KCO):
   a. Gas transfer per unit volume, often described as TLCO/VA
   b. Recorded in mmol/(min kPa l) and percentage predicted

Interpreting Gas Transfer Results

Low TLCO with Restrictive Spirometry

TLCO may be reduced in diffusion disorders such as ILD where there is structural loss in functional alveoli. KCO has relative preservation due to the heterogeneous pattern of most ILD and subsequent diversion of blood flow to less affected alveoli.

Low TLCO with Obstructive Spirometry

Alveolar capillary damage in emphysema results in reduced TLCO and KCO. Whilst actual lung volumes may be normal or increased, reduced helium gas mixing may result in a reduced VA measurement. Gas transfer is not used as a prognostic marker in COPD, but a TLCO percentage predicted significantly lower than FEV_1 may represent concurrent pathology such as pulmonary hypertension.

Low TLCO with Normal Spirometry

Pulmonary vascular disease, including pulmonary artery hypertension, chronic pulmonary emboli and vasculitis, can lead to a ventilation–perfusion mismatch and a reduction in TLCO. This can also occur in early ILD or falsely in anaemia and smokers.

Low TLCO with Increased KCO

This occurs where there is reduced functional lung volume, but normal diffusion. Post-pneumonectomy patients, for example, will have a reduced VA and TLCO, but an increased KCO from blood diversion to the remaining lung. Reduced lung expansion, as seen in kyphoscoliosis, neuromuscular disorders or inadequate inspiration due to poor technique, results in relative preservation of surface area, and thus VA at low lung volumes. This results in an increased TLCO/VA, and therefore KCO.

Increased TLCO and KCO

Gas transfer appears elevated in diffuse pulmonary haemorrhage (such as with pulmonary vasculitis). This is due to free red cells in the alveoli taking up CO and providing a falsely high reading.

References and Further Reading

Cooper BG. An update on contraindications for lung function testing. *Thorax* 2011;**66**:714–23.

Global Initiative for Chronic Obstructive Lung Disease (GOLD). goldcopd.org

Miller MR, Hankinson J, Brusasko V, *et al.* Standardisation of spirometry. *Eur Respir J* 2005;**26**:319–38.

Pellegrino R, Viegi G, Brusasco V, *et al.* Interpretive strategies for lung function tests. *Eur Respir J* 2005;**26**:948–68.

Shiner RJ, Steier J. *Lung Function Tests Made Easy.* Edinburgh: Elsevier/Churchill Livingstone; 2013.

Arterial Line Insertion

5.2.1

Oliver Sanders

Key Learning Points

1. Arterial lines offer beat-by-beat monitoring of a patient's blood pressure and allow for repeated arterial sampling – must-haves in critical care and major operative settings.
2. Careful consideration of the insertion site is necessary, especially when radial puncture is not available. The use of end-arteries could result in limb ischaemia in the event of complications.
3. The Allen's test is a simple and timely test for gross perfusion prior to arterial puncture; however, it is not without its shortcomings. Doppler ultrasound may be more effective, especially in anaesthetised patients.
4. There are several different techniques for arterial line insertion; however, the catheter-over-wire (Seldinger) technique is regarded as the safest.
5. A well-inserted and cared-for arterial line can remain *in situ* for several weeks, if required. Infection rates are lower than those of either peripheral or central venous catheters.

Keywords: arterial line, invasive monitoring, blood pressure

Indications

Arterial lines are inserted in the critical care setting, or prior to major surgical procedures where invasive cardiovascular and respiratory monitoring is required. They are used for continuous blood pressure monitoring and repeated arterial sampling; thus, they are essential in patients who are ventilated or require pharmacological blood pressure support. Arterial lines are more accurate than sphygmomanometric blood pressure measurements – especially in obese patients, they are more reliable when the blood pressure is very low, and they are essential for quantifying real-time response to vasoactive medications.

Contraindications to Line Insertion

- Absent pulse
- Inadequate collateral blood supply
- Local soft tissue infection
- Vascular disease/insufficiency, e.g. thromboangiitis obliterans or Raynaud's disease
- Previous vascular graft

Risks/Complications

- Haemorrhage
- Infection
- Distal tissue ischaemia
- Tissue necrosis
- Line fracture/embolus
- False aneurysm

Potential Insertion Sites
Radial Artery

The radial artery is by far the most common site for arterial line placement. It is easy to palpate, and most clinicians are comfortable with radial artery puncture. The hand is collaterally supplied by the ulnar artery, as ensured by the Allen's test (see below). If the arterial line blood pressure is to be corroborated by non-invasive means, the cuff should be placed on the contralateral arm so as not to give the artefactual impression of loss of cardiac output on the trace.

Brachial Artery

The brachial artery is an end-artery supplying the forearm, with almost no collateral supply. Therefore, complications of cannulation could cause devastating ischaemia. It is also affected significantly by arm position, so necessitates continuous elbow extension.

Femoral Artery

This provides a relatively safe alternative to the radial artery. However, a longer catheter is usually required, which is more prone to positional disturbance. Due to proximity to the groin, femoral arterial lines are also more prone to infection.

Dorsalis Pedis Artery

Dorsalis pedis mean arterial pressure readings may be higher than in the radial artery, by as much as 20 mmHg. Non-invasive corroboration is thus strongly encouraged. In the presence of a palpable posterior tibial pulse, this is thought to be a safe site for insertion and is not usually impeded by position variation.

Allen's Test

The Allen's test was first described in 1929 to demonstrate the collateral blood supply in the hands of vasculopathy patients. It thus provides an indication as to whether it is safe to proceed with radial arterial puncture, insomuch that ulnar artery blood supply to the hand should compensate for any loss of perfusion from the radial artery.

With the patient's hand tightly clenched in a fist, both the radial and ulnar arteries are compressed by the individual performing the procedure. The hand is subsequently opened, leaving the palm blanched and pale. With the radial artery still occluded, pressure is taken off the ulnar artery. If the normal pink colour of the palm returns in under 10 seconds, the collateral supply is considered adequate to proceed with radial puncture. Notably, whilst the Allen's test can be used as a guide, it cannot reliably quantify blood flow into the hand, and it is difficult to perform in a patient who is already anaesthetised. Doppler ultrasound does not share these shortfalls and may be used instead.

Procedure

There are many different techniques and cannulae available for arterial line insertion. However, here we describe the classic Seldinger insertion technique used for arterial line insertion into the radial artery.

- Explain the benefits and risks of the procedure to the patient, and gain consent (verbal consent is adequate in most instances).

- Ask the patient to extend their wrist, and make sure it is adequately supported, e.g. with a pillow.
- Identify the desired artery through palpation.
- Ensure the pressure transducer line is completely flushed through and ready for subsequent connection to the arterial cannula.
- Open the necessary equipment onto a sterile field, and clean the area thoroughly with chlorhexidine.
- Infiltrate the subcutaneous area with local anaesthetic (1–2 ml of 1% lidocaine will often suffice), ensuring not to inadvertently inject it into the artery. Allow sufficient time for the anaesthetic to take effect.
- With the wrist remaining in the extended position, use the introducer needle to puncture the palpable radial artery at approximately 30° to the skin.
- On successful puncture of the artery, pulsatile blood should flow from the introducer needle immediately. At this point, lower the hub of the introducer needle towards the skin to bring the introducer needle into the same plane as the vessel. Pulsatile flow should still be seen coming from the end of the introducer needle.
- With the introducer needle held fixed in position, insert the guidewire into the artery – flexible end first. There should be no resistance on guidewire insertion; resistance indicates the formation of a false passage or an extensive thrombus in the vessel lumen.
- Slide the introducer needle out of the skin and off the guidewire, whilst carefully maintaining the depth and position of the wire.
- Pass the arterial catheter over the guidewire and into the vessel. Some twisting/rotation of the arterial catheter may ease passage.
- With the arterial catheter inserted up to the winged hub, remove the guidewire and inspect for pulsatile flow coming out of the arterial catheter.
- Attach the transducer, and assess whether you can see an arterial waveform on the monitor. This will subsequently need 'zeroing'.
- Securely fix the cannula hub to the skin in the manner dictated by your hospital (e.g. Steri-strips, sutures, etc.), and cover with an appropriate dressing.
- Dispose of your sharps safely, and document the relevant points regarding your line insertion.

References and Further Reading

Roberts JR, Custalow CB, Thomsen TW. *Roberts and Hedges' Clinical Procedures in Emergency Medicine and Acute Care*, 7th edn. Philadelphia, PA: Elsevier; 2018.

Scheer B, Perel A, Pfeiffer UJ. Clinical review: complications and risk factors of peripheral arterial catheters used for haemodynamic monitoring in anaesthesia and intensive care medicine. *Crit Care* 2002;**6**:199–204.

Waldman C, Soni N, Rhodes A, Handy J. *Oxford Desk Reference: Critical Care*, 2nd edn. Oxford: Oxford University Press; 2019.

5.2.2

Use of Ultrasound for Vascular Localisation

Jonathan Barnes

Key Learning Points

1. Ultrasound guidance can, in trained hands, improve success of venous cannulation in difficult patients.
2. Different techniques exist, with none clearly superior to the other.
3. Find a technique that works for you and stick with it.
4. An understanding of vascular anatomy is essential to successful cannulation.
5. Differentiating between arteries and veins can be done in various ways and is an essential skill.

Keywords: ultrasound, cannulation, Seldinger, transverse, longitudinal

Introduction

Ultrasound use is now standard practice for insertion of central venous catheters. It is also a tool that is being increasingly utilised to assist with insertion of peripheral venous and arterial lines. Here we describe how to localise and identify the vasculature, and also briefly describe the different techniques for ultrasound-guided peripheral venous access.

Localisation of Vasculature

A good anatomical knowledge is the key to success for this technique. If you know where to look for the vessels, they will subsequently be easier to find.

Vessels appear as round, black structures in the transverse ultrasound plane, and as black tubes in the longitudinal view (Figure 5.2.2.1).

Arteries versus Veins

As vascular anatomy and structural relationships can be variable, it is imperative to be able to tell the difference between a vein and an artery.

- Structural differences
  - Arteries tend to have thicker walls than veins (increased echogenicity).
  - Arteries are normally round, whereas veins may be more oval-shaped.
  - Veins will be compressible (to complete flatness), whereas arteries are generally not. Be careful, however, as even arteries will be compressible if large amounts of pressure are applied.
  - Arteries are visibly pulsatile, whereas veins are not. Notably, however, veins may appear pulsatile if they are next to an artery where the pulse is transmitted from one vessel to the next.
- Colour flow
  - Turning on colour flow will allow you to see which way blood is flowing, thus allowing identification of whether it is an artery or a vein.
  - Blood flowing towards the transducer will appear red, whereas blood flowing away will appear blue. (This can be remembered by the acronym BART – Blue Away, Red Towards.) Importantly, red does not necessarily indicate an artery, nor blue a vein.
- Doppler flow
  - Placing Doppler flow over the vessel will allow visualisation of any pulsatile waveform. In the case of an artery, a clear arterial pressure versus time curve should be seen, and this will not be present for a vein.

Techniques for Ultrasound-Guided Peripheral Vascular Access

There are many different techniques utilised for ultrasound-guided peripheral vascular access. There is no clear evidence to suggest any one technique is superior

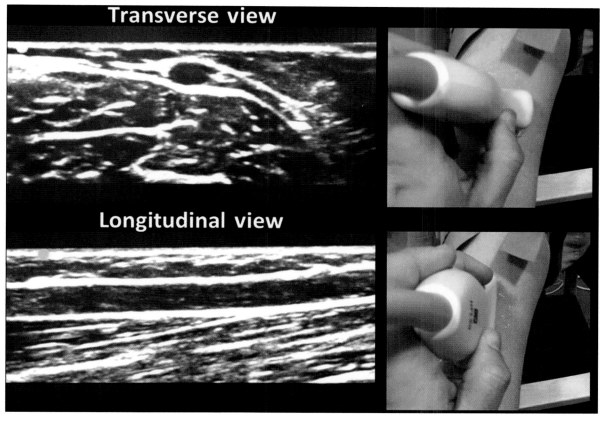

Figure 5.2.2.1 Different probe positions and vessel views. Transverse view (top) and longitudinal view (bottom).

to another. However, there is evidence that ultrasound-guided cannulation is more likely to be successful that non-ultrasound-guided in patients with difficult intravenous access.

The different techniques are briefly described below. In all instances, it is often useful to locate a larger vein (e.g. basilic) and aim to puncture it at a point at which it is close to the skin surface and has a straight orientation.

- Transverse out-of-plane puncture
  - Locate the vein using the probe in the transverse out-of-plane orientation.
  - Measure the depth to the centre of the vein, then puncture the skin approximately the same distance distal to the probe, aiming at a 30–45° angle.
  - If the probe and cannula are well aligned, the cannula will puncture the vein and can then be threaded as normal.

- Transverse in-plane puncture (the 'walking-it-in' approach)
  - Locate a vein and use a similar technique as above to locate a puncture site.
  - Move the probe distally, so that the cannula can be visualised as it punctures the skin.
  - Move the probe with the cannula as it moves through the subcutaneous tissue and into the vein.
  - Follow the tip up the vein, advancing the probe until the cannula tip is no longer seen, then advancing the cannula until the tip reappears (walk it in).

- Longitudinal in-plane puncture
  - This is a similar technique to the transverse out-of-plane technique, but it involves having the probe in the longitudinal orientation.

565

- ○ This view enables the cannula to be visualised as it punctures and then moves up the vein.
  - ○ This technique is particularly useful for ensuring you have not punctured the posterior wall; however, it can be challenging to obtain and maintain a good view.
- Seldinger
  - ○ Some studies have described using a Seldinger technique, whereby a hypodermic needle and an arterial line wire are utilised to insert a cannula.

References and Further Reading

McNamee J, Jeong J, Patel N. 2014. 10 Tips for ultrasound-guided peripheral venous access. *ACEPNow*. www.acepnow.com/article/10-tips-ultrasound-guided-peripheral-venous-access/

Stolz L, Stolz U, Howe C, Farrell IJ, Adhikari S. Ultrasound-guided peripheral venous access: a meta-analysis and systematic review. *J Vasc Access* 2015;**16**:321–6.

Central Venous Catheterisation

Oliver Sanders

Keywords: central venous catheter, CVC, invasive monitoring, central line, Seldinger technique

Introduction

Central venous catheterisation (CVC) is an essential skill for those working in the ICU. The indications, contraindications, complications, different sites for insertion and Seldinger method for insertion are outlined below.

Indications

- Central drug administration
- Repeated blood sampling
- Central venous pressure monitoring
- Lack of peripheral access
- Haemofiltration
- Parenteral nutrition
- Placement of temporary cardiac pacing wires
- Pulmonary catheters

Contraindications

There are no absolute contraindications to CVC. However, relative contraindications may guide the choice of site or positioning. These include:

- Local soft tissue infection
- Thrombophlebitis or obstructed/stenosed vein
- Severe coagulopathy
- Inability for the patient to lie flat/head down, e.g. raised intracranial pressure or an awake patient who tolerates this poorly
- Altered/deranged anatomy

Complications

Complications of central line insertion can be influenced by both the anatomical site and the device used. However, general complications which apply to CVC insertions include the following.

Immediate

- Arrhythmias
- Haemorrhage/haematoma formation
- Arterial puncture
- Vascular injury
- Pneumothorax
- Cardiac tamponade
- Haemothorax
- Foreign body embolisation
- Air embolus
- Lost/forgotten guidewire

Delayed

- Infection
- Thrombus
- Catheter fracture – either embolisation or retention following removal
- Vascular wall erosion

The number of unsuccessful attempts at catheterisation has been shown to be a strong predictor for the likelihood of complications – both immediate and delayed. The use of ultrasound has been found to maximise the chances of a successful insertion and to reduce the probability of complications.

Ultrasound

The use of ultrasound guidance is now standard practice for central venous cannulation. It has been shown to increase the probability of successful venous puncture on the first pass, and thus reduce complications. Ultrasound allows identification of the desired compressible vein (as well as differentiation from the adjacent non-compressible and pulsatile artery), visualisation of any abnormalities which may contraindicate vessel puncture at a given site (e.g. a thrombus or bifurcation in the vessel) and confirmation of the presence of the guidewire in the lumen of the vessel following puncture (which gives the user reassurance to continue safely).

In order to be used throughout the procedure, the ultrasound probe must be placed in a sterile dressing or plastic sheath (with a layer of sterile gel between the probe and the sheath, as well as between the sheath and the skin).

Sites

Internal Jugular Vein

Internal jugular vein (IJV) cannulation is associated with the greatest chance of first-pass cannulation of the vein. Use of this site, however, has the highest risk of arrhythmias, as the guidewire, or tip of the line, can enter the right atrium and irritate the endocardium. This route also normally requires the patient to be positioned in the Trendelenburg (head down) position, which can be problematic in those with cardiovascular instability or head injuries and raised intracranial pressure.

The IJV runs from just behind the earlobe to the sternoclavicular joint. Puncture can be made in the triangular space between the sternal and clavicular heads of the sternocleidomastoid, or deep to the posterolateral border of the muscle. The IJV lies laterally, but closely related, to the internal, then the common carotid artery, increasing the risk of arterial injury on blind puncture.

Optimum positioning for cannulation at this site is with the patient lying supine in the Trendelenburg position head, with the neck extended and facing the contralateral side. This position may be difficult for awake patients to tolerate, especially in those with respiratory

distress. Additionally, it is also advisable to forewarn and counsel patients who are claustrophobic about the necessity of placing sterile drapes over their face. The discomfort, however, can be minimised by an additional person holding the drape off their face.

Subclavian Vein

The subclavian vein is a continuation of the axillary vein, and becomes the brachiocephalic vein when it joins with the IJV at the thoracic inlet – posterior to the sternoclavicular joint. It begins at the apex of the axilla, and runs between the first rib and the posterior border of the clavicle. The anatomical course makes the use of ultrasound difficult, and complications such as pneumothorax are common at this site. Additionally, in the event of a significant bleed on cannulation (or on removal of a line), the vein itself is difficult to compress. The advantages of using the subclavian vein, however, are that patients find the line much more comfortable once it is sited and it is associated with less infection as the site is easier to keep clean.

Femoral Vein

Femoral vein puncture is often advocated in the emergency setting where access is desired quickly and there is fear that positioning an unstable patient in the Trendelenburg position may cause clinical deterioration. Its proximity to the groin, however, means that it is associated with far higher rates of site infections than the internal jugular and subclavian sites, and as a consequence, it requires more frequent removal and replacement. The optimum position for femoral vein cannulation is with the patient lying completely supine, with the desired leg externally rotated. The femoral vein is located medially to the palpable femoral artery within the femoral sheath.

Procedure

- Position the patient optimally for whichever puncture site has been chosen. Remember not to leave patients head down for long periods of time.
- Locate a preferable vein with ultrasound – as close to the skin as possible, and not obstructed by the adjacent artery. Check for pre-existing thrombosis, and ensure there is no local soft tissue infection which could precipitate bacteraemia.
- Ensure the area of skin which will become part of the sterile field is free from paraphernalia (e.g. jewellery, wires, ECG stickers, hair).

- Continuous ECG monitoring is required to monitor for arrhythmias.
- Open the equipment onto a sterile field on a trolley.
- Put on your surgical cap, face mask, sterile gown and gloves.
- Prepare the central line by flushing all lumens with saline through three-way taps or needle-free injection ports.
- Clean the skin with chlorhexidine wash, working in concentric circles from the centre outwards. Repeat three times to ensure the area is clean and sterile.
- Apply sterile drapes.
- Anaesthetise the site with subcutaneous lidocaine (orange needle).
- With the ultrasound probe (covered in a sterile dressing) held in the non-dominant hand, identify the vein, ensuring it is easily distinguishable from the adjacent artery.
- In the dominant hand, have a 5- or 10-ml syringe half-filled with saline attached to the introducing needle.
- Insert the needle into the vein, aiming for the area of maximum diameter (usually the middle), with suction continuously applied on the syringe. Blood will be easily aspirated once the tip of the needle is in the vein.
- With the needle held in a fixed position, remove the syringe and insert the guidewire to around 10 cm through the skin. The wire should enter with no resistance – if it does, then remove it and try again. Continuously monitor for arrhythmias.
- Retract the needle, leaving only the wire in the skin.
- Using ultrasound, check the wire is visible in the lumen – in both the cross-sectional and longitudinal planes.
- Make a small cut in the skin at the puncture site, with the scalpel blade faced away from the wire.
- Pass the dilator over the wire and, with the skin held taut, into the vein, taking care to follow the tract of the wire to avoid causing a kink. Remove the dilator once venous dilatation has occurred, and cover the area temporarily with some gauze (as dilated central veins bleed!).

- Pass the central line over the wire, ensuring that part of the wire is visible and being held at all times – either between the line and the skin or once it has passed through the line and out of the port.
- Advance the central line to the desired length (12 cm is usually adequate for right IJV insertion), keeping tension on the guidewire at all times.
- Remove the guidewire.
- Ensure all ports both aspirate and can be easily flushed.
- Fix the line to the skin with either sutures or adhesive dressings – as per trust policy. Ensure the skin is adequately anaesthetised if using sutures.
- Reposition the patient for comfort, and dispose of your sharps safely.
- Request a chest X-ray both to confirm the position of the line tip and to check for immediate complications such as pneumothorax.
- Document the procedure in the patient's notes, including that the line is safe to use (once confirmed).

Confirmation of Line Placement

Once a line is inserted, it must be checked to confirm both its anatomical location and that it is placed in a vein. At all sites, the line can be transduced, and a blood gas sample taken to ensure it is venous blood gas (VBG), as opposed to arterial blood gas (ABG), and for the internal jugular and subclavian locations, a chest X-ray should be taken. When confirming correct line placement on a chest X-ray, the tip should sit in the superior vena cava above the right atrium. It should be within approximately 5 mm of the projected border of the right heart, usually near the level of the carina. If the tip of the central line lies within the right atrium, there is a risk of perforation and cardiac tamponade, and as such, the line must be withdrawn to a safe distance and re-secured.

Arterial Puncture

Arterial punctures are a well-known complication of CVC insertion but may be minimised by using ultrasound. In most instances, an arterial puncture is obvious and given away by the high-pressure, pulsatile bright red blood exuding from the needle once the syringe is removed. If unsure, however, other means used for confirmation include applying a transducer directly to the puncture needle to determine the waveform and pressure, or taking a blood sample for point-of-care blood gas measurement (± comparison against a contemporaneous sample from an arterial line.)

In the event of arterial puncture with just the needle (in a non-coagulopathic patient), removal and application of sustained direct pressure are usually sufficient to stop the bleeding. If arterial cannulation using the wide-bore central line has occurred, a vascular surgeon's advice should be sought immediately.

References and Further Reading

Maecken T, Grau T. Ultrasound imaging in vascular access. *Crit Care Med* 2007;**35**(5 Suppl):S178–85.

Smith R, Nolan J. Central venous catheters. *BMJ* 2013;**11**:f6570.

Waldman C, Soni N, Rhodes A, Handy J. *Oxford Desk Reference: Critical Care*, 2nd edn. Oxford: Oxford University Press; 2019.

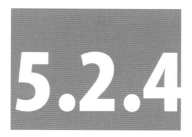

5.2.4

Pulmonary Artery Catheterisation: Insertion and Interpretation

Suehana Rahman

Key Learning Points

1. Pulmonary artery catheters are an invasive monitoring device used to measure cardiac output, mixed venous oxygen saturations and intra-cardiac pressures.
2. They are useful in the diagnosis and assessment of critically unwell patients in the context of unexplained shock, pulmonary artery hypertension and severe cardiogenic shock, and in the perioperative management of patients with severe cardiopulmonary disease undergoing major surgery.
3. Pulmonary artery catheters are used as both a diagnostic and a monitoring tool and, in themselves, are not a therapeutic intervention.
4. Accurate interpretation of the data produced is essential to its use.
5. Complications are largely related to catheter insertion and advancement.

Keywords: pulmonary artery catheter, cardiac output, pulmonary artery hypertension

Introduction

A pulmonary artery catheter (PAC) is a diagnostic and monitoring tool, used to measure right-sided intra-cardiac pressures, cardiac output (CO) and mixed venous oxygen saturation (SvO_2). Right heart catheterisation was first described in 1929, but its use was revolutionised in 1970 with the creation of a balloon-tipped catheter (also known as the Swan–Ganz catheter), which, when inflated, is carried into the pulmonary artery (PA) by continuous blood flow. The flotation procedure can thus be performed at the bedside and is guided by intra-cardiac pressure tracings. In the 1990s, use of the PAC declined, in part due to the negative publicity that arose following several studies that failed to show not only a lack of benefit with their use

on patient outcomes (e.g. PACMAN, 2005), but also an association with increased morbidity and mortality. More recently, however, there has been criticism of the way data from these studies have been interpreted, and their use is on the rise in specific circumstances. Notably, as a monitoring and diagnostic tool, patient outcomes are not dependent on the insertion of a PAC, but rather on the appropriate interpretation of the data produced and subsequent guidance of patient care.

Equipment Components

PACs are usually 110 cm in length and are available in sizes 5–8 G. They have up to five lumens and have markings at 10-cm intervals (Figure 5.2.4.1).

1. **Distal lumen.** This ends in the PA when the PAC is properly positioned, and is used to measure PA pressures and pulmonary artery wedge pressures (PAWPs), and to sample mixed venous blood.
2. **Proximal lumen.** This should ideally open in the right atrium (RA) (approximately 30 cm from the catheter tip) and can be used to measure the central venous pressure (CVP) and inject drugs/infusion fluids.
3. **Thermistor lumen.** The PAC contains two insulated wires leading to a thermistor 3.7 cm from the catheter tip. The proximal end is connected to a CO monitoring device.
4. **Balloon inflation lumen.** This is used to inflate the balloon at the catheter tip.
5. **Second proximal lumen.** This may be present and is usually dedicated to infusion of drugs.

Procedure

Preparation

1. The PAC is placed through a sterile sheath, and each of the ports flushed with normal saline.
2. The balloon is then inflated with 1.5 ml of air to check for both breaches in its integrity and

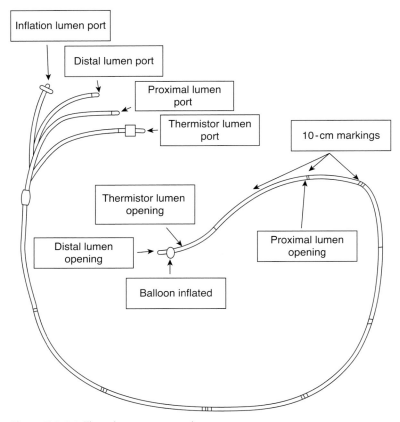

Figure 5.2.4.1 The pulmonary artery catheter.

symmetry of extension beyond the catheter tip. It is then deflated fully. The distal lumen is connected to a pressure transducer system for continuous monitoring during flotation.

3. Insertion of the PAC requires central venous access and involves advancing the catheter via an introducer until its tip is within the RA and is recording the CVP waveform.

Flotation

1. The balloon is inflated with 1.5 ml of air (taking note of any increased resistance, compared to the 'test' inflation, which would suggest that it is still within the introducer).

2. As the catheter is advanced, the inflated balloon is guided by the flow of blood across, first, the tricuspid valve into the right ventricle (RV) and then the pulmonary valve into the PA. When advanced further into the PA, with the balloon still inflated, it becomes 'wedged', so that the

catheter tip is isolated from the PA pressure and instead measures the PAWP. This is taken as an indirect measure of left ventricular end-diastolic pressure (Figure 5.2.4.2). The balloon should then be deflated and kept so until another PAWP measurement is required.

During flotation, each chamber is identified by its distinctive haemodynamic characteristics represented by varying pressure waveforms (Figure 5.2.4.3), and these should be acquired sequentially at expected distances from the insertion site.

Failure to identify the expected pressure waveforms may indicate catheter misdirection or coiling within the RV (which may lead to knotting if not identified and rectified). If suspected, the balloon should be deflated, the catheter withdrawn to the RA and flotation re-attempted. From the right internal jugular vein, RA pressure is usually identified at 20–30 cm, RV pressure at 30–40 cm, PA pressure at 40–50 cm and PAWP at distances slightly beyond 50 cm. Following the procedure,

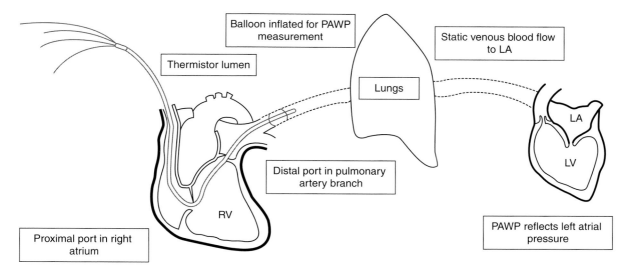

Figure 5.2.4.2 Insertion of a pulmonary artery catheter. LA = left atrium/atrial; LV = left ventricle; PAWP = pulmonary artery wedge pressure; RV = right ventricle.

Source: From Kersten LD: *Comprehensive Respiratory Nursing*, Philadelphia, 1989, Saunders.

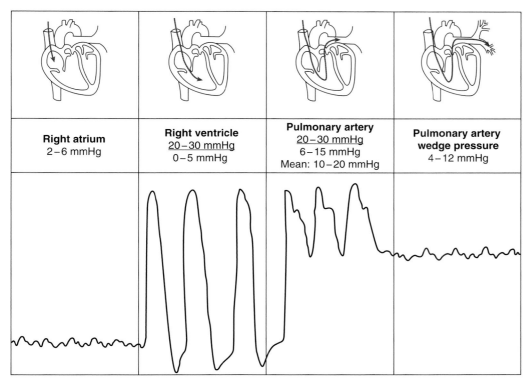

Figure 5.2.4.3 Sequential changes in pressure waveforms on advancement of the pulmonary artery catheter.

Source: From Wilkins RL, Dexter JR, Heuer AJ: *Clinical Assessment in Respiratory Care*, ed 6, St Louis, 2010, Mosby.

a chest X-ray should be performed and the catheter tip should be identified at no more than 3–5 cm from the midline or within 2 cm of the cardiac border.

Of note, the PAC should only be advanced with the balloon inflated, as otherwise there is an increased risk of valvular or myocardial injury caused by the unprotected catheter tip. Conversely, it should never be withdrawn with the balloon inflated.

Interpretation

Right Atrium

With the catheter tip in the RA, the initial pressure waveform will be that of the CVP, consisting of three peaks (*a*, *c* and *v*) and two descents (*x* and *y*).

Right Ventricle

As the catheter tip passes through the tricuspid valve, an RV pressure waveform is obtained, with an increase in systolic pressure and an up-sloping diastolic pressure tracing that occurs during diastolic RV filling. During this phase of the procedure, ventricular arrhythmias are common and usually self-limiting. If sustained, it should prompt either advancement into the PA or deflation of the balloon and withdrawal into the RA.

Pulmonary Artery

On crossing the pulmonary valve into the PA, an increase in the diastolic pressure should be seen in comparison to the RV, and a dicrotic notch observed representing pulmonary valve closure.

Pulmonary Artery Wedge Pressure

When the PAC is advanced further until the balloon occludes a branch of the PA, a PAWP waveform is attained. Normal wedge pressure waveforms contain the same characteristics as the RA pressure waveform (except with a delay of 150–200 ms), due to the fact that the wedged catheter tip measures left atrial pressures (LAPs) indirectly, and thus rely on the retrograde transmission of the LAP waveform.

Variations in intra-cardiac pressure tracings should be expected during the respiratory cycle and are caused by changes in intrathoracic pressure. End-expiratory pressures during both spontaneous and controlled mechanical ventilation should be used to provide the best estimates of filling pressure.

Clinical Use of Pulmonary Artery Catheters

Intra-cardiac Pressures

A PAC is a continuous pressure monitoring device that can provide useful information regarding temporal trends in intra-cardiac pressures and derived haemodynamic variables (Table 5.2.4.1). In the setting of RV failure, for example, the clinician may observe a pattern of increasing right atrial pressure (RAP) in the context of falling PA pressure. On the other hand, an increase in both RAP and PA pressure may indicate left ventricular (LV) failure, pulmonary hypertension or increased intravascular volume.

Table 5.2.4.1 Measured and derived variables obtained using pulmonary artery catheters

Measured variables			
Pressure variables	Reference range	**Derived variables**	Reference range
CVP/RA	2–6 mmHg	SV	60–100 ml
RV systolic	15–30 mmHg	SVI	33–47 ml/m^2
RV diastolic	0–5 mmHg	SVR	900–1200 dyne s/cm^5
PA systolic	15–30 mmHg	SVRI	1600–2400 dyne s/(cm^5 m^2)
PA diastolic	6–15 mmHg	PVR	80–120 dyne s/cm^5
PA mean	10–20 mmHg	PVRI	255–285 dyne s/(cm^5 m^2)
PA wedge	4–12 mmHg	Cardiac index	2.5–4 l/(min m^2)
Other variables			
SvO$_2$	65–75%		
Cardiac output	4–8 l/min		
Core temperature	36.5–37.5°C		

Abbreviations: CVP = central venous pressure; RA = right atrium; RV = right ventricle; PA = pulmonary artery; SvO$_2$ = mixed venous oxygen saturation; SV = stroke volume; SVI = stroke volume index; SVR = systemic vascular resistance; SVRI = systemic vascular resistance index; PVR = pulmonary vascular resistance; PVRI = pulmonary vascular resistance index.

Cardiac output

Thermodilution

Intermittent CO measurements can be obtained by creating temperature versus time washout curves in response to the injection of a bolus of room-temperature saline into the proximal RA port. As the blood passes the thermistor near the catheter tip in the PA, the decrease in temperature is measured and is inversely proportional to RV output. This may be equated to systemic CO if there is no intra-cardiac shunting or significant tricuspid regurgitation present.

Continuous Cardiac Output Monitoring

Some PACs use a heating filament attached at approximately 20 cm from the tip to warm the blood in the RA and RV. The resultant temperature change is sensed by the thermistor near the tip, and a warm thermodilution washout curve is used to calculate the CO.

Mixed Venous Oxygen Saturation

Many PACs now incorporate fibreoptic technology that allows monitoring of SvO_2 using reflectance oximetry. Sampling from the PA versus that from the RA, or central venous blood, is more accurate as it also incorporates coronary venous blood, which has a lower oxygen saturation due to higher myocardial oxygen extraction.

Other

PACs can also be used as multi-lumen infusion ports, and some provide atrial and ventricular pacing functions.

Complications

- Venous cannulation:
  - Bleeding
  - Pneumothorax
  - Haemothorax
  - Nerve injury
  - Infection
  - Venous thromboembolism
  - Venous air embolism
- PAC placement/manipulation:
  - Arrhythmias
  - Mechanical damage to the valves, RA, RV or PA
  - If wedged, continuous risk of pulmonary infarction or PA rupture
  - Knotting/kinking of the catheter. The PAC should not be advanced >10–15 cm without a change in the pressure waveform
  - Thrombosis
  - Infection
- Errors in monitoring:
  - Data misinterpretation and inappropriate management
  - PAWP not accurately reflecting LV filling pressure
    - Mitral stenosis/regurgitation
    - Left atrial myxoma
    - Pulmonary veno-occlusive disease
    - Cardiac tamponade

References and Further Reading

American Society of Anesthesiologists Task Force on Pulmonary Artery Catheterization. Practice guidelines for pulmonary artery catheterization: an updated report by the American Society of Anesthesiologists Task Force on Pulmonary Artery Catheterization. *Anesthesiology* 2003;**99**:988–1014.

Harvey S, Young D, Brampton W, *et al.* Pulmonary artery catheters for adult patients in intensive care. *Cochrane Database Syst Rev* 2006;**3**:CD003408.

Ikuta K, Wang Y, Robinson A, *et al.* National trends in use and outcomes of pulmonary artery catheters among Medicare beneficiaries, 1999–2013. *JAMA Cardiol* 2017;**2**:908–13.

Rajaram SS, Desai NK, Kalra A, *et al.* Pulmonary artery catheters for adult patients in intensive care. *Cochrane Database Syst Rev* 2013;**2**:CD003408.

Whitener S, Konoske R, Mark JB. Pulmonary artery catheter. *Best Pract Res Clin Anaesthesiol* 2014;**28**:323–35.

5.2.5 Principles of Defibrillation and Cardioversion

Jonny Coppel

Key Learning Points

1. Biphasic waveform defibrillators are used to depolarise cardiac muscle to restart the normal pacemaker functions of cardiac tissues.
2. Delays in defibrillation drastically reduce the chances of a successful outcome.
3. Communication and minimising peri-shock pauses are key to successful defibrillation.
4. Energy level settings should be determined by the manufacturer's instructions on a local machine.
5. Synchronised cardioversion can be used for arrhythmias with adverse features, with different initial energy settings being used for different types of arrhythmias.

Keywords: defibrillation, cardioversion, pad positioning, cardiac arrest

Introduction

The aim of defibrillation and cardioversion is to depolarise a sufficient mass of cardiac muscle simultaneously, enabling the sino-atrial node to resume automated control. Current defibrillators use biphasic, rather than monophasic, waveforms. The waveform describes the change of current flow over time during the defibrillation shock. In biphasic waveforms, the current passes from one electrode to another, and then back again once polarity reversal occurs. This is preferable to monophasic waveforms as lower energies are required for effective defibrillation.

Pad Positions

The order of positive and negative electrodes is not important. The chest must be dry, and jewellery and drug patches should be removed. No electrodes should be placed over breast tissue, and they must be at least four fingerbreadths away from an implantable cardioverter–defibrillator (ICD). The optimum position of the defibrillation pads is sternal–apical – one electrode is placed to the right of the sternum below the clavicle, the other in the V6 position. Alternative positions include:

1. **Bi-axillary position:** pads are placed on both lateral chest walls. This is useful in hairy chests
2. **Apico-posterior position:** one electrode is in the standard apical position, and the other is on the right upper back
3. **Anterior–posterior position:** one pad is placed anteriorly over the left precordium, and the other is posterior to the heart, just inferior to the left scapula. This is recommended for synchronised cardioversion of atrial fibrillation and atrial flutter.

Internal defibrillation can be used in certain circumstances where low-energy shocks can be delivered directly to the ventricles.

Defibrillation

Defibrillation is used to cardiovert ventricular fibrillation (VF) or pulseless ventricular tachycardia (pVT) in cardiac arrests. They are the most common initial rhythm in sudden cardiac arrest and carry a better prognosis than pulseless electrical activity (PEA) or asytole. Any delay in defibrillation for these rhythms reduces the patient's chance of survival by 7–10 per cent with every minute of delay, and the likelihood of a shockable first rhythm is highly correlated with the time of first rhythm analysis. Even if a shock is effective, there will still be a delay in recovery to a perfusing rhythm – hence, cardiopulmonary resuscitation (CPR) is essential until the next rhythm check.

Summary of Defibrillation Protocol in Advanced Life Support

During an arrest, once a defibrillator is set up and the pads are positioned, a quick look is carried out to assess the heart rhythm. If VF or pVT is noted, CPR is resumed whilst charging of the defibrillator occurs. Whilst charging, oxygen is removed (see below) and everyone, apart from the CPR provider, steps away from the patient. A shock is delivered immediately after the defibrillator is charged and the area is considered safe. CPR is immediately resumed, and the rhythm is checked at the end of the CPR cycle.

Optimising Defibrillation

Communication from both the arrest leader and the defibrillator operator to the rest of the team is key to safe and efficient defibrillation. It is important to emphasise that the quality of defibrillation is only as good as the quality of the CPR supporting it. The resuscitation leaders should ensure that CPR is stopped as close to defibrillation as is safe, and that it is resumed as quickly as possible after defibrillation. Every 5-second increase in pre-shock pauses almost halves the chance of successful defibrillation.

Oxygen

If oxygen is being delivered by a mask, remove the mask from the patient to a distance of at least 1 m away. If the patient has an endotracheal tube or a supraglottic airway device *in situ*, there is no increase in oxygen concentration in the zone of defibrillation, and so they do not need to be removed for the purposes of defibrillation.

Drugs in Defibrillation

When managing VF or pVT, 1 mg of adrenaline intravenously (IV) and 300 mg of amiodarone IV are administered after the third shock, with adrenaline being given after alternate shocks thereafter. Vascular access and drug administration should not delay CPR or defibrillation.

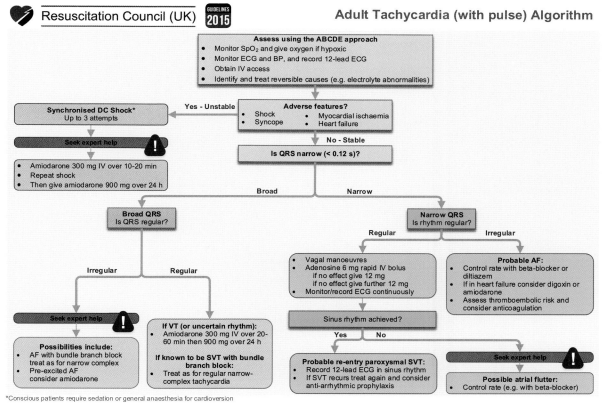

Figure 5.2.5.1 Adult tachycardia algorithm.

Energy Levels

For specific energy levels, you must refer to your local trust guidelines and to the manufacturer's instructions on your unit's defibrillator. As a general rule, the first shock should be of at least 150 J. In the future, in order to compensate for differences in chest wall impedance, there may be a move to use current, rather than energy, to guide defibrillation.

Implantable Cardioverter–Defibrillators

If an ICD is present but has failed to terminate an arrhythmia, continue normal ALS protocols whilst adjusting pad positioning as above. ICDs can unhelpfully discharge large numbers of shocks. Therefore, deactivation of the ICD by placing a magnet over it may be helpful. If return of spontaneous circulation (ROSC) is achieved, the functioning of the ICD, or any other implanted device, must be checked.

Cardioversion outside the Cardiac Arrest Situation

Outside the cardiac arrest situation, tachy- or brady-arrhythmias with associated adverse features (shock, syncope, heart failure, myocardial infarction) can be electrically cardioverted to normal sinus rhythm (Figures 5.2.5.1 and 5.2.5.2). Conscious patients should

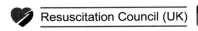 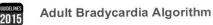

Figure 5.2.5.2 Adult bradycardia algorithm.

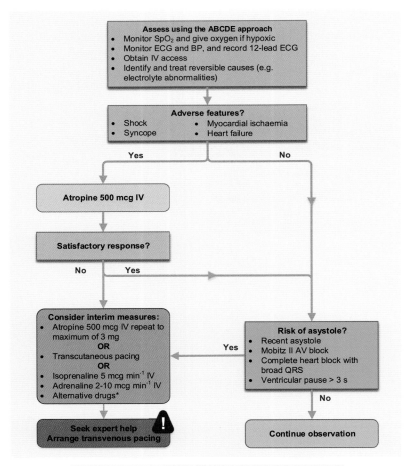

be anaesthetised or sedated when delivering the shock, though this is precarious in an unstable patient and an expert opinion should be sought. The cardioversion is synchronised, so that the shock is delivered during the peak of the QRS complex, in order to avoid delivering the shock when the ventricles are repolarising. If the latter occurs, there is a high chance of developing VF. There is often a delay between pressing the 'shock' button and the discharge, due to synchronisation. If synchronisation fails, choose another lead on the defibrillator and consider adjusting the amplitude. For a broad complex tachycardia or atrial fibrillation, start with 120–150 J and increase in increments if this fails. Atrial flutter and regular narrow complex tachycardia will often terminate with lower-energy shocks – start with 70–120 J. If three synchronized shocks fail to terminate the arrhythmia, give 300 mg of amiodarone IV over 10–20 minutes, then repeat the shock. A further 900 mg of amiodarone should be given over 24 hours.

Synchronised cardioversion is also indicated in an elective setting for converting some stable tachyarrhythmias resistant to pharmacological cardioversion. This is not discussed in this chapter.

Complications

Serious complications from cardioversion include VF, thromboembolisation and myocardial necrosis.

ST-segment elevation can be seen immediately after cardioversion and lasts for 1–2 minutes. If longer than 2 minutes, suspect myocardial injury.

References and Further Reading

European Society of Cardiology (ESC); European Heart Rhythm Association (EHRA); Brignole M, Auricchio A, Baron-Esquivias G, *et al.* 2013 ESC guidelines on cardiac pacing and cardiac resynchronization therapy: the task force on cardiac pacing and resynchronization therapy of the European Society of Cardiology (ESC). Developed in collaboration with the European Heart Rhythm Association (EHRA). *Europace* 2013;**15**: 1070–118.

Morrison LJ, Henry RM, Ku V, *et al.* Single-shock defibrillation success in adult cardiac arrest: a systematic review. *Resuscitation* 2013;**84**: 1480–6.

Nichol G, Sayre MR, Guerra F, Poole J. Defibrillation for ventricular fibrillation. *J Am Coll Cardiol* 2017;**70**:1496–509.

Resuscitation Council UK. Advanced Life Support, 7th edn. London: Resuscitation Council UK; 2016.

Soar J, Nolan JP, Bottiger BW, *et al.* European Resuscitation Council Guidelines for Resuscitation 2015 Section 3. Adult advanced life support. *Resuscitation* 2015;**95**:99–146.

5.2.6 Cardiac Pacing, Implantable Cardioverter–Defibrillators and Cardiac Resynchronisation Therapy

Edward Rintoul and Jeff Phillips

Key Learning Points

1. Knowledge of reason for insertion, functions and pacing location is essential for treating patients with a permanent pacemaker, especially if device malfunction is suspected.
2. When managing temporary pacing solutions, the minimum voltage should be at least double the capture threshold.
3. All implantable cardioverter–defibrillators (ICDs) have full pacemaker capabilities.
4. Magnets will turn off all anti-tachycardia therapies from an ICD, but not anti-bradycardia pacing.
5. External defibrillator pads must be connected if ICD therapies are turned off.

Keywords: pacemaker, temporary venous pacing, internal cardiac defibrillator

Introduction

Devices that may be encountered in the intensive care environment can be classified as either temporary or permanent transvenous, or miscellaneous.

Temporary

Transvenous right ventricular (RV) pacing is commonly inserted for acute symptomatic bradycardia (particularly third-degree heart block) in order to rapidly restore the heart rate. Transcutaneous external pacing may be required as an emergency bridging technique. However, the efficacy is variable and sedation is required.

Epicardial pacing is classically used post-cardiac surgery and involves attaching epicardial wires to the right atrium (RA) or right ventricle (RV), or both. Pacing wires are secured to the heart muscle under direct vision during surgery, and are subsequently removed after 4–5 days. Atrial wires provide haemodynamically superior pacing as A–V synchrony is preserved. However, the risk of cardiac tamponade on removal from the thin-walled chamber is higher, as compared to ventricular wires. They are of no use in atrial fibrillation where the intrinsic atrial rate is over 300/min, as the atrium is refractory to pacing and atrial pacing alone will fail if heart blocks exist post-surgery.

Permanent Transvenous

Permanent pacemaker (PPM) use is on the rise, with over 900 per million population inserted in England and Wales alike for 2015–2016. Venous access is usually attained via the left cephalic or axillary vein. The lead(s) are positioned endocardially (usually with a screw mechanism), and the proximal ends attached to a generator placed subcutaneously in an infra-clavicular pocket.

PPMs can be RA or RV, or both. They are used predominantly for heart blocks and sick sinus syndrome. Whilst sick sinus syndrome can be treated by an atrial lead only, atrioventricular (AV) node disease can follow, so RA and RV leads are usually used. As with temporary systems, permanent atrial fibrillation is a contraindication to atrial pacing wires. Importantly, long-term RV pacing can adversely affect systolic function.

Implantable cardioverter–defibrillators (ICDs) have the ability to deliver a shock in the event of ventricular arrhythmia, and the circuit is between the shock coil(s) on the RV lead and the ICD generator. Heart rate and additional algorithms determine malignant arrhythmias and treat with anti-tachycardia (overdrive) pacing, cardioversion or defibrillation. Overdrive pacing is successful in 70–90 per cent of ventricular tachycardias, requires less battery usage and is better tolerated by patients.

Cardiac resynchronisation therapy (CRT) involves biventricular pacing ± RA pacing. CRT is used for patients with impaired left ventricular (LV) systolic function, typically with ejection fraction <35 per cent and left bundle branch block. The purpose is to improve heart failure status and reverse LV remodelling by producing a more coordinated ventricular contraction. Therefore, these patients may not have a standard bradycardia indication for pacing. The left ventricle (LV) is paced from a lead positioned in the coronary sinus via the RA. Cardiac resynchronisation can be combined with a defibrillator (CRT-D) or used for pacing only (CRT-P). CRT-P is used in New York Heart Association (NYHA) IV patients in whom the risk of multiple shocks is high and quality of life often poor. The full list of indications for ICDs and CRT can be found in the National Institute for Health and Care Excellence (NICE) guidelines 2014 referenced further below.

Miscellaneous

A subcutaneous ICD and lead (S-ICD) is useful when a transvenous approach would be challenging. The shock coil is tunnelled subcutaneously along the sternal edge, and the box is placed in the left sub-axillary region. It can administer an 80-J shock but is limited by no overdrive pacing and no anti-bradycardia pacing (except post-shock pacing, which can be uncomfortable).

Leadless pacemakers are small bullet-shaped generators placed directly in the right ventricular (RV) wall indicated for patients with anatomically unsuitable veins.

Implantable loop recorders are subcutaneous cardiac rhythm monitors used in those with unexplained syncope or palpitations.

Each of the above devices can be confidently identified on a postero-anterior (P-A) chest X-ray.

Basic Pacing Concepts – Sensing and Capture

Permanent pacing systems will only be programmable by pacing specialists. However, the intensivist may have to recognise and change temporary pacemakers; thus, an understanding of function and terms is required. The two principal functions of a pacemaker are to:

1. Identify when the intrinsic heart rate falls below the lower rate limit or 'base rate' of the pacemaker, and

2. Successfully pace the relevant cardiac chamber when this occurs.

The first of these requires detection of the heart's intrinsic activity, known as 'sensing', and the second requires the delivered impulse to initiate depolarisation, known as 'capture'.

- **Threshold.** This is the minimum energy (in volts) required to reliably achieve capture. This is tested by pacing the chamber whilst reducing the voltage until a pacing spike is visible without a subsequent QRS complex ('loss of capture'). The minimum voltage required to achieve capture is the threshold value. The programmed output should be at least double the threshold.

- **Sensing.** This requires detection of relevant cardiac signals (e.g. the R wave), whilst others (e.g. T wave) are ignored. To do this, the device uses a high pass filter where only signals above a certain amplitude are registered. The upper limit of this filter is referred to as the device *sensitivity* (in millivolts). If the sensitivity value is too high, then relevant signals will be undetected and the device will pace inappropriately (under-sensing). This can cause pacing on T waves which is arrhythmogenic. If the sensitivity value is too low, then relevant signals will be recognised, but so too will extraneous ones. Pacing will thus be inappropriately inhibited (over-sensing), resulting in haemodynamic compromise if the patient's underlying rhythm is profound bradycardia. The programmed sensitivity should be no more than half of the QRS amplitude, and lead testing should include measurement of the intrinsic QRS signal so the sensitivity can be adjusted accordingly.

Modes of Operation

A pacemaker's mode of operation is denoted by a five-letter code (Table 5.2.6.1):

- **Position I** refers to the chamber paced.
- **Position II** refers to the chamber sensed.
- **Position III** refers to the pacemaker's response to sensed activity.
  - 'Inhibited' means that sensing in one chamber will suppress pacing in that chamber (e.g. if an R wave is sensed, then RV pacing will be inhibited).
  - 'Triggered' activity usually means sensing in one chamber will trigger pacing in the other. This is best demonstrated by A-sense V-pace – a sinus P wave is sensed in the atrium which then triggers ventricular pacing.

581

Table 5.2.6.1 Revised NASPE/BPEG generic code for pacemakers 2002

Position	I	II	III	IV	V
Category	Chamber(s) paced	Chamber(s) sensed	Response to sensing	Rate modulation	Multi-site pacing
	O = none	O = none	O = none	O = none	O = none
	A = atrium	A = atrium	T = triggered	R = rate modulation	A = atrium
	V = ventricle	V = ventricle	I = inhibited		V = ventricle
	D = dual (A + V)	D = dual (A + V)	D = dual (T + I)		D = dual (A + V)

Abbreviations: NASPE = North American Society of Pacing and Electrophysiology; BPEG = British Pacing and Electrophysiology Group.

- **Position IV** is a programmable feature that allows paced rate to be modulated according to patient activity.
- **Position V** predominantly refers to pacing simultaneously from two locations on an LV lead, as no bi-atrial systems exist commercially.

Management of Temporary Systems in the ICU

It is important to recognise if the pacing mode is appropriate for the hardware *in situ* and the patient's needs. For example, the DDD mode is always incorrect if there is only one pacing lead, and atrial pacing will be ineffective during atrial fibrillation. When interrogating devices, it is preferable to do so with patients in bed, as marked bradycardia can occur during testing which may cause haemodynamic compromise. All temporary systems should show a live display of device function (i.e. A-pacing/sensing, V-pacing/sensing) and it is not advisable to check underlying activity simply by pausing pacing, although this function does exist on some temporary pacing boxes. If pacing is occurring, then the base rate can be gradually lowered to see if the underlying rhythm emerges (as long as the patient is stable). Rhythm and ST changes can then be assessed, and a 12-lead ECG done.

Management of Permanent Systems in the ICU

The first consideration is whether the device is directly related to the patient's admission to the ICU. This is more likely in CRT and ICD patients, as the cardiovascular risks will already be higher. Advice from the pacing department is essential when interrogating the device, and the most recent follow-up documentation should be sought (which may be a challenge if done in another institution). There are five common device manufacturers, and the make should be communicated to the pacing team as each company has a different portable programmer. Pacing reports will provide information on pacing dependence, underlying pathology and implantation date, estimated battery life, mode programmed, sensing and capturing thresholds and arrhythmia history. ICD reports will also include therapies delivered for ventricular arrhythmias.

ICD therapies can be disabled by a pacing specialist using a portable programmer, and this may be necessary for procedures where noise may be detected by the device (e.g. diathermy). It may also be appropriate during resuscitation or if management of the patient becomes palliative. A magnet placed over the device generator will also inhibit anti-tachycardia therapies of an ICD but has no effect on bradycardia pacing. On removal of the magnet, therapies should be reactivated, but it is advisable to request a device check by a specialist.

When ICD therapies are switched off, ECG monitoring and external defibrillator pads must be used (positioned away from the ICD generator), as these patients are at high risk of ventricular arrhythmias. Central venous access may be challenging in those with cardiac devices, and guidewires may irritate the ventricle which can precipitate ventricular arrhythmias.

Magnets placed on PPM generators cause the device to switch to an asynchronous or 'fixed' pacing mode, e.g. VOO/DOO (depending on the device), though again normal function should resume when the magnet is removed. This can be useful if the patient has no underlying electrical activity and the device is over-sensing. However, placement of a magnet is not a benign event and if the patient has intrinsic activity, the 'magnet mode' can cause AV dyssynchrony or pacing on T waves.

References and Further Reading

Glikson M, Cosedis Nielsen J, Kronborg MB, *et al.*; ESC Scientific Document Group. ESC Guidelines on cardiac pacing and cardiac resynchronization therapy: developed by the Task Force on cardiac pacing and cardiac resynchronization therapy of the European Society of Cardiology (ESC). With the special contribution of the European Heart Rhythm Association (EHRA). *Eur Heart J* 2021;**42**:3427–520.

Holzmeister J, Leclercq C. Implantable cardioverter defibrillators and cardiac resynchronisation therapy. *Lancet* 2011;**378**:722–30.

National Institute for Health and Care Excellence. 2014. Implantable cardioverter defibrillators and cardiac resynchronisation therapy for arrhythmias and heart failure (review of TA95 and TA120). www.nice.org.uk/guidance/ta314/documents/arrythmias-icds-heart-failure-cardiac-resynchronisation-fad-document2

National Institute for Health and Care Excellence. 2014. Implantable cardioverter defibrillators and cardiac resynchronisation therapy for arrhythmias and heart failure. www.nice.org.uk/guidance/ta314

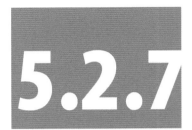

Needle Pericardiocentesis in Intensive Care

Peter Remeta

Key Learning Points

1. Cardiac tamponade is a life-threatening condition resulting from compression of the heart by accumulating fluid, blood, clots or pus within the pericardium.
2. The clinical picture is one of obstructive shock, characterised by equalisation of intra-cardiac pressures.
3. The amount of fluid required to cause cardiac tamponade varies and depends on the speed of accumulation, compliance of the pericardium and volume of fluid.
4. In a patient with clinical suspicion of tamponade, echocardiography is recommended as the first imaging technique to assess the size, location and haemodynamic impact of the pericardial effusion.
5. Cardiac tamponade is an indication for urgent pericardiocentesis or surgery.

Keywords: cardiac tamponade, pericardium, pericardiocentesis, echocardiography

Pathophysiology of Cardiac Tamponade

The pericardium is a relatively rigid sack. It contains up to 50 ml of pericardial fluid, which acts as a lubricant between the pericardial layers. A pericardial effusion can be classified by the:

- Time of onset: acute, subacute or chronic (when lasting >3 months)
- Distribution: circumferential or loculated
- Size: mild (<10 mm), moderate (10–20 mm) or large (>20 mm)
- Composition: exudate, transudate, blood, rarely air or gas (from bacterial infection)

The haemodynamic consequences of pericardial fluid accumulation will depend upon the amount of accumulated fluid, rate of accumulation, and compliance of the pericardium. If fluid accumulates gradually over a long period of time, the pericardium can stretch to hold over a litre without obvious haemodynamic consequences. Conversely, small volumes (e.g. as little as 50 ml) can cause cardiovascular compromise if they accumulate rapidly or are localised (such as post-cardiac surgery). When fluid accumulates, the increase in volume within the pericardium leads to an increase in intra-pericardial pressure, a decrease in atrial and ventricular transmural gradients, a decrease in stroke volume, equalisation of pressures in the atria and ventricles and subsequent tamponade.

Aetiology of Pericardial Effusion

- Malignancy (usually secondary; primary is very rare)
- Pericarditis (bacterial, viral, fungal)
- Autoimmune disease
- Metabolic (e.g. uraemia)
- Trauma (including aortic dissection or ruptured ischaemic myocardium)
- Iatrogenic – such as interventional cardiac procedures (some studies reported up to 6 percent incidence of tamponade), central venous catheter or pulmonary artery catheter insertion and post-cardiac surgery (up to 2 per cent will develop large effusions)

Diagnosis
History

A thorough history may provide clues as to the aetiology of the tamponade. These include asking about weight loss, decrease in exercise tolerance, progressive dyspnoea, peripheral oedema, recent infection, recent surgical/medical intervention or the presence of chest pain.

Clinical Examination

A patient with a tamponading heart will often be hypotensive, tachycardic and dyspnoeic, and will demonstrate signs of progressive cardiogenic shock (mottled, cold peripheries, venous congestion) and pulsus paradoxus (conventionally defined as an inspiratory decrease in systolic arterial pressure of >10 mmHg during normal breathing). An intubated patient in the ICU, often post-cardiac surgery or following an interventional procedure, may present with progressive hypotension requiring increased vasopressor or inotropic support. The classic signs of Beck's triad (elevated jugular venous pressure, muffled heart sounds and hypotension) are reported in <50 per cent of patients.

Investigations

- **ECG:** may demonstrate small-voltage pulsus alternans
- **Bloods:** arterial blood gases may reveal lactataemia and metabolic acidosis resulting from hypoperfusion and shock
- **Central venous catheter:** may demonstrate attenuated *y*-descent, and a pulmonary artery catheter (PAC) will reveal equalisation of atrial, pulmonary artery (PA) and pulmonary capillary wedge (PCW) pressures
- **Chest X-ray:** may reveal a large cardiac silhouette if the pericardial effusion is sizeable, but it can also be negative in an acutely developing tamponade or loculated effusion
- **CT chest, angiogram:** can be diagnostic

Box 5.2.7.1 Echocardiographic Criteria of a Tamponade

- Presence of an effusion
- 'Swinging heart'
- Late diastolic right atrial collapse
- Early diastolic right ventricular collapse
- Dilated inferior vena cava
- Significant respiratory variability (>25 per cent) of mitral inflow, tricuspid inflow or aortic outflow velocities
- Respiratory variation in ventricular chamber size

- **Echocardiography:** the gold standard for diagnosis and management (Box 5.2.7.1)

Indications for Pericardiocentesis

Pericardiocentesis in the ICU will be mostly therapeutic but may be considered for the purposes of providing a diagnosis. The presence of a pericardial effusion in a patient exhibiting signs of shock does not necessarily mean they are tamponading, and the echocardiographic signs detailed above should be looked for.

Elective and urgent pericardiocentesis is normally undertaken by interventional cardiologists. However, ICU physicians may be required to perform the procedures in the emergency setting (e.g. during cardiopulmonary resuscitation (CPR) or in institutions where 24-hour cardiology cover is not available).

Contraindications of Pericardiocentesis

There are no absolute contraindications in a peri-arrest situation.

Relative contraindications include coagulopathy, operator's inexperience and a loculated/septated effusion.

If the tamponade is associated with trauma, this is an indication for resuscitative thoracotomy. If a tamponade is associated with an aortic dissection, this is an indication for surgical treatment (unless life-threatening and there is no immediate access to surgical treatment).

Procedure
General Considerations

- Patient consent (if appropriate)
- Consider risk–benefit
- Check all equipment, including resuscitation equipment
- Ensure appropriate assistance and monitoring
- Attempt aseptic procedure (as much as possible in an emergency)

Equipment

- Pericardiocentesis set (Figure 5.2.7.1). This may not be available in an emergency on all ICUs, and a single-lumen catheter, small chest drain or central venous catheter could be used instead.
- Ultrasound. The choice of transducer probe depends on operator preferences and the view

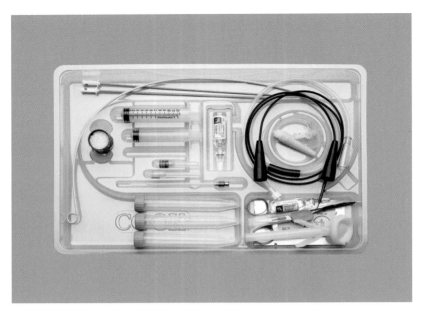

Figure 5.2.7.1 Pericardiocentesis set (Cook Medical).
Source: Permission for use granted by Cook Medical, Bloomington, Indiana.

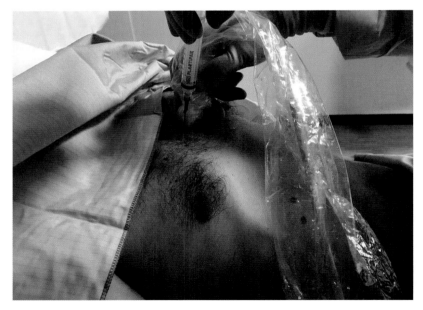

Figure 5.2.7.2 Parasternal approach.

required. It is usually a phased-array cardiac probe. A linear probe can be used for the parasternal approach, or an abdominal convex probe for subcostal views.

Technique

An ultrasound-guided real-time technique is recommended. The landmark technique may be considered when ultrasound is not available, but it has a much higher incidence of complications.

Three approaches are commonly performed and are often decided by the best view, the site of the largest collection and operator experience.

1. **Parasternal:** usually in the left fourth or fifth intercostal space, depending on the best view and the largest site of collection. Aim as close as possible to the sternum and upper border of the rib, to avoid the mammary artery (approximately 1 cm from the sternum). This approach is associated with an increased risk of pneumothorax (Figure 5.2.7.2).

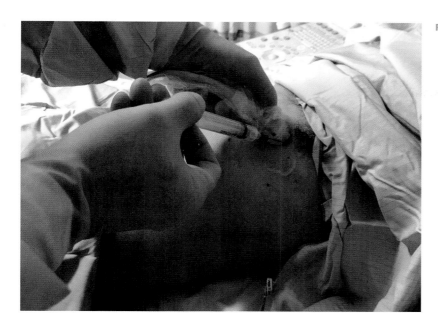

Figure 5.2.7.3 Apical approach.

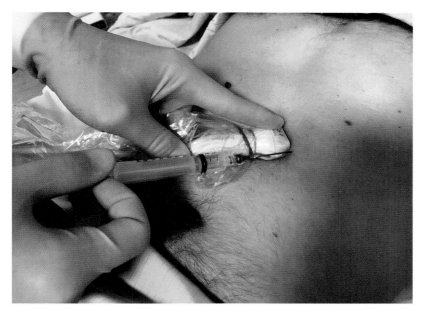

Figure 5.2.7.4 Subcostal approach.

2. **Apical:** usually in the fifth to seventh intercostal space. This approach is associated with a decreased risk of coronary injury, as vessels at the apex have the smallest diameter and it is the shortest distance from the chest wall to the pericardium (Figure 5.2.7.3).

3. **Subcostal:** the most common approach used in the past (pre-ultrasound era), and it is often accessible during CPR. It is associated with an increased risk of parenchymal injury (Figure 5.2.7.4).

Procedure

- Asepsis
- Local anaesthesia infiltration 1–2% lidocaine (if applicable)
- Insertion of needle under direct ultrasound guidance
- Confirmation of needle position with 3–4 ml of agitated saline
- Guidewire insertion – position within pericardium confirmed with ultrasound

587

- Dilation
- Drain insertion
- Securing the drain with sutures or dressing
- Drainage/staged drainage
- Sample for biochemistry, microbiology and cytology
- Consider antibiotic prophylaxis
- Chest X-ray/lung ultrasound to exclude pneumothorax
- Cardiology/cardio-surgical referral
- Echocardiographic follow-up

Complications of Pericardiocentesis

Increased use of ultrasound has made pericardiocentesis a much safer procedure. The overall reported incidence of complications is <6 per cent, with major complications accounting for <2 per cent. With the landmark technique, however, rates of major complications remain much higher at around 20 per cent.

Cardiac complications include coronary artery injury, myocardial perforation, myocardial laceration, intra-cardiac drain placement, air embolism, arrhythmia and worsening tamponade. Right ventricular failure has also been described with sudden decompression of large-volume effusions, and as such,

a staged decompression is recommended for drainage of large effusions.

Non-cardiac complications include pneumothorax, pneumopericardium, intercostal/mammary artery injury, liver injury, splenic injury and hollow viscus perforations.

References and Further Reading

Adler Y, Charron P, Imazio M, *et al*. 2015 ESC guidelines for the diagnosis and management of pericardial diseases. *Eur Heart J* 2015;**36**:2921–64.

Gluer R, Murdoch D, Haqqani HM, Scalia GM, Walters DL. Pericardiocentesis – how to do it. *Heart Lung Circ* 2015;**24**:621–5.

Holmes Jr DR, Nishimura R, Fountain R, Zoltan G. Iatrogenic pericardial effusion and tamponade in the percutaneous intracardiac intervention era. *JACC Cardiovasc Interv* 2009;**2**:705–17.

Porter TR, Shillcutt SK, Adams MS, *et al*. Guidelines for the use of echocardiography as a monitor for therapeutic intervention in adults: a report from the American Society of Echocardiography. *J Am Soc Echocardiogr* 2015;**28**:40–56.

Tsang TS, Enriquez-Sarano M, Freeman WK, *et al*. Consecutive 1127 therapeutic echocardiographically guided pericardiocenteses: clinical profile, practice patterns, and outcomes spanning 21 years. *Mayo Clinic Proc* 2002;**77**:429–36.

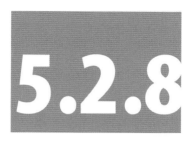

5.2.8

Cardiac Output Measurement and Interpreting the Derived Data

Charles M. Oliver

Key Learning Points

1. Cardiac output (CO) quantification is used clinically as a surrogate for tissue oxygenation in peri-operative and critical care patient management, and may be used to avoid injudicious fluid administration.

2. Devices estimate and monitor CO using the Fick principle, Doppler frequency shift and pulse pressure analysis.

3. Devices differ by invasiveness, provision of other indices and clinical information, required expertise and limitations and potential complications. Pulmonary artery catheters still remain the gold standard, but evidence supports the accuracy of other less invasive devices.

4. Selection of device is determined by the clinical setting, patient factors and clinician expertise.

5. Because CO is estimated, rather than measured directly, trends and response to interventions are more clinically meaningful than absolute values.

Keywords: cardiac output, perioperative, intensive care, clinical device, outcomes

Introduction

Cardiac output (CO) may be quantified and tracked in clinical practice using a variety of techniques and devices in order to inform therapeutic decisions, with the aim of optimising tissue oxygen delivery. Alongside CO, additional clinical information and physiological indices may be quantified and derived, the provision of which depends on the technique and device selected. Choice of the most suitable method of estimating and monitoring CO is therefore determined by the clinical setting, patient factors and clinician expertise.

Pulmonary Artery Catheters

Pulmonary artery catheters (PACs) are balloon-tipped, multi-lumen intravascular catheters (Figure 5.2.8.1). Flow-guided flotation of the catheter tip through the right heart permits CO quantification by means of dilution modelling, a derivation of the Fick principle. This is now most commonly performed using thermo-dilution, whereby the rate of change of temperature between blood in the right atrium and a pulmonary artery is measured by a thermistor sited at the catheter tip. Thermodilution is performed either by injecting a bolus of 4°C dextrose 30 cm proximal to the thermistor or by use of a continuously heated filament proximal to the thermistor (Figure 5.2.8.1).

CO can then be derived mathematically from the generated area under the curve (AUC) using a modified Stewart–Hamilton equation (Equation 5.2.8.1):

$$CO = \frac{\left[V \left(T_B - T_I \right) K_1 K_2 \right]}{\left[T_B(t)dt \right]} \qquad (5.2.8.1)$$

Where V = injectate volume

T_B = distal blood temperature

T_I = injectate temperature

K_1 and K_2 = mathematical constants

$T_B(t)$dt = the integral of blood temperature change

Dilution modelling using a PAC remains the gold standard method for cardiac output monitoring (COM), against which other techniques and devices are assessed. Advantages over other methods include the ability to directly measure right heart parameters, estimate left atrial filling pressure and quantify mixed venous oxygen saturation (using photometry), and provision of central venous access. However, pathologies, including tricuspid regurgitation and intra-cardiac shunts, may result in inaccurate CO estimation, and concern over potential risk of harm has resulted in a steep decline in their use outside specialist centres in recent decades.

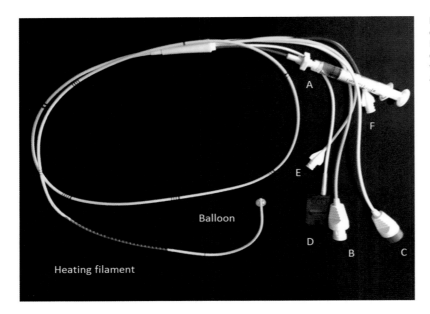

Figure 5.2.8.1 Pulmonary artery catheter. Connectors: A, balloon inflation; B, thermistor; C, heating filament; D, continuous oximetry; E, distal (right ventricular) injectate port; F, proximal (right atrial) injectate port.

Transoesophageal Echocardiography

Stroke volume (SV) through the left ventricular out-flow tract may be estimated, and CO then calculated by inbuilt software in contemporary transoesophageal echocardiography (TOE) machines. Advantages of TOE are that it also provides a vast array of dynamic information that may guide peri-operative and critical care management, including delineating causes of hypotension and quantifying treatment response. However, the requirement for an expert operator and the intermittent nature of CO estimation using this technique limit the clinical application of TOE for COM, even in specialist centres.

Doppler Devices

These devices utilise the Doppler equation with the Doppler frequency shift to quantify the velocity of blood flow in the descending aorta (Equation 5.2.8.2). This is commonly performed using an oesophageal 4-MHz continuous-wave ultrasound probe containing an array of adjacent emitting and receiving piezoelectric crystals. The change in frequency of waves reflected by moving blood cells is transformed using fast Fourier analysis to provide beat-by-beat estimates of velocity (stroke distance) using the Doppler equation:

$$V = \frac{c. \Delta f}{2 f_o. \cos\theta} \qquad 5.2.8.2$$

Where V = blood flow velocity

  c = speed of sound in body tissue (=1540 m/s)

  Δf = the frequency shift

  f_o = the emitted frequency

  θ = the incident angle.

A nomogram of population-averaged cross-sectional aortic areas is then referenced in order to estimate the volume of a column of blood, which is then used to estimate SV. Additional indices that may be estimated or derived include peak blood velocity (PV) and corrected flow time (FTc) available with CardioQ™, which may be interpreted as markers of left ventricular contractility and the balance between intravascular filling and vasomotor tone, respectively.

Accuracy of these parameters is reliant upon probe positioning (including minimising θ) and is influenced by physiological, surgical and pathological factors altering the proportion of left ventricular output conveyed through the thoracic descending aorta from 70 per cent. Aortic diameter values are not validated outside the following populations: age 16–99 years; height 149–212 cm and weight 30–150 kg (66–330 lb).

Pulse Pressure Analysis

Pulse pressure analysis COM devices analyse transduced arterial pressure waveforms, accessed via an indwelling arterial cannula. Proprietary algorithms are used to convert the transduced pressure–time function of the waveform into a volume–time function in order to estimate CO.

A host of devices exist, which are further differentiated by the required anatomical locations of arterial and venous cannulae, provision of additional physiological indices and use of dilution methods to calibrate pressure–volume conversion. PiCCO® and VolumeView™ require cannulation of a central vein and the femoral or brachial artery using proprietary catheters, whereas with LiDCO™, the location of arterial and venous cannulae is not restricted. These three devices use dilution techniques to calibrate arterial pressure waveforms against CO estimates (PiCCO and VolumeView use ice-cold water, and LiDCO uses lithium chloride), and repeat calibration is required periodically and in the presence of changes in systemic vascular compliance. Other devices, including Vigileo™ and LiDCOrapid®, estimate CO from pulse pressure waveforms without calibration against dilution-derived CO estimates.

Due to assumptions made by the algorithms used, CO estimates become unreliable in the presence of non-physiological or variable waveforms encountered in aortic valve pathologies, dysrhythmias, high-dose vasopressor use or mechanical assist devices. Uncalibrated estimates are unlikely to be sufficiently accurate to guide clinical decision-making in these clinical scenarios and calibrated estimates may need to be interpreted with caution.

Non-invasive Techniques

Two techniques can be used to continuously, but non-invasively, measure arterial blood pressure: applanation tonometry and the volume clamp. The 'volume clamp' used in Edwards' ClearSight™ is housed in a finger cuff. This closed-loop technique measures (at 1000 Hz) and maintains finger artery diameter at a constant value by means of an inflatable bladder. Arterial blood pressure may then be continuously, but non-invasively, measured. Derived parameters include CO, SV, stroke volume variation (SVV) and systemic vascular resistance (SVR).

Research Tools

Other methods of CO estimation include thoracic bio-impedance and bio-reactance, carbon dioxide rebreathing and suprasternal Doppler estimation.

References and Further Reading

Cecconi M, Dawson D, Casaretti R, Grounds RM, Rhodes A. A prospective study of the accuracy and precision of continuous cardiac output monitoring devices as compared to intermittent thermodilution. *Minerva Anestesiol* 2010;**76**:1010–17.

Reisner A. Academic assessment of arterial pulse contour analysis: missing the forest for the trees? *Br J Anaesth* 2016;**116**:733–6.

Sandham JD, Hull RD, Brant RF, *et al.* A randomized, controlled trial of the use of pulmonary-artery catheters in high-risk surgical patients. *N Engl J Med* 2003;**348**:5–14.

Vincent JL, Pelosi P, Pearse R, *et al.* Perioperative cardiovascular monitoring of high-risk patients: a consensus of 12. *Crit Care* 2015;**19**:224.

5.2.9

Echocardiography in Intensive Care

Andrew P. Walden and Karim Fouad Alber

Key Learning Points

1. Focussed echocardiography in the intensive care unit enables the physician to integrate echocardiographic findings as an extension of the clinical history and examination.
2. Ideally there are five views that should be assessed when performing a focussed intensive care echocardiography (FICE) scan.
3. The aim should be to acquire at least two acceptable views in order to confirm consistency in findings and avoid making judgements based on a single view that may have produced a spurious result.
4. The essence of FICE is for it to be utilised as a dichotomous decision-making tool designed to answer a series of questions in a patient with cardiovascular shock.
5. Common pathologies identified include dilated left ventricle, dilated right ventricle, hypovolaemia, pericardial effusion and pleural effusions.

Keywords: FICE, focussed echo, echocardiography, point-of-care ultrasound, POCUS

Introduction

Focussed echocardiography differs from department-based echocardiography in that it is designed to answer specific questions about the aetiology of cardiovascular shock and cardiac arrest. In the UK, the two main systematic approaches are focussed intensive care echocardiography (FICE) and focussed echocardiography in emergency life support (FEEL). Both FEEL and FICE use a binary protocol-driven approach to detect pathology. FICE is an accredited scanning

technique utilised in the ICU. It is important to understand the limitations of focussed echocardiography. It is not a substitute for full departmental echocardiography and is not used to diagnose valvular heart conditions or endocarditis. Where abnormalities beyond the scope of focussed echocardiography are found, one of the key recommendations is to refer on for a formal echocardiogram.

Focussed echocardiography in the ICU enables the physician to integrate echocardiographic findings as an extension of the clinical history and examination. Integrating this diagnostic test into the patient pathway ensures action as a result of the investigation without delay and also allows clinicians to monitor response to treatments such as administration of a fluid bolus. Without FICE, it is possible to embark on a course of treatment which may worsen a patient's condition. For example, over-resuscitation with fluid can often lead to right ventricular (RV) dilation, with a fall in cardiac output and renal capsule oedema, resulting in worsening renal function. This is easily identified using FICE. A FICE scan should be performed in any patient who has shock with or without a requirement for inotropes or vasopressors.

Lead placement and FICE views

ECG electrodes are attached to the patient for the duration of the scan to allow timing of the cardiac cycle (Figure 5.2.9.1).

Ideally there are five views that should be assessed when performing a FICE scan. The five views are:

1. Parasternal long axis
2. Parasternal short axis
3. Apical four-chamber view
4. Subcostal four-chamber view, with additional views of the inferior vena cava (to help with fluid status assessment)
5. Lung bases (to exclude pleural effusions)

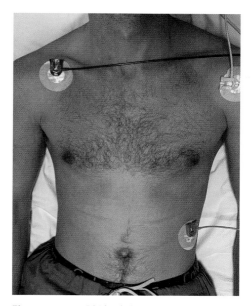

Figure 5.2.9.1 ECG lead placement.

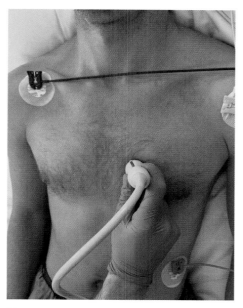

Figure 5.2.9.2 Parasternal long axis (PLAX).

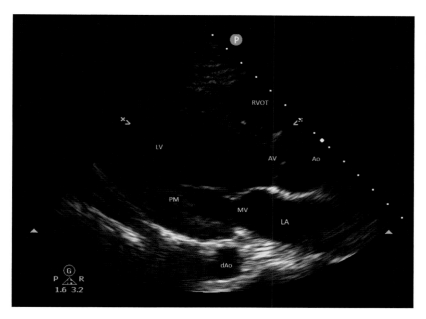

Figure 5.2.9.3 Parasternal long axis echocardiographic image. LA = left atrium; MV = mitral valve; PM = papillary muscle; LV = left ventricle; AV = aortic valve; Ao = aorta; RVOT = right ventricular outflow tract; dAo = descending aorta.

Parasternal Long Axis View

The probe is placed on left sternal edge, between the second and fourth intercostal spaces. The probe marker should be aiming towards the right shoulder. Examples of parasternal long axis views may be seen in Figures 5.2.9.2 and 5.2.9.3.

Parasternal Short Axis View

Rotate the probe clockwise 90°, with the marker aiming towards the left shoulder. Examples of parasternal short axis views may be seen in Figures 5.2.9.4 and 5.2.9.5.

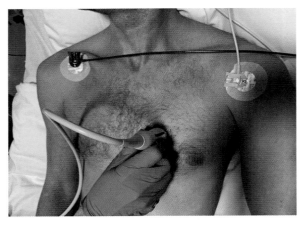

Figure 5.2.9.4 Parasternal short axis (PSAX).

Apical Four-Chamber View

The probe position is at the position of the apical impulse, with the probe marker aimed towards the left axilla. It often helps to position the patient in a left lateral position, with their left arm behind their head, in order to improve the sonographic window. Examples of apical four-chamber views may be seen in Figures 5.2.9.6 and 5.2.9.7.

The interventricular septum should be aligned vertically and both atrioventricular valves should be visible.

Subcostal Views

Position the patient supine. Hold the probe from above and place it below the xiphisternum, with the probe marker facing the patient's left. Warn the patient and proceed to apply gentle pressure to allow the probe to acquire an acoustic window beneath the ribcage. It can help to ask the patient to bend their knees in order to relax their abdominal muscles. Examples of subcostal four-chamber views may be seen in Figures 5.2.9.8 and 5.2.9.9.

Note the liver provides a good acoustic window. This view is often the quickest and most accessible in a cardiac arrest/peri-arrest scenario.

Whilst in the subcostal position, bring the right atrium into the middle of the view and rotate the probe 90° anti-clockwise to visualise the inferior vena cava (IVC) (Figure 5.2.9.10).

The inferior vena cava in the subcostal view can be visualised in B-mode ('brightness') (Figure 5.2.9.11), and in M-mode ('motion') (Figure 5.2.9.12).

The M-mode allows for high time resolution at the chosen ultrasound line for assessment of IVC variability.

The probe is positioned laterally/posterolaterally at the interface between the lung/diaphragm and the spleen/liver. Further assessment of a pleural effusion is often done more easily using a curvilinear probe, rather than using the phased-array probe. Lung bases may be seen in Figure 5.2.9.13.

The Essence of FICE

In practice, it may not be possible to always acquire all the views. This may be because the patient's anatomy does not provide favourable views, but

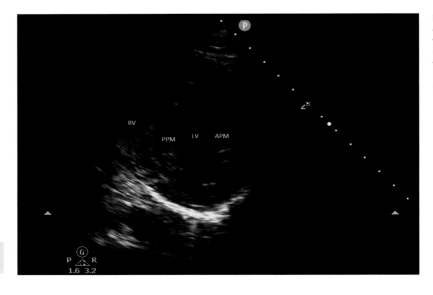

Figure 5.2.9.5 Parasternal short axis echocardiographic image with the left ventricle at the mid-papillary muscle level (right ventricle not fully visible). LV = left ventricle; PPM = postero-medial papillary muscle; APM = anterolateral papillary muscle; RV = right ventricle.

(a)

(b)

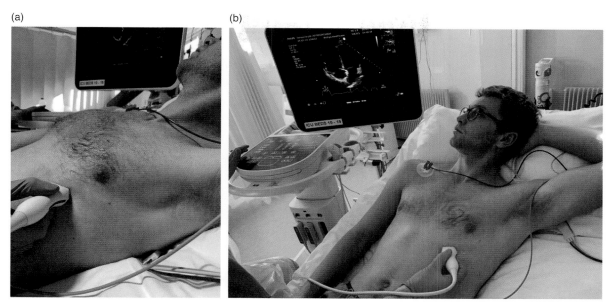

Figure 5.2.9.6 Apical four-chamber (A4Ch).

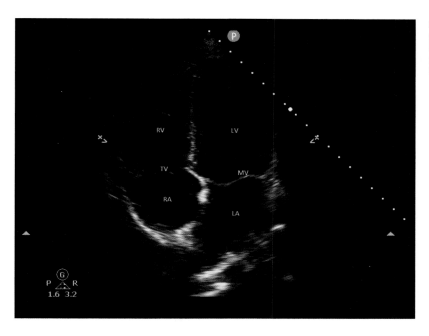

Figure 5.2.9.7 Apical four-chamber echocardiographic image. LA = left atrium; MV = mitral valve; LV = left ventricle; RV = right ventricle; TV = tricuspid valve; RA = right atrium.

also in intensive care, the patient may not be in the ideal position or able to obey commands easily. Furthermore, positive pressure ventilation may further obscure acoustic windows due to increased intrathoracic pressures. The aim should be to acquire at least two acceptable views in order to confirm consistency in findings and avoid making judgements based on a single view that may have produced a spurious result (e.g. due to foreshortening of a ventricle).

The essence of FICE is for it to be utilised as a dichotomous decision-making tool designed to answer

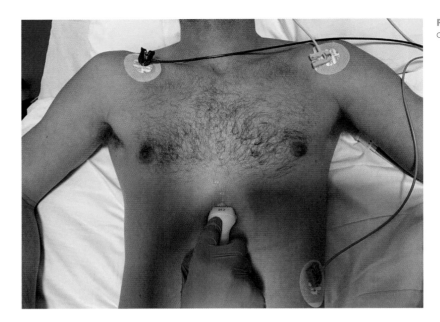

Figure 5.2.9.8 Subcostal (SC) four-chamber (or sub-xiphoid).

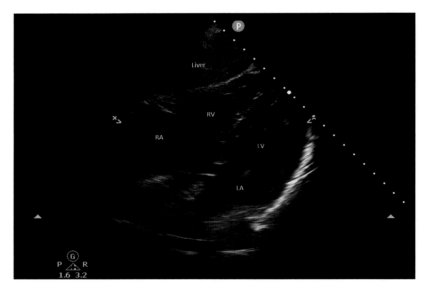

Figure 5.2.9.9 Subcostal four-chamber echocardiographic image. LA = left atrium; LV = left ventricle; RV = right ventricle; RA = right atrium.

the following questions in a patient with cardiovascular shock:

1. Is the left ventricle (LV) grossly impaired?
2. Is the LV dilated?
3. Is the right ventricle (RV) grossly dilated?
4. Is the RV severely impaired?
5. Is there evidence of severe hypovolaemia?
6. Is there a pericardial effusion?
7. Is there a pleural effusion?

Common Pathologies Identified
Dilated Left Ventricle

One of the most common and useful findings of focussed echocardiography is that of an impaired LV, a finding which often will lead to significant changes in clinical management. Gross left ventricular (LV) impairment and dilation can be reliably detected by visual assessment alone by the non-expert operator, and in the clinical context often helps confirm the

(a)

(b)

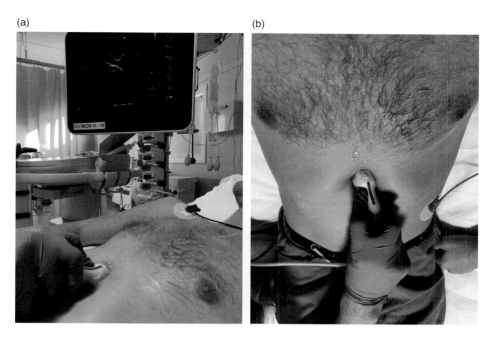

Figure 5.2.9.10 Subcostal inferior vena cava.

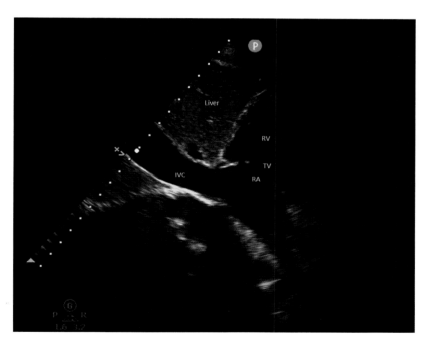

Figure 5.2.9.11 Subcostal inferior vena cava echocardiographic image (in B-mode).

presence of cardiogenic shock. A single measurement of the internal diameter of the LV in diastole can be taken in the PLAX view in order to detect a severely dilated LV (Figure 5.2.9.14). A cut-off value of 60 mm can be used, bearing in mind that formal LV dimension quantification will need correcting for gender and body surface area. Further quantitative assessment of the degree of LV impairment and/or presence of regional wall motion abnormalities (RWMAs) should be carried out by an appropriate British Society of Echocardiography (BSE)-accredited operator.

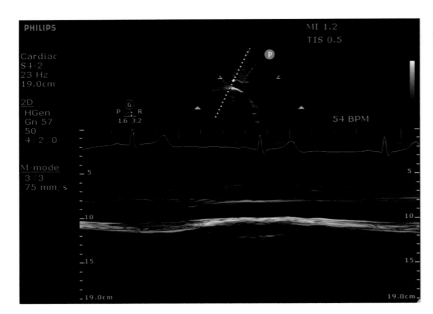

Figure 5.2.9.12 Subcostal inferior vena cava echocardiographic image (in M-mode).

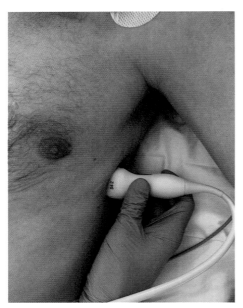

Figure 5.2.9.13 Lung bases.

Dilated Right Ventricle

RV dilation can also be detected by visual inspection and comparing it to the LV. In the A4Ch view, an RV that is greater than two-thirds, or approaching the same size as, the LV is likely to be dilated. In the PLAX view, the right ventricular outflow tract (RVOT) can appear as big as (or bigger than) the LV. Care should be taken in acquiring more than one view, as the RV

size estimation is prone to error due to probe positioning. In the PSAX view, the interventricular septum can often give a clue as to the aetiology of the dilated RV – with a 'flattened' or 'D-shaped' interventricular septum in systole consistent with a pressure-loaded RV, and in diastole with a volume-loaded RV. Figures 5.2.9.15 to 5.2.9.17 demonstrate the PLAX, PSAX and A4Ch views of a patient diagnosed with acute pulmonary embolism (PE). Note the flattened septum in the PSAX view.

The predominant systolic function of the RV is carried out by longitudinal shortening, and visual inspection of this can detect severe impairment. Furthermore, measurement of the tricuspid valve annular plane systolic excursion (TAPSE) can be carried out relatively easily using the M-mode in the A4Ch view, with a normal cut-off being >16 mm.

Hypovolaemia

Severe hypovolaemia can often result in a collapsing or 'empty' LV on parasternal views. The PSAX view will thus often show the papillary muscles come into contact in systole, resulting in a 'kissing' papillary muscles sign. The IVC will often be small (<2 cm) and will show a high degree of collapsibility (>50 per cent) on passive inspiration (Figure 5.2.9.18).

Pericardial Effusion

Pericardial effusions can be detected, as echo-poor (black) fluid collects around the heart in the pericardial

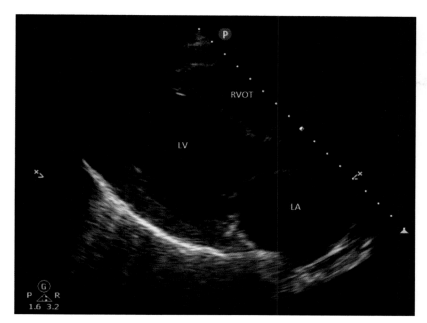

Figure 5.2.9.14 Dilated left ventricle on PLAX view. Note the thin-walled left ventricle and dilated left atrium, suggestive of a chronic aetiology for the left ventricular distensibility. LA = left atrium; LV = left ventricle; RVOT = right ventricular outflow tract.

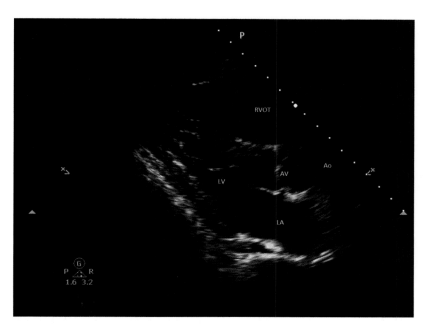

Figure 5.2.9.15 Dilated right ventricle – PLAX view.

space, and are often most readily detectable in the subcostal view. In the context of shock and other associated clinical signs, a diagnosis of tamponade can therefore be considered or excluded by the presence of a pericardial effusion (Figure 5.2.9.19). Although there are signs of 'tamponade physiology' on echocardiography, such as collapsing heart chambers (right atrium during systole or RV during diastole), these are beyond FICE and an expert opinion should be sought early if tamponade is suspected.

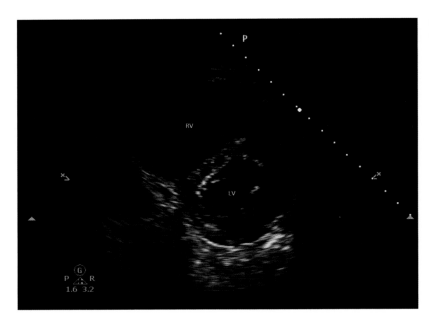

Figure 5.2.9.16 Dilated right ventricle – PSAX view.

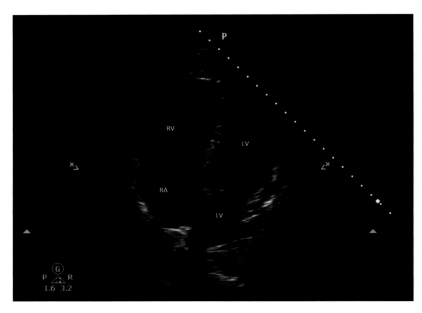

Figure 5.2.9.17 Dilated right ventricle – A4Ch view.

Pleural Effusions

Pleural effusions (Figure 5.2.9.20) can be detected starting from the lung bases and can be a useful sign in making a clinical assessment of the patient's volume status or the presence of cardiac failure. Larger effusions can also be detected in the parasternal views, and differentiating between pleural and pericardial fluid can be done by observing where the fluid tracks in relation to the descending aorta in the PLAX view – pericardial fluid will track above it and pleural fluid will track inferiorly to the descending aorta.

In conclusion, focussed echocardiography is a readily available and valuable tool available to physicians

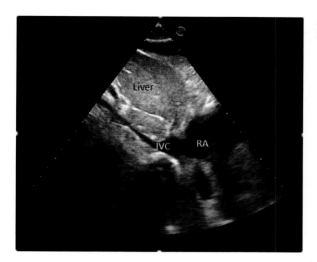

Figure 5.2.9.18 Subcostal IVC view of collapsed IVC in a hypovolaemic patient.

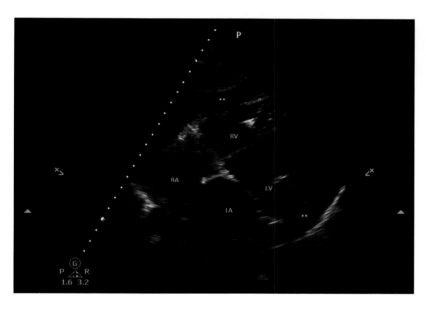

Figure 5.2.9.19 Subcostal four-chamber view in a shocked patient demonstrating a pericardial effusion surrounding the heart. Note there is a pacing wire in the right ventricle (bright echogenic focus). LA = left atrium; LV = left atrium; RA = right atrium; RV = right ventricle.

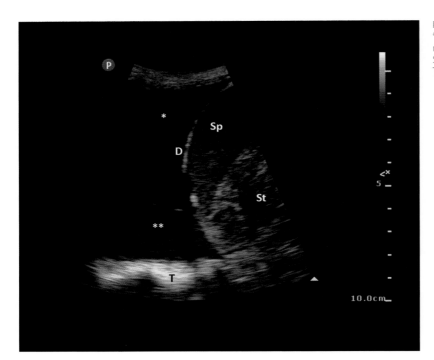

Figure 5.2.9.20 Pleural effusion. * Pleural effusion (dark). ** Echogenic material within effusion (plankton sign). Sp = spleen; St = stomach; D = diaphragm; T = thoracic vertebra (spine sign).

for the assessment of shocked and critically ill patients. It allows for rapid diagnosis of major causes of shock and for correct treatment to be instigated.

Acknowledgements

All images are produced by the author and subject to copyright.

References and Further Reading

Vieillard-Baron A, Millington SJ, Sanfilippo F, *et al.* A decade of progress in critical care echocardiography: a narrative review. *Intensive Care Med* 2019;**45**:770–88.

Wilson W, Mackay A. Ultrasound in critical care. *Contin Educ Anaesth Crit Care Pain* 2012;**12**:190–4.

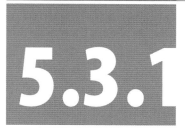

5.3.1

Principles of Performing a Lumbar Puncture (Intradural/'Spinal')

Jonathan Barnes

Key Learning Points

1. A lumbar puncture (LP) is a useful and extremely valuable investigation and should always be considered early.
2. LPs carry a morbidity risk, and patients should be screened for contraindications before performing the procedure.
3. Performing an LP in the sitting-up position is likely to be easier than in the lateral position; however, it does prevent all the tests from being done and may not be as well tolerated by the patient (particularly the acutely meningitic patient).
4. The risk of post-dural puncture headache can be minimised by using the smallest possible 'non-cutting' needle.
5. Ensure to send all samples that may be required and do not forget a paired serum glucose.

Keywords: lumbar puncture, meningitis, cerebrospinal fluid, post-dural puncture headache

Introduction

A lumbar puncture (LP), or spinal tap, is a procedure in which a needle is introduced through the dura in order to obtain a sample of cerebrospinal fluid (CSF). The needle passes through the dura into the subarachnoid space. The spinal cord terminates around L1. Therefore, LPs are normally performed at either L4/5, L3/4 or L2/3 (Figure 5.3.1.1).

Indications

There are several reasons why an LP may be performed. Essentially, these can be broadly categorised as follows:

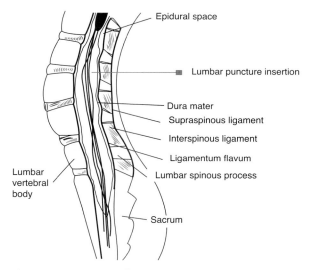

Figure 5.3.1.1 Anatomy for lumbar puncture.

*   To investigate for suspected central nervous system (CNS) infection (e.g. meningitis or encephalitis)
*   To investigate for suspected subarachnoid haemorrhage (SAH) – approximately 2% of SAH will be missed on CT scan
*   To investigate for suspected inflammatory disease in the CNS (e.g. any malignancy, including lymphoma, multiple sclerosis, etc.)
*   To diagnose and treat idiopathic intracranial hypertension (IIH)
*   To administer certain medications – either as a spinal anaesthetic or as intrathecal therapy (e.g. some chemotherapies)

Contraindications

*   Patient refusal
*   Infection/skin damage over insertion site
*   Raised intracranial pressure:
    *   For example, papilloedema, cranial nerve palsies, etc.

- Coagulopathy:[*]
  - Active oral anticoagulant use or international normalised ratio (INR) >1.4[**]
  - Low-molecular-weight heparin (LMWH) (prophylaxis) <12 hours
  - LMWH (treatment) <24 hours
  - Thrombocytopenia – platelets $<80 \times 10^9/l$[**]

Lumbar Punctures in the Emergency Setting

With the above in mind, it is vital to remember that an LP is an invaluable investigation in patients with suspected meningitis, and although appropriate precautions should be taken, it should not be delayed unnecessarily. The British Infection Association (BIA) guidelines state that:

- 'LP should not be delayed for the results of blood tests unless there is a high clinical suspicion of a bleeding diathesis'
- 'Patients should not have neuroimaging before their LP unless there is a clinical indication suggestive of brain shift'

Equipment and Technique
Equipment Required

- Sterile drapes pack
- Sterile gloves, gown, mask and hat:
  - Full asepsis is advocated for spinal anaesthesia by the Royal College of Anaesthetists, the American Society of Anesthesiologists and the American Society of Regional Anesthesia
  - As such, anaesthetists will normally also utilise full asepsis when performing an LP
  - Practice on regular wards, however, is often different, with many using only a non-sterile apron and gloves[***]
- Chlorhexidine spray:
  - The above listed groups advocate using 0.5% chlorhexidine, which should be kept well away from other equipment and allowed to dry

fully before puncture to minimise the risk of arachnoiditis
  - Again, however, practice on regular medical wards does differ and 2% solution is often used[***]
- Local anaesthetic:
  - 1% lidocaine – normally 2–5 ml is adequate, although more may be needed in bigger patients with a greater depth of subcutaneous tissue to anaesthetise
  - 5- or 10-ml syringe
  - Drawing-up needle (with filter)
  - Injecting needle – normally 23, 25 or 27 G
- Spinal needle:
  - Ideally a small-gauge non-cutting needle (with introducer)
- Manometer:
  - Ensure you have assembled your manometer and loosened the tap before the procedure
- Gauze swabs and dressing
- Sample bottles (see below)

Positioning

An LP may be performed with the patient either sitting up or in the lateral position, and both approaches have their advocates. Many find the sitting position easier; however, the effect of gravity will increase CSF pressure at the insertion point. Although this means that samples can normally be obtained faster, it also means that the pressure cannot be accurately measured. This position may also be less comfortable for the patient.

Whichever position is used, the key to success is to get the patient as curled up as possible, thus opening up the inter-spinous space.

Lateral Position (Either Left or Right Lateral)

- The patient lies in the left or right lateral position, with one pillow under their head (to keep the spine aligned) and one pillow between their legs.
- The knees and hips should be flexed as much as possible – the knees should be brought up towards the chest.
- The neck should be flexed, with the chin brought down on to the chest.

---

[*] The list of safe windows for regional anaesthesia in the presence of different anticoagulants is available through the Association of Anaesthetists of Great Britain and Ireland (AAGBI).

[**] These are generally regarded as the cut-offs. However, in certain situations, LPs may be performed outside of these ranges or may be avoided, even within the safe range.

[***] It is far beyond the scope of this book to resolve this ongoing debate. However, in general, being over-cautious is probably better than being under-cautious, although that is just the opinion of the authors.

Sitting

- The patient should be seated on the edge of the bed, with their legs on a chair or stool. They should be as far back on the bed as possible.
- The patient should be given a pillow to place under their arms, almost as if they are hugging it.
- The knees should be flexed and brought up as much as possible.
- The patient should drop their chin to their chest and curl up as much as possible – this is often described as the 'angry cat' or 'prawn' position.

Technique

1. Consent and position the patient. Collect all necessary equipment and utilise a trained assistant if possible.
2. Find the correct position for insertion:
   a. An imaginary line (Tuffier's line) can be drawn between the tops of the iliac crests. Tuffier's line should pass through the L4 vertebra.
   b. Using this line, by going one space below, the practitioner should find the L4/5 interspace, or L3/4 by going one space above.
   c. On palpation, the spinous processes can be felt as small, hard lumps, with the interspace between them.
   d. It may be useful to mark Tuffier's line, the midpoints of the spine, and even the spaces themselves on the patient before commencing the procedure – particularly in obese patients.
   e. Ultrasound can be used to identify the midline, each vertebral level, the interspace and the depth to the dura, and is becoming an increasingly popular technique.
3. Don hat and mask (if using), then wash your hands and don sterile gloves and gown (if using).
4. Apply chlorhexidine to the back, or if being applied from a non-sterile bottle (i.e. when using a spray bottle), this should be applied before scrubbing or by an assistant. It should always be allowed to dry.
5. Draw up lidocaine into your syringe using the filter needle, and then replace with your small-gauge hypodermic needle.
6. Palpate the patient's back. Feel for the interspinous space and puncture the skin at the inferior pole of

the space, angling slightly cephalad (i.e. just above the inferior spinous process).

7. Anaesthetise the skin and subcutaneous tissues:
   a. Initially raise a small wheal just below the skin.
   b. Then advance the needle into the interspinous space, aiming for the umbilicus.
   c. A firm feeling, almost like pushing a pin into a cork board, will be felt when (if) the needle enters the ligaments.
   d. From this point, aspirate (to ensure not in a blood vessel) and inject a small amount of local anaesthetic. Slowly withdraw the needle, repeating the process to anaesthetise the entire passage for the spinal needle.
   e. This process will anaesthetise the area around the needle. If a new puncture site, or a different spinal level, is subsequently required, the area should be re-anaesthetised.
   f. Advancing the local anaesthetic needle using the same approach as for the spinal needle can act as a useful guide for what angle will be needed for the LP itself.

8. Insert the spinal needle. Again, insert the needle at the inferior pole of the interspinous space; angle slightly cephalad, and aim towards the umbilicus. In the lateral position particularly, one must be careful to keep the needle perpendicular to the spine.
   a. If a non-cutting needle is being used, then the introducer should be inserted first, and then the blunt needle inserted through it.

9. As the needle enters the ligaments, the same cork-like feeling will be felt. A loss of resistance will be felt as the needle exits the ligaments, often described as a 'pop'. What is often described as a second 'pop' may be felt as the needle punctures the dura. This sometimes feels like pushing a sharp knife through a silk sheet, although in reality (particularly with small needles), this sensation is often not felt.

10. Next, withdraw the stylet from the needle and watch for the CSF to appear.
    a. If the CSF does not appear, try advancing the needle further (with the stylet back in).
    b. If this does not work, or if you encounter bone, withdraw the needle; adjust the angle, and re-advance. By always starting at the

inferior aspect of the interspinous space, one can be reasonably confident that the bone encountered is the spinous process of the inferior vertebrae. As such, it is sensible to try re-angling slightly upward. It is often possible to 'walk the needle' up off the bone and into the space.

  c. If the patient experiences a shooting pain in one leg/buttock, or can feel the needle off to one side, this suggests the needle is angled off towards that side, so re-adjust the other way.

11. Once the CSF has been obtained, attach the manometer (if lateral) to measure the pressure. A normal CSF pressure is around 12–20 cmH$_2$O.

12. Next fill your sample bottles. If these are sterile, you can handle them yourself; if not (which is normally the case), ask an assistant to hold the bottle below the spinal needle (without contaminating your sterile field) – 10–20 drops per sample is normally adequate for most samples.

13. Once all samples have been obtained, re-insert the stylet; withdraw the entire needle and apply the dressing.

  a. Re-inserting the stylet may reduce the risk of post-dural puncture headache (PDPH).

Samples to Send

For suspected meningitis, the BIA recommends recording/sending the following samples:

- CSF opening pressure
- CSF microscopy, culture and sensitivity
- Meningococcal and pneumococcal polymerase chain reaction (PCR)
- Protein and lactate
- Glucose (a paired serum sample should be sent at the same time)

Other tests often sent after an LP include:

- Virology – for suspected encephalitis
- Xanthochromia – for suspected SAH (this must be sent in an opaque bottle, or with the bottle kept in the dark)
- Cytology – for possible malignant disease
- Oligoclonal bands – for possible inflammatory disease

Other tests may be sent on specialist advice.

Interpreting Results in Suspected Meningitis

Table 5.3.1.1 gives a breakdown of CSF constituents in different forms of meningitis.

Complications

- PDPH –1 in 500 risk
- Infection (meningitis) – 1 per 100,000 to 150,000
- Spinal haematoma – 1 per 150,000 to 200,000
- Nerve injury leading to development of an area of pain, numbness or weakness:
  - Temporary – 1 per 1000
  - Permanent (duration over 6 months) – 1 per 10,000

Reducing the Risk of Post-dural Puncture Headache

Several strategies can be implemented to minimise the risk of patients developing a PDPH. These include:

- Using as small a needle as possible – many units now routinely use a 25-G needle or smaller
- Using a non-cutting needle (e.g. Whitacre or Sprotte needles) as these are associated with fewer PDPHs than cutting needles (e.g. Quinke needles)

Table 5.3.1.1 Interpretation of CSF features

Parameter	Normal	Bacterial	Viral	Tuberculosis	Fungal
Opening pressure (cmH$_2$O)	12–20	Raised	Normal/mildly raised	Raised	Raised
Colour	Clear	Purulent	Clear	Clear or cloudy	Clear or cloudy
White cell count (cells × 10^6/l)	<5	Raised (often >100)	Raised	Raised	Raised
White cell morphology	n/a	Neutrophils	Lymphocytes	Lymphocytes	Lymphocytes
Protein (g/l)	<0.4	Raised	Mildly raised	Raised	Raised
Glucose (mmol/l)	2.5–4.5	Low	Normal/mildly low	Low	Low
CSF-to-plasma glucose ratio	>0.66	Low	Normal/mildly low	Low	Low

- Replacing the stylet before removal
- Angling the bevel in line with the dural fibres – which are assumed to be longitudinal (bevel aiming upward in a lateral position and off to one side when sitting)

There is no evidence to support fluids, caffeine or prolonged bedrest following an LP to reduce the incidence of PDPH.

References and Further Reading

Association of Anaesthetists of Great Britain and Ireland. Safety guideline: skin antisepsis for central neuraxial blockade. *Anaesthesia* 2014;**69**:1279–86.

McGill F, Heyderman RS, Michael BD, *et al.* The UK joint specialist societies guideline on the diagnosis and management of acute meningitis and meningococcal sepsis in immunocompetent adults. *J Infect* 2016;**72**:405–38.

Oxford Medical Education. 2015. Lumbar puncture. www.oxfordmedicaleducation.com/clinical-skills/procedures/lumbar-puncture/

Perry S, Barnes J, Allen A. Tips from the shop floor: performing and interpreting a lumbar puncture. *Br J Hosp Med (Lond)* 2018;**79**:C183–7.

Plewa M, Dulebohn S. *Postdural Puncture Headache*. Treasure Island, FL: StatPearls Publishing; 2017. www.ncbi.nlm.nih.gov/books/NBK430925/

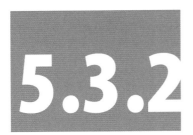

1. Patients with epidurals need careful and close monitoring.
2. It is the dose of local anaesthetic, not the volume, that is of most importance in ensuring adequate analgesia.
3. If the block is too low or absent, try topping up the epidural before removing it.
4. If the block is too high or off to one side, try changing the patient's position to use gravity to help you alter the block.
5. Always be wary of the hypotensive patient with an epidural. Do not assume it is always down to the epidural, but rather rule out other possible causes.

Keywords: epidural, analgesia, top-up, post-operative pain

Introduction

The epidural space is a potential space between the spinal ligaments and the dura. Epidural catheters are inserted using a Tuohy needle, which is advanced into the epidural space using a loss-of-resistance technique. A catheter is then left *in situ*, which allows subsequent administration of either a bolus or a continuous infusion of analgesia. Normally a mixture of local anaesthetic and opioid is administered together; however, other medications may also be used (Figure 5.3.2.1).

Indications

Epidurals are used in various settings, including for labour analgesia and chronic pain. In the ICU, epidurals will mostly be encountered in the post-operative setting where they are used to provide pain relief in patients who have had major thoracic, abdominal or pelvic surgery. In these cases, the epidural will most likely have been inserted pre-operatively by an anaesthetist.

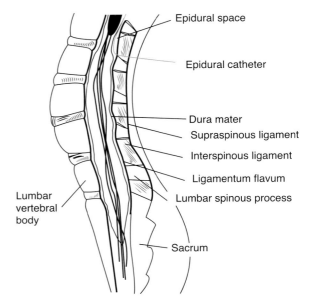

Figure 5.3.2.1 Epidural space.

Anatomy, Physiology and Pharmacology

Medications injected via the epidural catheter sit outside the dura and exert their effect on the spinal nerve roots. The desired effect is analgesia, and this requires blockade of the small sensory nerve fibres which transmit pain (C and Aδ fibres). Unfortunately, local anaesthetic is not discriminatory, and whilst small fibres are blocked first, other fibres may also be blocked, including the larger pre-ganglionic autonomic B fibres. In this instance, only the sympathetic fibres will be blocked (as the sympathetic chain arises from T1 to L2, whilst the parasympathetic nervous system has a cranio-sacral outflow), and this can lead to unopposed vasodilation and hypotension, which may, in the first instance, manifest as sweating and dizziness in the patient. If the epidural block level rises above T5, it may start to affect the cardio-acceleratory sympathetic fibres, leading to bradycardia. Patients may also experience motor weakness in their lower limbs (or in the case of a high block, upper limb weakness and difficulty breathing), and in this instance, it implies that the much thicker Aα fibres have also been blocked.

Epidural Regimes
Dosing

The two commonly used epidural dosing regimens are either a continuous epidural infusion or a patient-controlled epidural analgesia (PCEA) regime.

In labour analgesia, PCEA has been shown in a number of studies to lead to a reduced incidence of motor blockade, reduced overall medication consumption and a reduced incidence of further intervention. These results, however, have not been reliably reproduced in the post-operative population (in part as it requires an awake, communicative patient, which may not be the case in the ICU), and thus a continuous epidural infusion is often utilised.

Drug Choice

In general, a combination of a local anaesthetic and an opioid are used to provide analgesia. In most instances, a longer-acting local anaesthetic is used – normally bupivacaine, levobupivacaine or ropivacaine. There is some evidence to suggest an improved cardiac safety profile with the use of ropivacaine and levobupivacaine. However, there is no conclusive evidence to suggest using one over the other. For rapid provision of analgesia, such as on the labour ward or pre-operatively, a rapid-acting local anaesthetic such as lidocaine may be used. However, notably, the length of block is shorter.

Addition of an opioid has been shown to improve the analgesic effect of the block[*]. Highly lipid-soluble opioids, such as fentanyl or diamorphine, are often favoured as they are less likely to exhibit prolonged deposition in the epidural space, and thus there is less risk for delayed adverse effects such as respiratory depression.

It has been shown that the quality of analgesia attained is most dependent on the total dose of local anaesthetic administered, with the volume used being of lesser importance. Additionally, low-concentration, high-volume dosing is also associated with an increased incidence of hypotension.

---

[*] In the ICU, some units advocate the use of plain epidurals (i.e. without opioid), in an attempt to reduce the risk of delirium.

Assessment and Monitoring

The objective of an epidural is to achieve good analgesia specific to the area of pain. To assess the 'epidural level', a cold stimulus (e.g. ethyl chloride spray) should be applied initially to an 'unblocked' region well away from the surgical/injury site of interest. The patient should then be asked to confirm that they can feel cold sensation in that area. The cold stimulus should then be moved up the body, dermatome by dermatome, so that a clear area of sensory change can be demarcated. This should be performed bilaterally to assess for an asymmetrical block. Assessment for any degree of motor block for the corresponding myotomes should be made by asking the patient to move their limbs. Additionally, patients should also have continuous heart rate, blood pressure, respiratory rate, temperature and sedation score monitoring throughout.

Troubleshooting

Given the importance of a well-functioning epidural to patient care and comfort, it is important to understand how to troubleshoot a malfunctioning epidural. Several commonly encountered issues are described below.

Low Block Bilaterally

If the block is low, a bolus dose of medication may be administered. A hand-delivered bolus (as opposed to one given by the epidural pump) is often preferred, as greater hydro-dissection of the epidural space is thought to be achieved. Different regimens are suggested by different institutions. However, a typical drug choice would be 5 ml of 0.25% bupivacaine (with or without 50 µg fentanyl) or 5 ml of 'bag mix' (often 0.1% bupivacaine with 2 µg/ml fentanyl). Having given a bolus, it would then be normal to increase the rate of the continuous epidural infusion (CEI) by 1–2 ml/hr.

Reassessment of the patient 10–15 minutes post-bolus is mandatory, not only to assess for block improvement, but also to see if any side effects are evident. If there has been an improvement, continue with current management; if there is a partial improvement, consider a further bolus, or if there is no improvement, see below.

No Block Bilaterally

If there is no block, then first inspect the back. Ensure that the epidural catheter is still *in situ*, that it is still at the depth to which it was inserted and that the pump is still connected and running. Having done this, the steps outlined above should be followed. If there is still no block after a bolus, it would be reasonable to pull the catheter back by 1–2 cm (in a sterile manner) and try a further bolus as above. If this, however, fails to produce any block, then the epidural is likely not working and removal is warranted, followed by either immediate catheter re-insertion or provision of an alternative analgesic regimen (e.g. patient-controlled intravenous analgesia).

Unilateral Block or Patchy Block/Missed Segment

If the patient has a true unilateral block or demonstrates 'missed segments' on one side, lay the patient with the affected side down, and administer a bolus as above. Reassess in 15 minutes, and if an adequate block has not been established, consider pulling back the catheter by 1–2 cm and giving a further bolus, with the patient in a similar position.

High Block

If the epidural rises above T6, the cardio-acceleratory sympathetic fibres will be affected – often manifesting as a bradycardia. It is imperative that no further boluses are administered and the CEI should be stopped until the level has dropped by at least two segments[*]. Asking

---

[*] Some argue that the CEI should never be stopped as the level will drop too fast and may be difficult to re-establish. They would advocate instead reducing it to 1–2 ml/hr to maintain the patency of the epidural space, whilst allowing the level to drop. This, however, is an approach that should only be used cautiously by an experienced practitioner and in a highly monitored setting.

the patient to sit up, and thus using gravity, may also help matters.

Hypotension

Epidurals do cause hypotension due to blockade of the sympathetic nervous system. It is important, however, not to assume all hypotension in a critically unwell patient is epidural-related without considering other causes, e.g. sepsis and bleeding, etc.

If no other cause can be found, and the hypotension is therefore due to the epidural, then administer a fluid bolus and start/increase background fluids. If this is unsuccessful, then the options are either to stop the epidural or to commence a low-dose vasopressor infusion. If the epidural is working well, then the latter is normally favourable.

Disconnected Filter

If the epidural filter is witnessed to disconnect from the catheter, then it is reasonable to clean and cover each end with sterile wipes before reconnecting to a new sterile filter. If, however, there is an unwitnessed disconnection, this represents a significant infection risk and the epidural should be removed.

References and Further Reading

Hermanides J, Hollmann M, Lirk F. Failed epidurals; causes and management. *Br J Anaesth* 2012;**109**:144–54.

Sykes G. 2017. Epidural and spinal anaesthetics. Obstetric Excellence. www.obstetricexcellence.com.au/epidural-spinal-anaesthetics/

Vyver M, Halpern S, Joseph G. Patient controlled epidural analgesia versus continuous infusion for labour analgesia: a meta-analysis. *Br J Anaesth* 2002;**89**:459–65.

Abdominal Paracentesis

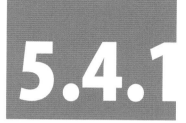

Jonathan Barnes

Key Learning Points

1. Abdominal drains should be inserted under ultrasound guidance.
2. Use the 'Z-track' technique to minimise complications.
3. Pay attention to volume replacement, particularly in the critically unwell patient.
4. Antibiotic administration should not be delayed in cases of suspected spontaneous bacterial peritonitis.
5. Differentiating transudative from exudative ascites is achieved by calculating the serum–ascites albumin gradient.

Keywords: paracentesis, ascitic drain, ascites, serum–ascites albumin gradient, spontaneous bacterial peritonitis

Introduction

Paracentesis is a procedure performed to drain fluid out of the peritoneal cavity.

Indications

Diagnostic

A simple ascitic 'tap' is performed as part of the investigation of ascites. The British Society of Gastroenterology (BSG) guidelines state that ascitic sampling should be performed in any patient presenting with cirrhosis and ascites admitted to hospital, and in all cirrhotic patients with ascites who show signs of infection or decompensation.

Therapeutic

Paracentesis with an ascitic drain is performed to relieve the symptoms of severe ascites. The BSG advises it as first-line therapy for large or refractory ascites.

Contraindications

Absolute

- Patient refusal
- Overlying skin infection (alternative puncture site should be sought)

Relative

- Coagulopathy/thrombocytopenia
  - Disorders of clotting are not an absolute contraindication, and many patients requiring paracentesis will have abnormal clotting and/ or platelet count. Caution, however, should be exercised in these patients
  - Routine use of fresh frozen plasma or platelet transfusion is not recommended
- Pregnancy
- Organomegaly

Technique for Insertion

Equipment Required

- Sterile gloves, gown and dressing pack
- 2% chlorhexidine wash/swabs
- Ultrasound
  - Ideally paracentesis should be performed under ultrasound guidance, ideally under direct vision. If an 'X marks the spot' technique is used, drain insertion should be performed immediately after marking, without moving the patient.
- Local anaesthetic
  - 5–10 ml of lidocaine with 25/27 G and 19/22 G needles
- 20-ml syringe
- Paracentesis drain
  - Various types of drains consisting of a rigid introducer and a catheter with a curled end

exist. Examples include pigtail drains and Bonanno catheters

- Scalpel
- Specimen bottles and drainage bag
- Suture kit and dressing

Technique for Insertion

1. Explain the procedure to the patient.
2. Position the patient. The patient should be supine, with the head resting on one pillow.
3. Clean the skin and prepare the sterile field.
   a. Remember to allow chlorhexidine to dry first.
4. Identify the insertion point.
   a. The point of insertion in an adult is approximately 10–15 cm superior and medial to the anterior superior iliac spine.
   b. Avoid the inferior epigastric artery, which runs along the lateral aspect of the rectus abdominis.
   c. Ultrasound will show a large fluid collection.
5. Anaesthetise the skin and subcutaneous tissue.
   a. Inject a few millilitres of local anaesthetic under the skin with your small needle.
   b. Applying negative pressure to the syringe, advance your larger needle perpendicular to the skin. Use a 'Z-track' approach, as this will help achieve good analgesia and minimise ascitic fluid leakage. This involves gently pulling down on the skin during insertion, to create an insertion channel that is staggered through the different layers.
   c. Advance until you breach the peritoneum; a small amount of ascites (straw-coloured fluid) will be aspirated – this helps confirm positioning.

   d. Withdraw your needle, injecting the local anaesthetic along your Z-track.
6. Make a small nick in the skin for your drain.
   a. Ensure your incision is large enough, or the drain will kink. However, too large an incision will increase the risk of complications. A few millimetres should suffice.
7. Insert your drain.
   a. Attach the 20-ml syringe to the drain.
   b. Using your Z-track approach and applying negative pressure to your syringe, advance the drain and introducer perpendicular to the skin, until you aspirate ascitic fluid (Figure 5.4.1.1).
   c. If the flow of fluid stops, then stop aspirating before retrying, as the negative pressure may have sucked in some bowel or omentum. If this is unsuccessful, the drain may have come out slightly, so advance a few millimetres and re-attempt aspiration.
8. Having entered the peritoneum, now advance your drain over the introducer.
   a. Gently advance the plastic drain into the peritoneal cavity, whilst preventing the sharp introducer from entering any further.
   b. It may be necessary to unclip the plastic drain from the introducer needle at the distal end to facilitate this.
9. Remove the introducer.
   a. The catheter should now be in the peritoneum. Slowly withdraw the introducer needle.
   b. There should be a flow of ascitic fluid from the drain.
   c. Do not panic over a slow or weak flow, as the drain may just require adjusting or patient repositioning.

Figure 5.4.1.1 The 'Z-track' technique.

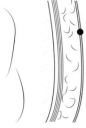

Mark insertion point

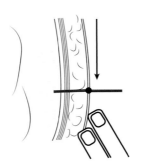

Apply traction to skin and insert drain

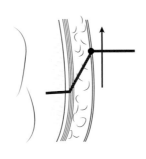

Release traction – Z-track achieved

10. Secure the drain.
    a. If you are using a pigtail drain, pull the pigtail cord to coil the drain and clip the threads to the drain.
    b. A simple anchor suture can now be used to secure the drain before applying a sterile dressing and a drainage bag.

Volume Replacement

Abdominal paracentesis is associated with large-volume shifts. This can lead to haemodynamic instability, especially if the patient is already unstable. How best to avoid and manage this has been an area of contention.

Although there is some weak evidence demonstrating that paracentesis of low volumes (<5 l) may be safe without volume replacement, expert consensus is that some form of volume expansion should be used for all patients undergoing paracentesis. The BSG recommends that 100 ml of 20% albumin should be given after each 3-litre aliquot of ascites drained.

Analysis of Fluid

Having inserted the ascitic drain, fluid can be removed for analysis. The most valuable clinical questions to answer are:

1. Does the patient have spontaneous bacterial peritonitis (SBP)?
2. What is the aetiology of the ascites?

Spontaneous Bacterial Peritonitis

Samples should be sent for microscopy, culture and sensitivities, and for a white cell count. A neutrophil count of $>250/\mu m^3$ is diagnostic of SBP, and empirical treatment should be started early as per local guidelines.

Aetiology of Ascites

To differentiate transudative ascites (cardiac failure, hepatic failure, portal vein thrombosis) from exudative ascites (intra-abdominal malignancy, pancreatobiliary inflammation, intra-abdominal infection), the serum–ascites albumin gradient (SAAG) should be calculated. An SAAG >11 g/l indicates an exudative cause.

Whilst the SAAG is standard practice, other techniques for diagnosing the aetiology of ascites exist, including 'ascites fluid viscosity' and the 'ascites-to-rectus abdominis muscle echogenicity ratio' (ARAER). In both techniques, a higher value indicates exudative ascites.

Other Samples

Samples may also be sent for:
- Amylase level (if pancreatic disease is suspected), glucose, lactate dehydrogenase (LDH), triglycerides, cytology, auto-antibodies and tuberculosis culture.

Complications

Acute Complications
- Bleeding, infection, damage to local structures (most notably bowel perforation) and haemodynamic instability due to large-volume removal

Chronic Complications
- Persistent leak of ascitic fluid

References and Further Reading

Aithal GP, Palaniyappan N, China L, *et al.* Guidelines on the management of ascites in cirrhosis. *Gut* 2021;**70**:9–29.

Moore K, Aithal G. Guidelines on the management of ascites in cirrhosis. *Gut* 2006;**55**:1–12.

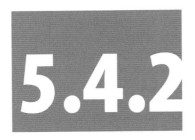

5.4.2

Sengstaken–Blakemore Tube Insertion

Jonathan Barnes

Key Learning Points

1. A Sengstaken–Blakemore tube (SBT) should only be employed as a rescue technique.
2. In practice, the four-lumen Minnesota tube is often encountered, not a classical SBT. However, insertion and aftercare are the same.
3. In most cases, only the gastric balloon will need inflating.
4. Monitor pressures regularly, and be careful to avoid complications.
5. An SBT is only a temporising measure, and having inserted one, it is vital to make a definitive management plan early.

Keywords: Sengstaken–Blakemore tube, Minnesota tube, variceal bleed, upper gastrointestinal bleed

Introduction

The double-balloon Sengstaken–Blakemore tube (SBT) was developed by its namesakes in 1950 to tamponade bleeding varices. The tube comprises a distal gastric balloon and a proximal oesophageal balloon. At the proximal end, there are three lumens – one for a gastric suction port and one to inflate each balloon. A Minnesota tube is a four-lumen version, with a fourth oesophageal suction port.

Use of the SBT is less common in modern clinical practice due to advances in endoscopic techniques. It is, however, still a vital piece of equipment which can tamponade bleeding in up to 90 per cent of acute variceal bleeds, and an understanding of how and when to perform the procedure is essential for the practising intensivist (Figure 5.4.2.1).

Indications

Indications for insertion of an SBT are acute and life-threatening variceal bleeding when endoscopic therapy is unavailable or when endoscopic and other

Figure 5.4.2.1 A Minnesota tube (the Sengstaken–Blakemore tube is the same, but without the oesophageal port).

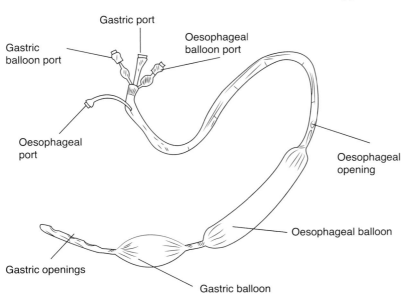

Gastric port

Oesophageal balloon port

Gastric balloon port

Oesophageal port

Oesophageal opening

Oesophageal balloon

Gastric openings

Gastric balloon

medical therapies (including haemostatic agents and vasoconstrictors) have failed. It is important, however, to remember that the SBT is only a tool intended to buy time until a more definitive treatment is available.

Contraindications

Contraindications include known unstable oesophago-gastric anatomy (e.g. post-surgery) or oesophageal strictures.

Technique for Insertion
Equipment Required

- SBT
  - Like a nasogastric tube, keeping these in the freezer will keep them more rigid and aid insertion
- Lubricating jelly
- Artery forceps or tube clamps, to clamp drainage port(s)
- Irrigating syringes, one for each port and one for each balloon
- Sphygmomanometer or manometer to measure balloon pressures
- Equipment for traction (see below)

Technique for Insertion

In the majority of cases, any patient with severe bleeding varices should be sedated and intubated for insertion of an SBT. Most people advocate insertion in the lateral decubitus position (as for endoscopy), although a 45° head-up position may also be used.

1. Prepare the tube by applying plenty of lubricating jelly, and then insert into the oesophagus via the mouth.
   a. When the SBT is cold and coiled, getting it to pass down the oesophagus can be challenging and use of a laryngoscope and Magill's forceps may be required, as per nasogastric tube placement (see Chapter 5.4.3, Nasogastric Tube Placement and Position Confirmation).
   b. The SBT can be passed via the nose, but this is often more complicated and is only indicated if, for some reason, the patient is not to be/cannot be intubated.

2. Pass the SBT down the oesophagus until it reaches the stomach.
   a. The tube should be inserted to at least 50 cm.
   b. Positioning should be checked via aspiration and/or chest radiography, as per nasogastric tube placement.

3. When confident that the tube is in the stomach, inflate the gastric balloon.
   a. Standard practice is to use air for balloon inflation in 50- to 100-ml aliquots
   b. The balloon pressure should be checked after each insertion. If the pressure rises above 15 mmHg, this suggests possible oesophageal placement, and the balloon should be deflated and repositioned.
   c. For an SBT, maximum inflation is normally up to 300 ml, whereas for a Minnesota tube, it is 500 ml.
   d. Some practitioners suggest using water-mixed radio-contrast for inflation, but this is not standard practice.

4. Once the balloon is inflated, clamp the tube and pull back on it. The tube should move back and then stop when it reaches the gastro-oesophageal junction (GOJ).

5. Now mark the position of the tube at the teeth.

6. Apply traction.
   a. For the balloon to effectively tamponade bleeding varices, it should apply continuous pressure to the GOJ.
   b. To achieve this, traction should be applied to the end of the tube.
   c. A common technique to do this involves attaching a weight (normally a 500-ml bag of intravenous fluid) to the end of the tube and hanging from a pulley.

In most patients, this will be effective in stopping the bleeding. However, if it does not, then this is the indication to also inflate the oesophageal balloon*. This should be performed by injecting small volumes of air into the balloon until the bleeding stops. The balloon pressure should be closely monitored, and bleeding will normally cease at a pressure of around 25–35 mmHg. The balloon should not be inflated above 40 mmHg pressure.

---

* An oesophageal balloon is avoided in the first instance due to the much higher complication rate.

Aftercare

An SBT is normally left in place on traction for 24 hours. If bleeding is ongoing, it may be left in for a further 24 hours (48 hours in total). If the oesophageal balloon has been inflated, attempt to reduce the pressure by 5 mmHg every 3 hours down to 25 mmHg, assuming bleeding does not restart. This will help prevent complications.

Complications

Although it is a lifesaving device, SBTs can also cause fatal complications. These include:

- Aspiration – this is the most common complication and most commonly occurs during insertion. It is avoided by intubating the patient first.
- Asphyxiation – this occurs due to tube migration and is again avoided by intubating the patient first.
- Oesophageal pressure necrosis and rupture – the oesophagus is extremely sensitive to damage. Perforation may occur directly from inflation of the oesophageal balloon or due to inadvertent inflation of the gastric balloon in the oesophagus.
- Pressure damage around the mouth.
- Pain.

References and Further Reading

Hanna S, Warren W, Galambos J, Millikan W. Bleeding varices: emergency management. *Can Med Assoc J* 1981;**124**:29–41.

Treger R. 2016. Sengstaken–Blakemore tube placement. Medscape. emedicine.medscape.com/article/81020-overview

Tripathi D, Stanley AJ, Hayes PC, *et al*. UK guidelines on the management of variceal haemorrhage in cirrhotic patients. *Gut* 2015;**64**:1680–704.

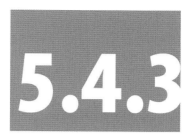

5.4.3

Nasogastric Tube Placement and Position Confirmation

Jonathan Barnes

Key Learning Points

1. There are different types of tubes for different indications.
2. For ease of insertion, keep the tubes in the fridge, ensure good lubrication and optimise head positioning.
3. Use the pH of the aspirate, and/or a chest radiograph, to check positioning.
4. On a chest radiograph, a correctly sited nasogastric tube should pass down the midline and bisect the carina, before passing below the diaphragm.
5. If initiating nasogastric feeding, start thinking about long-term feeding plans early, as in practice, these can take a while to sort out.

Keywords: nasogastric tube, Ryle's tube, enteral feeding

Introduction

A nasogastric tube (NGT), as the name suggests, is a tube inserted via the nose which passes through the oropharynx and oesophagus into the stomach, to allow either drainage of gastric contents or enteral feeding. The orogastric route may also be utilised.

Feeding tubes are fine-bore (6–8 Fr) polyurethane tubes, whereas drainage tubes are typically wide-bore (16–18 Fr) polyvinylchloride tubes, often termed 'Ryle's tubes'. Both types of tube can be inserted via either nostril and, in adults, typically require insertion to approximately 60 cm (Figure 5.4.3.1).

Indications

Feeding Tubes

These are inserted for:

- Feeding and medication administration in patients with:
  - An unsafe swallow (e.g. dysphagia or mal-coordinated swallow)
  - A depressed conscious level
  - A fragile anastomosis following upper gastrointestinal surgery
- Administration of gastric lavage (although this is rare in modern practice)

(a)

(b)

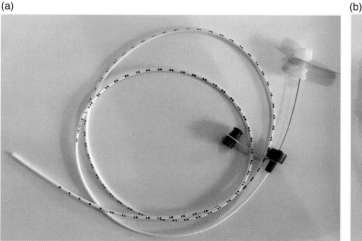
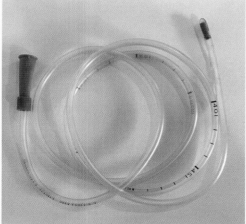

617

Figure 5.4.3.1 A fine-bore feeding tube (a) and a large-bore drainage tube (b).

Before starting nasogastric (NG) feeding, it is essential to ensure that the patient has a functioning gastrointestinal tract (GIT). It is also important to involve both the speech and language and the nutrition/dietitian teams early to make plans for the patient's long-term nutrition.

Drainage/Assessment

Drainage tubes may be inserted for:

- Decompression of bowel obstruction (including for symptomatic control)
- Assessment of upper gastrointestinal bleeding
- Aspiration of toxins

Contraindications

Absolute Contraindications to NGT

- Nasal and mid-face trauma
- Recent nasal/septal surgery
- Base of skull fractures
- Patient refusal

Relative Contraindications to NGT

- Friable oesophageal varices
- Strictures, trauma or recent surgery to the upper GIT
- Recent alkaline ingestion (due to risk of oesophageal damage)
- Coagulation abnormalities

Technique for Insertion

Equipment Required

- NGT
  - ○ Storing NGTs in the fridge can provide them with more rigidity, which may aid insertion
- Lubricant
- Equipment for securing the NGT
- Aspiration syringe
- Drainage bag
- Cup of water (in awake patient)
- Laryngoscope and Magill's forceps (in unconscious/anaesthetised patient)

The Conscious Patient

1. Explain the procedure; wash hands, and don gloves.
2. Position the patient.
   a. The patient should be sat upright, with the head slightly flexed.

b. When attempting a 'difficult' NGT insertion, it is useful to flex the head and neck during insertion. This occludes the airway and improves access to the oesophagus – effectively the opposite to the 'head-tilt, chin-lift' manoeuvre employed during resuscitation.

3. Examine the nostrils, and ask the patient to inhale through each in turn (occluding one, and then the other). Use the one which appears less occluded and is generally easier to inhale through.
4. Measure the NGT.
   a. Using the markings on the NGT (which typically occur every 1–5 cm), measure from the patient's nose to the xiphisternum via the earlobe.
   b. This indicates the required depth of insertion (normally around 60 cm in adults).
5. Apply lubricant to the distal 2–3 cm of the NGT.
6. Insert the NGT gently into the nostril and advance towards the back of the head in a horizontal plane, in keeping with the initial nasal passage.
   a. It may be necessary to rotate the tube slightly whilst passing it (clockwise, then anti-clockwise) to aid insertion.
   b. Do not angle the tube upwards or downwards.
7. After around 10–15 cm, the tube should be in the oropharynx. At this stage, the patient may complain of a sensation of an object in the throat.
8. Gently advance the tube from the oropharynx into the oesophagus.
   a. If safe to do so, it is useful to offer the patient a small sip of water, asking them to swallow as you advance the tube. This aids passage of the tube into the oesophagus.
9. Advance the tube to the required length.
10. The procedure should be stopped if:
    a. The patient becomes distressed and requests to stop
    b. There is evidence of significant nasal or pharyngeal bleeding
    c. The patient experiences respiratory difficulty
    d. The end of the tube emerges in the oral cavity, indicating it has coiled.

The Unconscious Patient

It is not uncommon for ICU physicians to be asked to insert an NGT under direct vision in an unconscious patient. This can be a challenging technique, especially if the patient is not sedated adequately. Additional sedation may be required to aid placement.

1. As before, wash hands, don gloves and inspect the nostrils. For this technique, the patient should be laid flat.
2. Gently perform laryngoscopy, attempting to move the endotracheal tube and tongue out of your field of vision, so you can achieve a view of the pharynx ± upper oesophagus.
3. Insert the NGT as before. The NGT should become visible as it enters the oropharynx.
4. It may be possible to directly advance the NGT into the oesophagus and then the stomach.
5. If this is not possible, use the Magill's forceps to gently clasp the NGT and advance it into the oesophagus.
   a. Grasp the tube as proximally as possible, with the forceps handles perpendicular to the blade of the laryngoscope.
   b. Advance the tube by gently rotating the forceps 90° anti-clockwise, accompanied by a gentle downward movement.
   c. Be careful not to grasp the uvula or damage other pharyngeal structures.

Technique for Checking NGT Placement

Assessment of NGT placement can be performed by pH testing of the aspirate or by radiographic interpretation. In many units, practice involves aspiration as first line, followed by a chest radiograph if this is inconclusive.

pH Testing

Having inserted the NGT, aspirate it and analyse the liquid using pH testing strips. A pH of between 0 and 5 indicates gastric placement. The NGT is safe to secure in place and use.

If an aspirate cannot be obtained, or if the pH is out of range, a chest radiograph should be requested.

A high pH may indicate non-gastric placement but also may occur in patients who are being treated with acid suppression therapy, even when the NGT is in the correct place.

X-ray Analysis

On a chest radiograph, a correctly sited NGT should pass down the midline and bisect the carina, before passing below the diaphragm (slightly to the left of the midline), with the tip visible in the gastric bubble. An example of an algorithm for assessment of NGT placement on chest radiographs is shown in Figure 5.4.3.2.

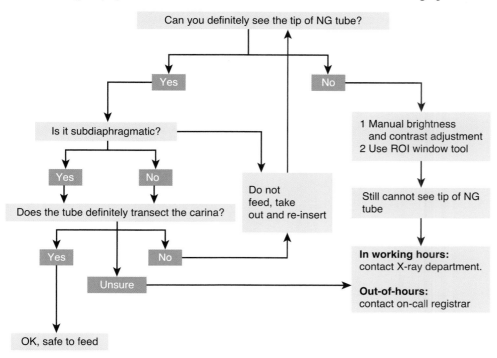

Figure 5.4.3.2 An example of an algorithm for assessment of nasogastric tube placement on chest radiographs.

Complications

Airway Complications

These include epistaxis, sore throat, sinusitis, damage to the uvula and pharyngeal structures and, after prolonged placement, nasal erosions.

Gastrointestinal Complications

These include gagging and vomiting, oesophageal perforation, damage to surgical anastomoses and, after prolonged placement, oesophageal strictures.

Complications of Misplacement

These include pulmonary aspiration, pneumonia, lobar collapse and intracranial placement in a skull base injury.

Alternatives to NGT Placement for Feeding

Other options for feeding could include:

- Nasojejunal tube (NJT)
- Percutaneous endoscopic gastrostomy (PEG)
- Radiologically inserted gastrostomy (RIG)
- Percutaneous endoscopic jejunostomy (PEJ)
- Total parenteral nutrition (TPN)

References and Further Reading

Oxford Medical Education. 2016. Nasogastric (NG) tube placement. www.oxfordmedicaleducation .com/clinical-skills/procedures/nasogastric-ng-tube/

Urinary Catheterisation

Oliver Sanders

5.5.1

Keywords: urinary catheter, urethral, bladder, output monitoring

Indications

Urinary catheterisation is necessary in most patients in the intensive care setting, especially in those who are sedated. The indications can be both diagnostic and therapeutic, and a patient may remain catheterised for minutes to years, depending on the indication.

Diagnostic

- Accurate measurement of the urine output in real time
- Obtaining an uncontaminated sample of urine
- Retrograde imaging of the lower urinary tract

Therapeutic

- Overcome urinary obstruction, either acute or chronic
- Prevention of complications of incontinence in bedbound patients
- Bladder irrigation

In the critical care setting, the two most universal indications are prevention of bed sores from incontinence and measurement of urine output which serves as a useful proxy for renal and (by extension) tissue perfusion, which is sensitive to fluctuations in mean arterial blood pressure.

Contraindications

There are very few contraindications to urinary catheterisation, and most apply to urethral catheterisation due to altered anatomy. The need for a catheter in the presence of any abnormal urethral anatomy, either acute or chronic, should be discussed with urologists. These changes could be the result of neoplastic, traumatic, inflammatory or congenital processes.

Risks/Complications

Early

- Bacteraemia
- Bleeding
- False passage creation
- Prostatic/urethral rupture
- Paraphimosis

Delayed

- Catheter-associated infections
- Strictures
- Bladder atrophy

Procedure

The following describes the general procedure applicable to both male and female catheterisation – with specific differences outlined.

- Inform the patient of the risks and benefits of the procedure, and gain consent for the procedure.
- Uncover the patient, exposing the external genitalia.

621

- Position the supine patient with knees bent and feet together, allowing the knees to fall to either side.
- Prepare the equipment onto a sterile field.
- With sterile gloves on, expose the urethral meatus by either spreading the labia or retracting the foreskin (if not circumcised).
- With the non-dominant hand fixed on exposing the meatus, use sterile gauze soaked in normal saline to clean the area – always wiping away from the meatus and not using the same gauze twice.
- Instil 10 ml of local anaesthetic lubricant gel into and around the meatus.
- Allow 2 minutes for the local anaesthetic to take effect, during which time you should change your sterile gloves.
- Introduce the catheter (which has already been attached to the catheter bag) slowly into the urethra.
- Continue to advance the catheter until urine is seen flowing into the bag. Note this may be delayed if the fenestrations at the tip are blocked by lubricant gel.
- Once urine is seen, advance the catheter a further 5 cm and inflate the balloon via the valved port with sterile water (a pre-filled syringe usually accompanies the catheter).
- Pull the catheter till a point of soft resistance.
- Clean any remaining gel from the patient. Return the foreskin to the natural position (if not circumcised), to avoid paraphimosis.
- Document the procedure, detailing the quantity and appearance of the urine. The urine should also undergo dipstick analysis at this point, and appropriate samples sent for microscopy, culture and sensitivity (MC&S).

Additional Points

Inflation of the balloon before it sits within the bladder often causes acute and severe pain in the awake patient, and may cause perforation or rupture. It is therefore advisable to wait until urine is observed before inflation. However, this may not be possible if the patient is anuric. It is therefore advisable to scan the bladder prior to catheterisation to assess the volume of urine within the bladder.

The choice of size and material of the catheter should be based on the estimated urethral diameter and the expected length of time for which the catheter is to stay in. Use of female-only catheters, which are shorter than universal devices, is outdated as there is a risk of prostatic rupture if inadvertently used in men.

Many trusts advocate the use of a prophylactic stat dose of intravenous antibiotic when inserting or changing a catheter due to an increased risk of translocation of bacteria. This should be confirmed with local trust guidance.

References and Further Reading

Hanno PM, Malkowicz SB, Wein AJ. *Clinical Manual of Urology*. New York, NY: McGraw-Hill; 2001.

Newman DK. The indwelling urinary catheter: principles for best practice. *J Wound Ostomy Continence Nurs* 2007;**34**:655–61.

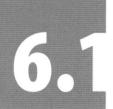

Management of Pre- and Post-operative Care of the High-Risk Surgical Patient

6.1

John Whittle

Key Learning Points

1. High-risk surgery is associated with significant inpatient mortality, and post-operative morbidity is associated with increases in long-term morbidity and mortality.

2. Perioperative care should be a team effort and proactive, rather than reactive.

3. Adequate risk assessment and ICU care triage are key to effective perioperative care.

4. Care bundles may reduce risk across a variety of surgeries and medical conditions through the aggregation of marginal gains.

5. Clear handover in the ICU can reduce medical error and improve patient safety.

Keywords: risk, triage, perioperative, optimisation, critical care

Introduction

High-risk surgery accounts for a disproportionate amount of in-hospital morbidity and mortality. In the UK, in 2006, patients admitted for high-risk surgery comprised only 12.5 per cent of admissions to hospitals but accounted for over 80 per cent of inpatient mortality.

Of those undergoing major surgery, between 10 and 17 per cent suffer major post-operative complications and up to half suffer short-term minor post-operative morbidity, resulting in increased usage of healthcare resources and delayed or failed recovery to preoperative function. Of those patients who go on to develop serious post-operative complications, up to 20 per cent go on to die within 30 days. The effects of post-operative complications persist post discharge from hospital, with a large number of patients suffering

reductions in physical function, as well as an increased mortality rate up to 5 years after the index surgery, even after the development of only one post-operative complication.

Whilst a large proportion of admissions to the ICU in the developed world result from high-risk surgery, only a small proportion of high-risk patients (15 per cent) are admitted to the ICU electively post-operatively.

Factors affecting post-operative outcomes are complex and result from the interaction of medical and physiological factors related to the baseline health of the patient, as well as factors related to the surgery itself and specific intra- and post-operative events.

Additionally, factors related to the specific health-care system in which the surgery takes place play a role, including surgical volume and availability and usage of intensive care beds.

Management of the elective high-risk surgical patient should be conceptualised as a continuum from the moment that surgery is considered through to discharge from hospital. Adequate risk assessment and ICU triage, as well as medical and physiological optimisation, should form the cornerstones of care, with subsequent intra- and post-operative care being adapted to account for patient-specific risks, as well as for global risks associated with the planned procedure. Appropriate ICU care forms only one part of a wider perioperative medicine approach to surgical risk.

This chapter will supply a brief overview of key concepts in this field and provide pointers for further in-depth reading.

Risk Scoring and ICU Triage

The first step in the care of the high-risk patient is identifying the individual at risk.

An expanding multiplicity of risk scoring systems have formed the bedrock of patient selection and assessment in recent years. Aside from better

623

informing shared decision-making, scoring systems have been used to help triage perioperative intensive care requirements.

Many individual perioperative risk factors, particularly specific co-morbidities such as diabetes or hypertension, have been associated with impaired post-operative outcomes. Similarly, patient factors, such as advanced age, frailty and poor nutritional status, are recognised as being independently predictive of operative outcome. In general, however, these factors have greater predictive power as part of a formalised risk score.

Many of these have been well validated and require varying amounts of physiological and biochemical data. Some, such as the Lee Revised Cardiac Risk Index, AKI risk index and ARISCAT (post-operative pulmonary complications), attempt to predict organ system-specific complications.

The best known and most commonly used is the ASA (American Society of Anesthesiologists) physical status classification system, which describes the general health of the patient, as well as their general burden of co-morbidities. It is simple to use and requires no laboratory data, and appears predictive of adverse outcome, though substantial inter-observer variation in scoring has been noted.

Other scoring systems in common use include P-POSSUM (Portsmouth Physiological and Operative Severity Score for the enUmeration of Mortality and morbidity) and SORT (Surgical Outcome Risk Tool). These encompass a range of variables, including patient- and surgery-specific data points, to produce a composite score. A predicted mortality of 5 per cent with P-POSSUM has been widely used to define high risk.

Assessment of the individual patient's functional status has further been incorporated into risk prediction models. Cardiopulmonary exercise testing (CPET) has gained popularity as an objective measure of individual patient-integrated physiology under conditions of controlled physical stress. Certainly, impaired aerobic fitness has been strongly associated with adverse perioperative outcomes, but the test requires specialist equipment and trained personnel. Other functional measures, such as self-reported activity scores and timed walk, have also been successfully used to predict post-operative outcome.

No large randomised trials exist to support the use of one risk prediction index over another in guiding perioperative management. However, data derived from rigorous risk assessment can be intelligently used in a pragmatic approach to patient care, especially in terms of triage to ICU and reduction in resource usage.

Pre-optimisation/Prehabilitation

Preoperative medical optimisation forms the bedrock of excellent perioperative care. Clear communication and documentation of goals of care as part of a shared decision-making approach informed by in-depth patient risk assessment and institutional protocols in the preoperative period will help minimise conflict in the post-operative period around haemodynamic targets, feeding strategies and antibiotic strategies, as well as reinforcing a patient-centred continuum of care across the perioperative period.

Preoperative cardiac investigations and management have been subject to a great deal of research. The American College of Cardiology (ACC)/American Heart Association (AHA) Task Force guidance is best placed to help guide the application of investigations such as cardiac catheterisation and stress echocardiography, as well as therapies such as perioperative beta-blockade. The POISE trials cast some doubt on the safety of elective beta-blockade in the perioperative period. In general, patients who are already on beta-blockade should be maintained on therapy during the perioperative period. Furthermore, targeted, titrated beta-blockade should be considered in those at highest risk of cardiac complications.

In general, patients identified as being at higher risk should be evaluated by a consultant anaesthetist with special interest in perioperative medicine. This individual is best placed to coordinate care throughout the perioperative period. Ideally, specific high-risk clinics should manage the care of high-risk patients. These clinics may be surgery-specific and involve several members of the multidisciplinary team, including the surgeon, anaesthetist, physiotherapist and specialist nurses. They may also offer advanced testing, such as CPET and echocardiography, at the time of clinic appointment. Elderly, frail patients may additionally benefit from engagement Perioperative Care of the Older Person (POPS) teams. These teams are in a unique position to manage polypharmacy and frailty assessment, and engage in preoperative decision-making, including risk assessment and discharge planning. In the post-operative period, these teams also specialise in transitioning patients back onto optimised longer-term medical therapy through to and beyond discharge.

Latterly, prehabilitation strategies have been trialled with some success. In general, prehabilitation entails a structured exercise programme tailored to the individual patient, often guided by CPET results. Over time, nutritional and cognitive interventions, among others, may be added to prehabilitation programmes in an attempt to optimise patient physiology prior to surgery.

Intraoperative Care

Good intraoperative care should form the basis of a continuum extending into the post-operative period, characterised by close attention to physiological optimisation in the context of judicious fluid management.

Establishment of adequate analgesia, including opiate-sparing techniques, can reduce post-operative morbidities such as ileus, delirium, chronic pain and pulmonary complications. Similarly, careful ventilator management, avoidance of absolute and relative hypotension and appropriate anaesthesia dosing (excessive depth of anaesthesia has been associated with delirium, hypotension and adverse outcomes across a variety of domains) can further contribute to reductions in immediate post-operative morbidity. Strategies and specific targets should be informed by preoperative risk assessments and will increasingly be guided by perioperative care bundles guiding care across the surgical pathway which are designed to modify risk. These bundles work on the principle of aggregation of marginal gains, are well accepted in intensive care practice and have shown promise across a variety of surgeries and medical conditions.

Handover to intensive care at the end of surgery should be structured and encompass both written and verbal components. An increasing body of evidence is developing in this field that highlights the importance of structured handover in patient safety. Many of the goals of preoperative care and intraoperative care, informed by the risk assessment, will be continued into the early post-operative period. Additionally, surgery-specific goals and plans will be handed over at this time. This is a clear opportunity to address key issues such as intraoperative events, mean arterial pressure (MAP), monitoring and fluid target goals, feeding, thromboprophylaxis and antibiotic strategy. Ideally, many of these issues will either be protocolised or, where a conflict appears to exist between medical goals and surgical goals, have been agreed upon during the preoperative period.

Perioperative Fluid Management

Fluid dosing is a subject of great complexity where both under- and over-administration are associated with adverse outcomes (ileus, pulmonary oedema, impaired wound healing, acute kidney injury). In general, perioperative cardiovascular management should be predicated on predefined treatment limits and/or targets. These will range from the simple (such as heart rate, urine output and MAP) to the complex, focussing on indices of cardiac output.

These limits should form the basis of a goal-directed therapy approach. The concept of goal-directed therapy grew from early observations by Shoemaker and colleagues that survivors of major surgery achieved higher values for cardiac output and oxygen delivery than non-survivors, and that active targeting of these values may result in a reduction in mortality. Since then, many trials have been carried out targeting various goals in both the intraoperative and early post-operative periods. Stroke volume optimisation and oxygen delivery augmentation have formed the basis of the majority of protocols. Latterly, a number of negative studies have cast doubt upon the efficacy of goal-directed therapy as a haemodynamic management strategy, though current evidence still appears to favour the approach, with the results of a large trial (OPTIMISE 2) being eagerly awaited.

Despite this, a rational, target- (or goal-) driven approach should be applied to fluid resuscitation that does not rely solely on indices such as heart rate and blood pressure which do not always reflect cardiac output and equally are not always predictive of fluid responsiveness. Goal-directed therapy protocols allow judicious fluid therapy, minimising variability in fluid prescribing and avoiding excess fluid therapy through thoughtless, non-parameter-driven bolusing. The value of goal-directed therapy is likely to be related to the fact that management is individually tailored to the requirements of each patient.

Post-operative Care

The principles for early post-operative care of the high-risk surgical patient may deviate from traditional intensive care in several ways. Traditional intensive care focuses on organ support; however, few post-operative patients, even among the highest risk, require this. Where organ support is necessary, it is likely to be single-organ for a limited period of time. Most post-operative strategies will target early mobilisation, effective fluid and analgesia management, early enteral feeding and prevention of common complications such as basal atelectasis and deep vein thrombosis. The greatest benefit of the ICU in this circumstance is the advanced monitoring available and the extended care from nursing and allied healthcare professionals. Indeed, this team approach should define the entirety of the perioperative journey for these higher-risk patients.

The guiding principle of post-operative care in the high-risk surgical patient remains the prevention of failure to rescue, hence preventing or reducing the impact of common complications such as acute kidney injury, delirium and cardiac arrhythmias. This can be conceptualised as proactive, rather than reactive, care focussing on preventing the development of complications, rather than on improving the care provided to manage complications. The physical location in which these therapies and protocols occur is partly irrelevant, the key being a loss of silo thinking. This approach has been described as 'intensive care without walls'.

Evidence for Intensive Care in High-Risk Surgical Patients

There are many components to safe perioperative care, and ICU admission is widely thought to be one of them. Differences in intensive care usage are widely cited as reasons for variation in post-operative outcomes. Indeed, in the Europe-wide EuSOS study, 73 per cent of patients who died were not admitted to the ICU at any stage after surgery. The greatest evidence for benefit lies in observational studies of patients refused admission to the ICU where admission to the ICU appeared to be associated with a mortality benefit. Furthermore, patients admitted to the ICU immediately after surgery appear to have better outcomes than those who are readmitted or have a delayed post-operative admission. However, not all studies have shown a mortality benefit in intensive care admission for higher-risk surgical patients.

Unfortunately, the benefits of post-operative intensive care admission are not testable in a randomised trial. Similarly, it is difficult to assess large data sets retrospectively for the reasons for intensive care admission (i.e. whether the patient was admitted as part of protocolised care or for specific medical risks). Objective data are, however, lacking for evidence-based criteria

for post-operative ICU admission and the intensive care bed remains a valuable commodity.

Patients may be admitted to the ICU because staff there are used to addressing increased monitoring needs, but evidence suggests that adequate staffing of surgical wards with qualified nurses also improves perioperative outcomes.

Conclusion

High-risk surgical patients continue to make up a substantial proportion of ICU admissions in most developed countries. Identification and optimisation of these patients prior to surgical interventions remains difficult. Pre-, intra- and post-operative variables all play a role in the development of considerable morbidity and mortality for high-risk patients. Appropriate decisions relating to the need for intensive care after surgery are key for high-quality patient care, yet adequate systems for triage remain elusive. The potential exists for underuse of critical care resources, with inappropriate lack of admission to an ICU for high-risk patients, as well as overuse, with unnecessary admissions leading to increased length of stay and costs. With the wealth of data now available regarding the perioperative status of many of these patients, further research is needed to help facilitate optimal care for post-surgical patients.

References and Further Reading

Fleisher LA, Fleischmann KE, Auerbach AD, et al. 2014 ACC/AHA guideline on perioperative cardiovascular evaluation and management of patients undergoing noncardiac surgery. A report of the American College of Cardiology/American Heart Association task force on practice guidelines. *Circulation* 2014;**130**:e278–333.

Pearse RM, Holt PJE, Grocott MPW. Managing perioperative risk in patients undergoing elective non-cardiac surgery. *BMJ* 2011;**343**:d5759.

Pearse RM, Moreno RP, Bauer P, et al. Mortality after surgery in Europe: a 7 day cohort study. *Lancet* 2012;**380**:1059–65.

Sobol JB, Wunsch H. Triage of high-risk surgical patients for intensive care. *Crit Care* 2011;**15**:217.

The Royal College of Anaesthetists. 2015. Perioperative medicine: the pathway to better surgical care. www.rcoa.ac.uk/sites/default/files/documents/2019-08/Perioperative%20Medicine%20-%20The%20Pathway%20to%20Better%20Care.pdf

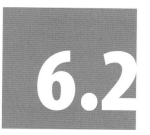

6.2 Management of the Critical Care Patient Following Cardiac Surgery

Nick Lees

Key Learning Points

1. The same principles of evidenced-based intensive care should be applied to cardiac surgical patients.
2. There is particular focus on invasive haemodynamic monitoring and immediate access to echocardiography.
3. Many elective patients can be managed aiming for early extubation and rapid discharge.
4. Inotropes and vasopressors are titrated according to assessment of left and right heart function and vascular resistance.
5. Complications include bleeding, tamponade, low cardiac output syndrome and arrhythmias.

Keywords: critical care, cardiac, surgery, perioperative

Introduction

Modern-day cardiac intensive care is managed by dedicated intensivists, directly applying the same evidence-based practices used in the general ICU. Despite the obvious increased focus on the heart and cardiovascular system and associated monitoring, these patients still require attention to basic ICU principles such as mechanical ventilation, renal replacement therapy, sepsis and nutrition.

Once a patient has been transferred to the ICU following cardiac surgery, the aims are to reverse any processes which contribute to instability or may delay extubation (e.g. hypothermia, electrolyte imbalances, coagulopathy and pain), whilst closely monitoring vital signs. Patients are usually still sedated and mechanically ventilated when leaving theatre, although patients having undergone less invasive procedures in the catheter laboratory, such as transcatheter aortic valve implantation (TAVI), may have just received sedation.

Handover

The initial handover from the anaesthetist and surgical team to the intensive care team is important. Bear in mind the anaesthetist has spent the last few hours with the patient, carefully titrating vasoactive and inotropic drugs, blood products and volume against trans-oesophageal echocardiography (TOE) assessments, so they should have a very good idea of the main concerns. The surgeon will be able to tell you in detail what has been done (i.e. which vessels were grafted in coronary artery surgery, valves replaced or repaired, etc.) and any difficulties that were faced. You should take note of whether or not cardiopulmonary bypass (CPB) was used, as there are specific complications associated with extracorporeal circulation. The past medical history is also important, as most cardiac patients have extensive medical co-morbidities, including diabetes, hypertension, chronic kidney disease and peripheral vascular disease, and consequently also take a lot of medications.

Some patients are suitable for 'fast-track' postoperative care – this means proactive management to facilitate early tracheal extubation (i.e. within 4 hours). Typically, these patients are preselected, are low risk, as calculated by scoring systems (e.g. EuroSCORE II), and have had relatively simple and quick surgery (e.g. coronary artery bypass graft (CABG) or aortic valve replacement). The anaesthetic technique is optimised to facilitate early extubation and usually involves lower doses of opioids, shorter-acting muscle relaxants and maintenance of normothermia. Benefits of fast-track are a reduction in time of mechanical ventilation and reduced ICU length of stay. Other 'more complex' patients may require a more prolonged period of monitoring and medical management before stopping sedation, and usually this is dictated by any complications or concern (e.g. unstable haemodynamics, poor gas exchange or bleeding). These patients are more likely to have had more complex surgery and longer time on

CPB and be higher risk (e.g. redo operations, aortic dissections, cardiac transplants and mechanical assist devices).

Examination

Once handover is complete, the patient should be exposed and examined. Surgical wounds and drains should be inspected, and invasive lines and their sites checked. Auscultation of the chest is important, as it is possible to diagnose significant or acute pathology such as haemo- or pneumothorax or signs of cardiac tamponade. Most patients are mildly hypothermic on arrival, so they may feel cool to touch. However, this is not necessarily indicative of a low cardiac output. Nearly all patients will have invasive monitoring, direct arterial pressure monitoring and a central venous catheter *in situ*. Pulmonary artery catheters (PACs) are often used in cardiac centres for higher-risk patients, both as means of directly measuring the pulmonary artery pressure, which is useful in situations like mitral valve surgery, cardiac transplantation and left ventricular assist device (LVAD), and also for cardiac output monitoring. Of note, the literature describing a lack of benefit for the PAC does not include cardiac surgical patients where staff are familiar with their use, and the direct and indirect measurements obtained are used to guide management. In addition, the much maligned central venous pressure (CVP) measurement is also useful, as elevated values are often indicative of worsening ventricular function or tamponade.

Cardiovascular System

An assessment should be made of the patient's cardiac output. Clinically this involves examination and assessment of skin perfusion and urine output. However, this may be measured by a PAC or other device, and clinically correlated by adequate mean arterial pressure, low right-sided pressures and a good urine output. Cardiac index (cardiac output divided by body surface area) is used more commonly than cardiac output, with values above 2.2 l/(min m²) being acceptable. Lactate values are often high after cardiac surgery (and are thought to be multifactorial in their origin, including related to systemic inflammation and pro-inflammatory cytokine production), and should be sequentially measured by blood gas analysis and seen to be falling. One state associated with lactic acidosis sometimes seen in cardiac surgery after CPB is the so-called 'vasoplegic syndrome', i.e. a severe drop in systemic vascular resistance refractory to, and requiring, high doses of vasopressors, but usually with an adequate cardiac index. This state is associated with an increase in morbidity and mortality.

In the post-operative setting, it is common to see disturbances of cardiac rate and rhythm, and patients are often paced using epicardial pacing wires placed intraoperatively. If not attached, a set of ventricular pacing wires are often left accessible on the skin for emergency use. If pacing wires are connected to a pacemaker box, the pacing mode, sensitivities, thresholds and underlying rhythm should be checked. It is common to pace at a rate of between 90 and 100 bpm postoperatively, so as to optimise the cardiac index. The atrial contraction component is particularly important to cardiac output in post-operative cardiac patients who tend to have worsened diastolic function, so atrial pacing or dual atrioventricular pacing is ideal. Atrial fibrillation occurs in at least 30 per cent of patients and is multifactorial in aetiology. Pharmacotherapy involves amiodarone (usually first line as it can be loaded with relative haemodynamic safety) or beta-blockers (if there is no contraindication). Direct current cardioversion should also be considered early on, and anticoagulation is important in the absence of surgical bleeding.

Inotropic drugs, if required, will most likely have been commenced already in the operating theatre. However, titration is done in the ICU thereafter. The choice of inotropic drug comes down to familiarity and institutional preferences, with little evidence to support one over the other. Commonly in cardiac surgery, adrenoreceptor agonists (noradrenaline, dobutamine) and phosphodiesterase inhibitors (milrinone, enoximone) are used alone or in combination (Table 6.2.1).

Weaning or increasing inotropic support should ideally be done using cardiac output monitoring and objective assessment of the heart and cardiovascular function. This may include mean arterial pressures, CVPs, pulmonary artery pressures, pulmonary artery wedge pressures and calculations or estimations of pulmonary and systemic vascular resistance and echocardiography. The values measured (both directly and derived) can help one decide upon fluid therapy, inotropic support and vasoconstrictors or vasodilator drugs, including pulmonary vasodilators such as inhaled nitric oxide. Sudden or sustained increases in support should mandate clinical examination, echocardiography and senior review, and consideration of states such as significant haemorrhage, left and/or right ventricular failure and tamponade.

Table 6.2.1 Inotropes and vasopressors used in cardiac intensive care

Drug	Mode of action	Notes
Adrenaline (epinephrine)	Most potent catecholamine. Acts via adrenergic receptors (α, β). Dose-dependent action	Profound increases in CO, HR, MAP and coronary blood flow Not usually first line, used in refractory shock states Myocardial oxygen demand/delivery ratio can be worsened Metabolic effects include increased plasma glucose and lactate concentrations
Dopamine	Precursor of noradrenaline. Acts via dopaminergic (DA1, DA2) and adrenergic (β and α) receptors. Dose-dependent action on receptors DA2, DA1, β, then α as dose increased	Doses of up to 5 µg/(kg min): primarily DA receptors are activated, causing a decrease in vascular resistance and a mild increase in cardiac output. No renal protective effect, but causes natriuresis At doses of 5–15 µg/(kg min), β-adrenoceptor effects lead to increases in CO and HR At higher doses, α-adrenoceptor effects predominate, causing an increase in vascular resistance
Dobutamine	Synthetic catecholamine. β1, β2 (binds in 3:1 ratio) and (weakly) α1 receptors	Dose-dependent increase in CO and a reduction in diastolic filling pressures and SVR Compared to dopamine, dobutamine tends to increase CO more, has little effect on MAP and tends to reduce ventricular filling pressures Tends to cause tachycardia Myocardial oxygen demand/delivery ratio can be worsened
Isoprenaline	Synthetic catecholamine. β1 and β2 activity, but without α activity	HR and contractility are increased (β1 activity). Decreased afterload and increased venodilation (β2) Mainly used as a chronotrope in patients with symptomatic bradycardia as an alternative to pacing
Levosimendan	Inotropic effects through Ca²⁺ sensitisation, without increasing intracellular cAMP or intracellular Ca²⁺ concentration Vasodilatory effects (e.g. coronary arteries) through K⁺ channel activation	Administered as 24-hour infusion, with or without loading dose. Long half-life (80 hours) of its active metabolite. Despite theoretical benefits, recent trials failed to show a mortality difference in patients given levosimendan preoperatively (LICORN), prophylactically (LEVO-CTS) or post-operatively (CHEETAH)
Milrinone, enoximone	Phosphodiesterase inhibitors leading to increase in cAMP	Positive inotropic effects (increased myocardial contractility and CO) plus a peripheral vasodilating action (decreased afterload and SVR) which may cause hypotension, especially if hypovolaemic. Can be mitigated by not using a loading dose Increases lusitropy (relaxation) No change or even improvement in myocardial oxygen demand/supply ratio Often used in cases of RV failure as it reduces RV afterload (PVR and PA pressures)
Noradrenaline (norepinephrine)	Precursor of adrenaline. Potent β1 and α activity, but minimal β2 effects	Mild inotropic and chronotropic effects at lower doses (β1). At higher doses, predominantly vasopressor actions (α), so increase in SVR and MAP. Will also increase PVR
Vasopressin	Acts on vascular smooth muscle V1 and oxytocin receptors, causing vasoconstriction	May also activate vascular smooth muscle V2 receptors, resulting in vasodilation
Methylene blue	Inhibitor of nitric oxide synthase and guanylyl cyclase	Useful in refractory hypotension in vasoplegic syndrome

Abbreviations: CO = cardiac output; HR = heart rate; MAP = mean arterial pressure; DA = dopamine; SVR = systemic vascular resistance; cAMP = cyclic adenosine monophosphate; RV = right ventricular; PVR = pulmonary vascular resistance; PA = pulmonary artery; Ca²⁺ = calcium; K⁺ = potassium.

The low cardiac output syndrome (LCOS) manifests itself as organ dysfunction and metabolic acidosis. It may develop after admission to the ICU, so staff should be vigilant, and deteriorating blood gases and physiology should again prompt clinical examination, echocardiography, instituting cardiac output monitoring and starting inotropic drugs. An improving picture will be demonstrated by adequate tissue oxygen delivery, as seen by falling serum lactate and adequate mixed venous oxygen saturations.

Cardiac tamponade is most commonly due to accumulation of blood in the pericardial space. This may develop as a consequence of blocked drains or occur after a bleeding episode once the drains have been removed. Bleeding may be from a surgical point or from general coagulopathy. It is characterised by a rise in CVP, systemic hypotension and end-organ dysfunction, i.e. cool peripheries, oliguria and rising serum lactate. Echocardiography can demonstrate a pericardial collection, and specific signs and criteria associated with tamponade due to altered ventricular filling.

Respiratory System

Blood gases should be optimised, and the lungs may require some recruitment and application of positive end-expiratory pressure (PEEP) – especially if they have been deflated during CPB and developed areas of collapse and atelectasis, or from pleural collections of blood.

Gut/Renal

The abdomen should be examined on a daily basis, and enteral nutrition commenced early on if the patient is not likely to be eating soon. H_2 antagonists or proton pump inhibitors are prescribed in most patients. Ileus and constipation are common post-operatively. Gut ischaemia is associated with LCOS and carries significant morbidity and mortality. Often this presents a few days after an episode of LCOS or sustained hypotension. Post-operative acute kidney injury (AKI) is common, and up to 30 per cent of CABG patients reach RIFLE (Risk, Injury, Failure, Loss of kidney function and End-stage kidney disease)/AKIN (Acute Kidney Injury Network) criteria for AKI. In many instances, this occurs on the back of chronic kidney disease.

Bleeding and Coagulopathy

Anaemia is common after cardiac surgery, and >50 per cent of patients receive a transfusion perioperatively. Transfusion has been shown to be associated with infection, low cardiac output, AKI and death. Severe post-operative blood loss and red blood cell transfusion in patients undergoing cardiac surgery are strongly associated with increased morbidity and mortality. Severe bleeding could be defined as >2 ml/(kg hr) chest drain blood loss for the first 3 hours post-operatively. As well as checking the full blood count and clotting screen, point-of-care analysis such as thromboelastography (TEG®) or rotational thromboelastometry (ROTEM®) is very helpful for rapid diagnosis of the coagulopathy. Management involves transfusion of packed cells and correcting the coagulopathy with appropriate blood products. Anti-fibrinolytics (tranexamic acid and, less commonly now, aprotinin) are almost universally used in cardiac surgery, and clotting factors such as fibrinogen concentrate and prothrombin complex concentrates are also commonly used, with the benefit of being administered in much smaller volumes and without the associated risks of blood product transfusion.

Reoperation due to bleeding after cardiac surgery is about 2–4 per cent, with risk factors including elderly patients, low body mass index (BMI) or body surface area (BSA), prolonged time on CPB, non-elective operations and preoperative use of anti-platelets or anticoagulant drugs. Patients who need to go back to theatre for bleeding have a higher risk of organ dysfunction, prolonged stay and more than double the rate of mortality.

The transfusion trigger in the stable, non-bleeding patient is usually at a haemoglobin level of 7–7.5 g/dl. However, a recent randomised controlled trial (TRICS III) demonstrated that a restrictive threshold (<7.5 g/dl) was not superior to the liberal (>9.5 g/dl) threshold with respect to post-operative morbidity.

Neurology

Delirium is often seen post-operatively. Risk factors include increasing age, previous stroke, length of surgery, atrial fibrillation and blood transfusion. Stroke occurs in around 2 per cent of patients, and as well as the usual vascular risk factors, it is associated with surgical manipulation of the aorta, intraoperative hypotension and post-operative atrial fibrillation.

Pain/Analgesia

Patients are managed with infusions of opiates, which should be appropriately loaded prior to reducing sedation. Morphine remains the most commonly used drug. Patient-controlled analgesia can be used once the patient is awake. Non-steroidal anti-inflammatory drugs (NSAIDs) tend to be avoided in cardiac patients, many of whom have renal insufficiency. Adverse events have been reported with the cyclo-oxygenase 2 (COX-2)-selective drugs.

Investigations in the Post-operative Setting

Routine bloods should be sent on arrival to the ICU, particularly full blood count and coagulation. Routine chest X-rays are often performed, and lung fields, pleural collections, invasive lines and drains should be checked. Intercostal chest drains are normally managed on low suction – initially to help expand the lungs and encourage drainage.

Echocardiography is readily available in the cardiac ICU, and bedside transthoracic echocardiography (TTE) or TOE should be performed if indicated. Notably with TTE, adequate windows are often obscured by surgical dressings, drains and mechanical ventilation, so if there is particular concern, then TOE should be used. The most common reasons for performing echocardiography would be to assess pericardial collections and assessment of left and right ventricular function, i.e. haemodynamic disturbances. Other reasons may include assessment of systolic anterior motion (SAM) of the mitral valve after mitral surgery or myectomy, monitoring placement of intra-aortic balloon pumps or extracorporeal membrane oxygenation (ECMO) cannulae, or to rule out thrombus prior to direct current (DC) cardioversion.

References and Further Reading

Griffiths SV, Conway DH; POPC-CB Investigators, *et al.* What are the optimum components in a care bundle aimed at reducing post-operative pulmonary complications in high-risk patients? *Perioper Med* 2018;7:7.

Pearse RM, Rhodes A, Grounds RM. Clinical review: how to optimize management of high-risk surgical patients. *Crit Care* 2004;8:503–7.

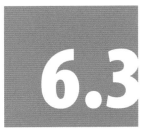

Management of the Critical Care Patient Following Craniotomy

Wilson Fandino

Key Learning Points

1. Most patients undergoing elective supra-tentorial craniotomy can be discharged safely to the neurosurgical ward.
2. The use of vasoactive agents and insulin infusions and the need for cardiovascular monitoring and intracranial pressure management are among the most common interventions requiring critical care admission.
3. Intraoperative complications requiring critical care admission include, but are not exclusive to, failed endotracheal extubation, cardiovascular instability, extensive blood loss and cerebral swelling.
4. Post-operative complications usually involve respiratory, cardiovascular or central nervous systems. Metabolic derangements and infectious diseases may also warrant treatment and close monitoring in critical care.
5. Use of opioids, when carefully titrated, is considered safe in neurological patients. Opioids should be always considered, because craniotomies are typically painful procedures.

Keywords: craniotomy, intraoperative complications, post-operative complications

Introduction

It is estimated that >25,000 craniotomies have been carried out in NHS England between April 2014 and March 2015. The most common pathologies requiring supra-tentorial or infra-tentorial craniotomy are summarised in Table 6.3.1.

In the UK, the indications for admission to the critical care unit (CCU) following a craniotomy are variable between neurosurgical units. Whilst some centres routinely send patients following craniotomy to a level

Table 6.3.1 Main indications for elective and emergency craniotomies

Elective procedures	· Tumour resection
	  ◦ Supra-tentorial
	  ◦ Infra-tentorial (posterior fossa)
	· Ventriculostomy
	· Vascular malformation obliteration (e.g. resection of arteriovenous malformation)
	· Clipping of unruptured cerebral aneurysm
	· Functional surgery (e.g. temporal lobectomy for epilepsy, insertion of deep brain stimulator)
	· Arnold–Chiari malformation decompression
	· Neurovascular decompression
	· Open brain biopsy

Emergency procedures	· Removal of haematoma
	  ◦ Epidural haematoma
	  ◦ Subdural haematoma: acute, subacute or chronic
	  ◦ Intracerebral haematoma: supra-tentorial haemorrhage
	· Removal of brain abscess
	· Posterior fossa haemorrhage
	· Clipping of ruptured cerebral aneurysm

2 CCU, some others allow a prolonged stay in the post-anaesthesia care unit (PACU). Admission of patients to level 3 CCU is typically reserved for patients with specific intraoperative or post-operative complications (see below). On the other hand, the cost of staying in the CCU can be 3–5 times as expensive as a standard neurosurgical ward; hence, there is a need for optimising the resources to guarantee equity of access for all patients. A thorough assessment on an individual basis and a better understanding of pre-operative risk factors and intraoperative and post-operative complications are essential to improve the efficiency of neuro-CCUs, whilst providing safe post-operative care.

Criteria for CCU Admission Following Craniotomy

Most patients undergoing elective supra-tentorial craniotomy do not benefit from routine CCU admission. In fact, many of them are safely extubated in the theatre and sent back to the neurosurgical ward after a short period of recovery in the PACU. Whilst this practice is strongly associated with a low rate of post-operative complications, the decision to admit the patient to the CCU relies on several factors, including: institutional practice, hospital infrastructure, nature of the procedure, type and location of the intracranial lesion, risk of post-operative seizures, predicted blood loss, coexisting co-morbidities and anaesthetic technique – most awake craniotomies do not require CCU admission. Among preoperative factors, age (>65 years), diabetes mellitus and craniotomy for vascular lesions appear to have a higher probability of CCU admission. On the other hand, CCU admission following emergency supra-tentorial craniotomy is usually required.

Interventions Requiring CCU Admission

Apart from 'standard' monitoring required following a craniotomy, there are some interventions that typically require CCU admission. These include blood pressure management with intravenous (IV) infusions, the need for insulin infusions, cardiovascular monitoring, intracranial pressure (ICP) monitoring and management of intracranial hypertension. Some other interventions, including external ventricular drain (EVD) insertion and use of hyperosmolar solutions, may not require routine CCU admission, provided that the ICP is controlled and there are no electrolyte derangements.

Complications Requiring CCU Admission

Intraoperative Complications

1. **Failed extubation:** prolonged operations, procedures with potential compromise of the airway reflexes (e.g. debulking of posterior fossa lesions may cause damage to neural structures, brainstem oedema and/or dysfunction of the cranial nerves) and craniotomies performed in the park-bench, sitting or prone position (which increase the risk of tongue swelling and oropharyngeal oedema) may impede a safe endotracheal extubation in the operating room. These potential CCU admissions are often known about in advance, and as such, the patient can normally be transferred post-operatively, whilst still intubated and ventilated, to the ICU in an elective manner. In other instances, the intended plan of immediate post-operative extubation fails,

thus necessitating re-intubation and unplanned CCU admission (e.g. upper airway oedema, acute respiratory failure, consciousness deterioration).

2. **Cardiovascular instability:** patients requiring high doses of vasopressors and those with extensive blood loss (particularly in the case of arteriovenous malformation and large meningioma resections) need continuous blood pressure ± cardiac output monitoring (e.g. PiCCO®, LiDCO®, Vigileo™).

3. **Extensive blood loss:** the majority of craniotomies do not require transfusion of blood products, with the exception of emergent and lengthy procedures (e.g. skull base and large vascular tumours) and vascular malformation obliterations. For the latter, some patients may require endovascular embolisation of the malformation as a first-stage procedure, to subsequently diminish the risk of intraoperative bleeding.

4. **Brain swelling:** prolonged procedures (which typically include resection of skull base tumours and large meningiomas with extensive manipulation of brain tissue) often stimulate oedema of the surrounding structures, thereby increasing the risk of failed endotracheal extubation.

Post-operative Complications

1. **Respiratory:** in general, respiratory complications are the most common indication for endotracheal re-intubation in the immediate recovery period of any procedure requiring general anaesthesia.

2. **Haemodynamics:** coexisting morbidities (myocardial infarction, cardiac failure, poor ASA (American Society of Anesthesiologists) physical status) and systemic complications (arterial hypotension or hypertension, massive bleeding) may prompt the use of vasopressor administration via a central line catheter (e.g. noradrenaline, dobutamine, vasopressin). Conversely, the use of IV medications for the treatment of hypertension (e.g. labetalol or esmolol) may be necessary in some specific circumstances. As both situations require greater degrees of haemodynamic monitoring than is normally achievable on the ward, CCU admission is warranted.

3. **Neurology:** post-operative haematoma, ischaemic stroke and extensive cerebral oedema are among the most common complications that can lead

to Glasgow Coma Score (GCS) deterioration, slow neurological recovery or new motor deficit. The occurrence of post-operative seizures is variable, depending on the underlying disease, the volume and location of the lesion and whether preoperative prophylaxis with phenytoin or levetiracetam was utilised. Up to 15–30 per cent of patients undergoing craniotomy for meningioma resection develop this complication, and large supra-tentorial lesions are at the highest risk. Young and male patients have been also reported to be at increased risk.

4. **Metabolic:** the syndrome of inappropriate anti-diuretic hormone secretion (SIADH), diabetes insipidus (DI) and cerebral salt wasting are relatively common in neurosurgical patients. In diabetic patients, prolonged fasting, surgical stress and administration of dexamethasone can also elicit acute decompensation. Post-operative nausea and vomiting (PONV), which is common in patients undergoing infra-tentorial craniotomy, and use of hypertonic solutions (i.e. mannitol and hypertonic saline) may also induce electrolytic derangements.

5. **Infectious:** systemic inflammatory response syndrome, sepsis, hospital-acquired pneumonia (HAP), cerebral abscess and meningitis are serious infective complications following a craniotomy.

Pain Management

Craniotomies are painful procedures, and a multi-modal approach should be utilised to treat anticipated pain. Long-lasting local anaesthetics can be infiltrated intraoperatively into the surgical incision and location of any cranial fixation pins. Additionally, it is the practice of some anaesthetists to perform a scalp block either at the beginning or at the end of the procedure.

Due to concerns regarding side effects, there is often reluctance to use high-dose opioids for post-operative analgesia of supra-tentorial craniotomies. Over-sedation is perhaps most often quoted, as it may impede a proper neurological assessment. However, the evidence supporting the avoidance of strong opioids in this context is weak, and most clinicians have realised that carefully titrated opiates can be used in a safe manner during the recovery period. Patient-controlled analgesia (PCA) with IV morphine or oxycodone is also used in many institutions in the UK and has been demonstrated to be safe.

Regimens used to treat post-operative pain are highly variable among countries and institutions. Codeine seems to be the preferred first-line opioid used in many institutions in the UK, but it is also important to optimise analgesia with scalp infiltration and non-opioid analgesics, including paracetamol and dexamethasone. In some institutions, the use of non-steroidal anti-inflammatory drugs (NSAIDs) is avoided, due to its effects on platelet function and increased risk of bleeding.

Recent evidence also supports the use of dexmedetomidine (a highly selective α_2 adrenergic agonist with anxiolytic, sedative and analgesic properties) for pain management following craniotomy. Further research is, however, needed to validate these results, especially as concerns exist about side effects such as bradycardia, hypotension and over-sedation.

Conclusion

Craniotomy is one of the most common procedures performed in the field of neurosurgery. Whilst it has long been believed that most elective patients require CCU admission post-operatively, several observational studies have demonstrated that many of these patients can be safely discharged from recovery to the neurosurgical ward. It is therefore important for the intensivist to carefully select patients who may have benefit from CCU admission, based on their coexisting diseases, nature of the procedure and intraoperative or post-operative complications.

References and Further Reading

Badenes R, Prisco L, Maruenda A, Taccone FS. Criteria for intensive care admission and monitoring after elective craniotomy. *Curr Opin Anaesthesiol* 2017;**30**:540–5.

Dunn LK, Naik BI, Nemergut EC, Durieux ME. Post-craniotomy pain management: beyond opioids. *Curr Neurol Neurosci Rep* 2016;**16**:93.

Hanak BW, Walcott BP, Nahed BV, *et al.* Postoperative intensive care unit requirements after elective craniotomy. *World Neurosurg* 2014;**81**:165–72.

Lonjaret L, Guyonnet M, Berard E, *et al.* Postoperative complications after craniotomy for brain tumor surgery. *Anaesth Crit Care Pain Med* 2017;**36**:213–18.

Reponen E, Korja M, Niemi T, Silvasti-Lundell M, Hernesniemi J, Tuominen H. Preoperative identification of neurosurgery patients with a high risk of in-hospital complications: a prospective cohort of 418 consecutive elective craniotomy patients. *J Neurosurg* 2015;**123**:594–604.

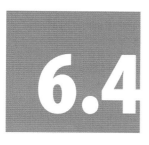

Management of the Critical Care Patient Following Liver Transplant

6.4

Mike Spiro and Jeremy Fabes

Key Learning Points

1. The demand for liver transplantation (LT) is expected to rise over time due to an increasing prevalence of end-stage liver disease (ESLD).
2. Perioperative management of LT patients, who are increasingly co-morbid, can be challenging.
3. Post-operative care in the ICU may minimise complications, particularly cardiovascular, renal and respiratory pathologies.
4. Management of post-operative coagulopathy and transfusion requires viscoelastic and other testing, beyond standard laboratory assays.
5. A low threshold of suspicion is required for detection of complications, especially of the hepatic vasculature.

Keywords: allograft, rejection, coagulopathy, hepatic arterial thrombosis

Introduction

The demand for liver transplantation (LT) is expected to rise over time due to the increasing prevalence of end-stage liver disease (ESLD). Perioperative management of LT patients, who are increasingly co-morbid, can be challenging. Management should involve consideration of every organ system, with a low threshold to involve surgeons early should concerns arise.

Cardiovascular

Subclinical coronary artery disease is common in ESLD patients. Pharmacological or exercise stress testing in at-risk patients has reasonable negative predictive value, but coronary revascularisation does not appear to improve perioperative outcomes. Cirrhotic cardiomyopathy with diastolic dysfunction and poor ability to increment contractility are common in ESLD, and tolerated in the pre-transplant high cardiac output, low systemic vascular resistance state.

Allograft survival requires effective graft perfusion and avoidance of hepatic venous stasis. However, myocardial ischaemia or increasing vascular tone following transplantation may precipitate cardiac decompensation, especially in cardiomyopathy. Maintenance of end-organ oxygen delivery with goal-directed fluid therapy, appropriate red cell transfusion and judicious vasopressor use to avoid excessive afterload can prevent this deterioration. Dynamic invasive monitoring, with pulmonary artery catheterisation in selected patients, guides volume, vasopressor and inotropic therapy, as well as assessing right heart function and left heart preload. Correction of acid–base balance, electrolyte levels and temperature control will also improve haemodynamic function. Where post-operative haemodynamics do not progressively improve, having excluded other complications, the quality of allograft function must be considered.

Following optimisation of circulating volume, avoidance of hypervolaemia is equally important to minimise the risk of pulmonary, renal and allograft oedema. Ongoing third-space losses due to post-operative inflammation must be replaced, but otherwise pursuit of a negative fluid balance as soon as possible often improves allograft haemodynamics and function.

Renal Failure

Chronic renal failure (CRF) in ESLD patients is common and increases global perioperative risk, especially cardiac events and acute renal failure. Acute kidney injury (AKI) following liver transplantation occurs in up to 50 per cent of patients, and the need for post-transplant renal replacement therapy is associated with an increased risk of early allograft dysfunction and mortality. Risk factors for renal dysfunction include intraoperative hypotension, lower-quality donor grafts

635

and graft failure, ischaemia–reperfusion injury, blood transfusion, preoperative renal disease and nephrotoxic exposure. Management of AKI and/or CRF in the ICU post-transplant follows routine practice, with determination and reversal of aetiology, avoidance of nephrotoxics, optimisation of fluid status and renal perfusion. Renal support during transplantation may be required.

The nephrotoxic calcineurin inhibitors tacrolimus and cyclosporine can be avoided until renal function improves by using T cell-specific antibodies or the renal-sparing purine synthesis inhibitor mycophenolate mofetil.

Hepatorenal Syndrome

The prevalence of hepatorenal syndrome (HRS) within the pre-transplant patient cohort may be as high as 50 per cent, and HRS unresponsive to medical therapy is an indication for LT, with good outcomes and subsequent improvement in renal function. Management of known HRS post-transplant differs from AKI/CRF, with a lower threshold to use vasopressin or terlipressin (with or without albumin support), to maintain renal perfusion and redress the splanchnic vasodilation that underlies HRS.

Ventilation

The increasing trend towards early extubation post-LT, either in theatre or in the ICU, does not appear to negatively impact on outcome and would be expected to improve allograft haemodynamics and avoid the recognised complications of prolonged intubation and ventilation. Patient selection is essential to avoid re-intubation for respiratory failure or early return to theatre due to borderline allograft function.

Acute respiratory distress syndrome (ARDS) is not uncommon following LT secondary to massive transfusion, transfusion-related acute lung injury (TRALI) and allograft reperfusion syndrome. Lung-protective ventilation strategies, as developed by ARDSNet, should be employed in all ventilated patients.

Allograft Function

Monitoring of graft function permits early identification of dysfunction or deterioration and intervention to prevent failure. Synthetic function is assessed through levels of clotting factors V and VII, the international normalised ratio (INR) and albumin, whilst graft survival can be followed through the degree of hepatocyte necrosis (alanine aminotransferase (ALT), aspartate aminotransferase (AST)), and cholestasis (alkaline phosphatase (ALP) and gamma-glutamyl transferase (γGT)). More dynamic tests of graft function include indocyanine green clearance and MEGX (monoethylglycinexylidide) testing.

Infection

Post-operative sepsis has only recently been overtaken by cardiac events as the major cause of death following LT. Infective sources include typical hospital-acquired infections, ventilator-associated pneumonia (VAP), immunosuppression-driven reactivation of latent infections and those derived from the donor organ or blood products. Pneumonia is commonly caused by typical VAP organisms, Gram-negative species, *Staphylococcus* and enterococci, as well as vancomycin-resistant *Enterococcus* (VRE). Multi-resistant organisms can be problematic and hard to treat. Typical fungal infections include *Candida* and *Aspergillus* and are most common during aggressive immunosuppressive management of acute graft rejection. The immunosuppressed state permits cytomegalovirus (CMV) infection from the graft; donor and recipient risk and antibody status must be assessed pre-operatively, and evidence of systemic CMV infection treated early with ganciclovir.

Preventative measures include tailored perioperative antibiotics and prophylactic fluconazole against *Candida* in some centres for higher-risk patients. Standard management of infection with identification, source control and targeted anti-infectives is employed, with a reduction or cessation in immunosuppression where required. Septic shock in the post-LT patient can be challenging to manage, with poor response to vasopressors.

Nutrition

Malnutrition and deranged metabolism are common in ESLD and increase the post-operative risk of infection and poor outcome. Glycaemic control may be deranged secondary to poor graft function, surgical stress, immunosuppressive agents and diabetes. Nutritional support is required during the catabolic post-surgical stress phase, especially with high-dose corticosteroid use. Enteric feeding is superior to parenteral, and trophic feed should be maintained, even in ileus. Nutritional assessment should encompass electrolyte, calorie and protein requirement.

Post-operative Complications in the ICU

Primary Graft Failure

Roughly 2 per cent of allografts will be unable to support the recipient's metabolic demands, with lower-quality grafts at higher risk. Clinical, synthetic and metabolic evidence of graft failure will be apparent. Management is supportive, with correction of coagulopathy, acid–base balance, electrolytes and hypoglycaemia. Re-transplantation prior to the onset of multi-organ failure is associated with significantly better outcomes.

Vascular

Hepatic artery thrombosis (HAT), whilst uncommon (approximately 1 per cent incidence), can lead to early allograft loss. The aetiology is multifactorial, with graft haemodynamics, the quality of arterial anastomosis and hypercoagulability contributing. Patients typically receive risk-profiled prophylactic anticoagulation to help prevent HAT. Routine duplex ultrasonography may detect early HAT, but poor sensitivity means a low threshold for suspicion must be maintained. Graft necrosis generates haemodynamic instability, with abrupt transaminitis, biochemical evidence of graft failure and coagulopathy. Urgent rescue interventions include radiological revascularisation or re-transplantation.

Portal vein thrombosis presents with evidence of allograft oedema, poor synthetic function and persistent ascites. Diagnosis is by duplex ultrasonography and angiography, with radiological or surgical correction.

Acute Rejection

T cell-mediated graft injury typically presents within the first 2 weeks post-transplant with transaminitis and cholestasis. Liver biopsy is diagnostic, and management with increased immunosuppression usually avoids re-transplantation.

Coagulopathy

Hepatic synthetic dysfunction drives coagulopathy through decreased levels of most pro-coagulant clotting factors, anti-thrombotic factors anti-thrombin III and protein C and S, as well as fibrinolytic factors such as plasminogen. For this reason, ESLD patients demonstrate varying degrees of both pro- and anticoagulant imbalance. Surgery will compound coagulopathy through factor consumption, haemodilution, hypocalcaemia and other perioperative changes.

Distinguishing post-operative coagulopathic bleeding from surgical causes is essential. Classical markers of clotting function are relatively inaccurate and in this setting may not reflect the bleeding risk or the need for blood products or factors. More accurate representation of coagulation is obtained from viscoelastic methods supported by factor assays (i.e. fibrinogen) and markers of factor function (i.e. functional fibrinogen). Targets for platelets, fibrinogen and thromboelastic indices will vary, depending on local protocols and the clinical scenario. Protocolised approaches to correction of coagulopathy based on viscoelastic testing demonstrate a reduction in blood product use and improved outcome. Minimisation of pro-coagulant factor use will reduce the risk of HAT and hepatic vein thrombosis.

Biliary

Biliary leak or obstruction is common post-LT. Low-volume biliary drainage, coupled with cholestasis and imaging demonstrating an obstructed biliary tree, is diagnostic. Management options are conservative or interventional, including endoscopic retrograde cholangiopancreatography (ERCP), percutaneous drainage or surgery.

Neurological

Common neurological sequelae of LT include seizures, intracranial haemorrhage and precipitation of new or worsening encephalopathy. Encephalopathy and seizure activity are often multifactorial, and risk is increased by pre-existing or new-onset metabolic and electrolyte dysfunction. Post-LT psychosis, whilst rare, can be profound and may be driven by high-dose steroids, the ICU environment or multiple drug interactions. New-onset neurological symptoms require exclusion of central nervous system infection and meningitis, especially CMV, fungal and classical microorganisms.

References and Further Reading

Beattie C, Gillies MA. Anaesthesia and intensive care for adult liver transplantation. *Anaesth Intensive Care Med* 2015;**16**:339–43.

Feltracco P, Barbieri S, Galligioni H, *et al.* Intensive care management of liver transplanted patients. *World J Hepatol* 2011;**3**:61–71.

Fernandez TMA, Gardiner PJ. Critical care of the liver transplant recipient. *Curr Anesthesiol Rep* 2015;**5**:419–28.

Kashimutt S, Kotzé A. Anaesthesia for liver transplantation. *BJA Education* 2017;**17**:35–40.

Management of the Critical Care Patient Following Heart Transplant

Nick Lees

Key Learning Points

1. Heart transplantation is a successful treatment for selected patients with severe heart failure.
2. Left ventricular assist devices are increasingly commonplace as a bridge to transplant.
3. After heart transplantation, invasive monitoring and careful assessment of the cardiac index are important, noting the differences in donor heart physiology.
4. Right ventricular dysfunction should be diagnosed and managed promptly.
5. Immunosuppression is started perioperatively, and these drugs require expert management.

Keywords: heart transplantation, left ventricular assist devices, right ventricular dysfunction, immunosuppression

Introduction

Cardiac transplantation is an effective treatment for selected patients with severe heart failure (HF) (New York Heart Association (NYHA) functional classes III and IV), with debilitating symptoms despite maximised medical and cardiac resynchronisation therapy. Over 100 adult heart transplants occur per year in the UK, with around 250 patients on the active waiting list at any one time.

It is important to understand the cause of a patient's HF, and the most common cause is dilated cardiomyopathy (DCM). Other aetiologies include ischaemic HF, adult congenital heart disease, severe valvular disease with secondary HF and other cardiomyopathies (e.g. idiopathic, restrictive, peripartum and chemotherapy-induced). Candidates for transplantation with HF usually follow a slow course, associated with gradual up-titration in medical therapy and worsening symptoms, but some present acutely, including younger patients with sudden decompensation and refractory cardiogenic shock. An increasing number of patients are being managed with left ventricular assist devices (LVADs) prior to transplantation ('bridge to transplant'). This is, in part, due to both lack of availability of donor hearts and improvement in technology and safety of the devices, but also in many cases to optimise potentially reversible organ dysfunction or pulmonary hypertension to allow eligibility for transplantation. LVADs may be short-term extracorporeal systems such as the CentriMag™ system, or durable and fully implantable continuous-flow devices such as the HeartWare™ ventricular assist system (HVAD™) or HeartMate® devices.

As a general rule, the ischaemic time after harvesting a donor heart is kept to <4 hours. However, the use of the Organ Care System (OCS™ Heart) allows warm perfusion and monitoring of the donor organ, thus prolonging the ischaemic time. The surgical technique for cardiac transplantation involves a median sternotomy, establishment of cardiopulmonary bypass, cardiectomy leaving the recipient's left atrial cuff behind and then implantation of the donor heart – normally in an orthotopic position with anastomoses of the left atrium, pulmonary artery, aorta and then the right atrium (Shumway–Lower technique).

Monitoring

Monitoring from theatres will include continuous ECG, arterial, central venous and pulmonary artery pressure monitoring, measurement of pulmonary artery wedge pressure (or a direct left atrial pressure line), intermittent or continuous cardiac output measurement, urine output measurement and immediate access to transoesophageal echocardiography (TOE).

Haemodynamics

Haemodynamic instability is common, with causative factors including ischaemia/reperfusion injury, post-bypass inflammatory response, elevated pulmonary vascular resistance and bleeding. The main post-operative priorities are to maintain an adequate cardiac index and to be vigilant for signs of worsening right ventricular (RV) function.

The haemodynamic strategy aims to optimise ventricular contractility with inotropes, whilst reducing afterload (especially on the right side), and as such inodilators such as the phosphodiesterase inhibitor milrinone are commonly used. Isoprenaline was traditionally used for its chronotropic and afterload-reducing effects but is less so now. Dopamine, dobutamine and adrenaline are also still commonly used, and vasopressors such as noradrenaline and vasopressin may be required to maintain an adequate mean arterial pressure (MAP), which is important in order to maintain adequate coronary artery perfusion. Inhaled pulmonary vasodilators are often started in theatre, and are usually continued for a short time post-operatively to reduce pulmonary vascular resistance and pulmonary hypertension, thus helping prevent RV failure. Achieving the right balance of inotropic/dilator support can be difficult, and is guided by visual inspection in theatre and echocardiographic assessment and by using information from invasive and cardiac output monitoring. Inotropes should be weaned off, as tolerated, over the first few days, and high or escalating inotropic requirement post-operatively is an ominous sign and should prompt immediate assessment of the patient. This should include TOE to check left and RV function and for any collection, and mechanical circulatory support may need consideration. Left ventricular failure is less common and a bad sign after a heart transplant, and hypotension and elevated pulmonary artery wedge or left atrial pressures are seen. Once again, TOE is important to make the diagnosis and guide further management.

If observations are stable (i.e. good cardiac index, low central venous pressue (CVP), low pulmonary artery wedge pressure (or left atrial pressure), inotropic support is not high and any acidosis is correcting), once the patient is normothermic, inhaled nitric oxide is weaned off gradually (paying attention to any rise in CVP or pulmonary artery pressure whilst doing so) and the patient can be woken and extubated.

Right Ventricular Failure

A common cause of early graft failure is RV failure, and signs include hypotension, rising CVP and pulmonary artery pressures, and worsening acidosis. Echocardiography will show a reduction in the RV systolic function, RV dilation and tricuspid regurgitation. Left ventricular function may be preserved. Treatment involves increasing inotropic support, starting or increasing inhaled pulmonary vasodilators, reducing excess preload by diuresis or haemofiltration and maintaining appropriate rate and rhythm with pacing and anti-arrhythmic drugs if necessary. There is little evidence to support one inotrope over another (and it largely comes down to institutional preference), but milrinone or enoximone are commonly used as first-line agents, alone or in combination with adrenaline. Systemic vasodilators, such as glyceryl trinitrate (GTN), are sometimes used, as they will lower PVR. However, the systemic blood pressure may drop adversely; hence inhaled selective pulmonary vasodilators are more useful. If the situation is not improving, there should be early consideration for mechanical circulatory support, including veno-arterial (VA) extracorporeal membrane oxygenation (ECMO) or a temporary right ventricular assist device (RVAD). Appropriate ventilatory support involves avoiding excessive intrathoracic pressures, so low inspiratory pressures are aimed for (as per usual good practice).

Rate and Rhythm
Donor Heart Physiology

Direct sympathetic and parasympathetic nervous system connections are absent in post-transplant donor hearts, and they do not re-innervate effectively. The resting heart rate is thus a little faster due to the absence of parasympathetic tone, and the heart rate variability response to exercise, for example, is reduced (Box 6.5.1). Heart rate increases in response to systemic catecholamines, but the level of response is reduced due to a lack of sino-atrial node innervation. The normal baroreceptor response is also impaired, and the transplanted heart therefore responds slowly to abrupt changes in blood pressure and filling volumes.

Box 6.5.1 Changes in the Transplanted Donor Heart
- Higher resting heart rate
- Impaired chronotropic and cardiac output response to exercise (heart rate slow to rise, then slow to fall afterwards)
- Altered diastolic function
- Higher stroke volume
- Impaired baroreceptor response
- Reduced/absent sensation of angina
- Supersensitivity to catecholamines

Management

Only drugs acting **directly** on the receptors in the heart (e.g. adrenoreceptors) will have an effect, so anticholinergics such as atropine will not work to increase the heart rate. The rate is thus dependent on the heart's intrinsic electrical activity and circulating catecholamines. Inotropic drugs like isoprenaline (traditionally used because of its inotropic, chronotropic and afterload-reducing properties) may be used, and temporary atrial and ventricular epicardial pacing is typically set at a rate of 100–110 bpm to maintain an adequate heart rate. Arrhythmias should be treated with pharmacotherapy such as amiodarone, avoiding negative inotropes in the early phase, or direct current (DC) cardioversion. Atrial fibrillation is often the first sign of rejection.

Fluids and Renal Function

The newly grafted heart is very sensitive to filling due to lack of compliance (diastolic dysfunction). Therefore, fluid challenges should be small and cautious, and guided by CVP and echocardiography if necessary. CVP is a useful trend monitor of RV function and ideally should be no more than 12 mmHg. Blood products should be leucocyte-depleted, and cytomegalovirus (CMV)-negative if donor and recipient are CMV-negative. Acute kidney injury (AKI) is common, and 5–10 per cent of patients may require haemofiltration. Risk factors for the development of AKI include reduced renal function pre-operatively, prolonged ischaemic time, elevated troponin release, prolonged time on cardiopulmonary bypass, previous cardiac surgery, mechanical circulatory support pre-operatively and blood product use. AKI also develops in the context of post-operative multi-organ failure or primary graft failure. Diuretics are commonly needed, especially as many patients have chronic fluid overload pre-operatively.

Bleeding

This is a particular concern, given the increasing number of patients with ventricular assist devices (VADs) *in situ* prior to transplant. As these patients have normally been taking anticoagulant and antiplatelet drugs pre-operatively, it increases the surgical complexity – which consequently then increases the duration of surgery. Similarly, patients on ECMO are usually heparinised and have platelet and clotting factor deficiencies, and this once again complicates matters. Blood and blood products are invariably required, as are anti-fibrinolytic drugs such as tranexamic acid. Clotting factors, such as prothrombin complex concentrate and fibrinogen concentrate, are particularly attractive options, as the infused volume is less. As a golden rule, cardiac tamponade must always be ruled out in any case of haemodynamic instability in the post-surgical patient.

Immunosuppression and Infection

Immunosuppressive therapy is given after heart transplantation, both as prophylaxis against rejection and also to treat breakthrough episodes of rejection.

De novo rejection is dependent on T cell activation, and primary prophylaxis is aimed at inhibiting the T cell activation cascade. Adequate prophylaxis cannot be achieved with any single agent with an acceptable level of toxicity, and most centres use a combination of a calcineurin inhibitor (CNI) (such as tacrolimus), corticosteroids and a proliferation inhibitor (such as mycophenolate or everolimus) for initial prophylaxis. Many centres use additional 'induction therapy' with an agent such as anti-thymocyte globulin (ATG) in the immediate post-operative period. Some immunosuppressants, particularly the CNIs, have a narrow therapeutic window and require therapeutic monitoring of blood levels, and drug interactions are common – again especially for the CNIs which are metabolised by the cytochrome P450 system in the liver. Other adverse effects of pharmacological immunosuppression include an increased risk of opportunistic infection, malignancy and chronic kidney disease. Prophylaxis against opportunistic CMV infection and *Pneumocystis jirovecii* should therefore be routinely administered, and this is usually achieved with valganciclovir and co-trimoxazole, respectively, whilst targeted prophylaxis against other infections such as toxoplasmosis and fungal disease may be needed, depending on the patient's risk profile and clinical course.

Acute Rejection

Hyper-acute rejection occurs within minutes to hours after implantation and reperfusion of the donor heart, and is due to the presence of preformed recipient antibodies against donor (ABO antigens or human leucocyte antigens (HLAs)). It is very uncommon as it can be prevented by ensuring ABO compatibility, and by doing an actual or virtual HLA cross-match. Treatment is by plasmapheresis and anti-B cell therapy. However, the condition is almost invariably fatal.

Acute rejection can be divided into cell (T cell) or antibody (HLA)-mediated rejection, and is suspected clinically with worsening cardiac function, with or without arrhythmias. Signs may vary from mild worsening of diastolic function to systolic dysfunction and heart failure. With adequate prophylactic maintenance immunosuppression, many patients will experience episodes of mild self-limiting rejection, but serious episodes account for 10 per cent of all deaths within the first 30 days following heart transplant. Serial echocardiographies are helpful in monitoring progress, and an endomyocardial biopsy should be performed as early as possible if there is suspicion of acute symptomatic cellular rejection. (Most centres still perform a number of routine surveillance endomyocardial biopsies in the first year after transplantation.) First-line treatment for acute rejection is with high-dose intravenous pulsed methylprednisolone (e.g. 1 g daily for 3 days), though additional treatment with an anti-T cell agent may be needed when there is serious cardiac dysfunction.

Antibody-mediated rejection is detected by the presence of donor-specific antibody in the serum and from specific features in the endomyocardial biopsy.

Treatment normally involves removal of circulating antibody by plasmapheresis or immunoadsorption, but may also include steroids and ATG. Additional treatments with agents such as rituximab and bortezomib are used to reduce antibody production by targeting B cells and plasma cells, and high-dose intravenous immunoglobulin may be used to replace depleted antibody levels and for its immunomodulatory effect.

Rejection causing haemodynamic compromise and cardiogenic shock should be managed as described above, together with supportive care for associated organ failures. Occasionally, short-term mechanical circulatory support (e.g. ECMO) may be required to buy time for drug therapy to impact upon the rejection process.

Non-cardiac Surgery in Heart Transplant Patients

Patients with heart transplant may present for non-cardiac surgery or require intensive care admission for other reasons. The considerations above relating to haemodynamics, risk of RV failure and immunosuppressive drugs/infections are the same. Transplanted hearts develop accelerated vascular atherosclerosis, so the risk of coronary ischaemia should be considered. Recipients have life-long follow-up with their transplant centre, so it is worth contacting them for advice and transfer if necessary.

References and Further Reading

International Society for Heart and Lung Transplantation. Professional practice guidelines and consensus documents. www.ishlt.org

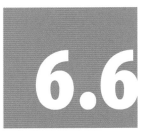

6.6 Management of the Critical Care Patient Following Lung Transplant

Nick Lees

Key Learning Points

1. Care should be taken to ensure non-injurious mechanical ventilation in newly transplanted lungs.
2. Effective analgesia may allow early extubation.
3. Complications include primary graft dysfunction.
4. Immunosuppression and aggressive management of infection are very important.
5. Extracorporeal support may be used before, during or after lung transplantation.

Keywords: critical care, lung transplant, post-operative

Introduction

Lung transplantation (LT) is an option for managing a wide range of severe chronic, end-stage lung disorders, with the potential to improve quality of life and survival for recipients declining in health despite maximal medical therapy. The most common indications are chronic obstructive pulmonary disease (COPD), idiopathic pulmonary fibrosis and cystic fibrosis (CF). Overall survival after LT is approximately 80 per cent at 1 year, 50 per cent at 5 years and 35 per cent at 10 years.

Referral to a specialist LT centre should occur early in patients with lung disease amenable to transplantation and a high risk of dying from their lung disease, who are on maximal medical therapy and without significant co-morbidities. Some patients who are on the list may acutely deteriorate, and in select cases, they may be suitable for bridge to transplant (BTT) with extracorporeal membrane oxygenation (ECMO).

Surgery and Monitoring

Surgery is now commonly performed without cardiopulmonary bypass (CPB), using a 'clamshell' thoracotomy approach or bilateral anterolateral thoracotomies.

If there is haemodynamic instability or concern about the patient being able to tolerate surgery and one-lung anaesthesia, then the surgery can be done on CPB. The lungs are implanted sequentially, with pneumonectomy followed by implantation of the donor lung and anastomoses to the main bronchus, pulmonary artery and left atrium. Standard setup and monitoring perioperatively include an arterial line, a central venous catheter, a pulmonary artery catheter, and a large-bore venous access. Transoesophageal echocardiography (TOE) is normally used during surgery. The main intraoperative risks include hypoxia and hypoventilation (i.e. one-lung anaesthesia in patients with end-stage lung disease), the potential for haemodynamic instability (especially during implantation of the left lung), right heart dysfunction, bleeding and primary graft dysfunction (PGD).

Management after Lung Transplant

Mechanical Ventilation

Patients are transferred to the ICU sedated and ventilated, to allow a period of monitoring before extubation. Capnography is mandatory. Ventilation should be protective and non-injurious, avoiding volu- and barotrauma, whilst achieving sufficient oxygenation and carbon dioxide clearance. It is good practice to avoid deep sedation and prolonged mechanical ventilation, both of which are associated with worse outcomes. If the post-operative recovery is uncomplicated, one should aim for early extubation within 24 hours.

For single LT, which is less commonly performed, low inflation pressures and minimal positive end-expiratory pressure (PEEP) should be used to prevent dynamic over-inflation of the more compliant native lung, as this could cause lung injury, mediastinal shift and haemodynamic instability.

Fluid Therapy and Haemodynamics

Most recipients have preserved ventricular function. However, particular attention should be given to right ventricular (RV) assessment and function which may deteriorate during prolonged surgery. Inotropes may be required. Inhaled pulmonary vasodilators (nitric oxide or prostacyclin) are usually started during the surgery, and should be weaned off within the first 12–24 hours post-operatively in uncomplicated patients to allow for prompt extubation. Fluids should be judicious and titrated to response, aiming to avoid a significant positive balance. However, many patients are significantly preload-responsive. This is especially true of CF recipients with chronic infection, as these patients invariably develop a clinically significant inflammatory response perioperatively and become vasodilated and hypotensive, often necessitating vasopressors such as noradrenaline and vasopressin.

Extracorporeal Life Support

There are a number of scenarios for the use of extracorporeal life support (ECLS) and ECMO in particular. ECMO may be used preoperatively as a 'BTT' in select patients on the waiting list who have acutely decompensated. Good outcomes can be achieved with these patients, especially if they are kept awake whilst on veno-venous (VV) ECMO and are able to engage in physiotherapy whilst waiting for transplant, as opposed to being on mechanical ventilation with the risk of deconditioning. ECMO can also be used at the time of surgery if there is primary graft dysfunction (PGD) and hypoxia, and this can be placed percutaneously in the groin (VV or veno-arterial (VA), depending on haemodynamics) and weaned off once there is recovery.

In the case of pulmonary arterial hypertension, a less common indication for transplant, there is RV dysfunction and the use of VA ECMO (or other mechanical circulatory support) is often required before, during and after the surgery.

Analgesia

LT is a potentially painful procedure involving thoracotomy; thus, in order to achieve early extubation, regional anaesthesia is most effective. Our practice is to use an opiate-based technique intraoperatively, and to place a thoracic epidural once in the ICU when the patient is stable with normal coagulation, lightly sedated and ready to wean. Paravertebral catheters are an alternative.

Immunosuppression

Immunosuppression generally consists of a three-drug regimen comprising a calcineurin inhibitor (tacrolimus or cyclosporine), a nucleotide-blocking agent (azathioprine or mycophenolate mofetil) and corticosteroids. The use of additional strong, early immunosuppressive drugs (induction therapy) is controversial and centre-dependent. Close monitoring of therapeutic drug levels and drug interactions that may affect levels is very important, plus adjusting for changes in pharmacodynamics such as gut failure and lack of enteral absorption and renal and hepatic dysfunction.

Complications after Lung Transplant
Respiratory

Primary graft dysfunction: PGD is a form of acute lung injury after LT, developing within the first 72 hours and associated with significant short- and long-term morbidity and mortality. The causes are multifactorial, including ischaemia–reperfusion injury, innate immune activation, oxidative stress and release of inflammatory mediators. It is characterised by severe hypoxaemia and lung oedema and diffuse pulmonary infiltrates are seen on chest X-ray without other identifiable causes. Treatment is supportive, with protective ventilation strategies akin to the management of acute respiratory distress syndrome (ARDS). Inhaled nitric oxide has been shown to improve oxygenation, selectively reduce pulmonary artery pressures and shorten the duration of mechanical ventilation through improvement in ventilation/perfusion (V/Q) matching. When maximal treatment fails, ECMO should be started as a bridge to recovery.

Anatomical and surgical problems: the bronchial anastomosis can become stenosed or break down, and risk factors for this include severe PGD, rejection, infection (especially *Aspergillus* and *Pseudomonas*) and prolonged mechanical ventilation. Diagnosis and surveillance are with regular bronchoscopy, and management comprises antibiotics/anti-fungals and therapeutic bronchoscopy procedures such as secretion clearance and stents.

Nerve damage may also occur during surgery. Damage to the phrenic nerve leads to diaphragmatic palsy and may present as a patient slow to wean from mechanical ventilation. This can be demonstrated on chest ultrasound, and treatment is generally conservative. However, diaphragmatic plication is an option in persistent cases. The vagus nerve may also be damaged, leading to gastroparesis and gastric reflux.

643

Cardiovascular

Causes of hypotension include bleeding, cardiac tamponade, vasodilation and RV failure. Clinical assessment and early echocardiography are important. There is an increased incidence of atrial tachy-arrythmias after LT, and this is associated with increased morbidity and mortality. Treatment should be with direct current (DC) cardioversion or drugs. However, amiodarone is associated with higher mortality in these patients, and only short courses given if possible.

Renal

Acute kidney injury (AKI) is a common complication after LT. Use of renal replacement therapy, which occurs in around 5 per cent of patients, is a marker of higher short- and long-term mortality. Risk factors for the development of AKI include diabetes, poor renal function preoperatively and primary pulmonary hypertension.

Rejection

As many as 55 per cent of LT recipients are treated for acute allograft rejection in the first year after transplantation. When symptomatic, the presentation is of dyspnoea, cough, sputum production, fever, increasing oxygen requirement, added sounds on lung auscultation and worsening of the chest X-ray appearance. Higher-grade rejection can lead to ARDS. Diagnosis is by transbronchial biopsy, which is useful in excluding an infectious cause. Treatment is supportive, as well as with increased immunosuppression (i.e. pulse methylprednisolone). Acute vascular or airway rejection are the main risk factors for the development of bronchiolitis obliterans syndrome (BOS), a condition of progressive airflow obstruction of the small airways in the lung and the most common cause of death after the first year.

Infection

Infection is a common cause of morbidity and mortality in the LT patient, and accounts for over 25 per cent of all post-transplant deaths. Patients are at increased risk of infection, both due to their continued immunosuppression and because of the effects caused by LT on local pulmonary defences such as mucociliary clearance. Infections may arise from the donor or recipient, and antibiotic prophylaxis is essential intra- and post-operatively. Antibiotics should be guided by previous recipient culture results, which, in the case of CF patients, often include chronic colonisation with multidrug-resistant organisms. Anti-fungal prophylaxis is also used, with *Aspergillus* representing a particular risk to the immunocompromised LT patient. Antiviral prophylaxis against cytomegalovirus is also routinely commenced, as this infection is a major cause of morbidity and mortality.

References and Further Reading

International Society for Heart and Lung Transplantation. Professional practice guidelines and consensus documents. www.ishlt.org

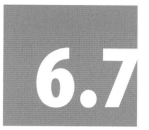

Pre- and Post-operative Management of the Critical Care Trauma Patient

6.7

Rebecca Brinkler and Anthony O'Dwyer

Key Learning Points

1. Patients are likely to have disturbances of acid–base balance, temperature, coagulation and haemodynamics on arrival.
2. Damage control surgery may be required to stabilise patients.
3. Care in the intensive care unit should centre around preventing secondary insult such as sepsis, venous thromboembolism, secondary brain injury and multi-organ failure.
4. The clinician may need to balance the mean arterial pressure between achieving adequate cerebral perfusion and avoiding further bleeding.
5. Patients are at significant risk of acute lung injury.

Keywords: trauma, injury severity, damage control resuscitation

Introduction

Trauma patients arriving in the ICU may come directly from the emergency department or via theatre. On admission, they are likely to have profound acid–base disturbance, significant hypothermia and coagulopathy, and be requiring organ support and further resuscitation. They will need full re-evaluation to detect missed injuries, and if they are not responding to resuscitation, they may require damage control surgery. Once stabilised from their initial injury, these patients are at risk of sepsis, venous thromboembolism, secondary brain injury and multi-organ failure. Treatment must then centre around preventing any further decline.

Severity of Injury

The most commonly used scoring system in trauma is the Injury Severity Score (ISS) (Table 6.7.1). This divides the body into six regions, each given a severity score using the Abbreviated Injury Scale (AIS) (Table 6.7.2).

The highest three scores are squared, and then added together to give a final ISS. The maximum ISS is 75. If any individual region scores 6, the ISS automatically becomes 75.

The ISS correlates linearly with mortality, morbidity and length of hospital stay, and so it is a useful prognostic tool (Table 6.7.3). However, as it relies on the AIS

Table 6.7.1 The six regions for the Injury Severity Score

Head and neck	Face
Chest	Abdomen
Extremity	External

Source: www.trauma.org

Table 6.7.2 The Abbreviated Injury Scale (AIS)

AIS score for each region	
1	Minor
2	Moderate
3	Serious
4	Severe
5	Critical
6	Maximal/unsurvivable

Source: www.trauma.org

Table 6.7.3 Injury Severity Score group and mortality

Injurity Severity Score	Percentage of major trauma patients	Percentage mortality of this Injurity Severity Score group
16–25	62.6	10.5
26–40	28.9	22.1
41–74	7.7	44.3
75	0.8	76.6

Source: Trauma and Audit Research Network (2009). *Modelling Trauma Workload: A project for the Department of Health.*

to generate a score, any error in the AIS will result in error in the ISS.

Problems and Treatment Strategies in the ICU

Respiratory Support

Trauma patients are at significant risk of acute lung injury, specifically acute respiratory distress syndrome (ARDS), transfusion-related acute lung injury (TRALI) and transfusion-associated circulatory overload (TACO).

Although TRALI is more likely to occur following transfusion of products with high plasma content, such as fresh frozen plasma (FFP), it has also been reported following transfusion of red blood cells and cryoprecipitate. It is clinically indistinguishable from ARDS (Table 6.7.4).

All patients with acute lung injury should receive lung-protective ventilation (<6 ml/kg). Use judicious transfusion of blood products, targeting transfusions to the requirements of the patient using near-patient testing (thromboelastography (TEG)*/rotational thromboelastometry (ROTEM)*) to reduce the risk of transfusion-related complications.

Cardiovascular Support

The aim is to restore micro-circulation and end-organ perfusion, ideally using fluid resuscitation with crystalloid or blood products, rather than vasopressors. Urine output, pH, lactate and base deficit give an indication of the state of micro-circulatory perfusion and may be better targets for resuscitation than haemodynamic values, as there may be significant dissociation between micro- and macro-circulation. Moderate hypotension should be tolerated, as over-resuscitation may lead to disruption of clot and further bleeding or haemodilution.

If patients are failing to respond, consider re-examining for missed injuries; 6.5 per cent of trauma-related deaths are due to undiagnosed injury. Ongoing bleeding may require further damage control surgery or management by interventional radiology.

Coagulopathy

Acute traumatic coagulopathy (ATC) occurs within minutes of injury, causing hyperfibrinolysis and a hypocoagulable state. It is thought to be due to tissue injury and tissue hypoperfusion triggering high levels of activated protein C. Metabolic acidosis, hypothermia and dilutional resuscitation compound this further, leading to trauma-induced coagulopathy (TIC). Coagulopathy is associated with longer ICU and hospital stay, increased incidence of multiple organ failure (MOF) and 3- to 4-fold higher mortality. Massive transfusion in trauma patients is associated with 50 per cent mortality.

Laboratory coagulation tests are poor predictors of bleeding, and transfusion should not be guided by these numbers. Rather, viscoelastic monitoring (TEG®, ROTEM®) should be used to allow targeted transfusion of blood and clotting products based on bedside analysis of the clot formation. This is likely to result in a better resolution of bleeding, with fewer blood products used.

Recombinant factor VIIa can be used in refractory coagulopathy, but it is still dependent on adequate levels of fibrinogen and platelets and is unlikely to work if the patient is acidaemic. In the CRASH2 study, tranexamic acid was shown to improve survival if given within an hour of admission to hospital, but survival was reduced if given after 3 hours.

Post-resuscitation, patients become pro-thrombotic with an increased risk of venous thromboembolism. Therefore, coagulopathy must be monitored carefully, and thromboprophylaxis considered once bleeding has stopped.

Table 6.7.4 Distinguishing ARDS, TRALI and TACO

	PaO$_2$/FiO$_2$ gradient	BNP (pg/ml)	PCWP (mmHg)	Other
ARDS	<200	<200	<18	
TRALI	<300	<200	<18	Within 6 hours of transfusion. May be febrile and hypotensive
TACO	Variable	>1200	>18	Within 2 hours of transfusion. Increased JVP, hypertensive

Abbreviation: ARDS = acute respiratory distress syndrome; TRALI = transfusion-related acute lung injury; TACO = transfusion-associated circulatory overload; PaO$_2$ = partial pressure of oxygen; FiO$_2$ = fraction of inspired oxygen; BNP = B-type natriuretic peptide; PCWP = pulmonary capillary wedge pressure.
Source: Shere-Wolfe R, *et al*. Critical care considerations in the management of the trauma patient following initial resuscitation. *Scandinavian Journal of Trauma, Resuscitation and Emergency Medicine* 2012;**20**:68.

Hypothermia

Environmental exposure at the time of injury causes hypothermia, but it is worsened by surgical exposure, administration of large fluid volumes and general anaesthesia. Whether arriving in the ICU from the emergency department or from theatre, these patients are likely to be still hypothermic. Hypothermia leads to dysrhythmias, worsens coagulopathy and increases infection risk. It must be treated aggressively.

Neuroprotection

Hypoxia and hypotension exacerbate brain injury and are associated with a worse long-term outcome. Maintaining the cerebral perfusion pressure (CPP) above 60 mmHg is associated with reduced mortality and morbidity. As CPP equals mean arterial pressure (MAP) minus intracranial pressure (ICP), it is advised to aim for a MAP >90 mmHg and an ICP <20 mmHg. Patients should be nursed with a 30° head-up tilt and be well sedated, aiming for a PaO_2 >8 kPa, and a $PaCO_2$ of 4.0–4.5 kPa. Neck ties should be avoided, and pyrexia, seizures and pain aggressively treated. ICP monitoring should be routinely used, and a head CT looking for correctable injuries should be conducted early.

If there is ongoing raised ICP, cerebrospinal fluid (CSF) drainage or mannitol can be considered, as can a decompressive craniotomy.

In contrast with damage control resuscitation, moderate hypotension results in a poor outcome in patients with severe traumatic brain injury. In a polytrauma patient, the clinician must balance the risk of clot disruption and further bleeding with a higher blood pressure against poor neurological outcome with a lower blood pressure.

Multi-organ Failure

The initial traumatic insult, along with hypotension and reperfusion, leads to systemic inflammatory response syndrome (SIRS). This, in itself, may lead to early MOF. The addition of a further insult – a 'second hit' – such as sepsis, transfusion, surgery, mechanical ventilation or fat embolism, adds to the initial injury and leads to late MOF.

Around 25 per cent of severe trauma patients (ISS >15) develop MOF. These patients have been shown to have a sixfold increase in mortality. They are also more likely to have a longer ICU stay and an increased need for assistance with activities of daily living after discharge.

The Denver, Sequential Organ Failure Assessment (SOFA) and Multiple Organ Dysfunction Score (MODS) scoring systems are all used for scoring post-injury MOF.

References and Further Reading

Bota DP, Melot C, Ferreira FL, et al. The Multiple Organ Dysfunction Score (MODS) versus the Sequential Organ Failure Assessment (SOFA) score in outcome prediction. *Intensive Care Med* 2002;**28**:1619–24.

Dewar D, Moore FA, Moore EE, Balogh Z. Postinjury multiple organ failure. *Injury* 2009;**40**:912–18.

Kushimoto S, Kudo D, Kawazoe Y. Acute traumatic coagulopathy and trauma-induced coagulopathy: an overview. *J Intensive Care* 2017;**5**:6.

Prout J, Jones T, Martin D. In: Trauma and stabilization. J Prout, T Jones, D Martin (eds). *Advanced Training in Anaesthesia*. Oxford: Oxford University Press; 2014. pp. 383–99.

Shere-Wolfe RF, Galvagno SM Jr, Grissom TE. Critical care considerations in the management of the trauma patient following initial resuscitation. *Scand J Trauma Resusc Emerg Med* 2012;**20**:68.

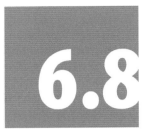

6.8 Management of the Critical Care Patient Following Major Abdominal Surgery

Anthony O'Dwyer and Rebecca Brinkler

Key Learning Points

1. Analgesia should be multi-modal and opioid-sparing.
2. Adequate resuscitation and management of effective circulation.
3. Intensive care unit-related complications should be prevented.
4. Nutritional support should be addressed.
5. Abdominal catastrophes should be recognised and prevented.

Keywords: abdominal surgery, anastomotic leak, gastrointestinal surgery, abdominal catastrophe

Introduction

Care for the patient after abdominal surgery (covering all intra-, retro- and extra-peritoneal organs, as well as the abdominal wall) is variable and often depends on the nature of the surgery. Encompassing elective, emergency or 'damage control' surgery (i.e. limiting contamination and vascular haemorrhage control), care is complex. Generally, patients requiring critical care admission require close attention to the management of pain, effective circulating volume, sepsis and anti-microbial therapy, nutrition, prophylaxis against ICU-related complications and the development of abdominal catastrophes. This chapter discusses these in brief.

Multi-modal, Opioid-Sparing Analgesia

Post-operative pain is deleterious to recovery for a variety of reasons, including raised circulating catecholamines, increased incidence of post-operative delirium, reduced motivation and mobilisation, restricted oral nutrition and diaphragmatic splinting with inability to perform lung exercises. In order to facilitate a swift and successful recovery, it is thus paramount that both adequate psychological and pharmaceutical support for pain control is provided. This should include:

- Involvement of an acute pain service
- Multi-modal (opioid-sparing) analgesia, including regular paracetamol ± non-steroidal anti-inflammatory steroids (NSAIDs):
  - Accelerates post-operative recovery
  - Reduces post-operative paralytic ileus
- Local anaesthetic techniques:
  - Regional blockade (e.g. tap block)
  - Thoracic epidural analgesia
  - Continuous wound infiltration (i.e. rectus sheath catheters)
  - Intravenous (IV) local anaesthetic infusions

Effective Circulating Volume/Adequate Resuscitation

Surgical tissue manipulation induces an inflammatory reaction, with consequent tissue oedema, activation of the renin–angiotensin–aldosterone pathway, raised anti-diuretic hormone (ADH) and salt and water retention. Abdominal surgery patients therefore have vast fluid requirements on day 1 (open surgery more so due to high evaporative loss), which slowly reduces with each post-operative day in passing. Typically, physiological recovery produces diuresis at around day 3. However, critically ill patients requiring ICU care for >48 hours are unlikely to follow that path and instead require tailored IV fluid therapy.

Fluid intake, losses and objective measures of perfusion should all be assessed, and fluid challenges should be guided by proactive monitoring and are administered above a maintenance infusion to achieve the best haemodynamic status. This could include using a cardiac output monitor to ascertain if the stroke volume increases by 10 per cent with a crystalloid bolus of 200–250 ml – repeated until <10 per cent improvement of stroke volume is seen, which suggests preload is optimised, and perfusion can be further optimised with inotropic support. Failure to account for this can lead to excessive iatrogenic fluid administration, with consequent cardiac dysrhythmias, myocardial ischaemia, increased work of breathing and mechanical ventilation.

Addressing the Need for Anti-microbial Treatment

Full details of sepsis management are beyond the scope of this chapter. However, the tenets of resuscitation, anti-microbial administration and source control remain. For abdominal surgery patients, the source of sepsis is most likely to be intra-abdominal and/or involve the operative site, which could include anastomotic leaks, perforations or an abscess. Points of consideration include the following:

- Broad-spectrum antibiotics should be administered until a specific source and pathogen are identified.
- Infected haematomas lack an independent blood supply, so antibiotics penetrate poorly and evacuation is therefore crucial.
- Consider anti-fungal cover for abdominal surgery (gastrointestinal (GI) perforation, pancreatitis or immunocompromised patients).
- Evaluate for intra-abdominal collections using abdominal CT (which can be difficult to interpret within the first 5 days post-operatively due to post-surgery inflammation, free gas from operation, etc.) or alternatives such as diagnostic peritoneal lavage, analysis of drain fluid for high white cell count, amylase, lipase, GI contents, etc.
- Have a low threshold to suggest exploration for 'non-improving' abdomen or radiologically guided drainage for source control.

Nutritional Support

Post-operatively, patients are hypermetabolic and hypercatabolic, with an estimated muscle mass loss of 1–2 per cent per day. Anabolism does not return until patients have entered the recovery phase, which may take days to weeks, depending on their clinical course. The post-abdominal surgery patient poses extra challenges, as the GI tract has suffered a direct insult, consequently compromising initiation and absorption of enteral feeding. The aims of treatment are to minimise GI losses and to provide safe and timely nutrition. Underfeeding is associated with weakness, infection, increased duration of mechanical ventilation and death; thus, in accordance with the surgeon, look to initiate early enteral nutritional support, if possible (e.g. <48 hours after ICU admission once fully resuscitated).

Regarding the route of nutrition administration, enteral nutrition has been shown to be superior to parenteral, with respect to reduced infective complications, reduced length of ventilatory support and lower associated financial costs. Top-up parenteral nutrition to prevent nutritional deficit can be utilised. However, other risks include complications related to central venous access and numerous nutritional/metabolic complications, including overfeeding, liver dysfunction, lipaemia, electrolyte imbalance and hypo-/hyperglycaemia. Total parenteral nutrition (TPN) is therefore generally only indicated for post-operative patients unable to tolerate enteral feeding, which could include:

- Non-functioning GI tract
- Proximal high-output or entero-cutaneous fistulae
- Short bowel syndrome
- Prolonged intestinal failure, e.g. radiation enteritis/necrotic bowel

TPN does not, however, need to be initiated immediately, and the EPANIC trial (early versus late parenteral nutrition in critically ill adults) in 2011 demonstrated faster recovery and fewer complications when initiation of parenteral nutrition was delayed until day 8 post-admission to the ICU.

Prophylaxis against ICU Complications

Patients having undergone abdominal surgery are at high risk of numerous ICU-related complications, especially respiratory complications (e.g. nosocomial pneumonia and macro- or micro-aspiration are prominent in abdominal surgery due to sedation-induced dependent atelectasis, diaphragmatic splinting and raised intra-abdominal pressure (IAP)). Enhanced recovery principles and standards of intensive care must therefore be adhered to, including:

- Stress ulceration prophylaxis
- Venous thromboembolism prophylaxis
- Normothermia
- Normoglycaemia (target glucose 6–10 mmol/l)
- Respiratory protection: nasogastric tubes, regular supraglottic suctioning, oral hygiene, extended lung re-expansion, protective lung ventilation and mobilisation and physiotherapy

Abdominal Catastrophes

As detailed, abdominal surgery poses a considerable risk of numerous complications, including accelerated

649

protein and fluid losses, wound infection, anastomotic leaks, entero-atmospheric fistulae formation and wound dehiscence with failure to close the anterior abdominal wall. Surgical stress inevitably results in a degree of capillary leak, which subsequently involves accumulation of ascites, visceral oedema, intra-abdominal hypertension and abdominal compartment syndrome (ACS). Monitoring and management of these sequelae are within the remit of the intensivist, and two such sequelae are detailed below and elsewhere in the book – abdominal compartment syndrome and anastomotic leak.

Abdominal Compartment Syndrome

This is described in detail elsewhere in the book and thus it is only mentioned in brief.

Small changes in IAP are well tolerated, but as pressures increase, regional blood flow and tissue perfusion become impaired.

Recognition and Diagnosis

- Standard measurement involves an intravesical Foley catheter
- Intra-abdominal hypertension = IAP >12 mmHg
- ACS = IAP >20 mmHg + organ dysfunction

Primary ACS is associated with abdominopelvic pathology, but ACS can arise secondary to extra-abdominal conditions (e.g. sepsis, capillary leak, major burns, massive fluid resuscitation). Associated complications may be seen in Table 6.8.1.

Management

- Non-operative:
  - Maintenance of intravascular volume and avoiding liberal fluid administration
  - Simple measures include nasogastric tube insertion for gastric decompression, avoiding constipation and potentially periods of muscle relaxation
  - Percutaneous drainage of abdominal collections
- Surgical decompression:
  - There is no specific IAP or consensus as to when to intervene with decompressive laparotomy; however, prompt intervention can reverse organ deterioration in 80 per cent of patients.

Anastomotic Leak

Defined as a leak of luminal contents from a surgical join between two hollow viscera; its prevalence is

Table 6.8.1 Complications of abdominal compartment syndrome

Renal	Increased renal vascular resistance (venous compression) • IAP >15 mmHg: threatens renal damage • IAP >25 mmHg: 65% have reduced urine output • IAP >35 mmHg: 100% have reduced urine output
Cardiovascular	Reduced CO secondary to reduced preload from a compressed IVC and hepatic vein with decreased LV compliance Secondary raised intrathoracic pressure leads to raised CVP, RAP and PCWP despite reduced CO
Respiratory	Diaphragmatic elevation and splinting reduce thoracic volume, lung compliance and thus ventilation Compressive atelectasis worsens V/Q mismatch, with resultant hypoxia, hypercarbia and acidosis
Gastrointestinal	Visceral hypoperfusion with secondary bacterial translocation and impaired abdominal wound healing
CNS	Worsening intracranial pressure in trauma patients

Abbreviations: IAP = intra-abdominal pressure; CO = cardiac output; IVC = inferior vena cava; LV = left ventricular; CVP = central venous pressure; RAP = right atrial pressure; PCWP = pulmonary capillary wedge pressure; V/Q = ventilation/pressure; CNS = central nervous system.
Source: Adapted from English W, McCormick B. *Abdominal compartment syndrome.* ATOTW 1st Dec 2008.

Table 6.8.2 Risk factors for anastomotic leak

Preoperative	Intraoperative
• Male • ASA >2 • Past medical history – diabetes, pulmonary disease, vascular disease, obesity • Smoker and alcohol excess • Corticosteroid use • Malnutrition and hypoalbuminaemia (<3.5 g/dl) • History of radiotherapy • Advanced tumour stage • Metastatic disease	• Distal rectal anastomosis • Positive histologic margin involvement in inflammatory bowel disease • Emergency surgery • Intraoperative contamination • Duration of surgery >4 hours • Blood loss >200 ml and intraoperative transfusion requirements • Inotrope use, intraoperative transfusion requirements • Preoperative antibiotics and selective decontamination reduce risk

Abbreviations: ASA = American Society of Anesthesiologists.
Source: McDermott FD, Arora S, Smith J, *et al.* Assoc Surgeons Great Britain and Ireland (ASGBI). *Prevention, diagnosis and management of colorectal anastomotic leakage.* Mar 2016

reported to be between 1 and 19 per cent. Associated risk factors are listed in Table 6.8.2.

Recognition and Diagnosis

The symptoms and signs are often non-specific, and as such, a high index of suspicion is required in any post-abdominal surgery patient, should they demonstrate any signs of deterioration. They may exhibit localised abdominal tenderness, raised inflammatory markers, gastrointestinal dysfunction (e.g. diarrhoea or rectal bleeding) and evidence of sepsis or less discernible signs such as new cardiac arrhythmias (e.g. atrial fibrillation), paralytic ileus or continual falls in albumin. Raised C-reactive protein (CRP) and procalcitonin are non-specific, but CRP >150 on post-operative days 3–5 should prompt further investigation.

Diagnostic imaging is not mandatory in the unwell patient with clinically evident abdominal sepsis (as this may delay definitive management). However, CT scanning and water-soluble contrast enema may be used.

Management

- Avoidance:
  - Goal-directed fluid management and limited vasopressor use
  - Avoid NSAIDs, which may be associated with an increased incidence of anastomotic leak in emergency colorectal operations
  - Immunonutrition supplementation for 5–7 days for malnourished patients, where possible, is prudent
- Conservative management for the stable patient, e.g. fluids, antibiotics and close observation in a high-dependency environment.
- Sepsis is the major cause of morbidity and should be managed promptly with source control:
  - Source control of sepsis should not be delayed after onset of hypotension. Mortality is 25 per cent if septic and <3 hours until source control, rising to 60 per cent if delayed by >12 hours.
  - Source control can be achieved through radiologically sited drainage or laparoscopy/laparotomy. Complete anastomotic

breakdown and/or multiple foci of intra-abdominal infection usually require laparotomy.

References and Further Reading

Bouze E, Pérez E, Muñoz P, *et al.* Continuous aspiration of subglottic secretions in prevention of ventilator-associated pneumonia in postoperative period of major heart surgery. *Chest* 2008;**134**:938–46

Caeser MP, Mesoten D, Hermans G, *et al.* Early versus later parenteral nutrition in critically ill adults. *N Engl J Med* 2011;**365**:506–17.

Clain J, Ramar K, Surani S. Glucose control in critical care. *World J Diabetes* 2015;**6**:1082–91.

de Lacerda Vidal CF, de Lacerda Vidal AK, de Moura Monteiro JG, *et al.* Impact of oral hygiene involving toothbrushing versus chlorhexidine in the prevention of ventilator associated pneumonia: a randomized study. *BMC Infect Dis* 2017;**17**:112.

English W. Abdominal compartment syndrome. *Update in Anaesthesia.* resources.wfsahq.org/wp-content/uploads/uia28-Abdominal-compartment-syndrome.pdf

English W, McCormick B. 2008. Abdominal compartment syndrome tutorial of the week. Number 120. resources.wfsahq.org/atotw/abdominal-compartment-syndrome-tutorial-of-the-week-number-120/

Garde M, Quintel M, Ghadimi M. Standard perioperative management in gastrointestinal surgery. *Langenbecks Arch Surg* 2011;**296**:591–606.

Harvey SE, Parrot F, Harrison DA, *et al.* Trial of the route of early nutritional support in critically ill adults. *N Engl J Med* 2014;**371**:1673–84.

Holst LB, Haase N, Wetterslev J, *et al.* Lower versus higher haemoglobin threshold for transfusion in septic shock (TRISS trial). *N Engl J Med* 2014;**371**:1381–91.

McDermott FD, Arora S, Smith J, *et al.*; Association of Surgeons of Great Britain and Ireland, The Association of Coloproctology of Great Britain and Ireland. 2016. Prevention, diagnosis and management of colorectal anastomotic leakage. www.acpgbi.org.uk/_userfiles/import/2017/02/Prevention-diagnosis-and-management-of-colorectal-anastomotic-leakage-ASGBI-ACPGBI-2016.pdf

National Institute for Health and Care Excellence. Nutrition support in adults. London: National Institute for Health and Care Excellence; 2006.

7.1

How to Identify and Attempt to Minimise the Physical and Psychosocial Consequences of Critical Illness for Patients and Families?

Alexa Strachan

Key Learning Points

1. Long-term physical and non-physical sequelae following critical care illness in patients are increasingly recognised.
2. Sequelae may include changes in cognition, psychology and physical well-being.
3. Meticulous attention to the 'ABCDEF care bundle' can help improve long-term function.
4. Individualised rehabilitation programmes should be developed for patients at risk of morbidity.
5. Services must be provided to support critical care patients beyond their acute admission.

Keywords: post-intensive care syndrome, rehabilitation programmes, follow-up, physical, psychological

Post-intensive Care Syndrome

'Post-intensive care syndrome' (PICS) is a condition described in survivors of intensive care that comprises impairment in 'physical, cognitive or mental health status' which persists beyond discharge from critical care. Critical care patients have higher mortality, compared to the general public, for a number of years following their discharge from hospital, and admission into critical care may have significant long-term sequelae for at-risk individuals.

Physical symptoms following critical care admission include loss of muscle mass and strength, stiffness,

fatigue, neuropathy and reduced mobility. Acquired neuromuscular weakness is the most common form of these impairments and can have a severe impact on long-term functional recovery.

Neurocognitive symptoms, such as delirium, short-term memory problems and amnesia, have been reported to occur in at least 25 per cent of patients. Risk factors include pre-existing cognitive dysfunction, delirium, acute cerebral pathology, hypoxia, hypotension, glucose dysregulation and sepsis. The incidence of psychological disability varies widely, but certainly symptoms of anxiety, depression and post-traumatic stress disorder are common. Thirty per cent of patients report psychological symptoms up to 24 months following discharge, with an associated impact on quality of life and physical function. Risk factors include sedation, benzodiazepine use, use of inotropes or vasopressors and disturbed memories of time spent in the ICU. The pathophysiology of cognitive and psychological disability has not been fully described. However, it is likely neurotoxic, with neuromodulatory and neuroinflammatory mechanisms implicated.

PICS also extends to recognise the negative impact of a critical care admission on the psychological health of family members (PICS-family (PICS-F)), which can occur regardless of outcome, typically presenting as mood disturbance or sleep disruption. The impact upon the family unit can be significant. Currently, there is little support for patients and families after discharge home, with families often needing to take on the role of carer for their loved one.

Up to 40 per cent of patients are unable to return to their pre-employment, with further implications for physical and psychological health.

Prevention of Physical and Psychosocial Consequences Following Critical Care Admission

Prevention of physical and non-physical consequences following a critical care admission must focus on eliminating causative factors, delirium management, addressing pain, appropriate use of sedation, reducing environmental stress, focusing on nutrition, sleep and mood management and regular communication with the patient and family. Early mobilisation and aggressive physical and occupational therapy play a vital role.

The 'ABCDEF care bundle' includes components described above. The acronym stands for assessment and management of pain, spontaneous awakening and breathing trials, choice of sedative/analgesic, delirium monitoring and management, early mobility and exercise and family engagement and empowerment. The care bundle coordinates the efforts of the multidisciplinary team and leads to improved functional outcomes, enabling participation in rehabilitation sooner.

The concurrent use of an ICU diary to record events by family members and medical staff may also reduce psychological distress by helping patients make sense of their admission and fill memory gaps by 'constructing an illness narrative'. Diaries may reduce the incidence of post-traumatic stress disorder (PTSD) in patients and have also been shown to be beneficial for families.

Structured Rehabilitation Plans

Following critical illness, physical and non-physical rehabilitation is a fundamental component of critical care to reduce such sequelae.

The National Institute for Health and Care Excellence (NICE) recommendations suggest adults admitted to critical care are screened for risk of morbidity (Table 7.1.1), and have specific physical and psychological rehabilitation goals agreed within 4 days of critical care admission or prior to discharge, whichever is the soonest.

Where possible, these goals should be made in conjunction with the patient and alongside families if appropriate. Rehabilitation goals can be short, medium or long term, and should be regularly reviewed and updated during the course of a critical care admission.

This agreed rehabilitation plan should be included in the formal handover of care from critical care to the general ward, and should be provided to facilitate

Table 7.1.1 Risk factors for physical or psychosocial morbidity in critical care patients

Physical	Non-physical
Anticipated long duration of critical care stay	Recurrent nightmares
Obvious significant physical or neurological injury	Intrusive memories of traumatic events that have occurred before admission or during critical care stay
Inability to self-ventilate on 35% oxygen or less	Acute stress reactions, including symptoms of new and recurrent anxiety, panic attacks, fear, low mood, and anger or irritability in the critical care unit
Presence of pre-morbid respiratory or mobility problems	Hallucinations, delusions and excessive worry or suspiciousness
Risk or presence of malnutrition, changes in eating patterns, poor or excessive appetite, inability to eat or drink	Expressing the wish not to talk about their illness or changing the subject quickly to another topic
Inability to get in and out of bed independently	Lack of cognitive functioning to continue to exercise independently
Inability to mobilise independently over short distances	

ongoing recovery in the community on discharge from hospital. It may be relevant to provide information to patients and/or carers on expected physical and cognitive recovery, nutritional support or psychological and emotional recovery. Information about managing activities of daily living, driving, returning to work or claiming benefits may be of use. Contact details of local support services may be of value to patients.

Long-Term Follow-Up

An additional review within 3 months after critical care discharge is recommended for patients admitted for >4 days to critical care with a risk of morbidity. This evaluation should screen for physical, psychological, cognitive, sensory and communication needs, alongside a social assessment to enable further support to be arranged. Following this review, patients should have the ability to self-refer to a follow-up clinic at any stage.

Cost Implications

There is substantial cost benefit in implementing these recommendations. Early focus on individualised rehabilitation goals may accelerate recovery, prevent morbidity and enable more timely discharge from hospital at a higher functional status.

References and Further Reading

Clancy O, Edginton T, Casarin A, Vizcaychipi MP. The psychological and neurocognitive consequences of critical illness. A pragmatic review of current evidence. *J Intensive Care Soc* 2015;**16**:226–33.

Hatch R, Young D, Barber V, Griffiths J, Harrison DA, Watkinson P. Anxiety, depression and post traumatic stress disorder after critical illness: a UK-wide prospective cohort study. *Crit Care* 2018;**22**:310.

Marra A, Ely EW, Pandharipande PP, Patel MB. The ABCDEF bundle in critical care. *Crit Care Clin* 2017;**33**:225–43.

National Institute for Health and Care Excellence. 2010. Costing report. Rehabilitation after critical illness costing report, February, 1–39.

National Institute for Health and Care Excellence. 2017. Rehabilitation after critical illness in adults. www.nice.org.uk/guidance/qs158/resources/rehabilitation-after-critical-illness-in-adults-pdf-75545546693317

Rawal G, Yadav S, Kumar R. Post-intensive care syndrome: an overview. *J Transl Intern Med* 2017;**5**:90–2.

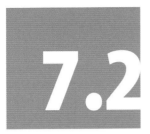

7.2 Principles of Assessment, Prevention and Treatment of Pain in Intensive Care

Harriet Kemp and Helen Laycock

Key Learning Points

1. Moderate to severe pain is common in ICU patients.
2. Assessment and management of pain can impact on psychological and physiological outcomes.
3. The American College of Critical Care published guidelines for the assessment and management of pain in the ICU.
4. Patients should be assessed regularly for pain using observational tools validated in the ICU environment.
5. Procedural pain should be considered for all interventions, even minor such as patient repositioning.

Keywords: pain, analgesia, pain assessment, procedural pain

Introduction

Pain is defined as 'an unpleasant sensory and emotional experience associated with actual or potential tissue damage'. Despite pain being the most commonly reported symptom by both medical and surgical ICU patients, it is often under-recognised and under-treated. Ineffective management has been shown to impact on both physical and psychological outcomes. There are guidelines for the assessment of pain in the critically ill, but assessment of ventilated patients, often with a decreased level of consciousness, poses a challenge. Additionally, there is limited evidence regarding best practice for therapeutic interventions to manage pain at rest and during the frequent interventions and procedures endured by ICU patients.

Importance of Pain Management

Ineffective pain management can lead to many deleterious consequences in ICU patients (Figure 7.2.1).

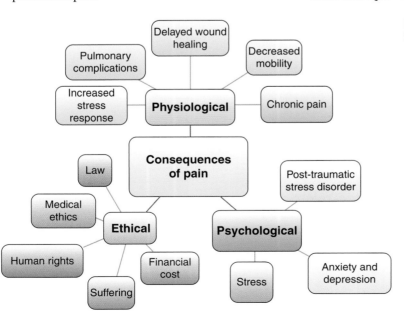

Figure 7.2.1 Consequences of pain in intensive care patients.

Physiological

- Metabolic: the correlation between pain scores and plasma levels of catecholamines, cortisol and glucose in the post-operative population indicates that pain can augment the stress response. In the critically ill population, this can worsen any existing physiological disturbance from an already severe inflammatory burden or concurrent pathology.
- Ventilation: pain can negatively impact on both spontaneously and mechanically ventilated patients by preventing deep inspiration and adequate respiratory physiotherapy. Patients are predisposed to atelectasis, hospital-acquired pneumonia and hypoxaemia. Regular pain assessment has also been shown to reduce the duration of mechanical ventilation and rates of pneumonia in the ICU population.
- Wound healing: reduced rates of wound infection have been linked to better pain control in post-operative patients.
- Chronic pain: the incidence of chronic pain 6 months following discharge from the ICU has been reported to be as high as 40 per cent. Chronic pain has a significant impact on physical and emotional rehabilitation. Patients who recall experiencing pain during their admission and those who had an episode of acute respiratory distress syndrome (ARDS) or sepsis are at higher risk of developing chronic pain. It is thought that altered excitability in the peripheral nervous system (peripheral sensitisation), changes in pain processing in the spinal cord and brain (central sensitisation) and inhibition of descending pain modulation pathways are responsible for this transition from acute to chronic pain.

Psychological

Inadequate pain management during ICU admission has been correlated with the development of anxiety, depression and post-traumatic stress disorder when assessed during long-term follow-up.

Economic

Economic analyses have revealed significant cost-saving per ICU hospitalisation when a protocolised pain management programme is introduced due to reduced length of stay, duration of mechanical ventilation, incidence of nosocomial infection and use of analgesic and sedative medication.

Pain Aetiology in the ICU

Common causes for pain in ICU patients and challenges faced by the ICU physician include:

1. **Sepsis:** pain intensity reported by medical patients with sepsis has been shown to be significant, potentially due to a hypernociceptive state as a result of acute inflammation
2. **Post-operative pain:** somatic, visceral and neuropathic pain can occur as a consequence of surgical intervention
3. **Trauma:** multiple injuries with cardiovascular instability, complicated by traumatic brain injury that can make pain assessment and management challenging
4. **Procedural pain:** common procedures such as repositioning of the patient, tracheal suctioning, drains and insertion of invasive monitoring are painful
5. **Chronic pain:** pre-existing conditions can be exacerbated during ICU admission, and regular analgesic prescriptions are ceased due to concerns of drug interactions or fears of their cardiovascular or neurological side effects
6. **Immobility:** pressure ulcers, muscle weakness and critical illness neuropathy are all potentially painful complications of prolonged immobility

Assessment of Pain in the ICU

Guidelines from the American College of Critical Care recommend pain should be assessed regularly in all patients, with assessment tools validated for use in the ICU population.

The gold standard for assessing pain is patient self-reporting such as a numerical rating scale. Intensity may not agree with the healthcare professional's perception of the level of pain that they assume should be associated with the injury. However, pain is subjective and can be influenced by previous pain experiences, personality traits and emotional state.

For many ICU patients, self-report is not possible due to barriers in communication or an altered conscious state. However, it is essential to assess for pain in sedated or unconscious patients, as even in those with a severely deranged level of consciousness, functional MRI still shows activation of the brain's pain matrix. The use of validated, pseudo-objective behavioural scales should be used in such cases. Two recommended observational tools validated for use in the

Table 7.2.1 The Behavioral Pain Scale (BPS)

Item	Description	Score[a]
Facial expression	Relaxed	1
	Partially tightened (e.g. brow lowering)	2
	Fully tightened (e.g. eyelid closing)	3
	Grimacing	4
Upper limbs	No movement	1
	Partially bent	2
	Fully bent, with finger flexion	3
	Permanently retracted	4
Compliance with ventilation	Tolerating movement	1
	Coughing, but tolerating ventilator	2
	Fighting ventilator	3
	Unable to control ventilator	4

[a] Scores from each domain are summed, giving a score ranging from 3 to 12.

Source: Adapted from Payen J, Bru O, Bosson JL, *et al.* Assessing pain in critically ill sedated patients by using a behavioural pain scale. *Critical Care Medicine.* 2001;**29**:2258–63.

ICU are the Behavioral Pain Scale (BPS) (Table 7.2.1) and Critical Care Pain Observation Tool (CPOT). Observational assessment tools score the patient's movement, facial expression and compliance with the ventilator to produce a score which can be used to measure baseline pain, as well as trends demonstrating the response to procedures or analgesic intervention.

Other surrogate measures, such as blood pressure and heart rate, have not been reliably correlated with pain experience in the ICU and should not be used.

Management

The response to all pharmacological and non-pharmacological interventions should be monitored with regular pain assessment. Analgesics regularly used in the ICU can have sedating side effects and may be used in combination with sedatives. Whilst it is recognised that lighter levels of sedation are associated with shorter length of stay and other beneficial outcomes, pain should be monitored and treated separately – the ideal regimen resulting in being able to manipulate sedation and analgesia independently. A multi-modal analgesic plan should be initiated early.

Pharmacological

- **Opioids:** for ICU patients, the recommended first-line analgesic agents are opioids. All opioids are equally effective when titrated to similar pain intensity endpoints. The most commonly used in Europe are fentanyl, morphine and sufentanil which can be administered as continuous infusions or boluses; however, combined infusion–bolus regimens can provide more tailored analgesia.
- **Paracetamol:** paracetamol can be used even in patients with severe liver disease, with an appropriately adjusted dose.
- **Non-steroidal anti-inflammatory agents:** ICU patients are at higher risk of developing non-steroidal anti-inflammatory drug (NSAID)-related side effects, including renal failure, gastrointestinal ulceration and cardiac events. The decision to use NSAIDs should be a risk–benefit assessment in the individual.
- **Alpha-2 agonists:** dexmedetomidine is used as a sedative agent in the ICU and demonstrates analgesic actions via alpha-2 agonism. There is no robust evidence that dexmedetomidine or clonidine provides superior analgesia, but they are useful as part of a multi-modal strategy in ICU patients.
- **N-methyl-D-aspartate (NMDA) antagonists:** ketamine can be used for procedural pain, such as dressing changes, and has the advantage of conferring cardiovascular stability. Psychotropic side effects occur less frequently if co-administered with sedative agents.
- **Gabapentinoids:** gabapentin or pregabalin can be used for likely neuropathic pain and should be continued, if the oral route is available, in those taking the medication prior to ICU admission.

Regional Anaesthesia in Intensive Care

For certain post-surgical populations, the use of epidurals or peripheral nerve blocks and catheters may be beneficial to improve analgesia and reduce respiratory complications. However, the benefit should be balanced with the risk of infection and coagulopathy in the individual.

Non-pharmacological

Simple, inexpensive non-pharmacological methods for reducing pain, such as correct positioning, massage, relaxation exercises and splinting, have limited side effects and can help the patient's family be involved with care.

Procedural Pain

Pain during common ICU procedures should not be underestimated, with approximately 80 per cent of ICU patients experiencing procedural pain. The Thunder II Project showed that patient turning, drain removal, tracheal suctioning, wound care and central venous catheter placement all caused significant pain and discomfort. As well as adequate background analgesia, procedural pain should be managed in a timely manner, pre-emptively, to allow the analgesic intervention of choice to have peak effect during the most painful components of the procedure. Local anaesthesia should also be considered for cutaneous puncture, even in sedated patients.

Pain management is an essential, but often underemphasised part of ICU patient care. Whilst the ICU setting provides a unique set of challenges for managing this common symptom, pain should be considered for every patient, at every assessment and before every intervention.

References and Further Reading

Devlin JW, Skrobik Y, Gelinas C, *et al.* Clinical practice guideline for the prevention and management of pain, agitation/sedation, delirium, immobility, and sleep disruption in adult patients in the ICU. *Crit Care Med* 2018;**46**:e825–73.

Kemp HI, Bantel C, Gordon F, Brett SJ, Laycock HC. Pain Assessment in INTensive care (PAINT): an observational study of physician-documented pain assessment in 45 intensive care units in the United Kingdom. *Anaesthesia* 2017;**72**:737–48.

Laycock HC, Ward S, Halmshaw C, Nagy I, Bantel C. Pain in intensive care: a personalized healthcare approach. *J Intensive Care Soc* 2013;**14**:312–18.

Payen J, Bosson JL, Chanques G, Mantz J, Labarere J; DOLOREA Investigators. Pain assessment is associated with decreased duration of mechanical ventilation in the intensive care unit: a post hoc analysis of the DOLOREA Study. *Anaesthesiology* 2009;**6**:1308–16.

Payen J, Bru O, Bosson JL, *et al.* Assessing pain in critically ill sedated patients by using a behavioural pain scale. *Crit Care Med* 2001;**29**:2258–63.

Sedation and Neuromuscular Blockade in Intensive Care

Edward Rintoul and Jeff Philips

Keywords: sedation, neuromuscular blockade, sedation holiday, ARDS

Sedation

The term sedation is imprecise, describing everything from anxiolysis to bordering on a general anaesthetic. This imprecision emphasises the need for clearly defining the required intentions when the decision to sedate a patient is made. In general, one should aim to use the minimum dose of sedative to achieve the objectives of the team without compromising patient safety. Over- and prolonged sedation are associated with worse outcomes. However, there are situations in intensive care medicine when deep sedation is required, and in these circumstances, it should be made very clear to the staff involved with the patient's care that this is the required objective.

Indications for Sedation

Indications include:

- Facilitating the use of otherwise distressing interventions, and minimising discomfort, e.g. tolerance of endotracheal tube and ventilation
- Management of anxiety or agitation
- Provision of amnesia during neuromuscular blockade

Use of sedation should always be in the context of a multi-modal approach to reduce a patient's physical, biological and psychological stress. Creating an environment that reduces these stresses may help to reduce or stop the need for sedation.

Prolonged sedation has adverse effects which may carry their own morbidity. Over-sedation may be responsible for prolonged mechanical ventilation, hypotension and underperfusion, greater immobility predisposing to deep vein thrombosis and critical illness polyneuropathy, immunosuppression, ileus of the gastrointestinal tract and an increase in delirium which can lead to the development of post-traumatic stress disorder.

Conversely, under-sedation can cause generalised discomfort and tracheal tube intolerance which leads to a hypercatabolic state, and increased sympathetic activity resulting in hypertension, tachycardia, increased myocardial oxygen demand, myocardial ischaemia, infection and psychological trauma.

Types of Sedative

It is not in the scope of this text to list all the pharmacological properties of drugs used to provide sedation in intensive care. Those who sedate patients in intensive care should, however, be fully versed in the benefits and problems associated with each drug, as well as in adjuncts to pharmacological sedation.

The ideal sedative should possess the properties seen in Box 7.3.1.

Box 7.3.1 Properties of an Ideal Sedative Agent

- Sedative, analgesic and anxiolytic properties
- Minimal cardiovascular and respiratory side effects
- Rapid onset and offset of action
- No accumulation in hepatic or renal dysfunction
- Inactive metabolites
- Stable in solution
- No interaction with other drugs
- Cheap

The ideal sedative agent unfortunately does not exist. Many drugs have been used throughout the years, including both inhalational and intravenous therapies. The most common combination now used is an intravenous anaesthetic agent (e.g. propofol) or a benzodiazepine, often in conjunction with an opioid. Other agents are also available to control agitation, delirium and pain, including the alpha-2 agonists clonidine and dexmedetomidine, ketamine and anti-psychotic agents such as risperidone or olanzapine.

Certain drug reactions are seen only in prolonged sedation. These include propofol infusion syndrome (PRIS) which is associated with high doses (>4 mg/(kg hr)) and long-term use (>48 hours). PRIS is characterised by progressive cardiac dysfunction, severe metabolic acidosis, hyperkalaemia, acute renal failure and rhabdomyolysis. The precise cause is unknown, but it is theorised that propofol triggers dysfunction in the mitochondrial respiratory chain which disrupts fatty acid oxidation, thereby causing a reduction in adenosine triphosphate (ATP) production and accumulation of free fatty acids. Discontinuation of propofol and instigation of supportive treatment should be commenced, and haemofiltration is recommended to eliminate propofol and its toxic metabolites.

It has been shown in multiple studies that over-sedation is associated with increased duration of mechanical ventilation, thus increasing exposure to associated risk factors for infection and length of stay in intensive care. The need for an optimal sedation level will vary between patients. However, the ideal is an awake, calm and cooperative patient, which, in practice, may be difficult to achieve.

Use of sedation holds ('sedation holidays') to assess neurological function allows titration of sedation. When used to optimise the level of sedation, randomised controlled trials (RCTs) have shown a reduction in the duration of mechanical ventilation

and intensive care stays. Guidance from the Intensive Care Society recommends the use of regular sedation breaks to be implemented where appropriate, except for patients in whom deep sedation is necessary or for those in whom optimal ventilation is difficult to achieve.

To optimise sedation in practice, clinicians and nurses require tools for evaluating the depth of sedation. There are multiple sedation scores which have been proposed and used in practice. Perhaps the most commonly used in the UK is the Richmond Agitation Sedation Scale (RASS) (Table 7.3.1).

Neuromuscular Blockade

The use of neuromuscular-blocking agents (NMBAs) in intensive care has decreased with heightened concern amongst clinicians regarding their adverse effects. These include critical illness weakness, increased incidence of patient awareness and prolonged mechanical ventilation. The quality of evidence supporting the use of NMBAs in intensive care is limited to weak recommendations, with the exception of use in acute respiratory distress syndrome (ARDS). In this instance, three multi-centre RCTs have demonstrated a reduction in mortality, improvement in oxygenation and fewer days

Table 7.3.1 The Richmond Agitation Sedation Scale

+4	Combative	Overtly combative or violent; immediate danger to staff
+3	Very agitated	Pulls on or removes tube(s) or catheter(s) or has aggressive behaviour towards staff
+2	Agitated	Frequent non-purposeful movement or patient–ventilator dyssynchrony
+1	Restless	Anxious or apprehensive, but movements not aggressive or vigorous
0	Alert and calm	Spontaneously pays attention to caregiver
−1	Drowsy	Not fully alert, but has sustained (>10 seconds) awakening, with eye contact, to voice
−2	Light sedation	Briefly (<10 seconds) awakens with eye contact to voice
−3	Moderate sedation	Any movement (but no eye contact) to voice
−4	Deep sedation	No response to voice, but any movement to physical stimulation
−5	Unarousable	No response to voice or physical stimulation

of mechanical ventilation in ARDS patients receiving NMBAs, compared to control groups receiving none. A recent multi-centre RCT has subsequently cast doubt on the efficacy of early use of NMBAs. Until further supporting evidence is available, it remains an indication for use of NMBAs.

Indications for Neuromuscular Blockade

- Acute respiratory distress with PaO_2/FiO_2 >20 kPa
- Therapeutic hypothermia for control of shivering
- Trial of neuromuscular blockade in profound hypoxaemia, respiratory acidosis or haemodynamic compromise
- Available evidence does not support routine neuromuscular blockade in status asthmaticus.

Non-depolarising NMBAs are competitive antagonists at nicotinic receptors and thus result in prolonged neuromuscular blockade. There are two classes – bis-benzylisoquinolinium and aminosteroid compounds. Aminosteroids have been loosely associated with an increased risk of critical care myopathy. However, this has not been demonstrated in any RCTs. The adverse effects of bis-benzylisoquinolinium compounds include cross-reactivity with muscarinic receptors and varying degrees of histamine release through direct action on mast cells. The pharmacodynamics and pharmacokinetic properties of NMBAs are not addressed further in this text.

Patients receiving continuous infusions of NMBA should be regularly assessed clinically for depth of neuromuscular blockade. This should include the use of a peripheral nerve stimulator with train-of-four (TOF) testing. However, sole reliance on TOF has not been shown to provide reliable or reproducible results for assessment of depth of neuromuscular blockade. Additionally, there is strong evidence to support routine lubrication of the eyes and ensuring eye closure to prevent corneal abrasions.

References and Further Reading

Murray M, DeBlock H, Erstad B, *et al*. Clinical practice guidelines for sustained neuromuscular blockade in the adult critically ill patient. *Crit Care Med* 2016;**44**:2079–98.

National Heart, Lung, and Blood Institute PETAL Clinical Trials Network; Moss M, Huang DT, Brower RG, *et al*. Early neuromuscular blockade in the acute respiratory distress syndrome. *N Engl J Med* 2019;**380**:1997–2008.

Price DR, Mikkelsen ME, Umscheid CA, Armstrong EJ. Neuromuscular blocking agents and neuromuscular dysfunction acquired in critical illness: a systematic review and meta-analysis. *Crit Care Med* 2016;**44**:2070–8.

Shehabi Y, Howe BD, Bellomo R, *et al*. Early sedation with dexmedetomidine in critically ill patients. *N Engl J Med* 2019;**380**:2506–17.

Whitehouse T, Snelson C, Grounds M (eds). 2014. Intensive Care Society review of best practice for analgesia and sedation in the critical care. www.ics.ac.uk/Society/Guidance/PDFs/Analgesia_and_Sedation

7.4 Intensive Care Unit-Acquired Weakness and Physical Rehabilitation

Mandy Jones, Alex Harvey and Eve Corner

Key Learning Points

1. Around 40 per cent of patients develop clinically detectable muscle weakness known as intensive care unit-acquired weakness (ICU-AW) that can lead to long-term functional deficit.

2. Accurate diagnosis of ICU-AW can be achieved through nerve conduction studies, electromyography, muscle biopsy and ultrasound of muscle cross-sectional area; however, more commonly, a clinical diagnosis is made using the Medical Research Council (MRC) Sum Score of muscle strength.

3. Prevention and timely management of sepsis is the optimal way to mitigate the risk of ICU-AW.

4. Minimising sedation, optimising pain relief, encouraging spontaneous breathing, early mobility and family engagement are the foundations of best quality care.

5. Rehabilitation should start early after admission to the intensive care unit and continue to at least 3 months after hospital discharge.

Keywords: mobilisation, weakness, physiotherapy, rehabilitation, physical therapy, sarcopenia

Intensive Care Unit-Acquired Weakness and its Functional Consequences

Intensive care survivors can present with functional disability and reduced quality of life, secondary to long-term muscle weakness, following resolution of critical illness after hospital discharge. Intensive care unit-acquired weakness (ICU-AW) is a global term used to describe neuromuscular dysfunction seen in critically ill patients, secondary to a systemic inflammatory response, prolonged mechanical ventilation and immobilisation. Recent work attributes this protracted muscle weakness to atrophy consistent with impaired myocyte regeneration.

ICU-AW is a clinical diagnosis given in the presence of diffuse, symmetrical proximal and distal peripheral muscle weakness (secondary to atrophy and reduced contractility) and failure to wean from mechanical ventilation, in the absence of a specific, direct attributing cause. The term ICU-AW incorporates pathology-specific critical illness myopathy (CIM), critical illness polyneuropathy (CIP) and the coexistence of both disorders – critical illness polyneuromyopathy (CIPNM). CIM is diagnosed when the criteria for ICU-AW are met, with electrophysiological evidence of reduced motor responses (proximal greater than distal), but maintained sensory responses; muscle fibre atrophy and/or necrosis may also be present. CIP is diagnosed when the criteria for ICU-AW are met, with electrophysiological evidence of reduced sensory and motor responses (more distal than proximal). CIPNM is diagnosed in the presence of limb weakness (distal greater than proximal) and digital sensory loss, with electrophysiological evidence of axonal sensorimotor neuropathy.

Development of ICU-AW can vary, dependent on the underlying critical illness. The incidence of ICU-AW is reported to be 40 per cent (95% confidence interval 38–42) in patients requiring mechanical ventilation for 7 days or more. It is reported that cytokine production secondary to critical illness produces microvascular, metabolic and electrical dysfunction, leading to the development of CIPNM. Independent risk factors for ICU-AW include severity of illness necessitating ICU admission, mechanical ventilation, duration of ICU stay, being female, sepsis/systemic inflammatory response syndrome (SIRS) and hyperglycaemia.

Initially, the presence of ICU-AW is associated with difficulty in weaning from mechanical ventilation

663

and an increased risk of hospital mortality. However, functionally, it poses a significant challenge to rehabilitation, as resultant muscle atrophy and weakness are often unresponsive to treatment strategies.

Assessment of ICU-AW

The diagnosis of ICU-AW is often a clinical one, and current guidelines recommend the Medical Research Council Sum Score which is used to grade muscle strength in 12 major muscle groups on a scale of 0 to 5 (giving an aggregate score out of 60). A score of <48 is considered diagnostic for ICU-AW in the absence of any other plausible aetiology. This is, however, a volitional test, meaning that the accuracy of assessment is dependent on the alertness and cooperation of the patient.

More advanced diagnostic techniques include nerve conduction studies (NCS) and electromyography (EMG) which allow earlier detection of ICU-AW than volitional measures. However, diagnostic thresholds are still to be established and the cost implications are far greater than a clinical examination. Ultrasound of the cross-sectional area of the rectus femoris is also a reliable diagnostic tool for ICU-AW, which is both non-volitional and non-invasive. This, however, requires technical expertise that may not be available. Finally, muscle biopsies are considered gold standard for the diagnosis of myopathies but come with the inherent risks associated with invasive procedures.

As well as assessing strength and neuromuscular function, it is also important to consider assessment of global function in critical care survivors. Previously, this had been difficult as the severity of weakness observed meant that there was a floor effect with established functional assessment tools from other specialties. However, a number of ICU-specific measurement systems are now available. Those with the most robust clinimetric properties are: the Chelsea Critical Care Physical Assessment tool (CPAx), the Functional Status Scale for ICU (FSS-ICU) and the Physical Functional Scale for ICU–score (PFIT-s). All of these tools allow grading of physical function from early in the ICU stay, thereby tracking recovery objectively.

Prevention and Rehabilitation of ICU-AW

Prevention and timely management of sepsis is the optimal way to mitigate the risk of ICU-AW. Further prevention strategies may include optimised glycaemic control. However, this is contentious as tightly controlled normoglycaemia is linked with mortality. Corticosteroids and neuromuscular-blocking agents have previously been associated with the development of ICU-AW, although the evidence is conflicting and unconvincing. The optimal nutritional strategies are currently unclear, with studies suggesting that high-protein feed in the first week of critical illness can hasten muscle wasting.

Preventing the iatrogenic effects of bed rest through minimising sedation, or no sedation in some cases, combined with early mobilisation, is both intuitive and safe, although evidence of long-term benefit is inconclusive.

Physical therapy often starts with relearning very low-level functional tasks, such as learning to roll in bed, learning to get from lying to sitting on the edge of the bed, sitting balance and standing practice, before progressing to walking. In the early days, it may take two or more therapists/nurses to facilitate these low-level tasks. Adjuncts, such as bed bicycles which allow passive, active-assisted and resisted cycling in the semi-recumbent position, tilt tables for passive movement into a standing position and neuromuscular electrical stimulation (NMES) to artificially contract the muscle, as well as manual handling equipment, such as standing hoists, are commonly used in the early days of rehabilitation. Notably, however, despite the intuitive nature of many of these interventions, the evidence is conflicting. If rehabilitation is started within 3 days of ICU admission, then it is likely to lead to functional improvements and may reduce length of stay. Issues with trial design may contribute to the inconsistent evidence base.

Focused strength training can be integrated into patients' rehabilitation plans as the muscles start to recover. However, when strength training is started early in the ICU stay, most patients are physically unable to complete these strength training tasks.

The optimum intensity of rehabilitation is also unknown. Wright and colleagues (2018) completed a high versus low intensity randomised controlled trial of early physical therapy within the ICU. High intensity was defined as 90 minutes of exercise per day, with emphasis on strength training, and low intensity (control) was 30 minutes per day. This was a negative trial, and the total time of rehabilitation in the high intensity group was just 23 minutes (interquartile range (IQR) 16–28) per day versus 13 minutes (IQR 10–17) per day in the low intensity group – both far below the target duration.

The ABCDEF Bundle

The ABCDEF bundle, which was developed as part of the Society of Critical Care Medicine's ICU Liberation campaign (www.sccm.org/ICULiberation/ABCDEF-Bundles), aims to improve pain management, reduce delirium and reduce the long-term consequences of a period of critical illness. The core components of this bundle are to have patients awake and off sedation, breathing spontaneously, pain-free, mobile and with family engagement. Early mobility and exercise feature as the individual 'E' element, with the purpose of identifying strategies for early mobilisation. Factors to consider before mobilising or exercising the critically ill patient are the patient's level of alertness, their cardiovascular stability and their ventilatory requirements. Mobilisation and exercise programmes must also take into account the risks versus the benefits of exercise and the patient's pre-morbid level of function.

Rehabilitation after Critical Illness

Survival after a period of critical illness is associated with physical, emotional and psychosocial morbidity and can result in significant limitations to everyday life. In an effort to optimise the patient's rehabilitation during and after a period of critical care, the National Institute for Health and Care Excellence (NICE) (2017) have published a quality standard in rehabilitation after critical illness in adults. This quality standard recognises the importance of continued rehabilitation after step down from the ICU.

The first of the four quality statements in this document focuses on the need for patients who are at an increased risk of developing physical and non-physical morbidity to have their rehabilitation goals agreed within 4 days of admission to critical care (or prior to discharge from the ICU if this comes sooner). These goals should be realistic, based on a comprehensive assessment, and should be agreed with the patient.

The transfer of the patient from critical care to the general ward is the focus of the next quality statement, and states that there should be a formal handover of their care, including their rehabilitation programme, to the general ward staff. This will help to prevent unnecessary delays to a patient's rehabilitation programme. In a study (n = 182) determining if patient mobility

achievements in an ICU are sustained after transfer to a general ward, it was found that patients experienced an average delay of 16 hours to regain or exceed chair level of mobility, and 7 hours to regain ambulation level.

Being discharged home can cause a great deal of anxiety for patients and their carers. As a consequence, the third quality statement stresses the importance of information about rehabilitation goals before discharge from hospital, so that patients can continue to work towards these goals after discharge.

The final quality statement emphasises the need for patients with a prolonged ICU stay, or those at risk of morbidity, to have a review 2–3 months after discharge from critical care, e.g. in a critical care follow-up clinic. This will ensure that any new problems are identified, and appropriate support can then be put in place.

Conclusion

ICU-AW is common and can lead to complex physical deficits. It should be identified as early as clinically possible, with the focus of care being mitigation of iatrogenic risk, minimal sedation, good pain relief, spontaneous breathing and mobilisation. If these can be achieved, it is likely to optimise functional outcome and minimise hospital length of stay. Important headway has been made in recent years to produce guidelines and quality standards in the rehabilitation of the critically ill, but the intensity and timing of physical interventions remain to be established.

References and Further Reading

National Institute for Health and Care Excellence. 2017. Rehabilitation after critical illness in adults. Quality standard [QS158]. www.nice.org.uk/guidance/qs158

Puthucheary ZA, Rawal J, McPhail M, *et al.* Acute skeletal muscle wasting in critical illness. *JAMA* 2013;**310**:1591–600.

Schaller S, Anstey M, Blobner M, *et al.* Early, goal-directed mobilisation in the surgical intensive care unit: a randomised controlled trial. *Lancet* 2016;**388**:1377–88.

Society of Critical Care Medicine. 2018. ICU Liberation Bundle (A–F). www.sccm.org/ICULiberation/ABCDEF-Bundles

Wright SE, Thomas K, Watson G, *et al.* Intensive versus standard physical rehabilitation therapy in the critically ill (EPICC): a multicentre, parallel-group, randomised controlled trial. *Thorax* 2017;**73**:213–21.

Follow-Up after Critical Illness

Joel Meyer and Andy Slack

Key Learning Points

1. Post-intensive care syndrome (PICS) affects between 40 and 60 per cent of critical illness survivors, and manifests as new impairments of cognitive, psychological and/or physical function.
2. Major risk factors for PICS include >72 hours of mechanical ventilation, prolonged ICU delirium, maternal/obstetric critical illness and baseline physical and mental health co-morbidities.
3. The typical service model of follow-up care includes a face-to-face outpatient review approximately 2–3 months following discharge home, with follow-up visits at 6 and 12 months where required.
4. Physical, cognitive, psychological and global clinical outcomes should be evaluated using domain-specific tools and assessments.
5. Critical care recovery clinics provide an important opportunity to reconnect with patients and 're-humanise' the ICU care delivered.

Keywords: post-intensive care syndrome, cognitive, psychological, physical, outcomes

Introduction

Modern critical care is producing more survivors. Vital organ function may be restored relatively quickly after reversible critical illness. However, the impact of illness, immobility and catabolic state upon nerves, muscle and the brain can be profound. Repair of these tissues tends to occur slowly and can only succeed once anabolism is restored.

Post-intensive care syndrome (PICS) affects between 40 and 60 per cent of critical illness survivors, and manifests as new impairments of cognitive, psychological and/or physical function. Timescales of clinical recovery vary considerably and extend into months or years. Individuals affected require assessment of impairments, guidance and intervention to achieve their maximal recovery and long-term outcome or to assist with adaptation to living with new disabilities.

The commitment to enhance post-critical care outcomes has been driven by national standards and gathered momentum through endeavours such as multi-centre recovery networks, systematic reviews of evidence, core outcome set development and expert panel consensus statements.

What is Meant by Recovery after Critical Illness?

Outcomes of importance to patients and their relatives are:

- Restoration of function and fitness
- Resumption of occupation(s)
- Sense of physical and mental well-being
- Quality of life, incorporating physical and non-physical components

Each of these outcomes correlates to individual, health service and societal economic gains.

Models of Follow-Up Care

Critical care recovery needs can be highly variable. For some, providing information about the anticipated timescale of recovery, signposting to sources of help and motivational goal setting are sufficient. At the other end of the spectrum, survivors at high risk of PICS (Box 7.5.1) may need multi-modal interventions and therapy referrals to address all or some of the PICS domains.

Box 7.5.1 Risk Factors for PICS

1. More than 72 hours of mechanical ventilation
2. Prolonged intensive care unit delirium
3. Maternal/obstetric critical illness
4. Baseline physical and mental health co-morbidities

The typical service model includes a face-to-face outpatient review approximately 2–3 months following discharge home, with follow-up visits at 6 and 12 months where required, as outlined in the National Institute for Health and Care Excellence (NICE) guidelines and Guidelines for the Provision of Intensive Care Services (GPICS) standards. Nurse-, therapist- and intensivist-led models may suit, depending on the case-mix. A systematic multidisciplinary approach reflecting the breadth of professional expertise given in the ICU and addressing diverse patient and family PICS domains at multiple time-points may be optimal (Figures 7.5.1 and 7.5.2).

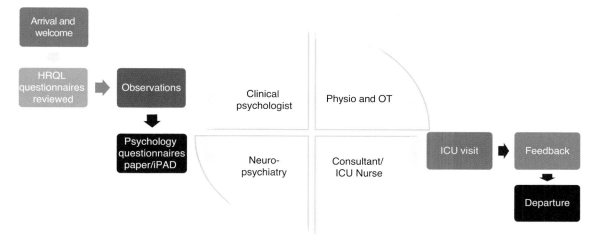

Figure 7.5.1 Proposed model for a comprehensive face-to-face multidisciplinary follow-up clinic. HRQL = health-related quality of life; OT = occupational therapy.

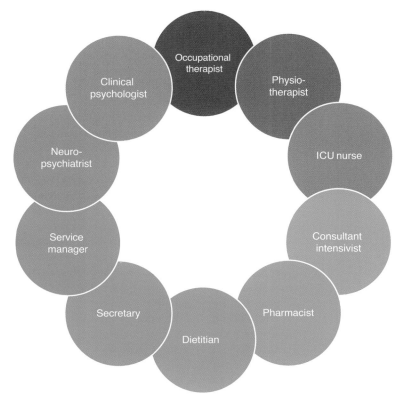

Figure 7.5.2 Multi-professional approach to critical care follow-up showing core and supplementary practitioners and supporting staff.

Other models of follow-up include inpatient ward-level consultations following ICU step-down, and these can enable anticipatory evaluation and intervention of evolving PICS features, as well as address anxieties related to decreased ward availability of staff and equipment. Outpatient virtual or telephone clinic models can also be used to circumvent potential travel and transport challenges in the target population that lives remotely from (specialist) ICUs.

Many critical care survivors need coordination of their care and safety netting to minimise care omissions and ensure referrals and review medications, whilst factoring in their pre-existing and newly diagnosed comorbidities or frailties which will modulate outcome. The critical care recovery phase may also provide their first opportunity for lifestyle interventions (diet, smoking, alcohol intake, driving safety), anticipatory care planning and behavioural change. These important interventions could ameliorate the high mortality in the first year following ICU discharge (approximately 20 per cent) and the high re-hospitalisation rate within 5 years post-discharge (approximately 25 per cent). High re-infection rates are observed within 1 year of ICU discharge, and 63 per cent of sepsis survivors require re-hospitalisation, compared to 30 per cent of controls (non-infectious diagnoses leading to ICU admission).

Numerous risk factors can be used to identify both ICU survivors in jeopardy of re-infection leading to re-hospitalisation in the first year (Box 7.5.2) and those at high risk of mortality (Box 7.5.3).

Box 7.5.2 Risk Factors for Re-infection Leading to Re-hospitalisation in the First Year

1. Initial presentation with sepsis
2. Admission from a nursing home
3. Prolonged length of stay in the intensive care unit
4. Indwelling catheter or foreign body
5. Low serum albumin

Box 7.5.3 Risk Factors Associated with 1-Year Mortality

1. Age
2. Co-morbidities
3. Clinical features on intensive care unit discharge (low systolic blood pressure, temperature, total protein, platelet count, white cell count)
4. Discharge levels of N-terminal pro-B-type natriuretic peptide (NT-pro-BNP), bioactive adrenomedullin (bio-ADM) and soluble ST2 (sST2)

Follow-Up Clinic Consultation

It is important to approach the consultation with the initial focus on the pre-critical illness status. The aim is to understand the person in terms of their social, occupational, driving, medical, surgical, psychiatric, medication and allergy histories. This has two key purposes – it builds rapport and allows an accurate comparison between the patient's pre-hospitalisation and critical illness recovery (current) status. In turn, these enable assessment of healthy and morbid trajectories for individuals suffering acute severe illness (Figure 7.5.3) and aid planning of appropriate interventions.

A time-framed explanation of the critical care admission is required to explain to the patient and caregivers about the diagnosis, level of organ dysfunction, interventions required (e.g. tracheostomy) and recovery phase. An enquiry about their memories of ICU focused specifically on any episode of delirium and hallucinations can be helpful, as it provides an opportunity to normalise their experience and ensure flashbacks are not intruding on their recovery. A visit to the ICU should be offered, and this can be planned during the current clinic visit or at a later date.

A systematic assessment is also required to evaluate the clinical features of PICS. This evaluation can be completed with face-to-face questions, or a multimodal approach can be employed with questionnaires offered either before the clinic (i.e. sent in the post with the appointment invitation) or upon arrival at the clinic (Figure 7.5.1). These questionnaires can be completed on paper or electronically on touchscreen devices (in clinic), and whilst they do provide a very useful way of avoiding consultation question fatigue, the reader may suffer with poor comprehension of the questionnaire when completing them alone. Common clinical outcomes and the tools or assessments used to evaluate domain-specific clinical outcomes are included in Table 7.5.1.

It is important to complete a focused examination, with particular focus on scars, wounds, hair, scalp and nails. It is not uncommon to encounter keloid scar formation, hair loss and wounds that have dehisced, have retained sutures (e.g. post-extracorporeal membrane oxygenation cannulae) or are slow to heal. During the consultation, an evaluation of the voice should be undertaken, assessing any new dysphonia or stridor. This is particularly key for patients who had a prolonged period of time with either endotracheal intubation or tracheostomy, or both.

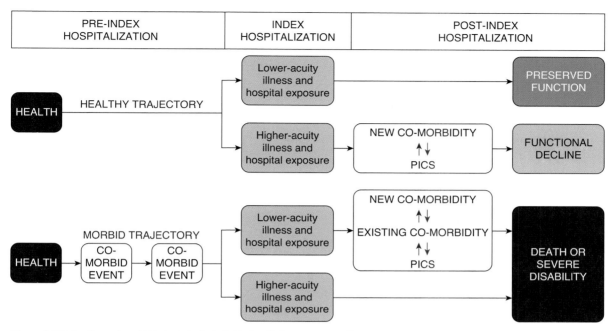

Figure 7.5.3 Healthy and morbid trajectories for individuals suffering acute severe illness.
Source: *American Journal of Respiratory and Critical Care Medicine* Volume 194 Number 2.

Table 7.5.1 Domain-specific clinical outcomes of interest and recommended measurement tools

Domain	Clinical outcomes	Tool/instrument
Physical	Weakness	Six-minute walk test and hand grip dynamometry[a]
	Fatigue	Exercise tolerance
	Sexual dysfunction	Clinical assessment
	Weight loss/gain/nutritional	Nutritional assessment
	Pain	EQ-5D and SF-36 version 2
	Global physical functions	Chelsea Critical Care Physical Assessment Tool (CPAx)
Cognitive	Memory	Montreal Cognitive Assessment (MoCA)[a]
	Attention	
	Execution	
Psychological	Post-traumatic stress disorder	Impact of Event Scale-revised (IES-r)
	Depression/anxiety	Hospital Anxiety and Depression Scale (HADS)
	Sleep dysfunction	
Global	Satisfaction with quality of life and personal enjoyment	EQ-5D, SF-36 version 2

[a] Assessment tool for the outcome did not reach the threshold for consensus but achieved the highest score.
Abbreviations: EQ-5D= EuroQoL-5 Dimension; SF-36 = Short Form 36; CPAx = Chelsea Critical Care Physical Assessment Tool; MoCA = Montreal Cognitive Assessment; IES-r = Impact of Event Scale-revised; HADS = Hospital Anxiety and Depression Scale.

Follow-Up Clinic Interventions

The intensivist's role is to identify outstanding medical and surgical interventions, investigations or treatments that are needed, based on a systematic assessment. Medicine reconciliation is important for identification of medications to be discontinued, commenced or dose-adjusted for changes in kidney function. Beta-lactam allergy status should be reviewed, and referral made to allergy specialist services, especially for patients at risk of re-infection. Given the high risk of re-infection and re-hospitalisation, vaccination administration with both the annual influenza vaccine and a single pneumococcal polysaccharide vaccine should be advocated, particularly in those younger patients who have had severe respiratory failure.

The interventions implemented should be patient-centred and address their primary concerns with any identified PICS features. There will be a requirement to consider hospital- versus community-based healthcare resources. Focussed follow-up and provision of information may be required as a consequence of their critical illness in the ICU, e.g. informing them that they had an acute kidney injury requiring renal replacement therapy and, therefore, they will be at increased risk of progressive chronic kidney disease, necessitating annual kidney function monitoring. Information should also be provided regarding entitlement for social services and income support, along with advice regarding fatigue management and engagement with employers. This is often best undertaken by occupational therapists, if available in clinic.

Assessment by a physiotherapist can identify global motor dysfunction, stiffness and impaired range of movement, as well as focal impairments of upper or lower limbs warranting further investigation. Duplication can be avoided by a combined physiotherapy and occupational therapy assessment.

The clinic provides an important opportunity to give advice about air travel and driving advice, including referral to the Driver and Vehicle Licensing Agency (DVLA) guidance which identifies notifiable conditions or anything that could affect the ability to drive safely.

The role of the clinical psychologist in clinic is invaluable for brief psychological interventions around acknowledging the impact of the critical illness, adapting to change, exploring anxiety triggers and motivational goal setting, as well as identifying patients at risk or requiring further mental health expertise.

Sexual dysfunction may not be a priority at the first clinic visit but may become more important as recovery progresses.

The output of the clinic evaluation is a comprehensive letter containing the multi-disciplinary assessments, a summary of all issues identified and a list of specific action points. Although addressed to the patient's general practitioner, ownership of the action plan by the intensivist is preferable; this often necessitates diligent coordination across both primary and secondary care providers. The plan is reviewed at subsequent 6- and 12-month appointments.

Future Directions

In 2005, only a minority of UK hospitals offered critical care services after critical illness. By 2018, this had changed, with the majority of UK centres providing aftercare services – an expansion which is also being mirrored internationally. There are compelling arguments that ICU clinicians should staff critical care recovery clinics, though others argue that intensivists are ill equipped to provide such aftercare. As intensivists who are actively involved in a critical care recovery clinic, it provides us an important opportunity to reconnect with patients and 're-humanise' the ICU care we deliver. Additionally, patients seem to find it important to discuss their ICU experience with the clinicians who directly cared for them.

More research is needed to help determine what interventions can usefully be implemented before, during and after ICU follow-up clinics. This will require closer collaboration with community services to ensure care plans are individualised and access to appropriate hospital and community physical intervention programmes is achieved, with the ultimate goal of reducing unscheduled healthcare utilisation and improving quality of life.

References and Further Reading

Azoulay E, Vincent JL, Angus DC, et al. Recovery after critical illness: putting the puzzle together – a consensus of 29. *Crit Care* 2017;**21**:296.

Cuthbertson BH, Wunsch H. Long-term outcomes after critical illness. The best predictor of the future is the past. *Am J Respir Crit Care Med* 2016;**194**:132–4.

Needham DM, Sepulveda KA, Dinglas VD, et al. Core outcome measures for clinical research in acute respiratory failure survivors. An International Modified Delphi Consensus study. *Am J Respir Crit Care Med* 2017;**196**:1122–30.

Schofield-Robinson OJ, Lewis SR, Smith AF, McPeake J, Alderson P. Follow-up services for improving long-term outcomes in intensive care unit (ICU) survivors. *Cochrane Database Syst Rev* 2018;**2**:CD012701.

Sevin CM, Jackson JC. Post-ICU clinics should be staffed by ICU clinicians. *Crit Care Med* 2019;**47**:268–72.

Wang T, Derhovanessian A, De Cruz S, et al. Subsequent infections in survivors of sepsis: epidemiology and outcomes. *J Intensive Care Med* 2014;**29**:87–95.

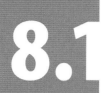

How to Manage the Process of Withholding or Withdrawing Treatment with the Multidisciplinary Team

Margaret Presswood

Key Learning Points

1. The presumption in favour of prolonging life is not absolute.
2. Skilful communication with the patient and those close to them is needed to establish which treatments are of ongoing benefit.
3. Treatments can be withheld/withdrawn when refused by a patient with capacity or when deemed not to be in the best interests of a patient who lacks capacity.
4. Do Not Attempt Cardiopulmonary Resuscitation (DNACPR) decisions need to be communicated to patients and those close to them, unless this will cause physical or psychological harm.
5. Devise an individualised end-of-life care plan before life-sustaining treatments are withdrawn.

Keywords: palliation, communication, capacity, multidisciplinary team

Introduction

The process of withholding or withdrawing treatment can be complex and fraught with ethical quandaries. Involvement of the patient, their family and the whole multidisciplinary team (MDT) (including the palliative care team) early on can aid decision-making.

Withholding or Withdrawing Treatment

Although psychologically it may be easier to withhold treatment than to withdraw treatment that has been started, there are no necessary legal or moral differences between the two actions.

Presumption in Favour of Prolonging Life

There is a presumption in law for medical teams to take all reasonable steps to keep a patient alive. But what constitutes 'reasonable' needs to be considered in the context of each case, bearing in mind the need to balance the competing clinical and resource needs of different patients and the patient's wishes.

Exceptions to the General Duty to Prolong Life

1. Patients with capacity who refuse life-prolonging treatment
2. Patients who lack capacity where life-prolonging treatment is not considered to be in their best interests

Decisions Need to Be Informed by Multidisciplinary Team Assessment

- Make a detailed assessment of the patient's condition, diagnosis and prognosis.
- Consult any locally or nationally agreed guidelines that exist, and seek advice from a senior clinician with experience of the condition where necessary.
- Consult with the wider MDT (e.g. the patient's general practitioner), and seek agreement on the most appropriate course of action.
- In emergency situations where there is insufficient information, there should be a presumption in favour of life-prolonging treatment.

Put Patients at the Heart of the Decision-Making Process

Put patients at the heart of the decision-making process to determine:

1. Whether the treatment can restore the patient to a way of living they would be likely to consider acceptable
2. Whether the patient is willing to accept the burdens and risks associated with receiving that treatment

When a Treatment Is Deemed to Clearly Offer no 'Clinical Benefit'

This may, for example, be when cardiopulmonary resuscitation will not be successful in restarting the patient's heart and breathing.

- The decision to withhold or withdraw the treatment rests with the medical team.
- You should sensitively inform a patient with capacity, and those close to or representing the patient if the latter lacks capacity, of the decision not to provide or not to continue the treatment and the reasons for it.
- Offer further discussion and, where necessary, a second opinion, but patients/families cannot insist that clinically inappropriate treatment is provided.
- A recent court ruling highlights the need to inform patients that a Do Not Attempt Cardiopulmonary Resuscitation (DNACPR) decision has been made, unless you have reason to believe that informing them will cause physical or psychological harm.

When the Overall Benefit of a Treatment Is Less Clear

In reality, the distinction between 'clinical benefit' and overall benefit to the patient is often not clear-cut. Skilful communication with the patient and those close to them is needed to decide on which treatments will provide overall benefit.

- **Assess whether the patient has capacity to contribute to the decision-making process**, according to the principles of the Mental Capacity Act 2005 (England and Wales) or the Adults with Incapacity (Scotland) Act and their Codes of Practice.
- If a patient has capacity:
  - Seek to understand the patient's understanding of their current condition, and establish their goals and expectations
  - Seek to understand their fears and what trade-offs they would be willing to make to achieve their goals
  - In light of what you have found and the MDT assessment, explain the appropriate options, setting out the potential benefits, burdens and risks of each (this may include withdrawal/withholding of particular treatments)
  - You may recommend a particular option that you believe is best for the patient, but you must not put pressure on them to accept your advice
  - The patient decides whether to accept any of the options
- If a patient lacks capacity:
  - Follow a similar process to that described above to establish which treatments would offer overall benefit to the patient and therefore are in their best interests. In this case, you need to consult with those close to the patient and members of the MDT to build a picture of what the patient would choose if they were able to express their wishes
  - Review any Advance Care Planning documentation (including any Advance Decision to Refuse Treatment), and assess whether it is relevant and legally binding for the treatment decisions being made
  - Check whether someone holds legal authority to decide which option would provide overall benefit for the patient (an attorney or other 'legal proxy')
  - When no legal proxy exists, the medical team takes responsibility for deciding which option would be in the patient's best interests. In England and Wales, an Independent Mental Capacity Advocate (IMCA) may be appointed if no close relatives or friends are available

Clinically Assisted Nutrition and Hydration

- Nutrition and hydration provided by tube or drip are regarded in law as medical treatment, and should be treated in the same way as other medical interventions.
- Nonetheless, some people see nutrition and hydration, whether taken orally or by tube or drip, as part of basic nurture for the patient that should almost always be provided.
- For this reason, it is especially important that you listen to, and consider, the views of the patient and of those close to them, and explain the issues to be considered, including the benefits, burdens and risks of providing clinically assisted nutrition and hydration (CANH).

Clinically Assisted Nutrition and Hydration in Patients in a Vegetative or Minimally Conscious State

Where a patient is in a prolonged disorder of consciousness for longer than 4 weeks following a sudden-onset brain injury, they require formal assessment, according to guidelines from the Royal College of Physicians (RCP), by professionals with appropriate training in this field. It is important to establish the patient's current condition and prognosis for functional recovery in order to inform an extensive best interests assessment process. Attempts must be made to identify all relevant people to be consulted about best interests decisions. If it is clear, following this process, that the 'best case scenario' in terms of recovery would not provide a quality of life that would be acceptable to the patient, withdrawal of CANH may be considered. The decision to withdraw CANH should be subject to a formal review by an independent second-opinion clinician.

Disagreement

If a disagreement arises, you should attempt to resolve the issues following the approach set out in the General Medical Council (GMC) guidance and it may be appropriate to offer a second opinion or, in rare cases, seek legal advice.

Care of the Patient during Withdrawal of Life-Sustaining Treatment

If the decision has been made to withdraw life-sustaining treatment and it is anticipated that the patient will die soon after treatment withdrawal:

- Continue sensitive communication with the patient and those close to them through every step of the withdrawal process. They will require intensive support during this time
- Consider whether organ donation is an option
- Devise a plan of care which considers place of care, symptom control and psychological, social and spiritual needs – which is tailored to the patient and their family's individual needs
- Consider referral to the specialist palliative care team for support with any of the above

References and Further Reading

British Medical Association. *Withholding or Withdrawing Life-Prolonging Medical Treatment*, 3rd edn. London: Blackwell Publishing; 2007.

British Medical Association. Clinically-assisted nutrition and hydration (CANH) and adults who lack the capacity to consent. London: British Medical Association; 2018.

British Medical Association, Resuscitation Council UK, Royal College of Nursing. 2016. Decisions relating to cardiopulmonary resuscitation, 3rd edn, 1st revision. www.resus.org.uk/sites/default/files/2020-05/20160123%20Decisions%20Relating%20to%20CPR%20-%202016.pdf

General Medical Council. Treatment and care towards the end of life: good practice in decision making. London: General Medical Council; 2010.

Royal College of Physicians. 2020. Prolonged disorders of consciousness following sudden onset brain injury: national clinical guidelines. www.rcplondon.ac.uk/guidelines-policy/prolonged-disorders-consciousness-following-sudden-onset-brain-injury-national-clinical-guidelines

Royal College of Physicians, British Society of Gastroenterology. Oral feeding difficulties and dilemmas: a guide to practical care, particularly towards the end of life. London: Royal College of Physicians; 2010.

Samanta J. Tracey and respect for autonomy: will the promise be delivered? *Med Law Rev* 2015;**23**:467–76.

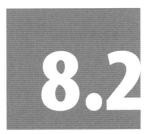

How to Discuss End-of-Life Care with Patients and Their Families/Surrogates

8.2

Edward Presswood

Key Learning Points

1. Recognise and overcome the barriers to good communication.
2. Treat patients as individuals.
3. Work in partnership with patients.
4. Listen to the patient's concerns.
5. Be honest and open, and act with integrity.

Keywords: communication, discussion, dying, capacity

Introduction

Doctors have a duty to be open and honest with patients. Doctors are sometimes reluctant to discuss end-of-life care with patients and relatives. The barriers to these discussions are:

1. A desire to not upset the patient
2. A desire to not upset the family
3. A lack of confidence in talking about dying
4. A feeling that the time is never quite right

Treat Your Patient as an Individual

Dying is a significant moment in a person's life. It is not merely a medical event; rather it is a moment that intertwines psychological, social and spiritual concerns. Therefore, when discussing end-of-life care, it is important to tailor the conversation to the individual patient and their family.

Capacity

The first step in having a conversation is establishing that the patient has capacity to make relevant decisions. In England and Wales, refer to the Mental Capacity Act and the Code of Practice.

If a patient lacks capacity, then find out if they have recorded an advance decision to refuse treatment (ADRT) or a statement of wishes, or nominated a lasting power of attorney (LPA) for their health and welfare.

Confidentiality

People who are dying have the same right of confidentiality as any other patient. You must respect their privacy.

Rapport

Rapport helps you to understand your patient. Rapport helps your patient to know that you care about them as an individual and will facilitate a trusting relationship. Rapport can be developed quickly, but try to build rapport with your patients before discussions about end-of-life care are needed.

Know All the Relevant Information

Before having a conversation about end-of-life care with a patient or his/her relatives, make sure that you know the details of the clinical history and current situation.

Optimise the Setting

Conversations about end-of-life care should take place in a quiet and private place. Make sure everyone who needs to be present has been informed about the meeting. Ask the nurse looking after the patient to join the conversation.

What Does the Patient Already Know?

Start conversations about end-of-life care by finding out what the patient or their family already know. Sometimes patients are already very well informed or their intuition about their deteriorating health is accurate. However, often patients and their family are not well informed and their expectations may be unrealistic. It is helpful to gauge how wide the 'information gap' is.

What Does the Patient Want to Know?

Most patients want to know the relevant information about their health. Many patients want to know their prognosis and want to be informed if they are dying. However, before discussing end-of-life issues, it is advisable to check with the patient what they actually want to know. Patients are entitled to decline the offer of information, or they might wish to defer the conversation. When a patient declines information, it is advisable to explain and document the potential consequences of them declining the relevant information.

Warning Shot

Prepare the patient and their relatives that the conversation is moving towards talking about death and dying. An example of a warning shot is: 'Unfortunately the bleeding into the brain has been severe, and I am very worried about what the future holds.'

Speak Honestly and Directly

Avoid euphemisms. Doctors sometimes use euphemisms in the hope that they will be less upsetting. However, euphemisms, such as 'passing away', are potentially ambiguous. In most cases, it is better to be direct and precise in the language that you use – for example: 'the pressure in the brain will continue to increase, and I think your relative is dying.'

Allow the Expression of Emotions

Patients and relatives may be upset or angry at the situation. Avoid platitudes. Avoid telling patients and relatives how they should feel or how they will feel later. It is often useful to be silent at this point. Allow the patient/relatives to lead where the conversation goes next.

Listen to Concerns and Answer Questions

Find out what the patient's and relatives' concerns are. Find out what their hopes and fears are.

Agree New Goals

Avoid the phrase: 'nothing more can be done.' There is a lot that needs to be done for a dying patient. Caring for a dying person is not about 'doing less'; rather it is about doing more of the things that matter most. Suggestions for new goals include:

1. Focusing on controlling symptoms and maximising comfort
2. Allowing the patient to die in their preferred location
3. Facilitating important conversations with their family
4. Helping the patient with legal affairs
5. Achieving a 'good' death – find out what this means to the patient/family
6. Helping the patient address any spiritual concerns or rituals
7. Discussing organ/tissue donation

Summarise

Summarise the key points of the conversation and offer a follow-up conversation.

Pitfalls to Avoid

Language

Remember that the words doctors use might have a different meaning for patients and relatives. For example, doctors should talk about withdrawing a **treatment**, rather than withdrawing **care**.

Collusion

Sometimes relatives might ask you to collude with them in not informing the patient of any bad news. Remember that your duty of care is to the patient, but recognise that the relatives are almost certainly motivated by compassion for the patient.

Denial

Sometimes patients and relatives do not accept the information that you give them. Denial is often a defence mechanism. Further exploration of their fears and scheduling a follow-up meeting can be helpful.

Resuscitation

Due to prominent legal cases, there can be misperception that agreeing a decision about cardiopulmonary resuscitation is the major component of end-of-life care discussions. You must comply with the law, but avoid making the conversation all about cardiopulmonary resuscitation.

Your Own Well-Being

Discussions about dying can have an emotional impact upon you and the rest of the team. Debriefing, reflection and clinical supervision may be helpful.

Tricky Cases

Some discussions about end-of-life care are very difficult. A multidisciplinary team approach may be helpful. Input from the palliative care team may be beneficial.

References and Further Reading

General Medical Council. Good medical practice. London: General Medical Council; 2013.

General Medical Council. Confidentiality: good practice in handling patient information. London: General Medical Council; 2017.

legislation.gov.uk. 2005. Mental Capacity Act 2005.

Office of the Public Guardian. Mental Capacity Act 2005 Code of Practice. London: The Stationery Office; 2013.

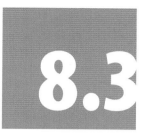

8.3

Managing Palliative Care of the Critically Ill Patient

Shankara Nagaraja

Key Learning Points

1. Palliative care is an approach that aims to improve the quality of life of patients and their families.
2. The limitation of therapy is considered when the burden of life-sustaining treatment outweighs the benefits.
3. At the point of withholding and withdrawal of life-sustaining treatment, the priority of care changes from 'cure' to 'comfort'.
4. A multidisciplinary and collaborative approach should be adopted for decision-making.
5. There should be access to spiritual care, including cultural and religious rituals.

Keywords: palliative care, critical illness, end-of-life care, advance directives

Introduction

End-of-life care refers to the care of patients when they are likely to die within the next 12 months, and of patients where death is imminent. Palliative care is an approach that improves the quality of life of patients and their families facing problems associated with life-threatening illness, and encompasses relief of pain and suffering from all domains – physical, psychosocial and spiritual. It also includes supporting those close to patients. Palliative care can be provided at any stage in the progression of a patient's illness, and not just in the last few days in their life.

'Good Death'

A 'good death' is one that is free from pain and suffering, and one where the patient retains a degree of control, autonomy and independence. The objective of critical care in these patients is to support them to live as well as possible until they die, and to do so throughout the process with upmost dignity.

Recognising the Dying Patient

Not all deaths in the critically ill can be predicted. However, whenever it becomes clear that the therapeutic trial has failed, recognising and communicating this to the patient and family allow the clinicians to concentrate on better palliative care.

The Decision-Making Process

- Patients with capacity have the right to choose between clinically appropriate treatment options. For patients lacking capacity, this choice must be made by the relevant decision-maker in accordance with the patient's best interests, as required by the Mental Capacity Act 2005. The past and present views of the patient, family and those close to the patient, as well as documents such as advance decision to refuse treatment (ADRT), must be considered to determine the best interests.
- A multidisciplinary and collaborative approach should be adopted for decision-making, with involvement of medical staff from critical care, the parent team (where appropriate) and nursing and allied health professionals, alongside the family.
- Effective communication with, and support of, the family and/or close friends must be maintained throughout.
- If asked for a treatment to be provided which the doctor considers clinically not appropriate and/ or not in the patient's best interests, the doctor should explain the basis for this view and explore the reasons for the request. If after discussion, the doctor still considers that the treatment would not be clinically appropriate and/or not in the patient's best interests, they are not obliged to provide it. As well as explaining the reasons for their decision,

677

the doctor should explain to the person the options available to them, including the option of seeking a second opinion, and/or applying to the court for an independent ruling should he or she wish to have that decision reviewed.

Decisions and Care at the End of Life

A 'good death' for the patient means avoidance of inappropriate prolongation of dying. Whilst legally and ethically there is no distinction between the acts of treatment withholding or withdrawal, clinicians find withdrawal harder.

For this reason, it is important to ensure and emphasise that it is the risky and burdensome treatment that is being withdrawn, and **not** the patient's care. The practices of treatment withdrawal differ. For intubated patients, terminal weaning or extubation is practised, depending upon expected patient discomfort and family circumstances. Opioids and benzodiazepines are titrated for patient comfort, applying the doctrine of 'double effect'. There should be access to spiritual care, including cultural and religious rituals. A quiet room with full access to the family is preferable.

Recognising Symptoms

For communicative patients, multiple symptom assessment scales have been studied. For patients who cannot report their symptoms, methods such as behavioural assessment scales or proxy symptom assessments can be undertaken. Alternatively, clinicians can use their judgement and experience to identify the sources of discomfort, assume the symptoms and treat as appropriate (Table 8.3.1). The specialist palliative care consultation should be considered when symptoms are hard to control, the needs are complex or the patient and family need psychological support.

Involving Family Members

Family members may want to be involved in simple caring interventions, such as mouth care, eye care, bed bath, and turning, or simply to be present with the patient. This may have a positive effect on both parties and should not be discouraged.

Religion and Spirituality

It is important to acknowledge and be responsive to the religious, cultural and spiritual needs of the patient and

Table 8.3.1 Alleviation of symptoms

Symptom	Options
Pain	Opioids: morphine, fentanyl NB: monitor bowel function; stimulant and osmotic laxatives may be used in conjunction
	Non-opioid analgesics: Paracetamol, ketamine Gabapentin and carbamazepine for neuropathic pain
Dyspnoea	1. Optimise underlying condition, e.g. inotropes and diuretics for heart failure 2. Non-invasive ventilation for specific conditions (if tolerated) such as chronic obstructive pulmonary disease and cardiogenic pulmonary oedema, but stop when no longer relieving the symptom 3. Appropriate positioning of the patient 4. Oxygen, air or a fan directed at the patient's face 5. Opioids – slow titration of rapid-acting agents 6. Benzodiazepines, in conjunction with opioids, e.g. lorazepam, midazolam
Thirst and xerostomia	1. Topical products with olive oil, betaine, xylitol, artificial saliva and salivary stimulants 2. Frozen gauze or ice 3. Heated humidifier if on high-flow oxygen
Excess secretions	Suctioning, hyoscine, glycopyrrolate
Restlessness/agitation	Midazolam, lorazepam, opioids, propofol
Delirium	Haloperidol

family. Main decisions such as treatment limitations and mode of treatment withdrawal are often dependent on these values for patients.

Communication

Empathic communication, skilful discussion of prognosis and effective shared decision-making improve family satisfaction. Family satisfaction has also been shown to be enhanced if a greater proportion of time is allowed for family speech.

Free and respectful communication within the critical care team, and between critical care and all other relevant teams, is vital before communication with the family. Disagreements within the critical care team will lead to mixed messages to the family. Organ donation should be considered when appropriate.

References and Further Reading

Aslakson RA, Randall Curtis J, Nelson JE. The changing role of palliative care in the ICU. *Crit Care Med* 2014;**42**:2418–28.

Braganza MA, Glossop AJ, Vora VA. Treatment withdrawal and end-of-life care in the intensive care unit. *BJA Education* 2017;**17**:396–400.

Downar J, Delaney JW, Hawry luck L, Kenny L. Guidelines for the withdrawal of life-sustaining measures. *Intensive Care Med* 2016;**42**:1003–17.

General Medical Council. Treatment and care towards the end of life: the duties of a doctor registered with the General Medical Council. London: General Medical Council; 2010.

Truog RD, Campbell ML, Curtis JR, *et al.* Recommendations for end-of-life care in the intensive care unit: a consensus statement by the American College of Critical Care Medicine. *Crit Care Med* 2008;**36**:953–63.

8.4 Brainstem Death Testing

Shankara Nagaraja

Key Learning Points

1. Brainstem death tests are a set of clinical tests of brainstem function.
2. There must be an established cause of irreversible brain damage.
3. The apnoea test is the final test.
4. The official time of death is the time of completion of first set of tests.
5. Exercise caution in patients treated with therapeutic hypothermia.

Keywords: brain death and diagnosis, brainstem death and diagnosis, apnoea test, brainstem reflex, brainstem death and test, neurological criteria of death

Definition of Death

Death is defined as the 'irreversible loss of those essential characteristics necessary for the existence of a living human person', and regarded as the 'irreversible loss of the capacity for consciousness and breathing'.

Testing to confirm brainstem death should only be undertaken if there is high-level clinical suspicion that the patient is dead and the patient's breathing and circulation are being artificially supported. The diagnosis of brainstem death can only be made if the following preconditions are met.

Established Cause of Irreversible Brain Damage

If such a diagnosis is not fully established, an extended period of continuous clinical observations and investigations should have established that there is no possibility of reversible or treatable underlying cause. This usually requires supplementary proof, e.g. imaging modalities such as CT scan or MRI brain.

Irreversible Coma

Patients must lack all evidence of responsiveness. Exclude or correct potentially reversible causes of coma (Table 8.4.1).

Table 8.4.1 Potential reversible causes of coma

Possible reversible causes	Considerations
Central nervous system depressant drugs, e.g. narcotics, hypnotics	• Review drug history • Allow >5 times the half-life of drugs for elimination, assuming normal hepatic and renal function • Beware of prolonged elimination of drugs in the presence of renal and hepatic failure • Use specific antagonist agents if available • Measure plasma levels of drugs if applicable
Hypothermia	• Core temperature >34°C whilst testing • Delay tests in patients undergoing therapeutic hypothermia
Correct confounding circulatory, metabolic and endocrine disturbances	• Mean arterial pressure >60 mmHg • Normocarbia (PaCO$_2$ <6 kPa) • Normoxia (PaO$_2$ >10 kPa) • Normal pH (pH 7.35–7.45) • Serum electrolytes within acceptable range for testing and compatible with normal mentation • Sodium: >115 mmol/l and <160 mmol/l • Potassium: >2 mmol/l • Magnesium: >0.5 mmol/l and <3 mmol/l • Phosphate: >0.5 mmol/l and <3 mmol/l • Glucose: >3 mmol/l and <20 mmol/l
No clinical suspicion of endocrine crises	• Rule out: myxoedema coma, thyroid crisis, Addisonian crisis

Excluding Potentially Reversible Causes of Apnoea

Potential reversible causes of apnoea may be seen in Table 8.4.2.

Demonstration of Coma, Apnoea and Lack of Brainstem Reflex Activity

This is established with clinical tests after the above three preconditions are met.

The Personnel

In the UK, brainstem death testing must be carried out by two medical practitioners registered with the General Medical Council (GMC) for >5 years, who are competent in conducting and interpreting these tests. At least one of these must be a consultant. They must not have any conflicts of interests and should not be part of the transplant team.

Brainstem Reflexes

The cranial nerves arising from the brainstem are tested to confirm the presence or absence of reflexes. The whole set of tests should be performed twice. Whilst one doctor performs the test, the other doctor observes the testing. The roles can be reversed for the second set of tests.

- **Pupillary reflexes (cranial nerves II and III)** – shine a bright light into each eye to test both direct and indirect reflexes.
- **Corneal reflex (cranial nerves V and VII)** – use a soft cotton swab to brush the cornea lightly to elicit eyelid movement.
- **Oculovestibular reflex (caloric reflex) (cranial nerves III, IV, VI and VIII)**
  - Inspect the tympanic membrane and ensure that the internal auditory canal is not obstructed.

Table 8.4.2 Potential reversible causes of apnoea

Possible reversible causes	Considerations
Neuromuscular-blocking agents	• Demonstrate adequate neuromuscular conduction
High cervical spine injury	• Exclude the injury with plain X-rays, CT and MRI • May need ancillary tests

  - Turn the head to 30° if there are no contraindications such as unstable cervical spine injury.
  - Slowly inject at least 50 ml of ice-cold water over 1 minute into each external auditory meatus, in turn. Observe the eyes for horizontal nystagmus. No eye movements should be seen.
- **Supraorbital pressure (cranial nerves V and VII)** – a deep, painful stimulus should not elicit motor responses in either the cranial or the somatic nerve distribution area.
- **Cough reflex (cranial nerve X)** – insert a suction catheter into the trachea up to the carina to stimulate cough reflex.
- **Gag reflex (cranial nerves IX and X)** – perform direct laryngoscopy and stimulate the posterior pharyngeal wall with a spatula to elicit a gag reflex or pharyngeal contraction.

The Apnoea Test

The apnoea test elicits the presence of an inspiratory attempt, by allowing the carbon dioxide level to rise whilst concurrently avoiding hypoxia, excessive hypercarbia or cardiovascular instability. As the test can cause secondary brain injury, this test should not be undertaken until bedside observations suggest that brainstem function has ceased irreversibly. Hence, this is the final test to be carried out.

- Undertake a recruitment manoeuvre (if needed) at the beginning and end of the test.
- Pre-oxygenate the patient with 100% oxygen.
- Check arterial blood gases (ABGs) to confirm that partial pressure of carbon dioxide ($PaCO_2$) and arterial oxygen saturation (SaO_2) correspond to the monitored end-tidal carbon dioxide ($ETCO_2$) and peripheral oxygen saturation (SpO_2).
- Adjust the ventilator settings to achieve a baseline $PaCO_2$ of at least 6 kPa and approximate pH 7.4. In patients with chronic carbon dioxide retention, allow $PaCO_2$ to rise above 6.5 kPa and approximate pH 7.4.
- Disconnect the patient from the ventilator.
- Maintain the patient's SpO_2 at >95 per cent, with either oxygen insufflation through the endotracheal tube at 5 l/min or through connection to a continuous positive airway pressure circuit.

- Observe the patient for any respiratory attempts. If, after 5 minutes of observation, no spontaneous respiratory attempt is seen, this suggests the absence of respiratory centre activity.
- Repeat the ABG to confirm that $PaCO_2$ has increased from the baseline level by at least 0.5 kPa.
- Reconnect the patient to the ventilator, and allow the return of blood gases and all other parameters to the pre-test level, in preparation for the second set of tests.
- Abort the test if blood pressure drops below 90 mmHg or SpO_2 drops below 85 per cent.

A significant number of patients may show reflex responses such as facial myokymia, Lazarus sign (arm flexion, shoulder abduction and hand raising) and spinal reflexes – either with or without tactile stimuli. These do not preclude the diagnosis of brainstem death.

Table 8.4.3 Ancillary tests used to support brainstem death

Ancillary test	Methods used
Blood flow in large cerebral arteries	• Four-vessel angiography • Transcranial Doppler • Magnetic resonance angiography • Spiral CT angiography
Brain tissue perfusion	• Xenon CT • Positron emission tomography
Brain electrical activity	• Electroencephalography • Evoked potentials

Brainstem death is confirmed after the second set of tests. However, the official time of death is when the first set of tests confirms the lack of brainstem reflexes.

Ancillary Tests

In some instances, brainstem death tests cannot be undertaken in their entirety to confirm brainstem death. Some examples might include extensive maxillofacial injuries, ocular trauma, suspected residual sedation and high cervical spinal cord injury. In these situations, ancillary tests can be undertaken to support the confirmation of brainstem death (Table 8.4.3).

References and Further Reading

Academy of the Medical Royal Colleges. A code of practice for the diagnosis and confirmation of death. London: Academy of the Medical Royal Colleges; 2008.

Bersten AD, Soni N (eds). *Oh's Intensive Care Manual*, 7th edn. Butterworth Heinemann Elsevier; 2014.

Cameron JE, Bellini A, Damian MS, Breen DP. Confirmation of brain-stem death. *Pract Neurol* 2016;**16**:129–35.

Oram J, Murphy P. Diagnosis of death. *Contin Educ Anaesth Crit Care Pain* 2011;**11**:77–81.

Webb AC, Samuels OB. Reversible brain death after cardiopulmonary arrest and induced hypothermia. *Crit Care Med* 2011;**39**:1538–42.

Physiological Support of the Organ Donor

8.5

Shankara Nagaraja

Key Learning Points

1. Any patient likely to progress to brain death is a potential organ donor.
2. Severe raised intracranial pressure and brain death are associated with various organ system consequences.
3. Optimising the physiological status of a potential donor is an active process and may require escalation of monitoring and therapies.
4. Donor management improves the quality of donated organs.
5. Care bundles for the management of brain-dead organ donors are available.

Keywords: brain death, brainstem death, organ donation, organ transplantation, donor management, donor optimisation

Introduction

The National Institute for Health and Care Excellence (NICE) advises that hospital staff should initiate discussions with a specialist nurse for organ donation (SNOD) when:

1. Intending to undertake brainstem death tests or withdraw life-sustaining treatment in patients with life-threatening conditions resulting in circulatory death, or
2. Admitting a patient with a catastrophic brain injury

Management of these patients' physiology in order to optimise the quality of donated organs will require a switch in focus from resuscitation of the brain to restoration of physiological and metabolic homeostasis of organs and tissues. This can make a huge difference to the success of subsequent organ retrieval and donation.

Pathophysiological Changes after Brainstem Death

Pathophysiological changes after brainstem death are commonly encountered and should be managed accordingly to optimise organ function.

Cardiovascular Changes

Increased intracranial pressure (ICP) leads to brainstem ischaemia and causes a hyperadrenergic state. This can result in dramatic changes in a patient's heart rate, blood pressure and peripheral vascular resistance, and may manifest as systemic and pulmonary hypertension, myocardial ischaemia, conduction abnormalities and arrhythmias. After brainstem infarction, loss of sympathetic activity can result in vasodilation and impaired cardiac output.

Respiratory Changes

Neurogenic pulmonary oedema can occur due to the combination of elevated pulmonary capillary hydrostatic pressure, left ventricular dysfunction and increased capillary permeability.

Endocrine Changes

Failure of the hypothalamic–pituitary axis leads to a decline in plasma hormone concentrations. Major hormonal imbalances are detailed in Table 8.5.1.

Table 8.5.1 Major hormonal imbalances

Hormone	Consequences
Anti-diuretic hormone deficiency	Diabetes insipidus Polyuria, dehydration, haemodynamic instability Hypernatraemia, hypomagnesaemia, hypocalcaemia
Reduced thyroid-stimulating hormone and free tri-iodothyronine	Progressive loss of cardiac contractility, poor peripheral perfusion, lactic acidosis
Impaired insulin secretion	Hyperglycaemia
Reduced cortisol levels	Impaired stress response, cardiovascular collapse

683

Other

Other pathophysiological changes encountered may include hypothermia (secondary to hypothalamic dysfunction), coagulopathy (secondary to release of tissue thromboplastin from ischaemic brain tissue) and a pro-inflammatory state (due to elevated pro-inflammatory cytokine concentrations and expression of leucocyte adhesion molecules in solid organs).

Stabilisation of a Brain-Dead Donor to Optimise Organ Function

After confirmation of brainstem death, emphasis of management in a patient should focus on optimisation of organ perfusion and function. This may involve the following.

Monitoring

Many authorities consider it appropriate to institute invasive monitoring in potential donors. If needed, preferred positions for invasive lines include the right internal jugular vein for central venous access, and the left brachial or radial artery for arterial lines. Serial lactate monitoring is advised, as is cardiac output monitoring if ejection fraction is <45 per cent.

Additional Investigations that May Be Warranted

- A 12-lead ECG and transthoracic echocardiography if cardiac transplant is expected
- A chest X-ray if a lung transplant is considered
- Troponin in all cardiac arrest cases

General Management

Continue with strict asepsis, venous thromboembolism prophylaxis (including low-molecular-weight heparin), correction of electrolyte disturbances, chest physiotherapy, antibiotics, enteral feeding, management of arrhythmias and precautions to reduce ventilation-associated pneumonia, whilst stopping all unnecessary drugs. Maintain normothermia. Targeted organ management includes the following.

Hormonal Resuscitation

- Methylprednisolone at a dose of 15 mg/kg (maximum 1 g) administered every 24 hours has been shown to reduce extravascular lung water and attenuate the effect of pro-inflammatory cytokines in many organs.

- Insulin titrated to ensure euglycaemia (6–10 mmol/l) has been shown to reduce pancreatic damage and osmotic diuresis.
- Early use of vasopressin is indicated for vasoplegia and/or diabetes insipidus (DI). If DI persists, desmopressin is indicated. The recommended dose of vasopressin is 1 IU bolus, followed by an infusion of up to 2.4 IU/hr, titrated to blood pressure. The dose of desmopressin is 1- to 4-µg bolus, with repeated doses of 1–2 µg 6-hourly.
- Intravenous dextrose solution can be used to replace water if the patient has DI.
- Tri-iodothyronine (T3) replacement at a dose of 4-µg bolus, followed by 3 µg/hr, is used to improve cardiac function and graft survival in haemodynamically unstable heart donors.

Respiratory

- Continue with lung-protective ventilation strategies, lung recruitment and minimal inspired oxygen (preferably <40 per cent). Transplant centres may request a broncho-alveolar lavage (BAL) and an arterial blood gas on 100% oxygen. Avoid high positive end-expiratory pressure (PEEP).

Cardiovascular

- Aim for restoration of intravascular volume, vascular tone and haemodynamic stability without causing fluid overload. A vasopressin infusion is considered the first-line agent to replace or minimise noradrenaline doses.
- Noradrenaline, adrenaline and phenylephrine are second-line agents. Even a modest dose of noradrenaline (>0.05 µg/(kg min)) is considered damaging to the myocardium. Use these agents with cardiac output monitoring.
- Some centres prefer dopamine as the second vasopressor. Discuss this with the retrieval team.
- Treat persistent hypertension (mean arterial pressure >95 mmHg) with infusions of short-acting agents such as esmolol, glyceryl trinitrate and sodium nitroprusside.
- Optimum haemodynamic targets are indicated in Table 8.5.2.

Haematology

- Blood transfusions and correction of coagulopathies are needed in patients with ongoing bleeding.

Table 8.5.2 Optimum haemodynamic targets

Haemodynamic targets	Value
Heart rate	60–120 bpm
Systolic blood pressure	>100 mmHg
Mean arterial pressure	60–80 mmHg
Central venous pressure	6–10 mmHg
Cardiac index	>2.1 l/(min m²)
Central or mixed venous oxygen saturation	>60%

- Keep the international normalised ratio (INR) <1.5, platelet count >50,000 and haemoglobin >7 g/dl. Avoid large platelet transfusions.

Renal
- Avoid excessive vasopressors with adequate fluid resuscitation.
- Systolic arterial pressure of 80–90 mmHg is adequate if only renal transplant is being considered. Avoid excessive vasopressors and nephrotoxic drugs.
- Maintain urine output at 0.50–2 ml/(kg hr).

Liver
- Restore liver glycogen with adequate nutrition.
- Maintain serum sodium at <155 mmol/l, as hypernatraemia may cause hepatocyte lysis and organ failure.

Optimising the physiological status of a potential donor can be initiated as soon as possible after consent or authorisation for organ retrieval is established. Donor optimisation care bundles are available on the NHS Blood and Transplant website. Implementing the protocols and care bundles improves both the number and the quality of organs retrieved, and decreases the donors lost due to instability.

References and Further Reading
Gordon JK, McKinlay J. Physiological changes after brain stem death and management of the heart-beating donor. *Contin Educ Anaesth Crit Care Pain* 2012;**12**:225–9.

McKeown DW, Bonser RS, Kellum JA. Management of the heartbeating brain-dead organ donor. *Br J Anaesth* 2012;**108**(Suppl 1):96–107.

NHS Blood and Transplant. Donor optimisation – guidance around selecting potential DBD donors. www.odt.nhs.uk/deceased-donation/best-practice-guidance/donor-optimisation/

NHS Blood and Transplant. 2012. Organ retrieval from donation after brain-stem death (DBD) donors in the UK. Donor Optimisation Extended Care Bundle. www.odt.nhs.uk/deceased-donation/best-practice-guidance/donor-optimisation/

Office of the Chief Health Officer, Ministry of Health NSW. 2016. Management of the adult brain dead potential organ and tissue donor. www1.health.nsw.gov.au/pds/ActivePDSDocuments/GL2016_008.pdf

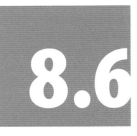

8.6 Management of Organ Donation Following Circulatory Death

Shankara Nagaraja

Key Learning Points

1. Controlled donation after circulatory death (DCD) follows a planned withdrawal of care.
2. The organ donation team should not be involved in treatment withdrawal decisions.
3. Critical pathways for DCD have been outlined by the World Health Organization.
4. Donation must never cause death of the patient.
5. After the death, interventions likely to restore cerebral circulation should not be undertaken.

Keywords: organ donation, circulatory death, treatment withdrawal

Introduction

Donation after circulatory death (DCD) refers to retrieval of organs for transplantation, after confirmation of death by circulatory criteria. Death here is defined as the 'irreversible cessation of neurological (pupillary), cardiac and respiratory activity', as opposed to brainstem death.

The steps in the DCD process described in Table 8.6.1 are specific for UK practice.

Controlled and Uncontrolled Donations

Controlled DCD follows a planned withdrawal of care, allowing time for mobilisation of retrieval teams, so multiple organs can be retrieved. These patients usually have suffered catastrophic brain injuries and, whilst not fulfilling the criteria for brainstem death, have severe injuries justifying withdrawal of care.

Uncontrolled donations occur when a person dies suddenly and unexpectedly – before consideration of organ donation is made. In this instance, donation is

Table 8.6.1 Modified Maastricht classification used to categorise donation after circulatory death

Category	Description	Type of DCD possible
I	Dead on arrival	Uncontrolled
II	Unsuccessful resuscitation	Uncontrolled
III	Anticipated cardiac arrest	Controlled
IV	Cardiac arrest in a brain-dead donor	Controlled
V	Unexpected arrest in ICU patient	Uncontrolled

Abbreviations: DCD = donation after circulatory death.
Source: Kootstra G, Daemen JH, Oomen AP. Categories of non-heart beating organ donors. *Transplant Proc* 1995; **27**: 2893–4.

usually restricted to kidneys and is normally only possible in centres where retrieval teams are readily available, i.e. transplant centres.

The Process of Controlled DCD

Critical pathways for DCD have been outlined by the World Health Organization (WHO). The following steps describe the principles and steps towards a controlled DCD in the UK.

1. The decision to withdraw treatment from a patient is done in the best interests of the patient and in accordance with the Mental Capacity Act and the General Medical Council guidelines. The organ donation team should not be involved in these decisions.
2. Potential donors include all patients where a decision to withdraw life-sustaining treatment is being made and death is considered imminent after treatment withdrawal. These patients should be discussed with the local transplant coordinators at the earliest possible opportunity, thus allowing them to review if the patient is on the organ donor register and the suitability of their organs for transplant.

3. Discussions relating to organ donation can only be undertaken after discussion with the patient's family and after their acceptance of treatment withdrawal.

4. The NHS Organ Donor Register is checked before approaching the family, and the approach is best done as a collaborative effort between senior medical staff and the specialist nurse for organ donation (SNOD). Once consent is obtained, the SNOD will coordinate both the processes of organ offering and retrieval and donor (and their family's) aftercare, in partnership with the hospital's clinical team.

5. If the patient meets the criteria for referral to the Coroner or Procurator Fiscal (Scotland), this should be undertaken.

6. Ideally withdrawal of treatment from the patient only takes place after the organ recipients are identified and admitted to transplant centres and the transplant team is deemed ready for organ retrieval. Continuing life-sustaining treatment to facilitate donation is considered to be in patients' 'broader' best interests, as long as it does not cause them harm or distress. That said, no treatment should be instituted against the patient's or family's wishes.

7. The location for treatment withdrawal can be in the theatre complex if transfer from the critical care unit is too protracted or complex. It should not, however, compromise the patient's dignity, privacy and comfort, nor should the family's access to their relative be restricted.

8. Treatment withdrawal is undertaken under the supervision of a senior clinician and can include terminal extubation and withdrawal of cardio-respiratory support. Patient comfort must be maintained at all times.

9. Donation may not proceed if the patient does not become asystolic for prolonged periods or develops prolonged and significant hypotension and hypoxia. The family needs to be made aware of this possibility.

10. Confirmation of death should be prompt, with a minimum of 5 minutes' observation to ensure that irreversible cardio-respiratory death has occurred. Absence of circulation may be confirmed with an arterial line, echocardiography or asystole on an electrocardiogram. Digital palpation of a central pulse is considered insufficient. Any return of cardiac or respiratory activity during the period of observation should prompt a further 5-minute observation period after subsequent asystole. These steps are safeguards to ensure that organ donation does not result in death of the patient – the 'Dead Donor Rule'.

11. Once the death is declared, the family is given up to 5 minutes with the patient, prior to their transfer to theatre for organ retrieval. The time is also used to complete the death certification.

12. After death, no interventions that might potentially restore cerebral circulation and function should be undertaken. Tracheal re-intubation and recruitment manoeuvres may be performed to facilitate lung donation; however, cyclical ventilation should not be started until cerebral circulation is excluded.

13. If donation does not proceed, a plan must be in place for subsequent care. The option of tissue donation must be considered.

Ischaemia Times

Two types of ischaemia in retrieved organs have been described – warm (functional) ischaemia and cold ischaemia. Warm ischaemia may be further classified into donor and recipient warm ischaemia. Donor warm ischaemia starts from the time of significant hypoxia (SpO_2 <70%) or hypotension (systolic blood pressure <50 mmHg) until cold perfusion begins. Unlike in donation after brainstem death (DBD), where cold perfusion occurs prior to organ retrieval, donor warm ischaemia of over 10 minutes is inevitable in DCD. Recipient warm ischaemia starts from removal of the organ from ice until reperfusion. Cold ischaemia refers to the time between the end of donor warm ischaemia and the onset of recipient warm ischaemia.

Longer ischaemia times make the quality of organs unacceptable for transplantation. The maximum acceptable functional ischaemia times before proceeding with organ retrieval (in minutes) are seen in Table 8.6.2.

Table 8.6.2 Acceptable functional ischaemia times

Organ	Time (minutes)	Other
Kidney	120	Additional 120 minutes in selected donors
Liver and pancreas	30	
Lung	60	Time to lung re-inflation

Patients from Emergency Department

The UK consensus statement recommends critical care admission for patients initially assessed in the emergency department, in whom organ donation is a possibility, whenever possible.

References and Further Reading

Department of Health, Intensive Care Society, NHS Blood and Transplant, British Transplantation Society. Donation after circulatory death. Report of a consensus meeting. London: Department of Health; 2010.

Dunne K, Doherty P. Donation after circulatory death. *Contin Educ Anaesth Crit Care Pain* 2011;**11**:82–6.

Kotloff RM, Blosser S, Fulda GJ, *et al.* Management of the potential organ donor in the ICU: Society of Critical Care Medicine/American College of Chest Physicians/Association of Organ Procurement Organizations Consensus Statement. *Crit Care Med* 2015;**43**:1291–325.

Manara AR, Murphy PG, Ocallaghan G. Donation after circulatory death. *Br J Anaesth* 2012;**108**(Suppl 1):i108–21.

Working Party of The British Transplantation Society. 2013. Transplantation from deceased donors after circulatory death. bts.org.uk/wp-content/uploads/2016/09/15_ BTS_Donors_DCD-1.pdf

9.1 Assessment and Management of the Sick Child

Andrew J. Jones and Thomas Brick

Key Learning Points

1. There are key physiological and anatomical differences between children and adults.
2. Despite the differences, the resuscitative process and 'ABC' approach are common to both patient groups.
3. Medications and fluid are administered to children based on their body weight.
4. The normal range for physiological parameters varies by age.
5. In-hospital cardiac arrest is usually due to hypoxia and will often follow a period of physiological deterioration.

Keywords: clinical assessment, paediatrics, weight, physiology

Introduction

The adult physician – when called upon to assist in the management of a critically ill child – needs to be aware of the anatomical, physiological and psychological differences between children and adults. However, perhaps with the exception of newborns, the resuscitative process is common to both. Adhere to the basic principles of critical care medicine, and do not delay essential interventions.

Differences

Weight

Weight is required for calculation of drug doses, fluid volumes and cardioversion. Weighing the child is rarely practical in the acute setting, and calculations are available to estimate weight based on age (Box 9.1.1).

Airway

The paediatric airway is anatomically quite different from the adult airway. In practice, important aspects

> **Box 9.1.1** Estimation of Weight Based on Age
>
> 0–12 months: weight (kg) = (0.5 × age in months) + 4
> 1–5 years: weight (kg) = (2 × age in years) + 8
> 6–12 years: weight (kg) = (3 × age in years) + 7

of airway management to be aware of include the following:

- When bag–mask ventilating, care should be taken to keep one's fingers away from the soft tissue of the chin to avoid compressing the floor of the mouth.
- In infants, a posterior-projecting epiglottis and anterior larynx make, in theory, a straight-bladed laryngoscope better for intubation. A curved blade is more appropriate once the child is above 6–10 kg. Experienced operators may opt to use a curved blade for all intubations.
- The cricoid ring is the narrowest part of the child's airway (not the larynx), and the cricoid has loosely bound epithelium which is vulnerable to trauma. Established practice has been to avoid cuffed tubes. However, there is evidence to suggest that high-volume, low-pressure microcuffs are no more harmful than uncuffed tubes. The risk–benefit is likely to be in favour of cuffed tubes, especially when high-pressure ventilation is needed. A cuffed tube will prevent the need to upsize the endotracheal tube (ETT) in the event of a large leak compromising ventilation.
- The trachea is short. The ETT should be sited in the mid-tracheal position. In a small infant, a change in tube length of 1 cm can mean the difference between an ideal tube position and an endobronchial intubation; therefore the ETT should be sited and secured with great care. Appropriate sizing may be calculated using the formulae in Box 9.1.2.

689

Box 9.1.2 Calculation of Endotracheal Tube Length

Size

Uncuffed endotracheal tube size (mm) = (age in years / 4) + 4

Cuffed endotracheal tube size (mm) = (age in years / 4) + 3

Length

Oral length (cm) = (age / 2) + 12

Nasal length (cm) = (age / 2) + 15

Breathing

The upper and lower airways are small, and therefore more prone to obstruction (resistance to flow is inversely proportional to the fourth power of the airway radius). This manifests clinically in conditions such as laryngotracheobronchitis (croup) and inflammation of the small airways in bronchiolitis. Even seemingly minor obstruction can result in respiratory failure – 1 mm of oedema can narrow a baby's upper airway by 60 per cent.

Target tidal volumes in relation to body weight remain constant, regardless of age (5–7 ml/kg). The chest wall is compliant – more so than in adults – which can lead to significant sternal and intercostal recession, resulting in increased work of breathing. Chest wall compliance also results in a less negative intrathoracic pressure, meaning the lung volume at end-expiration is close to the lung volume at which small airway closure starts (the closing volume). Invasively ventilated children require positive end-expiratory pressure (PEEP) – 5 cmH$_2$O is a good starting point – and applying continuous positive airway pressure (CPAP) during spontaneous ventilation can decrease work of breathing. Respiratory muscle fatigue can also be a problem in smaller children, as muscles of respiration have fewer type 1 fibres, so ventilatory support may be required early.

Circulation

Infants have a small, fairly fixed stroke volume (1.5 ml/kg in a neonate), and so variation in cardiac output is mostly dependent on heart rate. Ability to increase cardiac output at times of stress is thus relatively limited – an adult can both increase the stroke volume and double the resting heart rate, but a neonate with a resting heart rate of 150 bpm cannot. The fixed stroke volume can also blunt the response to fluid boluses in a younger child; from the age of 2 years and above, the response to fluid is similar to an adult's. Despite the

Table 9.1.1 Normal physiological parameters by age

Age	Heart rate (bpm)	Respiratory rate (breaths/min)	Blood pressure (systolic) (mmHg)
Newborn	90–180	40–60	60–90
1 month	110–180	30–50	70–104
3 months	110–180	30–45	70–104
6 months	110–180	25–35	72–110
1 year	80–160	20–30	72–110
2 years	80–140	20–28	74–110
4 years	80–120	20–26	78–112
6 years	75–115	18–24	82–115
8 years	70–110	18–22	86–118
10 years	70–110	16–20	90–121
12 years	60–110	16–20	90–126
14 years	60–100	16–20	92–130

Source: Taken from *Advanced Paediatric Life Support: A Practical Approach to Emergencies*, Sixth Edition. Martin Samuels and Sue Wieteska. 2016.

small stroke volume, the neonate has a cardiac index of 300 ml/(min kg). This decreases with age to 100 ml/(min kg) in teenagers and to 80 ml/(min kg) in adults.

Circulating blood volume at 70–80 ml/kg is higher than that of an adult. However, absolute blood volumes are small; what can appear to be a small amount of blood loss may lead to significant hypovolaemic shock. Neonates in the intensive care unit often need blood transfusions due to blood loss from routine sampling for laboratory investigations.

Systemic vascular resistance rises throughout childhood. Table 9.1.1 shows normal blood pressure values and other parameters.

Clinical Assessment

Outside of the paediatric intensive care unit (PICU) setting, a cardiac arrest is a rare event in children, with an out-of-hospital incidence of 8–10 per 100,000 and an estimated incidence amongst inpatients of 1 per 5000. Most in-hospital cardiac arrests will be because of progressive and persistent hypoxia due to a respiratory illness, and overall survival to hospital discharge following a cardiac arrest is about 40 per cent. It is therefore crucial that the clinical signs that herald an imminent arrest are promptly recognised and treated.

Careful observation of the child is essential, and it should be possible to form an instant impression of how sick a child is from the end of the bed.

It is reassuring if a child is crying lustily and vocalising normally. Listen for added airway noises. Stridor is a high-pitched noise on inspiration due to obstruction of the larynx or trachea. Stertor is a low-pitched snoring inspiratory noise usually due to pharyngeal obstruction, and may be accompanied by bubbling and gurgling of secretions. It may be observed, for example, in a child with cerebral palsy with impaired airway control and difficulty clearing secretions. Hypoxia in the context of new airway obstruction should be taken very seriously and may indicate an imminent need for intubation.

The level of tachypnoea or hypopnoea should be immediately obvious, and may be accompanied by signs of increased work of breathing such as nasal flaring and sternal, intercostal and subcostal recession. Grunting respiration is an attempt by the child to generate PEEP by approximating the vocal cords, and is usually a sign of severe lower respiratory tract disease. In bronchoconstriction, the volume of the wheeze does not necessarily indicate severity – more important are the respiratory effort, air entry, conscious level and degree of tachycardia. In the severest of bronchoconstriction, there may be no wheeze audible at all. Continuous pulse oximetry is essential in all critically unwell children, and saturations of <92% in a child who is receiving oxygen are concerning. Some children – such as those with neuromuscular conditions – may not exhibit the expected increased work of breathing in response to a respiratory infection. Tachypnoea and other respiratory signs may also be a sign of a circulatory or metabolic disease, e.g. sepsis or diabetic ketoacidosis (DKA).

When assessing circulation, evaluate perfusion by feeling the skin temperature and measuring the capillary refill time (CRT). Press on the sternum for 5 seconds, and colour should normally return in <2 seconds. This is not always reliable but is important when put together with other clinical signs. Measuring the heart rate and blood pressure is essential. Persistent tachycardia should not be attributed to pain or agitation without a thorough assessment. Hypotension is a late sign requiring immediate treatment.

Assessing neurological disability can be challenging. Pathological irritability or lethargy can be difficult to distinguish from normal childhood behaviours. However, any decrease in conscious level should be taken very seriously, and is worrying in the context of hypoxia or suspected organ hypoperfusion. Using the AVPU scale (Alert, responsive to Voice, responsive to Pain, Unresponsive), instead of a full Glasgow Coma Score (GCS), is perfectly acceptable. Pupillary responses are often forgotten but form an important part of the assessment.

References and Further Reading

Gupta P, Tang X, Gall CM, Lauer C, Rice TB, Wetzel RC. Epidemiology and outcomes of in-hospital cardiac arrest in critically ill children across hospitals of varied center volume: a multi-center analysis. *Resuscitation* 2014;**85**:1473–9.

Harless J, Ramaiah R, Bhananker SM. Pediatric airway management. *Int J Crit Illn Inj Sci* 2014;**4**:65–70.

Newth CJI, Rachman B, Patel N, Hammer J. The use of cuffed versus uncuffed endotracheal tubes in pediatric intensive care. *J Pediatr* 2004;**144**:333–7.

Samuels M, Wieteska S (eds). *Advanced Paediatric Life Support: A Practical Approach to Emergencies*, 6th edn. Chichester: Wiley Blackwell; 2016.

Spotting the Sick Child. Practical skills from clinical experience. www.spottingthesickchild.com/

Organisation of Paediatric Intensive Care and Paediatric Intensive Care Transport Services in the UK

Andrew J. Jones and Thomas Brick

Key Learning Points

1. In the UK, centralisation of services in the paediatric intensive care unit (PICU) has saved lives.
2. The development of paediatric intensive care transport services has accompanied the centralisation of paediatric intensive care.
3. Paediatric critical illness scoring systems (e.g. paediatric index of mortality (PIM) and paediatric risk of mortality (PRISM)) enable comparisons between units and across time to be made.
4. Current mortality in the paediatric intensive care unit (PICU) in the UK is around 3 per cent.
5. Nearly 6 in 10 PICU admissions in the UK are for children with life-limiting conditions.

Keywords: paediatric intensive care, paediatric intensive care transport, PIM score, PRISM score, funnel plots

Introduction

Paediatric intensive care developed in a fragmented fashion across the developed world from the 1960s. In the late 1990s, the UK began a process of centralisation of paediatric intensive care services, with the benefits of larger regional units having become apparent; high volume means that units develop broad experience of complex and unusual cases, a staff of specialist nurses and doctors can be maintained and staff training can take place in a coherent and organised manner. It is estimated that up to 450 children died annually in the UK during the 1990s due to lack of centralisation of paediatric intensive care services.

There are currently 32 paediatric intensive care units (PICUs) and 12 paediatric intensive care transport teams that report data to the Paediatric Intensive Care Audit Network (PICANet) in the UK and the Republic of Ireland. Annually, approximately 20,000 children under 16 years of age are admitted to PICUs in the UK and the Republic of Ireland. Over half of children admitted to PICUs are aged 1 or less. The median length of stay is typically short (<3 days), and mortality has reduced steadily over the past decade – from 5.5 per cent in 2003/2004 to 3.4 per cent in 2016.

Scoring Systems and Quality Metrics in PICU

Scoring systems in paediatric intensive care are used to describe severity of illness based on physiological variables (e.g. Pediatric Logistic Organ Dysfunction (PELOD) score), or risk of death based on a combination of physiological variables plus underlying disease (e.g. paediatric index of mortality (PIM) score, or paediatric risk of mortality (PRISM) score). For patients undergoing congenital cardiac surgery, scores based on the underlying diagnosis have been developed (e.g. Risk Adjustment for Congenital Heart Surgery (RACHS)). Scores enable comparison of performance across time and centres.

In the UK, all children admitted to PICU have key demographic and clinical information reported to PICANet. This allows calculation of a standardised mortality ratio (SMR) for each unit, which, in turn, enables comparisons to be made. In addition, the participating units report a selection of metrics to enable monitoring of the quality of care provided (e.g. staffing levels, emergency readmissions, transport team mobilisation time).

Graphics can be used to compare the performance of individual PICUs. Funnel plots for the SMR are frequently used – they demonstrate the SMR (ratio of observed deaths to expected deaths) for participating units (Figure 9.2.1). This is then plotted, and confidence limits calculated to allow for natural variation. The

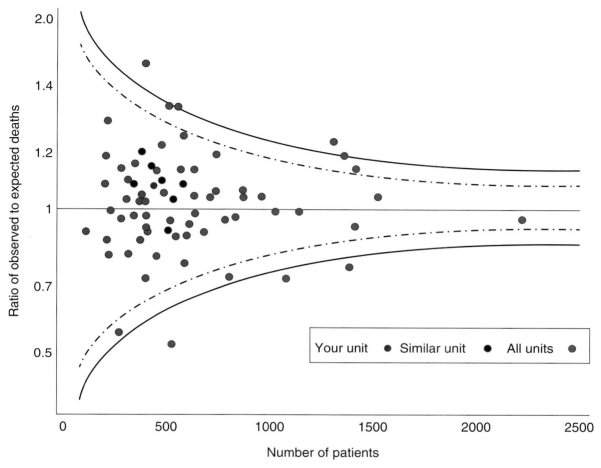

Figure 9.2.1 Example of a hospital mortality funnel plot. This funnel plot shows each unit plotted against total admissions on the *x*-axis and the ratio of observed to expected deaths on the *y*-axis. The dashed grey lines represent the inner control limits within which 95 per cent of units should lie if they are distributed by chance, and the solid grey lines represent the outer control limits within which 99.8 per cent of units should lie if they are distributed by chance.

Source: Adapted with the permission of the Intensive Care National Audit & Research Centre (INARC).

finding of SMRs which lie outside the confidence limits triggers an investigation to understand the causes.

Paediatric Intensive Care Transport Services

The development of paediatric intensive care transport services has accompanied the centralisation of paediatric intensive care. In most parts of the UK, retrieval by dedicated transport teams has replaced the practice of retrieval by the receiving intensive care unit. Dedicated teams offer a number of advantages – they encourage the development of expertise within the team they serve as a hub where referring hospitals can obtain advice, and they provide a bed-finding service

which is able to triage and allocate patients to the most appropriate receiving unit. A number of indicators can be used to measure the performance of such services: speed of retrieval, adverse physiological events during transport and the number of interventions required following arrival at the receiving unit. Morbidity and the incidence of adverse events are decreased with the use of specialised services.

Changing Patterns of PICU

Whilst mortality has decreased in PICU over the past three decades, the proportion of survivors with moderate to severe disability has increased. Long-stay patients utilise a large proportion of resources, and long PICU stays are associated with unfavourable outcomes. Children with life-limiting conditions make up nearly 60 per cent of admissions to UK PICUs, and these children are more likely to die in PICU than those without. Patterns of death are changing within PICUs (the length of stay of children who die in PICU has increased in the UK over the past decade), and a picture of early deaths due to treatment failure has been replaced by death after a long PICU stay. Survivors may be technology dependent; for example, the number of children who receive long-term ventilation in the UK has risen rapidly in recent years, in part due to the emergence of disease-modifying drugs altering the natural history of neuromuscular diseases (e.g. nusinersen for spinal muscular atrophy), but also due to changing parental expectations. These changes are happening against a backdrop of high-profile cases where the courts have been called upon to settle disagreements between parents and intensive care staff regarding ongoing futile treatment. The future of paediatric intensive care will be influenced not only by technological and organisational progress within the PICU, but also by the views of society with regard to resource allocation, parental autonomy and end-of-life care.

References and Further Reading

Fraser LK, Parslow R. Children with life-limiting conditions in paediatric intensive care units: a national cohort, data linkage study. *Arch Dis Child* 2018;**103**:540–7.

Namachivayam P, Shann F, Shekerdemian L, *et al*. Three decades of pediatric intensive care: who was admitted, what happened in intensive care, and what happened afterward. *Pediatr Crit Care Med* 2010;**11**:549–55.

Namachivayam P, Taylor A, Montague T, *et al*. Long-stay children in intensive care: long-term functional outcome and quality of life from a 20-yr institutional study. *Pediatr Crit Care Med* 2012;**13**:520–8.

Pearson G, Shann F, Barry P, *et al*. Should paediatric intensive care be centralised? Trent versus Victoria. *Lancet* 1997;**349**:1213–17.

PICANet. 2017. PICANet annual report 2017. www.picanet .org.uk/Audit/Annual-Reporting/

Ramnarayan P. Measuring the performance of an inter-hospital transport service. *Arch Dis Child* 2009;**94**:414–16.

Vos GD, Nissen AC, Nieman FHM, *et al*. Comparison of interhospital pediatric intensive care transport accompanied by a referring specialist or a specialist retrieval team. *Intensive Care Med* 2004;**30**:302–8.

Wilkinson D. Beyond resources: denying parental requests for futile treatment. *Lancet* 2017;**389**:1866–7.

9.3 Safeguarding and Non-accidental Injury

Andrew J. Jones and Thomas Brick

Key Learning Points

1. Safeguarding and child protection are the responsibility of all professionals involved in the care of children.
2. If a child is suspected of being at risk of harm, a referral to the local authority must take place.
3. Abusive head trauma is the most common form of death amongst children as a result of abuse.
4. Specific clinical findings are strongly associated with abusive head trauma in young children.
5. In the UK, a statutory process is in place to respond to the death of a child.

Keywords: safeguarding, child protection, child abuse, non-accidental injury, abusive head trauma, child death

Relevance to the Intensivist

All doctors who look after children must ensure that the welfare of the child is their paramount consideration (Children's Act 1989). The General Medical Council (GMC) states: 'all doctors must act on any concerns they have about the safety or welfare of a child or young person.' Since the Laming Inquiry into the death of Victoria Climbié, great emphasis has been placed on the importance of sharing information across agencies, overriding concerns about confidentiality. In short, safeguarding and child protection are everyone's business!

How Widespread Is Child Abuse?

It is impossible to ascertain the precise size of the problem, but a number of agencies collect data that inform the question. Of 14 million children in England in 2012, 370,000 were classed as in need and 43,000 were subject to a child protection plan (CPP), of which 42 per cent were due to neglect, 28 per cent due to emotional abuse, 12 per cent due to physical abuse and 5 per cent due to sexual abuse. Of the 4000–4500 annual child deaths in the UK, the vast majority are due to natural causes. However, it is estimated that every year, maltreatment of children is associated with 85 deaths per year in England. Children who go on to suffer serious harm or death have often already presented to healthcare services with signs of abuse which may have been missed. By implication, opportunities exist for the alert clinician to detect child abuse and prevent serious harm or death.

Types of Abuse
Physical Abuse

The question that must be forefront in the mind of the physician assessing a child with physical injuries is whether the explanation offered for the injuries matches the physical findings. Features which increase the risk of non-accidental injury are an inconsistent or evolving history, a suggested mechanism which is not appropriate for the developmental age of the child, a delay in presentation and if the quality of interaction between the parent and the child strikes the clinician as unusual. Young children are at risk of severe physical abuse, with age <2 years being a particular risk factor. A forensic approach by the medical team looking after a child who is suspected of having suffered a non-accidental injury is necessary. This will involve a detailed and contemporaneous history and a thorough physical examination, including a 'body map'. Findings should be recorded in detail sufficient for later use in social care or legal proceedings.

The two most common modes of physical abuse leading to involvement of the intensive care specialist are abusive head trauma (AHT) and abuse leading to abdominal or visceral injuries.

Abusive Head Trauma

AHT is the most common form of death amongst children as a result of abuse and mainly affects children

695

under 2 years, with the highest incidence in children <6 months of age. Brain injury results from shaking leading to acceleration/deceleration injuries with or without trauma, or secondary to trauma alone. In children who present with intracranial pathology (subdural haemorrhage, extradural haemorrhage, intra-parenchymal injury or cerebral oedema), the following findings are associated with AHT:

1. Bruising
2. Seizures
3. Apnoea
4. Long bone fractures
5. Retinal haemorrhages
6. Rib fractures

The presence of intracranial pathology with three of the six features is associated with an odds ratio of >100 for AHT versus non-AHT. In addition, the absence of a history of trauma is strongly associated with AHT.

The management of a child with significant intracranial injury follows the standard principles of paediatric neurocritical care.

In addition, a comprehensive workup is required to establish the cause. This will include a thorough history and clinical examination. The physical findings should be accurately recorded on a body map. The following investigations are key to ruling out alternative diagnoses and must be carried out meticulously:

- **Ophthalmological assessment:** the presence of retinal haemorrhages – specifically bilateral, multi-layer and numerous – is strongly associated with AHT and rarely found outside this population
- **Neuroimaging:** MRI brain and spine
- **Skeletal survey:** radiographs of long bones, ribs and the skull should be undertaken and reported by a paediatric radiologist
- **Haematological investigations:** platelet count, clotting screen (including factor assays) and platelet function assay
- **Microbiology:** bacterial and viral cultures of cerebrospinal fluid (CSF) (when appropriate) and blood
- **Metabolic investigations:** urine organic acids, blood carnitine and acylcarnitine (looking for glutaric aciduria type 1 which is associated with subdural haemorrhages), blood copper, calcium phosphate, alkaline phosphatase and vitamin D

Abusive Abdominal and Visceral Injuries

Abusive abdominal trauma is the second most common cause of death from child abuse, with mortality rates of 13–45 per cent. Mortality is highest in the neonatal age group. Organs most commonly injured are the liver, kidney and hollow viscera.

Fabricated or Induced Illness and Perplexing Presentations

A carer sometimes behaves in such a way as to convince healthcare professionals that the child in their care is sick. This may include poisoning (e.g. administration of insulin, salt, etc.) or invention or exaggeration of symptoms leading to unnecessary investigation or treatment. The pattern of presentation varies, but the child may present to the critical care physician with symptoms of poisoning, coma or seizures. Fabricated or induced illness (FII) should be considered when the clinical condition of the child is not explained by a recognisable illness. The diagnosis relies on meticulous history taking and examination, and advice should be sought from a specialist in paediatric child abuse.

Emotional Abuse, Neglect and Sexual Abuse

These can all occur in the critically ill child, although they might not be obvious at the time of presentation. Nevertheless, the clinician should remain aware of the possibility of their existence.

The Safeguarding Process – Roles, Responsibilities and Processes

If a professional has concerns that a child is being harmed, they must make a referral to the local authority, which will decide whether a child protection enquiry is to be undertaken. This is a process of information gathering in order to determine whether the child is at risk of significant harm. Three outcomes are possible:

1. No further action
2. 'Child in need' – a child who is unlikely to achieve or maintain a reasonable level of health or development, or whose health and development are likely to be significantly or further impaired, without the provision of services; or a child who is disabled
3. Child at risk of 'significant harm' – ill treatment or impairment of health or development

If the child is thought to be at risk of significant harm, a strategy discussion takes place involving the local authority, the police, health services, other relevant authorities and the referring agency to determine whether the child should be subject to a Section 47 enquiry. Within 15 days, a child protection conference must take place. This is attended by professionals working with the child and the family, and the purpose is to determine whether the child should be subject to a child protection plan (previously known as the 'child protection register') and what that plan should consist of. The plan must be reviewed within 3 months, then at 6-monthly intervals. Children should not remain subject to a child protection plan indefinitely, but instead the plan should address the underlying concerns and aim to reduce the risk to the child. If the level of risk cannot be adequately reduced, the local authority must consider additional measures, such as legal action to safeguard the child which may include placing the child in local authority care.

Following the death of a child, a local child death review meeting takes place. This is a multi-professional meeting which is attended by professionals who were involved in the care of the child during his or her life. All child deaths are subject to further review by an independent Child Death Overview Panel (CDOP), which considers modifiable factors that may have contributed to the death of the child. The information generated from this process feeds into the National Child Mortality Database, which is used to identify trends of patterns in child death in the UK and can ultimately be used to inform local and national policy. When abuse or neglect is implicated in the death or serious injury of a child, a Serious Case Review is held in order to analyse what has taken place, with the aim of learning lessons in order to reduce the risk of recurrence.

All NHS trusts must have a named doctor and nurse for safeguarding who will provide expert advice to fellow professionals within their organisation.

References and Further Reading

Agrawal S, Peters MJ, Adams GGW, Pierce CM. Prevalence of retinal hemorrhages in critically ill children. *Pediatrics* 2012;**129**:e1388–96.

Brandon M, Sidebotham P, Bailey S, *et al.* New learning from serious case reviews: a two year report for 2009–2011. London: Department of Health; 2012.

Hettler J, Greenes DS. Can the initial history predict whether a child with a head injury has been abused? *Pediatrics* 2003;**111**:602–7.

Keenan HT, Runyan DK, Marshall SW, Nocera MA, Merten DF. A population-based comparison of clinical and outcome characteristics of young children with serious inflicted and noninflicted traumatic brain injury. *Pediatrics* 2004;**114**:633–9.

Wolfe I, Macfarlane A, Donkin A, Marmot M, Viner R. Why children die: deaths in infants, children and young people in the UK. London: Royal College of Paediatrics and Child Health and National Children's Bureau; 2014.

9.4 Respiratory Failure

Andrew J. Jones and Thomas Brick

Key Learning Points

1. The anatomy and physiology of young children make them particularly vulnerable to respiratory failure.
2. Children who need intubating for upper airway obstruction require input from doctors competent in the management of the paediatric airway.
3. Respiratory failure is the most common indication for admission to the paediatric intensive care unit.
4. The principles of lung-protective ventilation apply in children.
5. High-frequency oscillatory ventilation is an effective rescue modality in children.

Keywords: respiratory failure, pARDS, bronchiolitis, croup, high-frequency oscillatory ventilation, mechanical ventilation, ECMO

Respiratory Anatomy and Physiology in Children

Respiratory illness requiring mechanical support is the most common indication for admission to a paediatric intensive care unit. Children are particularly vulnerable to respiratory failure, due to a combination of physiological and anatomical peculiarities outlined in Box 9.4.1.

Upper Airway Obstruction

Upper airway obstruction (UAO) refers to a restriction of airflow at the level of the pharynx, larynx and trachea. Children have small airways, and because resistance to flow is inversely proportional to the fourth power of the radius, a small degree of airway inflammation can result in significant respiratory compromise. The clinical presentation of UAO is with stridor, which should be distinguished from stertor or wheeze.

Airway obstruction can rapidly become life-threatening and requires the involvement of multiple disciplines (including anaesthesia and ear, nose and throat (ENT)) to ensure the airway is safely secured.

Laryngotracheobronchitis (Croup)

Croup is caused by inflammation of the subglottic airway due to infection, most commonly with parainfluenza virus. Presentation is with a barking cough and stridor. The typical age at presentation is between 6 months and 3 years – alternative diagnoses must be strongly considered outside of this age range. Croup severity can range from mild, self-limiting illness to a child with exhaustion, severe respiratory distress

---

Box 9.4.1 Physiological and Anatomical Differences between Adults and Children

- Increased metabolic demand – hence oxygen demand is higher compared with an adult
- Smaller airways are more liable to obstruction by mucus or oedema
- Compliant anatomical structures (larynx, trachea, bronchi)
  - Forced inspiration in upper airway obstruction leads to extra-thoracic tracheal collapse
  - Forced expiration in lower airways disease leads to high intrathoracic pressures, and therefore collapse
- Compliant chest wall leading to collapse
- Fatiguable diaphragm and intercostal muscles
- Alveolar immaturity: lower ratio of alveoli-to-body surface area in children than in adults; absence of airway channels allowing 'collateral ventilation' until 3–4 years of age
- Increased susceptibility to viral respiratory tract infections

and apnoea. Oxygen should not be given until the decision is taken to intubate the child, as it can mask impending airway obstruction. Croup can be treated with dexamethasone (0.6 mg/kg intravenous (IV), intramuscular (IM) or oral – whichever is least likely to perturb the child). Nebulised adrenaline (1:1000 0.5 ml/kg, max 5 ml) may be administered to allow time for steroids to take effect or to buy time whilst staff and equipment for intubation are organised. Repeated requirement for adrenaline nebulisation should prompt the involvement of a senior anaesthetist or intensivist.

Acute Epiglottitis

Acute epiglottitis has historically almost always been due to infection with *Haemophilus influenzae* type b (Hib), with a mortality of 6 per cent in children. Airway compromise is due to inflammation of supraglottic structures and can result in sudden respiratory arrest. Whilst rare nowadays (since the introduction of Hib vaccine), it should still be considered in the differential diagnosis for a child with stridor. Unlike in viral croup, the child will look toxic, irritable and restless, with a high fever. The onset is abrupt, and dysphagia with refusal to eat may be a feature. Classically, the child is described as leaning forward, with the mouth wide open, the tongue protruding, and drooling. Administer IV antibiotics (e.g. ceftriaxone) once the airway is secure.

Foreign Body Aspiration

If a foreign body lodges in the larynx or trachea, the child may present with severe respiratory distress leading to respiratory arrest. If the object makes its way into a bronchus, then the presentation may be more insidious with chronic cough and purulent sputum. It is most common between 6 months and 3 years of age, and any object can be aspirated, but latterly button batteries have proven particularly dangerous due to electrical damage to surrounding tissues. In 20 per cent of cases of foreign body aspiration, the chest X-ray will demonstrate the object itself, with unilateral hyperexpansion of the affected lobe if the obstruction is bronchial.

Subglottic Stenosis

This can be congenital or acquired. The acquired form, due to endotracheal tube (ETT) trauma, affects about 1–2 per cent of babies who have been ventilated on a neonatal intensive care unit. Whilst an affected child can be relatively asymptomatic, an intercurrent upper respiratory tract infection may precipitate UAO.

Intubating the Child with Upper Airway Obstruction

Indications

- Epiglottitis
- Decreased consciousness
- Rising $PaCO_2$
- Hypoxaemia (use SpO_2 <92% in 5 l/min oxygen by mask as a rough threshold)
- Apnoea

Preparation

- Minimal handling – conscious children will position themselves in order to optimise airway patency.
- Avoid distressing the child (e.g. avoid IV cannulation, nurse on parent's lap) – crying will disrupt laminar flow of air.
- Prepare for urgent intubation, should sudden airway obstruction occur.

Intubation

- The team should include the most experienced anaesthetist available and an ENT surgeon.
- Sit the child up.
- Deliver inhalational induction of anaesthesia with spontaneously breathing child.
- Patience – onset of anaesthesia may be slow.
- Apply positive end-expiratory pressure (PEEP) when tolerated.
- Achieve a deep plane of anaesthesia.
- Lay the child flat.
- Perform laryngoscopy once the child is deep enough under anaesthesia to tolerate.
- Use an uncuffed ETT – likely 0.5 size down from the calculated size. 'Croup tubes' are available in some centres. These are longer than standard ETTs and can be useful if severe airway narrowing mandates a very small tube in a large child (e.g. 3.5-mm ETT in a 5-year old).
- Intubate (orally, then perform tracheal toilet and consider changing to a nasal tube).
- Use muscle relaxation only once the airway has been secured.

699

In the intensive care unit, the child can be weaned off sedation and may well be tube-tolerant enough to self-ventilate with a Swedish nose (heat and moisture exchanger). In croup, the expected time to extubation is approximately 3 days. An air leak test does not predict extubation success. Dexamethasone should be continued until the child has been successfully extubated.

Paediatric Acute Respiratory Distress Syndrome

A paediatric-specific definition of acute respiratory distress syndrome (ARDS) was developed in 2015 (Table 9.4.1). It attempts to overcome a number of weaknesses in generalising adult definitions to children.

1. The oxygenation index (OI) (FiO_2 × mean airway pressure × $100/PaO_2$) is used to classify severity. This overcomes the influence that PEEP has on the partial pressure:fraction of inspired oxygen (PF) ratio. The oxygen saturation index (OSI) [(FiO_2 × mean airway pressure × 100)/SpO_2] can be used in children for whom an arterial blood gas is not available.
2. Children receiving non-invasive ventilation (NIV) are included in the paediatric ARDS (pARDS) definition, in which case the PaO_2/FiO_2 or SpO_2/FiO_2 ratio can be used (in children for whom no arterial blood gas is available).
3. In order to capture the heterogeneous population of children who develop pARDS, definitions encompass pre-existing chronic lung disease,

cyanotic congenital heart disease and left ventricular dysfunction.

A recent comprehensive study of pARDS suggests the primary aetiologies were pneumonia (35 per cent), aspiration (15 per cent), sepsis (13 per cent), near-drowning (9 per cent), concomitant cardiac disease (7 per cent) and other clinical conditions (21 per cent).

Mortality is high in pARDS (approximately 20–40 per cent) and it is influenced by both severity of respiratory failure and co-morbidity.

Diseases of the Lower Airway
Bronchiolitis

Bronchiolitis affects young infants, most commonly during winter epidemics, and is potentially life-threatening. It can present in children up to 2 years of age, although it is most commonly seen in children who are <1 year. Apnoea occurs in one in five paediatric intensive area unit (PICU) admissions. Risk factors for death are young age at presentation, low birthweight, prematurity and co-morbidities (e.g. chronic lung disease, congenital heart disease or immunodeficiency). Management is supportive. Children with bronchiolitis are at risk of hyponatraemia due to syndrome of inappropriate anti-diuretic hormone secretion (ADH) – fluid intake should be restricted; initial therapy should consist of isotonic fluids at 50–70 per cent of daily requirement. Although a number of therapies have been investigated in the treatment of bronchiolitis, no evidence exists for the routine use of the following

Table 9.4.1 Definition of paediatric acute respiratory distress syndrome

Inclusion	Within 7 days of known clinical insult			
	Chest imaging: new infiltrates consistent with acute pulmonary parenchymal disease			
Exclusion	Respiratory failure explained by cardiac failure, fluid overload or perinatal lung disease			
Oxygenation	Non-invasive ventilation (CPAP ≥5 cmH$_2$O)	Invasive mechanical ventilation		
		Mild pARDS	Moderate pARDS	Severe pARDS
	PaO_2/FiO_2 <300	4 < OI <8	8 < OI <16	OI >16
	SpO_2FiO_2 <264	5 ≤ OSI <7.5	7.5 ≤ OSI <12.3	OSI ≥12.3
Special populations	Children with cyanotic congenital heart disease, left ventricular dysfunction and chronic lung disease can be classified as pARDS if they meet criteria and the deterioration in oxygenation is not due to underlying disease			

Abbreviations: CPAP, continuous positive airway pressure; pARDS, paediatric acute respiratory distress syndrome; OI = oxygenation index; OSI = oxygen saturation index.

Source: Adapted from 'The Pediatric Acute Lung Injury Consensus Conference Group Pediatric Acute Respiratory Distress Syndrome consensus recommendation' (full reference below).

interventions: inhaled or systemic bronchodilators, glucocorticoids, nebulised hypertonic saline, Heliox®, leukotriene inhibitors or physiotherapy.

Bacterial Pneumonia

Differentiating bacterial pneumonia from viral lower respiratory tract infections in children presenting with respiratory failure and parenchymal infiltrates is challenging without recourse to invasive sampling. However, in the presence of fever, raised inflammatory markers and infiltrates on chest radiographs, presumptive treatment of community-acquired pneumonia should be initiated. Organisms depend on age.

- Under 1 month of age, perinatally associated organisms are implicated in the aetiology – group B *Streptococcus*, Gram-negative enteric bacteria, *Listeria*.
- In older infants and children, *Streptococcus pneumoniae* is the most commonly implicated organism.

HiB is nearly non-existent in regions where vaccination is widespread. Group A *Streptococcus* and *Staphylococcus* infections are more likely to result in severe disease and ICU admission. The role of atypical organisms (*Mycoplasma pneumoniae*, *Chlamydia trachomatis* and *Chlamydia pneumoniae*) in the pathogenesis of paediatric pneumonia is unclear, as these organisms are frequently isolated in asymptomatic children. A typical antibiotic choice would include a β-lactam and a macrolide, with anti-staphylococcal agents (e.g. clindamycin) added for complicated disease. Organisms implicated in hospital-acquired pneumonia include *Enterobacteriaceae*, *Staphylococcus aureus*, *Pseudomonas aeruginosa* and anaerobes. Empirical treatment combinations should include an aminoglycoside and Gram-positive cover (e.g. piperacillin–tazobactam, meropenem, ceftazidime).

Asthma

Asthma is one of the most common reasons for admission to hospital and to PICU in children. It is a disease of airway inflammation, with consequent airway oedema, bronchoconstriction and mucus plugging. Initial therapy is with inhaled bronchodilators (beta agonists and ipratropium bromide) and steroids. Sick children may require IV magnesium, salbutamol and aminophylline. Both salbutamol and aminophylline have a significant side effect profile. Salbutamol causes tachycardia and lactic acidosis, which may worsen work of breathing as the child attempts respiratory correction of lactic

acidosis. Aminophylline may cause tachyarrhythmia, hypokalaemia and seizures. Bronchodilator effectiveness is decreased under the age of 2, as the bronchiolar smooth muscle is underdeveloped, compared with that of an older child.

Clinical examination, blood gases and oxygen saturations guide therapy. A child who has a rising $PaCO_2$ and is hypoxic is worrying. Intubation and mechanical ventilation are not usually required and carry a risk of hypoxaemia, pneumothoraces and haemodynamic compromise from high intrathoracic pressures. If ventilated, muscle relaxation and low ventilator rates are used to avoid gas trapping (high $PaCO_2$ and acidaemia are well tolerated), and a pH of 7.1 is not unusual.

High-Flow Nasal Cannulae

The use of high-flow nasal cannulae (HFNC) uses heated, humidified air at a flow greater than the child's own peak inspiratory flow rate, and has become widespread in paediatric practice over the last decade. HFNC is used for the management of a number of diseases, including bronchiolitis, pneumonia, cardiac failure and asthma. It has a favourable safety profile, and its use is associated with reduced intubation rates in infants cared for in PICU. Suggested physiological mechanisms for the effectiveness of HFNC include pharyngeal dead space washout, reduction in airway drying and generation of PEEP. Experimental studies demonstrate that flow rates of at least 2 l/(kg min) generate a pharyngeal pressure of 4 cmH_2O, resulting in respiratory muscle unloading. The following flow rates may be used: 2 l/(kg min) for a child up to 10 kg, and 0.5 l/min for every additional kilogram, up to a maximum of 50 l/min.

Continuous Positive Airway Pressure

NIV is used in children for a number of indications: acute – established or existing respiratory failure, post-extubation respiratory distress, left ventricular support in cardiac failure; and chronic – obstructive sleep apnoea, neuromuscular disease and chronic lung disease.

Effective delivery of NIV results in alveolar recruitment (increased functional residual capacity) and improved oxygenation. Improved alveolar ventilation results in improved carbon dioxide clearance, hence decreases acidosis. Airway patency is maintained, and the work of breathing is improved. In addition, CPAP may abolish apnoea in infants with bronchiolitis.

701

Many interfaces exist. Short, soft nasal prongs are frequently used and usually well tolerated. Full-face masks make accessing the oral cavity for suctioning difficult. Children with an abnormal facial anatomy may be difficult to fit masks onto; nasopharyngeal CPAP via a single nasal prong (e.g. a cut-down, age-appropriate ETT) is an effective interface.

Mechanical Ventilation

The principles of mechanical ventilation are similar in children, and as in adult practice, we assume that children's lungs are vulnerable to damage from mechanical power, high driving pressures and high FiO_2. The principles of lung-protective ventilation apply equally to the management of pARDS; PEEP 10–15 cmH_2O in severe pARDS, tidal volume 3–6 ml/kg, inspiratory plateau pressure <28 cmH_2O, permissive hypercapnia (pH 7.15–7.30) and permissive oxygen saturation targets (88–92%) are recommended for those with severe pARDS. Prone positioning and neuromuscular blockade should be considered, and inhaled nitric oxide is indicated in situations of severe right ventricular failure or as a bridge to extracorporeal support.

High-Frequency Oscillatory Ventilation

High-frequency oscillatory ventilation (HFOV) delivers a constant distending pressure, with sinusoidal oscillatory flow, to deliver low tidal volumes. This results in improved oxygenation, with minimal haemodynamic consequences. Avoidance of an opening/closing cycle reduces the risk of atelectotrauma seen in conventional ventilation. Two recent randomised controlled trials comparing conventional lung-protective ventilation with HFOV in the treatment of ARDS in adults have shown harm or lack of benefit. However, despite a clear lack of evidence of clinical efficacy, HFOV remains in widespread use as a rescue therapy within the PICU population, both in the treatment of ARDS and with inhaled nitric oxide for the treatment of persistent pulmonary hypertension of the newborn.

Extracorporeal Membrane Oxygenation

The use of extracorporeal membrane oxygenation (ECMO) in neonatal and paediatric patients who are unresponsive to maximal conventional therapy, and who have potentially reversible lung disease, is well established. In the UK, approximately 100 neonates and 50 children receive ECMO for respiratory failure annually. UK outcomes are reported to the Extracorporeal Life Support Organization (ELSO). Contemporary international survival rates for children receiving respiratory ECMO reported to ELSO are as follows: 70 per cent for both viral and bacterial pneumonia, 65 per cent for ARDS and 63 per cent for non-ARDS acute respiratory failure.

References and Further Reading

Cheifetz IM. Pediatric ARDS. *Respir Care* 2017;**62**: 718–31.

Franklin D, Babl FE, Schlapbach LJ, *et al*. A randomized trial of high-flow oxygen therapy in infants with bronchiolitis. *N Engl J Med* 2018;**378**:1121–31.

Gelbart B, Parsons S, Sarpal A, Ninova P, Butt W. Intensive care management of children intubated for croup: a retrospective analysis. *Anaesth Intensive Care* 2016;**44**:245–50.

Harris M, Clark J, Coote N, *et al*. British Thoracic Society guidelines for the management of community acquired pneumonia in children: update 2011. *Thorax* 2011;**66**(Suppl 2):ii1–23.

Leinwand K, Brumbaugh DE, Kramer RE. Button battery ingestion in children: a paradigm for management of severe pediatric foreign body ingestions. *Gastrointest Endosc Clin N Am* 2016;**26**:99–118.

McIntosh K. Community-acquired pneumonia in children. *N Engl J Med* 2002;**346**:429–37.

Pediatric Acute Lung Injury Consensus Conference Group. Pediatric acute respiratory distress syndrome: consensus recommendations from the Pediatric Acute Lung Injury Consensus Conference. *Pediatr Crit Care Med* 2015;**16**:428–39.

Paediatric Sepsis

9.5

Andrew J. Jones and Thomas Brick

Key Learning Points

1. Sepsis remains a major cause of death in the paediatric population.
2. Mortality is higher in children with co-morbidities than in those without.
3. Volume resuscitation is still the mainstay of initial resuscitation.
4. Adrenaline is a rational choice as a first-line vasoactive agent.
5. Combining clinical examination with plasma lactate can be used to guide resuscitation.

Keywords: paediatric sepsis, septic shock, fluid resuscitation, goal-directed therapy, lactate

Definition and Recognition of Sepsis

Sepsis can be broadly defined as a dysregulated systemic response to infection. A clinically useful, validated definition of sepsis is not in widespread use in paediatric practice, and current definitions have limited clinical utility. The 'suspected infection plus a systemic inflammatory response (SIRS)', adapted for children from the adult 'Sepsis 2' definitions, lacks specificity and frequently leads to the diagnosis of sepsis in children with self-limiting viral illnesses. Adapting Sepsis 3 definitions to children may well prove more useful, and the concept of sequential organ failure has validity in critically ill children in the paediatric intensive care unit (PICU).

In practical terms, in addition to fever and tachycardia, additional evidence of organ dysfunction (e.g. tachypnoea, poor perfusion, hypotension, altered mental status, oliguria, hyperlactataemia) should trigger aggressive treatment of sepsis.

A range of tools to help trigger identification and initiation of treatment for sepsis are available, e.g. the 'Sepsis 6' tool. Due to the heterogeneity of institutions and environments, no tool is demonstrably superior to all others. Individual institutions should incorporate and adapt such tools into their inpatient and emergency work.

Patterns of Sepsis Presentation

The introduction of childhood immunisations against the most common bacteria responsible for sepsis in childhood has radically altered the epidemiology of paediatric sepsis in the UK. *Haemophilus influenzae* type b (Hib) and meningococcal C vaccinations in the 1990s have been followed by a 7-, then a 13-valent, pneumococcal vaccine and a meningococcal B vaccine for children. Adolescents have been offered meningococcal ACWY since 2015. As a consequence, previously well children are less likely to require ICU treatment for sepsis. Children admitted to PICU with severe sepsis are, however, likely to have co-morbid conditions (50 per cent have >2) and pre-existing disability (>50 per cent). A causative organism is identified in less than half of children with severe sepsis, and the likely causative aetiology often depends on age at presentation. Group B *Streptococcus* and Gram-negative organisms (both perinatally acquired) are seen in the neonatal period, whilst coagulase-negative *Staphylococcus* may be seen in neonates with an indwelling venous line. *Listeria monocytogenes* is acquired transplacentally, during or after delivery, and is a rare, yet well-recognised cause of sepsis and meningoencephalitis in the neonate. Older infants and young children remain susceptible to infection with strains of *Streptococcus pneumoniae* and *Neisseria meningitides* not covered by current vaccination schedules. *Staphylococcus aureus* is the most commonly isolated bacterium in worldwide studies of sepsis in children. Group A *Streptococcus* can cause severe septic shock, often coexisting with chickenpox. Infections with potentially multi-resistant organisms (e.g. *Pseudomonas*, *Klebsiella*, *Acinetobacter*, *Escherichia coli* and MRSA) are found in healthcare settings and present a challenge to the intensivist. Fungal infections (most commonly *Candida* species)

703

have been reported in between 5 and 13 per cent of children with severe sepsis and septic shock, in particular in high-risk groups (children with indwelling central venous catheters, and immunocompromised and low-birthweight children). In addition, viral infections (e.g. enterovirus, adenovirus, influenza and herpes simplex) can mimic bacterial sepsis in the infant and young child.

Haemodynamics of Paediatric Septic Shock

Unlike in adults where the predominant pattern of septic shock is one of vasoplegia with maintained cardiac output, septic shock in children displays a number of haemodynamic patterns. Typically, children with community-acquired septic shock present with low cardiac output and variable systemic vascular resistance. Children with septic shock due to an indwelling central venous catheter are more likely to present with vasoplegic 'adult'-type shock. Crucially, children can move between haemodynamic states throughout a single illness; therefore, the clinician is obliged to continually re-evaluate their patient and to tailor treatment accordingly. Note that even experienced clinicians are notoriously poor at accurate clinical assessment of cardiac output, and non-invasive cardiac output monitoring can be successfully used to ascertain haemodynamic patterns in paediatric septic shock.

Protocolised Management of Sepsis

Early administration of antibiotics and prompt reversal of shock are associated with improved outcomes in paediatric sepsis. A structured approach to the management of septic shock is detailed in the latest guidance from the American College of Critical Care Medicine (ACCM). The management algorithm for septic shock can be seen in Figure 9.5.1.

Current Controversies
Fluid Resuscitation in Septic Shock

Uncertainty exists in the choice of type, route, rate and volume of fluid resuscitation used in paediatric sepsis. Although fluid resuscitation remains central to the resuscitation of shocked children, fluid overload is associated with increased mortality in PICU. The publication of the FEAST (Fluid Expansion as Supportive Therapy) trial has fuelled controversy regarding optimal fluid volume in paediatric sepsis. In this large trial

of children in sub-Saharan Africa with severe febrile illness and impaired perfusion, mortality at both 48 hours and 4 weeks was increased in children randomised to receiving fluid boluses. The extent to which results of this trial are applicable to well-resourced environments where children have access to intensive care is unclear; however, it has underlined the need for high-quality studies in middle- and high-income countries.

Current consensus favours the use of isotonic crystalloids in the initial resuscitation of children with septic shock. No trial has yet established the superiority or otherwise of balanced crystalloids, compared with sodium chloride, as a resuscitation fluid in children. Some centres invoke a physiological rationale and favour human albumin solution in instances of capillary leak or when large fluid volumes are required. Again, however, there are no direct randomised controlled trial data in the paediatric population to inform this choice.

Choice of Vasoactive Agent

Use of adrenaline as the first-line vasoactive agent in children with fluid-refractory septic shock is supported by a number of small randomised, placebo-controlled trials demonstrating a survival advantage over dopamine. Ideally, inotropes are delivered by a central line, but in the absence of central venous access, delivery of inotropes by either the intraosseus or the peripheral route may be lifesaving.

Early Goal-Directed Therapy in Paediatric Sepsis

Mortality in paediatric sepsis has decreased dramatically over the last 20 years within the UK due to a number of factors, including widespread adoption of sepsis guidelines and centralisation of children's critical care and retrieval services. Targeting specific goals of therapy forms part of the surviving sepsis and ACCM guidance, and a single-centre trial of children with severe sepsis or septic shock in a middle-income country with high sepsis mortality demonstrated a survival advantage of tailoring therapy to target central venous oxygen saturation (ScVO$_2$). Recent large adult randomised trials of standard care versus early goal-directed therapy, however, do not support the use of targeting central haemodynamic goals in the treatment of septic shock. In paediatric practice, directing therapy at ScVO$_2$ is not routine – a recent international point prevalence study of children with sepsis or septic shock found that

Initial Resuscitation Algorithm for Children

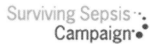

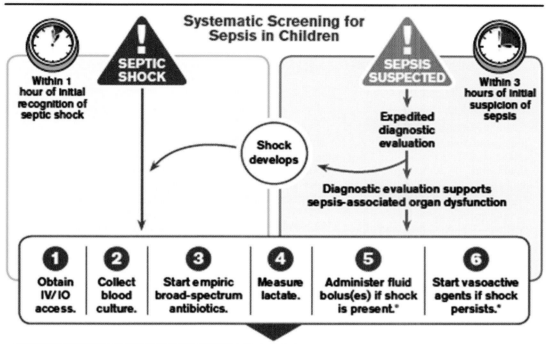

Systematic Screening for Sepsis in Children

SEPTIC SHOCK

SEPSIS SUSPECTED

Within 1 hour of initial recognition of septic shock

Within 3 hours of initial suspicion of sepsis

Expedited diagnostic evaluation

Shock develops

Diagnostic evaluation supports sepsis-associated organ dysfunction

1 Obtain IV/IO access.

2 Collect blood culture.

3 Start empiric broad-spectrum antibiotics.

4 Measure lactate.

5 Administer fluid bolus(es) if shock is present.*

6 Start vasoactive agents if shock persists.*

Respiratory support
Assess for Pediatric Acute Respiratory Distress Syndrome

Infectious source control

Continuous reassessment

Fluid and vasoactive titration*

Advanced hemodynamic monitoring if shock persists

- +/- hydrocortisone for refractory shock**
- Nutritional support
- Avoid hypoglycemia
- Antimicrobial stewardship

VA or VV ECLS for refractory shock or oxygenation/ventilation failure (after addressing other causes of shock and respiratory failure)

*See fluid and vasoactive algorithm. Note: Fluid bolus should be omitted from bundle if a) fluid overload is present or b) it is a low-resource setting without hypotension. Fluid in mL/kg should be dosed as ideal body weight.

**Hydrocortisone may produce benefit or harm.

Society of Critical Care Medicine

Fluid and Vasoactive-Inotrope Management Algorithm For Children

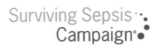

SEPTIC SHOCK

Healthcare Systems WITH Intensive Care ⟷ ⟷ **Healthcare Systems WITHOUT Intensive Care**

Abnormal Perfusion with or without Hypotension

- If signs of fluid overload are absent, administer fluid bolus, 10-20 mL/kg.
- Repeat assessment of hemodynamic response to fluid and consider fluid boluses, 10-20 mL/kg, until shock resolves or signs of fluid overload develop.
- Assess cardiac function.
- Consider epinephrine if there is myocardial dysfunction or epinephrine/ norepinephrine if shock persists after 40-60 mL/ kg (or sooner if signs of fluid overload develop).

Abnormal perfusion WITHOUT hypotension

- Do NOT give fluid bolus unless there are signs of dehydration with ongoing fluid losses (eg, diarrhea).
- Start maintenance fluids.
- Monitor hemodynamics closely.
- Consider vasoactive-inotropic support (if available).

Abnormal perfusion WITH hypotension*

- If signs of fluid overload are absent, administer fluid bolus, 10-20 mL/kg.
- Assess hemodynamic response to fluid and repeat fluid boluses, 10-20 mL/kg, until hypotension resolves or signs of fluid overload develop.
- Assess cardiac function (if available)
- Consider epinephrine/ norepinephrine if hypotension persists after 40 mL/kg or sooner if signs of fluid overload develop.

Fluid in mL/kg should be dosed as ideal body weight.

Shock resolved, perfusion improved

- Do not give more fluid boluses.
- Consider maintenance fluids.
- Monitor for signs/symptoms of recurrent shock.

| *Hypotension in healthcare systems WITHOUT intensive care is defined as either: | SBP < 50 mm Hg in children aged < 12 months | SBP < 60 mm Hg in children aged 1 to 5 years | SBP < 70 mm Hg in children aged > 5 years | OR | Presence of all 3 World Health Organization criteria: cold extremities, prolonged capillary refill > 3 seconds, weak/fast pulse |

www.sccm.org/SurvivingSepsisCampaign/Guidelines/Pediatric-Patients

Society of Critical Care Medicine
The Intensive Care Professionals

ESICM

Figure 9.5.1 Management of septic shock algorithm.

only 200 of 567 children had ScVO$_2$ measured. Lactate may be a more useful biomarker in paediatric sepsis; it is cheap and readily available, and has some utility in predicting outcome for children with severe sepsis in a range of settings. In addition, lactate clearance may reflect successful resuscitation, but it is neither sensitive nor specific enough to be used in isolation, and it must be integrated into a detailed clinical examination to guide management of sepsis.

Outcomes in Sepsis and Septic Shock

Mortality for children with severe sepsis and septic shock has improved over the past decades. In the United States, case fatality rates for children with severe sepsis declined from 10.3 to 8.9 per cent between 1995 and 2005. Infants have double the case fatality rate, compared with older children, largely due to deaths in the group of infants with very low birthweights. Death rates in Australia and New Zealand between 2002 and 2013 for children admitted to the ICU with sepsis were 5.6 per cent, and for septic shock 17 per cent. A UK study of deaths from sepsis in children referred for paediatric intensive care found mortality at 1 year was 21 per cent. Death rates were 54 per cent for children with co-morbidities, compared with 16 per cent for previously well children. Of the children who died, 55 per cent did so within the first 24 hours. Deaths after 24 hours were infrequent in children without co-morbidity, but much higher in those with co-morbidity. A recent pan-European cohort study of community-acquired sepsis in European PICUs found an in-hospital mortality rate of 6 per cent, increasing to 10 per cent in those with septic shock. Twenty-four per cent of previously healthy survivors were discharged with a disability.

References and Further Reading

Bhaskar P, Dhar AV, Thompson M, Quigley R, Modem V. Early fluid accumulation in children with shock and ICU mortality: a matched case-control study. *Intensive Care Med* 2015;**41**:1445–53.

Daniels R, Nutbeam T, McNamara G, Galvin C. The sepsis six and the severe sepsis resuscitation bundle: a prospective observational cohort study. *Emerg Med J* 2011;**28**:507–12.

Goldstein B, Giroir B, Randolph A; International Consensus Conference on Pediatric Sepsis. International pediatric sepsis consensus conference: definitions for sepsis and organ dysfunction in pediatrics. *Pediatr Crit Care Med* 2005;**6**:2–8.

Han YY, Carcillo JA, Dragotta MA, *et al.* Early reversal of pediatric-neonatal septic shock by community physicians is associated with improved outcome. *Pediatrics* 2003;**112**:793–9.

Maitland K, Kiguli S, Opoka RO, *et al.* Mortality after fluid bolus in African children with severe infection. *N Engl J Med* 2011;**364**:2483–95.

Weiss SL, Fitzgerald JC, Pappachan J, *et al.* Global epidemiology of pediatric severe sepsis: the sepsis prevalence, outcomes, and therapies study. *Am J Respir Crit Care Med* 2015;**191**:1147–57.

Weiss SL, Peters MJ, Alhazzani W, *et al.* Surviving sepsis campaign international guidelines for the management of septic shock and sepsis-associated organ dysfunction in children. *Intensive Care Med* 2020;**46**(Suppl 1):10–67.

9.6 Acute Neurological Disorders

Andrew J. Jones and Thomas Brick

Key Learning Points

1. Children with an acute neurological problem requiring intensive care will broadly present with seizures or decreased consciousness (or both).
2. The advanced paediatric life support (APLS) guidelines are regularly updated and provide guidance on treatment of status epilepticus.
3. It may be appropriate to extubate some children with seizures in the local hospital and avoid the need for transport to a paediatric intensive care unit.
4. It is not necessary to perform a lumbar puncture acutely.
5. Children requiring urgent neurosurgery are usually transported by the local team (rather than waiting for a specialist transport service).

Keywords: neurological disorders, status epilepticus, intraventricular shunts

Introduction

Neurological disorders account for 10 per cent of all admissions to paediatric intensive care units (PICUs) in the UK – the third largest diagnostic group after respiratory (29 per cent) and cardiovascular (28 per cent) disorders. There are a wide range of conditions and presentations, but in the critical care setting, it is useful to think about children presenting with neurological disorders as those with seizures and those with a decreased conscious level. A small subset of these children will require emergency neurosurgery.

Status Epilepticus

Status epilepticus, currently defined in advanced paediatric life support (APLS) guidelines as 'a generalised convulsion lasting 30 minutes or longer, or when successive convulsions occur so frequently over a 30-minute period that the patient does not recover consciousness between them', should be treated as an emergency. The death rate from a first episode of convulsive status epilepticus (CSE) is 3 per cent, comparable with that from infant respiratory failure.

Febrile seizures are the most common seizure disorder in children, with a prevalence of between 3 and 8 per cent. A febrile seizure describes convulsions associated with fever in the absence of central nervous system (CNS) infection or any electrolyte imbalance. By definition, they occur in children between 6 months and 6 years of age, and the median age of onset is 18 months. The trigger is normally a benign viral infection (human herpesvirus 6 accounts for 20 per cent of first febrile seizures). Febrile seizures are associated with normal neurodevelopmental outcomes, and the risk of developing epilepsy in later life is low. Most children with a febrile seizure – about 90 per cent – will convulse for <10 minutes. A febrile seizure is described as complex (as opposed to simple) if any of the following features are present:

- Duration of seizure longer than 15 minutes
- Multiple seizures within the last 24 hours
- Presence of focal seizures

Only 5 per cent of children will develop febrile status epilepticus.

Other causes of seizures in children are: breakthrough seizures in a child known to have epilepsy (possibly due to intercurrent illness), meningoencephalitis, metabolic or electrolyte derangement, poisoning or intoxication, stroke, a new space-occupying lesion and trauma (including non-accidental injury).

The incidence of a first episode of CSE from all causes is 17–23 episodes per 100,000 children per year. Febrile seizures account for 57 per cent of episodes, with 12 per cent caused by acute bacterial meningoencephalitis. The 1-year recurrence risk is estimated at 16 per cent.

Resuscitation should be addressed as for any acutely unwell child. Terminating the seizure is essential to prevent neuronal cell death and cerebral oedema, and usual practice is to institute anti-convulsant treatment after 5 minutes of CSE. The APLS guidelines for the convulsing child are constantly evolving. Current practice is to initially provide two doses of a benzodiazepine (intravenous (IV) lorazepam or buccal midazolam) within the first 10–15 minutes. The first of these is often given pre-hospital. If the seizure continues, the child should be given IV phenytoin 20 mg/kg over 20 minutes. Rectal paraldehyde is permitted whilst the phenytoin is being prepared, but should not delay starting the infusion. If the child is still fitting at 20 minutes after the start of the phenytoin infusion, then the next and final step is a thiopental rapid sequence induction (RSI).

An acute CT head is not required in all cases of status epilepticus, and is not necessary if the cause is thought to be a febrile seizure. New-onset focal seizures are an absolute indication to perform an urgent CT head. In practice, if aetiology is uncertain, a CT head is performed.

Other management points to consider include the following:

- Checking glucose early and correcting hypoglycaemia
- Broad anti-microbial cover should be commenced in all cases of febrile status epilepticus. A recommended regime to cover most treatable causes of infectious meningoencephalitis is ceftriaxone or cefotaxime, aciclovir and a macrolide
- If there is suspicion of raised intracranial pressure (ICP), then consider mannitol or hypertonic saline
- Checking electrolytes early – if serum sodium is <120 mmol/l, then use hypertonic saline to increase sodium until the seizure terminates
- Collecting urine for a toxicology screen if indicated
- A lumbar puncture does not need to be performed acutely, and should never be performed in a child with a decreased conscious level (regardless of CT findings)

Decision to Intubate

The indications to intubate are:

- Failure to respond to anti-convulsant therapy necessitating a thiopental RSI
- Benzodiazepine-induced coma with respiratory depression and/or airway compromise in a child who has stopped seizing
- To facilitate CT scanning

For the last two indications, it may be appropriate to extubate in the local hospital once the child has become more alert and providing there is return to neurological baseline and the CT head result is not of concern.

If the child is to be transferred to a PICU, then in most cases, a midazolam infusion will be commenced for sedation and seizure control. Ongoing paralysis should be avoided, if possible, so that seizure activity can be assessed. Maintain, where possible, neuroprotective intensive care measures (normothermia, normocarbia, avoidance of hypoglycaemia, etc.).

Intensive Care Management

On admission to a PICU, the following should be considered:

- Need for further neuroimaging
- Discontinuation of muscle relaxants (that may have been instituted for safe transfer)
- Review of anti-microbial therapy
- Anti-convulsant levels (if known epilepsy and on regular anti-convulsants)
- If seizures have terminated, assessment for discontinuation of sedation and early extubation
- Investigation and treatment of ongoing seizures, in conjunction with a paediatric neurologist

Coma

The Glasgow Coma Score (GCS) was devised for use in head-injured adults but has entered general use for all patients with a decreased conscious level, and has been adapted for children under 4 years old. It is an essential tool for objectively communicating the degree of coma but has limited predictive value in children.

Application of the GCS in children is by no means straightforward, and if the situation dictates a more pragmatic approach, then the AVPU scale can be employed (Alert, responds to Voice, responds to Pain, Unresponsive).

In children, the common causes of coma are hypoxia, shock and diffuse metabolic insults. Structural lesions account for <5 per cent of cases. Consider hypoxic–ischaemic encephalopathy, hypertension, infections, intoxication, electrolyte derangement, hypoglycaemia, inherited metabolic disease, post-CSE, cerebrovascular events, tumours and trauma. A detailed history will help narrow down the differential diagnosis.

The initial approach is to resuscitate and secure the airway if necessary. The child should be intubated if the

GCS is <9 (equivalent to P on the AVPU scale). Coma, with or without suspicion of raised ICP, is not a contra-indication to using ketamine as an induction agent. Once stabilised, the focus becomes treating the cause and preventing secondary brain injury.

Raised Intracranial Pressure

Signs of raised ICP are bradycardia (heart rate <60 bpm at age 4 weeks to 18 years), hypertension (mean arterial pressure >95th centile for age), unilateral or bilateral pupillary dilation or loss of reaction to light, an abnormal breathing pattern and abnormal posturing. These children should be intubated and managed as per the neuroprotective strategy described in Chapter 9.9, Trauma. Osmotherapy should be considered, and a CT head should be carried out urgently.

Neurosurgical Emergencies

Some causes of coma and/or seizures with raised ICP will be amenable to emergency neurosurgery. Such cases can be traumatic or non-traumatic, and include tumours and extradural, subdural and intracranial haemorrhages, abscesses and blocked intraventricular shunts. If the situation is time-critical, then the child must reach a neurosurgical centre as soon as possible – no more than 4 hours after the 'injury'. In such cases, the transfer will usually be carried out by the referring team (rather than by a specialist transport service).

A CT scan will be critical to decision-making, but the need for emergency neurosurgery and time-critical transfer should be considered based on clinical grounds, before the result of the CT scan is known.

Blocked Intraventricular Shunts

Some children with hydrocephalus (e.g. due to a neural tube defect or intraventricular haemorrhage associated with prematurity) will have been treated with surgical placement of a shunt system. The shunt is a hollow silicone tube which diverts cerebrospinal fluid from the ventricular system to, most commonly, the abdomen (a ventriculoperitoneal shunt) or, occasionally, the heart (a ventriculoatrial shunt). Shunts are prone to failure due to infection, obstruction or twisting or breaking of the connections, and if this occurs, the child will present with progressive decrease in consciousness and signs and symptoms of raised ICP (with or without fever). An urgent CT head and neurosurgical referral are required, and time-critical transfer to a paediatric neurosurgical centre may be indicated for emergent shunt revision.

References and Further Reading

Advanced Life Support Group, Samuels M, Wieteska S (eds). The child with a decreased conscious level. In: Advanced Life Support Group, M Samuels, S Wieteska (eds). *Advanced Paediatric Life Support*, 6th edn. Chichester: Wiley Blackwell; 2016. pp. 89–98.

Advanced Life Support Group, Samuels M, Wieteska S (eds). The convulsing child. In: Advanced Life Support Group, M Samuels, S Wieteska (eds). *Advanced Paediatric Life Support*, 6th edn. Chichester: Wiley Blackwell; 2016. pp. 99–106.

Chin RF, Neville BG, Peckham C, Bedford H, Wade A, Scott RC; NLSTEPSS Collaborative Group. Incidence, cause, and short-term outcome of convulsive status epilepticus in childhood: prospective population-based study. *Lancet* 2006;**368**:222–9.

Mangat HS, Patel C, Rodrigues D. Fifteen-minute consultation: assessment of a child with suspected shunt problems. *Arch Dis Child Educ Pract Ed* 2017;**102**:170–4.

PICANet. 2017. PICANet annual report 2017. Paediatric Intensive Care Audit Network. www.picanet.org.uk/Audit/Annual-Reporting/Annual-Report-Archive/

Reynolds S, Marikar D, Roland D. Management of children and young people with an acute decrease in conscious level (RCPCH guideline update 2015). *Arch Dis Child Educ Pract Ed* 2018;**103**:146–51.

Sadleir LG, Scheffer IE. Febrile seizures. *BMJ* 2007;**334**: 307–11.

9.7 The Collapsed Infant

Andrew J. Jones and Thomas Brick

Key Learning Points

1. The differential for a collapsed infant is broad and encompasses congenital heart disease, sepsis, surgical presentations, inborn errors of metabolism and trauma.
2. Treat first – diagnose at leisure; early support of the neonate's physiology is lifesaving.
3. Start prostaglandin if there is any suspicion of a duct-dependent cardiac lesion – it can always be stopped.
4. Start broad-spectrum empirical anti-bacterial drugs.
5. Sudden unexpected death in infancy describes all unexpected deaths in infancy. If, after thorough investigation, a cause cannot be found, the death is classified as having been caused by sudden infant death syndrome.

Keywords: paediatric sepsis, congenital heart disease, inborn error of metabolism, sudden unexpected death in infancy, SUDI, sudden infant death syndrome, SIDS

Introduction

This chapter offers an overview of the management of collapse in the infant period. This is a challenging clinical problem with a broad differential, for which an overview will be provided here. Further disease-specific details are provided in the relevant sections contained within this chapter.

The 'collapsed infant' is a useful description of the group of infants who present within the first few months of life with deranged physiology and non-specific symptoms, which may include temperature instability, respiratory distress, cardiovascular instability, irritability or lethargy, hypoglycaemia and metabolic acidosis.

Making a precise diagnosis may require specialist input, but whilst this is in progress, the clinician must focus on supporting the child's physiology according to an ABCDE approach (as outlined, for example, by the Advanced Life Support Group), but with some specific considerations. These are outlined below.

Initial Management

This is aimed at supporting the child's physiology. The search for a diagnosis should happen in conjunction with initiation of empirical treatment:

- Supplemental oxygen – only if required – to target saturations of >95%
- Early intravenous access – with use of intraosseous needles if at all delayed
- Fluid boluses – (10–20 ml/kg of crystalloid) in an attempt to restore perfusion
- Early intubation and ventilation
- Broad-spectrum antibiotics

Initial investigations should include: full blood count (FBC), urea and electrolytes (U&Es), liver function tests (LFT), clotting, C-reactive protein (CRP), chest X-ray (CXR), ECG if tachycardic (>220 bpm), four limb blood pressures and pre- and post-ductal oxygen saturations (taken, respectively, from the right hand and either foot), glucose, blood gas including lactate, blood cultures, urine microscopy culture and sensitivities and serum ammonia

A number of broad diagnostic categories may be identifiable.

Sepsis

Consider sepsis in the infant with risk factors (e.g. maternal group B streptococcal infection during pregnancy) and presenting with hypothermia or fever, shock and raised inflammatory markers.

The most common organisms to cause serious bacterial infection in the first month of life are group B *Streptococcus*. However, *Escherichia coli*, *Staphylococcus* and *Listeria monocytogenes* also need to be considered.

Coagulopathy and deranged liver function suggest neonatal herpes infection. A broad-spectrum cephalosporin, alongside ampicillin and aciclovir, is a typical combination. Blood cultures, FBC, CRP or procalcitonin and urine for microscopy, culture and sensitivity should be taken, but a lumbar puncture should be withheld until the child is stable with normal clotting and normal neurology.

Initial resuscitation with fluid boluses, prompt administration of antibiotics, early intubation and inotropic support with adrenaline infusion, followed by frequent reassessment, may be lifesaving.

Congenital Heart Disease

Congenital heart disease is responsible for 3–7.5 per cent of deaths in the first year of life. Detection of major congenital heart defects has improved due to widespread antenatal screening and increasing use of pulse oximetry at the time of the postnatal check. Nevertheless, congenital heart defects remain a significant cause of neonatal collapse. Presentation occurs at the time of ductal closure in children with duct-dependent pulmonary or systemic circulation.

Presentation can also occur with congestive cardiac failure associated with postnatal fall in pulmonary vascular resistance at 2–4 weeks of age. Myocarditis or cardiomyopathy must also be included in the differential of a neonate presenting with cardiac failure.

Signs

- Cyanosis that does not correct with oxygen therapy – suggestive of duct-dependent pulmonary circulation
- Shock – suggestive of duct-dependent systemic circulation
- Heart murmur
- Congestive cardiac failure (tachycardia, gallop rhythm, tachypnoea, hepatomegaly)
- Cardiomegaly visible on chest radiograph

Echocardiography carried out by a practitioner trained in paediatric cardiology provides a definitive diagnosis. However, this is only available in a limited number of specialist centres.

Inherited Metabolic Disorders

Inherited metabolic disorders encompass a wide range of diseases and include inborn errors of metabolism (IEM) and mitochondrial disorders.

Urea cycle defects, organic acidaemias and certain disorders of amino acid metabolism present with encephalopathy and biochemical abnormalities.

Initial presentation can often resemble sepsis, and indeed sepsis can coexist. Apnoea and seizures can be due to toxic metabolites, and respiratory distress a symptom of metabolic acidosis.

Some basic laboratory studies can help suggest a diagnosis in the acute setting:

- Blood gas
- Lactate
- Serum electrolytes
- Ammonia
- LFTs
- Blood glucose
- Urinary ketones

Urinary reducing substances, plasma and urine amino acids and urine organic acids can be sent to the laboratory in the acute setting, although results will take time and must not delay initial treatment.

Hyperammonaemia

Urea cycle defects may present with very high ammonia levels (>1000 µmol/l), whilst moderately raised levels of ammonia are seen in liver dysfunction from a range of causes. Infants with organic acidaemias are likely to have metabolic acidosis, as well as raised ammonia levels. Prolonged exposure to very high levels of ammonia confers a poor prognosis, and urgent treatment must be initiated.

Metabolic Acidosis

A metabolic acidosis with an elevated anion gap is seen in organic acidoses. The presence of lactic acidosis may suggest mitochondrial disease.

Initial Management

Hyperammonaemia should be treated initially with sodium benzoate and phenylbutyrate infusions, and urgent transfer to a paediatric intensive care unit that can provide haemofiltration must be arranged. More generally, whilst awaiting diagnosis, preventing catabolism should be attempted by stopping enteral (milk) feeds and infusing 0.9% saline with dextrose to provide 6–8 mg/(kg min) of dextrose, aiming for a blood sugar of 4–8 mmol/l. Some enzyme deficiencies are responsive to co-factors (e.g. thiamine, arginine, carnitine) which may be started at a specialist centre.

In the event of death of an infant with a suspected IEM, samples can be collected in order to establish a diagnosis, and may help parents plan future pregnancies. Urine, blood, plasma, skin, liver and muscle tissue should all be collected. If the neonate dies before transfer to a specialist centre, this should be done at the local hospital. Guidance from specialist paediatric metabolic physicians should be sought.

Surgical Emergencies

Consideration should be given to abdominal pathology as a cause of collapse in the infant. A collapsed infant with abdominal pain, distension or vomiting must trigger the physician to consider gut ischaemia as the cause, which may, in turn, be due to malrotation with midgut volvulus, intussusception, incarcerated hernia or intestinal obstruction. Bilious vomiting must be treated as evidence of a high intestinal obstruction. Necrotising enterocolitis is common in the preterm population and frequently presents with apnoea, shock, rectal bleeding and pneumatosis coli on the abdominal radiograph. Specific management includes nasogastric tube insertion and antibiotic therapy (e.g. penicillin, aminoglycoside and metronidazole), but definitive therapy is surgical, so rapid transfer to a paediatric surgical centre is important.

Trauma (Inflicted)

Trauma must be considered in an infant presenting with a decreased level of consciousness, external signs of physical injury, bleeding and shock. The aetiology may not be forthcoming, and imaging of the abdomen and head (computed tomography or ultrasound scan in a child with an open fontanelle) will be necessary to confirm the diagnosis.

Sudden Unexpected Death in Infancy and Sudden Infant Death Syndrome

Sudden unexpected death in infancy (SUDI) describes all unexpected deaths in infancy. If, after thorough investigation, a cause cannot be found, the death is classified as having been caused by sudden infant death syndrome (SIDS).

A number of factors have led to a reduction in the incidence of SIDS – partly due to improved diagnosis

Table 9.7.1 Risk factors for sudden infant death syndrome

Intrinsic risk factors
Male sex
Genetic polymorphism in serotonin transporter gene
Prematurity
Parental smoking, alcohol or drug use
Young maternal age
Socio-economic disadvantage
Extrinsic risk factors
Prone sleeping
Soft bedding
Bed sharing
Mild infection (including colds)

Source: Adapted from Kinney HC, Thach BT. The sudden infant death syndrome. *N Engl J Med* 2009;**361**:795–805.

resulting in fewer deaths being classified as unexplained, but also following public health initiatives, such as the Back to Sleep campaign, and a reduction in the incidence of maternal smoking. However approximately 200 infants die from SIDS in England and Wales annually. The causative mechanisms are thought to result from the interplay between external stressors and an infant with an immature cardiorespiratory and arousal defence mechanism. Risk factors may be seen in Table 9.7.1.

References and Further Reading

Advanced Life Support Group, Samuels M, Wieteska S (eds). *Advanced Paediatric Life Support*, 6th edn. Chichester: Wiley-Blackwell; 2016.

Burton BK. Inborn errors of metabolism in infancy: a guide to diagnosis. *Pediatrics* 1998;**102**:E69.

Kinney HC, Thach BT. The sudden infant death syndrome. *N Engl J Med* 2009;**361**:795–805.

Knowles R, Griebsch I, Dezateux C, Brown J, Bull C, Wren C. Newborn screening for congenital heart defects: a systematic review and cost-effectiveness analysis. *Health Technol Assess* 2005;**9**:1–152, iii–iv.

Congenital Heart Disease

9.8

Andrew J. Jones and Thomas Brick

Key Learning Points

1. Up to one-third of neonates with congenital heart disease will be discharged without a diagnosis.
2. Infants with congenital heart disease can present critically unwell in infancy.
3. Maintaining ductal patency with prostaglandin can be lifesaving in children with duct-dependent congenital heart disease.
4. Children undergoing staged single-ventricle palliation are at increased risk of death, and stabilisation requires some understanding of their underlying anatomy and physiology.
5. Children presenting with cardiogenic shock secondary to cardiomyopathy and myocarditis can be difficult to differentiate from children with septic shock. Initial management is supportive, aimed at maintaining adequate oxygen delivery.

Keywords: congenital heart disease, hypoplastic left heart, myocarditis, cardiomyopathy, prostaglandin

Introduction

Congenital heart disease (CHD) is present in approximately 6–8 per 1000 newborns. Approximately one-third will have a diagnosis that requires intervention in infancy. Antenatal screening and postnatal oximetry are able to detect an increasing proportion of affected infants, but up to 30 per cent will be discharged from hospital without a diagnosis.

Presentation in Infancy

Infants with critical CHD who have not been diagnosed before discharge from maternity services may present critically unwell in later infancy. The timing of the presentation depends on the anatomy of the lesion and the timing of arterial duct closure.

The presentation can be broadly categorised into one of the following three categories (Table 9.8.1):

1. Increasing cyanosis due to ductal closure in duct-dependent pulmonary circulation
2. Shock due to ductal closure in duct-dependent systemic circulation
3. Progressive heart failure

Diagnosis and Management of Infants with Suspected Congenital Heart Disease

The diagnosis of CHD must be considered in any infant presenting with shock, cyanosis or heart failure. The differential diagnosis is broad, and a general approach to stabilising the critically unwell infant is discussed in Chapter 9.7, The Collapsed Infant. How to differentiate

Table 9.8.1 Classification of congenital heart disease

Duct-dependent pulmonary circulation	Duct-dependent systemic circulation	Non-duct-dependent circulations
Pulmonary atresia with intact ventricular septum	Coarctation of the aorta	Total anomalous pulmonary venous drainage
Critical pulmonary stenosis	Aortic stenosis	Large ventricular septal defect
Tricuspid atresia	Hypoplastic left heart syndrome	Common arterial trunk
Severe neonatal Ebstein's anomaly	Interrupted aortic arch	Tetralogy of Fallot
Transposition of the great arteries[a]		

[a] In transposition of the great arteries, the pulmonary and systemic circulations are in parallel, and mixing is dependent on both the patency of the ductus arteriosus and adequate mixing at the atrial level.

Table 9.8.2 Differentiating cardiac cyanosis from respiratory disease

	Cyanotic congenital heart disease	Respiratory disease
Work of breathing	Minimal or none	Increased
Chest X-ray (lung fields)	Oligaemic in duct-dependent pulmonary blood flow Plethoric in pulmonary overcirculation	Collapse and consolidation
Chest X-ray (cardiac silhouette)	Cardiomegaly in heart failure or characteristic in specific lesions	Normal
Carbon dioxide	Normal	Raised
Response to high FiO$_2$	Limited improvement in oxygenation	Improvement in oxygenation

Abbreviation: FiO$_2$ = fraction of inspired oxygen.

cardiac cyanosis from respiratory disease can be seen in Table 9.8.2.

A definitive diagnosis of CHD is dependent on access to a practitioner trained in paediatric echocardiography. This is usually limited to regional centres, and urgent transfer is therefore indicated.

Clinical Examination

The presence of a harsh cardiac murmur, hepatomegaly, absent or weak femoral pulses or a marked difference between upper and lower limb blood pressures suggests a cardiac aetiology.

Differential cyanosis describes a situation when upper limb saturations (pre-ductal) are higher than lower limb saturations (post-ductal). The physiological basis for this is that pre-ductal circulation is supplied with oxygenated blood by the left ventricle, whilst postductal circulation is supplied with deoxygenated blood by the right heart via the ductus arteriosus. It occurs in critical coarctation of the aorta and interrupted aortic arch, but also in children with structurally normal hearts who have persistent pulmonary hypertension of the newborn.

Chest Radiograph

The chest radiograph can help differentiate between pulmonary and cardiac disease. Collapse and consolidation suggest pulmonary disease. The following features may help suggest a diagnosis:

1. Cardiomegaly: massive cardiomegaly is found in Ebstein's anomaly. Non-massive cardiomegaly is also caused by obstructed left-sided lesions, with consequent heart failure
2. Cardiac silhouette: an 'egg on a string' is seen in transposition of the great arteries (TGA), as the great arteries are in an anterior–posterior relationship, rather than side by side. A 'boot-shaped heart' is seen in tetralogy of Fallot (TOF),

as right ventricular (RV) hypertrophy leads to an upturned apex and the small pulmonary arteries result in a narrow mediastinum
3. Lung fields: oligaemic lung fields may be seen in lesions with obstruction to pulmonary blood flow (e.g. pulmonary stenosis, TOF). Plethoric lung fields may be seen in lesions with obstruction of pulmonary venous return (e.g. total anomalous pulmonary venous drainage, hypoplastic left heart with a restrictive atrio-septal defect) or in left-sided lesions which result in cardiac failure

Initial Management

Stabilisation and transfer of infants to a cardiac centre are essential for confirmation of diagnosis and ongoing intervention. The basis of initial management is organ support plus maintenance of ductal patency.

Prostaglandin

Alprostadil (prostaglandin E1) and dinoprostone (prostaglandin E2) are used to maintain ductal patency. Dosing should be started at 5–10 ng/(kg min), and can be increased to 100 ng/(kg min) under expert guidance. The risk of side effects (apnoea, hypotension and fever) rises as the dose is increased, and mechanical ventilation should be considered.

Infants with TGA or hypoplastic left heart syndrome who have a restrictive interatrial communication (resulting in inadequate intra-cardiac mixing) or with obstruction to pulmonary venous drainage (e.g. obstructed total anomalous pulmonary venous drainage (TAPVD)) may fail to improve following the initiation of prostaglandin. Urgent atrial septostomy is indicated in cases of inadequate intra-cardiac mixing, and urgent surgical repair may be necessary in obstructed TAPVD.

Mechanical Ventilation

A shocked neonate should be intubated, ventilated and sedated in order to maintain adequate oxygenation and ventilation, and to reduce oxygen consumption. In infants presenting with suspected cyanotic cardiac disease, supplemental oxygen should be used to target saturations of 80–85%. Delivering high fractions of inspired oxygen acts as a pulmonary vasodilator (and peripheral vasoconstrictor), and in univentricular circulation can result in overperfusion of the lungs at the expense of the systemic circulation. In left-to-right shunt lesions (e.g. atrioventricular septal defect, large ventricular septal defect), high fractions of inspired oxygen can result in worsening pulmonary oedema.

Cardiovascular Support

Fluid boluses (5–10 ml/kg of isotonic crystalloid) should be used to achieve adequate intravascular volume status. Vasoactive agents can be used to provide inotropy and chronotropy (e.g. dopamine 5–20 μg/(kg min) or adrenaline 0.05–0.3 μg/(kg min)). Diuresis is indicated in the setting of congestive heart failure due to a left-to-right shunt lesion. However, these lesions are unlikely to present with profound cardiovascular collapse, and as a consequence, the authors would not recommend diuresis in the setting of cardiovascular collapse.

Norwood Stage 1, Glenn or Fontan

Following discharge from hospital, approximately 7 per cent of children who have undergone a cardiac procedure will, at a later stage, either die or require admission for paediatric intensive care. Within this group, children who undergo staged palliation for a single-ventricle lesion are at particularly high risk of death. A basic understanding of the three-staged palliation for children with single-ventricle physiology is necessary to support the intensivist in providing initial stabilisation.

Norwood Stage 1

This involves reconstruction of the aortic arch, disconnection of the pulmonary trunk and creation of a shunt – either a Blalock–Taussig shunt (BTS) or a right ventricle-to-pulmonary artery conduit to provide pulmonary blood flow (Figure 9.8.1). An atrial septectomy is also necessary in order to allow pulmonary venous blood to return to the right ventricle. This operation is carried out within the first week of life.

Bidirectional Glenn

(Physiologically equivalent to hemi-Fontan or bidirectional cavopulmonary connection (BCPC).)

The superior vena cava is disconnected from the right atrium, and an end-to-side anastomosis to the right pulmonary artery is performed (Figure 9.8.2). The arterial shunt from the Norwood procedure is taken down. Lung perfusion is therefore dependent on venous return from the top half of the body.

Fontan

Venous return from the inferior vena cava is connected to the pulmonary arteries in order to complete the

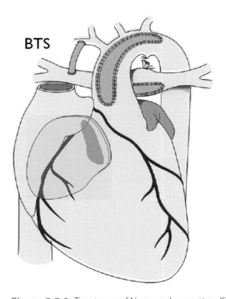
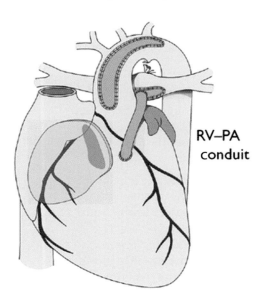

Figure 9.8.1 Two types of Norwood operation. BTS = Blalock–Taussig shunt; RV–PA conduit = right ventricle-to-pulmonary artery conduit.

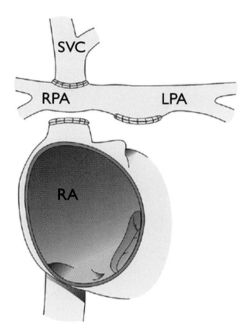

Figure 9.8.2 The bidirectional Glenn operation.

Fontan circulation (Figure 9.8.3). A fenestration may be left between the Fontan and the right atrium.

Acute Presentations

Children discharged following a Norwood stage 1 operation may present with symptoms attributable to their underlying anatomy (e.g. distortion, blockage or stenosis of the arterial shunt, pulmonary arteries or neoaorta), resulting in hypoxia or shock. In addition, common childhood illness can lead to profound haemodynamic disturbance; for example, respiratory disease can lead to increasing pulmonary vascular resistance resulting in profound cyanosis; a diarrhoeal illness resulting in hypovolaemia may lead to vasoconstriction and consequently to pulmonary overcirculation and shock. Management is to ensure adequate volume status, and to withhold supplemental oxygen unless saturations are below 70%. An inodilator can encourage systemic blood flow. Shunt occlusion due to thrombus (suggested by hypoxia and absence of a shunt murmur) should be treated with a heparin bolus.

Lung perfusion in both Glenn and Fontan circulations is driven by venous pressure. Any compromise to venous flow (anatomical disruption, thrombosis, decreased venous pressure due to hypovolaemia) or increased pulmonary vascular resistance (e.g. lung infection) can lead to profound cyanosis. Correction

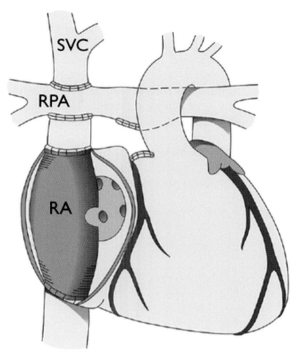

Figure 9.8.3 Fontan operation (total cavopulmonary connection).
Source: Yarlagadda, Vamsi V., and Ravi R. Thiagarajan. 'Cardiac Disease in Pediatric Intensive Care.' *Pediatric Intensive Care.* Oxford University Press, 2017. Pediatric Intensive Care, Chapter 7. Web.

of hypovolaemia and decreasing pulmonary vascular resistance with oxygen therapy are the mainstay of emergency management.

Myocarditis and Cardiomyopathy

Children with myocarditis or cardiomyopathy can present with symptoms which range from non-specific to congestive cardiac failure and acute cardiogenic shock. The history is often vague, although in myocarditis, a history of a preceding viral illness can sometimes be elicited. Children may present to the intensivist in shock, with marked tachycardia, tachypnoea, poor perfusion and hepatomegaly. Cardiomegaly and pulmonary oedema may be seen on the chest radiograph. ECG changes can include sinus tachycardia, non-specific ST changes, conduction abnormalities and ectopy. Echocardiography will demonstrate ventricular dysfunction, with a normal anatomy. The presence of ventricular dilation favours a diagnosis of dilated cardiomyopathy.

Differentiating between septic shock and cardiogenic shock can be difficult in the emergency

717

department. Initial stabilisation of these two groups of children shares a number of common features – intubation, ventilation and sedation decrease oxygen demand, and inotropic support improves ventricular contractility and cardiac output. Both groups are likely to receive empirical antibiotics. However, children with cardiogenic shock should receive judicious fluid resuscitation. Children presenting with ventricular arrhythmias, severe lactic acidosis and established organ dysfunction are at risk of complete cardiovascular collapse, in which case extracorporeal membrane oxygenation may be indicated.

References and Further Reading

Crowe S, Ridout DA, Knowles R, *et al.* Death and emergency readmission of infants discharged after interventions for congenital heart disease: a national study of 7643 infants to inform service improvement. *J Am Heart Assoc* 2016;**5**:e003369.

Feinstein JA, Benson DW, Dubin AM, *et al.* Hypoplastic left heart syndrome: current considerations and expectations. *J Am Coll Cardiol* 2012;**59**(1 Suppl):S1–42.

Wren C, Reinhardt Z, Khawaja K. Twenty-year trends in diagnosis of life-threatening neonatal cardiovascular malformations. *Arch Dis Child Fetal Neonatal Ed* 2008;**93**:F33–5.

Trauma

Andrew J. Jones and Thomas Brick

Key Learning Points

1. Trauma is the leading cause of death in children older than 1 year.
2. An isolated head injury is the most common presentation of major trauma.
3. Consider non-accidental injury in all children, particularly in those <2 years.
4. Have a high index of suspicion for cervical spine injury, and consider spinal cord injury without radiographic abnormality (SCIWORA) in younger children.
5. If cervical spine injury is suspected in the comatose child, immobilisation should be continued until adequate imaging and/or clinical assessment can be performed.

Keywords: trauma, primary survey, head injury, cervical spine

Introduction

In the developed world, trauma is the leading cause of death in children older than 1 year. About two-thirds of major paediatric trauma are isolated head injuries, and in Europe, blunt trauma is more common than penetrating injury. About three-quarters of all major paediatric trauma involves a motor vehicle.

Trauma services in the United Kingdom are centralised in regional major trauma centres (MTCs), but even in these specialised units, major paediatric trauma is rare. Only 5 per cent of all trauma cases involve children under 12 years; this equates to about one major paediatric trauma a day in the London area (8.6 million people).

Trauma affects children and adults differently. Children can compensate effectively for hypovolaemia and can lose up to 40 per cent of the circulating volume before hypotension manifests. Children have soft, compliant bones. The ribcage is less protective, and external forces are transmitted directly to underlying viscera (often without rib fracture). The abdominal musculature is less developed; the liver and spleen are relatively large and anterior, and in younger children, the bladder can sit partly in the abdomen – all of which make children more vulnerable to intra-abdominal injury.

A child's behavioural response to injury may also present a challenge. Children may not be able to express the degree and location of their pain.

The Primary Survey

The trauma assessment proceeds as it would for an injured adult, with problems addressed as they are identified.

An impression of airway patency can be gained by simple observation. Crying and screaming are a reassuring sign that the airway is clear and breathing is effective. Airway adjuncts should be used with caution – oral airways can precipitate vomiting and nasal airways may cause bleeding.

Indications for intubation include: distorted airway anatomy and/or copious oral bleeding, burns and/or suspicion of inhalation injury, respiratory failure, decreased conscious level and loss of airway reflexes (Glasgow Coma Score (GCS) <9) and severe distress and pain. Ketamine is the induction agent of choice for its cardiovascular stability. A traditional rapid sequence induction (RSI) may need modification in the younger child. Gentle ventilation may be required up until the point of intubation in order to prevent desaturation. A gastric tube is essential post-intubation to empty and decompress the stomach.

When assessing circulation, be aware that capillary refill time (CRT) and peripheral perfusion may be unreliable if the child is cold. The child is likely to be tachycardic, but this should not be automatically attributed to pain or distress. Hypotension is a late sign of hypovolaemia in children with shock, and persistent tachycardia may be an indication of significant haemorrhage.

As with adults, two points of intravenous (IV) access are required. This can be incredibly challenging – the threshold for recourse to intraosseous access should be low.

In significant haemorrhage, blood products should be given early and in preference to crystalloid. Aliquots of 10 ml/kg are recommended (to balance effective resuscitation with maintaining clot stability), but this may have to be revised in the face of ongoing massive bleeding. Ideally, give red cells, platelets and plasma in a 1:1:1 ratio.

Evidence does not exist to support a specific BP target. In some cases, traumatic brain injury (TBI) will mandate a higher BP. In the first instance, target a normal BP for age. Arterial access is desirable. Vasoactive drugs should not be used in the child who remains shocked due to blood loss. However, they do have a role in neurogenic shock, cardiac contusions and when targeting a higher BP in TBI. Tranexamic acid (an anti-fibrinolytic agent) is recommended in all trauma haemorrhage. The dose is 15 mg/kg (maximum 1 g), followed by an infusion.

Head Injury

The role of neurocritical care in TBI is to attenuate secondary brain injury. Secondary brain injury describes the inflammatory changes taking place over hours to days after a primary injury, which result in further cell death. In practice, this means the maintenance of adequate cerebral perfusion and oxygenation, and the prevention of raised intracranial pressure (ICP) due to oedema and/or the space-occupying effects of haematomas.

Initial resuscitation should proceed as normal, with meticulous attention to preventing hypoxia and hypotension. The National Institute for Health and Care Excellence (NICE) criteria exist for when to perform CT head in TBI, but in the severely injured child requiring intubation due to decreased GCS, CT will be performed as soon as the airway is secure and the child stable.

If CT demonstrates an intracranial lesion requiring urgent neurosurgery (e.g. an extradural haematoma), and the child is not in a neurosurgical centre, then transfer to an appropriate hospital should take place without delay by the referring team.

Following intubation, ongoing care should include the following.

- Sedate and paralyse with fentanyl, midazolam and vecuronium infusions; use boluses of sedation with procedures.

> **Box 9.9.1 Mean Arterial Pressure Targets**
>
> Age 0–2 years: target MAP >60 mmHg
> Age 2–6 years: target MAP >70 mmHg
> Age >6 years: target MAP >80 mmHg

- Ventilate to $PaCO_2$ of 4–5 kPa.
- Aim for oxygen saturations of >95% and PaO_2 of >13 kPa.
- Target a high mean arterial pressure (MAP) to maintain cerebral perfusion pressure (Box 9.9.1).
- Fluid-restrict to 50 per cent of maintenance; use isotonic maintenance fluid.
- Maintain normoglycaemia.
- Avoid hyperthermia.
- Treat seizures with phenytoin.
- If suspicion of raised ICP (e.g. unequal pupils, bradycardia, hypertension), give 3 ml/kg of 2.7% sodium chloride.

Once admitted to an appropriate paediatric intensive care unit (PICU), a decision must be taken about how to proceed. There are only three options.

1. Wake and assess
2. Insert an ICP monitor and continue neurocritical care
3. Urgent neurosurgery

In all cases, it must be considered whether the injury could be non-accidental, particularly in children under 2 years.

Cervical Spine Injury

Younger children have relatively large heads, with slack spinal ligaments and weak cervical musculature. This group is therefore more prone to cervical spine injury, and the injury commonly occurs at a higher level of the cervical spine (atlas, axis and C1/2) than might be expected in older children (C5/6). Spinal cord injury can occur in the absence of bony injury (spinal cord injury without radiographic abnormality (SCIWORA)). SCIWORA is defined as spinal cord injury with normal X-rays and CT, and is almost exclusively seen in children under 8 years. By 10 years, the spine can be considered 'adult'.

Spinal Protection

Injury to the cervical spine is assumed in any head-injured patient. Hard collars are being used less and less in children. Their application is no longer taught as a priority on advanced paediatric life support (APLS) courses, and they are not recommended for children under 5 years. Use manual in-line immobilisation for the initial assessment, then blocks and tape.

Clearing the Cervical Spine in Children under 10 Years

In children over 3 years who can communicate adequately, the NEXUS (National Emergency X-Radiography Utilisation Study) criteria can be used. Younger children who are alert will most likely clear their own spine. In intubated patients, where the cervical spine cannot be assessed clinically, clearing the spine is more difficult and subject to local guidelines. Lateral and anteroposterior (AP) cervical spine X-rays are required, proceeding to a CT scan if the X-ray films are inadequate or the history is suggestive of spinal injury. These imaging modalities cannot rule out spinal cord injury, and in most cases, immobilisation will continue until MRI or clinical assessment can be performed.

References and Further Reading

CRASH-2 Trial Collaborators; Shakur H, Roberts I, Bautista R, *et al*. Effects of tranexamic acid on death, vascular occlusive events, and blood transfusion in trauma patients with significant haemorrhage (CRASH-2): a randomised, placebo-controlled trial. *Lancet* 2020;**276**:23–32.

Hoffman JR, Mower WR, Wolfson AB. Validity of a set of clinical criteria to rule out injury to the cervical spine in patients with blunt trauma. National Emergency X-Radiography Utilization Study Group. *N Engl J Med* 2000;**343**:94–9.

Holcomb JB, Tilley BC, Baraniuk S, *et al*. Transfusion of plasma, platelets, and red blood cells in a 1:1:1 vs a 1:1:2 ratio and mortality in patients with severe trauma: the PROPPR randomized clinical trial. *JAMA* 2015;**313**:471–82.

Kochanek PM, Carney N, Adelson PD. Guidelines for the acute medical management of severe traumatic brain injury in infants, children, and adolescents – second edition. *Pediatr Crit Care Med* 2012;**13**(Suppl 1):S1–82.

London Ambulance Service. Annual report 2016/17. www.londonambulance.nhs.uk/wp-content/uploads/2020/01/London-Ambulance-Service-Annual-Report-2016-2017_.pdf

National Institute for Health and Care Excellence. 2014. Head injury: assessment and early management. www.nice.org.uk/guidance/cg176

Polke E, Lutman D; Children's Acute Transport Service. 2020. Transport considerations when transfer undertaken by local DGH team. cats.nhs.uk/wp-content/uploads/guideline-localteamtransfer.pdf

Acute Liver Failure, Inborn Errors of Metabolism and Diabetic Ketoacidosis

Andrew J. Jones and Thomas Brick

Key Learning Points

1. Children with acute liver failure (ALF) require rapid stabilisation and should be moved to a specialist centre as quickly as possible.
2. Once on a paediatric intensive care unit, ALF patients undergo standard neurocritical intensive care and a transplant assessment.
3. In ALF, children with encephalopathy more severe than grade 1 should be considered for intubation.
4. The mean arterial pressures targeted for encephalopathic patients vary with age.
5. In diabetic ketoacidosis, cerebral oedema is the most common cause of mortality and neurological observations should be performed regularly.

Keywords: acute liver failure, hepatic encephalopathy, transplant, metabolism, diabetic ketoacidosis

Introduction

Most critical care doctors have limited experience of looking after children with decompensated metabolic conditions or acute liver failure. These children are often very sick, and managing them can be a daunting experience. However, by sticking to the basics and promptly providing appropriate interventions, serious morbidity and death can be avoided.

Acute Liver Failure

Overview

Paediatric acute liver failure (PALF) is a clinical syndrome associated with massive necrosis of liver cells, or sudden, severe impairment of liver function, with or without hepatic encephalopathy (HE), developing in a child with no recognised chronic liver disease. The only curative treatment is liver transplant. Without it, mortality is 70 per cent.

The criteria for diagnosis are:

1. No known chronic liver disease
2. Biochemical evidence of acute liver injury
3. Coagulopathy that is not corrected by parenteral administration of vitamin K:
    a. HE must be present if uncorrected prothrombin time (PT) is between 15 and 19.9 seconds or the international normalised ratio (INR) is between 1.5 and 1.9
    b. HE is not required if PT is ≥20 seconds or the INR is >2.0

HE can be difficult to recognise in children, especially infants, and a separate grading scale is available for children under 4 years old (Table 9.10.1).

In infants, metabolic disease is the most frequent cause of PALF, whereas in children, viral hepatitis (in developing countries) or drug-induced PALF (in North America and the UK) are most frequently seen.

Management

The core tenet of acute management is stabilisation followed by transport to a centre specialising in paediatric liver disease for transplant assessment. Close liaison with the regional paediatric critical care transport service and the paediatric hepatology team will be required.

Once on an appropriate paediatric intensive care unit (PICU), the child will undergo standard paediatric neurocritical care and assessment for liver transplant. Some form of extracorporeal liver replacement may be employed as a bridge to transplant or native liver recovery. Molecular adsorbent recirculating system (MARS), haemofiltration and plasma exchange

Table 9.10.1 Hepatic encephalopathy grading scale for children under 4 years old

	Grade			
	I	**II**	**III**	**IV**
Symptoms		Inconsolable crying, inattention to tasks, child not acting like self to parents	Stupor, somnolence, combativeness	Coma **IVa** – responds to noxious stimuli **IVb** – no response
Signs		Normal or hyper-reflexic; other neurological signs are difficult to test	Hyper-reflexia, extensor reflexes, rigidity	Areflexia, flaccidity, decerebrate or decorticate posturing
Electroencephalography		Difficult to test and interpret	Markedly abnormal, triphasic waves	Markedly abnormal bilateral slowing, electric–cortical silence

Source: From Squires, James & Mckiernan, Patrick & Squires, Robert. (2018). Acute Liver Failure. *Clinics in Liver Disease*. 22. 10.1016/j.cld.2018.06.009.

are all options. The evidence does not demonstrate superiority of any one modality, and the choice of extracorporeal support will depend on unit preference and experience.

Airway and Breathing

Consider intubation if: grade 2 encephalopathy (to facilitate neuroprotection), fluid-refractory shock or pulmonary oedema. Avoid induction agents that cause hypotension (e.g. propofol and thiopentone). Due to risk of bleeding, do not perform a nasal intubation. If the child is encephalopathic, give 3 ml/kg of 2.7% hypertonic saline pre-induction. Aim for an SpO_2 of >96%. Use the minimum peak inspiratory pressure (PIP) for an end-tidal carbon dioxide ($ETCO_2$) of 4–5 cmH$_2$O.

Circulation

Use standard fluid resuscitation with 20 ml/kg aliquots. A central line will be needed (correct coagulation first; seek out the most skilled operator, and avoid the subclavian route). The first-line vasoactive drug is noradrenaline. If cardiac function is poor, consider adding adrenaline or dopamine. For refractory shock, use 2 mg/kg intravenous (IV) hydrocortisone. If encephalopathic, target mean arterial pressures of:

- >70 mmHg if over 4 years
- >60 mmHg if under 4 years
- >50 mmHg if <1 year

Fluids

Avoid hypotonic fluids and restrict maintenance to 60 per cent of daily requirements. Place a urinary catheter. Target a blood glucose of 4–7 mmol/l. If persistently hypoglycaemic, increase the glucose concentration.

Neurology

Provide standard neurocritical care. Use morphine/fentanyl and midazolam for analgesia and sedation. Treat seizures with IV phenytoin. If hypertensive or bradycardic, or if the pupils are dilated, assume that the intracranial pressure (ICP) is raised and treat with 2.7% sodium chloride (3 ml/kg) and/or mannitol (0.5 mg/kg). Note that fixed, dilated pupils in this context may be reversible. Consider ICP monitoring.

Haematology

Correction of coagulopathy is only necessary if the patient is bleeding or if an invasive procedure is planned. If correction is required, use vitamin K 1 mg/kg IV (up to a maximum of 10 mg), fresh frozen plasma (FFP) 10 ml/kg, cryoprecipitate 5 ml/kg and platelets 15 ml/kg. Ensure fibrinogen exceeds 1 g/l. If gastrointestinal bleeding is present (likely variceal), give an IV proton pump inhibitor and consider octreotide 1 µg/kg bolus followed by an infusion.

Other

N-acetylcysteine is used in all cases. It replenishes glutathione in paracetamol overdose, and has potential antioxidant and anti-inflammatory effects.

Inborn Errors of Metabolism

Inborn errors of metabolism (IEM) are a group of rare genetic diseases where an enzyme defect results in a blocked metabolic pathway. They can be baffling and intimidating, even to the experienced paediatric intensivist.

There are broadly two scenarios to consider:

1. The diagnosed child. A child with an existing diagnosis presents to the emergency department

with an intercurrent illness resulting in metabolic decompensation (accumulation of toxic substances). Resuscitation should proceed as normal, with reference to the child's emergency plan, which the parents should carry with them. If not, the British Inherited Metabolic Diseases Group (BIMDG) has a database of emergency regimes for specific diagnoses. Liaise with the regional metabolic diseases team.

2. The undiagnosed child (see also Chapter 9.7, The Collapsed Infant). For management of the 'collapsed' infant, a metabolic diagnosis should be considered in the differential diagnosis (along with sepsis, congenital heart disease and inflicted injury). Clues that might point to an IEM are: a few hours or days of being well, followed by deterioration, encephalopathy/seizures/apnoeas, severe lactic acidosis, hypoglycaemia, deranged liver function tests (LFTs) and hyperammonaemia (>150 µmol/l).

A diagnosis is not required to start management:

- Manage ABC – intubation may be required for encephalopathy or circulatory failure.
- If fluid boluses are required, use 0.9% sodium chloride.
- Discontinue enteral intake.
- Correct hypoglycaemia and prevent catabolism with 10% dextrose infusion (glucose of 6–8 mg/(kg min)).
- If hyperglycaemic, start insulin.
- Correct pH using bicarbonate.
- Hyperammonaemia – discuss with a specialist in paediatric metabolic medicine. May require IV infusions of 'ammonia-scavenging' drugs – sodium benzoate and sodium phenylbutyrate (which provide an alternative non-urea cycle pathway for nitrogen excretion). Rapid transfer to a PICU for haemofiltration will be necessary if ammonia is >500 µmol/l or if climbing rapidly. Rapid ammonia clearance can mitigate brain damage.

Diabetic Ketoacidosis

Diabetic ketoacidosis (DKA) is common to adult and paediatric practice. It is seen more frequently in children and young people, and can be life-threatening. In children, there are a few common pitfalls to look out for and avoid.

Children can present, like adults, with polyuria, polydipsia and malaise. Often the symptoms of an infectious illness are also present, and the index of suspicion for diagnosis in children needs to be high. Diagnosis requires a combination of hyperglycaemia, acidosis and ketosis.

The comprehensive management of DKA is described in a guideline available online from the British Society for Paediatric Endocrinology and Diabetes (BSPED).

If young people aged 16–18 years are being managed by an adult medical team, the adult guidelines should be followed. If a young person is being managed by paediatricians, the paediatric guideline should be followed.

For the acute presentation, the following (paediatric) management points should be considered.

- Metabolic abnormalities should be corrected slowly.
- Cerebral oedema is the most common cause of mortality, and neurological observations should be performed regularly.
- Risk factors for cerebral oedema include: pCO_2 <2 kPa, younger age, first presentation, elevated serum urea, rapid sodium (Na^+) correction, administration of bicarbonate.
- Intubation should be avoided, if possible. Hyperventilating the child after intubation is associated with a poorer outcome.
- Careful attention to fluid administration remains an important part of the management of DKA because of the risk of cerebral oedema. If present, shock should be treated with fluid boluses of up to 40 ml/kg. Hypocapnia leads to peripheral vasoconstriction and a prolonged capillary refill time (CRT); therefore, CRT is not a useful guide to the need for fluid resuscitation
- Start IV insulin at least 1 hour after starting IV fluids.
- Use corrected Na^+ to titrate rehydration. If corrected Na^+ is rising >5 mmol/l in 4 hours, this indicates too much fluid loss and the fluid rate should be increased by 25 per cent. If corrected Na^+ is falling >5 mmol/l in 4 hours, this indicates too much fluid gain. Decrease the fluid rate by 25 per cent. To calculate corrected Na^+:

Corrected Na^+ = measured Na^+ + 0.4 × (serum glucose in mmol/l − 5.5)

References and Further Reading

British Inherited Metabolic Diseases Group (BIMDG). bimdg.org.uk/site/index.asp

British Inherited Metabolic Diseases Group (BIMDG). Emergency guidelines. bimdg.org.uk/site/guidelines.asp

British Society for Paediatric Endocrinology and Diabetes. Guidelines. www.bsped.org.uk/clinical-resources/guidelines/

British Society for Paediatric Endocrinology and Diabetes. BSPED interim guideline for the management of children and young people under the age of 18 years with diabetic ketoacidosis. www.bsped.org.uk/clinical/docs/DKAGuideline.pdf

Champion M. An approach to the diagnosis of inherited metabolic disease. *Arch Dis Child Educ Pract* 2010;**95**:40–6.

Conn HO. Quantifying the severity of hepatic encephalopathy. In: HO Conn, J Bircher (eds). *Hepatic Encephalopathy: Syndromes and Therapies.* Bloomington, IL: Medi-ed Press; 1994. pp. 13–26.

Durand P, Debray D, Mandel R, *et al.* Acute liver failure in infancy: a 14-year experience of a pediatric liver transplantation center. *J Pediatr* 2001;**139**:871–6.

Kuppermann N, Ghetti S, Schunk JE, *et al.* Clinical trial of fluid infusion rates for pediatric diabetic ketoacidosis. *N Engl J Med* 2018;**378**:2275–87.

Lee WM, Stravitz RT, Larson AM. Introduction to the revised American Association for the Study of Liver Diseases Position Paper on acute liver failure 2011. *Hepatology* 2012;**55**:965–7.

Squires RH Jr, Shneider BL, Bucuvalas J, *et al.* Acute liver failure in children: the first 348 patients in the pediatric acute liver failure study group. *J Pediatr* 2006;**148**:652–8.

Wolfdorsf JI. The International Society of Pediatric and Adolescent Diabetes guidelines for management of diabetic ketoacidosis: do the guidelines need to be modified? *Pediatr Diabetes* 2014;**15**:277–86.

9.11 Analgesia and Sedation in the Paediatric Intensive Care Unit

Andrew J. Jones and Thomas Brick

Key Learning Points

1. There is significant variation in practice in choice of analgesic and sedative agents amongst paediatric intensive care units (PICUs).
2. There are validated pain and sedation scales for assessment of children.
3. Morphine is often used alone for both sedation and analgesia in neonates.
4. Propofol infusions are rarely used for sedation on PICU.
5. An intravenous bolus of ketamine at 1–2 mg/kg is the induction agent of choice for the critically ill, hypotensive child.

Keywords: analgesia, sedation, PICU, COMFORT scale

Introduction

The approach to pain relief and sedation can vary significantly amongst different paediatric intensive care units (PICUs) (and amongst different paediatric intensivists), and medicines such as midazolam that may once have been the mainstays of paediatric intensive care are now being replaced by newer agents. The child's disease state and developmental age will also influence the approach taken. There is no one-size-fits-all method. Instead, this section will focus on the commonly used agents and the broad principles of their use in children.

The prevention of pain and suffering is crucial to the management of critically unwell children. Children have the right to adequate pain relief, and a combination of pain, discomfort, anxiety and fear will result in an agitated child, jeopardising the effectiveness and safety of intensive care interventions (particularly invasive mechanical ventilation). A comfortable and adequately sedated child will have a reduced metabolic rate, reduced oxygen demand, a more normal sleep/wake cycle and reduced recall of traumatic interventions, and will be less likely to accidently extubate. Whilst medicines are normally required to achieve this, it is vital to also consider physical factors and the environment (e.g. noise and lighting), and the importance of parental contact and distraction. Watching television, for example, has been demonstrated to be an effective analgesic. Additionally, exchanging an endotracheal tube from oral to nasal can improve comfort, and children requiring intubation for airway pathology who do not require mechanical ventilation may breathe comfortably through a nasal tube without need for any sedative medicines.

Children often cannot effectively self-report pain symptoms, and so assessment can be challenging. It has been recognised that children receive analgesia less frequently, when compared to adults, and younger children receive analgesia less frequently than older children. Validated pain assessment scales exist, and in the non-verbal and/or intubated child on the PICU, such scales consider variables such as behaviour, presence of tears, facial expression and movements, as well as physiological measures such as heart rate. One such scale is the Toddler-Preschooler Postoperative Pain Scale (TPPPS).

Sedation scoring is required to prevent over- and under-sedation. The COMFORT scale (Table 9.11.1) takes into account blood pressure, heart rate, muscle tone, facial tension, alertness, agitation, respiratory response and movement. The child is observed over 2 minutes, a score assigned and sedation titrated accordingly. The aim for most children is for them to be sleepy, but easily rousable and cooperative. Disease state may dictate a deeper level of sedation; for example, a child with a severe head injury will require deep sedation, possibly with neuromuscular blockade.

Table 9.11.1 The COMFORT scale

	1	2	3	4	5
Alertness	Deeply asleep	Lightly asleep	Drowsy	Alert and awake	Hyperalert
Calmness/agitation	Calm	Slightly anxious	Anxious	Very anxious	Panicky
Respiratory response	No coughing or no spontaneous respiration	Spontaneous respiration	Occasional cough/resists ventilator	Actively breathing against ventilator or coughing regularly	Fights ventilator
Physical movement	None	Occasional, slight movements	Frequent, slight movement	Vigorous movements of extremities only	Vigorous movement of extremities, torso and head
Blood pressure	Below baseline	Consistently at baseline	Infrequent elevation of 15% or more (1–3 during observation period)	Frequent elevations of 15% or more (>3 during observation period)	Sustained elevation of ≥15%
Heart rate	Below baseline	Consistently at baseline	Infrequent elevations of 15% or more (1–3 during observation period)	Frequent elevations of 15% or more (>3 during observation period)	Sustained elevation of ≥15%
Muscle tone	Relaxed/none	Reduced muscle tone	Normal muscle tone	Increased tone/flexion of fingers and toes	Extreme rigidity/flexion of fingers and toes
Facial tension	Relaxed	Normal tone	Some tension	Full facial tension	Hyperalert

A score is made from 1 to 5 for each variable. Sedation is considered excessive in the range of 8–16, adequate (17–26) or insufficient (27–40). *Source:* Ambuel B, Hamlett KW, Marx CM *et al.* Assessing distress in pediatric intensive care environments: the COMFORT scale. *J Pediatr Psychol* 1992;**17**:95–109.

Analgesic Agents

Simple analgesics are important first-line agents. Paracetamol is widely used, is effective in combination with opioids and can also be administered via the oral, intravenous and rectal routes. Non-steroidal anti-inflammatory drugs (NSAIDs) have a more limited role on the PICU, and caution should be exercised in renal compromise, bronchospasm and clotting and platelet disorders. NSAIDs are effective for postoperative pain in children.

Morphine

In neonates, a morphine infusion is often used alone to provide both sedation and analgesia. Outside of the neonatal population, a morphine infusion is used primarily for analgesia and should be combined with another agent if sedation is required. Morphine has low lipid solubility, accounting for its slow onset of action. When administered as a single intravenous dose (0.1 mg/kg), its peak analgesic effect occurs at 20 minutes and it has a duration of action of about 4 hours. Clearance is slower in neonates, with a half-life of 6.5 hours, and even slower in preterm neonates (half-life of 9 hours). Clearance adjusts to adult values within the first 6 months of life. Histamine release

means morphine should be avoided in bronchospasm, and boluses of morphine can cause vasodilation and hypotension.

Fentanyl

This is a synthetic opioid with 100 times the potency of morphine. Its high lipid solubility means bolus doses (1–2 µg/kg) have a rapid onset of action (within 3 minutes). The half-life is 30–60 minutes. It is metabolised in the liver, and changes in hepatic blood flow can thus affect clearance. The neonatal liver has a low expression of CYP3A4, resulting in a longer half-life. A fentanyl infusion may be used as first-line analgesia on the PICU but is particularly useful in wheeze (as there is no histamine release) and in neurocritical care for its rapid onset following bolus administration and sympatholytic properties. It is not suitable for prolonged use, as accumulation in peripheral compartments can occur, leading to a longer context-sensitive half-time (i.e. the time for plasma concentration to halve increases with duration of the infusion).

Remifentanil

This is a synthetic opioid with equivalent potency to fentanyl, but a shorter half-life of 3 minutes (in all age groups) due to rapid degradation by plasma esterases. It is not in common usage on the PICU and, to date, has only been evaluated in very small randomised controlled trials. Its rapid onset and offset mean it may have some utility in procedural analgesia and in instances where a ventilated child requires a short period of analgesia and sedation before being woken up (e.g. following surgery or in neurological conditions where a brief window of increased consciousness is required for assessment).

Sedative Agents
Midazolam

This facilitates the action of gamma aminobutyric acid (GABA), an inhibitory neurotransmitter, by increasing the frequency of chloride channel opening. It is an anxiolytic, an anti-convulsant and a sedative, and historically has been the first-choice agent on the PICU for sedation. It has a cardio-depressant effect, particularly when given as a bolus, and therefore is used less commonly on the paediatric cardiac ICU. After an intravenous bolus, peak sedation occurs within 10 minutes and the duration of action is 30–120 minutes. When given as an infusion, the duration of action is longer, and after prolonged use, sedative effects may persist for 48 hours after discontinuation. As with other benzodiazepines, there is variability in efficacy between patients (with possible reduced sedative effect in younger children), and an intravenous infusion will require careful titration. The adverse effect profile of prolonged midazolam use includes tolerance, dependence and withdrawal symptoms after discontinuation, which has, in recent years, led to the search for alternative sedative agents.

Clonidine

This is an α_2 adrenoceptor agonist which exerts a sedative, analgesic and anxiolytic effect without causing respiratory depression. It has a role in treating opioid withdrawal and has been demonstrated to have an opioid- and benzodiazepine-sparing effect when given as an infusion in newborns. There is also evidence that an infusion of clonidine is an effective alternative to a midazolam infusion in providing sedation in children. Adverse effects include bradycardia and hypotension, with rebound hypertension if clonidine therapy is withdrawn abruptly.

Dexmedetomidine

This is also an α_2 agonist but is more selective for receptors in the central nervous system. An intravenous infusion can produce a patient who is sedated, but easily rousable. This is an attractive property and has particular utility for patients requiring short periods of mechanical ventilation. Adult data suggest reduced ICU delirium and mechanical ventilation duration with dexmedetomidine, when compared to midazolam. In children, dexmedetomidine has been shown to provide adequate sedation for mechanical ventilation, and may facilitate earlier extubation (when compared to fentanyl).

Propofol

Whilst the mainstay of sedation in many adult ICUs, it is rarely used on the PICU in the UK. This predominantly stems from concerns related to propofol infusion syndrome – in young children receiving an infusion for >3 days at a dose over 5 mg/(kg hr), there have been reports of metabolic acidosis, cardiac failure, rhabdomyolysis, hyperlipidaemia and hepatomegaly, which, in some cases, has resulted in death. Boluses, however, may be used for procedural sedation in older children.

Ketamine

This produces dissociative anaesthesia and has analgesic properties. Its use as a sedative is limited in older children by psychotic sequelae such as hallucinations and nightmares (which can be ameliorated by concomitant benzodiazepine use). It is also a useful adjunctive analgesic, often combined with opioids. Due to bronchodilator properties, it is a useful agent in asthma. An intravenous bolus of ketamine at 1–2 mg/kg is the induction agent of choice for the critically ill hypotensive child, as, in most cases, its sympathomimetic properties offset any negative inotropy and lead to an increase in heart rate and blood pressure. It should, however, be recognised that critically ill children may occasionally respond to ketamine with an unexpected decrease in blood pressure. This represents dwindling reserves of endogenous catecholamines and fatigue of sympathetic compensatory mechanisms, unmasking the negative inotropic effects of ketamine.

References and Further Reading

Ambuel B, Hamlett KW, Marx CM, *et al.* Assessing distress in pediatric intensive care environments: the COMFORT scale. *J Pediatr Psychol* 1992;**17**:95–109.

Bellieni CV, Cordelli DM, Raffaelli M, Ricci B, Morgese G, Buonocore G. Analgesic effect of watching TV during venipuncture. *Arch Dis Child* 2006;**91**:1015–17.

Hunseler C, Balling G, Rohlig C, *et al.* Continuous infusion of clonidine in ventilated newborns and infants. *Pediatr Crit Care Med* 2014;**15**:511–22.

Jenkins IA, Playfor SD, Bevan C, Davies G, Wolf AR. Current United Kingdom sedation practice in pediatric intensive care. *Pediatr Anesth* 2007;**17**:675–83.

Playfor SD. Analgesia and sedation in critically ill children. *Contin Educ Anaesth Crit Care Pain* 2008;**8**:90–4.

Saleh RH. Randomized controlled comparative trial between low dose dexmedetomidine sedation and that of fentanyl in children after surgical procedures in surgical pediatric intensive care unit. *Egyptian J Anaesth* 2016;**32**:137–42.

Striker TW, Stool S, Downes JJ. Prolonged nasotracheal intubation in infants and children. *Arch Otolaryngol* 1967;**85**:210–13.

Tarbel SE, Cohen IT, March JL. The Toddler-Preschooler Postoperative Pain Scale: an observational scale for measuring post-operative pain in children aged 1–5 years. A preliminary report. *Pain* 1992;**50**:273–80.

Wolf A, McKay A, Spowart C, *et al.* Prospective multicentre randomised, double-blind, equivalence study comparing clonidine and midazolam as intravenous sedative agents in critically ill children: the SLEEPS (Safety profiLe, Efficacy and Equivalence in Paediatric intensive care Sedation) study. *Health Technol Assess* 2014;**18**:1–212.

10.1 Principles of Transport of the Mechanically Ventilated Critically Ill Patient outside the ICU

Jonny Price and Scott Grier

Key Learning Points

1. All staff transferring critically ill patients must be appropriately trained.
2. Equipment should be standardised and allow the team to deal with common and unexpected events during transfer.
3. The decision to transfer a patient should be made by a senior clinician.
4. Proper preparation reduces risk.
5. Regular review of the patient during transfer ensures timely detection of deterioration and appropriate interventions.

Keywords: transport, intra-hospital, inter-hospital, critically ill

Introduction

Critically ill patients frequently require transportation around the hospital (intra-hospital), and occasionally between hospitals (inter-hospital). Regardless of the destination, the same approach to preparation, training, equipment and clinical governance should be taken.

Guidelines and National Organisation

National guidelines regarding transportation of critically ill patients exist in the UK. Inter-hospital transport services vary across the devolved nations of the UK. Neonatal and paediatric transportation is almost exclusively undertaken by specialist commissioned teams. Adult transportation is undertaken by specialist commissioned teams in Scotland and Wales, but performed on an ad hoc basis in England, largely by the transferring hospital. National guidelines demand that critical care networks and individual trusts have a robust governance system surrounding patient transfers.

Training and Staff

All staff involved in the transfer of critically ill patients should receive appropriate training and experience in a supernumerary capacity before independent practice. The Intensive Care Society (ICS) guidelines outline core and specialist competencies. Most transfers should be undertaken by two trained staff, usually a doctor and a nurse. The background and competency of each need to be appropriate to the patient being transferred, and risk assessment matrices exist to help in this decision-making process. A doctor with appropriate airway management competence should accompany all level 3 patients, and level 2 patients with potential airway or breathing issues.

Equipment

Emergency equipment should accompany a patient on any transfer. Many hospitals and some critical care networks have standardised 'transfer bags'. The contents should provide equipment necessary to manage common or unexpected events, e.g. advanced airway management, cardiac arrest or delivery of anaesthesia. Monitors should be suitable for purpose and visible, and contain sufficient power. Minimum monitoring includes ECG, oxygen saturations and non-invasive blood pressure. Waveform capnography must be used for ventilated patients. Invasive arterial blood pressure monitoring is frequently used and often preferable.

Sufficient oxygen supply must be guaranteed to undertake the transfer safely. Generally, twice the expected requirement (including driving gas for a ventilator) is recommended.

Inter-hospital transfers are best undertaken using a specialised transfer trolley with integrated attachments for the monitor, ventilator, syringe drivers and oxygen cylinders. These trolleys must be compatible with local ambulance providers to ensure that they are secure when in transit. If a dedicated trolley is not available, all equipment must be secured prior to departure, to prevent it from becoming a missile in the event of an accident.

Decision-Making

The decision to transfer an intensive care patient should be made by a senior clinician. The rationale for transfer should always be explained to the patient and/ or their family.

Patients require inter-hospital transfer for three main reasons:

1. Clinical – for specialist care or investigations
2. Non-clinical – inadequate resources at current location (e.g. no beds available)
3. Repatriation – ongoing care can be delivered in hospital closer to home (e.g. transfer to a local hospital from a major trauma centre)

Immediate (time-critical) transfers should receive a blue light response within 30 minutes, and urgent cases within 2 hours. Non-urgent transfers often use transport booked for a particular time.

Transport Modality

In the UK, most inter-hospital transfers are performed by road. Emergency response driving (blue lights and sirens) should facilitate passage through traffic. Aeromedical transfer is rare and requires specific training.

Preparation

Ideally, patients should be resuscitated and physiologically optimised prior to transfer. Some clinical scenarios (e.g. evacuation of an expanding acute extradural haematoma) require time-critical transfer for lifesaving treatment to achieve this. Patient warmth and dignity should be maintained throughout. Adequate, secure vascular access should be accessible. Accidental line or drain removal must be prevented. Prior to departure, the patient and all equipment should be secured. Attendants should be seated and wearing seat belts. Hospital notes and radiology and blood results should be shared according to local policies to ensure high-quality handover of information. Those escorting the patient should be appropriately dressed to ensure warmth and safety. A mobile telephone with contact details of both sending and receiving units is recommended. The team should plan for the return journey to their base hospital and carry means of financing this, if required.

Many critical care networks use a checklist to ensure adequate preparation prior to departure.

Undertaking the Transfer

The standard of care expected in critical care does not change during transfer.

Documentation should be completed, with most critical care networks using standardised forms. There is a nationally suggested core data set for these forms, and vital signs must be recorded. Practically, regular structured review of the patient enhances safety. We suggest the familiar 'ABCDE' approach. Should significant clinical deterioration occur en route, this should be communicated with the receiving site prior to arrival, especially if interventions are urgently required. Interventions should be minimised in a moving vehicle. The ambulance may be required to stop in a safe place to allow the clinical team to safely treat the patient whilst protecting their well-being. Formal verbal handover should occur on arrival at the receiving hospital (alongside transfer of patient notes and investigation results).

Points to Remember

Up to one in five critical care transfers involves a critical incident. Proper preparation and planning will help anticipate and manage many incidents. Vehicle accidents are not infrequent, and departments should ensure that staff are adequately insured in the event of a serious incident. The Association of Anaesthetists of Great Britain and Ireland (AAGBI) and ICS offer membership with personal accident insurance cover in the event of an accident during a patient transfer. Membership of a defence organisation is recommended.

References and Further Reading

Association of Anaesthetists of Great Britain and Ireland. 2009. Interhospital transfer. anaesthetists.org/Home/ Resources-publications/Guidelines/Interhospital-transfer-AAGBI-safety-guideline

The Faculty of Intensive Care Medicine. 2019. Guidance on: the transfer of the critically ill adult. www.ficm.ac.uk/ sites/default/files/transfer_critically_ill_adult_2019 .pdf

Welsh Assembly Government. 2016. Designed for life: Welsh guidelines for the transfer of the critically ill adult. www.wales.nhs.uk/sites3/Documents/962/ Guidelines%20for%20the%20Transfer%20of%20 the%20Critically%20Ill%20Adult_v5.pdf

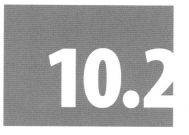

10.2

Pre-hospital (Helicopter) Emergency Medical Services

Marc Wittenberg and Dominik Krzanicki

Key Learning Points

1. The principles of emergency out-of-hospital care include attending the scene and initiating immediate medical care (primary retrieval), and transferring between geographical locations, often to more specialist tertiary medical centres (secondary retrieval).
2. Models of care delivery used by helicopter emergency medical services (HEMS) include both doctor–paramedic and paramedic-only response teams.
3. Both land and air service delivery have associated pros and cons.
4. HEMS systems are tightly governed and work to standard operating procedures.
5. Pre-hospital traumatic injury management broadly follows similar principles to those of in-hospital management; however, life-threatening injuries are managed on scene, sometimes with the addition of pre-hospital blood transfusion.

Keywords: pre-hospital care, HEMS, trauma

Introduction

Pre-hospital (helicopter) emergency medical services (HEMS) provide care to patients beyond the hospital environment. The specialty is usefully divided into primary and secondary retrieval.

Primary services attend the scene of a medical emergency or traumatic incident. They facilitate the delivery of immediate medical care, and then transfer the patient to a facility best suited to treating their condition. In the UK, these services can be both helicopter- and land-based, but operate under the umbrella of HEMS. There are over 20 air ambulance services that together provide geographical coverage for most of the UK.

Secondary retrieval involves transferring patients between medical facilities, so that the patients can receive definitive or tertiary-level care (e.g. burns, neurosurgery, paediatric/neonatal critical care). Patients will be variably stabilised and resuscitated, often with advanced monitoring and treatment modalities in progress. Secondary transfer can be performed by land or air (both rotary wing and fixed wing).

Some services focus solely on primary retrieval and others solely on secondary, and fewer will perform both functions. This chapter will focus on primary services within the UK, as transfer medicine is covered elsewhere.

Models of Care
Paramedic Only

Historically, helicopter services have operated as '*air ambulance services*'. These aircraft were manned as twin paramedic crews, with associated limitations in the scope of care that can be provided, as defined in the UK by the Joint Royal Colleges Ambulance Liaison Committee (JRCALC) guidelines. For example, although many paramedics are trained in endotracheal intubation, they are limited to cases where anaesthetic and/or neuromuscular-blocking agents are not required. Increasingly, however, second-generation supraglottic airway devices, such as the i-gel®, are being employed in lieu of an endotracheal tube for such scenarios.

A major advantage of this model of air ambulance services is that they can retrieve patients in a timely manner from difficult-to-access or remote locations, and the crews often have significant pre-hospital experience.

More recently, a small number of paramedics are being trained as critical care paramedics, with additional skills and knowledge that they are able to employ in independent practice, e.g. use of agents such as midazolam and ketamine for conscious sedation and conduct of thoracostomies for decompression of pneumothoraces.

733

Doctor–Paramedic

In contrast, HEMS models operate a doctor–paramedic model, whereby specially trained doctors are able to complement the paramedic, to bring an advanced skill set to patients, including, but not limited to, rapid sequence induction, advanced sedation and analgesia, blood transfusion and emergency thoracotomy.

The aim of such a service is to enable resuscitation room-level care to be delivered at the scene of the incident, thereby optimising the patient's outcome. In trauma, pre-hospital care is designed to optimise the airway, respiratory function and circulatory status of the patient, whilst at the same time minimising the delay between injury and definitive surgical intervention. This can sometimes mean conducting the intervention prior to the patient reaching the hospital, e.g. resuscitative thoracotomy or initiation of blood transfusion.

This level of service clearly comes at significant cost, including investment in training, equipment and the aircraft and vehicles themselves. An average cost per mission of a doctor–paramedic-crewed helicopter in the UK is in the region of £2700.

Although the service name implies exclusive use of aircraft, many urban services cannot fly and/or crucially land safely at night. For this reason, on many occasions, pre-hospital medical services are delivered to scene in fast-response cars when daylight is insufficient or weather conditions are unsuitable for air-based operations.

Benefits and Downsides of Rotary Wing (Helicopter) Transfer

Benefits

- Rapid delivery of an advanced medical team to the patient.
- Ability to access remote sites.
- Potentially faster transfer of patients to definitive care.
- Unique overview of trauma scenes from the air to assess mechanism and scale of incidents.

Downsides

- Cost of running helicopter services is significant.
- Transferring patients in helicopters involves a hostile environment with limited access to patients, noise, vibration and difficulties in adequate monitoring.

- Very difficult to deal with deterioration in flight.
- Helicopter services can be very susceptible to poor weather and light conditions, making it unsafe to operate.

Delivery of Care

Pre-hospital medicine can be very taxing for the most experienced physicians. The patient group represents the sickest or most critically injured group of patients; environmental conditions are often adverse, and the response team much smaller than one might expect in hospital. The specialty has borrowed heavily from the aviation industry with which it works so closely, to minimise risks, identify threats to good performance and mitigate against, as well as reduce, error under pressure.

Most services will work within a set of standard operating procedures (SOPs) to ensure that treatment is delivered consistently and allow practitioners to have a structured approach to patient management.

HEMS teams have to be able to deliver care within unfamiliar multidisciplinary teams (including ambulance personnel, fire crews, coastguard/lifeguard crews and the police). Teams apply great attention to detail to communications within and beyond the team, and are highly trained in non-technical skills, including crew resource management. Beyond that, however, they also have to communicate via radio and telephone with ambulance control, pilots and hospitals, to facilitate seamless and rapid transfer of patients.

In contrast to in-hospital practice which can be regarded as 'safe', the pre-hospital environment is very much more unstable. HEMS teams are equipped with personal protective equipment which satisfies both aviation and medical standards, as well as with other equipment, as required, including body armour, fall arrest harnesses, life jackets and helmets. Practitioners need to be aware of a wide variety of potential hazards relating to rail incidents, road incidents and chemical, biological, radiological and nuclear defence (CBRN) incidents.

Governance and Training

Medical standards in pre-hospital medicine are identical to those in hospital. It is completely unacceptable for there to be a difference in performance between a pre-hospital service and, for example, care delivered in a teaching hospital emergency department.

Clinical governance is crucial to allow services to identify adherence to SOPs, as well as to allow improvements to them. This governance is often in the form of regular (often weekly) morbidity and mortality (M&M) reviews, which robustly inspect individual missions to identify best possible care and any shortcomings.

Working within aviation allows teams to adopt a rigorous approach to safety – both logistical and medical. Incident reporting and safety management systems within pre-hospital medicine are widely held as a crucial pillar of high-quality practice.

HEMS systems adopt significant levels of training, often as highly immersive, medium-fidelity simulation or 'moulage'. Crews will be expected to undertake taxing training scenarios on a regular basis to be deemed 'flight-competent', and will be able to explore the difficult decisions and clinical dilemmas that they may face in practice, but within a safe environment. Such immersive simulation takes place much more frequently within pre-hospital medicine than it does in hospital, and has particular utility in training for low-frequency high-acuity scenarios, e.g. resuscitative hysterotomy.

Tasking

The decision as to which patients will benefit from advanced medical care in the form of a HEMS crew is complex and is one of the main determinants of success of a HEMS service. In most cases, tasking is performed by the ambulance service, whereby a dedicated paramedic (ideally a HEMS-trained paramedic) will be situated in the control room, screening all calls for the small percentage that would benefit from the attendance of a HEMS crew.

It must be borne in mind that HEMS operations are expensive, and not without risk, and once a crew is dispatched, they will be unavailable for other calls. Therefore, most dispatch systems operate within a set of criteria that will trigger a HEMS dispatch – which may necessitate further interrogation of the call(er) by the dispatching paramedic or, in some cases, immediate dispatch based purely on mechanism, e.g.:

- Road traffic accident (RTA) with patient ejected
- RTA with associated fatality
- RTA with person under vehicle
- Person under train
- Fall from height
- Amputation above wrist or ankle
- Emergency service request

In order to ensure successful tasking, it is expected that a proportion of missions (around 30 per cent) will end in a 'stand-down'. This is where either the mission is aborted en route, due to the fact that further information from the scene has meant that a HEMS crew is not required, or on scene where it transpires that perhaps the patient's condition is not as serious as first reported. In these cases, the patient is usually left in the care of the ambulance ground crews to be treated within their normal protocols.

Triage and Patient Destination

There has been a significant change within pre-hospital medicine with regard to where patients have been taken to. Evidence suggests that patients in certain groups will have better outcomes if they are taken directly to a specialist centre for management of their condition. This has prompted significant change for patients with neurosurgical and neurological emergencies, myocardial infarction, burns and trauma.

Advanced pre-hospital care medical teams will be able to bypass smaller, non-specialised departments to convey patients to more appropriate definitive care. Pivotal to this process is the fact that these teams can deliver advanced airway and other treatment interventions, allowing safe transfer to hospitals that involves a longer transfer time.

The benefits of selective primary transfer are such that many pathology types are now treated within networks, whereby ambulance services will directly triage patients to specialist receiving hospitals. This is notable for stroke, trauma and suspected myocardial infarction.

Mechanisms and Management of Traumatic Injury

Historically, the most common type of trauma patient was a young male who had been involved in an RTA. However, now in the UK, the most common type of major trauma (Injury Severity Score (ISS) >15) is an older person suffering a fall from standing height. In all cases, traumatic brain injury is the most common cause of death.

Traumatic Brain Injury

The principles of head injury management are similar to those in hospital (covered elsewhere), namely provision of adequate cerebral oxygenation and perfusion, avoidance of secondary brain injury and rapid transfer to a specialist centre.

However, one phenomenon particular to the pre-hospital setting is that of 'impact brain apnoea' (IBA).

It is characterised by cessation of breathing following a brain injury, and it is thought that the greater the impact, the longer the period of apnoea. In addition, a massive catecholamine surge occurs that manifests as hypertension followed by cardiovascular collapse.

It follows that 'hyper-acute' intervention is essential to minimise the impact of IBA, ideally performed by bystanders, potentially guided by the tasking paramedic. This is followed by prompt optimisation of the airway and correction of hypoxia and hypoventilation by pre-hospital practitioners.

Chest Injury

Life-threatening chest injuries are often occult in major trauma and difficult to diagnose in the pre-hospital environment. There should be a high index of suspicion based on the mechanism of injury and injury pattern. Injuries include:

- Pneumothorax (tension or open)
- Haemothorax
- Flail chest
- Cardiac tamponade

General management consists of administration of high-flow oxygen and early, effective analgesia to alleviate respiratory insufficiency.

Diagnosis of tension pneumothorax is challenging; however, in all patients with a clinical suspicion and signs of decompensation, the thorax should be decompressed. Needle thoracocentesis has a high failure rate, although it is within the skill set of paramedics. Advanced pre-hospital teams, especially in the setting of positive pressure ventilation, will opt for an open thoracostomy without an intercostal drain until definitive management is undertaken in hospital. Intercostal drains are an option pre-hospital, but usually exclusively in the context of a patient who is spontaneously ventilating with penetrating chest trauma. There is increasing utility in the application of diagnostic ultrasound to aid decision-making in these injuries.

In the setting of penetrating chest trauma, significant deterioration should prompt consideration of a resuscitative 'clam-shell' thoracotomy. Indications are as follows:

- Penetrating wounds to the chest or upper abdomen
- Cardiac arrest with loss of vital signs ≤15 minutes
- The suspected injury is suitable for temporary repair and control

Relative contraindications are:

- Cardiac arrest secondary to blunt trauma (there may be a caveat for very recent arrest to facilitate aortic compression)
- Loss of vital signs >15 minutes

Abdominal and Pelvic Injury

After head injury, haemorrhage is the leading cause of death in civilian trauma. Unlike bleeding from extremities where direct pressure or tourniquets can be employed, severe haemorrhage from the abdomen or pelvis secondary to blunt trauma can be difficult to diagnose and treat. Typically, a focussed history in the form of understanding the mechanism of injury and examination are sufficient to raise suspicion of injury and lead the HEMS practitioner to initiate treatment.

In the case of suspected pelvic injury, movement should be kept to an absolute minimum and the pelvic volume should be normalised by means of a pelvic splint. This promotes haemostasis and acts as a signal to teams further along the patient pathway not to excessively roll or move the patient. It is no longer appropriate to 'spring' or stress the pelvis. The clinical utility of this manoeuvre is minimal and it can promote further bleeding.

Definitive management of these patients is prompt transfer to an operating theatre/interventional radiology suite to control bleeding, with balanced damage control resuscitation initiated on scene and continued in transfer.

A significant number of patients with massive abdominal and pelvic bleeding will arrest before or on arrival to the emergency department. Resuscitative thoracotomy, to enable direct compression of the aorta in massive subdiaphragmatic haemorrhage, has been an intervention of last resort in this patient group, but with very poor outcomes and significant additional injury burden in those where it is successful at regaining circulatory control. More recently, the concept of placing an endovascular balloon in the aorta (percutaneously via the common femoral artery) to control haemorrhage and augment afterload in traumatic arrest and haemorrhagic shock has gained popularity. This is known as REBOA (resuscitative endovascular balloon occlusion of the aorta). This procedure is subject to a number of ongoing trials to determine both efficacy and complication burden.

Contemporary thinking in trauma medicine has essentially stopped the use of crystalloid in resuscitation of major traumatic haemorrhage. Many HEMS services now carry packed red cells to avoid crystalloid administration in such patients. It is recognised, however, that most of these patients also need clotting factors early in their resuscitation. As such, various methods of delivering these to patients are being investigated in the form of freeze-dried plasma, red cell and plasma component or prothrombin complex concentrates. Ultimately, there is a desire to administer whole blood to patients to include essential platelets in the resuscitation fluid.

References and Further Reading

Association of Ambulance Chief Executives. Annual report 2019–2020. www.associationofairambulances.co.uk/resources/AOAA-Annual%20Report%202016-FULL.pdf

Leech C, Porter K, Steyn R, *et al.* The pre-hospital management of life-threatening chest injuries: a consensus statement from the Faculty of Pre-Hospital Care, Royal College Surgeons of Edinburgh. *Trauma* 2017;**19**:54–62.

Moore LJ, Brenner M, Kozar RA, *et al.* Implementation of resuscitative endovascular balloon occlusion of the aorta as an alternative to resuscitative thoracotomy for noncompressible truncal hemorrhage. *J Trauma Acute Care Surg* 2015;**79**:523–30.

The Trauma Audit & Research Network (TARN). 2017. Major trauma in older people – 2017 report. www.tarn.ac.uk/content/downloads/3793/Major%20Trauma%20in%20Older%20People%202017.pdf

Walmsley J, Turner J. Stocklist—a study of clinical skills of critical care paramedics in the UK. *Emerg Med J* 2015;**32**:e5.

Wilson MH, Hinds J, Grier G, Burns B, Carley S, Davies G. Impact brain apnoea – a forgotten cause of cardiovascular collapse in trauma. *Resuscitation* 2016;**105**:52–8.

11.1

Leading the Daily Intensive Care Ward Round

Julian Howard

Key Learning Points

1. Insight into habitual barriers leads to an effective ward round.

2. The importance of location, which should be at the bedside, with the patient at the focus.

3. The importance of a structured approach, physical examination, checklists and goal setting.

4. The ward round should be multidisciplinary, promoting a culture of collaborative input, with all individual roles acknowledged and respected.

5. The ward round should be concluded by clarification of agreed goals for the day, defining individual responsibilities within the attending team and contemporaneous documentation.

Keywords: ward round, multidisciplinary, documentation, structured approach, responsibilities

Introduction

The business ward round is a key component of daily activity within the ICU. It allows the multidisciplinary team (MDT) to meet at the bedside and review a patient's condition, share information, address patient problems, plan and evaluate treatment and develop a coordinated plan of care. It can also facilitate joint learning through active participation of all members of the MDT by effective communication, and also enhance patient safety. When the patient is able to engage with the process, the ward round can have a significant impact upon both clinical and emotional outcomes for patients.

Unfortunately, there exists no 'gold standard' for best ward round practice and obviously the process is subject to local constraints with staffing resources. It is, however, possible to identify some key themes that should be mandatory for all practitioners. Core standards for ICUs support the concept of consultant-led multidisciplinary ward rounds occurring daily, with input from nursing, microbiology, pharmacy and physiotherapy. In practice, the microbiology round might be conducted separately away from the bedside, and physiotherapy rounds can be somewhat independent, as long as rehabilitation issues can be communicated easily to the clinical team.

The ward round should commence after nighttime handover and a review of current radiology for all patients. This allows immediate identification of which patients should be imaged routinely and the orders placed early in the day. Standardised location, time and composition of the healthcare provider team improve round effectiveness by facilitating greater availability of, and participation amongst, team members. It is recognised that measures of organisational culture, leadership, coordination and communication are associated with lower risk-adjusted length of stay in the ICU.

Composition of the team should include, as a minimum, the consultant, one ICU resident doctor, a senior nurse, a pharmacist and the bedside nurse. The main business ward round should not include the patient's family, who can be met with later in the day, either separately or during the evening ward round.

Barriers to Best Practice

1. Electronic patient records are progressively being implemented in many hospitals. Their design and implementation are optimised for individuals, rather than for groups, and unless the ward round is stage-managed, this can lead to difficulties, especially when screen size is inadequate and there are insufficient computers. Paper and electronic records present, and allow access to, the

information in completely different ways, and the latter is a far more complex system, affecting team interaction. Using paper records and a standard ICU chart, every team member can review all information, thus reducing errors. Restricted access to patient data for some within the team is a known obstacle to best care. Constant reminders may be necessary to maintain patient emphasis. The senior doctor's orientation towards the screen on display does little to direct the attention of those unable to see the screen. The consultant therefore loses the ability to guide the focus of the group. Dedication to screens inevitably detracts from physical examination of the patient, and also from normal social interaction. When new technologies are proposed, potential hazards should be identified and an evidence-based assessment undertaken, as occurs with other clinical innovations.

2. Substitution of the daily bedside ward round for a 'virtual' discussion remote from the patient is not acceptable. Side rooms should not be regarded as an impediment to best-quality practice, and rounds should still involve direct participation of the bedside nurse and patient.

3. A non-team-based hierarchical structure of those involved will restrict information exchange. All team members should be valued equally. The discussion environment should facilitate collaboration.

4. No rationale is provided for clinical decisions.

5. Patient goals are not documented.

6. Simple checklists are not utilised, thereby hindering a goal-oriented discussion.

7. There are continual interruptions from bleeps and mobile telephones.

Ward Round Structure

The leader of the ward round should introduce the team to the patient and the bedside nurse. They should enquire from the bedside nurse about current concerns and significant events. One doctor should perform a hands-on physical examination of the patient, including a neurological review if appropriate. (Coma or appropriate deep sedation should not preclude central nervous system (CNS) assessment, as lateralising signs, meningism and abnormal brainstem reflexes would always prompt further investigation.) The physical review should include both skin and invasive

vascular access devices, and question whether the lines are still required. The patient should always be exposed appropriately with privacy and dignity paramount. A stethoscope should be available for the round and be of adequate quality. Imaging can be considered an extension of the physical examination in ICU patients.

The senior doctor needs to review the ICU observation chart regarding physiological variables, and make decisions regarding changes in levels of support for major systems, i.e. ventilation, cardiovascular, renal, CNS and nutritional. The drug chart should be revised with the pharmacist on every round, as this practice has been shown to prevent prescription errors and reduce drug costs and also the risk of adverse drug events. In some units, the pharmacist has been given a full prescribing role. All drugs prescribed should be evaluated as to their ongoing usefulness. Do any drugs require monitoring of plasma levels, and when should these be taken, e.g. gentamicin and the Hartford nomogram?

During this period, all involved should have clear visual access to the data and information. The spatial configuration must be such that participation and visibility are maximised. The more people are empowered to participate, the less likelihood of an error in synthesising what is presented, and the culture should be one of systematic questioning by any team member.

A simple checklist can be reviewed with the group. A good example of this would be the 'FAST HUG' mnemonic (Feeding, Analgesia, Sedation, Thromboembolic prophylaxis, Head of bed elevation, stress Ulcer prevention and Glucose control). This approach rapidly identifies key aspects in the general care of all critically ill patients. The checklist can be expanded to include other evidence-based aspects of practice such as low tidal volume ventilation in acute lung injury and early mobilisation. Using checklists can also be a means of ensuring data collection for local quality improvement projects and standardising a routine and systematic process of care.

There should be a review of pain, sedation and delirium, with reference to validated assessment tools such as the Critical Care Pain and Observation Tool (CPOT), Richmond Agitation Sedation Scale (RASS) or Confusion Assessment Method for the ICU (CAM-ICU).

A note should be made of factors necessary for appropriate later discussion with the microbiologist if this individual is not present at the time. These might include maximum temperature within the last 24 hours, white blood cell (WBC) count, C-reactive protein (CRP), recent cultures and current anti-microbials.

It should be established when the patient's family was last updated or if this is required today, and whether any referrals to any other teams are necessary. Is the patient actually approaching 'end of life'? Is the patient fit for discharge? If a long-stay patient is progressing to imminent discharge, then it may be prudent to involve senior nursing staff from the destination ward and also the Outreach Team before the patient leaves the ICU. Before the plan for the day is formulated, enquiry should be made by the entire team as to whether any other key areas for review have been omitted. At all times, the atmosphere should be one whereby any team member can speak up openly if they have any safety concerns or issues of quality of care. This atmosphere can be created through leadership advocating a less steeped hierarchy and a shared perception of teamwork. Interprofessional tensions need to be minimised, and all team members trusted and respected with regard to their individual roles.

Finally, the plan for the day should be documented either manually or electronically. It should be visible at all times, either on a chart or on a screen by the patient. It should include simple goals for the bedside team, e.g. targets for RASS, peripheral oxygen saturation (SpO_2), partial pressure of oxygen (PaO_2), partial pressure of carbon dioxide ($PaCO_2$), mean arterial pressure (MAP), haemoglobin (Hb) and overall fluid balance. The plan should be prioritised towards the immediate problems. If the patient is undergoing a guided respiratory wean, then a period of overnight rest with increased ventilator support should be specified. Consideration should be given to organising an MDT and/or a family meeting, and the frequency and nature of future blood tests defined for the following 24 hours.

The team should be asked whether there are any concerns with the proposed plan. Is it realistic or are we losing focus and not actually addressing the 'bigger picture'? Any queries should prompt a rationale and discussion. It is imperative that communication is explicit and everybody involved understands their particular responsibilities once the plan has been finalised. Any uncertainties with regard to the patient trajectory should be acknowledged.

Although the daily business round is not a formal teaching round, there is often the opportunity to highlight significant learning points to all team members that can be explored later in greater depth.

Other Housekeeping Issues

During the encounter, the most senior doctor should be using their wisdom and experience to ensure that the patient is being progressed appropriately, and not being damaged by over-enthusiastic treatment measures. These are not uncommon and some examples are illustrated below.

1. Removal of fluid via continuous veno-venous haemofiltration (CVVHF), whilst the patient is receiving vasopressors, is usually detrimental to the circulation.

2. Simultaneous weaning of CVVHF in tandem with respiratory wean in a patient with multi-organ failure is often unsuccessful, as the respiratory progress can be slowed by oliguria and subsequent challenging fluid management off the filter, alongside deteriorating renal function. The real 'win' in this setting is to first liberate the patient from the ventilator, and to address other issues in a timely manner. ICU discharge cannot be effected whilst the patient is still ventilated!

3. Inappropriate management of oedema with diuretics, despite biochemical evidence that kidney function is deteriorating. A similar issue pertains in the context of acute lung injury where often the patient is being run 'dry', but obviously not at the expense of kidney damage. Renal failure has a significant effect on mortality that is not explained by underlying conditions alone, and should not be regarded as a treatable complication of serious illness.

4. Aggressive use of 'sedation holds' in an intubated patient who is weaning can sometimes result in pain and distress. The resulting increase in respiratory rate can often be misinterpreted as failure to cope, and the breathing support escalated, whereas the recommended approach would be to titrate analgesia and sedation to an appropriate target which permits the individual to be calm, comfortable and collaborative at all times, thus allowing progression of the wean and reduction of support.

5. Bedside attainment of blood pressure targets by simply dialling up the vasopressor infusion and ignoring the question 'Is my patient intravascularly deplete?'. The ward round should always critically review the patient's volume status, and emphasise the utility of a volume

challenge with a measured outcome, as assessed by a non-invasive cardiac monitoring device or even by a straight leg raise. Optimal fluid management continues to be difficult in many patients, and there should be a low threshold for utilisation of haemodynamic monitors throughout admission.

6. Forgetting to challenge continually the working diagnosis. At admission, the diagnosis can be uncertain, but the patient is treated as if the initial diagnosis is correct. Because the ICU environment is essentially supportive and acute, with a priority of effecting lifesaving physiological measures, sometimes a review of the patient's old notes can be overlooked. Later on, the patient's coexisting multiple pathologies may become more important and dictate both the immediate management plan and the future trajectory.

7. Inappropriate gain of medications on a rapid sequential basis. An example would be the prescription of anti-hypertensives to a patient who is actually agitated or uncomfortable and exhibiting an appropriate physiological response. Once prescribed, these drugs may follow the patient to the ward where colleagues may be reluctant to discontinue them because they have been prescribed by intensive care.

8. Untimely change of intravenous sedative infusion to intermittent nasogastric administration with rescue intravenous boluses for agitation in the context of an individual who is otherwise progressing. The patient can then become intermittently agitated and then grossly over-sedated. Nasogastric absorption can be variable, and the end-result can be a patient who is essentially stuck and all progress, including suitable rehabilitation, halted for many days. This is because an inappropriate progressive decision has been made.

9. Excessive and very detailed focus upon just one aspect of the patient's care. An example may be by spending the whole of the visit manipulating the ventilator, to the exclusion of a broad-based systems review involving other issues such as whether the patient is getting sufficient feed 5 days into their admission.

10. Considering extubation in a patient who either has a high secretion load or is very agitated. Under either of these circumstances, failure is likely.

11. Not increasing the overnight respiratory support (in order to secure a period of rest) for long-stay patients undergoing a slow-graded ventilator wean over many days.

12. Beware of making significant changes in routine support on the day of discharge. An example would be removal of the nasogastric tube and associated enteral feeding from a long-stay patient. Ward transition can be difficult for such individuals, particularly because of the reduction in nurse presence. In as little as a few days, basic nutritional requirements may be unfulfilled, leading to reversal of many days of progress whilst formerly in intensive care.

Conclusion

Context is paramount for successful ward round decision-making. We often make over 100 decisions during a business round and they are all formulated within a dynamic framework. Against a background of challenge, curiosity and our desire to advance the patient forward, we must also always be mindful of patient safety and the concept of non-maleficence. It is quite suitable on occasions to call a temporary halt to the weaning process, placing emphasis for the day upon rehabilitation and mobilisation. The decision therefore is 'no change'. This is especially true for long-term patients who are being managed on low levels of pressure support. Small decrements in the support at these levels can be significant for the individual. Time passing can aid recovery of muscle strength until the patient is ready to attempt further reduction of support. Ultimately, the MDT desires continual progress, rather than an alpine-like chart of 'one step forward – two steps back'.

Experience in leading the ward round informs upon the order and appropriateness regarding decision priorities and there can be no substitute for this. It is essential for the senior trainee in their advanced year to lead the process under observation, and this is one of the most valuable experiences they can have before graduating to consultant status.

The ward round is of central importance within the high-risk environment of the ICU, critical to providing high-quality safe care for patients in a timely, relevant manner. Good communication and a standardised structure are key features regarding its effectiveness.

References and Further Reading

Lane D, Ferri M, Lemaire J, Mclaughlin K, Stelfox H. A systematic review of evidence-informed practices for patient care rounds in the ICU. *Crit Care Med* 2013;**41**:2015–29.

Leape L, Cullen D, Clapp M, *et al*. Pharmacist participation on physician rounds and adverse drug events in the intensive care unit. *JAMA* 1999;**281**:267–70.

Morrison C, Jones M, Blackwell A, Vuylsteke A. Electronic patient record use during ward rounds: a qualitative study of interaction between medical staff. *Crit Care* 2008;**12**:R148.

Royal College of Physicians, Royal College of Nursing. 2012. Ward rounds in medicine –principles for best practice. www.colleaga.org/tools/ward-rounds-medicine-principles-best-practice

Royal College of Physicians, Royal College of Nursing. 2021. Modern ward rounds. www.rcplondon.ac.uk/projects/outputs/modern-ward-rounds

Vincent JL. Give your patient a fast hug (at least) once a day. *Crit Care Med* 2005;**33**:1225–9.

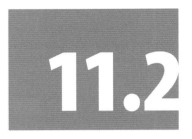

Principles and Compliance with Local Infection Control Measures

Julian Millo

Key Learning Points

1. Infection is a major cause for concern within critical care units.
2. Critically ill patients are particularly vulnerable to secondary infections.
3. Secondary prevention can be minimised by effective infection control measures.
4. Strict adherence to local infection control policies is appropriate.
5. Risks to healthcare workers need to be minimised.

Keywords: epidemiology, infection, colonisation, prevention, sepsis

Epidemiology of Infection in the ICU

Infection is a major problem for patients treated in intensive care. Despite extensive use of antibiotics, mortality is high. Increasing resistance to antibiotics is a major concern. In a worldwide prevalence study of infection in intensive care conducted in 2009, 51 per cent of nearly 14,000 patients were considered to be infected, and 71 per cent were receiving antibiotics. The most common sites of infection were the respiratory tract (62 per cent of cases), abdomen (20 per cent), bloodstream (15 per cent) and kidney or urinary tract (14 per cent). Microbiological cultures were positive in 70 per cent of infected patients. Commonly isolated pathogens included the Gram-positive organisms meticillin-sensitive *Staphylococcus aureus* (MSSA; 10 per cent of culture-positive patients), meticillin-resistant *S. aureus* (MRSA; 10 per cent), *Staphylococcus epidermidis* (also called coagulase-negative *S. aureus* or CONS; 10 per cent) and a smaller proportion of enterococci – some of which were resistant to the glycopeptide antibiotic vancomycin (vancomycin-resistant *Enterococcus* (VRE); 4 per cent). Gram-negative infections accounted for a greater proportion of cases of

infection (62 per cent). Causative Gram-negative organisms included *Escherichia coli, Enterobacter, Klebsiella* species (spp.), *Pseudomonas* spp., *Acinetobacter* spp. and numerous others. Antibiotic resistance due to extended-spectrum beta-lactamases (ESBLs) was noted in 3 per cent of cases of infection due to Gram-negative organisms. Anaerobes accounted for 5 per cent of cases of infection. By far, the most common cause of fungal infection was *Candida* spp. – isolated in 17 per cent of cases of infection. Infection was associated with longer length of stay (LOS) in the intensive care unit, longer hospital LOS and higher mortality (hospital mortality 33 percent versus 15 percent). In addition to these common causes of infection in intensive care, a range of other pathogens represent specific threats. Examples include *Clostridium difficile*-related disease, influenza, coronaviruses (e.g. severe acute respiratory syndrome (SARS), Middle Eastern respiratory syndrome (MERS)), viral haemorrhagic fevers (e.g. Ebola), tuberculosis (including multidrug-resistant tuberculosis) and *Candida auris*.

Mechanisms of Infection in the ICU

Colonisation, infection and sepsis represent a continuum of relationships between microorganisms and a given host. Individuals each have their own microbiome, the distribution and composition of which are influenced by exposure to microorganisms and antibiotic treatment. Colonisation is the presence of potentially pathogenic organisms. Infection is physiological disturbance due to microorganisms. Sepsis occurs when the host response to infection causes organ dysfunction or failure. Patients may become infected by microorganisms already present in their microbiome, most commonly with certain Gram-negative enteric bacteria. This can be termed 'autogenous' or 'endogenous' infection, and is the rationale for selective decontamination (*vide-infra*), a prospective treatment that can decrease the incidence of secondary infection in critically ill patients. Cross-infection is the transmission of infection from one patient to another. Important potential routes of transmission within the critical care unit include contact (particularly with the hands of healthcare workers) and airborne transmission. Droplet size influences both how long droplets remain airborne and the likely depth to which the respiratory tract will be penetrated. In concert with potential exposure to infective microorganisms, host defences are impaired by a number of mechanisms. Innate defences are breached by central venous catheters, and compromised by endotracheal tubes and sedative drugs. Severe illness causes post-acute impairment of host immunity, termed immunoparesis. Certain patient groups tend to be more susceptible to secondary infection. Risk factors include: extremes of age; high severity of illness scores; medications such as immunosuppression, corticosteroids or chemotherapy; patients with diabetes; and treatment with antibiotics. In addition to the patient, healthcare workers may contract infections, including by needlestick and splash injuries.

Approach to Infection Control

In 1847, the Hungarian physician Semmelweiss established the effectiveness of handwashing with an antiseptic agent to prevent puerperal sepsis, which, at the time, was a major cause of maternal mortality. His reward was to be hounded from the medical profession! In modern times, the success of national and international projects in reducing the incidence of nosocomial infections, such as catheter-associated bloodstream infections (CABSIs) and ventilator-associated pneumonia (VAP), was due, in part, to overcoming the reluctance of doctors to embrace infection control measures. Despite a number of advances, 6 per cent of hospital inpatients still acquire infection. Although deaths related to MRSA and *C. difficile* infections are decreasing, the incidence of *E. coli* infections is currently increasing. A proactive approach, openly demonstrating compliance with infection control measures, is appropriate. Monitoring and preventing healthcare-associated infection are mandated. For example, in 2016, the UK government announced an ambitious target of reducing Gram-negative bacteraemias by half by 2020.

Prevention of Infection in the ICU

The importance of prevention of infection was underlined in 2004 by the World Health Organization-sponsored 'World Alliance for Patient Safety' whereby 'Clean Care is Safer Care' was placed top of the Global Patient Safety Challenge. Effective hand hygiene practices were a key focus of this initiative. Evidence-based guidance promotes effective hand hygiene techniques, and the 'five moments for hand hygiene' prompts to perform hand hygiene frequently during patient care: before touching a patient, before a clean or aseptic procedure, after body fluid exposure/risk, after touching a patient and after touching a patient's surroundings.

Personal protective equipment (PPE), such as gloves, aprons or gowns, masks and protective eyewear, protects healthcare workers. Standard surgical masks, FFP3 masks and HEPA respirators afford increasingly greater degrees of protection against airborne pathogens. Sharps injuries are minimised by correct use of appropriate equipment and careful technique. If a sharps injury does occur, local policy should be followed. Appropriate vaccination decreases the risk to healthcare workers of both blood-borne and airborne infection. Clinical waste must be segregated and disposed of appropriately.

Cleaning, decontamination and sterilisation are complementary, yet distinct processes. Decontamination removes gross soiling and is a prerequisite to cleaning or sterilisation. Body fluid spillages (blood, faeces, vomit, urine and pus) may contain pathogens. Specific steps depend upon local protocols.

Isolation rooms within a critical care unit can protect both susceptible patients (e.g. those who are neutropenic) and staff and other patients from transmissible pathogens such as MRSA, influenza or tuberculosis. Traditional isolation rooms could be switched between positive and negative pressure. The modern configuration is a room accessed via an antechamber. Air within the antechamber is maintained at a higher pressure and flows into both the isolation room and the main critical care area.

References and Further Reading

Burke JP. Infection control – a problem for patient safety. *N Engl J Med* 2003;**348**:651–6.

Lim SM, Webb SA. Nosocomial bacterial infections in intensive care units. I: Organisms and mechanisms of antibiotic resistance. *Anaesthesia* 2005;**60**:887–902.

Malani PN. Preventing infections in the ICU: one size does not fit all. *JAMA* 2013;**310**:1567–8.

Russotto V, Cortegiani A, Graziano G, *et al.* Bloodstream infections in intensive care unit patients: distribution and antibiotic resistance of bacteria. *Infect Drug Resist* 2015;**8**:287–96.

11.3

Principles of Outcome Prediction, Prognostic Indicators and Treatment Intensity Scales and Limitations of Scoring Systems in Predicting Individual Patient Outcome

Andrew Selman, Peter Odor and Sohail Bampoe

Key Learning Points

1. Precise estimates of post-operative mortality and morbidity are difficult to obtain and both are recognised to vary greatly, depending on a patient's pre-operative functional status, the type and urgency of surgery and whether or not post-operative complications occur.

2. Risk scores apply a weighting to each factor, usually representing a component value for the score, with the resultant score corresponding with predicted risk.

3. Prognostic indicators may include population-based risk scores, individualised risk prediction models, objective functional capacity assessment and biomarkers.

4. Model discrimination describes how well a model discriminates between high- and low-risk patients, and is measured using a receiver operator characteristic curve (ROC) to calculate the area under the curve (AUC).

5. Technically, risk assessment tools are only valid for the specific patient population for whom the tool has been developed and on whom it has been tested.

Keywords: perioperative risk, post-operative complications, ASA, APACHE, SOFA, P-POSSUM, CPET

Why Assess Perioperative Risk?

Precise estimates of post-operative mortality and morbidity are difficult to obtain and both are recognised to vary greatly, depending on a patient's pre-operative functional status, the type and urgency of surgery and whether or not post-operative complications occur.

A small group of high-risk patients are responsible for over 80 per cent of perioperative deaths and prolonged hospitalisation, despite representing only 12.5 per cent of hospital admissions for surgery.

By identifying and quantifying risk in advance, we may be able to modify patient outcomes. Communicating this risk with patients can ensure that they are fully informed about those outcomes and their available treatment options. Potential harm could be avoided if high-risk patients decide upon lower efficacy, but lower-risk treatments, based upon risk prediction discussions. Resources, such as critical care, may be more effectively distributed.

How Do We Identify High-Risk Patients?

Risk scores are developed following a large-scale observational study of patients undergoing surgery, and multivariate regression analysis of measured factors determined to be independently associated with specific outcomes. Risk scores apply a weighting to each factor, usually representing a component value for the score, with the resultant score corresponding with predicted risk. Although these population-based risk scores allow comparisons to be made with other generalised groups of patients, they do not provide an individualised description of risk.

Population-Based Risk Scores
The American Society of Anesthesiologists (ASA) Score

The ASA score has undergone minor revision over the last 70 years, but the current version is very similar to the 1941 original – a five-point scale of systemic fitness. Application of the score involves subjective assessment of the presence and severity of a patient's pre-operative systemic disease. Survival following surgery has been shown to correlate with the ASA score across a number of different settings. Unfortunately, the ASA score makes no adjustment for demographic characteristics, nor for procedure-specific risk, and is poorly predictive of actual outcomes, with complications only being correctly predicted in a minority of patients. An alternative to the ASA score is the Charlson Comorbidity Index, which was originally developed to predict 10-year mortality in medical patients but has been validated for use in surgical patients too.

Organ-Specific Scoring Systems

The Goldman Cardiac Risk Index or the more recent Revised Cardiac Risk Index (or Lee's score) are common examples of organ-specific risk scores. The ARISCAT (Assess Respiratory Risk in Surgical Patients in Catalonia Tool) respiratory failure index predicts the likelihood of post-operative pulmonary complications after non-cardiac surgery. A score for risk of acute kidney injury following surgery has also been developed.

Physiological Risk Scores

The Acute Physiology and Chronic Health Evaluation (APACHE) is now in its third revised format. It can be used to assess perioperative risk, but needs to be done during the first 24 hours of admission and does not take into account the type of surgery. Therefore, it is mostly used in critical care to assess risk of mortality. Other examples are the Simplified Acute Physiology Score (SAPS) and the Mortality Prediction Model (MPM).

Systems Scoring Multiple Organ Dysfunction

The Sequential Organ Failure Assessment (SOFA), previously known as Sepsis-related Organ Failure Assessment, uses six physiological variables to score the level of organ dysfunction related to sepsis, but is also validated for assessing organ dysfunction not related to sepsis. The score is then converted into a percentage for morbidity and mortality. The Multiple Organ Dysfunction Score (MODS) also uses six physiological variables to give a score in the same way as SOFA.

Individualised Risk Prediction Models

The Portsmouth Physiological and Operative Severity Score for the enUmeration of Mortality and morbidity (P-POSSUM) is the physiology and operative severity score for the enumeration of mortality and morbidity. POSSUM was developed in 1991, with the 'P' added in 1998 to denote Portsmouth when it was updated to correct for an over-predicted mortality percentage in low-risk groups. It takes into account 12 physiological variables and six surgical variables, and is regularly used in general surgical patients.

The Surgical Outcome Risk Tool (SORT) is a pre-operative risk prediction tool used to predict risk of death within 30 days of surgery for non-neurosurgical and non-cardiac surgery. Its variables are type of surgery, severity and urgency, ASA score, whether the surgery is in one of the three higher-risk groups (thoracic, vascular or gastrointestinal), whether the patient has cancer and three age classifications.

A common risk prediction model used in the United States is the American College of Surgeons National Surgical Quality Improvement Program (ACS NSQIP®). This considers surgical and physiological data to calculate a percentage risk for multiple types of complication, as well as mortality and readmission. It uses data from >3.2 million operations in 668 hospitals across the United States, but it only includes patients in the United States, and so its applicability to patients in the UK is unclear.

Objective Functional Capacity Assessment

Functional capacity assessment involves measurement of global or organ-specific performance, in order to predict post-operative outcome. Traditional functional capacity can be subjectively assessed using metabolic equivalents (METs). This approach is recommended by the American Heart Association and the European Society of Cardiology. One MET is equivalent to 3.5 ml/(kg min), which is the rate of oxygen consumption of a healthy 40-year-old male weighing 70 kg, at rest. The number of METs is quantified as the maximum physical activity a patient can achieve. Being unable to achieve at least 4 METs (climbing two flights of stairs) puts a patient at increased risk of post-operative morbidity and mortality. The obvious limitation to this score is in patients who are unable to achieve this because of non-cardiorespiratory limitations to exercise.

Cardiopulmonary exercise testing (CPET) is a functional assessment carried out on an exercise bike, with periods of increasing cardiovascular work, whilst recording multiple variables. It is popular because it assesses pulmonary, cardiac and circulatory function, all at the same time, and quantifies the patient's functional ability to adapt to increased metabolic demands. The results are presented in a nine-panel plot of the data obtained, the most commonly used being the anaerobic threshold and maximum utilisation of oxygen. It is a useful pre-operative risk stratification tool for predicting post-operative outcome but needs further evaluation in some surgical subspecialties.

Biomarkers

Using biomarkers when assessing perioperative risk is a newer approach. There is evidence that use of N-terminal fragment of B-type natriuretic peptide (NT-pro-BNP), troponin and high-sensitivity C-reactive protein (hsCRP) is helpful in predicting adverse outcomes. Despite this, it is not yet clear how we should manage patients with elevated levels or which patients will benefit most from intervention.

Assessment of Frailty

Frailty is a state of vulnerability leading to poor resolution of homeostasis after a stressor event. It is the result of cumulative functional decline of the body's organ systems with age, and scores attempt to predict the level of physical independence retained or dependence acquired following surgery. These are likely to play an important role in risk stratification of patients in an increasingly ageing population.

Limitations of Scoring Systems

The principle behind testing risk prediction models is known as model validation and uses the concepts of model calibration and discrimination. Model calibration, how well the prediction agrees with the actual outcome, uses goodness of fit and is defined as a p-value. Model discrimination describes how well a model discriminates between high- and low-risk patients and is measured using an ROC to calculate the AUC.

Technically, risk assessment tools are only valid for the specific patient population for whom the tool has been developed and on whom it has been tested. Many of the scoring systems are designed for specific patient populations, such as elderly patients with hip fracture, and therefore, tool performance is linked to the clinical context. Even the more generally applicable tools are still population-specific, meaning that the NSQIP model developed in the United States will not necessarily produce accurate predictions for patients in the UK, since it has not been validated yet.

References and Further Reading

Bilimoria KY, Liu Y, Paruch JL, *et al.* Development and evaluation of the universal ACS NSQIP surgical risk calculator: a decision aid and informed consent tool for patients and surgeons. *J Am Coll Surg* 2013;**217**:833–42.e1–3.

Ferreira FL, Bota DP, Bross A, Mélot C, Vincent JL. Serial evaluation of the SOFA score to predict outcome in critically ill patients. *JAMA* 2001;**286**:1754–8.

Moran J, Wilson F, Guinan E, McCormick P, Hussey J, Moriarty J. Role of cardiopulmonary exercise testing as a risk-assessment method in patients undergoing intra-abdominal surgery: a systematic review. *Br J Anaesth* 2016;**116**:177–91.

Protopapa KL, Simpson JC, Smith NCE, Moonesinghe SR. Development and validation of the Surgical Outcome Risk Tool (SORT). *Br J Surg* 2014;**101**:1774–83.

Prytherch DR, Whiteley MS, Higgins B, Weaver PC, Prout WG, Powell SJ. POSSUM and Portsmouth POSSUM for predicting mortality. *Br J Surg* 1998;**85**:1217–20.

Vincent JL, Moreno R, Takala J, *et al.* The SOFA (Sepsis-related Organ Failure Assessment) score to describe organ dysfunction/failure. On behalf of the Working Group on Sepsis-Related Problems of the European Society of Intensive Care Medicine. *Intensive Care Med* 1996;**22**:707–10.

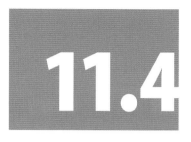

11.4

Scoring Systems for Severity of Illness in Critical Care

Katie Samuel and Sam Bampoe

Key Learning Points

1. Predictive scoring systems can use physiological, clinical and laboratory data to predict critical care patient mortality.
2. Their use extends to enabling standardisation of research cohorts, comparing and auditing critical care units and triaging critical care provision.
3. The most commonly used general scoring systems worldwide are APACHE (Acute Physiology and Chronic Health Evaluation) II and SOFA (Sequential Organ Failure Assessment) scores.
4. All systems need to be validated for calibration and discrimination, and have the potential to become less accurate over time.
5. No one system is better than any other – all have advantages and disadvantages.

Keywords: severity of illness, predictive scoring systems, APACHE, SAPS, Mortality Prediction Model

Introduction

In order to assess the severity of illness in intensive care patients, a number of predictive scoring systems can be employed. These systems not only can be used to predict patient outcomes, but have use in standardising research groups, comparing and auditing the quality of patient care between units, as well as triaging critical care provision in major incidents.

The available scoring systems have been developed and validated in multi-centre studies using data from ICUs, and generally use physiological and laboratory data, in combination with clinical information, to provide numerical illness severity scores. These are calculated using model-specific algorithms and mostly provide an estimate of in-hospital mortality. Various

factors have been shown to contribute to patient mortality after admission to the ICU (e.g. increasing age, severity of acute illness, pre-existing malignancy); these therefore carry a weighted value.

Validity

To use scoring systems appropriately in clinical practice, they need to have been appraised for validity. This is done by assessing model calibration (the correspondence between a range of predicted and actual mortalities in a population) and discrimination (the individual sensitivity and specificity of a prediction).

Calibration can deteriorate over time; new patient interventions evolve, and the case-mix of admitted patients changes. This tends to lead to an overestimation of mortality for any given score, which similarly reduces discrimination. Updating predictive systems periodically is therefore needed to maintain their validity.

Scoring Systems

There are a large number of predictive scoring systems that have been created – the most commonly used are discussed below.

Acute Physiologic and Chronic Health Evaluation (APACHE I, II, III, VI)

The APACHE score is the most widely used physiology-based score worldwide. Initially created in 1981, it has undergone modification to reduce the number of variables needed for ease of use, whilst maintaining its discriminatory value. APACHE II is most commonly used, scoring a patient on 12 physiological variables, chronic health conditions and type of admission, which are collected within 24 hours; the 'worst' scoring variable within this time is used. Each variable is given a weighted score, with a maximum score of 71 – for reference, a score of 25 represents a predicted mortality of 50 per cent, and a score of over 35 represents a predicted mortality of 80 per cent (Table 11.4.1).

Table 11.4.1 APACHE II scoring parameters

Parameter	Points
Age	0–6
Temperature	0–5
Mean arterial pressure	0–4
Heart rate	0–4
Respiratory rate	0–4
PaO_2/A–a gradient	0–4
Arterial pH	0–4
Sodium	0–4
Potassium	0–4
Creatinine (acute or chronic)	0–8
Haematocrit	0–4
White cell count	0–4
Glasgow Coma Score	0–15
Chronic organ insufficiency[a] (with/without emergency admission)	0–5

[a] Liver: cirrhosis, portal hypertension, gastrointestinal bleed related to portal hypertension, hepatic encephalopathy; cardiovascular: New York Heart Association class IV heart failure; respiratory: chronic disease causing severe exercise restriction, chronic hypoxia, hypercarbia, secondary polycythaemia, pulmonary hypertension, respiratory dependency; renal replacement therapy; immunosuppression.

Simplified Acute Physiology Score (SAPS I, II, III)

Based on physiological parameters such as the APACHE scoring system, SAPS uses values measured within the first 24 hours of ICU admission. The most commonly used SAPS II uses dichotomous scoring variables for co-morbidities, as well as for physiological data, by categorising ranges of continuous measurements (e.g. a systolic blood pressure of 70–99 mmHg scores 5 points). SAPS uses fewer scoring parameters than APACHE and therefore is useful in facilitating quick and efficient data collection (Table 11.4.2).

Mortality Prediction Model (MPM I, II, III)

MPM uses only physiological variables (no laboratory data) taken at the time of ICU admission, again in a dichotomous fashion, apart from age. The predictive score can be repeated serially (e.g. at 72 hours) to gauge disease progression.

Sequential Organ Failure Assessment (SOFA)

Although originally produced to sequentially describe the degree of organ dysfunction in septic patients,

Table 11.4.2 SAPS II scoring parameters

Parameter	Points
Heart rate	0–11
Systolic blood pressure	0–13
Temperature	0–3
PaO_2/FiO_2 (only if invasively/non-invasively ventilated)	6–11
Urine output	0–11
White cell count	0–12
Urea	0–10
Potassium	0–3
Sodium	0–5
Bicarbonate	0–6
Bilirubin	0–9
Glasgow Coma Score	0–26
Age	0–18
Chronic disease[a]	0–17
Admission type (medical/elective/emergency surgical)	0–8

[a] Metastatic cancer, haematological malignancies, acquired immune deficiency syndrome.

SOFA has since been validated for use in other causes of organ dysfunction, including haematopoietic stem cell transplant and cardiac surgery. It uses measurements of six organ systems to give a weighted score, with a maximum of 24:

- Respiratory – PaO_2/FiO_2 ratio and respiratory support
- Cardiovascular – amount of vasoactive medications
- Central nervous system – Glasgow Coma Score
- Renal – serum creatinine and urine output
- Coagulation – platelet number
- Liver – serum bilirubin

The SOFA score is measured as the worst value within the first 24 hours, and then every 48 hours afterwards. This allows a sequential assessment of organ dysfunction, with not only the highest and mean scores being predicative of mortality, but also an increase of 30 per cent in score being associated with over 50 per cent mortality.

Quick SOFA (qSOFA) is a simplified version validated to identify septic patients in non-ICU settings (e.g. emergency department). A point is scored for:

- Respiratory rate >22 breaths/min
- Altered mentation, and
- Systolic blood pressure <100 mmHg.

Scoring 2 or more is reported as leading to poorer outcomes.

Table 11.4.3 Comparison of commonly used illness severity predictive scoring systems

Scoring system	Commonly used version	Outcome measures	Advantages	Disadvantages	Study population
APACHE	APACHE II	Mortality (APACHE IV – LOS)	Accurate and well established	High number of input variables for versions I, III and IV	5800 patients, USA Excluded burns, uncomplicated myocardial infarction
SAPS	SAPS II	Mortality	Easier data extraction – fewer measured variables Validated internationally	Cannot predict LOS	13,100 patients, USA and Europe Excluded <18 years, burns, coronary care, cardiac surgery
MPM	MPM II	Mortality	Easiest data extraction (no laboratory data needed)	Cannot predict LOS Most susceptible to poor validity over time	6500 patients, USA and Europe Excluded <18 years, burns, coronary care, cardiac surgery
SOFA		Mortality	Most accurate for septic patients Gives sequential data	No percentage of predicted mortality given	1400 patients, worldwide Excluded <13 years, admissions <48 hours following uncomplicated surgery

Abbreviation: LOS = length of stay.

Considerations and Limitations

No one model has been proven better than another – all have their advantages and disadvantages (Table 11.4.3).

Ease of use is a consideration when choosing which model to use – those with a larger number of variable inputs will be more time-consuming to collate. As electronic clinical records are becoming more commonplace, once the time and cost of setting up an automatic data entry system has been considered, the ongoing calculation of any method of risk prediction is undemanding.

Risk prediction calculators were not widely and freely available in the past, which has contributed to the preference for some models over others. Now the majority are easily found in the public domain. Some subscription models do allow for customisation to better reflect units' case-mix.

Limitation in using risk prediction tools needs to be considered to avoid inappropriate interpretation of results. The original validated population for each tool may not be generalisable to all worldwide healthcare institutions or patients (e.g. obstetric and burns patients). Individual units' case-mix may therefore limit the application of some models. In addition, if patients are transferred from other hospitals or units, a lead-time bias can occur whereby their mortality is actually higher than predicted by some scoring systems (APACHE II in particular).

Disease-Specific Scoring systems

Besides generalised ICU scoring systems, there are also disease- and organ-specific scoring systems. These have use in assessment of disease severity, triggering referral to the ICU and aiding clinical decisions in appropriateness of critical care provision.

These include:

- Model for End-Stage Liver Disease (MELD) – prognosis of chronic liver disease (used in place of the older Child–Pugh Score)
- Modified Glasgow Score – acute pancreatitis severity
- Trauma Injury Severity Score (TRISS) – probability of survival from trauma
- Intracerebral Haemorrhage (ICH) Score – prognostication after ICH
- Rockall Score – severity and prognosis of upper gastrointestinal bleeding.

References and Further Reading

Bouch DC, Thompson JP. Severity scoring systems in the critically ill. *Contin Educ Anaesth Crit Care Pain* 2008;**8**:181–5.

Breslow MJ, Badawi O. Severity scoring in the critically ill: Part 1—interpretation and accuracy of outcome prediction scoring systems. *Chest* 2012;**141**:245–52.

Breslow MJ, Badawi O. Severity scoring in the critically ill: Part 2: maximizing value from outcome prediction scoring systems. *Chest* 2012;**141**:518–27.

Kelley MA. 2021. Predictive scoring systems in the intensive care unit. www.uptodate.com/contents/predictive-scoring-systems-in-the-intensive-care-unit

Vincent J-L, Moreno R. Clinical review: scoring systems in the critically ill. *Crit Care* 2010;**14**:207.

11.5 Managerial and Administrative Responsibilities of the Intensive Care Medicine Specialist

Alison Pittard

Key Learning Points

1. The role of the intensive care medicine specialist as a manager, or leader, contributes to the efficiency of the intensive care unit.
2. These non-clinical responsibilities evolve over the lifetime of the specialist's career.
3. A significant proportion of the managerial and administrative work occurs as part of normal daily activities.
4. The lead clinician or clinical director will assume most of the strategic responsibilities, but some of these, and those directly related to service delivery, may be delegated.
5. Local/national healthcare legislation and the ethical framework within which medicine is practised will affect strategic decision-making.

Keywords: management, safety, strategy, legislation, administration

Introduction

Intensive care medicine (ICM) is a very practical, 'hands-on' specialty, yet there is a huge managerial and administrative burden that underpins the delivery of a high-quality service. Some of this is overt, but much of it occurs as part of normal daily activity, with the extent of responsibility dependent on the grade of doctor. In addition to this are the non-specialist requirements that the organisation, the NHS or the government demands of all doctors. In this chapter, the latter will be mentioned for completeness, but unless they are of particular significance in ICM, they will not be explored.

The Responsibility Spiral

The role of the intensivist as a manager, or leader, is embedded in curricula, and acquisition of these skills contributes to the efficiency of the ICU. Initially, the responsibilities of an ICM specialist are mainly clinical, e.g. maintenance of legible, contemporaneous medical records, safe prescribing, following guidelines, continuity of care through detailed handover practices and discharge summaries. The skills underpinning this performance, such as good communication, teamwork/leadership and quality and safety, are part of the Generic Professional Capabilities framework. They form the foundations upon which the specialist develops and becomes more involved in the running of the unit and shaping its progress. As experience continues, the specialist will become more confident, e.g. in writing coroner's reports or police statements. The principles of healthcare legislation, such as child protection, mental health and surrogate decision-making, become real as does the associated administrative burden. The specialist may begin to influence guidelines through local committees, appraising the literature and utilising expert knowledge to promote quality and safety. Such a managerial role may lead on to involvement at a regional or national level. Whatever the geography, it is a managerial/administrative responsibility of the ICM specialist and should be recognised as important.

The Lead Clinician/Clinical Director

This is a well-recognised responsibility of the ICM specialist, usually a senior medical member of the clinical ICU team. This non-clinical role enhances the quality of patient management and the efficacy of the ICU, and is a core standard in the UK. Guidelines for the Provision of Intensive Care Services (GPICS) establish the important non-clinical responsibilities, but depending on local circumstances, some may be delegated to other team members to share the burden.

Strategic

- **Design and planning** – this requires an understanding of the requirements for the structure, function and financing of the service, departmental budgeting, healthcare economics and the ability to develop a business case. Knowledge of current governmental building regulations is essential when considering critical care design.

- **Resource management** – healthcare is a finite resource requiring effective and efficient management to ensure maximum benefit. The GPICS has defined the optimum staffing establishment for all healthcare professionals and non-clinical staff in the ICU. Workforce planning, vital if patient safety and quality of care are to be maintained, requires interaction with local workforce managers, regional service delivery managers and national bodies such as the Faculty of Intensive Care Medicine and Department of Health. Equipment is another resource that must be managed effectively to ensure optimum selection. When considering resource allocation, it is important to consider the ethical principles underpinning this, and the legislative framework within which healthcare in the UK is provided.

- **Quality assurance** – there are a number of different levels to this, from a personal clinician's responsibility to an organisational one. All doctors must engage in an annual appraisal process and be revalidated every 5 years. This also encompasses maintaining one's health, reporting mistakes/errors and fostering an open culture to learn from such events. It is also important for individuals to be aware of the team around them and, in an area where patients are critically unwell and dependent on highly skilled personnel and complex technology, recognise and act upon impaired function. The lead clinician, in conjunction with others, will identify occupational and safety hazards and either implement mechanisms to prevent harm or raise them with risk management.

Delivery

- **Leadership** – as well as being a member of the multidisciplinary team, the ICM specialist has a leadership role. Both within and outside the ICU, e.g. hospital wards or in the emergency department, it is important to consider the risk–benefit and cost-effectiveness of treatment, gain the trust of other members of the team, manage competing priorities and be capable of triage management. Conflict can arise, and to resolve this in a mutually acceptable way requires good negotiating skills.

- **Clinical audit and quality improvement** – advances in medical research and national guidelines should be critically appraised and, where appropriate, their integration into clinical practice facilitated. It is the responsibility of the ICM specialist to ensure the clinical care they provide is safe and effective, patient-centred, timely and equitable. Engagement in local and national critical incident reporting processes is also fundamental for maintaining patient safety and quality of care.

It is important to realise that the ICM specialist does not need a management title to have an administrative responsibility. The knowledge, skills and behaviours required to be a good leader are embedded in training programmes, being recognised as a core component of our daily work. Some will want a more formal role, but the majority contribute without realising.

References and Further Reading

Department of Health. 2013. Health Building Note 04–02. Critical care units. www.england.nhs.uk/publication/critical-care-units-planning-and-design-hbn-04-02/

General Medical Council. Generic Professional Capabilities Framework. www.gmc-uk.org/education/standards-guidance-and-curricula/standards-and-outcomes/generic-professional-capabilities-framework

The Faculty of Intensive Care Medicine. 2019. Guidelines for the Provision of Intensive Care, edn 2. www.ficm.ac.uk/sites/default/files/gpics-v2.pdf

The Faculty of Intensive Care Medicine. 2019. The CCT in Intensive Care Medicine – Part III. Syllabus. www.ficm.ac.uk/sites/default/files/cct_in_icm_part_iii_-_syllabus_2019_v2.4.pdf

Valentin A, Ferdinande P; ESICM Working Group on Quality Improvement. Recommendations on basic requirements for intensive care units: structural and organizational aspects. *Intensive Care Med* 2011;**37**:1575–87.

11.6 Communication in Intensive Care

Orlanda Allen and Dev Dutta

Key Learning Points

1. Patients and their representatives (family or friends) have identified effective communication as a critical component of high-quality care whilst in the ICU.
2. Support for patients' advocates is, in some instances, just as important as the care of the patients themselves.
3. Do not underestimate the importance of prior preparation before meeting a family.
4. Given the dynamic ICU environment and the multi-professional nature of the care, clear documentation is imperative.
5. A medical record is a legally binding document.

Keywords: communication, intensive care unit, healthcare professionals, preparation, medical records, documentation

The Importance of Communication in ICU

The ICU is a complex environment in which care providers are trained to carry out standard interventions and treatments aimed at reversing serious illness. Patients and their representatives (family or friends) have identified effective communication as a critical component of high-quality care whilst in the ICU. Critically ill patients often require intensive support and, as a consequence, may not be able to make decisions or express their personal wishes regarding care. In these circumstances, their representatives can find themselves unexpectedly in the position of having to act as advocates for patients. For many, this can be fraught with anxiety and negative emotions, especially if the patient's wishes regarding artificial life support interventions have not been previously established.

Effective Communication with Patients and Their Representatives

Support for patients' advocates is, in some instances, just as important as the care of the patients themselves. Family dynamics can be complex, and providers must anticipate and be able to manage these various sensitivities. Communication skills can be acquired and developed, based on a number of principles outlined below.

Planning for Meetings with Patients and Their Advocates

Preparation

- Appropriate time frame available for discussion
- Suitable environment, e.g. privacy, comfort, with appropriate facilities (adequate seating, drinks, tissues, etc.)
- Awareness of family disputes
- Gathering all relevant information
- Update of patient condition and further history taking

Meeting Attendees

- Patient, when possible, bedside meeting appropriate
- Patient advocates, e.g. legal surrogate decision-makers and important people (next of kin) or other patient representatives
- Intensive care team
- Interpreter for non-English speakers
- Bedside nurse acting as family advocate
- Social worker or pastoral care worker if appropriate
- Religious/spiritual support if appropriate

Meeting Management

- Objectives of the meeting set
- Open disclosure

- Knowledge; previous history, previous statements about medical care, current ICU prognosis, likelihood of recovery
- Exploring complex choices and decision-making
- Change in therapeutic goals and expectations
- Second opinions if needed
- Conflict resolution between healthcare professionals and family members
- Discussion of palliation if appropriate
- Discussion of organ and tissue donation

Maintaining Accurate, Legible Legal records

Documentation is an extremely important form of communication. Given the dynamic ICU environment and the multi-professional nature of the care, clear documentation is imperative.

A medical record is a legally binding document and the following need to be rigorously observed.

- Handwriting must be legible, and appropriate coloured ink used to facilitate photocopying or scanning of documents.
- Records must be accurate and written in such a way that the meaning is clear. They must demonstrate a full account of the assessment made, care planned and provided and any action taken or not.
- All entries must be dated – day/month/year, timed and signed.
- All entries providing information on care and condition of the patient must be recorded as soon as possible after an event has occurred.
- In the event of an error being made, an incorrect entry must be corrected by striking it through with one line, and applying the author's initials, the time and date by the correction. The original entry must still be legible. Errors must not be amended or deleted using correction fluid, scribbling out or writing over them.

References and Further Reading

British Medical Association Board of Medical Education. *Communication Skills for Doctors: An Update*. London: British Medical Association; 2004.

Gillon S, Wright C, Knott C, McPhail M, Camporota L. *Revision Notes in Intensive Care*. Oxford: Oxford University Press; 2016.

Medical Protection Society. *MPS Guide to Medical Records*. London: Medical Protection Society; 2008.

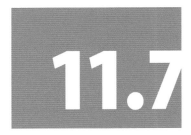

Professional Relationships with Members of the Healthcare Team

11.7

Orlanda Allen and Dev Dutta

Key Learning Points

1. Clear and effective communication is crucial between healthcare teams.
2. A clear and informative handover is essential for ensuring the continuity of excellent patient care.
3. The role of an intensivist not only involves the delivery of care on an intensive care unit, but rather extends across the whole hospital at all hours.
4. Patient-centred care and safety are your primary concerns.
5. The intensivist is also a key player in creating a positive working environment that both respects and encourages the input and contribution of other team members in making the best decisions for patient care.

Keywords: teamwork, multidisciplinary, handover, patient-centred, supporting colleagues

Teamwork and Collaboration

In the ICU, the doctor benefits from being a member of a patient-centred team providing a wide range of professional skills. Good communication amongst all members of the team is essential. This is facilitated by regular multidisciplinary team (MDT) meetings scheduled once or twice a week, and must include all healthcare professionals involved in the patient's care. Patients and their representatives will have contact with several different members of the team at various times, and from their perspective, a coordinated and consistent response is reassuring. Inadequate communication within the MDT has been repeatedly identified as an underlying factor when communication with patients and their representatives has broken down or been poorly managed.

Ensuring Continuity of Care through Effective Handover of Clinical Information

A clear and informative handover is essential for ensuring the continuity of excellent patient care. All patient benefits gained in a shift can be undone if poor, or worse still no, communication occurs between medical professionals.

Handovers should be:

- Of sufficient duration
- Multidisciplinary and, whenever possible, must include senior clinician involvement
- Designated as 'bleep-free', except for life-threatening emergencies
- At all shift changes, e.g. 5 p.m., 8 p.m., 8 a.m.
- Supervised by the most senior clinician present
- Succinct and include only relevant information, ideally supported by IT systems
  A verbal handover should also be given for:
- Patients with anticipated problems, to clarify management plans and ensure appropriate reviews
- Outstanding tasks, together with a required timelines for completion

Supporting Clinical Staff outside ICU and Contribution of Appropriate Supervision, Training and Delegation

The role of an intensivist not only involves the delivery of care on an ICU, but rather extends across the whole hospital at all hours. This may include:

- Identification of deteriorating ward-based patients and early intervention

- Identification of patients requiring formal admission to areas of higher levels of support
- Follow-up of recently discharged patients to reduce the risk of readmission
- Support for ward staff where immediate care needs may be beyond their skill sets
- Initiation of palliative care/end-of-life measures, where appropriate, on deteriorating patients

Patient-centred care and safety are your primary concerns, and it is easy to forget that tasks and jobs that we find easy to perform, and perhaps expect to be done promptly on an ICU, are not so easily accomplished on a busy ward where one nurse may be looking after 15 different patients – each with their own demands. Take time to ensure that the staff involved with ward patient care are able to carry out any tasks required of them, and in a time frame you deem fit, and utilise the whole MDT.

Additionally, the role carries a wide range of other responsibilities, from teaching juniors new skills through to supervision of many different professionals and specialties, including medical teams within the ward environment. Providing both leadership and support, through training, appropriate delegation of tasks and reassurance in decision-making, allows colleagues and team members the confidence to develop their roles and responsibilities. The intensivist is also a key player in creating a positive working environment that both respects and encourages the input and contribution of other team members in making the best decisions for patient care.

References and Further Reading

British Medical Association. Safe handover, safe patients. Guidance on clinical handover for clinicians and managers. London: British Medical Association; 2004.

General Medical Council. Good medical practice. www .gmc-uk.org/ethical-guidance/ethical-guidance-for-doctors/good-medical-practice

Lanceley A, Savage J, Menson U, Jacobs I. Influences on multidisciplinary team decision making. *Int J Gynaecol Cancer* 2008;**18**:215–22.

Pendleton D, Schofield T, Tate P, Havelock P. *The Consultation: An Approach to Learning and Teaching.* Oxford: Oxford University Press; 1984.

11.8 Legal and Ethical Issues in Intensive Care

Chris Danbury

Key Learning Points

1. The capacity to make an autonomous decision is central to all of modern medicine.
2. Valid consent requires the voluntary decision of an individual with capacity who has been given adequate information.
3. When a patient lacks the capacity to consent, then the justification for treating them is best interests.
4. Mediation is a process where the two (or more) sides of a dispute have a structured conversation to try and find a mutually acceptable resolution.
5. The results of mediation showed that between 60 and 90 per cent of disputes settled without the need to go to court.

Keywords: ethics, capacity, consent, best interests, conflict resolution

Introduction

Law and ethics play a big part in intensive care medicine. Our patients are frequently unconscious and there are often time-critical decisions to be made about the treatment they receive. There are a number of key themes that need to be considered by the practising intensive care physician. There are other textbooks considering the subject in a more detailed way.

Capacity

The capacity to make an autonomous decision is central to all of modern medicine. In England and Wales, it is underpinned by the Mental Capacity Act 2005. This Act states in Paragraph 2 that:

> A person must be assumed to have capacity unless it is established that he lacks capacity.

This flows from common law decisions taken over a great many years.

In 1972, Lord Reid in *S* v. *McC*: *W* v. *W* [1972] AC 25 said, on p. 43:

> … English law goes to great lengths to protect a person of full age and capacity from interference with his personal liberty. We have too often seen freedom disappear in other countries not only by coups d'état, but by gradual erosion: and often it is the first step that counts. So it would be unwise to make even minor concessions.

In re F (Mental Patient: Sterilisation) [1990] 2 AC 1, Lord Goff of Chieveley said on p. 72:

> I start with the fundamental principle, now long established, that every person's body is inviolate.

Lord Donaldson of Lymington, MR said in re T (Adult: Refusal of Treatment) [1993] Fam. 95, on p. 113:

> … the patient's right of choice exists whether the reasons for making that choice are rational, irrational, unknown or even non-existent.

This includes life-sustaining treatment, as Dame Butler-Sloss said in *Ms B* v. *An NHS Hospital Trust* [2002] EWHC 429:

> I am therefore entirely satisfied that Ms B is competent to make all relevant decisions about her medical treatment including the decision whether to seek to withdraw from artificial ventilation. Her mental competence is commensurate with the gravity of the decision she may wish to make.

In order to have capacity, a person must be able to:

1. Understand the information relevant to the decision
2. Retain that information for as long as is necessary to take the decision
3. Use the information as part of the process of making the decision

4. Communicate their decision (whether by talking, using sign language or any other means)

If a person has capacity to make decisions, then those decisions must be respected, even if the intensive care physician considers that the decision is unwise.

Consent

Consent to treatment follows from capacity. Consent is the respect we give to an autonomous person. Valid consent requires the voluntary decision of an individual with capacity who has been given adequate information. Failure to give that information may be considered to be negligent, as seen in the case of *Montgomery* v. *Lanarkshire Health Board* [2015] UKSC 11 (UKSC (2015) 11 March 2015):

> … Although [the doctor's] evidence indicates that it was her policy to withhold information … from her patients … the 'therapeutic exception' is not intended to enable doctors to prevent their patients from taking an informed decision. Rather, it is the doctor's responsibility to explain to her patient why she considers that one of the available treatment options is medically preferable to the others, having taken care to ensure that her patient is aware of the considerations for and against each of them.

This is a difficult area as patients will often be affected by drugs, disease process and other factors which may affect their ability both to have capacity and to be able to give consent to the treatment in the ICU.

The court's approach is to usually maximise future opportunities. Therefore, it is unlikely that any remedy or sanction will be applied to a clinician who treats a patient to stabilise them, in order for them to be able to subsequently participate in the decision-making process about the patient's future care.

Simply put: treat first, worry about the rest when there is time – later!

Best Interests

When a patient lacks capacity to consent, then the justification for treating them is best interests.

This can be a difficult concept to understand. As the Mental Capacity Act Code of Practice says, the decision-maker (the intensivist in this situation) **must** take into account:

- the person's past and present wishes and feelings
- these may have been expressed verbally, in writing or through behaviour or habits.

- any beliefs and values (e.g. religious, cultural, moral or political) that would be likely to influence the decision in question.
- any other factors the person themselves would be likely to consider if they were making the decision or acting for themselves.

As well, the intensivist should 'consult other people for their views about the person's best interests and to see if they have any information about the person's wishes and feelings, beliefs and values'. The wording of the Act says that the consultation should occur if it is reasonable and appropriate to do so. In the context of an ICU, if the relative is there in person, it is difficult to conceive of a situation where it would be unreasonable or inappropriate to talk to that relative, no matter how difficult or unpleasant the discussion may be. Therefore, for all intents and purposes, the Act places an obligation on us to talk to relatives in order to aid us determine the best interests of our patient.

Recently, case law has guided us on how the courts would consider a disagreement between relatives and doctors about best interests. Although relating to a brain-dead child, Mr Justice Hayden said in A (A Child), Re (Rev 1) [2015] EWHC 443 (Fam):

> I am very clear that should a difference of view arise between treating clinicians and family members in circumstances where assisted ventilation is continuing, any dispute, if it cannot be resolved otherwise, should be determined in the High Court, not under coronial powers.

More recently, Mr Justice Peter Jackson said in M (Withdrawal of Treatment: Need for Proceedings) 2017 EWCOP 19 about whether there was a requirement to go to court:

> … the decision about what was in M's best interests is one that could lawfully have been taken by her treating doctors, having fully consulted her family and having acted in accordance with the Mental Capacity Act and with recognised medical standards. These standards will doubtless evolve …

The message appears clear – if there is no disagreement between clinicians and family about what is the best interests of the patient, then decisions can be made, including end-of-life decisions. However, if there is disagreement, and then ultimately if there is no alternative way of resolving the disagreement, then the Court of Protection must decide.

Conflict Resolution

How likely is it to go to court? In 2014/15, there were 258,956 critical care admissions. The case-mix programme from the Intensive Care National Audit & Research Centre (ICNARC) suggests that ICU mortality in the UK is approximately 18 per cent. Therefore, there were around 46,600 deaths in ICUs in the UK in 2014/15. From the Ethicus study, we know that at least 70 per cent of deaths in the ICU involve some decision-making by the treating team. The decision is usually to either withhold or withdraw treatment, knowing that the patient will die as result of that decision. The data further suggest that over 90 per cent of these patients go on to die in the ICU. So there is a small group of patients who do survive despite the decision to withhold or withdraw. The Conflicus study reported that 'Although ICU directors reported few conflicts, families and ICU physicians and nurses perceived conflicts for up to 80 per cent of patients requiring treatment-limitation decisions'. Therefore, using the data above from 2014/15, there was probably some degree of conflict/disagreement in around 26,000 of the 46,000 deaths in ICUs in the UK.

Mediation may be part of the answer. Mediation is a process where the two (or more) sides of a dispute have a structured conversation to try and find a mutually acceptable resolution. The mediator oversees this and acts as a neutral third party. Mediation has a long history in various forms. There are a number of different potential benefits to mediation.

- Cost – generally the cost of mediation is a fraction of the cost of going to court.
- Confidentiality – as we have seen in the case of Charlie Gard, going to court potentially means massive publicity. Mediation is strictly confidential, with the parties bound to keep what is discussed in the mediation private. The mediator cannot be forced to give evidence if a trial occurs in the event of a failed mediation. In legal terms, the mediation is without prejudice.
- Control – the parties involved in mediation have control over what happens. There is a lot more flexibility over the result. In court, the judge has control and the law determines what remedy is applied.
- Compliance – in the event of a successful mediation, it is much more likely to stick, as both sides have found the result acceptable. Although in a great deal of mediations, both sides find the acceptable result uncomfortable.

- Support – the mediator has experience of the type of situation in which the parties find themselves. This can be very helpful for the parties who are unlikely to have experienced anything like this before.

There is an increasing amount of literature for mediation. For example, the '*Elder and Guardianship Mediation: A Report prepared by The Canadian Centre for Elder Law*' has reviewed the situation in North America. Although this is looking at elderly adults who lack capacity, the overlap between these adults and patients in the ICU is clear. The paper reviews mediation which has been used in circumstances where there is disagreement between decision-makers and the family/attorneys responsible for the individual, including mediating clinical disagreements. The results are interesting. As might be expected, knowledge of both medicine and the law by the mediator was considered very important and pre-mediation meetings, where the mediator talked individually to each of the parties, were invaluable. The results of mediation showed that between 60 and 90 per cent of disputes settled without the need to go to court. Interestingly, 90 per cent of participants found the experience useful, even amongst those parties who did not settle.

Mediation is well established in English law, albeit largely outside of medicine. In the family division of the High Court, mediation in the financial settlement of divorces is mandatory, and the Civil Division requires mediation in disputes valued in excess of £100,000. This year, NHS Resolution have started mediating clinical negligence cases following a successful pilot project.

References and Further Reading

Azoulay E, Timsit J-F, Sprung CL, *et al.* Prevalence and factors of intensive care unit conflicts: the Conflicus study. *Am J Respir Crit Care Med* 2009;**180**:853–60.

Canadian Centre for Elder Law. 2012. Report on elder and guardianship mediation. papers.ssrn.com/sol3/papers.cfm?abstract_id=2008347

Danbury C, Newdick C, Waldmann C, Lawson A (eds). *Law and Ethics in Intensive Care*. Oxford, NY: Oxford University Press; 2010.

Health and Social Care Information Centre. 2010. Hospital Episode Statistics. Adult Critical Care in England – April 2014 to March 2015. files.digital.nhs.uk/publicationimport/pub19xxx/pub19938/adul-crit-care-data-eng-apr-14-mar-15-rep.pdf

Sprung CL, Cohen SL, Sjokvist P, *et al.* End-of-life practices in European intensive care units: the Ethicus study. *JAMA* 2003;**290**:790–7.

11.9

The Legal Framework

Jo Samanta and Dev Dutta

Key Learning Points

1. Professional regulation and legal framework closely interact in providing care of patients in intensive care.
2. Legal and ethical issues closely interplay with common law, statute and public law.
3. The Mental Capacity Act and safeguarding process have introduced a robust decision-making process.
4. Clinicians have to be aware of the legal framework whilst making treatment refusal and life-sustaining treatment decisions.
5. Patients with capacity can refuse or influence any treatment, but cannot demand any specific treatment.

Keywords: legal framework, Mental Capacity Act, law, safeguarding

Introduction

Caring for patients in intensive care is subject to the general law, as well as to legal and ethical issues that are specific to this area. It is potentially extensive and engages the common law (e.g. negligence actions), statute (e.g. Mental Capacity Act), public law (e.g. judicial review) and European law (human rights). The law is underpinned by a complex web of professional regulation, local governance and formal complaints systems. It is an important area, as evidenced by recent statistics.

The Hospital Adult Critical Care Activity in England for 2015–16 may be seen in Box 11.9.1.

Assessment of Capacity

A fundamental issue to be considered at the start of the decision-making process is whether a patient has decision-making capacity. In law, the presumption is that adults have decision-making capacity unless proved otherwise (Section 1(2) Mental Capacity Act 2005).

> **Box 11.9.1** NHS-Funded Adult Critical Care Activity in England
>
> Hospital Adult Critical Care Activity 2015–16 (published 23 February 2017):
>
> - 271,079 records of adult critical care periods in 2015–16 (an increase of 4.4 per cent from 2014 to 2015)
> - People aged 50 years and over accounted for 77 per cent of admissions
> - Males made up more than half of all records

> **Box 11.9.2** Assessment of Capacity
>
> Assessment of capacity is a two-stage process:
>
> 1. Does the person have an impairment of, or a disturbance in, the functioning of the mind or brain?
> 2. Is the person unable to:
>   a. Understand the relevant information
>   b. Retain the information
>   c. Use or weigh the information
>   d. Communicate the decision?
>
> Source: Sections 2(1) and 3(1) Mental Capacity Act 2005.

Assessment of capacity is a two-stage process, as shown in Box 11.9.2.

For patients who are critically ill, the presumption of capacity might be rebutted easily because of sedation or a low Glasgow Coma Score, although determining capacity in other situations might be less certain. An objectively unwise decision does not necessarily mean that a person lacks capacity. Accurate and timely record-keeping regarding capacity assessment is required and will underpin clinical decisions, as well as potential Deprivation of Liberty Safeguards (DoLS) considerations.

Competent Adults
Consent to Treatment

Valid consent is a founding principle of medical law and is based on respect for autonomy. Consent must

Box 11.9.3 The Requirements of Valid Consent

- Person needs capacity
- Consent must be voluntary
- Disclosure of material risks
- Treatment must be lawful and not against public policy

be given voluntarily by patients with decision-making capacity after being given sufficient information to make a decision. The requirements of valid consent are listed in Box 11.9.3.

Doctors have a legal duty to take reasonable care to disclose material risks of clinically indicated treatment. Material risks do not relate solely to percentages and include factors such as the nature of risks, the effects of their occurrence, potential benefits, alternatives and risks of those alternatives (*Montgomery* v. *Lanarkshire Health Board* [2015] UKSC 11). Detailed professional guidance is available which emphasises the partnership approach to consent and other forms of decision-making.

Refusal of Treatment

Adults with capacity can refuse even lifesaving medical treatment (Re B (adult: refusal of medical treatment*)* [2002] EWHC 429).

Treatment Demands

Adults with capacity can influence the treatment they receive by consenting to, or refusing, clinically indicated treatment. Although patients may request specific treatment, there is no right to dictate and requests are conceded only where these align with clinical judgement.

Adults who Lack Capacity

Capacity is decision-specific and may be temporary or permanent. Decisions made for, or on behalf of, persons who lack capacity must be made in their best interests (Section 1(5) Mental Capacity Act 2005) using the 'least restrictive principle'. Decision-makers must act in what they 'reasonably believe' is in the person's best interests.

Best Interests

All decisions must be made in the person's best interests, rather than in the interests of others. A person's best interests can be determined as shown in Box 11.9.4.

Box 11.9.4 The Best Interests Test

A person's best interests are determined with reference to:

- All circumstances
- The likelihood of capacity being regained
- The person's past and present wishes and feelings
- Beliefs and values
- Any other factors the person would be likely to consider

Source: Section 4 Mental Capacity Act 2005.

Box 11.9.5 Determining Best Interests

Where practicable and appropriate in determining best interests, decision-makers should consult:

- Anyone identified by the person as someone to be consulted
- Anyone who cares for the person or is interested in their welfare
- Any attorney or deputy who has authority to be consulted regarding the best interests of the person

Source: Section 4(7) Mental Capacity Act 2005.

For 'unbefriended' patients (those with no known friends or family to consult regarding their best interests, apart from professional caregivers), it may be necessary to appoint an Independent Mental Capacity Advocate (IMCA). IMCAs have the right to ask for additional clinical opinions and request further information, as well as challenge clinical decisions that are not considered to be in the person's best interests (Box 11.9.5).

Advance Care Plans

On occasion, intensivists will be confronted with patients who lack capacity but who have an advance care plan in place that is intended to inform decision-makers of their past views and opinions regarding clinical treatment. The implications of this will depend upon the type of advance care plan that is in place (Box 11.9.6). Best interests do not apply to a patient who has a valid and applicable advance decision to refuse the treatment being considered (Sections 24–26 Mental Capacity Act 2005). However, advance decisions are rare in practice (around 4 per cent of the population in the UK). In addition, or alternatively, a health and welfare attorney may have been appointed. Decision-makers acting under a lasting power of

Box 11.9.6 Advanced Care Plans

- Advance refusals of treatment
  - Must be valid and applicable to the treatment being considered
- Lasting powers of attorney for health and welfare decisions
  - Must make decisions in the person's best interests
- Statements of wishes
  - Not binding but must be taken into account in decisions

Source: Sections 4(6), 9, 10, 11, 24, 25, 26 Mental Capacity Act 2005.

attorney or deputyship must make decisions in the person's best interests. Although statements of wishes are not binding in law, these must be taken into account as part of the decision-making process (Section 4(6)(a) Mental Capacity Act 2005).

Prolonged Disorders of Consciousness

For patients with prolonged disorders of consciousness (PDOC), including vegetative and minimally conscious states, the presumption of capacity will be rebutted. In intensive care situations, it is likely that all efforts will be directed at saving life where possible and to transfer following clinical stability. Practice Direction 9E used to state that serious medical treatment decisions (including withdrawal or withholding of clinically assisted nutrition and hydration) should be referred to the Court of Protection. However, the recent redraft of the Practice Directions no longer refers to serious medical treatment decisions. Clarification of the widely assumed common law requirement is expected from the Supreme Court following the recent case of *Re Y* (2017) EWHC 2866. Removal of this requirement will bring these decisions in line with other serious treatment decisions that are made in the best interests of patients and only irreconcilable differences are referred to the court.

Do Not Attempt Cardiopulmonary Resuscitation

Cardiopulmonary resuscitation is an emergency intervention for cardiac arrest which aims to resynchronise a heart with dysregulated cardiac rhythm to maintain oxygenation, whilst the cause of the arrest can be established and treated. Its likelihood of success is improved by the immediacy of efforts to resuscitate. Cardiac arrest is the first part of the dying process for everyone, but the circumstances and timing will be variable and the potential success will be dependent upon facts and circumstances. Do Not Attempt Cardiopulmonary Resuscitation (DNACPR) is an anticipatory decision that if a patient suffers a cardiac arrest, efforts to restore the circulation by means of cardiopulmonary resuscitation will not be made on patients for whom resuscitative efforts will be inappropriate. For example:

1. Where a person with capacity makes an informed decision not to be resuscitated in the event of a cardiac arrest
2. Where resuscitation is likely to be futile
3. Where the burden of cardiopulmonary resuscitation outweighs the potential benefit

A key ethical and legal consideration is whether patients need to be informed of cardiopulmonary resuscitation, if this treatment will not be offered on the basis of futility or the burdens would outweigh the benefits. This issue was considered in *Tracey* v. *Cambridge University NHS Trust* [2014] (Box 11.9.7).

Box 11.9.7 *Tracey* v. *Cambridge University NHS Trust* [2014]

Mrs Tracey was admitted to critical care following a road accident. She had terminal lung cancer. She informed her carers that she wished to be involved in all decisions regarding her care. When being removed from the ventilator, a DNACPR was completed without Mrs Tracey's or her family 's involvement. The daughter objected vociferously on the basis that no one had been involved in the decision. Following a marked deterioration in her condition, unsuccessful attempts were made to discuss the implications of cardiopulmonary resuscitation. Mrs Tracey did not wish to engage in further discussions about end-of-life care. A second DNACPR was completed following family consultation, following which Mrs Tracey died. An application for judicial review was brought against the hospital, alleging that the decision-making process and lack of consultation had breached Mrs Tracey's Article 8 rights in failing to consult her, or her family, or to notify her of the decision that had been made. It was held that patient involvement in decisions about cardiopulmonary resuscitation should be presumption, even if resuscitation would be futile. No involvement was permissible where there was a real risk of actual physical or psychological harm.

Source: *Tracey* v. *Cambridge University NHS Trust* [2014] EWCA Civ 822.

Futile Medical Treatment

Treatment is described as 'futile' when no clinical benefit is expected to be gained from medical intervention and is used to justify selective non-treatment of patients with a very poor clinical prognosis. From a medical perspective, futility can be categorised as either 'physiological' or 'qualitative'. Physiological futility is a technical decision that treatment will not achieve its physiological aims. Qualitative futility is a normative concept which balances anticipated burdens against anticipated benefits. As such, considerations of qualitative futility can be important for determining whether or not life-prolonging treatment should be continued. Box 11.9.8 illustrates how conceptions of futility were examined in *Aintree* v. *James* [2013].

Gross Negligence Manslaughter

Intensive care environments are subject to the same requirements as general patient care environments in that clinical negligence will be proven where there is a duty of care, that the standard of care was breached, in that the standard expected was not reached in the circumstances, and finally that actionable damage was caused by the breach of duty.

A criminal action can be brought against a doctor where a negligent act or omission causes the patient's death. The key case is *R* v. *Adomako* [1995]. In this case, the anaesthetist failed to notice a disconnected oxygen pipe. The patient died after suffering a cardiac arrest. It is apparent that a doctor's extreme subjective recklessness or incompetence is such that it warrants criminal sanction. The House of Lords laid down a four-stage test to determine gross negligence manslaughter: (1) the existence of a duty of care; (2) a breach of that duty, which (3) caused or significantly contributed to the death; (4) which should be characterised as gross negligence, and is therefore a crime. In *R* v. *Sellu* [2016], evidence was accepted by the jury that delays in initiation of emergency surgery and failure to resuscitate and refer to intensive care all had a decisive influence on the patient's death.

> ### Box 11.9.8 In *Aintree* v. *James* [2013] – Conceptions of Futility Examined
>
> 1. Futility is wider than the goal of curing, or palliating, the patient's condition
> 2. Wider and more aggregate conceptions of benefit
> 3. The question to be asked is whether treatment would confer 'some benefit'
>
> Source: *Aintree University Hospitals* v. *James* [2013] UKSC 67.

Similarly, in *R* v. *Bawa-Garba* [2015], a doctor was found guilty of gross negligence manslaughter when she failed to diagnose a child's sepsis and delayed resuscitation, when she mistook the patient for another child who had a DNACPR order in place. This case, however, has been controversial and raised several other issues of complex healthcare environments.

Resources and Rationing

Intensive care is a scarce resource and must therefore be rationed. There is no national guidance for resource allocation, but General Medical Council guidance provides that lifesaving treatment should not be rationed since there are a finite number of beds and intensive care consultants must decide who to admit. The NHS is unable to fund every form of clinically indicated treatment, and decisions to fund certain interventions means inevitably that other therapies cannot be resourced. It is difficult for patients to challenge decisions to withhold treatment on the basis of lack of resources, as patients do not have an enforceable right to healthcare. For this reason, challenges against decisions not to provide treatment are usually framed under public law – by judicial review. A successful action requires the applicant to establish some illegality, irrationality or procedural impropriety during the decision-making process on the part of the NHS body.

Financial considerations and government economic policy can be taken into account in service provision, as in an early case of judicial review – *R* v. *Cambridge DHA ex p B* [1995] 2 All ER 129 (Box 11.9.9).

> ### Box 11.9.9 *R* v. *Cambridge DHA ex p B* [1995]
>
> - The Health Authority decided not to fund further treatment for a girl with leukaemia.
> - Her father's action for judicial review was unsuccessful.
> - Medical opinion was divided – some believed further treatment was futile, whilst others felt that it could be beneficial.
> - The court held that in a perfect world, any treatment that might offer a chance of survival would be provided, but that it would be:
>
> … shutting one's eyes to the real world if the court were to proceed on the basis that we do live in such a world. … difficult and agonising judgements have to be made as to how a limited budget is best allocated to the maximum advantage of the maximum number of patients.
>
> Source: *R* v. *Cambridge DHA ex p B* [1995] EWCA Civ 43.

However, some judicial actions have succeeded. In *R (Rogers)* v. *Swindon NHS PCT* [2006] EWCA 392, a woman with breast cancer requested Herceptin®, a new unlicensed drug, on the basis of efficacious early trials. The policy of the Primary Care Trust (PCT) was to fund this treatment only in 'exceptional' cases – her request was declined. The Court of Appeal found that the PCT's decision was unlawful, as it had not defined the circumstances which would represent 'exceptional'. On the evidence, the PCT operated a policy of never funding Herceptin®. Since cost was not referred to as a relevant factor, they could not rely on resource constraints as a reason for denying treatment.

The principle that emerges is that lawful decisions will involve fact-sensitive, individualised decision-making processes, whereas blanket exclusionary policies may be amenable to judicial review.

In the recent case *N* v. *A CCG* [2017] UKSC 22, the Supreme Court confirmed that the court can make decisions only between options that are available (Box 11.9.10). The issue concerned the role of the court where there was a dispute between healthcare funders and a family about the services provided to a person who lacked capacity to decide.

References and Further Reading

Brazier M, Cave E. *Medicine, Patients and the Law*, 6th edn. Manchester: Manchester University Press; 2016.

Danbury C, Newdick C, Lawson A, *et al*. *Law and Ethics in Intensive Care*. Oxford: Oxford University Press; 2010.

General Medical Council. 2010. Treatment and care towards the end of life: good practice in decision making. www.gmc-uk.org/ethical-guidance/ethical-guidance-for-doctors/treatment-and-care-towards-the-end-of-life

General Medical Council. 2020. Decision making and consent guidance. www.gmc-uk.org/guidance/ethical_guidance/consent_guidance_index.asp

Laing J, McHale J. *Principles of Medical Law*, 4th edn. Oxford: Oxford University Press; 2017.

legislation.gov.uk. 2005. Mental Capacity Act 2005. www.legislation.gov.uk/ukpga/2005/9/contents

Newdick C. *Who Should We Treat? Rights, Rationing and Resources*. Oxford: Oxford University Press; 2005.

NHS. Mental Capacity Act. www.nhs.uk/conditions/social-care-and-support-guide/making-decisions-for-someone-else/mental-capacity-act/

Resuscitation Council UK. Guidance: DNACPR and CPR decisions. www.resus.org.uk/library/additional-guidance/guidance-dnacpr-and-cpr-decisions

Box 11.9.10 *N* v. *A CCG* [2017]

- MN was profoundly disabled in his early twenties, with severe learning and physical disabilities and a rare epileptic condition resulting in frequent seizures and a risk of sudden death.
- MN was cared for in a care home around 6 miles away from his parents.
- The dispute concerned whether MN could be accompanied to visit his parents at their home and whether his mother could assist the staff with MH's intimate care when she visited. The care home was unwilling to permit this.
- The Clinical Commissioning Group (CCG) responsible for funding was not prepared to invest the additional resources required for home visits to take place.
- The court held that it did not have power to order the CCG to fund what the parents wanted.
- Nor did it have power to order care providers to do that which they were unwilling or unable to do.

Source: *N* v. *A CCG* [2017] UKSC 22.

11.10

CoBaTrICE: The Importance of Learning Opportunities and Integration of New Knowledge in Clinical Practice

Alison Pittard

Key Learning Points

1. CoBaTrICE is an international, competency-based programme for training in intensive care medicine.
2. Traditional educational methods are no longer effective or efficient due to limitations on time.
3. A supportive environment where learning and professional development occur alongside delivery of clinical care should be fundamental.
4. All encounters in the clinical environment should be seen as potential learning opportunities and utilised proactively.
5. Rapidly assessing learner needs and providing specific feedback on performance is key.

Keywords: training, education, opportunities, learning, CoBaTrICE

Introduction

Historically, medical education, and particularly intensive care medicine (ICM), was one of experiential learning in an apprenticeship style, supplemented by didactic classroom teaching. The specialty continually advances and this, along with a limit on working hours, a dynamic and demanding clinical environment and external regulation, means that traditional teaching methods are no longer sufficient. The breadth and depth of knowledge, skills and behaviours expected of the modern ICM clinician is incorporated into a curriculum, formalising acquisition of competencies to achieve high-level outcomes. Approaches to teaching and learning that take these into account must be incorporated to ensure education is efficacious and efficient.

What Is CoBaTrICE?

CoBatrICE is an international Competency Based Training programme in ICM for Europe and other regions. The programme developed with support from the European Society of Intensive Care Medicine (ESICM), using a modified Delphi and nominal group consensus technique, and incorporates competencies felt to be important for ICU clinicians to acquire in order to ensure high-quality education, and hence patient care. In 2006, the foundations for the first programme were established. In 2010, The Faculty of Intensive Care Medicine (FICM) was tasked with creating a standalone Certificate of Completion of Training (CCT) curriculum in the UK and this is primarily based on CoBaTrICE. Curricula continually evolve to facilitate the incorporation of new knowledge, update existing competencies and remove those that are no longer appropriate. The original 2011 curriculum was updated in 2014, and again in 2018. An outcomes-based curriculum has been published in 2020 to meet the new requirements from the General Medical Council (GMC).

Educational Approaches

ICM is very much a practical specialty and knowledge underpins the behaviours and skills used in the clinical setting. Acquisition of knowledge occurs in a number of ways and should be tailored to the needs of the individual learner. 'Passive' learning, such as conferences, lectures and journal reading, is ideal for delivering core knowledge. There are online resources that learners can access and the FICM has its own e-learning for ICM (e-ICM) for this purpose, which can be found on its website at ficmlearning.org. 'Active' learning, the application of this knowledge and the practice of both the art and science of ICM, is best cultivated at the bedside. For this reason, every encounter in the ICU should be a potential learning opportunity. Due to the nature of the workload in ICM, it is difficult to plan teaching/learning opportunities. Therefore, a proactive approach and discussion of clinical cases allow new knowledge to be expressed, shared and implemented into clinical practice. Many strategies exist to facilitate teaching when time is limited, reinforcing the concept that even small amounts of focussed teaching can be beneficial to the learner.

Integration in Clinical Practice

A supportive environment where learning and professional development occur alongside delivery of clinical care should be fundamental in any specialty. ICM is a multidisciplinary specialty and it is possible, by proactively identifying appropriate learning opportunities and linking to specific competencies, to develop the entire team. This targeting is much easier with outcomes-based curricula.

There are common themes that should be considered when looking at delivering efficient and effective teaching. All of these are affected by internal, external and patient factors. To support and organise effective learning, it is important to be aware of these factors to enhance the learning experience.

Learning Needs

It is important to rapidly identify the needs of the learner. This avoids wasting time teaching areas that are already known or that the trainee is not ready for. Of course, the trainee must be aware of their own needs, but with use of their training portfolio and educational contract, this should be relatively easy. Methods of establishing these needs could be asking during a pre-ward round team brief what training needs there were for the day, asking a question prior to an encounter to assess the current level of knowledge and understanding or a brief period of observation.

Opportunities

Every encounter is a learning opportunity and should be utilised to direct teaching to learners' needs. The handover ward round is a good example of one process creating multiple opportunities. These include clinical management, diagnostics, data interpretation, communication and leadership skills and teamwork.

Talking to relatives is a task usually undertaken by a single individual, but it is also a valuable encounter educationally. Where time and workload permit, allowing a trainee to observe a senior clinician can be beneficial and equip the trainee with new ideas that can be incorporated into their own practice. The educator can also observe the trainee in a similar situation to evaluate their level of competence and facilitate formative feedback.

Acquisition of procedural skills is more complex, as a balance needs to be achieved between providing opportunities for trainees and ensuring patient safety. Increasing use of simulation and observation and performance in an elective setting prior to undertaking high-risk procedures in the critically ill can help to create a good balance.

Outcome

Specific feedback on performance is a powerful tool that, if delivered correctly, influences future behaviour and promotes self-reflection. Feedback given immediately at the bedside has the advantage of being patient-focussed and is highly valued by trainees, who associate this with high-quality teaching.

Conclusion

Technical advances and increasing demands create challenges for ensuring adequate training/education. Evidence-based approaches for improving the efficacy and efficiency of ICM education should be integrated into training programmes. There is no standardised way of incorporating education into clinical practice, and therefore, the approach taken by individual units should not disrupt work flow or compromise patient safety or quality of care. What is clear is that a move away from didactic bedside teaching and introducing small amounts of time focussed on teaching in the clinical arena are much more efficient.

References and Further Reading

CoBaTrICE Collaboration; Bion JF, Barrett H. Development of core competencies for an international training programme in intensive care medicine. *Intensive Care Med* 2006;**32**:1371–83.

General Medical Council. Excellence by design. www.gmc-uk.org/education/standards-guidance-

and-curricula/standards-and-outcomes/excellence-by-design

Huggins K. Lifelong learning: the key to competence in the intensive care unit? *Intensive Crit Care Nurs* 2004;**20**:38–44.

Joyce MF, Berg S, Bittner EA. Practical strategies for increasing efficiency and efectiveness in critical care education. *World J Crit Care Med* 2017;**6**:1–12.

The Faculty of Intensive Care Medicine. E-ICM. www.ficm .ac.uk/news-events-education/e-icm

Index